THIRD EDITION

# Therapeutic Choices



*E*

**JEAN GRAY, MD, FRCPC**

*ASSOCIATE EDITORS*

**ANNE M. GILLIS, MD, FRCPC**

**GORDON E. JOHNSON, PhD**

**JEFFREY A. JOHNSON, PhD**

**STUART M. MacLEOD**
**MD, PhD(Pharmacol), FRCPC**

**JAMES McCORMACK, BSc(Pharm), PharmD**

**WILLIAM McLEAN, PharmD, FASHP, FCCP**

**CHRISTOPHER PATTERSON**
**MD, FRCPC, FACP**

**ROBERT E. RANGNO, BSc, MSc, MD, FRCPC**

**MICHAEL J. RIEDER, MD, PhD, FRCPC**

Canadian Pharmacists Association
Association des pharmaciens du Canada

Canadian Cataloguing in Publication Data

Main entry under title:

Therapeutic choices

3rd ed.
Includes bibliographical references and index.
ISBN 0-919115-89-6

1. Therapeutics—Handbooks, manuals, etc.
I. Gray, Jean (Jean Dorothy), 1942– II. Canadian Pharmacists Association.

RM121.5.T44 2000 615.5 C00-900771-7

# Editorial Board

# Practitioner Review Board

# Contributors

Sueda Akkor
*Vancouver, B.C.*

Upton Allen
*Toronto, Ont.*

Fred Y. Aoki
*Winnipeg, Man.*

S.A. Awad
*Halifax, N.S.*

Tony R. Bai
*Vancouver, B.C.*

Benoit Bailey
*Montréal, P.Q.*

Rosemary Basson
*Vancouver, B.C.*

Israel Belenkie
*Calgary, Alta.*

C. Laird Birmingham
*Vancouver, B.C.*

Ari Bitnun
*Toronto, Ont.*

M. A. Boctor
*Saskatoon, Sask.*

Bruce Carleton
*Vancouver, B.C.*

S. George Carruthers
*London, Ont.*

Andrew Chalmers
*Vancouver, B.C.*

Hugh Chaun
*Vancouver, B.C.*

Nikhil Chopra
*Halifax, N.S.*

Anthony W. Chow
*Vancouver, B.C.*

John Collins
*Hamilton, Ont.*

Janet Cooper
*Ottawa, Ont.*

Robert Côté
*Montreal, P.Q.*

Marie J. Craig-Chambers
*Newmarket, Ont.*

Jean-Pierre DesGroseilliers
*Ottawa, Ont.*

Orna Diav-Citrin
*Jerusalem, Israel*

David Diemert
*Montreal, P.Q.*

Simon Dobson
*Vancouver, B.C.*

Paul Dorian
*Toronto, Ont.*

Jean Ethier
*Montreal, P.Q.*

Ernest L. Fallen
*Hamilton, Ont.*

Brian G. Feagan
*London, Ont.*

Richard N. Fedorak
*Edmonton, Alta.*

Louis A. Fernandez
*Halifax, N.S.*

Laura A. Finlayson
*Halifax, N.S.*

J. Mark FitzGerald
*Vancouver, B.C.*

Jonathan A.E. Fleming
*Vancouver, B.C.*

Alastair J. Flint
*Toronto, Ont.*

A. Mervyn Fox
*London, Ont.*

Jane Garland
*Vancouver, B.C.*

Glenn H. Gill
*Halifax, N.S.*

G. Barry Gilliland
*Saskatoon, Sask.*

Anne M. Gillis
*Calgary, Alta.*

Ronald Gold
*Toronto, Ont.*

Elliot M. Goldner
*Vancouver, B.C.*

Gillian Graves
*Halifax, N.S.*

Daniel B. Gregson
*London, Ont.*

Lyn Guenther
*London, Ont.*

David A. Hanley
*Calgary, Alta.*

John G. Hanly
*Halifax, N.S.*

Jenny Heathcote
*Toronto, Ont.*

David J. Hirsch
*Halifax, N.S.*

Vincent C. Ho
*Vancouver, B.C.*

L. John Hoffer
*Montreal, P.Q.*

John P. Hooge
*Vancouver, B.C.*

Jeffrey A. Johnson
*Edmonton, Alta.*

Gary I. Joubert
*London, Ont.*

Sidney H. Kennedy
*Toronto, Ont.*

J.S. Keystone
*Toronto, Ont.*

James Kissick
*Kanata, Ont.*

Sandra Knowles
*Toronto, Ont.*

Gideon Koren
*Toronto, Ont.*

Gunnar Kraag
*Ottawa, Ont.*

Joanne M. Langley
*Halifax, N.S.*

Elizabeth J. Latimer
*Hamilton, Ont.*

David C.W. Lau
*Calgary, Alta.*

Raymond P. LeBlanc
*Halifax, N.S.*

Mary Anne Lee
*Calgary, Alta.*

Robert S. Lester
*Toronto, Ont.*

Timothy P. Lynch
*London, Ont.*

C. MacLean
*Halifax, N.S.*

J. Dick MacLean
*Montreal, P.Q.*

W. Stuart Maddin
*Vancouver, B.C.*

Elizabeth Mann
*Halifax, N.S.*

Thomas J. Marrie
*Edmonton, Alta.*

David G. McCormack
*London, Ont.*

James McCormack
*Vancouver, B.C.*

Peter J. McLeod
*Montreal, P.Q.*

Rob Miller
*Halifax, N.S.*

Julio S.G. Montaner
*Vancouver, B.C.*

Valentina Montessori
*Vancouver, B.C.*

Mark Montgomery
*Calgary, Alta.*

D. William Moote
*London, Ont.*

Lynne Nakashima
*Vancouver, B.C.*

Claudio A. Naranjo
*Toronto, Ont.*

Lindsay E. Nicolle
*Winnipeg, Man.*

Robert P. Nolan
*Toronto, Ont.*

Richard W. Norman
*Halifax, N.S.*

Richard I. Ogilvie
*Toronto, Ont.*

Sagar V. Parikh
*Toronto, Ont.*

John D. Parker
*Toronto, Ont.*

John O. Parker
*Kingston, Ont.*

Paul M. Peloso
*Saskatoon, Sask.*

Ross A. Pennie
*Hamilton, Ont.*

Stephen J. Phillips
*Halifax, N.S.*

R. Allan Purdy
*Halifax, N.S.*

Paul Rafuse
*Halifax, N.S.*

Kenneth Rockwood
*Halifax, N.S.*

Ghislaine O. Roederer
*Montreal, P.Q.*

Coleman Rotstein
*Hamilton, Ont.*

André Roussin
*Montreal, P.Q.*

R. Mark Sadler
*Toronto, Ont.*

R.D. Schwarz
*Halifax, N.S.*

John W. Sellors
*Hamilton, Ont.*

Eldon A. Shaffer
*Calgary, Alta.*

Catherine Shea
*Dartmouth, N.S.*

Neil H. Shear
*Toronto, Ont.*

Robert Sheldon
*Calgary, Alta.*

Jay Silverberg
*Toronto, Ont.*

Mathieu Simon
*Québec, P.Q.*

Michael B.H. Smith
*Craigavon, N. Ireland*

David P. Speert
*Vancouver, B.C.*

A. Jon Stoessl
*Vancouver, B.C.*

Mark G. Swain
*Calgary, Alta.*

R.P. Swinson
*Hamilton, Ont.*

Stephen R. Tan
*Toronto, Ont.*

W. Grant Thompson
*Nepean, Ont.*

A.B.R. Thomson
*Edmonton, Alta.*

J. Carter Thorne
*Newmarket, Ont.*

Eldon Tunks
*Hamilton, Ont.*

Alexander G.G. Turpie
*Hamilton, Ont.*

Hillar Vellend
*Toronto, Ont.*

David Warren
*London, Ont.*

C. Peter N. Watson
*Toronto, Ont.*

Sharon Whiting
*Ottawa, Ont.*

N. Blair Whittemore
*Montreal, P.Q.*

W.L. Wobeser
*Kingston, Ont.*

Donna M.M. Woloschuk
*Winnipeg, Man.*

James M. Wright
*Vancouver, B.C.*

D. George Wyse
*Calgary, Alta.*

# Canadian Pharmacists Association

President: *Garry King, BSP*
Executive Director: *Jeff Poston, PhD, MRPharmS*
Senior Director, Publications: *Leesa D. Bruce*
Editor-in-Chief: *Carol Repchinsky, BSP*

Managing Editor: *Frances Hachborn, BScPhm*
Clinical Editor: *Carol Repchinsky, BSP*
Assistant Editor: *Dianne Baxter*
Editorial Administrator: *Murielle Danis*

Manager, Publication Technology: *Darquise Leblanc*
Design and Production: *Lucienne Prévost*
Desktop Publisher: *Kathleen Régimbald*

The editors wish to thank Kate Reid, Sheryl Neilson and Angela Polsinelli for their assistance.

Original Cover Design: *Purich Design Studio*
Indexer: *Heather Ebbs, Editor's Ink*
Printed by: *Webcom Limited*

# Table of Contents

Foreword xiii
How to Use *Therapeutic Choices* xiv

**Psychiatric Disorders** ***(Christopher Patterson)***

1. Acute Agitation, *Alastair J. Flint* 1
2. Anxiety Disorders, *R.P. Swinson* 7
3. Attention Deficit Hyperactivity Disorder, *A. Mervyn Fox* 16
4. Dementia, *Kenneth Rockwood and Catherine Shea* 25
5. Depression, *Sidney H. Kennedy and Sagar V. Parikh* 33
6. Insomnia, *Jonathan A.E. Fleming* 43
7. Psychoses, *Jane Garland* 52
8. Drug Withdrawal Syndromes, *Claudio A. Naranjo* 63

**Neurologic Disorders** ***(Jean Gray)***

9. Chronic Spasticity and Muscle Cramps, *John P. Hooge* 74
10. Headache in Adults, *R. Allan Purdy* 80
11. Headache in Children, *Sharon Whiting* 92
12. Acute Pain, *Benoit Bailey* 101
13. Back Pain, *Eldon Tunks* 110
14. Neuropathic Pain, *C. Peter N. Watson* 118
15. Pain Control in Palliative Care, *Elizabeth J. Latimer* 125
16. Bell's Palsy, *Mary Anne Lee* 133
17. Parkinson's Disease, *A. Jon Stoessl* 137
18. Seizures, *R. Mark Sadler* 147

**Eye Disorders** ***(Christopher Patterson)***

19. Cataract Surgery Postoperative Care, *Raymond P. LeBlanc* 158
20. Glaucoma, *Paul Rafuse* 161
21. Red Eye, *Sueda Akkor* 168

**Cardiovascular Disorders** ***(Anne M. Gillis)***

22. Prevention of Ischemic Stroke, *Robert Côté* 174
23. Hypertension, *S. George Carruthers* 180
24. Dyslipidemias, *Ghislaine O. Roederer* 191
25. Acute and Postmyocardial Infarction, *Ernest L. Fallen* 202
26. Angina Pectoris, *John O. Parker and John D. Parker* 215
27. Congestive Heart Failure, *Israel Belenkie* 229
28. Supraventricular Tachycardia, *Anne M. Gillis and D. George Wyse* 241
29. Ventricular Tachyarrhythmias, *Paul Dorian* 253
30. Acute Stroke, *Stephen J. Phillips* 263

31. Venous Thromboembolism, *Alexander G.G. Turpie* 273
32. Intermittent Claudication, *Richard I. Ogilvie* 281
33. Raynaud's Phenomenon, *André Roussin* 285
34. Syncope, *Robert Sheldon* 289
35. Systemic Thromboembolism, *Anne M. Gillis* 295

**Respiratory Disorders *(Michael J. Rieder)***

36. Allergic Rhinitis, *D. William Moote* 298
37. Viral Rhinitis, *Timothy P. Lynch* 306
38. Adult Asthma, *David G. McCormack* 312
39. Asthma in Infants and Children, *Mark Montgomery* 320
40. Chronic Obstructive Pulmonary Disease, *Tony R. Bai* 329
41. Croup, *Michael B.H. Smith* 338
42. Smoking Cessation, *Robert P. Nolan* 343

**Gastrointestinal Disorders *(James McCormack)***

43. Chronic Liver Diseases, *Mark G. Swain* 350
44. Viral Hepatitis, *Jenny Heathcote* 362
45. Gastroesophageal Reflux Disease, *Eldon A. Shaffer* 373
46. Peptic Ulcer Disease and Upper Gastrointestinal Bleeding, *A.B.R. Thomson* 382
47. Inflammatory Bowel Disease, *Brian G. Feagan* 396
48. Irritable Bowel Syndrome, *W. Grant Thompson* 408

**Genitourinary Disorders *(James McCormack)***

49. Lower Urinary Tract Symptoms and Benign Prostatic Hyperplasia, *Richard W. Norman* 414
50. Urinary Incontinence and Enuresis, *S.A. Awad and R.D. Schwarz* 422

**Musculoskeletal Disorders *(William McLean)***

51. Fibromyalgia, *Andrew Chalmers* 430
52. Chronic Fatigue Syndrome, *Elizabeth Mann* 435
53. Polymyalgia Rheumatica, *Nikhil Chopra and John G. Hanly* 439
54. Hyperuricemia and Gout, *Gunnar Kraag* 444
55. Rheumatoid Arthritis, *Marie J. Craig-Chambers and J. Carter Thorne* 454
56. Osteoarthritis, *Paul M. Peloso* 467
57. Osteoporosis, *David A. Hanley* 476
58. Sports Injuries, *James Kissick* 487

**Skin Disorders *(Jean Gray)***

59. Acne, *Rob Miller* 493
60. Rosacea, *W. Stuart Maddin* 501

61. Sunburn, *Lyn Guenther* 507
62. Burns, *David Warren* 513
63. Pressure Ulcers, *Stephen R. Tan* 520
64. Psoriasis, *Jean-Pierre DesGroseilliers* 530
65. Atopic Dermatitis, *Robert S. Lester* 538
66. Pruritus, *Laura A. Finlayson* 543
67. Scabies and Pediculosis, *Sandra Knowles and Neil H. Shear* 552
68. Bacterial Skin Infections, *Vincent C. Ho* 558

**Endocrine Disorders *(Gordon Johnson)***

69. Contraception, *Gillian Graves* 569
70. Dysmenorrhea, *Glenn H. Gill* 578
71. Endometriosis, *G. Barry Gilliland* 584
72. Menopause, *John Collins* 595
73. Sexual Dysfunction, *Rosemary Basson* 602
74. Diabetes Mellitus, *M.A. Boctor* 612
75. Thyroid Disorders, *Jay Silverberg* 629

**Blood Disorders *(James McCormack)***

76. Common Anemias, *N. Blair Whittemore* 639

**Fluid and Electrolyte Disorders *(Michael J. Rieder)***

77. Dehydration in Children, *Gary I. Joubert* 648
78. Hypovolemia, *Peter J. McLeod* 655
79. Edema, *David J. Hirsch* 659
80. Hypercalcemia, *Donna M.M. Woloschuk* 666
81. Potassium Disturbances, *Jean Ethier* 674

**Infectious Diseases *(Stuart MacLeod)***

82. Acute Otitis Media in Childhood, *Ross A. Pennie* 684
83. Streptococcal Sore Throat, *David P. Speert* 694
84. Bacterial Meningitis, *Ari Bitnun, Upton Allen and Ronald Gold* 699
85. Prevention of Bacterial Endocarditis, *Hillar Vellend* 707
86. Community-acquired Pneumonia, *Thomas J. Marrie* 711
87. Tuberculosis, *J. Mark FitzGerald and Thomas J. Marrie* 719
88. Acute Osteomyelitis, *Simon Dobson* 729
89. Septic Shock, *Anthony W. Chow* 737
90. Sexually Transmitted Diseases, *John W. Sellors* 748
91. Urinary Tract Infection, *Lindsay E. Nicolle* 762
92. Malaria Prophylaxis, *W.L. Wobeser and J.S. Keystone* 768
93. Traveler's Diarrhea, *J. Dick MacLean and David Diemert* 775
94. Herpesvirus Infections, *Fred Y. Aoki* 782
95. HIV Infection, *Valentina Montessori and Julio S.G. Montaner* 788

96. Opportunistic Infections in HIV-positive Patients, *Daniel B. Gregson* 798
97. Infections in the Cancer Patient, *Coleman Rotstein* 810

**Eating and Nutrition-related Disorders *(Robert Rangno)***

98. Nutritional Supplements for Adults, *L. John Hoffer* 821
99. Obesity, *David C.W. Lau* 827
100. Eating Disorders, *C. Laird Birmingham and Elliot M. Goldner* 836

**Cancer Chemotherapy Toxicity *(James McCormack)***

101. Chemotherapy-induced Nausea and Vomiting, *Lynne Nakashima* 843
102. Management of Other Side Effects of Chemotherapy, *Louis A. Fernandez* 852

**Symptom Control *(Robert Rangno)***

103. Nausea, *C. MacLean* 861
104. Constipation, *Hugh Chaun* 867
105. Diarrhea, *Richard N. Fedorak* 874
106. Fever in Children, *Joanne M. Langley* 882
107. Thermoregulatory Disorders in Adults, *Mathieu Simon* 885
108. Cough, *Tony R. Bai* 892
109. Persistent Hiccoughs, *James M. Wright* 898

**Appendices *(Robert Rangno)***

I. Dosage Adjustment in Renal Impairment, *James McCormack, Bruce Carleton and Janet Cooper* 901
II. Drug Exposure During Pregnancy and Lactation, *Orna Diav-Citrin and Gideon Koren* 916
III. Pharmacoeconomic Considerations, *Jeffrey A. Johnson* 925
IV. Glossary of Abbreviations 929
V. Microorganism Abbreviations Used in *Therapeutic Choices* 935

**Index** 937

# Foreword

Both the Editorial Board and the Canadian Pharmacists Association have been gratified by the interest and enthusiasm expressed for the first two editions of *Therapeutic Choices*. Reflecting the input of both the readers and our Practitioner Review Board, the third edition has continued to emphasize evidence-based decision making and has expanded the number of chapters containing pharmacoeconomic analyses. New topics include Acute Stroke, Hypertensive Crisis (included with Hypertension), Bell's Palsy, Systemic Thromboembolism, Irritable Bowel Syndrome, Polymyalgia Rheumatica, Endometriosis, Sexual Dysfunction (expanded from Erectile Dysfunction in the second edition), Obesity, Nausea and Thermoregulatory Disorders in Adults. Many chapters included in previous editions have new authors. Once again, we ask that readers make CPhA aware of other topics that should be included in subsequent editions.

*Therapeutic Choices* has intentionally been created with a disease-oriented approach. The discussion about drugs reflects common and accepted practice. For this reason, CPhA has not asked authors to provide a conflict of interest disclosure statement. The Editorial Board has extensively reviewed all materials submitted to ensure that the information in each chapter is objective and unbiased.

Carmen Krogh had the original vision for this book. Frances Hachborn, Carol Repchinsky, Lucienne Prévost and Dianne Baxter translated this vision into reality for this edition. The members of the Editorial Board have been more than colleagues — in assisting with developing the book, identifying authors, editing and providing guidance and new ideas. My gratitude is extended to the staff at CPhA, the Editorial Board and the Practitioner Review Board for their continued enthusiasm and dedication.

Jean Gray

# How to Use *Therapeutic Choices*

The third edition of *Therapeutic Choices* consists of 109 chapters and 5 appendices. Each topic presents essential therapeutic information in easily readable algorithms and tables. Because of size constraints, each chapter contains a suggested reading list. Readers wishing more detailed references may contact the Canadian Pharmacists Association, 1785 Alta Vista Dr., Ottawa, ON K1G 3Y6.

Drug therapy is discussed using generic drug names. Brand name inclusion in the chapters is not intended as an endorsement of that brand name. Many Canadian brand names are listed in the tables to the chapters. These are not all inclusive and are not listed in any order of preference.

The true cost of a specific therapy involves a number of elements including the manufacturers' list price, the mark-up and the dispensing fee, the length of drug therapy and costs related to drug administration. Prices used to determine cost of therapy in this book are the acquisition costs in Ottawa at the time of writing. The drug costs in the tables do not involve a dispensing fee or mark-up.

Costs shown are relative and are indicated by the "$" symbol; actual costs are shown occasionally. For most conditions, calculations were made with the cost of the lowest priced product at the dosage specified by the author for a given period. The treatment period selected for most chronic conditions is 30 days. However, treatment periods vary, and the legend accompanying each table should be consulted.

Readers of *Therapeutic Choices* requiring more detailed information on pediatric therapy should consult specialized texts.

Fifteen chapters include pharmacoeconomic considerations written by a pharmacoeconomist. They appear in a shaded box at the end of each of these chapters. General principles of pharmacoeconomics are discussed in Appendix III.

An appendix of drugs requiring dosage adjustment in patients with compromised renal function is provided (Appendix I). In the tables, a small icon (  ) appears after the drug name if dosage adjustment should be considered.

## Description and Limitations of Information

*Therapeutic Choices* contains selected information representing the opinions and experience of individual authors. The authors, editors and publishers have tried to ensure the accuracy of the information at the time of publication. Users of *Therapeutic Choices* should be aware that the text may contain information, statements and dosages for drugs different from those approved by the Therapeutic Products Programme, Health Canada. The manufacturers' approval has not been requested for such information. Users are advised that the information presented in *Therapeutic Choices* is not intended to be all inclusive. Consequently, health care professionals are encouraged to seek additional and confirmatory information to meet their practice requirements and standards as well as the information needs of the patient.

CHAPTER 1

# Acute Agitation

*Alastair J. Flint, MB, ChB, FRCPC, FRANZCP*

Agitation refers to a range of behavioral disturbances including aggression, combativeness, noisiness, restlessness, hyperactivity and disinhibition. It can be a manifestation of a psychiatric disorder, a medical or neurological disorder, or drug intoxication or withdrawal.

## Goals of Therapy

- To prevent harm to patients and caregivers
- To calm the patient and relieve his or her distress
- To facilitate psychiatric, medical or surgical management of the patient

## Investigations

- Obtain a history with specific attention to:
  - nature and duration of symptoms and precipitating factors
  - past history of agitation/aggression (severity, frequency, consequences, precipitants and ameliorators including previous treatment response)
  - known psychiatric, medical and neurological conditions
  - medication and drug (including alcohol) history
- Obtain collateral information from a reliable informant when the patient is not able to provide an accurate history
- Mental status examination, including an assessment of the patient's cognitive function
- Physical examination to check vital functions and look for physical conditions that could be contributing to the agitation. Conditions to think about include:
  - neurological (head injury, seizures, stroke, encephalopathy, degenerative disorders, brain abscess or tumor)
  - metabolic/endocrine (electrolyte imbalance, hypoglycemia, hypoxia, thyrotoxicosis, uremia)
  - cardiovascular (congestive heart failure, myocardial infarction)
  - infections (encephalitis, meningitis, pneumonia, septicemia, urinary tract infection)
  - constipation/fecal impaction
  - urinary retention

- drug toxicity (alcohol, anticholinergics, benzodiazepines, hallucinogens, psychostimulants, sympathomimetics) or drug withdrawal

- Laboratory tests, including drug screen, guided by the history and physical examination

## Therapeutic Choices (Figure 1)

### Safety Measures

- Prevent harm to patients and caregivers.
- Do not compromise your ability to escape from a dangerous situation.
- Attempt to calm the patient verbally; if this fails, do not persist but call for help. Ensure sufficient manpower to manage an aggressive patient; a strong patient may require 5 or more people. If possible, use staff who have expertise in managing aggressive patients. Designate a leader to assign the different tasks.
- A patient who is chemically or physically restrained should not be left unattended. Ensure regular monitoring of his or her vital signs.

### Nonpharmacologic Choices

- Whenever possible, identify the disorder(s) contributing to the agitation and attempt to make a diagnosis before instituting pharmacotherapy.
- Tailor treatment to the diagnosis.
- Correct physical and/or environmental contributors as soon as possible.
- Temporary physical restraint or seclusion when appropriate.
- Attempt to explain why the patient is being medicated or physically restrained. Provide reassurance.
- Carefully document the behavioral disturbance and the rationale for your interventions.

### Pharmacologic Choices

#### *Delirium*

Delirium is best managed by the timely diagnosis and treatment of the causative condition(s). This includes tapering or discontinuing nonessential medications.

Psychosis and agitation, often requiring antipsychotic medication, are present in many delirious patients. Because of its minimal anticholinergic and hypotensive effects, **haloperidol** is the antipsychotic of choice in the symptomatic treatment of delirium. Recommended doses are 0.5 to 1 mg BID-TID PO or IM in the

Figure 1: **Management of the Acutely Agitated Patient**

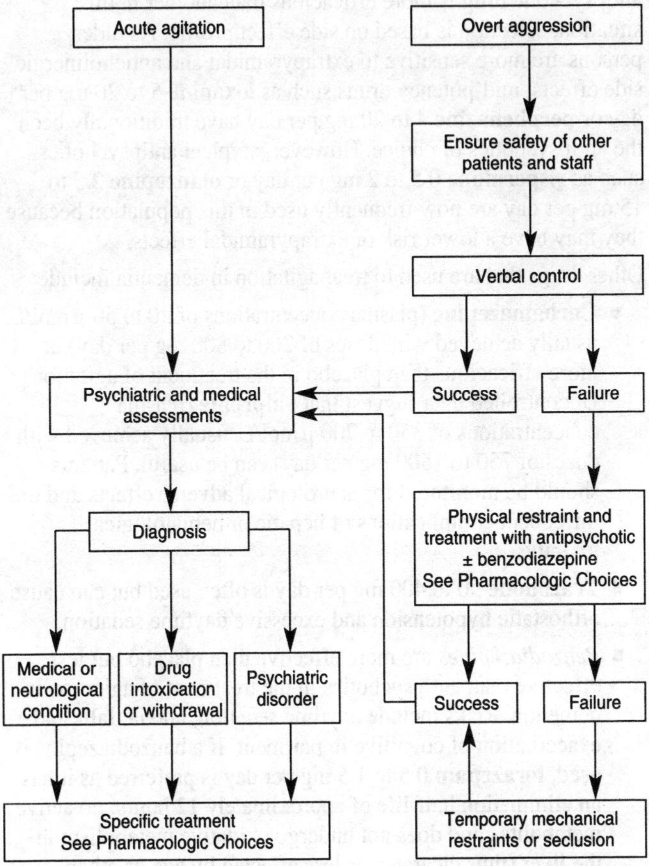
Acute agitation
Overt aggression
Ensure safety of other patients and staff
Verbal control
Psychiatric and medical assessments
Success
Failure
Physical restraint and treatment with antipsychotic ± benzodiazepine See Pharmacologic Choices
Diagnosis
Medical or neurological condition
Drug intoxication or withdrawal
Psychiatric disorder
Success
Failure
Specific treatment See Pharmacologic Choices
Temporary mechanical restraints or seclusion

elderly and 2 to 5 mg BID-TID PO or IM in younger adults. Haloperidol can be given IV to patients who are unable to take medication by mouth and for whom multiple IM injections are inadvisable (e.g., patients in intensive care units).

In general, benzodiazepines are reserved for the specific treatment of alcohol or benzodiazepine withdrawal delirium (Chapter 8). Benzodiazepines are not recommended in other types of delirium because they may worsen cognitive impairment, psychomotor impairment and behavioral disinhibition.

### *Dementia*

Assess the patient for medications, physical problems (including constipation or pain), or depression that could be contributing to the agitation and remedy as many of these factors as possible.

Antipsychotics are the most extensively studied drugs for the treatment of agitation in dementia. There is no evidence that one antipsychotic drug is more efficacious than another in this situation; selection is based on side effect profile. As older persons are more sensitive to extrapyramidal and anticholinergic side effects, mid-potency drugs such as **loxapine** 5 to 20 mg per day or **perphenazine** 4 to 20 mg per day have traditionally been the antipsychotics of choice. However, atypical antipsychotics such as **risperidone** 0.5 to 2 mg per day or **olanzapine** 2.5 to 15 mg per day are now frequently used in this population because they may have a lower risk of extrapyramidal effects.

Other drugs that are used to treat agitation in dementia include:

- **Carbamazepine** (plasma concentrations of 20 to 50 μmol/L, usually achieved with doses of 200 to 800 mg per day) is more efficacious than placebo in the treatment of agitation. Uncontrolled data suggest that **valproate** (plasma concentrations of 350 to 700 μmol/L, usually achieved with doses of 750 to 1500 mg per day) can be useful. Patients should be monitored for neurological adverse effects and the infrequent complications of hepatic or hematological toxicity.
- **Trazodone** 50 to 400 mg per day is often used but can cause orthostatic hypotension and excessive daytime sedation.
- *Benzodiazepines* are more effective than placebo but less effective than antipsychotics in the treatment of agitation in dementia. Risks include daytime sedation, ataxia, falls and exacerbation of cognitive impairment. If a benzodiazepine is used, **lorazepam** 0.5 to 1.5 mg per day is preferred as it has an elimination half-life of approximately 12 hours, no active metabolites and does not undergo oxidative metabolism in the liver (thus clearance is less affected by age or other drugs).
- Beta-blockers, buspirone and lithium have also been used. As there are no placebo-controlled data regarding the efficacy or safety of these drugs in elderly patients with dementia, none can be recommended.

### *Schizophrenia*

Typical antipsychotics (e.g., haloperidol) remain the mainstay of treatment for acute agitation or aggression associated with schizophrenia because they can be administered IM and there is greater flexibility in their dosing. High-potency (e.g., haloperidol) or mid-potency (e.g., loxapine) antipsychotics are preferred because they are less likely to cause hypotension, anticholinergic toxicity, confusion or excessive sedation. In a young agitated schizophrenic patient, the typical dose of **haloperidol** is 5 to 15 mg per day and of **loxapine** it is 25 to 50 mg per day, although higher doses may at times be required. Benzodiazepines are often used as an adjunct in order to reduce the daily dose requirement of neuroleptic, provide sedation and control akathisia (neuroleptic-induced restlessness). **Lorazepam** 1 to 2 mg BID-TID is a reasonable choice since it can be given IM as well as PO, has a rapid onset of action and does not accumulate in the body.

Rapid neuroleptization may be required for a patient who is markedly agitated or violent. In this situation, a combination of haloperidol and lorazepam is commonly used (Table 1).

Table 1: **Rapid Neuroleptization**

A combination of **haloperidol** 5 mg and **lorazepam** 1–2 mg can be given IM and repeated at 30 to 60 minute intervals until the agitation/aggression is controlled. Older patients should receive one half or less of these dosages.

A PRN order for **benztropine** 2 mg PO/IM up to 3 doses in 24 hours should be available in case the patient develops dystonia (younger patients, especially men, are at highest risk of dystonia).

Closely monitor vital signs and neurological status. Neuroleptic malignant syndrome (characterized by muscle rigidity, fever, altered level of consciousness, autonomic instability, elevated white blood count, elevated creatine kinase) may occasionally complicate rapid neuroleptization; the risk is increased in patients who are dehydrated.

### Mania

*Mood stabilizers* (lithium, carbamazepine, valproate) are the mainstay of treatment for mania and bipolar disorder. Plasma levels of **lithium** used for the treatment of acute mania (1.0 to 1.2 mmol/L in younger adults and 0.8 to 1.0 mmol/L in the elderly) are typically higher than those used for the maintenance treatment of bipolar disorder (0.8 to 1.0 mmol/L in the young and 0.5 to 0.8 mmol/L in the elderly). Recommended plasma levels of **carbamazepine** are 20 to 50 μmol/L and of **valproate** are 350 to 700 μmol/L. Adjunctive treatment with *antipsychotic* medication is frequently required in acute mania, especially if psychosis or severe behavioral disturbance is present. High-potency or mid-potency antipsychotics are recommended, but the patient should be carefully monitored for neurological adverse effects which may be more common and/or severe with the combination of a mood stabilizer and a neuroleptic than with either drug alone. **Lorazepam** or **clonazepam** is frequently used as an alternative to antipsychotic medication if the patient is agitated but not psychotic or aggressive.

### Agitated Depression

Psychomotor agitation is a common complication of severe major depression. Antidepressant medication or ECT is the definitive treatment, but in the early stages of management, adjunctive treatment with a benzodiazepine or a neuroleptic can be useful.

### *Intoxication with Illicit Drugs*

A number of illicit drugs such as amphetamines, cocaine, PCP and hallucinogens can cause psychomotor agitation and/or aggression either directly or by inducing violence as a function of a paranoid psychosis. **Haloperidol** alone or in combination with **lorazepam** is commonly used as emergency treatment. Dosing guidelines, including the use of rapid neuroleptization, are similar to those for patients with schizophrenia.

## Therapeutic Tips

- Whenever possible, identify the disorder(s) contributing to the agitation and tailor treatment accordingly.
- The best predictor of violence is a history of violence.
- Ensure that there is sufficient manpower to manage an aggressive patient; a strong patient may require 5 or more people.
- A patient who is chemically or physically restrained should not be left unattended.
- Agitation in elderly patients can usually be managed with lower doses of psychotropic medication than in younger patients.

### *Suggested Reading List*


American Psychiatric Association. Practice guideline for the treatment of patients with Alzheimer's disease and other dementias of late life. *Am J Psychiatry* 1997;154 Suppl:1–39.

Buckley PF. The role of typical and atypical antipsychotic medications in the management of agitation and aggression. *J Clin Psychiatry* 1999;60 (Suppl 10):52–60.

Fava M. Psychopharmacologic treatment of pathologic aggression. *Psychiatr Clin North Am* 1997;20:427–451.

Flint AJ, Van Reekum R. The pharmacologic treatment of Alzheimer's disease: a guide for the general psychiatrist. *Can J Psychiatry* 1998;43:689–697.

Lavine R. Psychopharmacological treatment of aggression and violence in the substance using population. *J Psychoactive Drugs* 1997;29:321–329.

CHAPTER 2

# Anxiety Disorders

*R.P. Swinson, MD, FRCPsych, FRCPC*

## Goals of Therapy

- To decrease symptomatic anxiety
- To decrease anxiety-based disability
- To prevent recurrence
- To treat comorbid conditions

## Classification of Anxiety Disorders*

Panic disorder with or without agoraphobia
Agoraphobia without history of panic disorder
Social phobia
Specific phobia
Obsessive–compulsive disorder
Post-traumatic stress disorder
Acute stress disorder
Generalized anxiety disorder
Anxiety disorder due to a general medical condition
Substance-induced anxiety disorder
Anxiety disorder not otherwise specified

** As per DSM-IV-R (1994).*

## Investigations

- Thorough history with attention to:
  - nature of symptoms and onset
  - nature and extent of disability
  - presence of physical and psychological comorbid conditions

*Note:* Comorbid mood disorders, especially depression, should be treated as the primary condition.

- Interview questions (Table 1) assist in obtaining an accurate diagnosis
- Physical examination to exclude endocrine or cardiac disorders and to look for signs of substance use
- Laboratory tests:
  - CBC, liver function tests, gamma-glutamyl transpeptidase (GGT), thyroid indices (supersensitive TSH), ECG

*Note:* Physical disorders should be treated before one makes a definitive diagnosis of an anxiety disorder.

Table 1: **Interview Questions to Establish Specific Anxiety Diagnosis***

| Questions | Further Information |
|---|---|
| Do you have sudden episodes of intense anxiety? | Establish nature of attack. |
| Do you have difficulty going to places to which you used to be able to go? | Inquire about crowded places, line-ups, movies, highways, distance from home. |
| Do you have difficulty talking to people in authority or speaking in public? | Establish situations (one-on-one or groups). |
| Are you afraid of blood, small animals or heights? | Establish precise feared situation. |
| Do you repeat actions that you feel are excessive? | Ask about washing, counting, checking and hoarding. |
| Do you have thoughts that keep going in your mind that you can't stop? | Ask nature of thoughts (illness, harm, sex). |
| Have you experienced any emotionally stressful events? | Establish the nature (accident, sexual, torture) and timing of the trauma. |
| Do you worry a lot of the time? | Ask about worries related to health, family, job and finances. |

* *To be relatively sure of the diagnosis of a specific anxiety disorder, follow the order of the questions as presented. Panic attacks are diagnosed first, followed by phobic disorders, obsessive-compulsive disorder, post-traumatic stress disorder and generalized anxiety disorder. Anxiety disorders that do not fit into the above categories are atypical. An accurate diagnosis is essential before instituting pharmacologic therapy.*

## **Therapeutic Choices** (Figure 1)

### Nonpharmacologic Choices

- Caffeine or other stimulant use should be controlled.
- Alcohol use should be minimal; it should not be used to control anxiety.
- Short-acting benzodiazepine use should be reduced as much as possible; ideally, it should not be continued on a PRN basis for longer than 4 days.
- Stress reduction, including relaxation training and time management, is often helpful initially.
- Specific cognitive behavioral therapy (CBT) may be required; a psychiatric consultation should be obtained for any patient who does not improve within 6 to 8 weeks of adequate drug therapy.

Relatively mild anxiety states in reaction to life circumstances are often time-limited, and many patients will respond to anxiety management strategies without medication. Support, problem-solving and relaxation techniques will frequently be helpful as the environmental crisis resolves. However, specific anxiety or mood disorders may develop from the original reaction.

Figure 1: **Management of Anxiety Disorders**

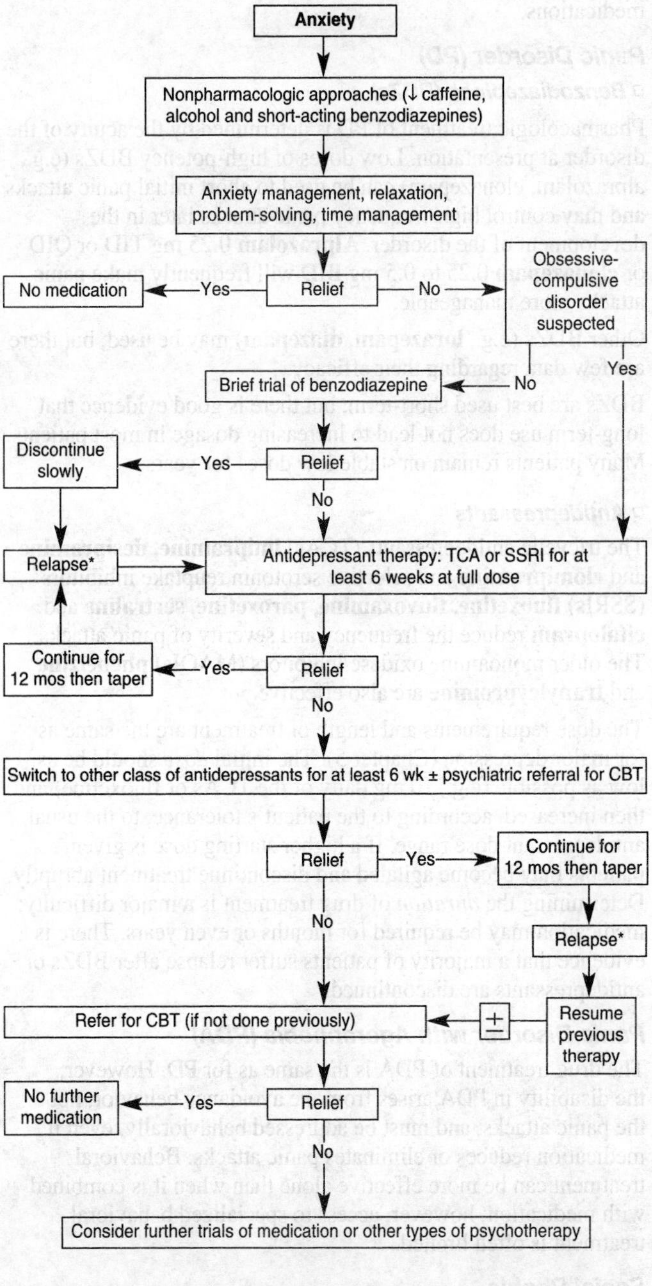
Anxiety
Nonpharmacologic approaches (↓ caffeine, alcohol and short-acting benzodiazepines)
Anxiety management, relaxation, problem-solving, time management
No medication
Yes
Relief
No
Obsessive-compulsive disorder suspected
Yes
Brief trial of benzodiazepine
No
Discontinue slowly
Yes
Relief
No
Relapse*
Antidepressant therapy: TCA or SSRI for at least 6 weeks at full dose
Continue for 12 mos then taper
Yes
Relief
No
Switch to other class of antidepressants for at least 6 wk ± psychiatric referral for CBT
Relief
Yes
Continue for 12 mos then taper
No
Relapse*
Refer for CBT (if not done previously)
±
Resume previous therapy
No further medication
Yes
Relief
No
Consider further trials of medication or other types of psychotherapy

* *If patient has relapsed twice, long-term therapy is indicated.*

*Abbreviations: TCA = tricyclic antidepressant; SSRI = selective serotonin reuptake inhibitor; CBT = cognitive behavioral therapy.*

## Pharmacologic Choices (Table 2)

The anxiety disorders respond differentially to the available medications.

### *Panic Disorder (PD)*

#### ❑ *Benzodiazepines (BDZs)*

Pharmacologic treatment of PD is determined by the acuity of the disorder at presentation. Low doses of high-potency BDZs (e.g., alprazolam, clonazepam) can be used to abort initial panic attacks and may control high-frequency panic attacks later in the development of the disorder. **Alprazolam** 0.25 mg TID or QID or **clonazepam** 0.25 to 0.5 mg BID will frequently make panic attacks more manageable.

Other BDZs (e.g., **lorazepam, diazepam**) may be used, but there are few data regarding their efficacy.

BDZs are best used short-term, but there is good evidence that long-term use does not lead to increasing dosage in most patients. Many patients remain on stable low doses for years.

#### ❑ *Antidepressants*

The tricyclic antidepressants (TCAs) **imipramine, desipramine** and **clomipramine** and selective serotonin reuptake inhibitors (SSRIs) **fluoxetine**, **fluvoxamine**, **paroxetine**, **sertraline** and **citalopram** reduce the frequency and severity of panic attacks. The older monoamine oxidase inhibitors (MAOIs) **phenelzine** and **tranylcypromine** are also effective.

The dose requirements and length of treatment are the same as for major depression (Chapter 5). The initial *dose* should be as low as possible (e.g., 10 mg daily of the TCAs or fluoxetine) and then increased, according to the patient's tolerance, to the usual antidepressant dose range. If a higher starting dose is given, patients may become agitated and discontinue treatment abruptly. Determining the *duration* of drug treatment is a major difficulty; medication may be required for months or even years. There is evidence that a majority of patients suffer relapse after BDZs or antidepressants are discontinued.

### *Panic Disorder with Agoraphobia (PDA)*

The drug treatment of PDA is the same as for PD. However, the disability in PDA arises from the avoidance behavior, not the panic attacks, and must be addressed behaviorally, even if medication reduces or eliminates panic attacks. Behavioral treatment can be more effective alone than when it is combined with medication; however, access to specialized behavioral treatment is often limited.

### *Social Phobia*

This excessive fear of being criticized or negatively evaluated by others presents as shyness, avoidance of social contact or difficulty dealing with authority figures. It is particularly important to rule out major depression and alcohol use. CBT or other psychotherapy is usually necessary to deal with significant social phobia.

Drug treatment varies according to the type of social phobia. Simple stage fright or fear of public speaking may respond to low-dose **propranolol** (10 mg) taken 30 minutes before the event. Very low doses of **lorazepam** (0.5 to 1 mg) may also be used. More complex or pervasive social phobia can be treated with the same antidepressants used for PD (i.e., **tricyclic antidepressants** and **SSRIs**). MAOIs may also be used; **moclobemide** (in antidepressant doses) is the initial choice, given the safety of the reversible inhibitors of monoamine oxidase-A (RIMAs). The dose of moclobemide often requires titration to the upper end of the dosage range.

### *Specific Phobia*

There is usually no indication for medication to treat the fear of heights, animals or blood. As few as 2 to 3 hours of behavioral treatment can be successful.

### *Obsessive–Compulsive Disorder (OCD)*

A chronic disorder that often begins in childhood or adolescence, OCD can be extremely disabling. CBT is often helpful, but drug therapy is indicated for many patients. The most effective medications are **clomipramine** (a nonselective serotonin reuptake inhibitor) or the **SSRIs**, in the usual antidepressant range. It may take 6 to 8 weeks to produce any change in symptoms; an adequate trial at full dosages for at least 6 weeks is required. There is no evidence to suggest that SSRIs vary in efficacy, but patients may be able to tolerate one drug better than others in the same group. SSRIs may be better tolerated than clomipramine, but the initial agitation experienced with SSRIs may cause some patients to discontinue treatment. **Phenelzine** or **tranylcypromine** may be tried if SSRIs are not beneficial. Treatment, if successful, may continue for years.

Benzodiazepines alone are not helpful in treating OCD.

### *Post-traumatic Stress Disorder (PTSD)*

There is no definitive treatment for PTSD, a mixture of anxiety, avoidance, mood change, insomnia and physical pain. Medication is part of a multimodal treatment program that depends on the nature, severity and frequency of the trauma. Although *benzodiazepines* are often used, there is little evidence of their efficacy. *Antidepressants* may help with mood, anxiety and pain; selection is often based on the side effect profile. *SSRIs* in antidepressant doses are the first choice. **Amitriptyline**, **doxepin** or **clomipramine** is given in low dosage for pain relief but must be given in full antidepressant dosage to affect mood changes.

Table 2: **Drugs Used in the Management of Anxiety Disorders**

| Drug | Indication(s)* | Dosage | Adverse Effects | Comments | Cost† |
|---|---|---|---|---|---|
| **Benzodiazepines** | PD, PDA, GAD | | Drowsiness (tolerance develops with continued therapy), dizziness, ↓ concentration, retrograde amnesia, physical dependence. Rarely, paradoxical anger or hostility. | Discontinue gradually to avoid rebound anxiety. Contraindicated in pregnancy and in patients with a known history of abuse. Dose escalation is rare in patients taking BDZs for chronic anxiety. Use lower doses in elderly. Warn patients re: concomitant use of alcohol, other CNS depressants (↑ effect). | |
| *alprazolam* Xanax, generics | | *PD, PDA:* 0.25 mg TID–QID, up to 1 mg QID | | | \$–\$\$ |
| *clonazepam* Rivotril, generics | | 0.25–0.5 mg BID | | | \$ |
| **Tricyclic Antidepressants** | PD, PDA, PTSD, GAD, SP; OCD – clomipramine | | CNS effects (agitation on initiation of therapy, confusion, drowsiness, headache), anticholinergic effects (dry mouth, blurred vision, constipation, etc.), weight gain, nausea, cardiovascular effects (tachycardia, arrhythmias, orthostatic hypotension), anorgasmia. | May ↑ effect of anticholinergic drugs, CNS depressants, warfarin. Do not use MAOIs concurrently. May take 2–3 mos for maximum effect. | |
| *clomipramine* Anafranil, generics | | 75–225 mg/d | | | \$–\$\$\$ |
| *desipramine* Norpramin, generics | | 75–300 mg/d | | | \$–\$\$\$\$ |
| *imipramine* Tofranil, generics | | 75–300 mg/d | | | \$ |

| | | | | | |
|---|---|---|---|---|---|
| **Selective Serotonin Reuptake Inhibitors** | PD, PDA, OCD, PTSD, SP | | **All:** Agitation (on initiation of therapy), nausea, anorgasmia. | Serotonergic syndrome with MAOIs (hypertension, tremor, agitation, hypomania). | |
| *citalopram* Celexa | | 20–60 mg/d | Insomnia, diarrhea. | | $$–$$$$ |
| *fluoxetine* Prozac, generics | | 20–80 mg/d | Insomnia, headache, ↓ appetite, diarrhea. | Inhibition of cytochrome P450 enzymes results in many drug interactions. | $$–$$$$$ |
| *fluvoxamine* Luvox, generics | | 150–300 mg/d | Anticholinergic effects, sedation. | Avoid concurrent use of fluoxetine or fluvoxamine with astemizole and terfenadine. | $$$–$$$$$ |
| *paroxetine* Paxil | | 20–60 mg/d | Anticholinergic effects, sedation. | | $$$–$$$$$ |
| *sertraline* Zoloft | | 50–200 mg/d | Insomnia, diarrhea. | | $$$–$$$$$ |
| **Serotonin-Norepinephrine Reuptake Inhibitors** | GAD | | Nausea, insomnia, dizziness, asthenia. | Do not use with MAOIs. | |
| *venlafaxine* Effexor | | 37.5–225 mg/d | | | $$–$$$$ |
| **Monoamine Oxidase Inhibitors** | PD, PDA, OCD (refractory) | | Insomnia, dizziness, orthostatic hypotension, edema, sexual dysfunction. | Dietary restrictions (tyramine-containing foods) are necessary. | |
| *phenelzine* Nardil | | 45–90 mg/d | | Sympathomimetics may ↑ BP; SSRIs, TCAs, levodopa may ↑ effects and side effects. | $$–$$$ |
| *tranylcypromine* Parnate | | 20–60 mg/d | | Do not use with meperidine (agitation, hyperpyrexia, circulatory collapse may occur). | $$–$$$$ |

*(cont'd)*

Table 2: **Drugs Used in the Management of Anxiety Disorders** *(cont'd)*

| Drug | Indication(s)* | Dosage | Adverse Effects | Comments | Cost† |
|---|---|---|---|---|---|
| **Reversible Inhibitors of Monoamine Oxidase-A**<br>*moclobemide*<br>Manerix | SP | 300–600 mg/d | Nausea, insomnia. | Do not use with meperidine, TCAs, SSRIs. | $$–$$$$ |
| **Azapirones**<br>*buspirone*<br>Buspar, generics | GAD | 5 mg BID–TID, up to 60 mg/d | Nausea, headache, dizziness, restlessness/insomnia. | Avoid use with MAOIs.<br>Not as rapid an onset as with BDZs. | $$–$$$$$ |
| **Other**<br>*propranolol*<br>Inderal, generics | SP (specific task anxiety) | 10 mg, 30 min before task PRN | Hypotension. | | $ |

* *PD = panic disorder; PDA = panic disorder with agoraphobia; GAD = generalized anxiety disorder; OCD = obsessive–compulsive disorder; PTSD = post-traumatic stress disorder; SP = social phobia.*

† *Cost of 30-day supply – includes drug cost only.*
*Legend: $ < $20 $$ $20–40 $$$ $40–60 $$$$ $60–80 $$$$$ > $80*
*Dosage adjustment may be required in renal impairment – see Appendix I.*

### *Generalized Anxiety Disorder (GAD)*

A state of chronic worry that usually continues for years once it has begun, GAD tends to be diagnosed more often when there is little attention to the specific anxiety symptoms. Patients with GAD frequently exhibit mood change, social anxiety and obsessional traits that must be addressed; a combination of anxiety management and medication therapy is thus indicated.

*Low-dose BDZ*s for several weeks at a time can be used for symptom relief. *Antidepressants* of all classes are helpful including **venlafaxine**, a serotonin-norepinephrine reuptake inhibitor.

**Buspirone** has low abuse potential and is less sedating than BDZs. Like antidepressants, it is relatively slow to have effect. There is no cross-tolerance with BDZs; care must be taken when switching from long-term BDZ therapy to avoid precipitating withdrawal symptoms if the BDZ is discontinued abruptly.

## Therapeutic Tips

- Short-term interventions may help.
- If BDZs are not quickly effective (within 2 weeks) at low doses, discontinue and switch to an antidepressant.
- If one antidepressant does not work in adequate dose and after adequate time, switch to one from another class.
- If the second antidepressant fails, refer the patient to a specialized anxiety or mood clinic.

## *Suggested Reading List*

Antony MM, Swinson RP. *Anxiety disorders and their treatment: A critical review of the evidence-based literature*. Ottawa: Health Canada, 1996:1–101.

Davidson JR, Dupont RL, Hedges D, Haskins JT. Efficacy, safety and tolerability of venlafaxine extended release and buspirone in outpatients with generalized anxiety disorder. *J Clin Psychiatry* 1999;60:528–535.

Gould RA, Otto MW, Pollack MH, Yap L. Cognitive behavioral and pharmacological treatment of generalized anxiety disorder: a preliminary meta-analysis. *Behavior Therapy* 1997;28:295–305.

Last CG, ed. *Anxiety across the lifespan: a developmental perspective.* New York: Springer, 1993.

Salvador-Carulla L, Segui J, Fernandez-Cano P, Canet J. Costs and offset effect in panic disorders. *Br J Psychiatry* 1995:166 (suppl 27):23–28.

Steketee GS. *Treatment of obsessive compulsive disorder.* New York: Guilford, 1993.

CHAPTER 3

# Attention Deficit Hyperactivity Disorder

*A. Mervyn Fox, MB, BS, FRCPC, DCH*

Attention deficit hyperactivity disorder (ADHD) is a cognitive-behavioral syndrome characterized by inattention, impulsivity, distractibility, poor organizational skills, inability to perform for delayed rewards, poor listening and fidgetiness. Only 50% of patients show hyperactivity. Sleeplessness, daydreaming, dawdling, resistance to change and difficulties in school, especially in arithmetic, are characteristic. The primary neurological dysfunction appears to be in the right cortico-frontal-striate circuitry and there is a strong familial tendency. However, symptoms may also be secondary to a variety of developmental, neurological and emotional disorders, chaotic home environments, family stressors and child abuse. Most children with ADHD have learning disabilities.

Accurate diagnosis requires time, since no universally accepted diagnostic test exists. The combination of semi-structured interview probing for core symptomatology and standardized behavior rating scales completed by parents and teacher is the most consistent diagnostic process. DSM-IV requires evidence of significant functional impairment in at least two settings such as home and school.[1] Diagnosis requires that the child, rather than the parents or teachers, is significantly distressed and disadvantaged by the symptoms. Successful intervention is measured by an improvement in the child's wellbeing rather than in a reduction of the stress experienced by adults.

## Goals of Therapy

- To reduce symptoms
- To improve family function and child's self-esteem
- To improve child's academic attainments, especially in written assignments, spelling and arithmetic
- To improve child's benefit from behavior management, special education or social skills training

[1] *American Psychiatric Association. Diagnostic and Statistical manual of mental disorders, 4th ed.: DSM–IV. Washington, D.C.: American Psychiatric Association, 1994:78–85.*

## Investigations

- Comprehensive interview with special attention to:
  - age at onset and duration of symptoms
  - situations which elicit or reduce symptoms
  - family, educational, neurological and neuropsychiatric history with special reference to bipolar affective disorder
  - symptoms of likely comorbid conditions including oppositional defiant disorders,* conduct disorder,† learning disability
- Physical examination to:
  - screen for anemia, thyroid dysfunction, hearing loss and middle ear dysfunction, visual acuity, neurologic disorders or dysmorphic syndromes‡
  - establish baselines for height and weight
- No routine laboratory, electrophysiological or neuroimaging investigations
- Obtain reports from school teachers, psychologists and special education consultants
- Medication history for drugs that may exacerbate symptoms (e.g., phenobarbital, tranquilizers, decongestants, antihistamines)

Note that normal behavior in the office does not exclude the diagnosis.

## Therapeutic Choices

Pharmacologic **and** nonpharmacologic measures are usually used simultaneously (Figure 1). The child may not respond to nonpharmacologic adjuncts until medication has been initiated.

### Nonpharmacologic Choices (Figure 1)

Foods that aggravate symptoms should be avoided.
Going to school without breakfast is a common cause of classroom inattention. Sleep habits should be reviewed.

* ***Oppositional defiant disorder*** *is characterized by long-standing and repetitive incidents including loss of temper, arguments with adults, deliberate provocation and defiance, irritability, anger and resentfulness, spite and swearing to a degree markedly different from others of the same mental age. ODD more often reflects prior disciplinary and other experiences rather than biological mechanisms.*

† ***Conduct disorder*** *is characterized by persistent violations of the rights of others with severe infractions of societal norms. Typical symptoms include persistent use of violence to achieve interpersonal objectives, theft, fire setting, cruelty to animals and major property damage.*

‡ ***Dysmorphic syndromes*** *are associated with detectable variations of the size or proportions of body parts, especially of the face and limbs, which reflect either underlying anomalies of the development of the brain or other organs secondary to metabolic or genetic disorders, or malformations due to an atypical physical environment in utero. A familiar example is Down syndrome.*

The younger the child, the more important it is to recommend nonpharmacologic approaches first. Hyperactive behavior is commonplace in healthy toddlers aged 2 to 3 years and is often seen in gifted, curious and enquiring children. Side effects and treatment failures are more common in preschool children and may deter parents from consenting to medication in the school years, when the indications and benefits are clearer.

## Pharmacologic Choices (Table 1)

First, decide on type of therapeutic trial and expected outcomes (shaded box below and Figure 1).

| Patient Characteristics | Type of Trial |
|---|---|
| Questionable diagnosis<br>Comorbidity present<br>Unreliable family<br>Multiple pre-existing "side effects" | Placebo trial<br>Blind to family and school |
| Classroom symptoms predominate<br>Few family concerns | Drug/placebo<br>Blind to school |
| Pervasive symptoms<br>Secure diagnosis | Titrate dose to response |

### *Stimulants*

**Methylphenidate** or **dextroamphetamine** are each effective in over 80% of accurately diagnosed ADHD; 96% of cases will respond to at least one stimulant. Thus virtually all patients can be managed effectively with stimulants; recourse to second-line drugs should be reserved for those with significant comorbidity or major side effects which do not respond to dosage reduction.

**Methylphenidate** is the first choice because its quick action and short half-life allow benefits to be recognized early and side effects to wear off quickly. Start with 5 to 10 mg with breakfast, (5 mg under age 9) increasing by 5 to 10 mg weekly until benefit is no longer obtained, side effects occur, or each dose approaches 1 mg/kg body weight. Add second or third doses as necessary at 3- or 4-hour intervals. Many children manage on one daily dose, others need three or four. Typically 0.3 mg/kg/dose is effective but individual titration is essential. Academic achievement may improve with smaller doses than may be necessary for control of behavior.

"Rebound symptoms" due to fluctuating blood levels can usually be controlled by adjustments in timing of methylphenidate. If this is impossible or the mid-morning dose is unacceptable to the child, **dextroamphetamine** 10 mg (controlled-release spansule) is generally more effective than sustained action methylphenidate.

Figure 1: **Management of Attention Deficit Hyperactivity Disorder**

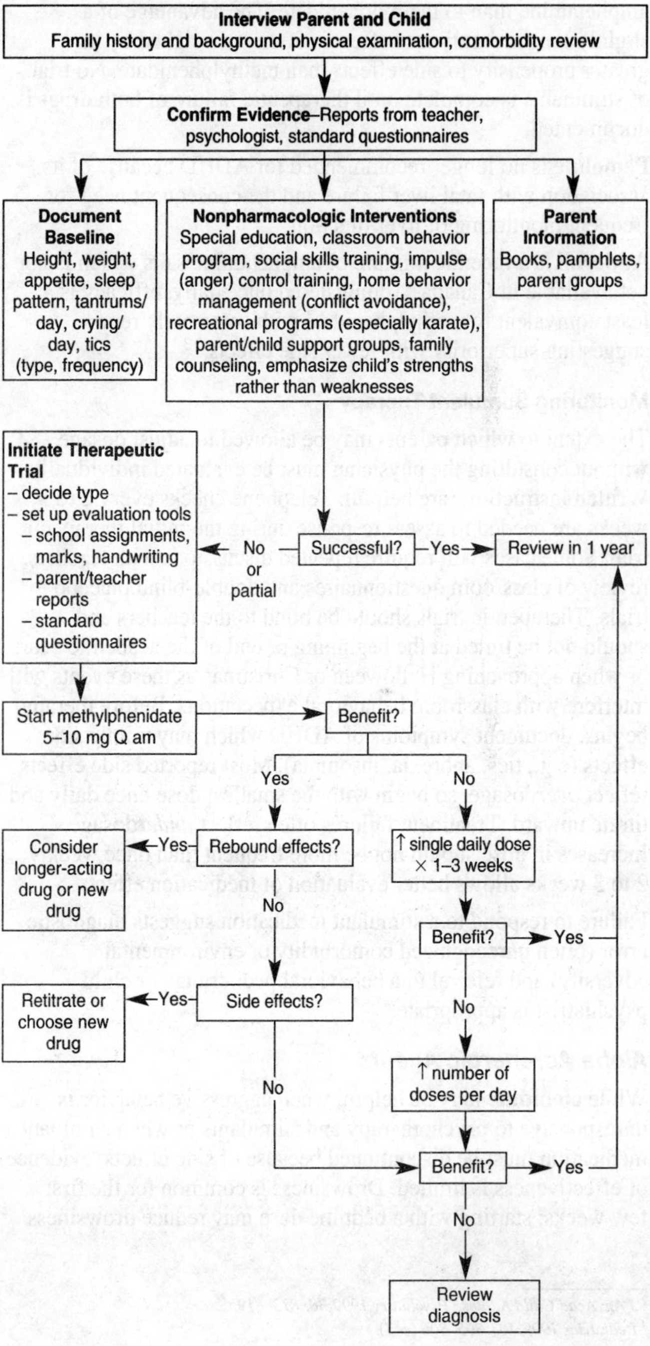
Interview Parent and Child
Family history and background, physical examination, comorbidity review
Confirm Evidence–Reports from teacher, psychologist, standard questionnaires
Document Baseline
Height, weight, appetite, sleep pattern, tantrums/day, crying/day, tics (type, frequency)
Nonpharmacologic Interventions
Special education, classroom behavior program, social skills training, impulse (anger) control training, home behavior management (conflict avoidance), recreational programs (especially karate), parent/child support groups, family counseling, emphasize child's strengths rather than weaknesses
Parent Information
Books, pamphlets, parent groups
Initiate Therapeutic Trial
– decide type
– set up evaluation tools
– school assignments, marks, handwriting
– parent/teacher reports
– standard questionnaires
No or partial
Successful?
Yes
Review in 1 year
Start methylphenidate 5–10 mg Q am
Benefit?
Yes
No
Consider longer-acting drug or new drug
Yes
Rebound effects?
↑ single daily dose × 1–3 weeks
No
Benefit?
Yes
Retitrate or choose new drug
Yes
Side effects?
No
No
↑ number of doses per day
Benefit?
Yes
No
Review diagnosis

Because of its street value and potential for abuse, dextroamphetamine should be prescribed cautiously, especially in adolescence. Some patients may respond better to dextroamphetamine than to methylphenidate. The advantage of a slightly longer duration of effect is often outweighed by its greater propensity to side effects than methylphenidate. No trial of stimulants is complete until therapeutic failure of both drugs is documented.

**Pemoline** is no longer recommended for ADHD because of its association with fatal liver failure and the consequent need for frequent monitoring of liver function.

**Adderall** is a racemic mixture of amphetamine salts which is not yet available in Canada. Administered once daily, efficacy is at least equivalent to methylphenidate with some early reports suggesting superiority with fewer side effects.[2,3]

#### Monitoring Stimulant Therapy

The extent to which parents may be allowed to adjust dosage without consulting the physician must be evaluated individually. Written instructions are helpful. Telephone checks every 2 to 3 weeks are needed to assess response during the initial therapeutic trial. Some cases will require repeated discussions with teachers, review of classroom questionnaires and double-blind placebo trials. Therapeutic trials should be blind to the teachers and should not be timed at the beginning or end of the academic year, or when approaching Halloween or Christmas as these events will interfere with classroom behavioral expectations. Before therapy begins, document symptoms of ADHD which may mimic side effects (e.g., tics, anorexia, insomnia). Most reported side effects reflect *over*dosage, so begin with the smallest dose once daily and titrate upward. Treatment failures often reflect *under*dosage. Increases in dose should not be more frequent than once weekly; 2 to 3 weeks allows better evaluation of medication effects.

Failure to respond to a stimulant medication suggests diagnostic error (often unrecognized comorbidity or environmental adversity) and referral to a behavioral pediatrician or child psychiatrist is appropriate.

### *Alpha Adrenergic Agents*

While **clonidine** may be helpful when aggressive behavior is unresponsive to psychotherapy and stimulants or when stimulant medication must be discontinued because of side effects, evidence of effectiveness is limited. Drowsiness is common for the first few weeks; starting with a bedtime dose may reduce drowsiness

---

[2] *J Am Acad Child Adolesc Psychiatry 1999;38: 813–819.*

[3] *Pediatrics 1999;103:805–806 (e43).*

Table 1: **Drugs Used in Attention Deficit Hyperactivity Disorder**

| Drug | Dosage | Adverse Effects | Comments | Cost* |
|---|---|---|---|---|
| **Stimulants** | Pharmacokinetics reflect wide individual variations; titrate dose against response. | Common, usually transient, continue trial: weepiness, headache, abdominal pain (if not taken with food), mild anorexia, mild insomnia. | First-line therapy: methylphenidate, dextroamphetamine. | |
| *methylphenidate* Ritalin, Ritalin SR, generics | Usual: 0.3 mg/kg given once daily – TID<br>Range: 0.15–1 mg/kg/dose | Transient, stop and re-evaluate: growth failure, psychotic reactions, insomnia, platelet changes.<br>Overdose symptoms, stop and retitrate: weight loss, sedation, "glassy eyes", insomnia, hyperactivity.<br>Significant, may be permanent, stop and re-evaluate: tics, neurologic symptoms, exacerbation of symptoms (may aggravate Tourette's syndrome). | Avoid concurrent use of methylphenidate and dextroamphetamine with MAOIs.<br>Methylphenidate: uncertain effects on seizure disorders; discontinue if seizures occur. May ↑ plasma levels of phenytoin, TCAs.<br>Dextroamphetamine: do not use in cardiovascular disease. | 10 mg/d<br>$ |
| *dextroamphetamine* Dexedrine | Usual: 0.15 mg/kg given once daily – TID<br>Range: 0.15–0.3 mg/kg/dose | | | 5 mg/d<br>$ |
| *pemoline* Cyclert | Usual: 1–2 mg/kg once daily<br>Range: Up to 112.5 mg/d | | Pemoline: no longer recommended. Removed from market due to reports of fatal hepatotoxicity | † |

*(cont'd)*

Table 1: **Drugs Used in Attention Deficit Hyperactivity Disorder** *(cont'd)*

| Drug | Dosage | Adverse Effects | Comments | Cost* |
|---|---|---|---|---|
| **Antidepressants** | | | | |
| *imipramine*<br>Tofranil, generics | Usual: Up to 5 mg/kg/d once daily<br>Range: 25–75 mg HS | Orthostatic hypotension, arrhythmias (potential for fatal arrhythmias in overdose), anticholinergic effects, drowsiness, tremor, weight gain. | Do ECG to exclude conduction defects before prescribing.<br>Do not use with MAO inhibitors; may cause mania, excitation, hyperpyrexia.<br>Barbiturates, carbamazepine, rifampin may ↓ effect. | $ |
| *desipramine*<br>Norpramin, generics | Usual: Up to 3.5 mg/kg/d, given once daily – TID<br>Range: 25–50 mg/dose | Desipramine may be better tolerated. | Cimetidine, fluoxetine, neuroleptics may ↑ effect and toxicity. | $–$$ |
| **Alpha Adrenergic Agents** | | | | |
| *clonidine* ❥<br>Catapres, generics | Usual: 4–5 µg/kg/d, divided QID | Hypotension, sedation, dry mouth, could exacerbate depression. | Avoid concurrent use with amitriptyline, desipramine and imipramine.<br>Safety in large numbers of patients unknown. | $ |
| **Neuroleptics** | | | | |
| *thioridazine*<br>Mellaril, generics | Usual: 1–3 mg/kg/d, given once daily – TID | Sedation, anticholinergic effects, tardive and withdrawal dyskinesias, hypotension. | Use with caution in epileptic children or those with cardiovascular disease. | $ |

❥ *Dosage adjustment may be required in renal impairment – see Appendix I.*
† *Removed from market September 1999. Available in exceptional cases through Health Canada's Special Access Program.*

* *Cost of 30-day supply – includes drug cost only.*
*Legend: $ < $10 $$ $10–20*

and improve sleep problems. Clonidine may be used if prominent tics precede treatment or arise during stimulant therapy (and do not improve with reduced dosage). A family history of or comorbidity with Tourette's syndrome is a relative rather than an absolute contraindication to stimulants. Because serious but probably coincidental side effects have been attributed to the combination of clonidine and methylphenidate, the combination is not recommended to be prescribed by family physicians. Baseline blood pressure should be obtained and the patients warned of the possibility of hypertension if the drug is suddenly discontinued.

### *Antidepressants*

Antidepressants are less successful than stimulants in improving cognitive aspects of ADHD, but equally effective in reducing inappropriate behavior. Consider tricyclic antidepressants, **desipramine** or **imipramine** if stimulants fail or must be discontinued because of rebound symptoms or side effects (especially insomnia), or if there is a comorbid mood disorder. However, depressed patients with ADHD respond at least as well to stimulants as to antidepressants.

Although **SSRIs** lack evidence of efficacy in ADHD, they may be more effective than tricyclics in true mood disorders. Therefore, the combination of SSRI and stimulant is recommended for ADHD with comorbid mood disorder. SSRIs may be considered in adolescence if there is a risk of substance abuse. (See Chapter 5 for prescribing information).

**Bupropion** may prove a useful addition to the available treatments for hyperactivity, inattention and aggression, including antisocial conduct disorders, especially where stimulant side effects are severe, or there is a high level of anxiety. However, evidence to date is only suggestive.[4,5]

### *Neuroleptics*

There are no accepted criteria for the diagnosis of ADHD in preschool children, in whom other developmental, temperamental and environmental factors are more likely to cause hyperactivity. Involvement in a good early childhood education program and improving parenting skills are preferred to medication in all but extreme cases threatening family integrity. If the diagnosis is questionable but the symptoms intolerable, neuroleptics may be preferred to stimulants in preschool children, as stimulant side effects may be sufficient to deter parents from their use when the child is older and more likely to benefit.

---

[4] *J Am Acad Child Adolesc Psychiatry 1998;37:1271–78.*
[5] *J Am Acad Child Adolesc Psychiatry 1996;35:1314–1321.*

## Therapeutic Tips

- Parents and teachers are exposed to inaccurate information regarding diagnosis and management of ADHD, especially the benefits and side effects of medication. Physicians should provide factual oral and written material, connect the family with knowledgeable support groups, and help parent and child to reach their own conclusions.
- Remember that every prescription of medication must be conducted as an individual therapeutic trial.
- It must be made clear that good and inappropriate behaviors remain the child's responsibility. Medication is neither a controlling straitjacket nor a magic wand.
- Drug holidays are unnecessary unless anorexia results in growth failure. Fluctuating behavioral competence may increase the child's sense of demoralization. Children have as much to learn from their parents as at school (organizational skills, ability to defer gratification, self-discipline and self-esteem).
- Successful stimulant therapy should be continued as long as there is clear benefit, often into adult life. At least once a year medication should be withdrawn for 1 week to evaluate the need for prescription. Some children learn by experiencing normal attention and impulse control and manage well after 1 to 2 years.
- Although stimulants are helpful in increasing academic productivity, may improve speed and neatness of handwriting, and sometimes reading comprehension, they will not affect learning disabilities, which **must** be independently diagnosed in order for early and appropriate special educational intervention to be made.

## *Suggested Reading List*


American Academy of Child and Adolescent Psychiatry. Summary of the practice parameters for the assessment and treatment of children, adolescents and adults with ADHD. *J Am Acad Child Adolesc Psychiatry* 1997;36:1311–1317.

Cantwell DP. Attention deficit disorder: a review of the past 10 years. *J Am Acad Child Adolesc Psychiatry* 1996;35: 978–987.

Fox AM, Mahoney W (editors). *Children with school problems: a physician's manual.* Ottawa: Canadian Pediatric Society 1998.

Fox AM, Rieder MJ. Risks and benefits of drugs used in the management of the hyperactive child. *Drug Safety* 1993;9:38–50.

Spencer T, Biederman J, Wilens T, et al. Pharmacotherapy of attention-deficit disorder across the life cycle. *J Am Acad Child Adolesc Psychiatry* 1996;35:409–432.

CHAPTER 4

# Dementia

*Kenneth Rockwood, MD, FRCPC and*
*Catherine Shea, MD, FRCPC*

Dementia is a syndrome of acquired global impairment of cognitive function sufficient to interfere with normal activities. The most common causes are Alzheimer's disease, vascular dementia, a mixture of the two and Lewy body dementia. Dementias are progressive deteriorating illnesses in which treatment options are different at different stages of the illness.

## Goals of Therapy

- To slow disease progression (chiefly Alzheimer's disease and vascular dementia)
- To treat behavioral and psychological symptoms
- To alleviate caregiver burden

## Investigations

### Dementia

- History of memory impairment and potentially reversible causes. Cognitive impairment can be assessed using the Mini-Mental State Examination[1] (MMSE) and functional disability using the Functional Assessment Questionnaire (FAQ)[2]
- Physical examination to identify the cause and to look for potentially reversible causes
- Laboratory tests: CBC, electrolytes, kidney function, TSH, calcium
- CT scan for young patients (< 60 years), new onset, rapid progression, post-head injury, focal or lateralizing signs, history of cancer, use of anticoagulants, early urinary incontinence and gait disorder, or unusual cognitive symptoms[3]

### Behavioral and Psychological Symptoms

Behavioral disturbances can be part of the illness or have medical and/or environmental precipitants:

- History of concomitant symptoms, environmental precipitants or medication changes

[1] *J Psychiatry Res 1975;12:185–189.*
[2] *Psychopharmacol Bull 1988;24:653–659.*
[3] *Can Med Assoc J 1999;160(Suppl 12).*

Figure 1: **Management of the Elderly Patient with Behavioral Problems**

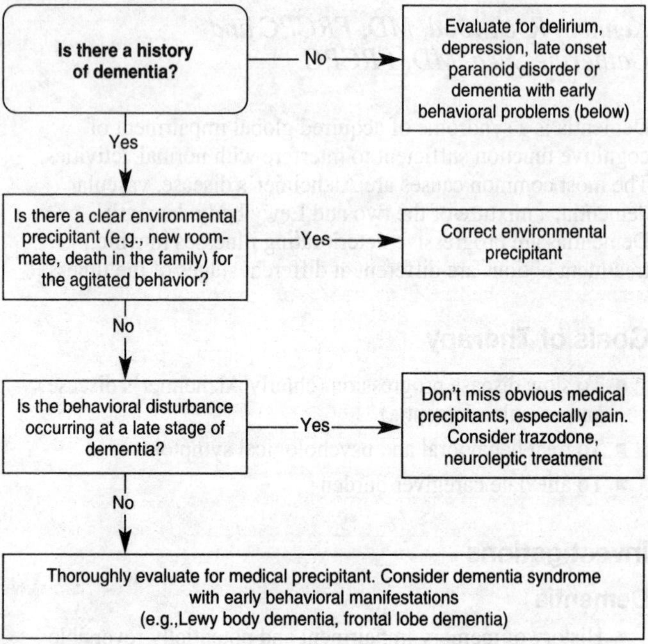
Is there a history of dementia?
No
Evaluate for delirium, depression, late onset paranoid disorder or dementia with early behavioral problems (below)
Yes
Is there a clear environmental precipitant (e.g., new room-mate, death in the family) for the agitated behavior?
Yes
Correct environmental precipitant
No
Is the behavioral disturbance occurring at a late stage of dementia?
Yes
Don't miss obvious medical precipitants, especially pain. Consider trazodone, neuroleptic treatment
No
Thoroughly evaluate for medical precipitant. Consider dementia syndrome with early behavioral manifestations (e.g.,Lewy body dementia, frontal lobe dementia)

- Examination for focal or lateralizing signs or meningismus. Both sets of signs will usually be absent; thus toxic or metabolic causes should be evaluated, particularly signs of infection, congestive heart failure
- Laboratory tests: CBC, electrolytes, urea, creatinine, glucose, urinalysis, chest radiograph

Lack of **stage congruence** of the symptoms suggests a medical cause for agitated behavior. In Alzheimer's disease, psychosis and behavioral symptoms tend to occur in the later stages. If seen early, a more aggressive medical investigation is warranted. Environmental precipitants should be sought (Figure 1). A careful psychiatric history should be elicited because psychiatric syndromes which have occurred earlier in the patient's life may recur and can guide treatment.

## Therapeutic Choices

### Nonpharmacologic Choices

Family and other caregivers should be involved in all nonpharmacologic therapy.

- Before disease progression hampers competence, durable power of attorney and advance health care directives should be explored.
- Because individuals with dementia are at increased risk for accidents (falls, burns), environmental hazards should be removed.
- Patients should be counseled against driving after the initial stages of disease.

## Pharmacologic Choices (Table 1)

### Dementia

**Donepezil** is a cholinesterase inhibitor which is indicated in mild to moderate Alzheimer's disease (MMSE scores 10–26). Significant benefits in cognition and function have been demonstrated.[4,5] While clinically detectable, these benefits are often small. A minority of patients do particularly well. Successful treatment is not reversal of all symptoms, but rather consists of stabilization of some problems, improvement in others and progression in the remainder. Patient's responses vary and assessment must be individualized. Follow-up to detect side effects after 2 weeks of initiating or increasing treatment, and every 3 months to monitor treatment effects is advised. Duration of the trials has been at most 6 months under double-blind conditions and a dose response effect has been shown in only one trial.[5]

**Rivastigmine** is the second cholinesterase inhibitor to be approved for Alzheimer's disease.[6] Although the drugs have distinct modes of action, no comparative trials of efficacy and safety exist. Until more familiarity with these drugs is achieved, close attention to prescribing recommendations is advised.

Despite many trials, clinically significant beneficial effects of **ergoloid mesylates** in Alzheimer's disease have not been demonstrated.

**Vitamin E**, in a dose of 2000 IU per day of alpha tocopherol, appeared to slow the progression of dementia.[7] Few side effects were apparent beyond an increased incidence of falls.

Long-term use of **nonsteroidal anti-inflammatory drugs** may be protective for Alzheimer's disease.[8] Similar evidence is accumulating for estrogen use.[8] Nevertheless, there are insufficient data to recommend the routine use of either of these classes of drugs in dementia prevention or treatment.

---

[4] *Neurology 1998;50:136–145.*
[5] *Geriatr Cog Disord 1999;10:237–244.*
[6] *BMJ 1999;318:633–638.*
[7] *N Engl J Med 1997; 336:1216–1222.*
[8] *Can Med Assoc J 2000;162:65–72.*

Table 1: **Drugs Used in the Treatment of Dementia**

| Drug | Dosage | Adverse Effects | Cost* |
|---|---|---|---|
| *donepezil* ➔ Aricept | Initial: 5 mg/d<br>Target: 10 mg/d<br>Adjust dose after 6 wks | Nausea, vomiting, diarrhea, fatigue, muscle cramps, anorexia. | $$$ |
| *rivastigmine* Exelon | Initial: 1.5 mg BID<br>Target: 6–12 mg/d<br>Adjust dose monthly | Side effects are similar to donepezil. | $$$ |
| *vitamin E* | 2000 IU/d | Generally well tolerated. Nausea, diarrhea, intestinal cramps, fatigue, weakness, headache. | $ |
| *trazodone* Desyrel, generics | Initial: 25–50 mg QHS<br>Maximum: 400 mg/d in divided doses | Drowsiness, nausea, vomiting, headache, dry mouth, priapism. | $ |
| *risperidone* ➔ Risperdal | Initial: 0.5 mg/d<br>Target: 1 mg/d<br>Maximum: 2 mg/d | Extrapyramidal symptoms, insomnia, constipation, GI upset. | $ |

➔ *Dosage adjustment may be required in renal impairment – see Appendix I.*
* *Cost of 30-day supply – includes drug cost only.*
*Legend: $ < $50 $$ $50–100 $$$ $100–150*

In the largest study of disease progression to date, **selegilene** proved more effective than placebo, but no more effective than Vitamin E alone in delaying death, institutionalization and progression to severe dementia.

Treatment with **ginkgo biloba** has shown a statistically significant difference in measures of cognition in a one-year, double-blind study, but the size of the effect was small and not detected clinically.[9] There is also question about the actual content of the active compound in commercially available preparations.

## Behavioral and Psychological Symptoms

### *Antidepressants*

Many patients in the early stages of dementia suffer from depression. Occasionally, depression manifests as cognitive impairment. Antidepressant therapy may be beneficial. **Selective serotonin reuptake inhibitors** are less likely than tricyclic antidepressants to cause anticholinergic side effects or to worsen orthostatic hypotension, which is common in this population. If used, a tricyclic with a low potential for anticholinergic effects, such as **desipramine or nortriptyline**, should be chosen. (Refer to Chapter 5 for dosing information.)

#### *Trazodone for Behavioral and Sleep Disturbances*

Trazodone, a serotonergic agonist, is often used successfully to manage agitated behavior.[10] Start with a low dose of 25 to 50 mg, usually first given at night and increased every few days until the desired effect is achieved (maximum dose of 400 mg per day). Trazodone is also used to treat disrupted sleep–wake cycles and "sun downing'' (worsening of behavior as darkness falls).

### *Neuroleptics*

For behavioral disturbances associated with dementia, especially aggression, or if psychotic symptoms are evident, **risperidone** is effective at a dose of 0.5 mg to 2 mg per day, with 1 mg per day being optimal.[11,12] Periodic reassessment is essential; even in the absence of therapy, the natural history is gradual diminution of these problems. Typical neuroleptics (**thioridazine**, **loxapine** or **haloperidol**) have long been used, despite modest evidence for benefit.[13] Tardive dyskinesia, a potentially irreversible movement disorder, is a consequence of their indiscriminate use. As the elderly demented brain is exquisitely sensitive to neuroleptics, initial doses should be small (e.g., risperidone 0.5 mg per day).

---

[9] *JAMA 1997;278:1327–32.*

[10] *Psychopharmacology. New York: Raven, 1995:1427–1436.*

[11] *J Clin Psychiatry 1999;60:107–115.*

[12] *Neurology 1999;53:946–955.*

[13] *J Am Geriatr Soc 1990;38:553–563.*

### *Benzodiazepines*

Data on the efficacy of benzodiazepines for behavioral problems are conflicting. Although use can result in oversedation and worsening cognition, benzodiazepines are sometimes indicated for severe agitation. Low doses of a short-acting agent without active metabolites (**lorazepam** 0.5 to 1 mg, **oxazepam** 5 to 10 mg, **temazepam** 15 mg) may be tried. In an acute situation, to manage severely agitated patients, **lorazepam** 0.5 to 1 mg can be mixed in the same syringe with **haloperidol** (0.5, 1 or 1.5 mg) and given IM every 8 hours for a maximum of 3 days.

### *Others*

Beta-blockers (particularly **pindolol**), **carbamazepine, divalproex, lithium** and **buspirone** have also been used successfully in case reports, but better evidence is lacking. These agents seem to work best when the problem behavior mimics the psychiatric syndrome for which the drug is efficacious, e.g., lithium for cycling and manic features.

### *Vascular Dementia: Slowing Disease Progression*

Vascular risk factors should be modified, particularly to ensure good control of hypertension. **Acetylsalicylic acid** has been reported to slow progression of multi-infarct dementia.[13] There is very limited evidence for modest benefit from **pentoxifylline.**[14]

### *Dementia with Lewy Bodies*

Because of the neuroleptic sensitivity syndrome in diffuse cortical Lewy body disease, neuroleptics should be avoided. These patients often present with hallucinations and early parkinsonism, which can be worsened by neuroleptics.[15] There is anecdotal evidence for using donepezil in Lewy body dementia.[16] Prescribing considerations are similar to Alzheimer's disease.

### *Prevention of Dementia*

Cardiovascular risk factors increase the chance of all causes of late-life dementia, including Alzheimer's disease. Evidence from the Syst-Eur trial suggests that the incidence of dementia can be halved in elderly patients treated for systolic hypertension.[17]

## Therapeutic Tips

- Tips for using antidepressants in dementia include:
  – Start low.
  – Monitor for side effects.

---

[13] *J Am Geriatr Soc 1989;37:549–555.*
[14] *J Am Geriatr Soc 1992;40:237–244.*
[15] *Neurology 1996;47:1113–1124.*
[16] *Int Psychogeriatr 1998;10:229–238.*
[17] *Lancet 1998;352:1347–1352.*

- Increase until the recommended dosage range is reached.
- Once the lower end of the recommended dosage range has been reached, continue increasing the dose as side effects permit until the patient benefits, or the maximum dose has been reached.
- Maintain for 4 to 6 weeks after the first indication of symptomatic improvement (e.g., improved mood, appetite, sleep or energy) *before* deciding that the drug is ineffective, or that only a partial response has been achieved.

■ Tips for using neuroleptics in dementia include:
- Start low, go slow.
- Treat to a designated endpoint, usually an improvement in symptoms, not their complete resolution.
- Neuroleptic-induced akathisia (increased motor restlessness) may be misinterpreted as lack of drug effect. The dose then is increased, increasing motor restlessness. This cycle of worsening akathisia and increased neuroleptic use can result in extrapyramidal rigidity to the point of immobility.

## Pharmacoeconomic Considerations

*Jeffrey A. Johnson, PhD*

With the recent introduction of the first drug therapies for Alzheimer's Disease (AD), there has been considerable attention to the economic burden of the disease, as well as the evaluation of the pharmacoeconomic impact of the new therapies. In Canada, the annual societal cost of caring per AD patient increased with severity, ranging from $9,451 for mild disease to $36,794 for severe disease.

Initial economic evaluations indicate that donepezil may be cost-effective due to reductions in progression of disease and reduced institutionalization. While use of donepezil may result in increased costs for informal caregiver's time at home, the overall reduction in health care costs and increased health-related quality of life (HRQOL) suggest that donepezil would be a cost-effective therapeutic choice. The pharmacoeconomic evidence suggests that the cost-effectiveness of donepezil increases if prescribed earlier in the disease, for less advanced AD (i.e., MMSE > 10). The economic evaluations of donepezil were both based on the same 24-week phase 3 clinical trial; further information on the longer term duration of effect will be required to validate these pharmacoeconomic modeling studies.

Economic evaluations of tacrine and propentoylline in AD have also been conducted in other countries, and have indicated marginal economic benefit, but these products are not available in Canada.

***Suggested Reading:***

*Hux MJ, O'Brien BJ, Iskedjian M, et al. Relation between severity of Alzheimer's disease and cost of caring. Can Med Assoc J 1998;159:457–465.*

*Neumann PJ, Hermann RC, Kuntz KM, et al. Cost-effectiveness of donepezil in the treatment of mild to moderate Alzheimer's disease. Neurology 1999;52:1138–1145.*

*O'Brien BJ, Gorree R, Hux M, et al. Economic evaluation of donepezil for the treatment of Alzheimer's Disease in Canada. J Am Geriatr Soc 1999;47:570–578.*

## Suggested Reading List

Alexopoulos GS, Silver JM, Kahn DA, Frances A, Carpenter D. Treatment of agitation in older persons with dementia. *Postgrad Med* 1998;103:April Supplement.

Carrier L, Brodarty H. Mood and behaviour management. In: Gauthier S, ed. *Diagnosis and management of Alzheimer's disease*. 2nd ed. London: Martin Dunitz, 1999.

Forette F, Rockwood K. Therapeutic interventions in dementia. In: Wilcock GK, Bucks R, Rockwood K, eds. *Diagnosis and management of dementia*. Oxford: Oxford University Press, 1999.

Patterson CJS, Gauthier S, Bergman H, et al. Management of dementing disorders. Conclusions from the Canadian consensus conference on dementia. *Can Med Assoc J* 1999;160(Suppl 12):S1–S15.

CHAPTER 5

# Depression

*Sidney H. Kennedy, MD, FRCPC and*
*Sagar V. Parikh, MD, FRCPC*

## Goals of Therapy

- To relieve symptoms of depression
- To prevent suicide
- To restore optimal functioning
- To prevent recurrence

## Classification (Tables 1 and 2)

Table 1: **Criteria for a Major Depressive Episode***

Depressed mood and/or loss of interest or pleasure (irritability)
plus
at least four of the symptoms below for the same two-week period
(must represent a change from previous functioning)

| Physical | Psychological |
|---|---|
| Change in sleep | Feelings of worthlessness or guilt |
| Change in appetite or weight | Difficulty concentrating or making decisions |
| Fatigue | Recurrent thoughts of death or suicidal ideation |
| Change in activity level (agitated or slowed down) observed by others | |

Not due to medical or drug induced conditions or normal bereavement

* *As defined by Diagnostic and Statistical Manual of Mental Disorders, fourth ed. (DSM-IV). Washington, DC: American Psychiatric Association, 1994.*

## Therapeutic Choices

### Nonpharmacologic Choices

- Adherence to treatment and favorable response are strongly influenced by initial health education. One visit for "psycho-education" alone or with video and reading materials is strongly recommended. Five key points to stress: take medication daily; whom to call for questions about side effects or other issues; antidepressants must be taken for 2 to 4 weeks for a noticeable effect; continue to take medication even if feeling better; do not stop taking the antidepressant without checking with the physician.
- Both *cognitive–behavioral* (CBT) and *interpersonal* (IPT) *psychotherapies* are as effective as antidepressants in mild to moderate depression; antidepressants appear to be more effective in moderate to severe depression.
- All can be combined with antidepressant medications.

Table 2: **Common Depressive Syndromes**

| Syndromes | Essential Features | Treatment Implications |
|---|---|---|
| **Major Depression** | | |
| Typical | Depressed mood or loss of interest and four other depressive symptoms | Antidepressants and focused psychotherapies. |
| Atypical | Overeating/weight gain<br>Oversleeping, rejection sensitivity<br>Mood reactivity preserved | SSRIs, MAOIs are preferred;<br>TCAs may be less effective. |
| "Anxious" | Prominent anxiety symptoms in addition to major depressive symptoms | Initial dose should be low, but may ultimately require a higher dose for longer duration. |
| Seasonal | Fall onset, spring offset<br>Recurrent | Light therapy is optimal; SSRIs may be as effective. |
| Melancholic | Unreactive mood<br>Worse in morning<br>Excessive guilt | Electroconvulsive therapy, TCAs and SNRI recommended. |
| Psychotic | Hallucinations<br>Delusions | Electroconvulsive therapy or combination antidepressant with neuroleptic therapy. |
| **Dysthymia** | Chronic depressive illness for two or more years, fewer and less severe symptoms than major depression | Antidepressants, but may be less effective than with major depression.<br>Consider SSRIs. |
| **Bipolar Depression*** | Prior history of mania or hypomania<br>Mixed episodes may occur | Try to avoid antidepressants.<br>Mood stabilizers preferred, e.g., lithium, valproate, carbamazepine. |

* *Can J Psychiatry 1997;42 Suppl 2: 67S–100S.*

## Pharmacologic Choices (Table 3)

### *Selective Serotonin Reuptake Inhibitors (SSRIs)*

*Greater tolerability* and *easy dosing* contributed to the rapid adoption of SSRIs as first-choice antidepressants. Although efficacy is considered comparable to established and novel antidepressants (4 to 6 weeks is still required for a therapeutic trial; about 65% of patients respond), the well-tolerated side effect profile greatly expands the population that may be treated

Table 3: **Antidepressant Drugs**

| Drug | Daily Dosage Starting* | Usual† | High‡ | Adverse Effects | Drug Interactions | Cost^π |
|---|---|---|---|---|---|---|
| **SSRIs** | | | | | | |
| *citalopram* Celexa | 10–20 mg | 20–40 mg | 60 mg | Nausea, dry mouth, somnolence, sweating. | **For all SSRIs:** MAOIs may cause severe reaction – tremor, agitation, hypomania, hypertension. Drugs that inhibit cytochrome P-450 enzymes may ↑ SSRI levels. All SSRIs inhibit certain cytochrome P-450 isoenzymes involved in drug metabolism, resulting in many potential drug interactions. | $$ |
| *fluoxetine* Prozac, generics | 10–20 mg | 20–40 mg | 60–80 mg | Nausea, nervousness, anorexia, insomnia. | | $$–$$$$ |
| *fluvoxamine* Luvox, generics | 50–100 mg | 150–200 mg | 400 mg | Nausea, drowsiness, sweating, anorexia. | | $$$ |
| *paroxetine* Paxil | 10–20 mg | 20–40 mg | 60 mg | Nausea, drowsiness, fatigue, sweating, dizziness. | | $$$–$$$$ |
| *sertraline* Zoloft, generics | 25–50 mg | 50–100 mg | 150–200 mg | Nausea, tremors, diarrhea, dry mouth. | | $$$ |
| **MAOIs** | | | | | | |
| *phenelzine* Nardil | 15–30 mg | 30–75 mg | 90–120 mg | **For both agents:** Edema, postural hypotension, insomnia, sexual dysfunction. | **For both agents:** Sympathomimetics may ↑ BP; meperidine may cause agitation, hyperpyrexia, circulatory collapse; TCAs, levodopa may ↑ effects and side effects; tyramine-containing food may cause hypertensive crisis. Avoid combination with SSRIs. | $–$$$ |
| *tranylcypromine* Parnate | 10–20 mg | 20–60 mg | 60–80 mg | | | $$–$$$ |

*(cont'd)*

Table 3: **Antidepressant Drugs** *(cont'd)*

| Drug | Starting* | Daily Dosage Usual[†] | High[‡] | Adverse Effects | Drug Interactions | Cost[π] |
|---|---|---|---|---|---|---|
| **TCAs** | | | | | | |
| *amitriptyline* Elavil, generics | 25–50 mg | 75–200 mg | 250–300 mg | **For all TCAs:** Anticholinergic (dry mouth, blurred vision, constipation, urinary hesitancy, tachycardia, delirium), antihistaminergic (sedation, weight gain), orthostatic hypotension, lowered seizure threshold. | **For all TCAs:** Combination with MAOIs may result in mania, excitation, hyperpyrexia. Barbiturates, carbamazepine and rifampin may decrease effect. Cimetidine and neuroleptics may increase effect and toxicity. Possible interaction with antiarrhythmics: may increase effect of either drug. May decrease antihypertensive effect of clonidine. May augment hypotensive effect of thiazides. | $ |
| *clomipramine* Anafranil, generics | 50–75 mg | 100–250 mg | 300–450 mg | | | $$–$$$$ |
| *desipramine* Norpramin, generics | 50–75 mg | 100–200 mg | 300–450 mg | | | $$–$$$ |
| *doxepin* Sinequan, generics | 50–75 mg | 100–250 mg | 300–450 mg | | | $–$$$ |
| *imipramine* Tofranil, generics | 50–75 mg | 100–250 mg | 300–450 mg | | | $ |
| *maprotiline* Ludiomil, generics | 50–75 mg | 100–250 mg | 300–450 mg | | | $–$$ |
| *nortriptyline* Aventyl, generics | 25–50 mg | 75–150 mg | 200 mg | | | $$–$$$ |
| *protriptyline* Triptil | 10–20 mg | 20–40 mg | 40–60 mg | | | $$–$$$$ |
| *trimipramine* Surmontil, generics | 50–75 mg | 100–250 mg | 300–450 mg | | | $–$$ |

| | | | | | | |
|---|---|---|---|---|---|---|
| **Other** | | | | | | |
| *nefazodone* Serzone | 100–200 mg | 300–500 mg | 600 mg | Dizziness, amblyopia, dry mouth, nausea, drowsiness. | May displace protein-bound drugs. May augment hypotensive effect of antihypertensives. May inhibit metabolism of triazolam, alprazolam, midazolam, cyclosporine, nifedipine, lidocaine, erythromycin. | $$$–$$$$$ |
| *venlafaxine* Effexor XR | 37.5–75 mg | 112.5–225 mg | 225–300 mg | Nausea, drowsiness, nervousness, dizziness, dry mouth, may ↑ BP if dose > 300 mg/d. | Drugs that inhibit cytochrome P-450 may ↑ venlafaxine levels. May interact with MAOIs. | $$$$–$$$$$ |
| *moclobemide* Manerix | 200–300 mg | 450–600 mg | 900 mg[#] | Nausea, insomnia, dizziness. | Avoid sympathomimetics, meperidine. Caution with opioids, antihypertensives, antipsychotics, SSRIs, selegiline, excessive tyramine, alcohol. Reduce dose with cimetidine. | $$–$$$ |
| *bupropion* SR Wellbutrin SR | 75 mg | 150–300 mg | 375–450 mg | Agitation, insomnia, anorexia, contraindicated if history of seizures. | May ↑ levels of cyclophosphamide, ifosfamide and orphenadrine. | $$–$$$ |

** Lower starting dose indicated where previous side effect experience or polypharmacy; often applies to elderly patients.*
*† For SSRIs upper starting dose may be usual dose, e.g., fluoxetine 20 mg or sertraline 50 mg; otherwise increments every 5–7 days.*
*‡ Higher doses often exceed manufacturer's recommended upper doses and usually result in more disabling side effects. These doses should be used with caution.*
*π Cost of 30-day supply – includes drug cost only.*
*Legend: $ < $20 $$ $20–40 $$$ $40–60 $$$$ $60–100 $$$$$ > $100*
*# Exceeds manufacturer's recommended maximum dose of 600 mg.*

effectively. Sexual dysfunction (anorgasmia in women and delayed ejaculation in men) is more common with all SSRIs than was initially recognized. **Citalopram**, the newest SSRI, shares the same efficacy and side effect profile as the other SSRIs.

### *Tricyclic Antidepressants (TCAs)*

Long the mainstay of antidepressant pharmacotherapy, tricyclics are less favored now because of frequent side effects, especially cardiotoxicity, and lethality in overdose. In general, they are equivalent to newer agents in efficacy and less expensive. However, clomipramine was found to be superior to several new agents in the treatment of hospitalized depressed patients.[1]

*Secondary amine TCAs* include **desipramine**, **nortriptyline** and **protriptyline**. The severity of anticholinergic and antihistaminergic side effects is less than with the *tertiary amines* (**amitriptyline**, **imipramine**, **doxepin**, **clomipramine** and **trimipramine**). **Maprotiline** is a related *tetracyclic* antidepressant with similar efficacy and side effects, although there is an increased risk of seizures at high doses (above 200 mg).

For most cyclic antidepressants, it is best to "start low and go slow." A usual starting dose is 50 mg given at night, building to 100 mg after 3 to 5 days and increasing weekly, depending on tolerability and antidepressant response. The average dose can be approximated by calculating 3 mg/kg body weight. In elderly, cachexic or medically ill patients, lower starting doses (10 to 25 mg) are more appropriate and can be gradually increased to 1.5 mg/kg body weight.

### *Classical Monoamine Oxidase Inhibitors (MAOIs)*

Use of phenelzine and tranylcypromine is limited by concerns about hazardous drug–drug and food–drug interactions. However, many TCA nonresponders are responsive to MAOIs. Historically, **phenelzine** in doses of 30 to 90 mg per day has been the drug of choice in atypical depression. **Tranylcypromine** 20 to 60 mg per day may be superior to imipramine in treating bipolar depression. Because of the irreversible enzyme inhibition, food and drug cautions must be followed for 2 weeks after the last dose of MAOI.

### *Reversible Inhibitors of Monoamine Oxidase-A (RIMA)*

RIMAs do not require dietary precautions and have less hazardous drug–drug interactions than MAOIs. The only RIMA available in Canada is **moclobemide**. In the treatment of outpatient depression, clinical trials suggest comparable efficacy to TCAs and SSRIs and a lower rate of adverse effects.

---

[1] *Psychopharmacology 1986;90:131–138.*

Moclobemide is prescribed in divided doses between 300 and 600 mg daily, although higher doses have been used for partial responders when side effects are minimal or absent. Nausea may be an early but brief adverse effect; insomnia may persist. Sexual dysfunction is rare.

### *Serotonin–Norepinephrine Reuptake Inhibitors (SNRI)*

**Venlafaxine** may be effective in refractory patients. It may be more effective than other antidepressants for melancholic depression but this deserves further study.[2,3] Nausea is a common initial side effect although it occurs less frequently with the extended release formulation.

### *Other Antidepressants*

**Bupropion** modulates norepinephrine and dopamine systems. It is useful as a first-line agent for major depression and appears to be a preferred antidepressant for bipolar depression.[4] Bupropion should not be prescribed for patients who have a history of bulimia nervosa, head injury or seizure disorder because of an increased risk of seizures. It also has a favorable profile with regard to sexual dysfunction.

**Trazodone** and **nefazodone** have serotonin reuptake inhibiting and $5HT_2$ receptor antagonism effects. Both offer comparable efficacy to existing SSRIs. The role of trazodone is limited mainly because of excessive sedation at therapeutic doses; lower doses (50 to 100 mg) may provide a useful hypnotic effect in combination with other antidepressants. Like moclobemide and bupropion, nefazodone causes less sexual dysfunction than other antidepressants.

**Amoxapine** is an older antidepressant that is metabolized to a loxapine-like antipsychotic compound; this has resulted in extrapyramidal side effects and tardive dyskinesia.

Two new antidepressants are expected to be available in Canada in 2000. Like venlafaxine, **mirtazapine** has dual noradrenergic and serotonergic actions and may produce a greater percentage of full responders during treatment. Sedation and weight gain are noted side effects. **Reboxetine** is a selective noradrenergic inhibitor with some evidence of greater arousing and energy enhancing properties compared to SSRIs. Dry mouth and insomnia are among the most common effects.

Several *augmentation* and *combination* therapies have been evaluated in refractory depression and are best carried out in consultation with mood disorder specialists[5]: lithium carbonate,

---

[2] *Psychopharmacology 1996;9:139–143.*
[3] *Br J Psychiatry 1999;175:12–16.*
[4] *J Clin Psychiatry 1994;55:391–393.*
[5] *Can J Psychiatry 1989;34:451–456.*

triiodothyronine ($T_3$), L-tryptophan, buspirone, pindolol or methylphenidate in combination with TCA, MAOI or SSRI drugs. Combination desipramine–fluoxetine or bupropion–SSRI has also been reported to be successful in refractory patients.

*ECT* is efficacious in 80 to 90% of depressed patients, superior to any single antidepressant drug therapy. However, relapse and recurrence rates are high in the absence of other prophylactic treatment.

### Duration of Antidepressant Treatment

Evidence supports the continuing use of antidepressant therapies for a minimum period of 1 year. When the intervals between depressive episodes become briefer and the disability associated with each depressive episode worsens, the duration of treatment should be further extended. After one episode, treat for 1 year and after two or more episodes, treat for at least 2 years. Cognitive-behavioral and interpersonal therapy have been effective in preventing relapse beyond the duration of therapy.

## Therapeutic Tips

- Choose one or two agents from several antidepressant classes (SSRI, SNRI and other) and use them consistently.
- Provide structured psychoeducation with initial prescription.
- Reinforce the importance of continuation and maintenance therapy.
- Plasma drug levels are not useful with SSRI, MAOI, RIMA and other new antidepressants. Plasma monitoring with some TCAs, i.e., desipramine, imipramine, amitriptyline and nortriptyline is helpful when noncompliance, toxicity or non-response is suspected.
- Switch or augment if no response at highest tolerable dose after 6 to 8 weeks.
- Review alcohol and drug abuse history in nonresponders.
- Refer for psychiatric consultation if there is psychotic symptoms, acute suicidal ideation or failure of 3 treatment trials.
- After recovery and a suitable period of prophylaxis, taper the antidepressant slowly over 1 to 2 months.

## Pharmacoeconomic Considerations

*Jeffrey A. Johnson, PhD*

A recent Canadian economic evaluation of the therapeutic choices for major depression indicated that a treatment strategy of starting an SSRI first, which may be replaced by a TCA if the SSRI is unsuccessful, is preferred over a TCA-*only* strategy. That is, an SSRI-first strategy is both more effective and less costly. Further, the SSRI-first strategy is equally effective, but more costly than a TCA-*first* strategy (i.e., replacing with an SSRI if TCA is unsuccessful). When HRQOL outcomes are considered, the results are even more favorable toward the SSRIs. These evaluations were based on clinical studies of only 4 to 12 weeks' duration, but were modeled for 9 months. Use of SSRIs has also been shown to be associated with reduced costs in acute overdose situations. The true cost-effectiveness of the drug therapies for depression will depend on the success of treatment in the longer term. Including patient preferences in the evaluation appears to favor the use of the newer agents, with less bothersome side effects. While the introduction of SSRIs has resulted in an increase in expenditures in drug therapy for depression, more evidence is required to determine the most appropriate balance of costs and outcomes of the use of tricyclics and SSRIs.

***Suggested Reading***

*Canadian Coordinating Office for Health Technology Assessment. Selective serotonin reuptake inhibitors (SSRIs) for major depression. Part II: the cost-effectiveness of SSRIs in treatment of depression. Ottawa: Canadian Coordinating Office for Health Technology Assessment (CCOHTA); 1997.*

*Revicki DA, Palmer CS, Phillips SD, Reblando JA, Heiligenstein JH, Brent J, Kulig K. Acute medical costs of fluoxetine versus tricyclic antidepressants: A prospective multicentre study of antidepressant drug overdoses. PharmacoEconomics 1997; 11:48–55.*

*Mamdani MM, Parikh SV, Austin PC, Upshur EG, Use of antidepressants among elderly subjects: Trends and contributing factors. Am J Psychiatry 2000; 157:360–367.*

## *Suggested Reading List*

Andrews JM, Nemeroff CB. Contemporary management of depression. *Am J Med* 1994;97 (Suppl 6A):24S–32S.

Canadian Network for Mood and Anxiety Treatments. *Guidelines for the diagnosis and pharmacological treatment of depression.* First Edition Revised. Toronto: CANMAT, 1999.

Paykel ES, Priest RG. Recognition and management of depression in general practice: consensus statement. *BMJ* 1992;305:1198–2002.

Preskorn SH. Comparison of tolerability of bupropion, fluoxetine, imipramine, nefazodone, paroxetine, sertraline and venlafaxine. *J Clin Psychiatry* 1995;56:17–25.

Rakel RE. Depression. *Prim Care* 1999;26:211–224.

CHAPTER 6

# Insomnia

*Jonathan A.E. Fleming, MB, FRCPC*

## Goals of Therapy

- To promote sound and restorative sleep when external (e.g., stress, noise, jet lag) or internal (e.g., pain, anxiety) factors disrupt natural sleep
- To reduce significant daytime impairment (dysphoria, fatigue, decreased alertness, etc.) associated with sleep loss
- To potentiate the effectiveness of behavioral interventions in managing patients with primary, chronic insomnia

Insomnia is a common symptom in a number of psychiatric, medical and sleep disorders. First determine if the complaint is primary (e.g., chronic psychophysiological insomnia), the focus of this chapter, or secondary (e.g., insomnia associated with a mood disorder or chronic pain). Secondary insomnia usually responds to treatment of the underlying disorder (e.g., a nocturnal dose of a sedating antidepressant).[1]

## Investigations

- A complete sleep history (Table 1) is **essential:**
  - to quantify current sleep performance and daytime impairment (to measure the effects of any intervention)
  - to rule out other sleep pathologies including those where hypnotics are contraindicated and potentially lethal (e.g., obstructive sleep apnea)
- Psychiatric work-up to rule out associated mental disorders (especially mood and anxiety disorders, drug and alcohol use)
- Medical work-up to rule out associated medical disorders (especially those associated with nocturnal discomfort or pain)
- Medication and drug history (including caffeine, nicotine, alcohol and recreational drug use)
- Self-rating scales for depression and anxiety symptoms (e.g., Zung Depression Scale) are useful screening tools for evaluating the presence of depressive or anxiety disorders causing insomnia

[1] *For more information on secondary insomnia, refer to Kryger ME et al, (Eds), Principles and Practice of Sleep Medicine. 2nd ed. Toronto, W.B. Saunders, 1994.*

Figure 1: **Management of Primary Insomnia**

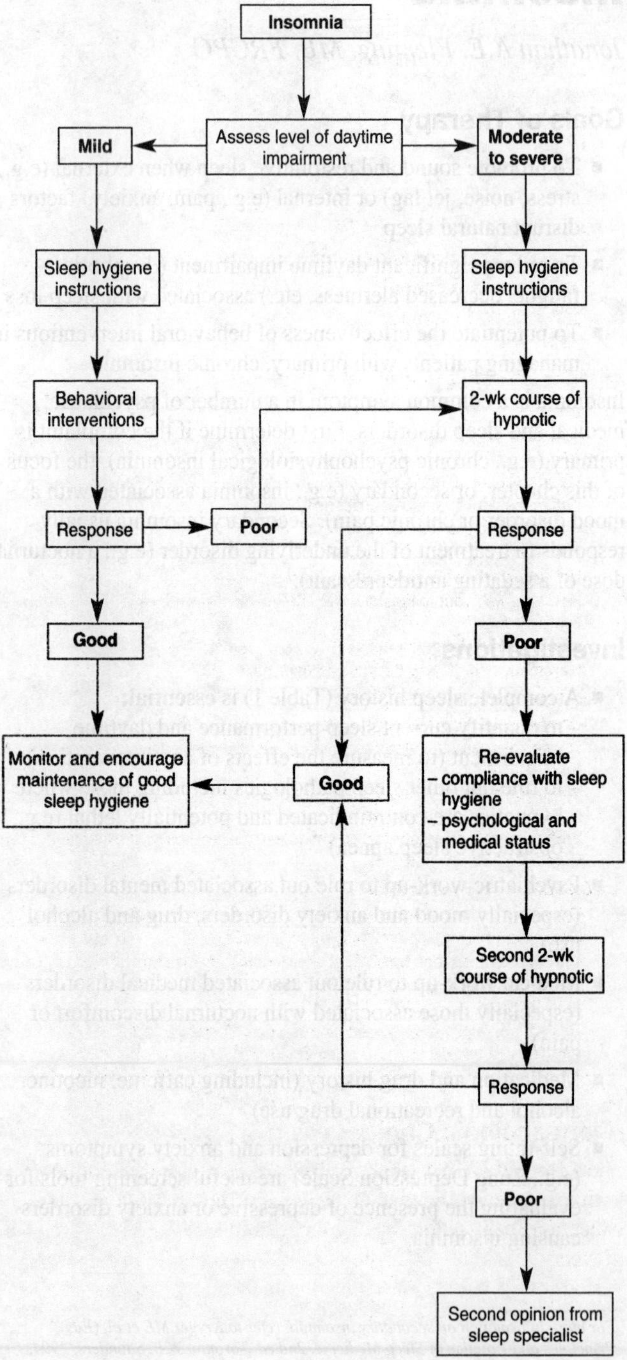
Insomnia
Assess level of daytime impairment
Mild
Moderate to severe
Sleep hygiene instructions
Sleep hygiene instructions
Behavioral interventions
2-wk course of hypnotic
Response
Poor
Response
Good
Poor
Monitor and encourage maintenance of good sleep hygiene
Good
Re-evaluate
– compliance with sleep hygiene
– psychological and medical status
Second 2-wk course of hypnotic
Response
Poor
Second opinion from sleep specialist

## Therapeutic Choices (Figure 1)

### Nonpharmacologic Choices

- Instruct patient in sleep hygiene (Table 2); monitor and encourage compliance throughout treatment and follow-up.
- Relaxation exercises (available as audio recordings for home use).
- Sleep restriction, stimulus control or other behavioral approaches, alone or with pharmacologic interventions.
- Aerobic exercise, a useful modifier of stress and dysphoric moods, also promotes deeper and more restful sleep; patients with insomnia should be encouraged to decrease daytime rest periods and increase exercise.

Table 1: **The Sleep History**

**1. Time data** (answers to these questions can also be collected as part of a sleep diary)

Did you nap or lie down to rest today? If yes, when and for how long?
What time did you go to bed last night?
What time did you put out the lights?
How long did it take you to fall asleep?
How many times did you awaken last night?
How long was your longest awake period; when was it? What time did you finally awaken?
What time did you get out of bed?
How many hours sleep did you get last night?

**2. Questions about the sleep period**

Do physical symptoms, such as pain, prevent you from falling asleep?
Do mental or emotional symptoms (e.g., worry or anxiety) prevent you from falling asleep?
When you awaken during the night, what awakens you? (Snoring? Gasping for air? Dreams/nightmares? Noise?)
When you get up for the day, do you have any symptoms? (Headache? Confusion? Sleepiness?)

**3. Questions for the bed partner**

Does your partner snore, gasp or make choking sounds during the night?
Does your partner stop breathing during the night?
Do your partner's legs twitch, jerk or kick during the night?
Has your partner's use of alcohol, nicotine, caffeine or other drugs changed recently?
Has your partner's mood or emotional state changed recently?
What do you think is the cause of your partner's sleep problem?

### Pharmacologic Choices (Table 3)

Short courses (2 to 4 weeks) of hypnotics are useful combined with good sleep hygiene (Table 2). A comprehensive evaluation, education (nature of sleep, importance of sleep hygiene especially preventing extended sleeping such as naps or nocturnal sleep periods of >8 hours) and careful monitoring of progress are important. With these measures, the use of the preferred agents, the benzodiazepines or non-benzodiazepines such as zaleplon and

Table 2: **Sleep Hygiene Guidelines**

1. Keep a regular sleep–wake schedule, 7 days per week.
2. Restrict the sleep period to the average sleep time you have obtained each night over the preceding week.
3. Avoid lying in, extensive periods of horizontal rest or daytime napping; these activities usually affect the subsequent night's sleep.
4. Get regular exercise every day: about 40 minutes of an activity with sufficient intensity to cause sweating. If evening exercise prevents sleep, schedule the exercise earlier in the day.
5. Avoid caffeine, nicotine, alcohol and other recreational drugs, all of which disturb sleep. If you must smoke do not do so after 7:00 p.m.
6. Plan a quiet period before lights out; a warm bath may be helpful.
7. Avoid large meals late in the evening; a light carbohydrate snack (e.g., crackers and warm milk) before bedtime can be helpful.
8. Turn the clock face away and always use the alarm. Looking at the clock time on awakening can cause emotional arousal (performance anxiety or anger) that prevents return to sleep.
9. As much as possible, keep the bedroom dark and soundproofed. If you live in a noisy area, consider ear plugs.
10. Use the bedroom only for sleep and intimacy; using the bed as a reading place, office or media center conditions you to be alert in a place that should be associated with quiet and sleep. If you awaken during the night and are wide awake, get up, leave the bedroom and do something quiet until you feel drowsy-tired, then return to bed.

**NB:** Pharmacologic (or any) interventions will be less effective if these guidelines are not followed. In mild cases of insomnia, sleep hygiene guidelines, practised consistently and together, may be sufficient to reinstate a normal sleep pattern.

zopiclone, in patients with primary insomnia is usually straightforward.

### *Benzodiazepines (BDZs)*

All BDZs have sedative properties that allow their use as hypnotics, but they differ significantly in potency and pharmacokinetics. All may cause confusion and ataxia, especially in the elderly and in medically ill people. For pharmacodynamic and pharmacokinetic reasons, as well as the greater research and clinical experience with BDZ hypnotics in sleep-disturbed populations, they are preferred over BDZ anxiolytics. When insomnia is secondary to prominent anxiety symptoms, a long-acting BDZ given at night may promote sleep and manage daytime anxiety symptoms. It is inappropriate to use an anxiolytic BDZ during the day to manage anxiety and a hypnotic BDZ at night.

**Temazepam** is a good all-purpose hypnotic with a half-life sufficient to cover the whole sleep period without causing hangover effects. It has fewer rebound effects than more potent BDZs such as lorazepam.

Confidence in **triazolam**, once the most frequently used hypnotic in Canada, has been undermined by successive reductions in the recommended dose and widespread reports of rare but disturbing behavioral effects. Its pharmacokinetics make it more suitable for managing initial (first third of the night) rather than maintenance (last third of the night) insomnia. Only short treatment courses (≤ 7 days) are recommended.

Although the number of comparative studies is relatively small, **oxazepam** is as effective as the hypnotic BDZs. Because of its slow absorption, it should be given 60 to 90 minutes before retiring. There are fewer trials (compared to other BDZ hypnotics) studying the effects of **lorazepam** on insomnia. As with other high-potency, short-acting BDZs, lorazepam may cause worse rebound effects on discontinuation than lower potency BDZs.

**Flurazepam** and **nitrazepam** are longer-acting BDZs marketed as hypnotics. Due to their long half-lives, they accumulate with repeated dosing and produce more hangover effects than short-acting BDZs. In the elderly, they cause higher cortical impairment resulting in confusion and falls. Their use, particularly in the elderly, is not recommended.

### *Zopiclone*

Although not a BDZ, this drug acts at the BDZ receptor and so has similar therapeutic and side effects. However, higher cortical effects and significant interaction with low doses of alcohol are absent. Tolerance to the hypnotic effect may be delayed, and rebound insomnia may be reduced compared to BDZs. Zopiclone is preferred in those who must avoid cognitive and amnesic effects.

### *Zaleplon*

The pyrazolopyrimidine, zaleplon, is a non-benzodiazepine sedative–hypnotic which acts as a selective agonist at the benzodiazepine omega-1 (Type 1) receptor. It has an unusually short elimination half-life of about 1 hour, short duration and rapid onset of action. Zaleplon 10 mg significantly reduces sleep latency with little effect on stages of sleep. It appears to be well tolerated, being free of significant residual or discontinuation effects. Although experience is limited, zaleplon promises to be useful in managing sleep-onset insomnia.

### *Chloral Hydrate and Barbiturates*

The toxicity and drug interaction profile of chloral hydrate make it less safe than BDZs. Tolerance to its hypnotic effect typically develops within 2 weeks. Its use is not recommended. The barbiturates are contraindicated in the management of insomnia due to their unacceptable safety profile.

### *L-Tryptophan*

The Canadian supply of L-tryptophan has not been associated with the development of the eosinophilia–myalgia syndrome

Table 3: **Drugs Used to Manage Primary Insomnia**

| Drug | Night-time Dose | Comments | Cost* |
|---|---|---|---|
| *temazepam* Restoril, generics | Starting 15 mg<br>Maximum 30 mg | Good all-purpose hypnotic. Does not accumulate. | $ |
| *triazolam* Halcion, generics | Starting 0.125 mg<br>Maximum 0.25 mg | Anterograde amnesia (especially with higher dosages, concurrent use of alcohol) and other potency and dose-related side effects (rebound insomnia, daytime anxiety) have limited its use. Useful for initiating sleep. Absence of hangover effects (does not affect daytime alertness) is a major advantage. | $ |
| *oxazepam* Serax, generics | Starting 15 mg<br>Maximum 30 mg | Slowly absorbed — onset of action is delayed; should be taken 60–90 min before retiring. No hangover effects. | $ |
| *lorazepam* Ativan, generics | Starting 0.5 mg<br>Maximum 1 mg | May cause more rebound insomnia on withdrawal than temazepam or oxazepam. May cause amnesia with higher dosages. | $ |
| *zaleplon* Starnoc | Starting 5 mg (geriatric)<br>Usual adult 10 mg<br>Maximum 20 mg | Headache most common side effect. Minimal hangover, memory impairment or rebound insomnia. Rifampin: ↓ zaleplon concentration 80%. Cimetidine: ↑ zaleplon concentration 85%. | $$$$ |

| | | | |
|---|---|---|---|
| *zopiclone*<br>Imovane, generics | Starting 3.75 mg (geriatric)<br>Usual adult 7.5 mg<br>Maximum 7.5 mg | Does not accumulate. Free of cognitive effects; major adverse effect is bitter/metallic taste. May cause less rebound on withdrawal. Minimal additive effects with low doses of alcohol. | $$$ |
| *L-tryptophan*<br>Tryptan, generics | 1–3 g 20 min before bedtime | Alternative to benzodiazepines. May cause the serotonin syndrome (shivering, diaphoresis, hypomanic behavior and ataxia) alone or when combined with other medications, especially MAO inhibitors and serotonin reuptake inhibitors. Erratic response. | $$$$ |

* *Cost of 14-day supply – includes drug cost only.*
*Legend: $ < $2   $$ $2–5   $$$ $5–10   $$$$ > $10*

(a potentially lethal disorder) that has been described in the US. In high dosages (> 1 g), L-tryptophan has a hypnotic effect, but it is not as predictable as that seen with traditional hypnotics. It may be useful when one wishes to avoid BDZs.

### *Melatonin*

Use of melatonin (1 to 5 mg) in primary insomnia remains controversial. More studies are required to determine if the slow release form has a role in maintenance insomnia of middle and old age. It is not available in Canada and quality of preparations available in the United States is uncontrolled.

## Therapeutic Tips

- Sedative–hypnotics should always be started at the lowest dose and used for the shortest possible time. If after 2 courses of hypnotic therapy the patient continues to experience disrupted sleep and daytime impairment, the clinician should confirm compliance with sleep hygiene measures, carefully re-evaluate the patient's psychiatric and medical status and consider referral to a sleep specialist.
- Set realistic treatment goals with the patient, mainly to minimize daytime impairment; a chronic poor sleeper will not be turned into a good sleeper overnight.
- The degree of daytime impairment directs the intervention: if there is an acute change in daytime functioning, a short course of hypnotics may be indicated; if the daytime impairment is mild or chronic, a behavioral intervention (e.g., sleep restriction) should be tried first.
- Sleep diaries (Table 1) are often helpful in delineating the initial complaint, monitoring progress and facilitating withdrawal.
- It is inappropriate to use the sedative side effect of another medication (e.g., antihistamines, antidepressants) to avoid using a BDZ when the latter is the treatment of choice.
- Warn about combined effects when hypnotics are used with other CNS depressants (e.g., alcohol).
- If a short course of a hypnotic has been used, plan to withdraw it at a low-stress time (e.g., a weekend). Two nights before the planned withdrawal, the patient should shorten the sleep time (while staying on the medication) by 20 minutes. This modest degree of sleep deprivation will promote physiological sleepiness, which should counterbalance any sleep disruption associated with withdrawal. This shortened sleep period should be maintained for 1 week.

- Remain vigilant for the emergence of a mood disorder (which should always be treated with antidepressants rather than hypnotics alone) as protracted insomnia may be the prodrome of an affective illness. Furthermore, one year of continued sleep disturbance increases the risk of a mood disorder in the subsequent year.

### *Suggested Reading List*

Eddy M, Walbroehl GS. Insomnia. *Am Fam Physician* 1999;59:1911–1916.

Gillin JC, Byerley WF. The diagnosis and management of insomnia. *N Engl J Med* 1990;322:239–248.

Kupfer DJ, Reynolds CF. Management of insomnia. *N Engl J Med* 1997;336:341–346.

Morin CM, Colecchi C, Stone J, Sood R, Brink D. Behavioral and pharmacological therapies for late-life insomnia—a randomized controlled trial. *JAMA* 1999;281:991–999.

Spielman AJ, Caruso LS, Glovinsky PB. A behavioral perspective on insomnia treatment. *Psychiatr Clin North Am* 1987;10:541–553.

CHAPTER 7

# Psychoses

*Jane Garland, MD, FRCPC*

## Goals of Therapy

- To control specific psychotic symptoms: hallucinations, delusions, disordered thinking and behavior
- To reduce agitation in acute psychosis
- To prevent relapse of chronic psychotic illness

## Investigations

- Thorough history including longitudinal history of psychotic symptoms, drug abuse, drug sensitivities, medical conditions, mood symptoms, response to antipsychotics, including adverse effects
- Specific diagnosis:
  - differentiate acute delirium, organic psychotic disorder or mania from chronic schizophrenia or schizoaffective disorder
  - rule out drug withdrawal delirium and drug intoxication (hallucinogens, amphetamines, cocaine, alcohol, anticholinergics)
- Physical examination:
  - to determine medical conditions that could produce or exacerbate an acute psychotic picture
  - to detect conditions such as parkinsonism and postural hypotension that may be exacerbated by antipsychotics
- Laboratory tests: baseline CBC, TSH and liver function tests; ECG in patients over 40

## Therapeutic Choices (Figures 1 and 2)

### Nonpharmacologic Choices

- Reduce environmental stressors and stimulation.
- Educate family and caregivers regarding symptoms and treatment.
- Ensure adequate hydration, nutrition and safety.
- Avoid alcohol, psychoactive substances.
- As patient improves, introduce educational approaches to coping strategies, vocation and regularity of lifestyle.
- Frequent, brief contacts with physician and other health care providers give support, increase compliance and enable early detection of psychotic relapse.

## Figure 1: **Management of Acute Psychotic Symptoms**

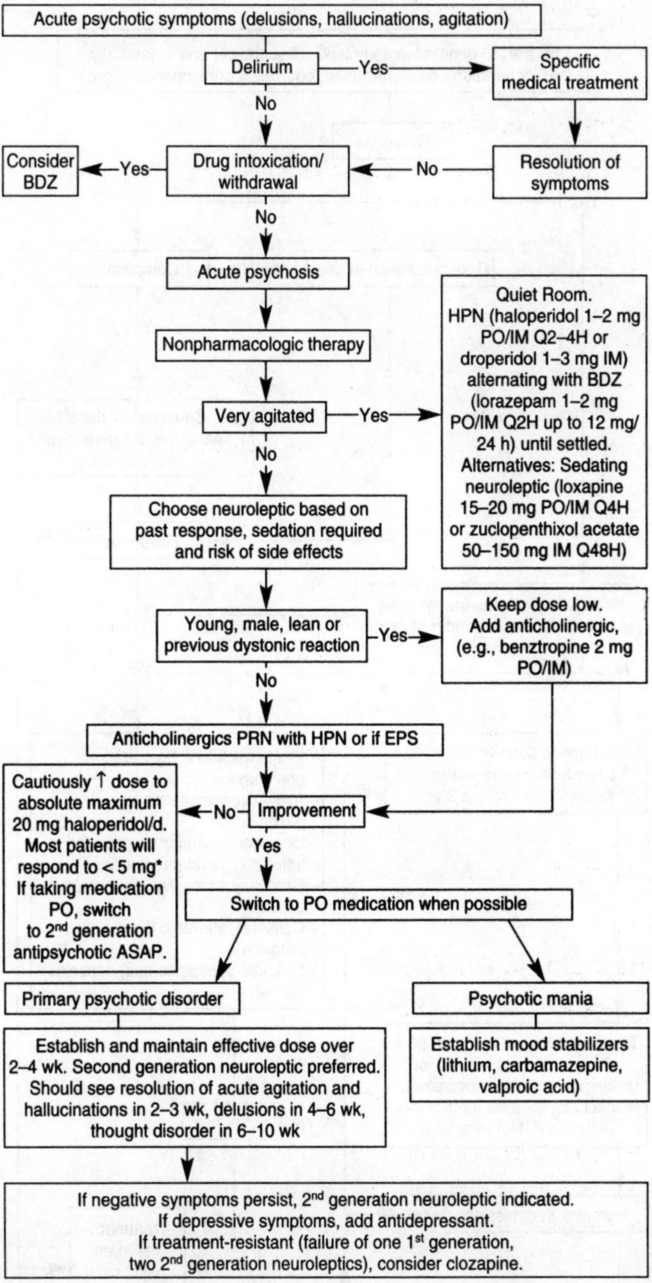
Acute psychotic symptoms (delusions, hallucinations, agitation)
Delirium
Yes
Specific medical treatment
No
Consider BDZ
Yes
Drug intoxication/ withdrawal
No
Resolution of symptoms
No
Acute psychosis
Nonpharmacologic therapy
Very agitated
Yes
Quiet Room. HPN (haloperidol 1–2 mg PO/IM Q2–4H or droperidol 1–3 mg IM) alternating with BDZ (lorazepam 1–2 mg PO/IM Q2H up to 12 mg/ 24 h) until settled. Alternatives: Sedating neuroleptic (loxapine 15–20 mg PO/IM Q4H or zuclopenthixol acetate 50–150 mg IM Q48H)
No
Choose neuroleptic based on past response, sedation required and risk of side effects
Young, male, lean or previous dystonic reaction
Yes
Keep dose low. Add anticholinergic, (e.g., benztropine 2 mg PO/IM)
No
Anticholinergics PRN with HPN or if EPS
Cautiously ↑ dose to absolute maximum 20 mg haloperidol/d. Most patients will respond to < 5 mg* If taking medication PO, switch to 2nd generation antipsychotic ASAP.
No
Improvement
Yes
Switch to PO medication when possible
Primary psychotic disorder
Psychotic mania
Establish and maintain effective dose over 2–4 wk. Second generation neuroleptic preferred. Should see resolution of acute agitation and hallucinations in 2–3 wk, delusions in 4–6 wk, thought disorder in 6–10 wk
Establish mood stabilizers (lithium, carbamazepine, valproic acid)
If negative symptoms persist, 2nd generation neuroleptic indicated. If depressive symptoms, add antidepressant. If treatment-resistant (failure of one 1st generation, two 2nd generation neuroleptics), consider clozapine.

*Abbreviations: BDZ = benzodiazepine, HPN = high potency neuroleptic, EPS = extrapyramidal symptoms.*
** Can J Psychiatry 1999;44:164–167.*

Figure 2: **Maintenance Treatment for Subacute Psychosis or Chronic Schizophrenia**

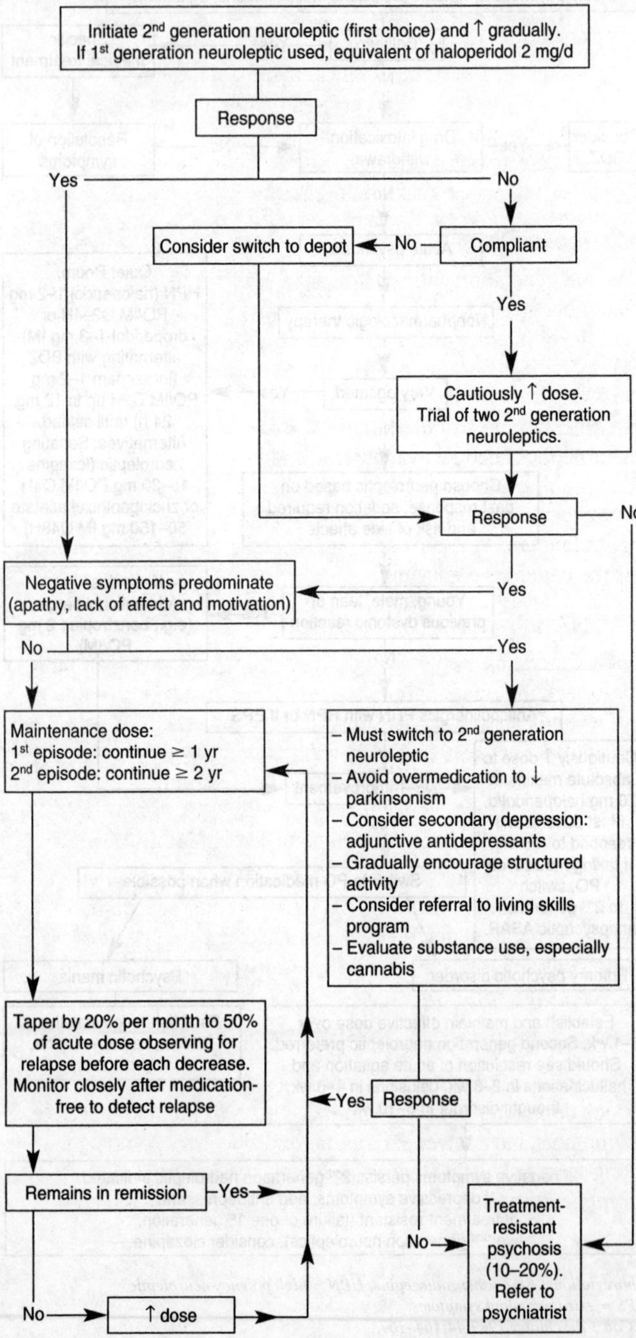
Initiate 2nd generation neuroleptic (first choice) and ↑ gradually.
If 1st generation neuroleptic used, equivalent of haloperidol 2 mg/d
Response
Yes
No
Consider switch to depot
No
Compliant
Yes
Cautiously ↑ dose.
Trial of two 2nd generation neuroleptics.
Response
No
Yes
Negative symptoms predominate (apathy, lack of affect and motivation)
No
Yes
Maintenance dose:
1st episode: continue ≥ 1 yr
2nd episode: continue ≥ 2 yr
– Must switch to 2nd generation neuroleptic
– Avoid overmedication to ↓ parkinsonism
– Consider secondary depression: adjunctive antidepressants
– Gradually encourage structured activity
– Consider referral to living skills program
– Evaluate substance use, especially cannabis
Taper by 20% per month to 50% of acute dose observing for relapse before each decrease. Monitor closely after medication-free to detect relapse
Yes
Response
Remains in remission
Yes
No
Treatment-resistant psychosis (10–20%). Refer to psychiatrist
No
↑ dose

## Pharmacologic Choices (Table 1)

### Antipsychotics

#### *Indications for Antipsychotics*

Antipsychotics are indicated for:

- acute exacerbation of chronic schizophrenia
- acute psychotic symptoms in bipolar disorder and depression
- acute agitation and psychosis in delirium
- maintenance treatment of chronic schizophrenia

#### *Choice of Drug*

Second generation antipsychotics are more clinically effective and more cost effective both in the acute phase of treatment[1,2] and in community treatment.[3] Current clinical guidelines consider them drugs of first choice.[4] However, in acute psychosis (Figure 1) and in treatment noncompliance (Table 2), first generation neuroleptics are still used until IM forms of second generation neuroleptics become available. Compliance is important in determining practical effectiveness, and is affected by dosage frequency, cost and side effect profile. Informed consent regarding tardive dyskinesia (TD) must be documented as soon as the patient is competent.

#### *First Generation Antipsychotics*

First generation antipsychotics (e.g., **chlorpromazine**, **loxapine**, **haloperidol**) are thought to produce their primary therapeutic effect and extrapyramidal side effects by blocking dopamine receptors. They also block other receptors (serotonergic, cholinergic, adrenergic and histaminic) to varying degrees, producing sedation, and autonomic and cardiovascular side effects, especially orthostatic hypotension and tachycardia.

"Positive symptoms" of schizophrenia (i.e., hallucinations, delusions, thought disorders, paranoia) are more responsive to first generation neuroleptics than the negative symptoms (i.e., amotivational state, apathy, poor self-care, social withdrawal, poverty of speech).

#### *Second Generation Antipsychotics*

**Clozapine**, **olanzapine**, **risperidone** and **quetiapine** selectively block dopamine and serotonin receptors. All improve negative symptoms, have fewer extrapyramidal side effects and a lower long-term risk of TD than typical agents. Clozapine is effective in *treatment-resistant psychosis*. Due to risks of agranulocytosis

---

[1] *Am J Psychiatry 1999;156:863–868.*
[2] *Clin Ther 1999;21:1105–1116.*
[3] *Pharmacoeconomics 1999;15:469–480.*
[4] *Can J Psychiatry 1998; 43 Suppl 2:25S–40S.*

Table 1: **Drugs Used in Psychosis**

| Drug | CPZ Equivalence* | Potency† | Notable Adverse Effects | Drug Interactions | Comments | Cost‡ |
|---|---|---|---|---|---|---|
| **First Generation Antipsychotics** | | | | | | |
| *chlorpromazine* Largactil, generics | 100 mg | Low | All: sedation, autonomic and cardiovascular effects, especially orthostatic hypotension, tachycardia (↑ with LPN), tardive dyskinesia, seizures (1%), ↑ prolactin, weight gain.<br>EPS, including parkinsonism, akinesia, akathisia (↑ with HPN).<br>Chlorpromazine: orthostatic hypotension notable.<br>Thioridazine: retinal damage with doses > 800 mg/d.<br>Pimozide: cardiac conduction effects with doses > 8 mg. | Serum level of antipsychotics may be ↑ by TCAs.<br>Serum level of antipsychotics ↓ by carbamazepine (↑ liver metabolism), antacids (↓ absorption).<br>Cardiac effects: phenothiazines, pimozide prolong QT interval; interaction with other drugs (e.g., astemizole, terfenadine, antiarrhythmics) may promote this.<br>Effects of levodopa may be inhibited. | Whenever possible, neuroleptic dosage should be reduced, or a lower potency drug should be considered to reduce EPS.<br>CPZ and methotrimeprazine: useful if sedative effect desirable.<br>Haloperidol: high potency and low cardiac toxicity; is available PO/IM/depot/IV form.<br>Pimozide: effective in delusional disorder, tics.<br>Loxapine: useful if sedation required and in elderly. Has low cardiac toxicity. | $ |
| *thioridazine* Mellaril, generics | 90–100 mg | Low | | | | $ |
| *methotrimeprazine* Nozinan, generics | 75 mg | Low | | | | $ |
| *loxapine* Loxapac, generics | 10–15 mg | Intermediate | | | | $$–$$$ |
| *perphenazine* Trilafon, generics | 10 mg | Intermediate | | | | $ |
| *trifluoperazine* Stelazine, generics | 3–5 mg | High | | | | $ |
| *fluphenazine HCl* π Moditen HCl, generics | 2 mg | High | | | | $ |
| *haloperidol* π Haldol, generics | 2 mg | High | | | | $ |
| *pimozide* Orap | 1 mg | High | | | | $ |
| *flupenthixol* π Fluanxol | 1 mg | High | | | | $ |

**Second Generation Antipsychotics**

| | | | | | | |
|---|---|---|---|---|---|---|
| *clozapine* Clozaril | 50 mg | Low | Agranulocytosis (1–2%), seizures (5%), excessive salivation, weight gain. | Fluvoxamine and erythromycin ↑ clozapine levels. BDZs: ↑ respiratory depression. | Useful in treatment-resistant patients and for negative symptoms. Prescribed only by psychiatrist. Very low EPS. | $$$$$$ |
| *olanzapine* Zyprexa | 3 mg | Intermediate | Weight gain. Dizziness, sedation. | | Very low EPS | $$$$$ |
| *quetiapine* Seroquel | 100 mg | Low | Sedation, weight gain. May ↑ risk of cataracts. | Phenytoin ↓ clearance of quetiapine. Avoid alcohol. | Low EPS. | $$$ |
| *risperidone* Risperdal | 1.5 mg | High | Hyperprolactinemia, pronounced hypotension, weight gain, restlessness. | | Low EPS | $$$ |

* *CPZ equivalence is the equipotent dosage of any antipsychotic compared to 100 mg of chlorpromazine.*

† *Potency refers to the affinity for dopamine $D_2$ receptors. High-potency neuroleptics (HPN) are more likely to cause neuromuscular effects (e.g., EPS); low-potency neuroleptics (LPN) are more likely to cause non-neuromuscular effects.*

π *Depot form available. See Table 2.*

‡ *Cost of 30-day supply of 300 mg/d CPZ equivalence – includes drug cost only.*

*Legend: $ < $50   $$ $50–100   $$$ $100–150   $$$$ $150–200   $$$$$ $200–250   $$$$$$ > $250*

(1 to 2%, requiring weekly WBC monitoring) and seizures (5%) as well as high cost, clozapine is reserved for treatment-resistant patients.

### Dosing

Traditional dosing of antipsychotics has been too high.[5] Doses greater than 5 mg haloperidol/day are rarely necessary and are associated with poor patient acceptance and clinical outcome. Typical dose range for newer agents is the equivalent of 300 mg CPZ, i.e., 4.5 mg risperidone, 10 to 15 mg olanzapine or 300 to 400 mg of quetiapine. For acute treatment, refer to Figure 1. For subacute treatment (Figure 2), initiate equivalent of 1 to 2 mg haloperidol or risperidone/day and increase at intervals of two weeks, for a total of 6 to 8 weeks. If no response occurs, neuroleptic may be changed; for treatment-resistant psychosis, refer to a psychiatrist.

Once therapy is stabilized, simplify to once-daily dosing if possible; for noncompliance, consider depot preparations (Table 2).

### Maintenance Treatment

Continuous treatment reduces the relapse rate in chronic schizophrenia from 70 to 20% in a year (this is even further reduced with use of second generation agents). The lowest effective daily dose (about 300 mg CPZ or equivalent) of oral or depot medication should be used to prevent relapse. Following a single psychotic episode, after a year of symptom remission, systematic tapering by 20% per month until 50% of the acute dose is reached, may be considered. With repeated episodes, tapering should be attempted after at least 2 months during which residual symptoms have returned to baseline. At the first sign of relapsing symptoms, the patient should be immediately restabilized on higher dose. Patients should be monitored closely for early prodromal symptoms and signs of relapse.

### Special Considerations

In the ***elderly*** lower doses should be used. Second generation agents are effective with reduced TD risk. Cardiac toxicity is less with loxapine than other first generation agents.

In ***pregnancy*** no teratogenic effects have been documented for neuroleptics, but their risk/benefit should be considered, and the drugs should be avoided in the first trimester.

In ***neonates*** hypertonia has been noted following prepartum antipsychotics.

In ***children***, olanzapine and clozapine have been studied in open trials for schizophrenia. Risperidone has been studied for

[5] *Can J Psychiatry 1999; 44: 164–167.*

Table 2: **Depot Neuroleptics**

| Drug | Usual Dose IM* | Frequency | Cost† |
|---|---|---|---|
| *fluphenazine decanoate* Modecate | 12.5–37.5 mg | Q3 wk | $ |
| *haloperidol decanoate* Haldol LA | 100–200 mg | Q4 wk | $ |
| *flupenthixol* Fluanxol | 20–40 mg | Q2 wk | $–$$ |
| *zuclopenthixol acetate* Clopixol-Acuphase | 50–150 mg | Q2–3 days | $$$$$ |
| *pipotiazine* Piportil | 150–300 mg | Q4 wk | $$$-$$$$$ |

** A small dose (10% of usual daily dose) should be given to test for allergies.*
*† Cost of 4-week supply – includes drug cost only.*
*Legend: $ < $25 $$ $25–50 $$$ $50–75 $$$$ $75–100 $$$$$ > $100*

pervasive developmental disorder. Second generation agents are preferred as long-term TD risk is a major concern. Haloperidol and pimozide are effective in tic disorders.

### Side Effects

***Tardive dyskinesia*** (TD) occurs after chronic exposure to dopamine-blocking agents and is characterized by involuntary movements of mouth, face, trunk or extremities. The incidence increases with total neuroleptic exposure; it is about 5% per year of first generation neuroleptic exposure and 20 to 25% in chronically treated schizophrenic patients. The rates are higher with intermittent therapy, drug holidays or affective disorders. The risk is higher in the elderly, females and in the presence of neurological disorders.

TD may be masked by neuroleptics and may emerge with dose reduction or withdrawal. Withdrawal-emergent TD often improves significantly with time.

Treatment is generally unsatisfactory but can include continued suppression with neuroleptics, benzodiazepines, adrenergic agents such as propranolol and clonidine, and experimental use of buspirone. As use of second generation neuroleptics such as clozapine, olanzapine and risperidone may reduce risk, consider switching to one of these agents if TD arises.

***Neuroleptic malignant syndrome***, a serious side effect of neuroleptic therapy, occurs with an incidence of 1 to 4%. It is characterized by muscle rigidity, fever, autonomic instability, labile blood pressure, clouded consciousness, elevated WBC and elevated creatine kinase. Risk factors include use of high-potency neuroleptics and dehydration. Treatment is primarily supportive (hydration and cooling) but may include amantadine, dantrolene sodium or bromocriptine.

Other serious side effects include ***cardiac conduction disturbances***, which occur with all antipsychotics in higher doses (e.g., pimozide in doses over 8 mg/day). ***Seizures*** occur at a rate of 1% with all neuroleptics. ***Liver damage*** may occur with phenothiazine derivatives. *Note:* Neuroleptic-induced ***hyperprolactinemia*** stimulates growth of breast cancer in animals.

### Laboratory Monitoring

Laboratory investigations are indicated when adverse effects are suspected and may include liver enzymes, thyroid function tests, bilirubin and CBC. Clozapine requires continuous weekly monitoring of WBC. A low incidence of agranulocytosis occurs with phenothiazine derivatives.

Because there is no consistent relationship between plasma levels and clinical response, monitoring of plasma levels is reserved for nonresponsive patients and for identification of drug interactions that may raise neuroleptic levels excessively.

### Adjunctive Medications (Table 3)

**Antiparkinson agents** are used with high-potency neuroleptics, either prophylactically or PRN to control *extrapyramidal motor effects*, especially in patients at high risk (young, male, previous history).

**Benzodiazepines** are used in acute psychosis for *sedation* and to achieve a *reduction in required neuroleptic dose*. They may be helpful in controlling *akathisia* (intense restlessness with resultant pacing and agitation) and *reducing incidence of acute dystonias* during initiation of emergency antipsychotic treatment.

**Propranolol** or **amantadine** have some efficacy in *akathisia*. Antidepressants such as **imipramine** or **fluoxetine** may be considered for secondary *depression*.

## Therapeutic Tips

- A higher dose of antipsychotic agent does not speed resolution of acute psychosis.
- Compliance is key to successful resolution of psychosis and prevention of relapse.
- Successful relapse prevention requires combined psychoeducation and pharmacotherapy.
- It is important to distinguish negative symptoms of schizophrenia from extrapyramidal side effects of medication (e.g., akinesia) and secondary depression.
- Adjunctive mood stabilizers should be considered for bipolar or schizoaffective symptoms.

Table 3: **Adjunctive Medications Used in Psychosis**

| Drug | Dose (Titrate PRN) | Comments | Cost* |
|---|---|---|---|
| **Drugs for Management of Parkinsonism** | | | |
| *benztropine* Cogentin, generics | 1–2 mg TID PO/IM | IM benztropine or diphenhydramine can be used for acute dystonia. PO benztropine or procyclidine for tremor and rigidity. Side effects include dry mouth, blurred vision, constipation, confusion. Toxic in overdose. Amantadine may be helpful for akathisia. | $† |
| *procyclidine* Kemadrin, generics | 2.5–5 mg TID PO | | $ |
| *trihexyphenidyl* generics | 2–5 mg TID PO | | $ |
| *diphenhydramine* Benadryl, generics | 25–50 mg QID PO/IM | | $-$$† |
| *amantadine* Symmetrel, generics | 100 mg up to BID | | $$ |
| **Drugs for Management of Akathisia** | | | |
| *propranolol* Inderal, generics | 10–40 mg/d | Monitor for hypotension. Contraindicated in asthma. Caution in diabetes. | $ |
| Benzodiazepines | | | |
| *lorazepam* Ativan, generics | 0.5–2 mg Q4H PO/IM | Side effects include excessive sedation, impaired memory and poor concentration. | $† |
| *clonazepam* Rivotril, generics | 0.25–2 mg Q6–8H PO | | $–$$ |
| *alprazolam* Xanax, generics | 0.25–1 mg Q4H PO | | $–$$ |

*Dosage adjustment may be required in renal impairment – see Appendix I.*

† *Cost for oral tablets; IM formulations may be higher.*

* *Cost of 30-day supply – includes drug cost only.*

*Legend:* $ < $20   $$ $20–40

- Informed consent, regarding risks and benefits, must be documented once the patient's mental state renders him/her competent to provide it.

## Pharmacoeconomic Considerations

*Jeffrey A. Johnson, PhD*

The atypical antipsychotics, clozapine, olanzapine and risperidone have higher drug acquisition costs compared to conventional agents, but may be cost-effective choices in the treatment of schizophrenia. Clozapine has been considered cost-effective, but likely only in the management of treatment-resistant schizophrenia, despite the additional monitoring costs. In the treatment of chronic schizophrenia, most pharmacoeconomic analyses indicate that treatment with olanzapine or risperidone does not significantly increase, and may even decrease, the overall direct costs of care for schizophrenia.

The major economic advantage of the atypical agents over older, more conventional agents is the reduction in institutionalization. Reductions in adverse effects with the newer agents may also provide a benefit when HRQOL is considered, although measuring this benefit directly in the patient population may be difficult. An important consideration of the pharmacoeconomic literature is that the new therapeutic choices are usually compared with the older agents, such as chlorpromazine or haloperidol; there is little evidence to indicate which of the atypical agents is the more cost-effective choice for chronic schizophrenia (i.e., olanzapine versus risperidone).

***Suggested Reading***

*Chouinard G, Albright PS. Economic and health state utility determination for schizophrenic patients treated with risperidone or haloperidol. J Clin Psychopharmacol 1997;17:298–307.*

*Oh P, Einarson TR, Iskedjian M, Addis A, Lanctot K. Pharmacoeconomic evaluation of risperidone and clozapine in chronic and treatment-resistant schizophrenia. Ottawa: Canadian Coordinating Office for Health Technology Assessment (CCOHTA); 1997.*

*Foster RH, Goa KL. Olanzapine. A pharmacoeconomic review of its use in schizophrenia. Pharmacoeconomics 1999;15:611–640.*

*Foster RH, Goa KL. Risperidone. A pharmacoeconomic review of its use in schizophrenia. Pharmacoeconomics 1998;14:97–133.*

## Suggested Reading List

Canadian Psychiatric Association. Canadian Clinical Practice Guidelines for the Treatment of Schizophrenia. *Can J Psychiatry* 1998;43(Suppl 2, revised).

Conley RR, Love RC, Kelley DL, Bartko JJ. Rehospitalization rates of patients recently discharged on a regimen of risperidone or clozapine. *Am J Psychiatry* 1999;156:863–868.

Calvin PM, Knezeck LD, Rush AJ, Toprac MG, Johnson B. Clinical and economic impact of newer versus older antipsychotic medications in a community mental health center. *Clin Ther* 1999;21:1105–1116.

Hamilton SH, Revicki DA, Edgell ET, Genduso LA, Tollefson G. Clinical and economic outcomes of olanzapine compared with haloperidol for schizophrenia. Results from a randomized clinical trial. *Pharmacoeconomics* 1999;15:469–480.

Zhang-Wong J, Zipursky RB, Beiser M, Bean G. Optimal haloperidol dosage in first-episode psychosis. *Can J Psychiatry* 1999;44:164–167.

CHAPTER 8

# Drug Withdrawal Syndromes

*Claudio A. Naranjo, MD*

Alcohol, stimulant (cocaine and amphetamine), opioid and benzodiazepine withdrawal are discussed in this chapter. See Chapter 41 for management of nicotine withdrawal.

## Definition[1]

- The development of a substance-specific syndrome due to the cessation of (or reduction in) substance use that has been heavy and prolonged
- The substance-specific syndrome causes clinically significant distress or impairment in social, occupational or other important areas of functioning
- The symptoms are not due to a general medical condition and are not better accounted for by another mental disorder

## Goals of Therapy

- To relieve acute symptoms
- To prevent complications
- To smooth transition into a rehabilitation program
- To prevent relapse

## Investigations

- Interview
- Specialized assessment instruments or scales (self-administered or interviewer-administered) [e.g., Clinical Institute Withdrawal Assessment for Alcohol (CIWA-Ar),[2] CIWA-Benzo[3]]
- Physical examination
- Laboratory tests for presence of all suspected psychoactive substances in urine, blood and/or breath
- Rule out organic complications (e.g., infection)

---

[1] *Diagnostic and Statistical Manual of Mental Disorders, 4th Ed, 1994.*
[2] *Br J Addict 1989;84:1353–57.*
[3] *J Clin Psychopharmacology 1989;9:412–416.*

## Therapeutic Choices (Figure 1)

### Nonpharmacologic Choices

- Monitoring signs and symptoms.
- Reassurance, supportive nursing care.
- Reality orientation.
- Psychosocial treatment program.

### Pharmacologic Choices

- Treat specific symptoms of withdrawal and associated complications.
- Substitute abused drug with one of same or similar class (an agonist) that is not likely to be abused.
- Substitute abused drug with one which blocks its reinforcing effects (an antagonist).

### *Alcohol Withdrawal Syndrome (AWS)*

***Diagnostic Criteria*** (Table 1)

***Assessment:*** The symptoms and severity of the AWS vary with the intensity and duration of the preceding alcohol exposure. Severity can be assessed with the CIWA-Ar. Symptoms of a mild reaction are tremor, insomnia and irritability lasting 48 hours or less. In a severe AWS, these are followed by hallucinations, seizures and delusions. Acute withdrawal symptoms may be followed by a protracted withdrawal syndrome with persistent alterations in physiology, mood and behavior lasting for up to a year.[4]

Abstinence may be forced by illness or injury. Adequate assessment of AWS risk can lead to appropriate prophylaxis, preventing a variety of post-surgical complications and AWS in 75% of patients.[5]

***Management:*** Nonpharmacologic interventions are generally effective for mild AWS (CIWA-Ar score ≤ 20). Patients in moderate to severe withdrawal (CIWA-Ar score > 20) should receive medication (Table 2).

***Long-term Rehabilitation:*** Following successful withdrawal from alcohol, the treatment goal may be abstinence or moderation (drinking < 12 drinks per week, and ≤ 4 drinks per day for males or ≤ 3 drinks per day for females). Medications should be administered only within the context of a relapse prevention (cognitive-behavioral or psychosocial) program in intellectually intact individuals who are motivated (or required, as in judicial programs) to reduce their alcohol consumption. The alcohol-

---

[4] *Diagnostic and Statistical Manual of Mental Disorders, 4th Ed, 1994.*

[5] *Anesthesia and Analgesia 1999;88:946–954.*

Figure 1: **Management of Drug Withdrawal Syndromes**

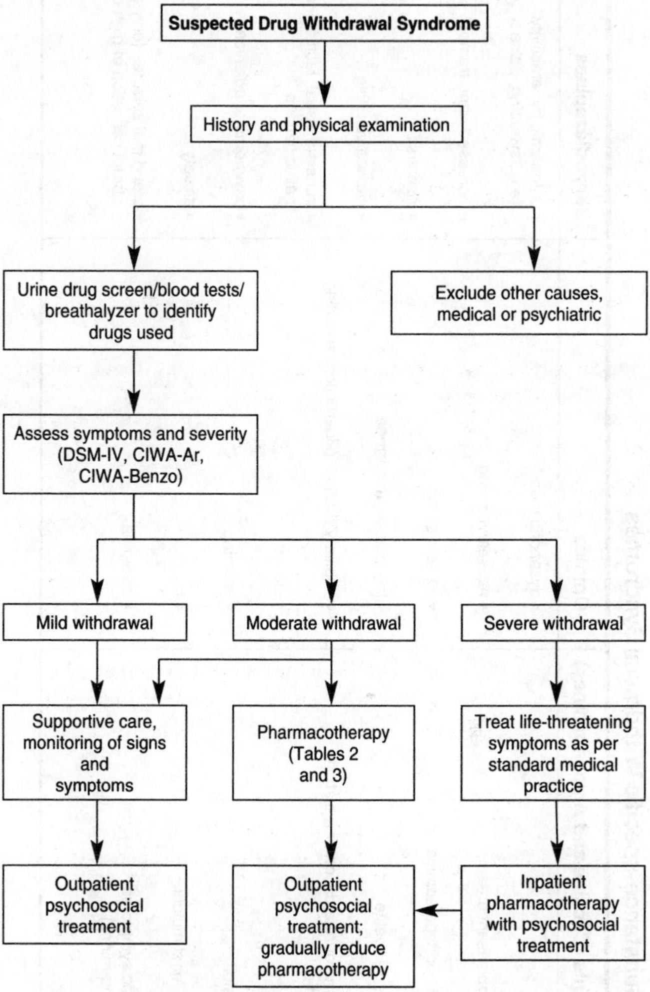
Suspected Drug Withdrawal Syndrome
History and physical examination
Urine drug screen/blood tests/ breathalyzer to identify drugs used
Exclude other causes, medical or psychiatric
Assess symptoms and severity (DSM-IV, CIWA-Ar, CIWA-Benzo)
Mild withdrawal
Moderate withdrawal
Severe withdrawal
Supportive care, monitoring of signs and symptoms
Pharmacotherapy (Tables 2 and 3)
Treat life-threatening symptoms as per standard medical practice
Outpatient psychosocial treatment
Outpatient psychosocial treatment; gradually reduce pharmacotherapy
Inpatient pharmacotherapy with psychosocial treatment

sensitizing drugs, **disulfiram** and **calcium carbimide**, inhibit hepatic aldehyde dehydrogenase, causing increased blood acetaldehyde levels after alcohol ingestion. The result is a very unpleasant episode of flushing, tachycardia, weakness and nausea. When the goal is abstinence, these drugs have a limited role.

**Naltrexone**, a long-acting opioid antagonist, is indicated for alcohol dependence. Although efficacy beyond 12 weeks of treatment has not been established, administration for at least 6 months is advisable due to the high risk of relapse within this time period.

Table 1: **Diagnostic Criteria for Substance-specific Withdrawal Syndromes**

| Alcohol | Stimulants (Cocaine and Amphetamines) | Opioids | Benzodiazepines |
|---|---|---|---|
| • autonomic hyperactivity (e.g., sweating, pulse > 100 bpm) | • fatigue | • dysphoric mood | • autonomic hyperactivity (e.g., sweating, pulse > 100 bpm) |
| • increased hand tremor | • vivid, unpleasant dreams | • nausea/vomiting | • increased hand tremor |
| • insomnia | • insomnia or hypersomnia | • muscle aches | • insomnia |
| • nausea/vomiting | • increased appetite | • lacrimation, rhinorrhea | • nausea/vomiting |
| • transient visual, tactile or auditory hallucinations | • psychomotor retardation or agitation | • pupillary dilation, piloerection, sweating | • transient visual, tactile or auditory hallucinations |
| • psychomotor agitation | • anxiety | • diarrhea | • psychomotor agitation |
| • anxiety | • depression | • yawning | • anxiety |
| • grand mal seizures | • craving for stimulant | • fever | • grand mal seizures (only after abrupt cessation of high doses) |
| • depression | • psychotic symptoms (amphetamines) | • insomnia | |

Table 2: **Pharmacologic Management of Alcohol Withdrawal**

| Symptom/Severity of Withdrawal | Drug | Dose and Route | Interval | Comments | Cost* |
|---|---|---|---|---|---|
| Neurological symptoms | Thiamine | 25–50 mg IV | Daily for 3 days | To treat/prevent neurological complications, e.g., Wernicke's encephalopathy. Some clinicians administer thiamine to all patients experiencing alcohol withdrawal. Can administer PO after first dose. | $$ |
| Mild to moderate | Lorazepam | 2 mg SL | Q2H | Administer 3 doses, with supportive care. | $ |
| Moderate to severe | Diazepam<br>Chlordiazepoxide | 20 mg PO<br>100 mg PO | Q1–2H | The initial dose can be repeated every 1–2H until patient shows signs of improvement or mild sedation; median dose is usually 60 mg of diazepam or 300 mg of chlordiazepoxide. | $<br>$ |
| Extreme | Diazepam | 2.5 mg/min IV | Slow infusion | Rarely needed; most patients respond to adequate dosing with oral diazepam. In those rare cases when needed, should be administered until patient is calm (subsequent dosages must be individualized on the basis of the clinical picture). | $$ |
| Hallucinations, thought disorder, severe agitation | Haloperidol | 0.5–5.0 mg IM, IV or PO | Q2H | Until controlled or to a maximum of 5 doses; appropriate doses of diazepam should be used concurrently. | $$ |

*(cont'd)*

Table 2: **Pharmacologic Management of Alcohol Withdrawal** *(cont'd)*

| Symptom/Severity of Withdrawal | Drug | Dose and Route | Interval | Comments | Cost* |
|---|---|---|---|---|---|
| Seizure | | | | | |
| History of seizure disorder or previous withdrawal seizures | Phenytoin | Maintenance: 100 mg PO<br>Loading: 200–300 mg PO | Q8H | Phenytoin detected in blood, maintenance dose: 100 mg; not detected in blood: loading dose: 200–300 mg, maintenance dose: 100 mg. | $ |
| Repeated seizures requiring acute therapy | Phenytoin | Loading dose: 1 g IV | Infuse at 50 mg/min | Loading dose is 10 mg/kg. Do not dilute in saline or dextrose solution. | $$$$ |
| | | Maintenance: 100 mg PO | Q8H | | $ |
| Status epilepticus | Diazepam | 5 mg/min IV | Infuse | Until seizures cease or 25–30 mg total has been given. | $$ |
| Long-term reduction in alcohol intake | Naltrexone | 50 mg/day | 12–24 weeks | Use as part of a comprehensive treatment program.<br>Contraindicated in acute hepatitis or liver failure.<br>Hepatotoxicity may occur with very high doses (> 300 mg/day). | $159 for 30 days |

* *Cost for a single administration – drug cost only.*

*Legend: $ < $1 $$ $1–10 $$$ $10–20 $$$$ $20–30*

**Acamprosate**, which affects glutamate and GABA to reduce craving and unpleasant effects of alcohol abstinence, is expected to become available.

Patients with comorbid depression or anxiety may benefit from **antidepressants** and **anxiolytics**, particularly if the alcohol dependence was secondary to depression or anxiety.

Generally, follow-up "booster" sessions are required after completion of a cognitive-behavioral or psychosocial relapse prevention program for the long-term maintenance of abstinence or moderation of alcohol use. Self-help groups, e.g., Alcoholics Anonymous (AA), are available in many communities.

## *Stimulant (Cocaine and Amphetamine) Withdrawal Syndrome*

***Diagnostic Criteria*** (Table 1)

***Assessment:*** Symptoms of cocaine withdrawal are subjective, generally psychological and frequently subtle. Most will decrease steadily over several weeks. Craving for cocaine is the most long-lasting symptom, and can lead to cocaine-seeking behavior and subsequent relapse for up to 1 year after withdrawal.

Amphetamine withdrawal may also include psychotic symptoms such as paranoia and visual and auditory hallucinations. Withdrawal symptoms tend to decrease steadily over several weeks or longer with amphetamines.

***Management:*** Medications should be used within the context of psychosocial treatment. Comorbidity, polydrug use (particularly heroin) may influence efficacy of treatment. Currently, there is no standard accepted pharmacologic treatment for stimulant withdrawal. Dopamine agonists (**bromocriptine, amantadine**) and tricyclic antidepressants (**desipramine, imipramine**) have been shown to reduce craving and some symptoms of withdrawal (Table 3). Neuroleptics are contraindicated as they may increase drug craving.

***Long-term Rehabilitation:*** Intensive psychosocial treatment (> 2 times/week), particularly outpatient abstinence-oriented cognitive behavioral therapy, is the usual initial therapeutic choice. Legal, financial or medical problems (e.g., HIV infection, pregnancy) must be addressed if present. Adjunctive pharmacotherapy is indicated for patients who do not respond to an adequate trial of psychosocial treatment. No medication has been shown to be consistently efficacious in the long-term maintenance of cocaine abstinence. **Desipramine** may relieve comorbid or subsequent depression. **Bromocriptine** has been shown to relieve craving in some studies. **Buprenorphine**, a mixed opioid agonist–antagonist, is under investigation in methadone-maintained cocaine-dependent patients following positive results in preliminary studies.

### Opioid Withdrawal Syndrome

***Diagnostic Criteria*** (Table 1)

***Assessment:*** The symptoms of opioid withdrawal are not life-threatening and generally last about 2 weeks if craving for the abused drug can be overcome.

***Management:*** The best way to avoid craving and subsequent relapse is to make the abused drug completely unavailable. Many opioid abusers can undergo withdrawal in a supportive environment without medications. However, there are effective pharmacologic strategies to reduce the acute symptoms of opioid withdrawal and facilitate long-term abstinence (Table 3). The treatment of choice has been oral administration of **methadone**, a long-acting pure opioid agonist. Many patients begin to experience renewed, but milder, withdrawal symptoms when the dose of methadone drops to below 20 or 30 mg/day. **Clonidine**, a nonopioid antihypertensive medication, can assist in methadone substitution by suppressing nausea, vomiting, cramps and sweating. However, it does little for the muscle aches, insomnia and drug craving symptoms of withdrawal, and its hypotensive effect makes it more suitable for inpatient use, where blood pressure can be monitored.

**Buprenorphine** has been found to be as efficacious as methadone but is not yet available in Canada.

Another protocol involves sequential treatment with **clonidine** and **naltrexone** (an opioid antagonist). Pretreatment with clonidine prevents naltrexone-precipitated withdrawal while the administration of naltrexone ensures a smooth transition into long-term opioid antagonist treatment. Naltrexone acts by blocking the psychological and physiological effects of the abused opioid such that no euphoric effects will be experienced if the drug is used. An opioid-free interval of 5 to 10 days or pretreatment with clonidine is necessary to avoid precipitated withdrawal. Naltrexone has a long duration of action, allowing infrequent dosing. It does not prevent drug craving.

***Long-term Rehabilitation:*** Oral **methadone** may be administered for up to 180 days, or longer depending on patient needs, with gradual decreases of the dose from 60 mg/day to discontinuation.

The nonpharmacologic components of treatment may be continued long-term. Self-help groups, e.g., Narcotics Anonymous (NA), are available in many communities.

### Benzodiazepine (BDZ) Withdrawal Syndrome

***Diagnostic Criteria*** (Table 1)

***Assessment:*** A withdrawal syndrome is more likely with higher doses, use more than 1 year, and with short to intermediate half-life BDZs (e.g., lorazepam). The diagnosis of a true withdrawal syndrome must be well established before initiating therapy.

Table 3: **Pharmacologic Management of Cocaine and/or Opioid Withdrawal**

| Drug | Administration | Comments | Cost* |
|---|---|---|---|
| **Cocaine** | | | |
| Dopamine agonists: | | | |
| *bromocriptine* | 0.625–2.5 mg PO QID for 30 days | Reduced symptoms of withdrawal and craving. | $–$$ |
| *amantadine* | 100 mg PO TID for 30 days | | $$ |
| *pergolide mesylate* | .05–1.5 mg PO TID for 7 days† | | $$–$$$$$ |
| *desipramine* | 200–300 mg/d PO for 12 wks† | Improved depressive withdrawal symptoms in some studies. | $$ |
| **Opioids** | | | |
| *methadone* | 10 mg PO Q2–4H to stabilization (usually 10–40 mg), then taper by 5 mg/d over 1 wk | For acute withdrawal symptoms. | $ |
| | 60 mg/d PO for 180 days or longer | For long-term maintenance. | $$ |
| *clonidine* | 0.5–1.5 mg/d PO for 8 days, then taper over 3 days | Suppresses nausea, vomiting, cramps, sweating. | $$ |
| *buprenorphine* | 4–16 mg/d sublingual for 4–12 wks | Abruptly discontinue. | ‡ |
| *clonidine/naltrexone* | Clonidine 1 mg/d PO on day 1, taper over 6 days; naltrexone 25 mg/d PO on day 1, increase to 100–150 mg/d over 6 days | Needs careful monitoring for hypotension and precipitated withdrawal. Leads into naltrexone relapse prevention. | $$$$/ $$$$$ |
| **Cocaine and Opioid Abusers** | | | |
| *buprenorphine* | 4–16 mg/d PO suppresses opioid withdrawal symptoms; 12–16 mg/d may be needed for cocaine withdrawal | Promising results treating cocaine withdrawal in methadone-maintained cocaine abusers; still under study. | ‡ |

** Cost for 7 days' treatment — drug cost only.*

*Legend: $ <$5 $$ $5–25 $$$ $25–50 $$$$ $50–75 $$$$$ $75–100*

*† Duration of study, not necessarily the recommended clinical treatment regimen.*

*‡ Not available in Canada.*

*Dosage adjustment may be required in renal impairment—see Appendix I.*

Withdrawal symptoms must be distinguished from "recurrence" or "rebound" of anxiety, panic disorder or insomnia. Recurrence usually develops slowly after drug discontinuation and remains at a steady level until drug therapy is reinitiated; rebound is more intense and of short duration; the withdrawal syndrome begins soon after drug discontinuation, particularly if the drug had a short half-life, but eventually resolves.

***Management:*** The withdrawal syndrome usually resolves spontaneously and without complications, depending on the dose and half-life of the drug and duration of use. Patients who have used a BDZ for > 12 weeks should have the dose gradually reduced and replaced by a medication with a long half-life and cross-tolerance to BDZs, e.g., diazepam. Patients in withdrawal are usually administered a loading dose of approximately 50% of the reported daily dose of BDZ in diazepam equivalents (Table 4), which is reduced by 10 to 20% per day to discontinuation. Patients who were using low doses (< 60 mg diazepam equivalents) can usually be managed ambulatory. Patients who have used high doses of BDZ or are in acute withdrawal should be hospitalized to facilitate assessment and prevent complications such as seizures, particularly if there is a history of serious withdrawal reactions. After loading with **diazepam** 20 mg Q1H PO, a slower tapering schedule of 5 to 10% each day is recommended. Response to treatment can be monitored with sensitive instruments such as the CIWA-Benzo scale.

***Long-term Rehabilitation:*** The few available data on relapse to BDZ use indicate that approximately 50% of patients remain abstinent after at least 1 year. However, some patients may replace the BDZ with other medications such as chloral hydrate, neuroleptics (e.g., chlorpromazine) or antidepressants (e.g., fluoxetine). The non-BDZ anxiolytic, **buspirone**, has less abuse

Table 4: **Dose Equivalents of Benzodiazepines**

| Benzodiazepine | Elimination half-life | Dose equivalent (mg) |
|---|---|---|
| Alprazolam | Intermediate | 0.25 |
| Bromazepam | Intermediate | 3.0 |
| Chlordiazepoxide | Long | 25.0 |
| Clorazepate | Long | 3.75 |
| Diazepam | Long | 5.0 |
| Flurazepam | Long | 15.0 |
| Lorazepam | Intermediate | 1.0 |
| Nitrazepam | Long | 5.0 |
| Oxazepam | Intermediate | 30.0 |
| Temazepam | Intermediate | 15.0 |
| Triazolam | Short | 0.25 |

and dependence potential and produces fewer withdrawal symptoms upon discontinuation than BDZs.

## *Suggested Reading List*

American Psychiatric Association. Practice guidelines for the treatment of patients with substance use disorders: alcohol, cocaine, opioids. *Am J Psychiatry* 1995; 152(11, supplement):1–59.

Ball JC, Ross A. *The effectiveness of methadone maintenance treatment. Patients, programs, services, and outcome*. New York: Springer-Verlag, 1991.

Haack MA. Treating acute withdrawal from alcohol and other drugs. *Nurs Clin North Am* 1998;33:75–92.

Schaffer A, Naranjo CA. Recommended drug treatment strategies for the alcoholic patient. *Drugs* 1998;56:571–585.

Sellers EM. Alcohol, barbiturate and benzodiazepine withdrawal syndromes: clinical management. *Can Med Assoc J* 1988;139:113–118.

CHAPTER 9

# Chronic Spasticity and Muscle Cramps

*John P. Hooge, MD, FRCPC*

## *Chronic Spasticity*

Chronic spasticity is the result of disorders of motor pathways in the brain (commonly stroke, head injury or cerebral palsy) or the spinal cord (commonly spinal cord injury or multiple sclerosis). It is one part of the upper motor neuron syndrome in which the patient is disabled by a complex combination of positive and negative symptoms. It can be harmful (reducing functional use of limbs, causing painful spasms and leading to contractures) or helpful (the patient with weakness or paralyzed legs may rely on spasticity of extensor muscles to transfer or stand).

## Goals of Therapy

- To improve active function or passive movement of limbs
- To improve comfort
- To reduce extensor or flexor spasms
- To prevent contractures

## Therapeutic Choices (Figure 1)

### Nonpharmacologic Choices

**Rehabilitation assessment:** Since spasticity does not occur in isolation, but as one part of the upper motor neuron syndrome, treatment should be tailored to each patient's needs. The rehabilitation team can assist in determining treatment goals. Interventions that help reduce spasticity may include positioning, stretching, casting, seating modifications and other treatments.

**Surgery:** Various orthopedic and neurosurgical procedures may help severe persistent spasticity that is unresponsive to other treatments.

### Pharmacologic Choices

All medications should be started at a low dose and increased gradually with monitoring for effects and side effects (Table 1).

**Baclofen** and **tizanidine** have similar efficacy and are the drugs of choice for spasticity of spinal cord origin and in multiple sclerosis. Baclofen may be less effective for spasticity of cerebral origin and use may be limited by sedation. It should not be

Figure 1: **Management of Chronic Spasticity**

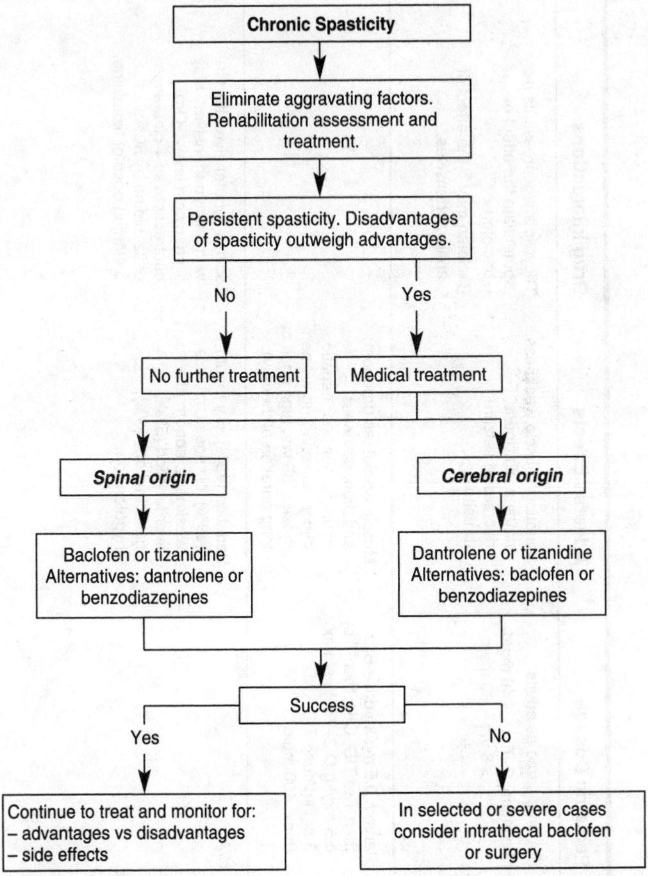
Chronic Spasticity
Eliminate aggravating factors. Rehabilitation assessment and treatment.
Persistent spasticity. Disadvantages of spasticity outweigh advantages.
No
Yes
No further treatment
Medical treatment
Spinal origin
Cerebral origin
Baclofen or tizanidine Alternatives: dantrolene or benzodiazepines
Dantrolene or tizanidine Alternatives: baclofen or benzodiazepines
Success
Yes
No
Continue to treat and monitor for: – advantages vs disadvantages – side effects
In selected or severe cases consider intrathecal baclofen or surgery

stopped suddenly because abrupt withdrawal can cause hallucinations, confusion or convulsions.

In some patients with very severe spasticity, oral baclofen may have little or no effect. **Intrathecal baclofen** via catheter from a programmable pump to the lumbar subarachnoid space can be very effective,[1] but is expensive.

**Tizanidine** is an alpha-adrenergic agonist related to clonidine. It can reduce spasticity of spinal or cerebral origin and causes increased weakness less often than baclofen. Liver function should be monitored at baseline and at months 1, 3 and 6 of tizanidine treatment.

---

[1] *J Neurosurg 1993;78:226–232.*

Table 1: **Drugs Used in Chronic Spasticity**

| Drug | Adult Dosage | Pediatric Dosage | Adverse Effects | Drug Interactions | Cost* |
|---|---|---|---|---|---|
| *baclofen* Lioresal, generics | Starting: 5 mg BID or TID ↑ 5–15 mg Q 3–7 d up to 80 mg/d divided TID (**NB:** some patients can tolerate and benefit from doses up to 120 mg/d) | Starting: same as adults Maximum: 2–7 yrs – 40 mg/d > 8 yrs – 60 mg/d | Sedation, muscle weakness, nausea, dizziness, decreased seizure threshold. | Tricyclic antidepressants may potentiate the effect of baclofen. Baclofen may ↑ the effect of antihypertensives. | $$ |
| *dantrolene* Dantrium | Starting: 25 mg daily or BID; then ↑ by 25 mg Q 3–7 d up to 400 mg/d divided TID–QID | Starting: 0.5 mg/kg/dose BID; then ↑ to TID, QID; then ↑ by 0.5 mg/kg Q 3–7 d to a max 3 mg/kg/dose TID–QID (max. 400 mg/d) | Muscle weakness (frequent), sedation, dizziness, nausea, diarrhea, hepatic injury (especially in women, those > 35 yrs, high dose or long duration of therapy). | | $$ |
| *tizanidine* Xanaflex | Starting: 2–4 mg daily; ↑ by 2–4 mg Q2–4 d up to 36 mg/d divided TID | N/A | Sedation (49%), dry mouth (49%), dizziness, muscle weakness, abnormal liver function (5%), hallucinations (3%), hypotension. | Additive hypotensive effect with antihypertensives. May ↑ phenytoin levels. Oral contraceptives ↓ clearance of tizanidine by 50%; ↓ starting dose of tizanidine. | $$$$ |

| | | | | | |
|---|---|---|---|---|---|
| **Benzodiazepines**<br>*diazepam*<br>Valium, generics | Diazepam:<br>Starting: 2–5 mg/d; then ↑ by 2–5 mg Q 3–7 d up to 60 mg/d divided BID–TID | Diazepam:<br>0.1–0.8 mg/kg/d divided BID–TID<br>Begin low and ↑ | Sedation, muscle weakness, confusion, drug dependence. | Drug effects are potentiated by alcohol and CNS depressant drugs, clarithromycin and erythromycin. | $ |
| *clonazepam*<br>Rivotril, generics | For nocturnal spasms:<br>Diazepam: 5–10 mg HS<br>Clonazepam: 0.5–2 mg HS | | | | $ |

** Cost of 30-day supply – includes drug cost only.*
*Legend: $ < $10 $$ $10–100 $$$ $100–200 $$$$ $200–300*

➊ *Dosage adjustment may be required in renal impairment – see Appendix I.*

Since it has a different mechanism of action than baclofen, tizanidine can be administered with baclofen, potentially allowing dose reductions of both drugs and increasing the reduction of spasticity.

**Dantrolene** is the only antispasticity drug to act peripherally on the muscle fiber. It commonly produces muscle weakness, which limits its usefulness unless the patient has good strength but is restricted by spasticity, or is completely paralyzed. Dantrolene may be more effective in spasticity of cerebral origin than baclofen. Its potential for hepatotoxicity is significant, especially in women, those > 35 years and those receiving high doses for prolonged periods; AST and ALT should be monitored during treatment. If there is no clear benefit after 45 days of treatment, the drug should be discontinued.

**Diazepam** and **clonazepam**, the benzodiazepines most commonly used for spasticity, effectively reduce spasticity of cerebral and spinal origin. Their usefulness is limited by sedation.

## Therapeutic Tips

- Spasticity frequently increases in response to any noxious stimulus in the body (e.g., urinary tract infections or calculi, pressure sores, ingrown toenails and other skin irritations). Before treating spasticity with medication, these conditions should be ruled out or treated if present.
- The advantages and disadvantages of spasticity to the patient should be considered before deciding to treat with medication.
- Drugs for spasticity may reduce muscle tone, deep tendon reflexes, clonus and muscle spasms but often do little or nothing to aid function, ambulation or activities of daily living.
- Muscle spasms occurring during the night can interrupt sleep. Diazepam or clonazepam can be very helpful in reducing these nocturnal spasms.

## *Muscle Cramps*

Ordinary muscle cramps are usually painful, asymmetric, occur at rest, frequently at night and most often affect the gastrocnemius muscle and small muscles of the foot. They occur when a muscle already in its most shortened position involuntarily contracts.

## Goals of Therapy

- To prevent or relieve the cramp and associated pain

## Investigations

- History and physical examination with attention to:
  - contributing factors, e.g., prolonged or excessive muscle use, high heat, salt depletion, hemodialysis or use of drugs (nifedipine, clofibrate, salbutamol, penicillamine, excessive alcohol)
  - muscle weakness, sensory symptoms or fasciculations suggesting an underlying neurological disorder
  - symptoms of tetany – paresthesias of the mouth, hands, legs and carpopedal spasm
- Laboratory investigations:
  - sodium if salt depletion is suspected
  - calcium, magnesium, potassium if tetany is suspected

## Therapeutic Choices

### Nonpharmacologic Choices

- To relieve cramps – passive stretching of the involved muscle.
- To prevent cramps – conditioning exercises and stretching exercises of the involved muscles.

### Pharmacologic Choices

**Quinine sulfate** is the drug of choice for ordinary muscle cramps. Side effects are rare at the usual dose of 200 to 300 mg HS, but higher doses can cause cinchonism (nausea, vomiting, tinnitus and deafness), visual toxicity or cardiac arrhythmias. Quinine-associated thrombocytopenia occurs rarely, is potentially life threatening, unpredictable and not dose related. A therapeutic trial of 3 to 6 weeks should be tried. If successful, re-evaluate the need for treatment in 3 to 6 months.

## *Suggested Reading List*

Alonso RJ, Mancall EL. The clinical management of spasticity. *Semin Neurol* 1991;11:215–219.

Glenn MB, Whyte J. *The practical management of spasticity in children and adults.* Philadelphia: Lea and Febiger, 1990:1–7, 201–226.

Gracies J, Elovic E, McGuire J, Simpson D. Traditional pharmacologic treatments for spasticity. Part II. General and regional treatments. *Muscle Nerve* Suppl 1997;6:S92–120.

McGee SR. Muscle cramps. *Arch Intern Med* 1990;150:511–518.

Parziale JR, Akelman E, Herz DA. Spasticity: pathophysiology and management. *Orthopedics* 1993;16:801–811.

CHAPTER 10

# Headache in Adults

*R. Allan Purdy, MD, FRCPC*

## Goals of Therapy

- To relieve or abolish pain and associated symptoms (e.g., nausea/vomiting)
- To prevent recurrent symptoms in primary headache disorders (e.g., migraine, tension-type and cluster)
- To diagnose and manage serious causes of headache (e.g., tumor, arteritis, infection, hemorrhage)
- To prevent complications of medication usage

## Investigations

- A thorough history and physical are most important for a correct diagnosis. Note characteristics of the headache:
  - onset: sudden, gradual, recurrent or chronic
  - quality: severe or mild to moderate intensity
  - temporal profile: progressive or self-limited
  - associated symptoms: nausea, vomiting, sensitivity to light, noise or odors, systemic or other neurologic signs or symptoms
  - interference with activities of daily life (e.g., migraine)
- The physical examination should be normal; if any abnormalities are found (especially visual, motor, reflex, sensory, speech or cognitive), investigation is warranted
- CT/MRI scans are not routine but must be done if any organic etiology is suspected (see box below)

### Red Flags for Serious Headache

- **Age of Onset** – middle aged to elderly patient
- **Type of Onset** – severe and abrupt
- **Temporal Sequence** – progressive severity or increased frequency
- **Significant change in headache pattern**
- **Neurologic Signs** – stiff neck, focal signs, reduced consciousness
- **Systemic Signs** – fever, appears sick, abnormal examination
- **CAUTION:** If headache does not fit typical pattern, a serious diagnosis can be missed

Figure 1: **Diagnosis and Initial Assessment of Headache**

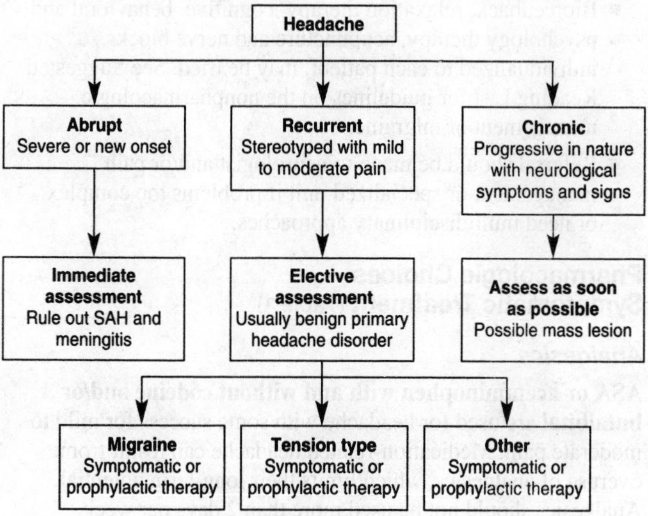
Headache
Abrupt
Severe or new onset
Recurrent
Stereotyped with mild to moderate pain
Chronic
Progressive in nature with neurological symptoms and signs
Immediate assessment
Rule out SAH and meningitis
Elective assessment
Usually benign primary headache disorder
Assess as soon as possible
Possible mass lesion
Migraine
Symptomatic or prophylactic therapy
Tension type
Symptomatic or prophylactic therapy
Other
Symptomatic or prophylactic therapy

*Note: Any headache not recognized as migraine, tension headache or known cause is in the "other" group. Investigate if no response to usual treatments.*

*Abbreviations: SAH = subarachnoid hemorrhage.*

- Lumbar puncture if subarachnoid hemorrhage, encephalitis, high- or low-pressure headache syndromes or meningitis is suspected
- Laboratory tests (on an individual basis)
  – ESR for suspected temporal arteritis
  – endocrine, biochemical, infection work-up
  – search for malignancy if indicated
- Facial pain may need a thorough assessment by a dental specialist familiar with headaches and facial pain and/or an ENT specialist if sinus or other ENT disorders are suspected

## Therapeutic Choices (Figure 1)

If serious structural CNS causes for headache and facial pain have been ruled out, the primary headache disorders and some forms of facial pain can be managed as follows.

### Nonpharmacologic Choices

- Explanation and reassurance are most important.
- Triggers, especially in migraine, should be avoided.
- Rest in a dark, noise-free room, application of ice and sleep can help.

- Informal psychotherapy from family doctor, and if psychiatric comorbidity present, referral to psychiatrist.
- Biofeedback, relaxation therapy, cognitive–behavioral and psychology therapy, acupuncture and nerve blocks, individualized to each patient, may be tried. See Suggested Reading List for guidelines on the nonpharmacologic management of migraine.
- Referral should be made to neurologist and/or pain management or specialized unit if problems too complex or need multidisciplinary approaches.

## Pharmacologic Choices

### Symptomatic Treatment (Table 1)

#### *Analgesics*

**ASA or acetaminophen with and without codeine and/or butalbital** are used for headache with some success for mild to moderate pain. Medication-related headache can result from overuse of analgesics, which limits their long-term potential. Analgesics should not be used more than 2 days per week. Butalbital compounds and opioids have limited use in benign headache disorders because of potential for dependency.

#### *Ergot Derivatives*

**Ergotamine** acts on 5-HT receptors and is classically used for migraine and cluster but use is limited by side effects. It is available in many formulations and routes of administration. Ergotamine may produce rebound headaches if used more than 2 days per week.

**Dihydroergotamine (DHE)** has similar actions to the triptans but also interacts centrally with dopamine and adrenergic receptors, accounting for some of its side effects. It can be used to treat acute intractable headache or withdrawal from analgesics. It produces no dependence.

#### *Triptans*

The triptans currently available to abort migraine include **sumatriptan, naratriptan, zolmitriptan** and **rizatriptan**. All act on serotonin (5HT) subclass 1B and 1D receptors on extracerebral blood vessels and neurons respectively; the latter three act centrally as well. The supposed mechanism of action is to prevent neurogenically sterile inflammatory responses around vessels and constrict blood vessels. The newer agents may alter pain transmission centrally at the level of the trigeminal nucleus of the medulla, an action that may or may not have clinical benefits.

Subcutaneous sumatriptan has the fastest onset of action and remains the most efficacious triptan for a severe migraine attack. It is also useful in an acute cluster headache. Naratriptan has maximal efficacy at 4 hours with less recurrence than the others, and near placebo rates of side effects. Naratriptan may be best for moderately severe migraine attacks and for individuals who have a low tolerance for side effects or have high recurrence rates of pain.

There is little to distinguish efficacy at 2 hours, recurrence rate at 24 hours and side effects of the other formulations of sumatriptan from zolmitriptan or rizatriptan. Some patients taking rizatriptan may obtain more complete relief of pain up to 2 hours. However, the benefits in individual patients may vary as well as differences in patient preference for various formulations (i.e., injection, nasal spray, tablet or fast melt tablets). Overall there is now good evidence that all the triptans are efficacious, generally well tolerated and safe. All are contraindicated in patients with cardiac disorders, sustained hypertension, basilar and hemiplegic migraine.

### *Butorphanol Tartrate*

Butorphanol is an opioid receptor agonist-antagonist with potent analgesic effects and rapid onset. It is available as a nasal spray to treat acute migraine. It may be of use in infrequent attacks of severe migraine when other treatments are not beneficial. It has some risk of abuse and can precipitate withdrawal in individuals addicted to opioids. Its major side effects are dysphoria, drowsiness, nausea and dizziness.

### *Others*

**Corticosteroids** can be useful in many headache disorders, including status migraine, cluster headache and cerebral neoplasms with edema (especially metastatic lesions). Steroids in temporal arteritis relieve headache and prevent blindness.

**Phenothiazines** (e.g., **prochlorperazine** or **chlorpromazine**) have been used in the emergency room for treatment of migraine and other intractable headaches.

If no success is obtained with the above treatments for acute migraine, **ketorolac** IM may be effective. **Meperidine** administered IV or IM should be regarded as a treatment of last resort. **Indomethacin** has been found useful in chronic paroxysmal hemicrania and related disorders.

**Antinauseants** (e.g., **dimenhydrinate** 50 to 100 mg PO PRN) and antiemetic/prokinetic agents (e.g., **metoclopramide** 10 mg PO or IV and **domperidone** 10 to 20 mg PO) are useful as adjunctive or primary therapy in headache disorders associated with nausea and vomiting.

Table 1: **Medications for Symptomatic Treatment of Headache**

| Drug | Dosage per Attack | Selected Adverse Effects | Comments | Cost*/Dose |
|---|---|---|---|---|
| **Analgesics** | | | | |
| *ASA/acetaminophen* with *codeine* and/or *butalbital* 282, 292; Tylenol w/Codeine (#2, 3, 4); Fiorinal plain, C1/4, C1/2; generics | ASA, acetaminophen 650–1300 mg Q4H × 2<br>Codeine varies with formulations<br>Butalbital as per formulation | GI upset with ASA/NSAIDs.<br>Dependence and tolerance to barbiturates and narcotics.<br>Potential liver and kidney dysfunction for acetaminophen with chronic use of high doses or in acute overdose. | Analgesics may be simple or compounds with or without narcotics or barbiturates.<br>Symptomatic treatment only.<br>Use only 2 d/wk. Great risk of rebound headache (less for naproxen). Naproxen sodium useful in perimenstrual attacks. | $ |
| *ibuprofen* Motrin, Advil, generics | Ibuprofen 400–800 mg Q6H × 2 | | | $ |
| *ketorolac* Toradol | 30–60 mg IM (max 120 mg/24 h) | Somnolence | Repeat dosages must be individualized. | $–$$ |
| *naproxen* Naprosyn, Anaprox (sodium), generics | Naproxen sodium 275–550 mg Q2–6H<br>Naproxen 250–500 mg Q2–6H | | | $ |
| *opioids* (many formulations) | Opioids require individual consideration | | | $ |
| **Ergot Derivatives** | | | | |
| *ergotamine* Ergomar | **Ergotamine and caffeine tablets:** 2 × 1 mg tablets at onset and 1 mg Q1H × 3 | Chest pain, tingling, nausea, vomiting, paresthesias, cramps, vasoconstriction.<br>Ergot dependence producing ergotism. | Use only 2 d/wk. Contraindicated in pregnancy, cardiac disorders, hypertension, sepsis, peripheral vascular disease, peptic ulcer disease, renal or liver disease. Caution in elderly. | $ |
| *compounds* Cafergot, Cafergot-PB, Megral, (many formulations, routes: PO, SL, inhaled and rectal suppositories) | **Ergotamine and caffeine suppositories:** 1/2 of a 2 mg supp at onset (maximum 3 mg within 24 h) | | | $ |

| | | | | |
|---|---|---|---|---|
| *dihydroergotamine (DHE)* parenteral and nasal (Migranal) formulations | DHE: 0.5–1 mg SC, IM or IV. May repeat at 1 h; max: 4 doses/24 h. Preceded by 10 mg metoclopramide IV or 5 mg prochlorperazine IV<br>Deliver IV meds **SLOWLY**<br>See Raskin Protocol for use in intractable headache (*Neurology* 1986;36:995–997) | Same as for ergotamine but less frequent and less prolonged.<br>Watch for hypotension, rarely. | Not as potent a vasoconstrictor as ergotamine, mainly venoconstrictor. Same contraindications as ergotamines; no dependence. Good for attacks beginning in ER and in treating medication-associated headaches. | $<br>plus cost of administration and parenteral antiemetics if given IV |
| | Nasal: 1 spray 0.5 mg in each nostril, may repeat in 15 min if no effect. Max: 2 mg/d | Rhinitis, nausea, taste disturbance. | Convenient. Bypasses GI tract. | $ |
| **Triptans** | | | | |
| *naratriptan* Amerge tablet | 1–2.5 mg PO may repeat in 4 h max: 5 mg/24 h | Chest discomfort, fatigue, dizziness, paresthesias, drowsiness, nausea, throat symptoms. All triptans have a similar side effect profile except for naratriptan which may have less adverse effects.<br>Taste disturbance, nausea with nasal spray.<br>Also faster onset than oral. | Do not use if **any** cardiac-like symptoms. Contraindicated in ischemic heart disease, sustained hypertension, pregnancy, basilar or hemiplegic migraine, or with MAO inhibitors (except naratriptan), ergotamine-containing products. Caution with SSRIs. Do not use a triptan within 24 h after another triptan. Avoid combination of rizatriptan with propranolol (↑ AUC of triptan). | $$$ |
| *rizatriptan* Maxalt tablet, wafer | 5–10 mg PO may repeat in 2 h max: 20 mg/24 h | | | $$$ |
| *sumatriptan* Imitrex tablet, SC autoinjection, nasal spray | 25–100 mg PO may repeat in 2 h max: 200 mg/24 h<br>6 mg SC may repeat in 1 h max: 2 injections/24 h<br>5–20 mg IN may repeat in 2 h max: 40 mg/24 h | | | Injection $$$$$<br>Tablets $$$<br>Nasal $$$ |
| *zolmitriptan* Zomig tablets | 2.5–5 mg PO may repeat in 2 h max: 10 mg/24 h | | Maximum dose of zolmitriptan 5 mg/24 h if also on fluvoxamine or cimetidine. | $$$ |

** Cost per dose – includes drug cost only.*

*Legend: $ < $5 $$ $5–10 $$$ $10–20 $$$$ $20–30 $$$$$ > $30*

Table 2: **Medications for Prophylactic Treatment of Headache**

| Drug | Daily Dosage Range | Selected Adverse Effects | Comments | Cost* |
|---|---|---|---|---|
| **Beta-blockers** | | | | |
| *atenolol*<br>Tenormin, generics | 50–150 mg | Fatigue, impotence, bradycardia and hypotension, GI symptoms, bronchospasm, CHF, depression. | Contraindicated in asthma, insulin-dependent diabetes, heart block or pregnancy. Avoid abrupt withdrawal. Consider long-acting formulations. Nadolol has fewer CNS side effects and is excreted by kidneys. | $–$$ |
| *metoprolol*<br>Lopresor, Betaloc, generics | 100–200 mg | | | $ |
| *nadolol*<br>Corgard, generics | 20–160 mg | | | $ |
| *propranolol*<br>Inderal, generics | 40–240 mg | | | $ |
| **Calcium Channel Blockers** | | | | |
| *flunarizine*<br>Sibelium | 5–10 mg (QHS) | Bradycardia, hypotension, constipation (verapamil), weight gain, extrapyramidal effects, drowsiness, depression (flunarizine). | Long latency to onset. Many patients have side effects. Contraindicated in hypotension, heart failure and arrhythmia. Avoid if severe constipation, especially verapamil. Do not use flunarizine in depressed patients or patients with extrapyramidal disorders. | $$–$$$$ |
| *verapamil*<br>Isoptin, generics | 240–320 mg | | | $$ |
| **Antiepileptics** | | | | |
| *valproate*<br>Depakene | 500–1500 mg/d | Nausea, alopecia, tremor, weight gain, ↑ hepatic enzymes. | Start low dosage 250–500 mg/d. Do CBC, liver function tests initially; if ↑, ↓ dosage; if 2–3 × normal, stop medication. | $–$$$ |
| *divalproex sodium*<br>Epival | 500–1500 mg/d | Neural tube defects can occur. Avoid with ASA or warfarin. | | $$–$$$$ |

| | | | | |
|---|---|---|---|---|
| **Tricyclic Analgesics** | | | | |
| *amitriptyline* Elavil, generics | 10–150 mg (QHS) | Weight gain, drowsiness, anticholinergic symptoms (e.g., dry mouth, constipation), lower seizure threshold, confusion. | Dose can be cumulative, adjustments needed. Contraindicated if significant cardiac disease, glaucoma, prostate disease or hypotension. Start low dosage in elderly or in patients sensitive to these agents. | $ |
| *doxepin* Sinequan, generics | 25–100 mg (QHS) | | | $ |
| *nortriptyline* Aventyl, generics | 10–150 mg (QHS) | | | $–$$$ |
| **Serotonin Antagonists** | | | | |
| *pizotyline* Sandomigran | Pizotyline: Start with 0.5 mg QHS, gradually ↑ to TID; if necessary to 3 or 6 mg/d (usual dose: 1–6 mg) | Weight gain, retroperitoneal cardiac and pulmonary fibrosis with methysergide; drowsiness, weight gain with pizotyline. | Consider QHS dosing of pizotyline at increasingly higher doses. **NEVER** use methysergide for more than 6 mos without a 1 mo drug holiday. ↓ dosage gradually before discontinuation. Methysergide not a first-line medication, many contraindications to use; review every time medication prescribed. | $–$$$$ |
| *methysergide* Sansert | Methysergide: Start with 2 mg QHS, gradually ↑ to TID; if necessary ↑ to 8 mg/d (usual dose: 4–8 mg) | | | $$–$$$$ |
| ***Others*** | | | | |
| *lithium* (renal icon) Carbolith, Lithane, generics | 300 mg TID | GI upset, tremor, polyuria, hypothyroidism. | Used in chronic cluster headache. Contraindicated in renal dysfunction, dehydration, CHF. ACE inhibitors and Angiotensin II receptor blockers: ↓ Li clearance. NSAIDs and thiazide diuretics: ↑ serum Li levels. | $ |

*(renal icon) Dosage adjustment may be required in renal impairment – see Appendix I.*

* *Cost of 30-day supply – includes drug cost only.*
*Legend: $ < $20 $$ $20–40 $$$ $40–60 $$$$ > $60*

## Prophylactic Treatment (Table 2)

### *Beta-blockers*

Beta-blockers are commonly used and efficacious in migraine prophylaxis; their mechanism of action is uncertain. Effective drugs lack partial agonist activity, but CNS penetration, membrane stabilization and cardioselectivity do not influence efficacy. **Metoprolol** has the best evidence to support its use but there is more experience with **propranolol**. **Nadolol** does not appreciably cross the blood-brain barrier and can be used in hopes of reducing central side effects.

### *Calcium Channel Blockers*

These drugs may work by modulating neurotransmitter function rather than producing vasodilation or protecting against hypoxia. **Verapamil** is useful in migraine and cluster headache prophylaxis. **Flunarizine** is nonselective for cardiac receptors and has good efficacy in migraine.

### *Tricyclic Analgesics*

**Amitriptyline, nortriptyline** and **doxepin** are effective for migraine and tension-type headache, acting as analgesics at doses lower than those required for affective disorders. They do not produce dependence and are relatively safe medications.

### *Valproate/Divalproex Sodium*

These agents are effective in migraine prophylaxis and may work by modulating GABA receptors in the peripheral trigeminovascular system. Guidelines for use have been published.[1] Teratogenicity (neural tube defects) occur. ASA should be avoided with valproic acid because of effects on hemostasis and coagulation.

### *Serotonin Antagonists*

**Methysergide** is a potent prophylactic medication for migraine and cluster headaches. It has potentially serious long-term side effects which can be avoided by limiting duration of treatment. Although less potent than methysergide, **pizotyline** (pizotifen) is helpful in migraine if tolerated at maximal dosage. These drugs may work by antagonizing 5-$HT_2$ receptors of the smooth muscle of blood vessels, causing vasoconstriction but this is questionable.

### *Others*

Oral **magnesium** (600 mg/d), **riboflavin** (400 mg/d) and the herb **feverfew** have shown some efficacy in migraine prophylaxis but more trials are needed.

---

[1] *Headache 1996;36:547–555.*

**Lithium** 300 mg TID is useful in the prophylactic treatment of chronic cluster headache.

**Carbamazepine** and **phenytoin** are used to treat facial pain. These antiepileptic medications have potentially significant side effects and drug interactions but can benefit some patients. Teratogenic effects (neural tube defects) have been reported with carbamazepine.

## Chronic Daily Headache and Medication-induced Headache

Chronic headache occurs daily or almost daily for 6 months or longer. The commonest cause of these headaches are *transformed migraine and chronic tension-type headache.* In the former there is history of migraine attacks and over several years the migraine attacks become more frequent. Soon the migraine characteristics give way to chronic daily headache with a daily or near-daily background headache that often resembles a typical "tension-type headache." People with chronic tension-type headache may have no history of distinct migraine. Patients with these disorders frequently use excessive amounts of abortive agents, including ergots, acetaminophen, ASA and opioid analgesics. They can have *rebound headaches* as a result of *medication-induced headache,* while some may have symptoms of depression or other psychological comorbidities. Most will improve in days or a few weeks with the discontinuation of these medications, especially mixed analgesics.

It is generally believed that analgesics, especially opioids, should not be used for more than two days per week in primary headache disorders such as migraine or tension-type headache or they will cause development of chronic daily headache. Further, if chronic daily headache develops, other useful abortive and prophylactic medications usually have less efficacy.

Management includes recognition of these disorders, tapering and stopping the offending agent(s) and starting a prophylactic medication such as **amitriptyline** or another agent listed in Table 2. During withdrawal, particularly in patients with transformed migraine, abortive agents such as **DHE** or a **triptan** should be employed for treatment of the migraine headaches that emerge. Short-term admission to hospital may be required to use the Raskin protocol (using DHE)[2,3] and give support. If psychological comorbidities, including depression, are present they must be managed and treated. Referral to a multidisciplinary pain management clinic should be considered for cases failing to respond to therapy.

---

2 *Neurology 1986;36:995.*

3 *Neurol Clin 1990;8:850–865.*

## Therapeutic Tips

The management of headache is as much an art as science; the science is improving, but the art remains important. Communicating with patients to let them know their headache is real, and that they have a specific diagnosis, is of paramount importance. Patients' expectations should be determined and management options explained to them. After serious causes are excluded, the interaction with the patient is the first and most important therapeutic choice.

- Abortive treatment without exceeding recommended dosages should be given as soon as possible.
- Use of analgesics more than 2 days per week should be avoided.
- Calendar or diary of headaches is very useful in follow-up assessment.
- A record of medications, their usefulness, dosage and side effects should be kept.
- If migraine occurs more than 3 to 4 times per month, prophylactic medications should be tried for several months and then discontinued.
- Different medications may need to be tried.
- Follow-up is most important in managing chronic headache.
- Reassurance and explanation are most important in the long term.
- Always offer hope to patients with chronic headache even if no cure is available; most primary headaches can be controlled.

## Pharmacoeconomic Considerations

*Jeffrey A. Johnson, PhD*

Given the considerable morbidity and health care resource utilization by patients with migraine headache, this condition has been considered most often in terms of the pharmacoeconomic impact. Effective migraine treatment is clearly the most cost-effective in terms of both direct and indirect costs. For the prophylaxis of migraines there are many older low-cost medications (e.g., amitriptyline and imipramine, or propranolol and atenolol) that have equal or better effectiveness than newer, more expensive agents. However, there is little published evidence for the relative cost-effectiveness of these agents. Similarly, there are many useful therapeutic choices for acute migraine treatment, with a wide cost range among these drugs. Oral and subcutaneous sumatriptan have favorable economic impact when compared to oral caffeine/ergotamine in migraine. From the societal perspective, sumatriptan was both more effective and less costly when drug and other health system costs, recurrent headaches and personal productivity losses were all considered. Even when evaluated from the narrower health systems perspective, oral and subcutaneous sumatriptan resulted in incremental health benefits as reasonable incremental costs. Differences in patient preferences for formulations for the newer triptans (i.e., nazatriptan, zolmatriptan or rizatriptan) is a consideration; however, there is no evidence that any one offers an economic benefit over the others.

***Suggested Reading***

*Adelman JU, Von Seggern R. Cost considerations in headache treatment. Part 1: prophylactic migraine treatment. Headache 1995;35:479–487.*

*Von Seggern R, Adelman JU. Cost considerations in headache treatment. Part 2: acute migraine treatment. Headache 1996;36:493–502.*

*Evans KW, Boan JA, Evans JL, Shuaib A. Economic evaluation of oral sumatriptan compared with oral caffeine/ergotamine for migraine. PharmacoEconomics 1997;12:565–577.*

## ***Suggested Reading List***

Goadsby P. A triptan too far? *J Neurol Neurosurg Psychiatry* 1998;64:143–147.

Mathew NT, ed. Advances in headache. *Neurology Clinics* 1997;15(1).

Pryse-Phillips WEM, Dodick DW, Edmeads JG, et al. Guidelines for the diagnosis and management of migraine in clinical practice. *Can Med Assoc J* 1997;156:1273–1287.

Pryse-Phillips WEM, Dodick DW, Edmeads JG, et al. Guidelines for the nonpharmacologic management of migraine in clinical practice. *Can Med Assoc J* 1998;159:47–54.

Ramadan MM, Schultz LL, Gilkey SJ. Migraine prophylactic drugs – proof of efficacy, utilization, and cost. *Cephalalgia* 1997;17:73–80.

CHAPTER 11

# Headache in Children

*Sharon Whiting, MBBS, FRCPC*

Headaches occur commonly in children and adolescents. They may occur as a primary disorder such as migraine or accompany systemic disorders or infectious diseases. It is estimated that 25% of children will have experienced a significant headache by age 10.

## Goals of Therapy

- To make an accurate diagnosis of headache
- To relieve or abort pain and associated symptoms
- To prevent further headaches

## Investigations (Figure 1)

- The history is the key to the diagnosis of headache and should be obtained from both parent and child
  - specific questions: where pain began, progress, duration, frequency, relieving and aggravating factors (especially sleep loss, excitement, certain foods, relief with activity) and associated symptoms such as vomiting and photophobia
  - specific neurological symptoms: seizures, visual disturbance, difficulty with balance, personality change, weakness
  - analgesic use
  - interference with school and social life
  - symptoms suggestive of renal, cardiac or dental disease
  - general: pregnancy, labor, delivery, growth and development, behavior, academic function

*Note*: During the interview, observe interaction between parent and child.

- Physical examination:
  - blood pressure, vital signs, palpation of sinuses, examination of teeth, neck stiffness, examination of optic fundi
  - height, weight, head circumference
  - a thorough neurological examination including cranial nerves, muscle tone, power and reflexes, and tests of coordination
- Investigations:
  - sinus x-rays if sinusitis
  - CT followed by lumbar puncture with measurement of opening pressure if pseudotumor cerebri suspected

– lumbar puncture if infectious process suspected
– CT and/or MRI if abnormal neurological examination, decreased visual acuity, recent behavior change, increasing severity and frequency of headaches, headache does not fit a known pattern

Figure 1: **Identifying the Temporal Profile of the Headache**

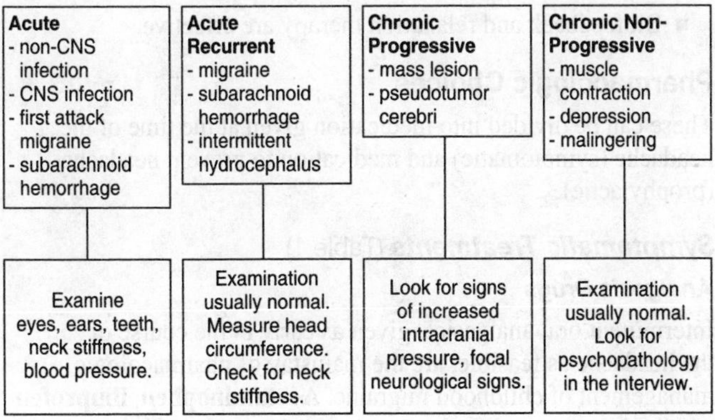
Acute
- non-CNS infection
- CNS infection
- first attack migraine
- subarachnoid hemorrhage
Acute Recurrent
- migraine
- subarachnoid hemorrhage
- intermittent hydrocephalus
Chronic Progressive
- mass lesion
- pseudotumor cerebri
Chronic Non-Progressive
- muscle contraction
- depression
- malingering
Examine eyes, ears, teeth, neck stiffness, blood pressure.
Examination usually normal. Measure head circumference. Check for neck stiffness.
Look for signs of increased intracranial pressure, focal neurological signs.
Examination usually normal. Look for psychopathology in the interview.

## Therapeutic Choices

### *Tension Headache*

#### Nonpharmacologic Choices

- Psychological evaluation.
- Relaxation therapy.
- Biofeedback.

#### Pharmacologic Choices

- Simple analgesics (acetaminophen, ASA) and NSAIDs are effective (Table 1).
- Amitriptyline (Table 2) is effective in patients with a component of depression.

### *Medication–induced Headache*

Analgesic headache induced by medications such as acetaminophen and NSAIDs is now recognized to occur in pediatric patients. Treatment involves education and gradual withdrawal of analgesic drugs. Use of a prophylactic agent (Table 2) should be considered.

## *Migraine*

### Nonpharmacologic Choices

After exclusion of mass lesion or other causes:

- Reassure and explain.
- Discuss triggers of migraine, e.g., lack of sleep, too much sleep, excitement, foods, stress, menstruation.
- Encourage sleep at the time of headache and medication early in the course of the headache.
- Biofeedback and relaxation therapy are effective.

### Pharmacologic Choices

These can be divided into medication given at the time of the headache (symptomatic) and medication to prevent headache (prophylactic).

#### *Symptomatic Treatments* (Table 1)

##### *Analgesic Drugs*

Intermittent oral analgesics, given as early in the course of the headache as feasible, are the mainstay of pharmacologic management of childhood migraine. **Acetaminophen**, **ibuprofen** and **ASA** at appropriate doses are effective.

Combination drugs such as ASA with caffeine and butalbital, with or without codeine (Fiorinal), play secondary roles should the initial agents fail. These sedating drugs have abuse potential and should be reserved for adolescents for brief periods only. Care must be taken to avoid unnecessary opioids.

##### *Antiemetics*

Nausea and vomiting occur in up to 90% of young migraine sufferers and besides being disabling, inhibit oral administration of analgesics. Antiemetics alone (e.g., **chlorpromazine**, **prochlorperazine**, **metoclopramide**) are surprisingly effective in elimination of all symptoms including the headache. Chlorpromazine with chloral hydrate to induce sleep is an effective combination in childhood migraine.

##### *Ergotamine and Dihydroergotamine*

Ergotamine compounds have very limited use in pediatrics for the following reasons:

- Auras are uncommon and inconsistent; therefore, warning indicators that trigger the time to treat with ergot are often unreliable
- Ergot can exacerbate gastrointestinal upset
- Ergots are contraindicated in complicated migraine syndromes because of the risk of increasing vasospasm

In severe intractable headache, dihydroergotamine can be used IV in combination with an antiemetic in the emergency department.

#### *Triptans*

While there are some studies of 5-HT agonists in pediatrics, they are not currently approved for children. The value of sumatriptan in children is not well established and it may be less effective in children.

### *Prophylactic Agents* (Table 2)

#### *Serotonin Antagonists*

**Pizotyline,** a less potent prophylactic medication than methysergide, is helpful in migraine. Methysergide is not used in pediatric headache because of potentially serious long-term side effects.

#### *Beta-blockers*

The beta-blocker **propranolol** has been commonly used and is effective in some cases. It is contraindicated in reactive airway disease, diabetes mellitus and bradyarrhythmias. Depressive symptoms are an under-reported but common effect in adolescents.

#### *Antihistamines*

**Cyproheptadine,** an antihistamine with antiserotonergic and calcium channel blocking properties, is firmly entrenched as a prophylactic agent, although it has never been subject to controlled study. Its use in older children and adolescents is limited by sedative properties and associated weight gain.

#### *Calcium Channel Blockers*

**Flunarizine** has been shown to significantly reduce headache frequency and severity in children.

#### *Antidepressants*

**Amitriptyline** has shown efficacy of 50 to 55% in adults. No controlled trials in children have been reported.

#### *Nonsteroidal Anti-inflammatory Agents*

These medications reduce headache frequency and severity in adults when used as prophylaxis, presumably through prostaglandin inhibition. A series in adolescent children showed a 60% reduction in headache frequency and severity using **naproxen sodium.**

#### *Anticonvulsants*

Carbamazepine and valproic acid have been studied in adults but not in children. Phenobarbital and phenytoin are no longer used.

Table 1: **Drug Treatment of Headache in Children**

| Drug | Daily Dosage Range | Adverse Effects | Comments | Cost* |
|---|---|---|---|---|
| **Analgesics** | | | | |
| *acetaminophen* | 10–15 mg/kg/dose Q4H | All: Gastrointestinal upset. | Medication most often used at time of headache. | $ |
| *ASA* | Age ≥ 12 yrs: 500–650 mg PRN | | Because of the concern of Reye's syndrome, ASA should not be used in the context of fever or a viral illness. | $ |
| *ibuprofen*<br>Motrin, Advil, generics | 5–10 mg/kg/dose 4 times daily | | | $ |
| *naproxen sodium*<br>Anaprox, generics | Age > 2 years: 5–7 mg/kg/dose Q8–12H | | | $ |
| **Combination Therapy** | | | | |
| *butalbital, caffeine, ASA*<br>Fiorinal, generics | 1–2 tablets 4 times daily | Gastrointestinal upset; dependence and tolerance to barbiturates and opioids. | Reserved for adolescents. No more than 2 days/week. Risk of tolerance, addiction and misuse. | $ |
| *orphenadrine citrate, ASA, caffeine*<br>Norgesic | 1–2 tablets 4 times daily | | | $–$$ |
| **Antiemetics** | | | | |
| *chlorpromazine*<br>Largactil, generics | 1 mg/kg PO/IM to a maximum of 25 mg Q8H | Hypotension. | Can be used with PO chloral hydrate 25–50 mg/kg PO Q8H. | $ |
| | 0.1 mg/kg IV Q10–15 minutes to a maximum of 30 mg | | Can cause hypotension when given IV. Use in the emergency department. | $ |
| *prochlorperazine*<br>Stemetil, generics | 2.5–5 mg twice daily PO<br>10 mg IV | Extrapyramidal dysfunction. | Use IV in adolescents in the emergency department. | $<br>$ |
| *metoclopramide*<br>Maxeran, Reglan, generics | 1–2 mg/kg (<10 mg) PO<br>10 mg IV | Extrapyramidal dysfunction. | Use IV in adolescents in the emergency department. | $<br>$$ |

| | | | | |
|---|---|---|---|---|
| **Ergot Derivatives**<br>*dihydroergotamine* | | | | |
| Dihydroergotamine (DHE) | 0.1–0.25 mg/dose IV. May be repeated Q20 minutes × 3. Give metoclopramide 0.2 mg/kg/dose 30 minutes prior to IV dihydroergotamine (maximum 20 mg). | Flushed feeling. Tingling in extremities. Nausea and vomiting. | Useful in patients with severe and prolonged migraine headache. This protocol to take place in hospital. Contraindicated in complicated migraine, coronary heart disease, abnormal blood pressure, abnormal ECG. | $–$$ |
| Migranal | Nasal spray: 1 spray into each nostril. May repeat in 15 min. | Nausea, taste disturbance, rhinitis. | | $$$ |
| **Triptans**<br>*naratriptan, rizatriptan, sumatriptan, zolmitriptan* | | | Not currently indicated for children under age 18. | |

** Cost per dose (based on 20 kg) – includes drug cost only.*
*Legend: $ < $1 $$ $1–5 $$$ $5–10*

Table 2: **Prophylactic Treatment of Headache in Children**

| Drug | Daily Dosage Range | Adverse Effects | Comments | Cost* |
|---|---|---|---|---|
| **Beta-blockers**<br>*propranolol*<br>Inderal, generics | 0.6–1.5 mg/kg/d PO | Fatigue, bradycardia, hypotension, depression. | Contraindicated in asthma, diabetes, heart block, bradyarrhythmias, pregnancy. Avoid abrupt withdrawal. | $ |
| **Serotonin Antagonists**<br>*pizotyline*<br>Sandomigran | 0.5–1.5 mg/d PO | Sedation and weight gain. | Start medication slowly and increase over 1–3 weeks. | $–$$ |
| **Calcium Channel Blockers**<br>*flunarizine*<br>Sibelium, generics | 5 mg/d PO | Bradycardia, hypotension, depression. | May take several weeks before effective. Do not use in depressed patients or those with extrapyramidal disorders. | $$ |
| **Tricyclics**<br>*amitriptyline*<br>Elavil, generics | 10–150 mg/d | Weight gain, drowsiness. Anticholinergic symptoms such as dry mouth and constipation. | Contraindicated in significant cardiac disease or hypotension. | $ |

| | | | | |
|---|---|---|---|---|
| **Antihistamines** | | | | |
| *cyproheptadine* Periactin, generics | Age 2–6 years: 2 mg Q8–12H (maximum 12 mg/d)<br>Age 7–14 years: 4 mg Q8–12H (maximum 16 mg/d) | Drowsiness, weight gain. | | $–$$ |
| **Nonsteroidal Anti-inflammatory Agents** | | | | |
| *naproxen sodium* ➔ Anaprox, generics | 275–550 mg twice daily | GI upset. | Use in adolescents. | $$ |
| **Anticonvulsants** | | | | |
| *valproic acid* | 10–30 mg/kg/d in 2 or 3 divided doses | Anorexia, weight gain, hepatic dysfunction, pancreatic dysfunction. | Use mainly in adolescents. | $ |

** Cost of 30-day supply – includes drug cost only.*
*Legend: $ < $20 $$ $20–40*

*➔ Dosage adjustment may be required in renal impairment – see Appendix I.*

## Therapeutic Tips

- There are very few controlled trials of pharmacologic management of childhood migraine; hence, anecdotal experience prevails. Most young patients with migraine do not require daily medication but need *access to reliable analgesia at home and at school.*
- Children are debilitated by nausea and vomiting and benefit greatly from *antiemetics. Rest and sleep* are usually very helpful.
- *Consider prophylactic agents* for children who cycle through periods of time when they experience such frequency of headache that their *lifestyle is disrupted* or when isolated or infrequent events are *severe and complex.*
- *Calendars* are helpful in identifying triggers, headache patterns, frequency and severity and are invaluable for management and evaluation of response to therapy.
- Prophylactic medication should be considered, using medications with the least side effects first. Pizotyline or propranolol are the *drugs of first choice*. Cyproheptadine is usually used in younger children. For adolescents, propranolol, amitriptyline, naproxen sodium and flunarizine are used in that order.
- The prognosis for children with migraine is favorable with 50% of patients reporting improvement within 6 months after medical intervention, regardless of treatment methods used.
- Most children respond to reassurance, general advice and simple remedies for attacks when they occur.

## *Suggested Reading List*

Rothner A. Headaches in children and adolescents. *Child Adolesc Psychiatr Clin North Am* 1999;8:727–745.

Forsyth R, Farrell K. Headache in childhood. *Pediatr Rev* 1999;20:39–45.

Singh B, Roach E. Diagnosis and management of headache in children. *Pediatr Rev* 1998;19:132–135.

CHAPTER 12

# Acute Pain

*Benoit Bailey, MD, MSc, FRCPC*

The undertreatment of pain has been demonstrated in several studies. Treatment should be tailored to the level of pain the patient is experiencing; an analgesic effective for a type of pain in one patient may not necessarily be helpful in another with the same type of pain. For mild to moderate pain, the first step should be the use of a nonopioid analgesic alone or in combination. If the pain is still present or worsening, include a weak opioid alone or in combination with a nonopioid analgesic. If the pain is still present or worsening, use a stronger opioid alone or with a nonopioid analgesic. For severe pain, starting with a strong opioid is usually more appropriate (Figure 1).

## Goals of Therapy

- To recognize the patient that is experiencing pain
- To relieve the pain until the cause is treated
- To identify and treat the cause of pain

## Investigations

- Observe the patient for behavioral signs of pain (e.g., agitation, crying, teeth gritting, withdrawal from activity)
- Solicit self-reports of the pain
- Inquire about the history and perform a physical examination to determine the cause and severity of the pain
- Use a pain scale as needed to assess pain
- Inquire about medication history for self treatment and possible allergy or adverse drug reactions to analgesics
- Laboratory investigations as appropriate to determine the cause of the pain

## Therapeutic Choices

### Nonpharmacologic Choices

Patients presenting with acute pain should be assessed rapidly with calmness, empathy and reassurance. Encourage patients to verbalize their pain at all stages of treatment. Measures to decrease pain should be initiated immediately (immobilizing a fracture, dressing on burns, applying cold or heat or other techniques such as relaxation, imagery and distraction) until pharmacologic treatment is started. Do not wait until a full assessment is made to start pharmacologic treatment.

Figure 1: **Management of Acute Pain**

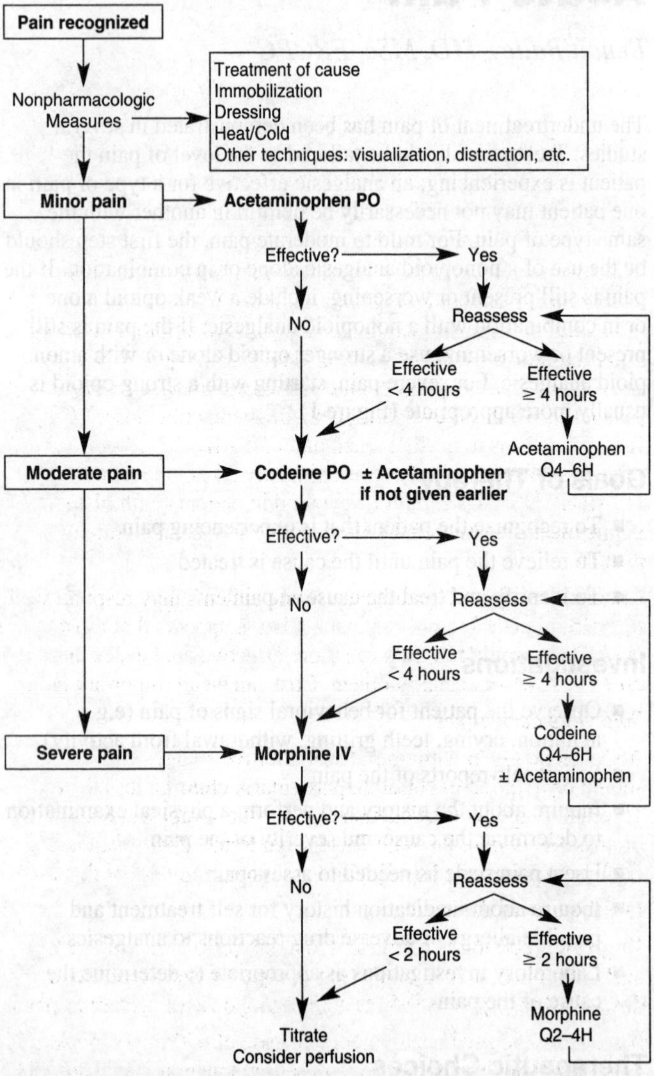
Pain recognized
Nonpharmacologic Measures
Treatment of cause
Immobilization
Dressing
Heat/Cold
Other techniques: visualization, distraction, etc.
Minor pain
Acetaminophen PO
Effective?
Yes
No
Reassess
Effective < 4 hours
Effective ≥ 4 hours
Acetaminophen Q4–6H
Moderate pain
Codeine PO ± Acetaminophen if not given earlier
Effective?
Yes
No
Reassess
Effective < 4 hours
Effective ≥ 4 hours
Codeine Q4–6H ± Acetaminophen
Severe pain
Morphine IV
Effective?
Yes
No
Reassess
Effective < 2 hours
Effective ≥ 2 hours
Morphine Q2–4H
Titrate
Consider perfusion

## Pharmacologic Choices (Table 1)

### *Oral Pain Management*

#### Nonopioid Analgesics

**Acetaminophen** can be used for *mild to moderate pain*. Its advantages include equal analgesic and antipyretic action to ASA and fewer adverse reactions and drug interactions than NSAIDs. However, it has no anti-inflammatory action. It can be used with opioid analgesics for additive analgesic effect.

**Nonsteroidal anti-inflammatory drugs (NSAIDs)** are a heterogeneous group of medications with analgesic, antipyretic and anti-inflammatory action that can be used for *mild to moderate pain*. Classic NSAIDs are divided into 5 classes: salicylates, fenamates, propionic acid derivatives, oxicams and acetic acid derivatives. Recently, NSAIDs which selectively inhibit cyclooxygenase (COX-2 inhibitors) have become available. COX-2 inhibitors have fewer gastrointestinal adverse effects and do not increase bleeding time but their place in the treatment of acute pain is unclear. A single dose of a COX-2 inhibitor appears as effective as a single dose of other NSAIDs.

The adverse effects of NSAIDs are limited with single or few doses and are qualitatively similar to ASA. Chronic use is associated with gastrointestinal symptoms (ulceration, bleeding and perforation) and renal failure. ASA, unlike other NSAIDs, irreversibly inhibits platelet function for the lifetime of the platelet (8–10 days) even after a single therapeutic dose. Platelet function returns to normal when other NSAIDs have been eliminated from the body (approximately 24 hours for most NSAIDs). NSAIDs should be avoided in patients with history of peptic ulcer disease, renal failure, congestive heart failure or asthma.

Choosing an NSAID is difficult. Some patients may respond well to a certain class but not to others. Also, it appears that most NSAIDs in single full dose are more effective analgesics than full doses of ASA or acetaminophen. Cost can be an important factor.

***Salicylate derivatives***

**ASA** can be given with opioids for additive analgesic effect. It should be avoided in children, particularly children less than 16 years of age with chickenpox or flu-like symptoms because of possible association with Reye's syndrome. **Diflunisal** and **choline magnesium trisalicylate** are other members of this class.

***Propionic acid derivatives***

**Ibuprofen** 200 mg is equivalent to a dose of 650 mg of ASA or acetaminophen; a dose of 400 mg is superior and longer acting. A dose of 10 mg/kg is as safe as a 15 mg/kg dose of acetaminophen.

**Naproxen** 250 mg is equivalent to a dose of 650 mg of ASA; a dose of 500 mg is superior. Both doses are longer acting than ASA.

***Acetic acid derivatives***

**Tolmetin**, **indomethacin**, **diclofenac**, **sulindac** and **ketorolac** are available in this class.

### Opioid analgesics

Opioids can be used for the treatment of *moderate to severe pain*. However, for severe pain the parenteral route is preferred because of its faster onset of action. Opioids may be substituted using equipotent doses (Chapter 15). However, the adverse effects of

Table 1: **Analgesics for the Treatment of Acute Pain**

| Drug | Dosage | | Comments | Cost* |
|---|---|---|---|---|
| **Nonopioid Analgesics** | | | | |
| **Acetaminophen** | Pediatric: | 10–15 mg/kg/dose PO Q4H | Oral suspension available. | $ |
| Tylenol, many others | | 15–20 mg/kg/dose PR Q4H<br>max: 5 doses/d | | $$ |
| | Adult: | 325–650 mg PO or PR Q4H<br>max: 4 g/d | | $–$$ |
| **ASA** | Analgesic and antipyretic: | | | |
| Aspirin, many others | Pediatric: | 10–15 mg/kg/dose PO Q4H<br>max: 5 doses/d | | $ |
| | Adult: | 325–650 mg PO Q4H<br>max: 4 g/d | | $ |
| | Anti-inflammatory: | | Monitor levels with anti-inflammatory doses. | |
| | Pediatric: | 60–100 mg/kg/d PO divided Q6–8H | | |
| | Adult: | 500–1000 mg Q4–6H | | |
| **Ibuprofen** | Analgesic and antipyretic: | | | |
| Motrin, Advil, generics | Pediatric: | 10 mg/kg/dose PO Q6–8H<br>max: 40 mg/kg/d | Oral suspension available. | $ |
| | Adult: | 200–400 mg PO Q6–8H<br>max: 1.2 g/d | | $ |
| | Anti-inflammatory: | | | |
| | Pediatric: | 30–50 mg/kg/d PO divided Q6–8H<br>max: 2.4 g/d | | |
| | Adult: | 400–800 mg PO Q6–8H<br>max: 3.2 g/d | | |

| | | | |
|---|---|---|---|
| **Naproxen** ❥<br>Naprosyn, generics | Analgesic and antipyretic:<br>Pediatric: 5–7 mg/kg/dose PO Q8–12H<br>max: 1.25 g/d | Oral suspension available. | $ |
| | Adult: 500 mg initially, then 250 mg PO Q6–8H<br>max: 1.25 g/d | | $ |
| | Anti-inflammatory:<br>Pediatric: 7–20 mg/kg/d PO divided Q12H<br>max: 1.25 g/d<br>Adult: 250–500 mg PO Q12H<br>max: 1.25 g/d | | |
| **Tolmetin** ❥<br>Tolectin, generics | Anti-inflammatory:<br>Pediatric: 15–30 mg/kg/d PO divided Q6–8H<br>max: 30 mg/kg/d | | $ |
| | Adult: 400–600 mg PO Q8H<br>max: 2 g/d | | $$ |
| **Ketorolac** ❥<br>Toradol, generics | Pediatric: 0.2–1 mg/kg/dose IM or IV Q4–6H<br>max: 30 mg/dose<br>Adult: 10–30 mg IM or IV Q4–6H<br>max: 120 mg/d | Dose not well established. Limited information available. | $$$ |
| **Opioid Analgesics** | | | |
| **Codeine**<br>generics | Pediatric: 0.5–1 mg/kg/dose PO Q4–6H<br>max: 60 mg/dose | Oral suspension available. | $ |
| | Adult: 15–60 mg PO Q4–6H<br>max: 60 mg/dose | | $ |

*(cont'd)*

Table 1: **Analgesics for the Treatment of Acute Pain** *(cont'd)*

| Drug | Dosage | Comments | Cost* |
|---|---|---|---|
| **Opioid Analgesics** *(cont'd)* | | | |
| **Morphine**<br>Statex, MS•IR, M.O.S., generics | Immediate-release oral:<br>Pediatric: 0.2–0.5 mg/kg/dose PO Q4–6H<br>Adult: 10–30 mg PO Q4–6H | | $ |
| Kadian, MS Contin, M-Eslon, M.O.S.-SR, Oramorph SR | Sustained-release oral:<br>Pediatric: 0.3–0.6 mg/kg/dose PO Q12H<br>Adult: 15–30 mg PO Q12H | Rarely used for acute pain. | $$ |
| | Pediatric:<br>Intermittent IV: 0.1–0.2 mg/kg/dose Q2–4H<br>Continuous IV infusion: 0.01–0.05 mg/kg/h<br>– Breakthrough pain during infusion: 0.01–0.05 mg/kg/dose | Titrate to effect. | $ |
| | Adult:<br>Intermittent IV: 2.5–10 mg IV Q2–4H<br>Continuous IV infusion: 1–10 mg/h<br>– Breakthrough pain during infusion: 2.5–5 mg/dose | Titrate to effect. | $ |
| **Meperidine**<br>Demerol, generics | Pediatric: 1–1.5 mg/kg/dose IV Q3–4H<br>max: 100 mg/dose | | $ |
| | Adult: 50–100 mg IV Q3–4H<br>max: 100 mg/dose | | $ |
| **Fentanyl**<br>generics | Pediatric: 0.5–4 mcg/kg/dose IV Q1–2H<br>Adult: 50–100 mcg IV Q1–2H | Titrate to effect. | $$$$ |

** Cost per dose (assuming 20 kg for children and 70 kg for adults) – includes drug cost only.*
*Legend: $ < $0.50 $$ $0.50–1.00 $$$ $1.00–5.00 $$$$ > $5.00*

*Dosage adjustment may be required in renal impairment – see Appendix I.*

codeine and meperidine can limit this process. Adverse effects include constipation (codeine may be the worst offender), nausea, sedation, respiratory depression and (if used for long period of time) tolerance, dependence and withdrawal symptoms.

**Codeine** is frequently given concomitantly with acetaminophen or ASA for additive analgesic effect without increasing the adverse effects. Some patients are resistant to the analgesic effect of codeine. The use of codeine, particularly in the elderly, should be accompanied by stool softeners and/or bulk-forming laxatives.

**Morphine** is available in several immediate-release dosage forms and in sustained-release preparations. However, sustained-release preparations should rarely be given for the treatment of acute pain. Because of less adverse effects compared to codeine, morphine can be titrated to achieve pain-free status.

**Hydroxymorphone**, **hydrocodone**, **oxycodone**, **meperidine**, **propoxyphene** and **pentazocine** are other available oral opioids.

### *Parenteral Pain Management*

Parenteral administration of analgesics includes the subcutaneous, intramuscular and intravenous routes. The intravenous route is preferred because it is pain free and onset of action is predictable.

#### Nonsteroidal anti-inflammatory drugs (NSAIDs)

**Ketorolac** is an NSAID that can be given IM or IV for the treatment of *moderate to severe pain*. A dose of 30 mg is comparable to a moderate dose (12 mg) of morphine. It has the same adverse effect profile as the oral NSAIDs. The pharmacologic effect cannot be titrated but it can be used when opioids are contraindicated. Ketorolac is effective for the treatment of renal colic.

#### Opioid analgesics

**Morphine** is the standard to which other opioids are compared. Its advantages over meperidine include longer duration of action and metabolism not affected by liver and renal disease. It can be administered as continuous infusion or as patient controlled analgesia (PCA), a pump that is programmed to deliver a preset amount of drug by continuous infusion or repeated boluses and smaller breakthrough bolus doses.

Use of **meperidine** in patients with renal failure should be avoided because an active metabolite (normeperidine) will accumulate and cause seizures in some patients. This same metabolite causes the adverse CNS effects of meperidine (tremors, hyperreflexia, hallucinations). Meperidine should also be avoided in patients with liver disease and those who have received monoamine oxidase inhibitors in the past 14 days. Usually, meperidine should not be given for pain that is expected to last more than 3 hours where morphine is a better choice.

**Fentanyl** is a synthetic opioid which has a duration of action of only 30 to 60 minutes, limiting its usefulness for the treatment of pain unless given by infusion (no advantage over morphine and much more costly) but making it an ideal analgesic for brief procedures. It has almost no hemodynamic effects and does not induce histamine release, unlike morphine and meperidine. Rapid administration can lead to chest wall rigidity that can potentially interfere with ventilation.

### *Topical and Local Anesthesia*

Infiltrative techniques using **lidocaine** are the most frequently used for minor procedures. A dose of 3 to 5 mg/kg (maximum 300 mg) can be used for direct infiltration or regional nerve block. Coadministration of **epinephrine** allows an increase of lidocaine dose to 5 to 7 mg/kg unless epinephrine is contra-indicated (i.e., if tissue vascularity is poor or if distal vasculature is involved). If allergy is suspected to amide type local anesthetics (e.g., lidocaine, bupivacaine), an ester type (e.g., procaine, tetracaine, benzocaine) can be used because of the absence of cross-reactivity.

For small facial lacerations, a mixture of tetracaine 0.5 to 1%, epinephrine (adrenaline) 0.25 to 0.5% and cocaine 1 to 4% (**TAC**) can be applied topically (3 mL – maximum cocaine 6 mg/kg), but the restricted status of cocaine limits its usefulness. A mixture of lidocaine 0.4%, epinephrine 0.1% and tetracaine 0.05% (**LET**) (2 mL) is as effective topically as TAC.

On intact skin, eutectic mixture of local anesthetics (**EMLA**), a mixture of prilocaine and lidocaine, is effective but utility is limited by the time required for adequate local anesthesia (45 to 60 minutes). In order to be effective, a large amount should be applied with an occlusive dressing well before the procedure (for minor procedures, 2.5 g/site; for major procedures, 2 g/10 $cm^2$).

### *Inhalation Pain Management*

**Nitrous oxide** ($N_2O$) at a concentration of 30 to 50% can be used as an analgesic. Advantages include rapid onset of action and short duration of action. Contraindications include: altered level of consciousness, severe maxillofacial injuries, chronic obstructive pulmonary disease, acute pulmonary edema, pneumothorax, shock, decompression sickness, bowel obstruction and major chest injury. It can produce lightheadedness, drowsiness, nausea, vomiting and excitement.

## Therapeutic Tips

- Choose the route of administration and medication according to the severity of the pain, rapidity of onset of action and duration of action.

- The use of sedatives can also be considered, particularly for procedures, but should not replace analgesics.
- Always wait the appropriate amount of time according to the onset of action of the analgesic to perform a procedure or evaluate if the analgesic was effective.
- Monitor the level of consciousness and presence of other adverse effects after administration of the analgesic.
- The need for analgesics should be constantly reassessed.
- Avoid the use of opioids on an as-needed basis. A regular schedule of administration is more effective.
- Keep **naloxone** on hand when administering opioids parenterally in case of overdosage. An overdosage will not occur as long as the patient has pain.
- Consult specialized acute pain services as needed.

Table 2: **Naloxone for Treatment of Opioid-induced Respiratory Depression**

| |
|---|
| Adults and children > 5 yrs or > 20 kg weight:<br>0.4 to 2 mg IV Q2–3 min |
| Children birth-5 yrs or ≤ 20 kg weight:<br>0.1 mg/kg Q2–3 min |
| Maximum: 10 mg<br>May need to repeat in 1 to 2 hours, depending on half-life of opioid.<br>Continuous infusion may be used for overdoses of long-acting opiates. Starting dose is 2/3 of the initial dose that was effective for the patient, administered per hour by infusion *OR* 0.4–0.8 mg/h in adults and 0.05–0.15 mg/kg/h in children. Titrate to effect. |

## Suggested Reading List

Acute Pain Management Guideline Panel. *Acute pain management: operative or medical procedures and trauma*. Clinical Practice Guideline. AHCPR Publ. No 92–0032. Rockville, MD: Agency for Health Care Policy and Research, Public Health Services, US Department of Health and Human services, February, 1992.

Anon. Drugs for pain. *Med Lett Drugs Ther* 1998;40:79–84.

Ducharme J. Emergency pain management: A Canadian association of emergency physicians consensus document. *J Emerg Med* 1994;12:855–866.

Follin SL, Charland SL. Acute pain management: operative or medical procedures and trauma. *Ann Pharmacother* 1997; 31:1068–1076.

McQuay H, Moore A, Justins D. Treating acute pain in hospital. *BMJ* 1997;314:1531–1535.

CHAPTER 13

# Back Pain

*Eldon Tunks MD, FRCPC*

This chapter summarizes the nonsurgical management of low back pain (LBP).

## Goals of Therapy

**Acute LBP**

- To promote rapid recovery and reduce distress

**Subacute/recurrent LBP**

- To assess appropriately and prevent chronicity
- To prevent or minimize work absence

**Chronic LBP**

- To promote or restore healthy behavior, fitness and appropriate role functions by defining and treating medical and psychological factors associated with persistent/recurrent pain, according to evidence-based principles

## Investigations

Assessment/red flags:

### *Acute LBP* (Figure 1)

- For herniated nucleus pulposus:
  – positive SLR (straight leg raising) (leg pain at <60°)
  – weak dorsiflexion of ankle (L4-5), or great toe (L5-S1 or L4-5)
  – reduced ankle reflex (L5-S1)
  – reduced light touch in L4, L5 or S1 dermatomes of foot/leg
- For cancer:
  – age >50
  – bedrest does not relieve pain
  – failure to improve after >1 month therapy
  – previous cancer history
  – unexplained weight loss
  – positive laboratory tests including imaging
- For spinal osteomyelitis:
  – intravenous drug abuse
  – infection of skin or urinary tract
  – fever
  – vertebral tenderness
  – positive laboratory tests including imaging

Figure 1: **Management of Acute Low Back Pain**

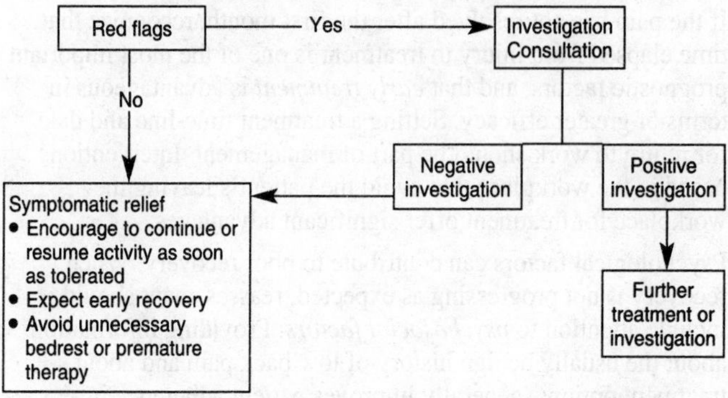
Red flags
Yes
Investigation Consultation
No
Negative investigation
Positive investigation
Symptomatic relief
• Encourage to continue or resume activity as soon as tolerated
• Expect early recovery
• Avoid unnecessary bedrest or premature therapy
Further treatment or investigation

- Compression fracture:
  - age >70
  - corticosteroid use
  - history of a fall/trauma
  - positive laboratory tests including plain x-rays
- Cauda equina syndrome:
  - acute urinary retention or overflow incontinence
  - loss of anal sphincter tone/fecal incontinence
  - perineal numbness
  - weakness of legs
  - emergency laboratory assessment and imaging

When red flags are present, further investigation and/or referral for consultation are indicated.

### *Subacute LBP*

When there is lack of expected progress or lack of resolution, the patient should be re-evaluated. (See above for red flags.) When red flags are present, imaging and consultation is appropriate. After the first 4-6 weeks, EMG may be helpful when there are clinical findings of nerve root embarrassment.

## Therapeutic Choices

### Nonpharmacologic Choices

### *Acute LBP*

**0 to 30 days: Promoting earlier recovery**

For acute or recurrent back pain of less than 3 weeks, provide symptomatic relief, encourage the patient to continue or resume activity as soon as tolerated, and expect early recovery. Avoid unnecessary bedrest for uncomplicated back pain, and also avoid premature physical therapy. This results in the shortest sick leave.

### *Subacute LBP*

**30 to 90 days: Restoring function**

If the pain has not resolved after the first month, recognize that time elapsed from injury to treatment is one of the most important prognostic factors, and that *early treatment* is advantageous in terms of greater efficacy. Setting a treatment time-line and date for return to work should be part of management. Interventions based in the workplace that avoid the patient's leaving the workplace for treatment offer significant advantages.

Psychological factors can contribute to poor recovery. When recovery is not progressing as expected, reassessment should include attention to *psychosocial factors*. Providing information about the usually benign history of low back pain and about treatment options, generally improves patient adherence in recovery process.

There are many potential modalities of treatment. *Physical therapy* modalities are more efficacious than no treatment. However, there is little to recommend one conservative treatment over another, except that active exercise appears to be more beneficial than treatment by passive modalities, and bedrest for uncomplicated back pain is not therapeutic.

**Approximately 3 to 6 months: Interrupting progress toward chronic pain** (Figure 2)

For recurrent back pain, or persistent back pain of 3 months or more, reassessment is appropriate. This should include screening for psychosocial complications.

If there is marked functional disability associated with pain that is recurrent or persisting for 3 months, treatment appropriate at this time includes a *coordinated program of active exercise* with graded quotas, patient education, collaborative goal-setting with the patient to promote functional activity, liaison with major stakeholders, a clear target for work re-entry, work re-entry guidelines to patient and employer and worksite modification if relevant. If the coordinated program is unsuccessful, referral to a multidisciplinary chronic pain clinic may be appropriate.

Red flags for *psychosocial factors* include (but are not limited to): complaint of constant extreme pain, pain in many parts of the body, patients believing that they will never return to work, self-report of very high levels of functional disability, history of long/repeated work absenteeism, longstanding psychiatric distress, or an adversarial posture associated with compensation/litigation, although compensation/litigation by itself has a less definite effect on outcomes.

If several significant red flags for psychosocial factors are detected, associated with persistent or recurrent pain, it is appropriate to investigate further and treat any Axis I psychiatric

Figure 2: **Management of Persisting Low Back Pain***

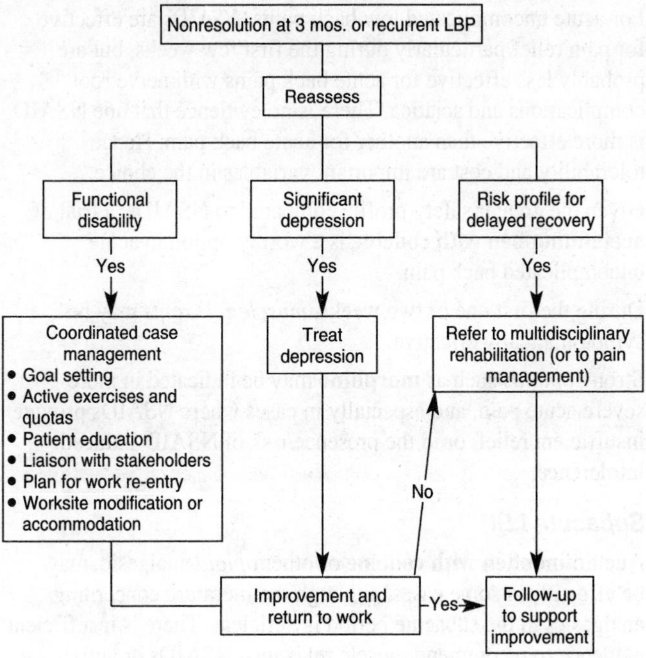
Nonresolution at 3 mos. or recurrent LBP
Reassess
Functional disability
Significant depression
Risk profile for delayed recovery
Yes
Yes
Yes
Coordinated case management
• Goal setting
• Active exercises and quotas
• Patient education
• Liaison with stakeholders
• Plan for work re-entry
• Worksite modification or accommodation
Treat depression
Refer to multidisciplinary rehabilitation (or to pain management)
No
Improvement and return to work
Yes
Follow-up to support improvement

* *Adapted from Crook J, Tunks E. Pain Clinics. In: Lane NE, Wolfe F, eds. Musculoskeletal Medicine. Rheum Dis Clin North Am. Philadelphia: WB Saunders Press. 1996;22(3):599–611.*

disorder (e.g., depression), and in some cases to refer to a comprehensive rehabilitation program (or possibly to a multidisciplinary chronic pain management clinic).

### ***Chronic LBP – Persistent pain after six months or more*** (Figure 2)

When pain with functional impairment has persisted for several months despite attempted treatment, a comprehensive *rehabilitation* focus (or possibly a multimodal chronic pain management program), including two or more of cognitive-behavioral therapy, active exercise, functional restoration, patient goal-setting, patient education, psychosocial intervention and training in coping skills, is preferred over single modality or less intensive treatments. Even "back school" or "patient education" tends to be ineffective at this point, unless an active exercise and/or functional restoration focus is included. In any treatment of persistent pain, engaging the patient to collaborate actively in setting treatment goals and quotas and in monitoring progress is a key ingredient.

## Pharmacologic Choices (Table 1)

### *Acute LBP*

For acute uncomplicated low back pains, *NSAIDs* are effective for pain relief particularly during the first few weeks, but are probably less effective for acute back pains with nerve root complications and sciatica. There is no evidence that one NSAID is more effective than another for acute back pain. Hence tolerability and cost are important variables in the choice.

Given the greater safety profile compared to NSAIDs, a trial of **acetaminophen with codeine** is a worthy option in acute uncomplicated back pain.

During the first one or two weeks, *muscle relaxants* may be symptomatically effective.

Strong *opioids* such as **morphine** may be indicated in more severe acute pain, and especially in cases where NSAIDs provide insufficient relief, or in the presence/risk of NSAID-induced intolerance.

### *Subacute LBP*

**Acetaminophen with codeine** or other *opioid* analgesic, may be effective in some cases, although the literature concerning analgesics in the subacute period is deficient. There is insufficient evidence to recommend muscle relaxants, NSAIDs or antidepressants for subacute back pain.

### *Chronic LBP*

Some patients with persistent low back pain respond to analgesics containing *opioids*. If opioids are to be used in more than small doses, and for a longer period of time, *sustained-release preparations* are probably preferable. It is appropriate to consider opioid analgesics if pain is a significant barrier to function, an unremitting source of distress and if there are no significant contraindications. When in doubt, obtaining a consultation is appropriate.

*Recurrent or persistent problems after multidisciplinary chronic pain clinic programs*

There is little evidence that patients who have “failed” treatment in a comprehensive rehabilitation program (or in a chronic pain management program) will benefit from a second attempt, unless barriers to progress are first identified and addressed. Barriers might include, for example, an Axis I disorder (especially major depression, dysthymia or anxiety disorder), a significant attitude problem (such as unwillingness to set goals for change “despite pain”), a significant obstacle within the job environment, or a previously undetected medical/surgical problem.

Table 1: **Drugs Used in the Treatment of Back Pain**

| Drug | Dosage | Comments | Cost |
|---|---|---|---|
| **Analgesics** | | | |
| **NSAIDs** | | See Chapter 55 for more information. | |
| *ibuprofen* ◗ Motrin, Advil, generics | 600–1200 mg/d PO divided Q6–8H | No evidence that one NSAID is superior to another for back pain. | $ |
| *naproxen* ◗ Naprosyn, generics | 500–1000 mg/d PO divided Q8–12H | | $ |
| *acetaminophen with codeine 15/30/60 mg* Tylenol preparations, various manufacturers | 1–2 tabs QID max: 8 tabs/d | | $–$$ |
| **Opioids** | | | |
| *morphine sustained-release* ◗ Kadian, M-Eslon, MS Contin, Oramorph SR, M.O.S.-SR | Initial: 15 mg Q12H PO | Start low. Titrate dosage against pain gradually enough to manage adverse effects (e.g., sedation, constipation). Upper limits of clinically appropriate dosage have not been identified. MS Contin and Codeine Contin have been tested in randomized controlled trials for back pain. | $$–$$$$$ |
| *codeine sustained-release* Codeine Contin | Initial: 50 mg Q12H PO | | $–$$$ |
| **Muscle Relaxants** | | | |
| *cyclobenzaprine* Flexeril, generics | 10–30 mg/d PO divided TID | Can be given as one PM dose. | $–$$ |
| *orphenadrine* Norflex | 100–200 mg/d PO divided BID | Can be given as one PM dose. | $–$$ |

*(cont'd)*

Table 1: **Drugs Used in the Treatment of Back Pain** *(cont'd)*

| Drug | Dosage | Comments | Cost |
|---|---|---|---|
| **Tricyclic Antidepressants** | | | |
| *amitriptyline* Elavil, generics | Initial: 10–25 mg QHS, ↑ by 10–25 mg QHS weekly until effect | Adverse effects include hypotension, dry mouth, blurred vision, drowsiness, confusion, weight gain, constipation, urinary retention, ↓ seizure threshold, ECG changes. Do not use with MAOIs. SSRIs: ↑ serum levels of TCAs. | $ |
| *desipramine* Norpramin, generics | Initial: 10 mg QAM, ↑ to 25–75 mg/d | | $ |

* *Cost of 30-day supply – includes drug cost only.*
*Legend: $ < $20 $$ $20–40 $$$ $40–60 $$$$ $60–80 $$$$$ > $80*

❥ *Dosage adjustment may be required in renal impairment – see Appendix I.*

### Therapeutic Tips

- A significant minority of chronic pain sufferers have *comorbid depression, anxiety, or dysthymia* (chronic depression/anxiety), often "masked" by the pain presentation. Key questions can reveal the underlying mood disorder; insomnia, nightmares, irritability, withdrawal, panic or anxiety during the day or night, or persistent tearfulness, poor concentration, lack of enjoyment (anhedonia), poor appetite, weight loss or gain, irritability, frequent thoughts that "life is not worth living." Comorbid mood disorders often respond to antidepressants, so that coping with pain improves.
- For some but not all chronic pain conditions, *tricyclic antidepressants* may have an analgesic or coanalgesic effect, even when depression is not a diagnosis.

## *Suggested Reading List*

Basmajian JV, Banerjee SN, eds. *Clinical decision making in rehabilitation*. New York: Churchill Press, 1996.

Bigos SJ, Bowyer O, Braen G, et al. *Acute low back problems in adults*. Clinical Practice Guide Number 14. Rockville, MD: Agency for Health Care Policy and Research, Public Health Service, US Dept. of Health and Human Services; 1994 December. AHCPR Publication No. 95–0642.

Lane NE, Wolfe F, eds. Musculoskeletal medicine. *Rheum Dis Clin North Am* 1996;22(3).

Sternbach RA. *Mastering pain. A twelve step program for coping with chronic pain*. New York: Ballantyne Books, 1987.

Tunks E, Crook J, Crook M. Natural history and efficacy of treatment of chronic pain arising from musculoskeletal injury. In: Sullivan T, ed. *Injury and the new world of work*. Vancouver: UBC Press, 2000.

CHAPTER 14

# Neuropathic Pain

*C. Peter N. Watson MD, FRCPC*

Neuropathic pain implies pain in the distribution of a nerve or group of nerves. The term "neuralgia" suggests a paroxysmal, brief, lancinating quality.

## Goals of Therapy

- To diagnose lesions causing neuropathy that may require surgery (herniated discs and tumors) by appropriate imaging (CT and MR).
- To reduce pain from severe or moderate to mild and tolerable. Both patient and physician should understand that total pain relief is not realistic for most of these difficult problems.
- To balance pain relief against acceptable side effects
- To plan gradual drug withdrawal after initial control of pain (which may resolve spontaneously, e.g., postherpetic neuralgia)

## Investigations

- History for:
  - the temporal profile and characteristics of the pain
  - depression, insomnia, disability and previous treatments
  - history of chemical dependency, especially if opioids are considered
- Physical examination:
  - to determine areas of sensory loss (hypoesthesia) and skin sensitivity characteristic of neuropathy, i.e., causalgia, allodynia, hyperpathia, hyperalgesia[1]
  - to determine other neurological findings which might indicate a progressive lesion requiring imaging and surgery
  - to determine concurrent conditions that contribute to the pain problem, e.g., metabolic, vascular, myofascial, psychogenic
- Other investigations:
  - imaging with CT or MR scanning if a space-occupying lesion is suspected
  - diagnostic sympathetic blockade if complex regional pain syndrome is suspected

---

[1] *Causalgia – a burning pain due to injury of a peripheral nerve.*
*Allodynia – pain resulting from a non-noxious stimulus to normal skin.*
*Hyperpathia – abnormally exaggerated subjective response to painful stimuli.*
*Hyperalgesia – abnormally increased pain sense.*

Figure 1: **Pharmacologic Management of Neuropathic Pain**

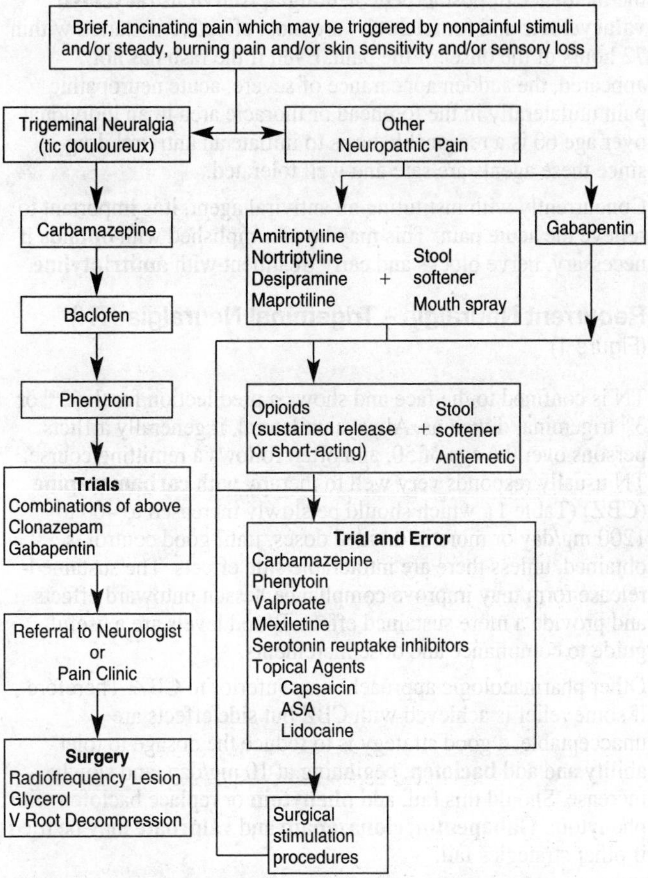
Brief, lancinating pain which may be triggered by nonpainful stimuli and/or steady, burning pain and/or skin sensitivity and/or sensory loss
Trigeminal Neuralgia (tic douloureux)
Other Neuropathic Pain
Carbamazepine
Amitriptyline
Nortriptyline
Desipramine
Maprotiline
+
Stool softener
Mouth spray
Gabapentin
Baclofen
Phenytoin
Opioids (sustained release or short-acting)
+
Stool softener
Antiemetic
Trials
Combinations of above
Clonazepam
Gabapentin
Trial and Error
Carbamazepine
Phenytoin
Valproate
Mexiletine
Serotonin reuptake inhibitors
Topical Agents
Capsaicin
ASA
Lidocaine
Referral to Neurologist or Pain Clinic
Surgery
Radiofrequency Lesion
Glycerol
V Root Decompression
Surgical stimulation procedures

– during pharmacotherapy, blood levels help to assess compliance and guide dosage

## Therapeutic Choices

### Acute Neuralgia – Herpes Zoster (HZ)

The varicella-zoster virus, dormant in dorsal root ganglia, is reactivated by such factors as trauma, decreased immunological competence and lymphoma. HZ occurs more commonly in persons over age 50. Severe pain, stabbing and dysesthesia are soon followed by vesicular eruption in the affected dermatomes (thoracic dermatomes in about 50% of cases, and cranial in about 15%). Motor deficits occur in more severe cases. When it affects the forehead, observation for eye complications is essential.

The risk of chronic postherpetic neuralgia increases with age and with severity of the eruption. Early treatment of HZ may reduce the incidence of postherpetic neuralgia. Antivirals (**acyclovir**, **valacyclovir** and **famciclovir**) are most effective if started within 72 hours of the onset of the pain. Even if the rash has not appeared, the sudden appearance of severe, acute neuropathic pain unilaterally in the forehead or thoracic area in an individual over age 60 is a reasonable basis to initiate an antiviral drug since these agents are safe and well tolerated.

Concurrently with instituting an antiviral agent, it is important to relieve the acute pain. This may be accomplished with **opioids** if necessary, nerve blocks and early treatment with **amitriptyline**.

### Recurrent Neuralgia – Trigeminal Neuralgia (TN)
(Figure 1)

TN is confined to the face and shows a predilection for the 2nd or 3rd trigeminal divisions. Always unilateral, it generally afflicts persons over the age of 50, and often follows a remitting course. TN usually responds very well to therapy with **carbamazepine** (CBZ) (Table 1), which should be slowly increased to 400 to 1200 mg/day or more in divided doses, until good control is obtained, unless there are intolerable side effects. The sustained-release form may improve compliance, lessen untoward effects and provide a more sustained effect. Blood levels are a useful guide to compliance and dose increments.

Other pharmacologic approaches are inferior to CBZ. Therefore if some relief is achieved with CBZ but side effects are unacceptable, a good strategy is to reduce the dosage to tolerability and add **baclofen**, beginning at 10 mg/day, and slowly increase. Should this fail, add **phenytoin** or replace baclofen with phenytoin. **Gabapentin, clonazepam** and **valproate** may be tried if other strategies fail.

Should medical therapy fail, neurosurgical options, e.g., decompression of the gasserian ganglion, or ablative procedures to the gasserian ganglion have a high success rate in experienced hands.

### Chronic Neuralgia

The following conditions are grouped together because the pharmacologic approaches are similar.

#### *Nerve Root Compression: Cervical and Lumbar Radiculopathy*

Although many low back pains and sciatic pains are not attributable to herniated disc and compromised nerve roots, disc material may be extruded through the ligamentum flavum. This sequestrum causes nerve root compression (cervical and lumbar radiculopathies). In the acute phase, anti-inflammatories (**NSAIDs**) may be effective. Where necessary, additional pain relief can be achieved with strong **opioids** (Table 1), an appropriate regimen of rest and avoidance of further aggravation.

This pain often settles with conservative management. Consider surgical treatment: if medical treatment fails over 6 to 12 weeks and if neuroimaging with CT or MR shows a surgically treatable lesion; if acute pain is excruciating and intractable; if a neurological deficit and a correctable lesion are present. Signs of a progressive neurological deficit should prompt surgical consultation as early as possible. Investigation is needed if pain does not resolve within a reasonable time frame, or if this is the first episode in an elderly person (because of possible malignancy or other serious illnesses).

### *Complex Regional Pain Syndrome (CRPS)*

CRPS, the new term for reflex sympathetic dystrophy or sympathetically maintained pain may cause neuropathic pain and neurovascular and dystrophic changes. It may result from penetrating or crush injuries to nerve but sometimes occurs after stroke or myocardial infarction. Characteristics include burning pain, hyperalgesia, hyperpathia and allodynia, sweating, rubor and coldness of the limb.

If symptoms persist, after a few months one may see widening of the painful area, cool cyanotic skin, a glossy appearance to the skin, altered hair growth and progressive loss of function.

Some will go on to dystrophic changes, osteoporosis, nail changes, subcutaneous thinning with pointed digits, and further loss of function with contractures or frozen shoulder and continued severe pain. A larger proportion of chronic cases lose the neurovascular picture and end up with more of a chronic diffuse myofascial pain with poor function.

While CRPS was thought to be due to sympathetic overactivity, evidence now points to a disorder of upregulation of adrenergic receptors. Although sympathetic blocks often provide temporary relief, sympathectomy does not necessarily result in permanent resolution. Bier blocks using guanethidine are ineffective. Physical therapy, corticosteroids, sympathectomies and repeated sympathetic blocks have limited success. At follow-up, two-thirds are likely to have continued pain, and only about one-quarter return to fully normal activity. Some of these patients may require chronic opioid therapy.

### *Chronic Peripheral Neuropathic Pain: Postherpetic Neuralgia (PHN), Diabetic Neuropathy and Phantom Limb Pain*

**Tricyclic antidepressants, gabapentin** and **opioids** (oxycodone) (Table 1) are proven therapies for PHN. The standard therapy has been **amitriptyline** but gabapentin is an alternative first-line choice. **Nortriptyline**, **desipramine** and **maprotiline** may be tried in sequence as some patients may respond better to one of

Table 1: **Drugs Used in Neuropathic Pain**

| Drug | Dosage | Adverse Effects | Cost* |
|---|---|---|---|
| **Antidepressants** | Begin 10–25 mg QHS. Increase by same dose weekly to relief or side effects. Give with mouth spray and stool softener. | dry mouth, constipation, drowsiness, blurred vision, urine retention (in elderly male), weight gain, confusion, tachycardia | |
| *amitriptyline* Elavil, generics | | | $ |
| *desipramine* Norpramin, generics | | | $ |
| *nortriptyline* Aventyl, generics | | | $ |
| *maprotiline* Ludiomil, generics | | | $ |
| **Anticonvulsants** | | | |
| *carbamazepine* Tegretol, generics; Tegretol CR | Start with 100 mg BID to TID. Increase by 100 mg every few days to side effects or relief. Blood levels may be guide to compliance and dosage increases. Consider controlled-release preparations. | drowsiness, ataxia, dizziness, nausea, hyponatremia | $ (Tegretol, generics); $ (Tegretol CR) |
| *gabapentin* ◗ Neurontin | Start with 300–400 mg/d. Increase every few days to BID and TID. Max dose may be 3600 mg/d. | drowsiness, ataxia, GI upset, fluid retention | $$$–$$$$ |
| *phenytoin* Dilantin | 100–300 mg QHS. Depending on age. Blood levels may guide therapy and assess compliance (therapeutic range 40–80 µmol/L). | ataxia, drowsiness, nausea | $ |
| **Baclofen** ◗ Lioresal, generics | Start 10 mg BID. Maximum 20 mg TID. | drowsiness | $$–$$$ |
| **Opioids** | Start low and go slow. Increase to relief or unacceptable side effects. | | |
| *oxycodone* Percocet, Percodan, OxyContin, generics | 5–10 mg Q6H | nausea (antiemetic), constipation (stool softener), drowsiness (reduce dose) | $–$$ |
| *morphine* ◗ MS Contin, M-Eslon | 10–15 mg Q12H | | $$ |
| *hydromorphone* Dilaudid, Hydromorph Contin | 1–2 mg Q6H | | $ (Dilaudid); $$ (Hydromorph Contin) |
| *fentanyl patch* Duragesic | 25 µg/h Q 3 days | | $$$ |

* *Cost of 30-day supply – includes drug cost only*

*Legend:* $ < $10   $$ $10–50   $$$ $50–100   $$$$ >$100

◗ *Dosage adjustment may be required in renal impairment–see Appendix I.*

these agents. A stool softener and mouth spray of artificial saliva will pre-empt the common side effects of constipation and dry mouth. If pain is severe, **opioid** therapy (Table 1) may be prescribed. Psychological dependence, tolerance and physical dependence are not major problems when opioids are used for chronic, severe, nonmalignant pain. Guidelines are suggested in Table 2.

**Lidocaine** 5% topical gel has been shown to relieve PHN and may soon be available as a transdermal patch.

Other treatments, such as topical **capsaicin** or **SSRI antidepressants**, are unproven or of modest efficacy. However, a trial and error approach may be helpful in refractory patients for a possible analgesic response, placebo benefit, general antidepressant effect, while awaiting the possibility of spontaneous pain resolution and for psychological support.

Surgical treatment has no role in PHN and other neuropathic pains in the majority of patients.

## Therapeutic Tips

- While patients frequently say they have used amitriptyline or carbamazepine or other agents, these drugs have often been used in too high or too low a dose and for too short a period of time. It is useful to re-institute these drugs according to the guidelines (start low, go slow, increase to side effects or relief, treat side effects if possible).

### Table 2: **Guidelines for Opioid Therapy of Nonmalignant Pain**

1. Consider after other reasonable therapies have failed.
2. Perform a complete pain and psychosocial history and physical examination. A history of substance abuse, tension-type headaches and pain that appears largely determined by psychologic factors is a relative contraindication to the use of opioid therapy.
3. A single physician who sets up a contract with the patient should be responsible for opioid prescriptions. The agreement should specify the drug regimen, possible side effects, the functional restoration program and that violations will result in the abrupt termination of opioid therapy.
4. The opioid analgesic of choice should be administered around the clock without a provision of "rescue doses" for breakthrough pain. Drug administration should include a titration phase to minimize side effects. If a graded analgesic response to incremental doses is not observed, the patient may not be opioid-responsive and opioid treatment should probably be terminated.
5. The patient should be seen monthly for the first few months and every two months thereafter. At each visit the patient should be assessed for analgesia, opioid-related side effects, compliance with functional goals and presence of aberrant drug-related behavior.
6. The goal of opioid therapy is to make the pain tolerable. For some patients with nonmalignant pain (i.e., postherpetic neuralgia), the administration of an opioid analgesic can make the difference between bearable and unbearable pain.

- Gabapentin is an anticonvulsant which is showing promise in neuropathic pain. The incidence of intolerable side effects is low. High doses may be necessary.
- Be sure the patient understands the goals of therapy: reduction in pain from moderate or severe, to mild at the price of some side effects, which may be tolerable or treatable.
- A rating scale, such as a scale of 0 to 10 where 0 is no pain and 10 the worst pain imaginable, may be used to evaluate pain relief.
- After a period of relief of 1 to 3 months it may be possible to reduce or stop the drugs. Gradual reduction is preferable.
- If opioids are used, guidelines are important and should be worked through with the patient (Table 2).
- A trial and error approach of scientifically unproven treatments is reasonable if standard therapy fails.
- Repeated visits can provide important psychological support and hope for desperate patients as trial and error approaches are also utilized.
- If chronic neuralgia is being managed in general practice, semi-annual or annual visits with a pain specialist help to provide support to the family practitioner for contentious approaches such as opioids, as well as the chance of a novel therapy for the patient.

## Suggested Reading List

Backonja M, Beydoun A, Edwards KR, et al. Gabapentin for the symptomatic treatment of painful neuropathy in patients with diabetes mellitus. *JAMA* 1998;280:1831–1836.

Merskey H, Bogduk N. *Classification of chronic pain.* 2nd ed. Seattle: IASP Press, 1994.

Moulin DE. Opioid analgesics for chronic nonmalignant pain. *The Canadian Journal of CME* 1996;8:137–144.

Rowbotham M, Harden N, Stacey B, et al. Gabapentin for the treatment of postherpetic neuralgia. *JAMA* 1998;280: 1837–1842.

Watson CPN, ed. *Herpes zoster and postherpetic neuralgia.* New York: Elsevier, 1994.

Watson CPN, Babul N. Efficacy of oxycodone in neuropathic pain: a randomized trial in postherpetic neuralgia. *Neurology* 1998;50:1837–1841.

CHAPTER 15

# Pain Control in Palliative Care

*Elizabeth J. Latimer, MD, CCFP, FCFP*

Palliative care is the active and compassionate care of the patient when the goals of cure and prolongation of life are no longer paramount.

## Goals of Therapy

- To relieve pain and other symptoms while maintaining as alert a sensorium as possible
- To support patient and family
- To enhance the quality of life remaining

## Investigations

- A careful *pain history* and *physical examination* to determine the nature, etiology and severity of the pain (Figure 1)
  - *neuropathic pain* is often described as burning or hot (dysesthetic) or shooting and electric shock-like (lancinating)
  - *bone pain* is aching and may increase on movement
  - *liver capsular stretch* is a deep aching that may be referred to the shoulder and have a pleuritic component
  - if able, the patient should **quantify** the pain on a 0–5 scale (5 being the worst pain imaginable and 1 being minimal)
  - the level of pain at the time of analgesic dosing, the level of pain relief achieved at maximum effect and the duration of the best relief achieved should be noted
- A detailed *medication history*
- *Laboratory tests:* minimum required for diagnosis

## Therapeutic Choices (Figure 1)

### Nonpharmacologic Choices

- *Team approach* to total patient care (physical, emotional, spiritual).
- *Relaxation and imagery* to enhance well-being.
- *Physical and occupational therapy* to maximize function and reduce strain.

Figure 1: **Approach to Pain Management**

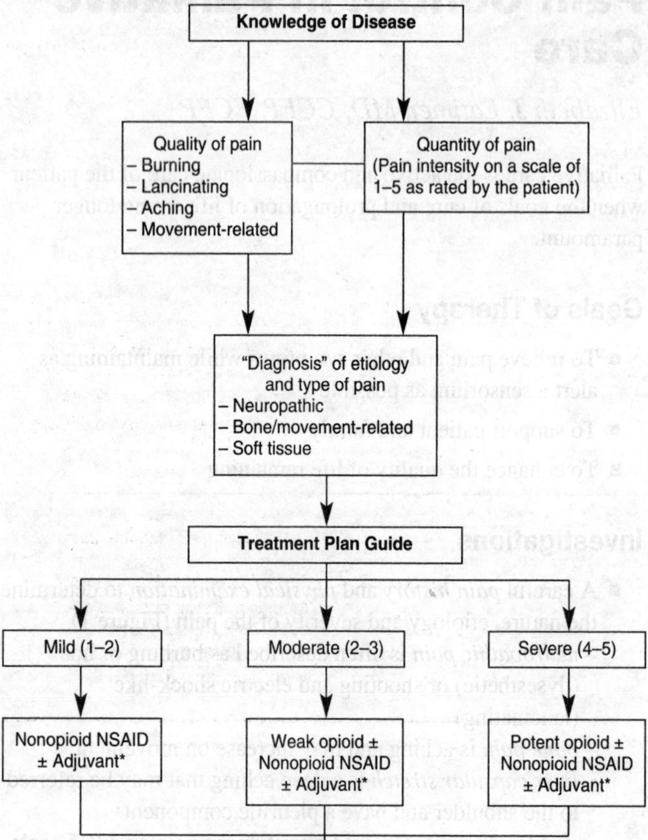
Knowledge of Disease
Quality of pain
– Burning
– Lancinating
– Aching
– Movement-related
Quantity of pain
(Pain intensity on a scale of 1–5 as rated by the patient)
"Diagnosis" of etiology and type of pain
– Neuropathic
– Bone/movement-related
– Soft tissue
Treatment Plan Guide
Mild (1–2)
Moderate (2–3)
Severe (4–5)
Nonopioid NSAID ± Adjuvant*
Weak opioid ± Nonopioid NSAID ± Adjuvant*
Potent opioid ± Nonopioid NSAID ± Adjuvant*
Reassess relief and modify plan PRN

* *Depending on etiology and quality of pain, appropriate adjuvant (tricyclic antidepressant, anticonvulsant, corticosteroid) is added (Table 4).*

- *Disease-directed treatment* to enhance symptom control, e.g., radiotherapy (bone pain, tumor pressure), chemotherapy (generalized bone pain), antibiotics (infection), anticholinergics (troublesome secretions), antianginals (ischemic cardiovascular pain).
- *Transcutaneous nerve stimulation* for pain relief.
- *Acupuncture and hypnosis* for pain and other symptoms and general distress.

## Pharmacologic Choices (Table 1)

### *Analgesics*

Analgesics are given regularly around the clock and orally when possible. Alternative routes are used if there is swallowing difficulty or vomiting or in the latter stages of illness. A *program of analgesia* is usually required, combining opioids, medications to control side effects of opioids and adjuvant analgesics (Tables 1, 2, 3 and 4). Patient and family teaching is required. The use of a dosette system is recommended.

Table 1: **Treatment Plan for Pain Control in Palliative Care**

| Degree of Pain | Analgesic | Example and Dose |
|---|---|---|
| Mild (1–2)* | Nonopioid | Acetaminophen 650 mg QID–Q4H<br>ASA plain or enteric-coated 650 mg PO QID–Q4H<br>NSAIDs ➊: dose varies |
| Moderate (2–3)* | Weak opioid | Codeine 30 to 60 mg PO Q4H (added to the above) |
| Severe (4–5)* | Potent opioid | The following are starting doses:<br>Morphine ➊ elixir or tablets 10–15 mg PO Q4H (↑ in 5–10 mg increments)<br>Hydromorphone 2 mg PO Q4H (↑ in 2 mg increments) |

** Refers to pain intensity on a 0–5 point scale as rated by the patient.*

➊ *Dosage adjustment may be required in renal impairment – see Appendix I.*

### *Opioid Analgesics* (Table 2)

Opioid analgesics are the mainstay of pain control. Physicians should be familiar with one or two drugs for regular prescribing, using others for specific situations. **Morphine** and **hydromorphone** are the opioids of choice in palliative care. If codeine phosphate 60 mg PO Q4H does not relieve pain, morphine 10 to 15 mg or hydromorphone 2 to 4 mg PO Q4H should be started. Because the medication is new to the patient, dosing may be on a Q4H PRN basis for the first 24 hours, then Q4H regularly thereafter.

There is no ceiling dose of opioid analgesics. Dose requirements are highly individual, ranging from a few to several hundred milligrams Q4H; escalation should be titrated against pain relief achieved and level of side effects, particularly sedation. Dramatic or continued increases in analgesic requirements indicate the need to reassess the patient to rule out new complications (e.g., pathological fracture, epidural cord compression). *Initial doses of opioids should be lowered* in patients with impaired renal or hepatic metabolism or those who have not recently been taking potent opioids and who have not developed tolerance to the side effects.

*Breakthrough pain* should be treated with half the regular dose of analgesic. For example, a regular dose of hydromorphone 16 mg would require a standard order for 8 mg Q1–2H PRN for breakthrough pain.

Short-acting (4 hour half-life and Q4H dosing) preparations of **morphine** and **hydromorphone** are used to achieve analgesia. Sustained-release formulations (oral, transdermal, or rectal) can follow for ease of dosing. **Transdermal fentanyl** patches are effective for patients who are unable to use oral analgesics. Hydromorphone may cause less confusion in the *elderly* and those with *renal impairment* than morphine, and is viewed by some as the drug of choice in this group.[1]

Fortunately, true *morphine allergy* (anaphylaxis) is rare but does occur. Anileridine or fentanyl may be used in this situation. Meperidine can be used but is a poor alternative.

**Meperidine** is not recommended for regular use in chronic pain because of its short duration of action, poor oral absorption and potential accumulation of the metabolite normeperidine, which can cause CNS excitation and seizures. **Heroin** has no proven superiority over morphine in equianalgesic doses.

### *Alternative Routes for Opioid Analgesia*

Opioids can be given by oral, parenteral, transdermal or rectal routes; match route to individual patient need. *Equivalent doses* are noted in Table 2. Subcutaneous doses are usually given intermittently by in-place butterfly needles which eliminate the need for repeated injections. Continuous infusion pumps are required in about 5% of cases (high doses, severe pain problem, need for bolus extra dosing).

If suppositories are not available, individual **rectal doses** can be created by placing oral tablets inside gelatin capsules and inserting rectally.

### *Use of Adjuvant Analgesics* (Table 4)

Particular pain syndromes may require special analgesic modalities in addition to opioids.

Careful reassessment of relief achieved with appropriate adjustments in therapy is necessary for effective management.

---

[1] *Mayo Clin Proc 1994;69:384–390.*

Table 2: **Opioid Analgesics**

| Opioid | Equianalgesic Dose | Interval | Dosage Forms | Comments | Cost* |
|---|---|---|---|---|---|
| **Weak** | | | | **For all Opioids** | |
| *codeine*<br>various | 180–240 mg PO<br>120 mg SC† | 4 h | Oral elixir: 3 mg/mL<br>Tablets: 30, 60 mg<br>Injection: 30, 60 mg/mL<br>Oral combinations with acetaminophen or ASA | **Adverse Effects**<br>Nausea and vomiting, constipation, sedation or drowsiness, confusion, psychotomimetic effects, respiratory depression, myoclonus, urinary retention, dry mouth. See Table 3 for management of adverse effects. | $–$$$ |
| **Potent** | | | | | |
| *morphine*<br>M.O.S., MS•IR, Morphitec, Statex, Morphine HP, generics | 20–30 mg PO, PR<br>10–15 mg SC† | 4 h | Oral solution: 1, 5, 10, 20, 50 mg/mL<br>Tablets: 5, 10, 15, 20, 25, 30, 40, 50, 60 mg<br>Injection: 2, 10, 15, 50 mg/mL<br>Suppository: 5, 10, 20, 30 mg | **Drug Interactions**<br>CNS depressants including narcotics, sedatives, tranquilizers, alcohol may ↑ CNS depression. | Soln $<br>Tab $<br>Inj $<br>Supp $$$$ |
| *morphine*<br>*(sustained-release)*<br>M-Eslon, M.O.S.-SR, MS Contin, Oramorph SR, | 60–90 mg PO, PR | 12 h | SR tablets: 15, 30, 60, 100, 200 mg<br>SR capsules: 10, 30, 60, 100 mg<br>SR suppositories: 30, 60, 100 & 200 mg | For fentanyl and meperidine: MAO inhibitors. | $–$$ |
| Kadian | 120–180 mg PO | 24 h | SR capsules: 20, 50, 100 mg | | |
| *hydromorphone*<br>Dilaudid, Dilaudid-HP, generics | 4–6 mg PO, PR<br>2–3 mg SC† | 4 h | Oral solution: 1 mg/mL<br>Tablets: 1, 2, 4, 8 mg<br>Injection: 2, 10, 20, 50 mg/mL<br>Suppository: 3 mg | | Soln $<br>Tab $<br>Inj $$–$$$<br>Supp $$$$ |

*(cont'd)*

Table 2: **Opioid Analgesics** *(cont'd)*

| Opioid | Equianalgesic Dose | Interval | Dosage Forms | Comments | Cost* |
|---|---|---|---|---|---|
| *hydromorphone* ☛ (sustained-release) Hydromorph Contin | 12–18 mg PO | 12 h | SR capsules: 3, 6, 12, 24 & 30 mg | | $$ |
| *fentanyl* Duragesic | Based on total daily morphine dose (or equianalgesic dose of other opioid)<br>50 µg/h patch is approximately equivalent to a total daily morphine dose of 180 mg PO or 90 mg SC†<br>Patch is usually changed Q 72 h | | Transdermal patch: 25, 50, 75, 100 µg/h | | $$$ |
| *anileridine* ☛ Leritine | 75 mg PO<br>25 mg SC† | 3–4 h | Tablets: 25 mg<br>Injection: 25 mg/mL | Anileridine and meperidine should not be used routinely because of short duration of action and potential for side effects in higher doses. Main indication is use in case of true morphine allergy. | Tab $$<br>Inj $$$$ |
| *meperidine* ☛ Demerol, generics | 300 mg PO<br>75 mg IM, SC† | 3–4 h | Tablets: 50 mg<br>Injection: 50, 75, 100 mg/mL | | $ |

† *The SC route is almost always preferred. The IM route is more painful and unnecessary.*
☛ *Dosage adjustment may be required in renal impairment – see Table 1.*

* *Cost per day of doses equianalgesic to 360 mg/d of oral morphine – includes drug cost only.*
*Legend: $ < $4 $$ $4–8 $$$ $8–12 $$$$ > $12*

## Table 3: **Management of Opioid Adverse Effects**

| | |
|---|---|
| Nausea and vomiting | **Haloperidol** 1–2 mg PO/SC BID–TID (may be given as a single daily dose)<br>If persistent, add **metoclopramide** 10–20 mg PO/SC/IV TID–QID<br>If there is a clear vestibular component (motion-type sickness) **dimenhydrinate** 50–100 mg PO/PR Q8H–Q6H or **scopolamine** 0.4 mg SC Q4H or 1.5 mg transdermal Q72H |
| Constipation | Regular doses of stool softener + stimulant laxative (e.g., **docusate** 100–200 mg + **sennosides** 2–3 tablets or **bisacodyl** 10–15 mg PO BID–TID)<br>The softener may be replaced with **lactulose** 30 mL BID–TID<br>**Bisacodyl suppositories, phosphate enemas** or **oil retention enemas** may be required at intervals<br>**Magnesium hydroxide/mineral oil** mixture 30 mL + **cascara** 5 mL daily–BID may be used at intervals in addition to regular regimens |
| Confusion and/or agitation | **Haloperidol** 1–2 mg PO/SC BID–TID (may be given as a single daily dose) |
| Multifocal myoclonus | May occur when opioid doses ↑ or clearance ↓ or in presence of other metabolic disturbances. Opioid dose should be ↓ slightly; consider rehydration if appropriate in the clinical context. If severe, switch to another opioid and give 50–60% of the equianalgesic dose. **Lorazepam** 1–2 mg SL, **midazolam** 0.5–1.0 mg SC Q3–4H PRN (or regularly) or **diazepam** 5 mg PO/PR Q8H–Q6H PRN (or regularly) for myoclonus |

*Dosage adjustment may be required in renal impairment – see Appendix I.*

## Table 4: **Adjuvant Analgesics**

| Type of Pain | Adjuvant |
|---|---|
| Neuropathic pain | |
| *Dysesthetic/ burning pain* | Add tricyclic antidepressant* (**imipramine** or **amitriptyline**) 25 mg PO BID–TID; may ↑ gradually up to 150 mg/d (may be given as a single bedtime dose if tolerated) |
| *Lancinating/ shock-like pain* | Add **carbamazepine*** 100–200 mg PO TID–QID |
| *If severe* | **Dexamethasone** 4 mg PO/SC/IV TID–QID (may need as much as 24–32 mg/d in some cases) |
| Bone pain | Add NSAID with cytoprotective agent (e.g., **naproxen** 500 mg PO/PR BID with **misoprostol** 200 μg PO BID) |
| *If severe* | **Dexamethasone** 4 mg PO/SC/IV TID–QID (may need as much as 24–32 mg/d in some cases)<br>**Bisphosphonates** may be helpful in multiple bone metastases. |
| Closed space pain | **Dexamethasone** as described above |
| Pleuritic pain | NSAID as described above |

* ***Note:*** *Doses of tricyclics and carbamazepine* ***should be lowered by 50%*** *in frail or elderly patients or in hepatic or renal impairment; dose increments should be made cautiously.*

*Dosage adjustment may be required in renal impairment – see Appendix I.*

### *Suggested Reading List*

Doyle D, Hanks GWC, MacDonald N. *Oxford textbook of palliative medicine.* 2nd ed. New York: Oxford University Press, 1998.

Librach SL, Squires BP. *The pain manual: principles and issues in cancer pain management.* Toronto: Pegasus Health Care International, 1997.

CHAPTER 16

# Bell's Palsy

*Mary Anne Lee, MD, FRCPC*

## Definition

Bell's palsy is an idiopathic, lower motor neuron paralysis of the facial nerve affecting 20 to 30 per 100,000 per year. The sexes are equally affected. The incidence increases until age 40 and then remains static until the 8th decade when it again increases. Approximately 5 to 10% of patients may have a recurrent palsy affecting the same or opposite side. The incidence of Bell's palsy appears to be greater in individuals with diabetes or hypertension and also in pregnant women. Recent evidence suggests that the herpes simplex virus-1 may be the etiologic agent.[1] Approximately 7% of patients experience a complete spontaneous recovery with no therapeutic intervention. Unfortunately, those who are not going to experience complete recovery often cannot be identified early in their course.

## Goals of Therapy

- To promote complete recovery of function through prevention of denervation
- To protect the eye from corneal ulcers
- To control pain

## Investigations (Table 1)

- Complete history and physical examination to exclude other causes of peripheral facial palsy

Table 1: **Differential Diagnosis of Bell's Palsy**

- Ramsay Hunt syndrome — check for vesicles in the ear
- Facial nerve tumors — cerebellopontine angle tumors
  — parotid tumors
- Infection of middle ear or mastoid
- Lyme disease
- Neurosarcoidosis
- Brain stem lesions such as multiple sclerosis — check for other brain stem signs

[1] *Ann Intern Med 1996;124:27–30.*

- EMG and facial nerve conduction studies — will help with prognosis but are not necessarily helpful for deciding on treatment since abnormalities often are not present during the first few days
- Skull x-ray and CT scan if trauma is suspected
- MRI — in selected cases with atypical features such as slow progression or associated neurologic signs and symptoms
- Laboratory Tests
  - CBC, blood sugar, ESR

## Therapeutic Choices (Figure 1)

### Pharmacologic Choices (Table 2)

#### *Eye care*

- Lubricating ophthalmic drops or ointment.
- Tape eyelid at night.

#### *Analgesics*

- Ibuprofen or acetaminophen with or without codeine.
- Rarely more potent narcotics such as meperidine or morphine are needed.

#### *Corticosteroids and Antivirals*

**Prednisone** 1 mg/kg for 5 days, then taper over 5 days. If facial paralysis is complete, then 1 mg/kg for an additional 5 days and then taper. Steroids have been used empirically for many years for treatment of Bell's palsy but only one double-blind controlled study has proven efficacy.[2] Treated patients were less likely to develop denervation (5.7% vs 19.5%) and achieved a better grade of recovery.

**Acyclovir** — a single study compared acyclovir 800 mg TID for 10 days to prednisone 1 mg/kg for 10 days and then tapered over 6 days.[3] Prednisone alone proved to be superior to acyclovir alone (93.6% of the prednisone group achieved a good to excellent recovery compared to 83.3% of the acyclovir group). Treatment with acyclovir, however, was superior to the natural history of untreated Bell's palsy with only 70% of untreated patients experiencing a good to excellent outcome.

**Prednisone and acyclovir** — a double-blind, randomized study compared acyclovir and prednisone to placebo and prednisone.[4] The combination of acyclovir (400 mg 5 times a day for 10 days) and prednisone (30 mg BID for 5 days and then tapered over the next 5 days) was superior to prednisone alone. Eighty-seven

[2] *Laryngoscope 1993;103:1326–1333.*
[3] *Laryngoscope 1998;108:573–575.*
[4] *Ann Otol Rhinol Laryngol 1996;105:371–378.*

Figure 1: **Management of Bell's Palsy**

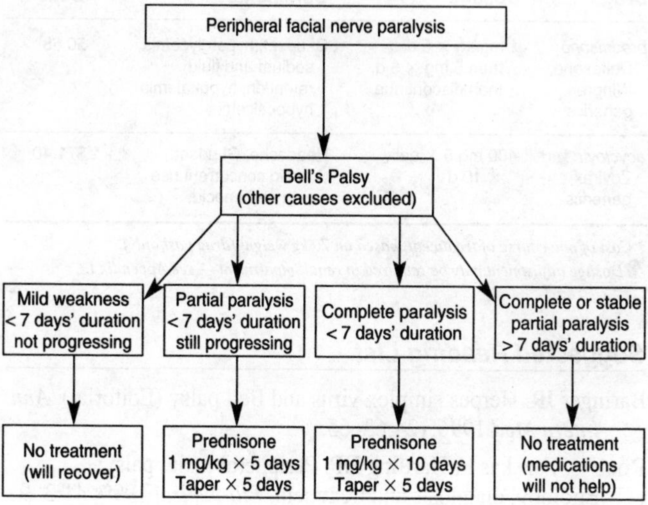
Peripheral facial nerve paralysis
Bell's Palsy (other causes excluded)
Mild weakness < 7 days' duration not progressing
Partial paralysis < 7 days' duration still progressing
Complete paralysis < 7 days' duration
Complete or stable partial paralysis > 7 days' duration
No treatment (will recover)
Prednisone 1 mg/kg × 5 days Taper × 5 days
Prednisone 1 mg/kg × 10 days Taper × 5 days
No treatment (medications will not help)

percent of the acyclovir-prednisone group had a good to excellent recovery as compared to 72% of the prednisone-placebo group.

## Therapeutic Tips

- No treatment is needed for mild weakness that is no longer evolving.
- Prednisone should be used in all other cases of Bell's palsy unless there is a contraindication to steroid use, such as diabetes or peptic ulcer disease. It should be started as early as possible, preferably by day 3 and certainly before day 7.
- The use of acyclovir alone is not indicated.
- The combination of acyclovir and prednisone has been shown to be superior to prednisone alone in a small, double-blind, controlled study but further combination studies are warranted before this can be considered the standard of care for Bell's palsy. As well, the optimal dose of acyclovir is not established. The cost of acyclovir and potential side effects should be considered.

Table 2: **Drugs for Treatment of Bell's Palsy**

| Drug | Dosage | Comments | Cost* |
|---|---|---|---|
| *prednisone* Deltasone, Winpred, generics | 1 mg/kg × 5 d, then 5 mg × 5 d, then discontinue | GI upset, hyperglycemia, sodium and fluid retention, hypokalemia, hypocalcemia | $0.68 |
| *acyclovir* ❥ Zovirax, generics | 400 mg 5 × daily × 10 d | Headache, GI upset. Avoid concurrent use with probenecid. | $71.40 |

** Cost of one course of treatment, based on 70 kg weight (drug cost only).*

❥ *Dosage adjustment may be required in renal impairment — see Appendix I.*

## Suggested Reading List

Baringer JR. Herpes simplex virus and Bell palsy (Editorial). *Ann Intern Med* 1996;124:63–65.

Roob G, Fazekas F, Hartling HP. Peripheral facial palsy: Etiology, diagnosis and treatment. *Eur Neurol* 1999; 41:3–9.

CHAPTER 17

# Parkinson's Disease

*A. Jon Stoessl, MD, FRCPC*

## Goals of Therapy

- To control symptoms. Presently there is no neuroprotective (i.e., treatment which slows the underlying disease process) strategy available. Thus, symptomatic therapy should be initiated when dictated by sufficient disability to justify its use; when this occurs will differ from one individual to another.
- To optimize current function.
- To minimize long-term complications.
- To build a partnership between the patient and the physician. Inform patients about side effects, mechanisms and limitations of their medications so they may report back in an accurate fashion, allowing appropriate adjustments to be made.

## Investigations

- In most cases, this is clinical, based on the presence of rest tremor, rigidity and bradykinesia. Although postural instability occurs later in the disease, its presence as an early feature is generally suggestive of an alternate diagnosis.
- Drug-induced parkinsonism should be excluded by history. Potential culprits include antipsychotic agents, antiemetic neuroleptics (e.g. metoclopramide, prochlorperazine) and reserpine.
- In addition to looking for the cardinal features of Parkinson's, exclude abnormalities of eye movements, long tract signs and evidence of autonomic dysfunction, as well as cognitive impairment and hallucinations.
- Patients with atypical features should have imaging studies, and in young patients, Wilson's disease should be excluded with a serum ceruloplasmin level and slit lamp examination.

## Therapeutic Choices

### Nonpharmacologic Choices

- Counselling to aid with understanding the disease and its treatment, cope with the impact on the patient's and caregivers' lives, and assist with depression.
- Physical therapy for help with ambulation and balance.

- Speech language assessments for speech and swallowing disturbances.

## Pharmacologic Choices (Figure 1, Table 1)

### *Levodopa*

This is still the gold standard of therapy for Parkinson's. (However, see dopamine agonists as monotherapy for early disease.) Levodopa is converted to dopamine by surviving dopaminergic neurons, and probably by nondopaminergic neurons as well. Benefit is usually seen early, but as disease progresses, higher doses may be required and complications may emerge, often in the form of fluctuations in motor function and involuntary movements or dyskinesias. There is a strong theoretical basis to suggest that these complications are related to pulsatile stimulation of dopamine receptors and are less likely to emerge if receptors are stimulated in a more continuous fashion. For this reason, many prefer to *initiate* therapy with a controlled release form of levodopa/carbidopa (Sinemet CR), although the clinical evidence for this approach is suboptimal. CR preparations are advantageous once fluctuations have appeared. Levodopa should always be administered in conjunction with a peripheral decarboxylase inhibitor (carbidopa in Sinemet; benserazide in Prolopa), in order to minimize peripheral side effects and maximize the beneficial central effects. The passage of levodopa into the brain is dependent upon a large neutral amino acid transport system; thus levodopa absorption may be subject to competition from dietary amino acids.

Figure 1: **Management of the Previously Unmedicated Parkinson's Patient**

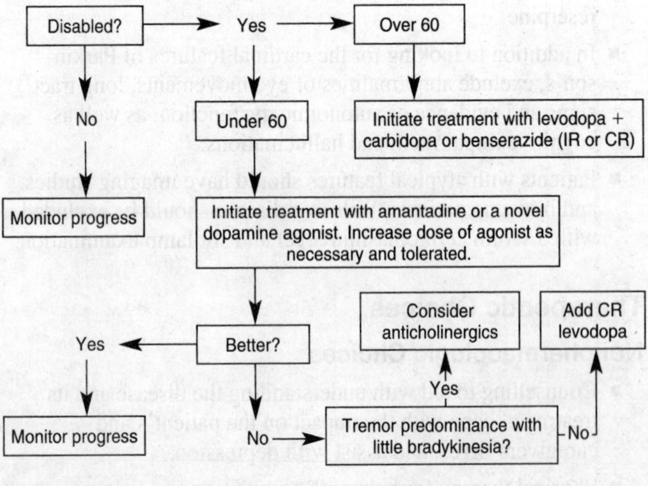
Disabled?
Yes
Over 60
No
Under 60
Initiate treatment with levodopa + carbidopa or benserazide (IR or CR)
Monitor progress
Initiate treatment with amantadine or a novel dopamine agonist. Increase dose of agonist as necessary and tolerated.
Consider anticholinergics
Add CR levodopa
Yes
Better?
Yes
Monitor progress
No
Tremor predominance with little bradykinesia?
No

*Abbreviations: IR = immediate release; CR = controlled release*

Table 1: **Drugs Used in the Treatment of Parkinson's Disease**

| Drug | Dosage | Adverse Effects | Drug Interactions | Cost* |
|---|---|---|---|---|
| **Levodopa**<br>*levodopa/carbidopa*<br>Sinemet, generics<br>Sinemet CR | **Levodopa/carbidopa (regular) – levodopa/benserazide**<br>initial: 50/12.5 mg BID<br>usual: 100/25 mg–150/37.5 TID-QID | Nausea, vomiting, orthostatic hypotension, dyskinesias, hallucinations, confusion. | Neuroleptics ↓ effect of levodopa.<br>Antihypertensives, diuretics, tricyclic antidepressants may ↑ hypotensive action. | Sinemet, Prolopa $$ |
| *levodopa/benserazide*<br>Prolopa | **Levodopa/carbidopa (controlled release)**<br>initial: 100/25 mg BID<br>usual: 200/50 mg QID | | | Sinemet CR $$$ |
| **Dopamine Agonists** | | | | |
| *bromocriptine*<br>Parlodel, generics | initial: 1.25 mg BID<br>usual: 10 mg TID | Nausea, vomiting, orthostatic hypotension, hallucinations, psychosis, erythromelalgia, pleural fibrosis (do a baseline chest x-ray before initiating therapy). | Antihypertensives, diuretics, tricyclic antidepressants may ↑ hypotensive action of dopamine agonists. | $$$$ |
| *pergolide*<br>Permax | initial: 0.05 mg daily<br>usual: 0.5–1.5 mg TID | | | $$–$$$$ |
| *pramipexole*<br>Mirapex | initial: 0.125 mg TID<br>usual: 0.5–1 mg TID | Orthostatic hypotension, somnolence, confusion, hallucinations, nausea, vomiting. | Neuroleptics ↓ effect of dopamine agonists. | $$$$ |
| *ropinirole*<br>Requip | initial: 0.25 mg TID<br>usual: 3–6 mg TID | | Ciprofloxacin ↑ levels of ropinirole. | $$$$–$$$$$ |

*(cont'd)*

Table 1: **Drugs Used in the Treatment of Parkinson's Disease** *(cont'd)*

| Drug | Dosage | Adverse Effects | Drug Interactions | Cost* |
|---|---|---|---|---|
| *selegiline (deprenyl)*<br>Eldepryl, generics | 2.5 mg daily–5 mg BID | Insomnia.<br>Give before 1 p.m. | Avoid use with meperidine, dextromethorphan, SSRIs and dextroamphetamine. | $–$$ |
| *tolcapone*<br>Tasmar | 100 mg TID | Dyskinesia, nausea, sleep disorder, anorexia, dystonia, diarrhea, hepatic failure. | Potentiates levodopa. | Restricted use. |
| **Anticholinergic Agents** | | | | |
| *benztropine*<br>Cogentin, generics | 1 mg BID–2 mg BID | Dry mouth, blurred vision, constipation, urinary retention, aggravation of glaucoma, confusion, memory impairment. Avoid in elderly. | Amantadine may ↑ anticholinergic effects. | $ |
| *ethopropazine*<br>Parsitan | 25 mg BID–50 mg TID | | | $ |
| *procyclidine*<br>Kemadrin, generics | 5 mg TID | | | $ |
| *trihexyphenidyl*<br>generics | Initial: 1 mg BID<br>Usual: 2 mg TID | | | $ |
| *amantadine* ◗<br>Symmetrel, generics | usual: 100 mg BID | Same as anticholinergics. Also livedo reticularis, ankle edema. Use with caution in elderly. | Anticholinergic agents may ↑ effects. | $ |

◗ *Dosage adjustment is required in renal impairment – see Appendix I.*
* *Cost of 30-day supply of usual dose – includes drug cost only.*
*Legend:* $ < $50   $$ $50–100   $$$ $100–150   $$$$ $150–200   $$$$$ > $200

Although there is a longstanding controversy regarding the potential disadvantages of levodopa therapy, it is fairly clear that levodopa is not actually toxic to nigral dopamine neurons (use does not hasten the progression of Parkinson's disease). However, long-term use, particularly in high doses and a pulsatile fashion, does contribute to the emergence of motor complications, which may be disabling and difficult to control. Thus, levodopa should be used only when necessary, but not withheld when needed. Failure to respond at any stage to adequate doses (at least 1000 mg daily) of levodopa suggests a diagnosis other than Parkinson's. Sinemet CR has a duration of action which is approximately 25–30% longer than that of immediate release preparations, but bioavailability is also less by a similar degree, so that higher doses are required.

### *Dopamine agonists*

These agents, which directly stimulate dopamine D2 receptors, are extremely useful as adjuncts to levodopa. Unlike levodopa, they are not dependent upon enzymatic conversion to an active agent and not subject to competition from dietary amino acids. They have a longer duration of action than levodopa and may be less likely to elicit dyskinesias than comparably effective doses of levodopa. The prototypic agent is **bromocriptine**, which is still a useful agent. **Pergolide** is another ergot derivative which is more potent and has a longer duration of action than bromocriptine.

**Ropinirole** and **pramipexole** are two novel, highly selective non-ergot derived dopamine agonists. Although they share all the side effects of dopaminergic stimulation with the older agents, because they are not ergot derivatives, they are not prone to cause erythromelalgia (vasculitic, painful red swelling of the legs) or pleural fibrosis. As adjuncts to levodopa therapy, they appear to be comparable to the older agents, although possibly better tolerated. The use of these new agents has recently been associated with sudden onset of sleep. Although fatigue is a common manifestation of Parkinson's and sedation is a well recognized side effect of both levodopa and the dopamine agonists, these "sleep attacks" have occurred in some patients while they were driving.

The new dopamine agonists may revolutionize the treatment of newly diagnosed Parkinson's. Initiation of therapy with an agonist rather than with levodopa is associated with a lower incidence of dyskinesias over the long term. However, bromocriptine has been relatively ineffective as monotherapy, most patients requiring the addition of levodopa within a matter of months. Both ropinirole and pramipexole may be effective as *monotherapy* for longer—possibly 3 to 5 years. A study comparing initiation of therapy with ropinirole versus levodopa reported a dramatically lower incidence of dyskinesias in patients whose initial therapy was ropinirole, *even in those who required the later addition of levodopa.* Thus, at least in younger patients, who are likely to be more tolerant of dopamine agonists and who are more prone to developing motor complications in response to levodopa, initiation with ropinirole or pramipexole seems to be the most appropriate. Like all dopamine agonists, these drugs may cause confusion, hallucinations, nausea and postural hypotension and should be used with caution in the frail elderly. Their use has been associated with sudden onset of sleep, and driving may accordingly be restricted.

### *Anticholinergics*

While these agents may be useful in young patients with tremor-predominant disease, they otherwise no longer play a major role in the treatment of Parkinson's disease. They have only a minor impact on bradykinesia, which is the most disabling aspect of Parkinson's, and a great propensity to cause confusion and hallucinations, particularly in the elderly.

### *Amantadine*

Amantadine has been regarded as a relatively mild agent which might forestall the requirement for levodopa therapy by a few months. It may act by stimulating release of dopamine from surviving neurons, and possibly by anticholinergic mechanisms as well. Its use has seen a recent resurgence, based on the recognition that it is a weak antagonist at excitatory amino acid receptors. There are at least theoretical grounds to believe that it might delay disease progression, if Parkinson's is related to excitotoxic mechanisms. Its use is associated with increased survival in patients with Parkinson's. Recent reports suggest that amantadine may not only potentiate the benefits of levodopa, but may also help to suppress levodopa-induced dyskinesias.

### *Selegiline*

Selegiline is a selective monoamine oxidase type B (MAO-B) inhibitor which is used as an adjunct to levodopa, and may potentiate or prolong its action. The mechanism for its effect is controversial as dopamine neurons themselves predominantly express MAO-A and the symptomatic effects of selegiline may relate to increased levels of the trace amine 2-phenyl-ethyl-amine rather than dopamine itself. There may also be effects on dopamine release and/or reuptake. The use of selegiline as an adjunct to levodopa has largely become superfluous since the availability of controlled release preparations, COMT inhibitors and novel dopamine agonists.

The use of selegiline was associated with a delayed requirement for levodopa in patients with early Parkinson's, initially interpreted as evidence for a neuroprotective effect. Longer term evaluation has led to the realization that the majority of this effect was symptomatic and if there is any neuroprotective effect, it is likely to be extremely small. A 1995 report that use of selegiline was associated with increased mortality has not been substantiated. However, selegiline can lead to sleep disturbance, confusion, hallucinations, an increase in dyskinesia and autonomic dysfunction (both hyper- and hypotension).

### COMT Inhibitors

In addition to decarboxylation, levodopa is subject to O-methylation by the ubiquitous enzyme catechol-O-methyltransferase (COMT). Blockade of this process in the periphery results in a prolongation of the area under the curve for plasma levodopa concentration, without much change in the maximal concentration. COMT inhibitors, which have no useful role when given without levodopa, are therefore extremely helpful for smoothing out predictable fluctuations in motor function. Their use is associated with increased dyskinesia and potentiation of other dopaminergic effects. The only agent available in Canada was **tolcapone**, which was withdrawn because of rare but occasionally fatal hepatic failure. Tolcapone is still available under special authorization for those patients who have previously received it and whose parkinsonism cannot be adequately managed with other available therapies. **Entacapone**, a similar agent with a shorter duration of action, but which does not appear to be prone to cause hepatic dysfunction, has not yet been approved for use in Canada.

### Management of complications

Peripheral side effects such as *nausea*, *vomiting* and *postural hypotension* are associated with levodopa, the dopamine agonists and amantadine. These may respond to **domperidone** (10 mg QID, AC and HS). If postural hypotension continues to be a significant problem, **fludrocortisone** (0.1 to 0.4 mg/day) or **midodrine** (7.5 to 30 mg/day) may be used. Advanced Parkinson's may also be associated with other evidence of autonomic dysfunction, which presumably arises as a result of the disease process itself. This includes bladder disturbance and erectile dysfunction, which must be assessed on an individual basis and may require more detailed laboratory investigation. Sphincter-detrusor dyssynergia is a common basis for urinary dysfunction and may respond to alpha adrenergic blockade (which may, however, potentiate postural hypotension). Erectile dysfunction may respond to sildenafil, but this drug should be avoided in patients with unstable cardiac disease; nitrate use is an absolute contraindication.

*Fluctuations and dyskinesias* are best managed by efforts to prevent their emergence (see above). Once they occur, efforts should be made to smooth out the delivery of levodopa (by use of controlled release preparations, dose adjustments and COMT inhibitors) and if possible to minimize levodopa and maximize the use of a dopamine agonist (Figure 2). Surgery may be helpful (see below).

*Toxic psychosis* may be a psychiatric complication. Intercurrent illness should be excluded. Anticholinergics, selegiline and amantadine should be withdrawn. Then the dose of dopamine agonist and finally of levodopa should be cautiously reduced, recognizing that parkinsonism may get worse. Dramatic reduction of antiparkinson medication can lead to a neuroleptic malignant-like state, with severe rigidity, immobility, fever and autonomic instability. If problems persist, low doses of an atypical neuroleptic such as **clozapine** (usually < 75 mg/day), may be helpful. Olanzapine and quetiapine are also used, although there is less evidence. In patients without cognitive impairment, ECT may be used (this may not only help control the psychosis and ameliorate depression, but also typically results in improvements in the motor disorder as well).

*Depression* is a common manifestation of Parkinson's and frequently responds well to medication. Some of the **SSRIs** may exacerbate parkinsonism or dyskinesia, but they are frequently well tolerated. **Venlafaxine, tricyclic antidepressants** and ECT are also helpful. The MAO-A inhibitor moclobemide and bupropion should theoretically elevate dopaminergic function and be helpful in this setting, but experience is limited.

Figure 2: **Management of the Levodopa-treated Patient with Motor Complications**

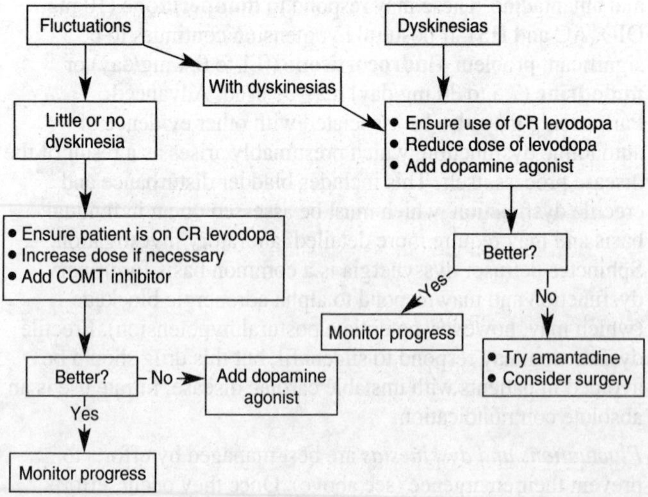

Fluctuations
Dyskinesias
With dyskinesias
Little or no dyskinesia
• Ensure use of CR levodopa
• Reduce dose of levodopa
• Add dopamine agonist
• Ensure patient is on CR levodopa
• Increase dose if necessary
• Add COMT inhibitor
Better?
Yes
No
Monitor progress
• Try amantadine
• Consider surgery
Better?
No
Add dopamine agonist
Yes
Monitor progress

### *Surgery*

A detailed consideration of surgical options for Parkinson's is beyond the scope of this chapter. However, pallidotomy may be of value for patients with a history of levodopa-responsiveness, but who are unable to tolerate adequate doses of medication because of dyskinesias (or occasionally because of psychosis). Although other manifestations of the Parkinson's may improve, the most consistent and long-lasting benefit is seen in dyskinesias contralateral to the operated side. Bilateral ablative procedures should generally be avoided. Implantation of a high frequency stimulating electrode into the internal segment of the globus pallidus has effects very similar to pallidotomy, but the effect is reversible; thus undesired effects of bilateral lesions can be avoided. Bilateral stimulation of the subthalamic nucleus is currently undergoing evaluation and appears promising for reversing most aspects of parkinsonism. Dyskinesias are alleviated predominantly because a successful procedure allows marked reductions in levodopa dose. Experimental human fetal transplantation procedures appear promising.

## Therapeutic Tips

- Not all therapy involves the use of drugs. Consider other needs, including communication, physical therapy and emotional wellbeing.
- Symptomatic medication should be introduced when dictated by disability, at a time which must be individually defined.
- For younger patients, therapy should be introduced with one of the newer dopamine agonists or amantadine. Levodopa should be added when needed. For older patients, levodopa is usually the appropriate first-line therapy.
- Medication should be prescribed in the minimum amount needed to manage disability. Efforts should be made to stimulate dopamine receptors in as smooth a fashion as possible (i.e., avoid high, infrequent doses).
- Monitor patients at regular intervals for complications, including postural hypotension, other autonomic problems, psychiatric complications, swallowing disturbance, motor fluctuations and involuntary movements. Adjust existing medication or add other medication as appropriate.

### *Suggested Reading List*

Factor SA, Friedman JH. The emerging role of clozapine in the treatment of movement disorders. *Movement Disorders* 1997;12:483–496.

Lang AE, Lozano AM. Parkinson's disease. *N Engl J Med* 1998;339:1130–1143.

Olanow CW, Koller WC. An algorithm (decision tree) for the management of Parkinson's disease: treatment guidelines. *Neurology* 1998;50 (Suppl. 3):S1–S57.

Rascol O, Brooks DJ, Korczyn A, et al. A five-year study of the incidence of dyskinesia in patients with early Parkinson's disease who were treated with ropinirole or levodopa. *N Engl J Med* 2000;342:1484–1491.

CHAPTER 18

# Seizures and Epilepsy

*R. Mark Sadler, MD, FRCP*

## Goals of Therapy

- To decide if treatment with antiepileptic drugs (AEDs) is indicated for the patient presenting with the first seizure
- To prevent seizure recurrence in patients with an established diagnosis of epilepsy (i.e., patients with recurrent seizures)
- To prevent or minimize adverse effects of AEDs
- To promote an optimum quality of life

## Investigations (Figure 1)

### *History*

- A detailed history of the patient's "spells" obtained from the patient and a witness is the single most important factor in making a diagnosis.
- Is there an aura? The presence of a warning suggests that the seizures are partial (focally originating) and therefore evokes focal brain pathology; the nature of the aura suggests the anatomical site of seizure onset. Lack of an aura indicates partial seizures that spread very rapidly *or* that the seizures are of the primary generalized variety.
- Inquire about history of intracranial sepsis, significant head trauma, stroke, family history of seizures or other neurologic diseases, any systemic disorders that may affect the central nervous system (e.g., malignancies, fluid and electrolyte disorders), drugs (prescribed or recreational), recent sleep deprivation, symptoms of raised intracranial pressure.

### *Clinical features*

- *Simple partial seizures* (with motor or sensory features) exhibit no impairment of consciousness
- *Complex partial seizures* are focally originating seizures consisting of impaired awareness, a duration of 1 to 2 minutes, a blank stare, frequently accompanied by motor automatisms (e.g., lip smacking and chewing movements), and brief postictal confusion
- *Absence* (*"petit mal"*) seizures are a primary generalized seizure type, last only seconds, recur daily, have no warning, no postictal confusion and almost always onset in childhood or adolescence

- *Primary or secondarily generalized tonic-clonic* (*"grand mal"*) seizures have a fairly uniform sequence of impaired consciousness, motor features (tonic and clonic phases), often urinary incontinence, duration of 1–2 minutes, and postictal stupor, confusion and headache
- *Atonic seizures* consist of an abrupt loss of consciousness, falling, no other motor features, and return to awareness in seconds. These seizures occur as part of a clinical scenario in patients with childhood onset epilepsy, significant intellectual handicaps and other seizure types. Atonic seizures virtually never begin in otherwise intellectually and physically intact adults
- *Myoclonic seizures* are usually a primary generalized seizure type consisting of brief, bilateral "shock-like" jerks
- Do the clinical features suggest one of the entities (e.g., syncope or psychogenic pseudoseizures) commonly mistaken for epileptic seizures?

**Physical examination**

- Look for evidence of any systemic disorder that can affect the central nervous system.
- Look for focal or lateralizing findings in the neurologic examination (hemianopia, motor weakness, hemisensory disturbance, reflex asymmetry).
- Assess potential injuries sustained during a convulsion (e.g., tongue laceration, shoulder dislocation, vertebral compression fracture).

**Laboratory Investigation**

For the patient presenting with the *first seizure,* consider:

- CBC, electrolytes, renal function
- Chest x-ray if metastatic disease is a consideration
- Electroencephalogram (EEG) to support the clinical impression of seizures and to determine if the seizure is partial (focally originating) or primary generalized
- Computed tomography (CT) head scan. Adults should have a CT scan unless the patient is otherwise well and their EEG demonstrates generalized spike-and-wave discharges (which indicates one of the primary generalized seizure syndromes that are not accompanied by gross structural brain abnormalities). Most patients should have a CT scan before a lumbar puncture (see below).
- Lumbar puncture if the presenting clinical features suggest intracranial sepsis (meningitis, encephalitis, brain abscess).

- Magnetic resonance imaging (MRI) scan if the patient has partial seizures of unknown etiology and negative CT scan.

For the patient with *known epilepsy treated with AEDs* and presenting with a *seizure recurrence*, assess: factors that may precipitate loss of seizure control (medication noncompliance, intercurrent illness with fever and vomiting), sleep deprivation, alcohol and other nonprescription drug use; addition (or sudden withdrawal) of a drug that may promote seizures or may cause a drug interaction with AEDs

- Measure AED serum levels

## Therapeutic Choices

### Nonpharmacologic Choices

- Avoid sleep deprivation.
- Alcohol consumption should be kept to a minimum. Cocaine, amphetamines, and phencyclidine must be forbidden because of their proconvulsant properties.

### Pharmacologic Choices

The choice of an AED depends on the seizure type (Table 1), potential for drug interactions and side effects (Table 2), cost (Table 2) and physician comfort level with the drug.

- Select a single AED.
- Start the AED at a fraction of the initial target dose to minimize the risk of dose-dependent adverse effects (exceptions are ethosuximide, phenytoin and phenobarbital).
- Inform patient of potential risks of treatment.
- Evaluate the patient after the initial target dose has been achieved. Make a small dose reduction if dose-related adverse effects (AEs) are problematic. The dose should be slowly increased if seizures have recurred.
- A second AED should be added if the maximum tolerated dose of the first AED has failed to achieve satisfactory seizure control. The first AED should be gradually withdrawn after the maintenance dose of the second drug has been achieved. Polytherapy is usually reserved until monotherapy with 2 to 3 drugs has failed.

Figure 1: **Management of Seizures and Epilepsy**

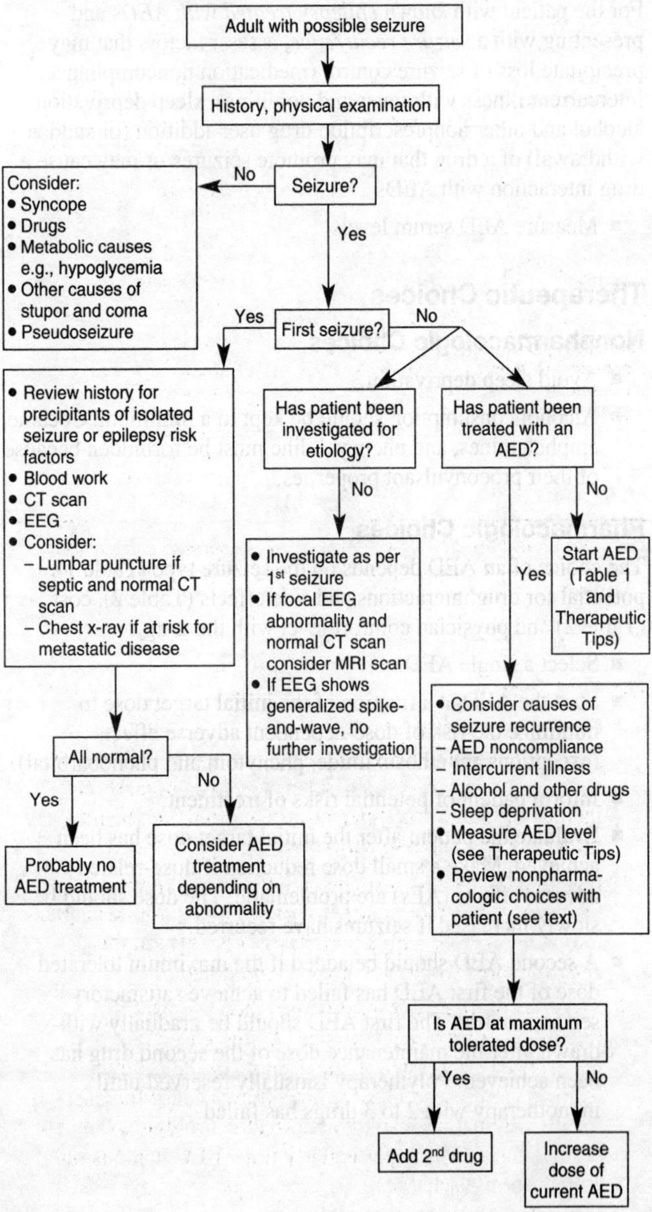
Adult with possible seizure
History, physical examination
Seizure?
No
Consider:
• Syncope
• Drugs
• Metabolic causes e.g., hypoglycemia
• Other causes of stupor and coma
• Pseudoseizure
Yes
First seizure?
Yes
• Review history for precipitants of isolated seizure or epilepsy risk factors
• Blood work
• CT scan
• EEG
• Consider:
– Lumbar puncture if septic and normal CT scan
– Chest x-ray if at risk for metastatic disease
All normal?
Yes
Probably no AED treatment
No
Consider AED treatment depending on abnormality
No
Has patient been investigated for etiology?
No
• Investigate as per 1st seizure
• If focal EEG abnormality and normal CT scan consider MRI scan
• If EEG shows generalized spike-and-wave, no further investigation
Has patient been treated with an AED?
No
Start AED (Table 1 and Therapeutic Tips)
Yes
• Consider causes of seizure recurrence
– AED noncompliance
– Intercurrent illness
– Alcohol and other drugs
– Sleep deprivation
• Measure AED level (see Therapeutic Tips)
• Review nonpharmacologic choices with patient (see text)
Is AED at maximum tolerated dose?
Yes
Add 2nd drug
No
Increase dose of current AED

Table 1: **Therapeutic Choices for AEDs*†**

| Seizure Type | 1st Choice Monotherapy | Alternate Monotherapy or Add On |
|---|---|---|
| **Generalized Tonic-Clonic** | carbamazepine<br>phenytoin<br>valproic acid | clobazam<br>lamotrigine<br>topiramate |
| **Absence** | ethosuximide<br>valproic acid | clobazam<br>lamotrigine<br>topiramate |
| **Myoclonic and Atonic** | valproic acid | clobazam<br>lamotrigine<br>topiramate |
| **Partial (simple or complex) with or without 2° generalization** | carbamazepine<br>phenytoin | clobazam<br>gabapentin<br>lamotrigine<br>phenobarbital<br>primidone<br>topiramate<br>valproic acid<br>vigabatrin |

* *AEDs are listed alphabetically; the order in the list does not imply a rank order.*
† *Guberman A, Bruni J. Clinical Handbook of Epilepsy. Guelph: Meducom International Inc., 1997.*

### *The First Seizure*

- Most patients present with a primary or secondarily generalized tonic-clonic seizure. It is important to determine if the event was *truly* the first seizure. Common errors include failure to recognize prior nocturnal convulsions and prior nonconvulsive seizures.
- Not all patients with a single convulsion will have a recurrence. The recurrence risk over 2 years after a single idiopathic seizure with a normal EEG is 24%. In this situation most would not advocate treatment.
- The risks of treatment must be weighed against the likelihood of seizure recurrence. An increased risk of recurrence is suggested if one or more of the following features are present: clear remote known cause for a seizure; focally originating seizure; abnormal neurologic examination; abnormal EEG (particularly if the EEG demonstrates epileptiform discharges).
- The decision to treat patients with AEDs after a single seizure must be individualized.

Table 2: **Antiepileptic Drugs***

| Drug (Usual Adult Dose) | Selected Adverse Effects† | Advantages | Disadvantages | Comments | Cost‡ |
|---|---|---|---|---|---|
| *carbamazepine* Tegretol, generics 800–1200 mg/d | Rash 5–10%, rarely can be very serious; ↑ liver enzymes; blood dyscrasia common; transient neutropenia; extremely rarely aplastic anemia; low serum sodium. | BID dose with controlled release (CR) preparations; linear pharmacokinetics. | Liver enzyme inducer; drug interactions; only oral form available; may worsen absence seizures; may produce or exacerbate myoclonus. | Start at 100 mg BID and increase by 200 mg/day q 3–4 days. Controlled release preparation may be better tolerated and improve compliance. | $ |
| *clobazam* Frisium 20–40 mg/d | Irritability; depression. | Very safe; daily or BID dosing; broad spectrum; rapid onset; few drug interactions. | Tolerance (initial good response followed by loss of seizure control). | Can be very useful as "add-on" for patients "nearly" seizure free. | $ |
| *ethosuximide* Zarontin 750–1000 mg/d | GI upset. | Few drug interactions. | For absence seizures only. | Confers no protection for generalized tonic-clonic seizures. | $ |
| *gabapentin* Neurontin 1200–3600 mg/d | † | No drug interactions; well tolerated; safe; not metabolized, can use in liver failure. | TID dosing. Not for 1° generalized seizures. | Very expensive at high doses. Best used as "add on" drug. | $$$–$$$$$ |

| | | | | | |
|---|---|---|---|---|---|
| *lamotrigine*<br>Lamictal<br>300–400 mg/d | Rash 5–10% which rarely can be very serious; insomnia. | BID dosing; broad spectrum; no enzyme induction (few interactions); some patients more "alert". | Very slow dose titration (see product monograph); metabolism markedly inhibited by valproic acid; only oral form available. | Very expensive at high doses; increasing use as monotherapy; increasing use for 1° generalized seizures. | \$\$\$–\$\$\$\$ |
| *phenobarbital*<br>generics<br>90–120 mg/d<br>*primidone*<br>Mysoline, generics<br>500–1000 mg/d | Sedation prominent; skin rash 5%; some patients intolerant of low dose primidone; depression; diminished libido. | Long t1/2; daily dosing for phenobarbital; inexpensive (phenobarbital); parenteral form of phenobarbital easy to use (emergencies). | Potent liver enzyme inducers; metabolism inhibited by valproic acid; QID dosing for primidone (to maintain high primidone/phenobarb ratio); primidone slow dose titration. | Declining use because of adverse effect profile.<br>Primidone metabolized to phenobarbital but parent compound has significant antiseizure properties. | \$ |
| *phenytoin*<br>Dilantin<br>300–400 mg/d | Skin rash 5–10%, rarely very serious; ↑ liver enzymes; blood dyscrasias; gingival hyperplasia; dose-related encephalopathy. | Daily or BID dosing; parental form; inexpensive; easy to give loading dose but follow manufacturer's instructions carefully. | Saturation kinetics; enzyme inducer; many drug interactions; long term cosmetic effects. | Saturation kinetics complicates dosing. | \$ |
| *topiramate* ◗<br>Topamax<br>200–400 mg/d | Cognitive problems common; kidney stones; weight loss; headache; fingers/toes paresthesias. | BID dosing; broad spectrum; safe; few drug interactions. | Slow titration; ↓ efficacy of oral contraceptives; expensive. | Potent AED with broad spectrum of activity but cognitive effects commonly limit use. | \$\$\$–\$\$\$\$ |

*(cont'd)*

Table 2: **Antiepileptic Drugs*** *(cont'd)*

| Drug (Usual Adult Dose) | Selected Adverse Effects† | Advantages | Disadvantages | Comments | Cost‡ |
|---|---|---|---|---|---|
| *valproic acid* Depakene, generics *divalproex sodium* Epival, generics 750–1500 mg/d | Nausea; weight gain; tremor; hair loss; blood dyscrasias; hepatotoxicity rarely; edema rarely; menstrual irregularities; teratogenicity (spina bifida) (1–2%). | Often may use BID dosing; broad spectrum; no enzyme induction; very low incidence of rash; cognitive effects generally less than other older AEDs. | Drug interactions (but does not reduce oral contraceptive efficacy). | Drug of first choice for patients with mixed 1° generalized seizures (generalized tonic-clonic, myoclonus, absence). | \$–\$\$ |
| *vigabatrin* Sabril 2000–4000 mg/d | Low incidence of psychosis, depression; irreversible visual field problems. | BID dosing; well tolerated; few drug interactions; easy to use; (linear pharmacokinetics); does not exhibit skin, blood, liver adverse effects. | May worsen absence seizures, myoclonus; expensive at high doses. | Recent reports of visual field defects has limited use of this drug. | \$\$\$–\$\$\$\$ |

** Consult product monograph for details of dosing, preparations, titration schedules, drug interactions and a complete list of adverse effects.*

*† Virtually all AEDs can produce sedation, fatigue, cognitive impairment, dizziness and ataxia in a dose-dependent fashion.*

*‡ Cost of 30-day supply—includes drug cost only.*

*Legend: \$ <\$50 \$\$ \$50–100 \$\$\$ \$100–150 \$\$\$\$ \$150–200 \$\$\$\$\$ >\$200.*

*Dosage adjustment may be required in renal impairment—see Appendix I.*

### *Women with Epilepsy*

- There is an increased risk of oral contraceptive (OC) failure in women taking enzyme enhancing AEDs. (The OC should contain >35 micrograms of estradiol.)
- Discuss pregnancy plans *prior* to conception.
  - Is AED treatment still required?
  - Withdraw least helpful AEDs if the patient is treated with AED polytherapy (determined by the history of which drug seemed to be more or less helpful when added).
  - Avoid valproic acid if there is a positive family history of neural tube closure defects.
  - There is no data to indicate which of the commonly used AEDs is unequivocally "best" or "least harmful." The best AED is the drug that best controls the patient's seizures.
  - Women of childbearing potential should receive continuous folate supplementation (2 to 4 mg/day) to possibly reduce the risk of teratogenic effects (neural tube defects) associated with AEDs.
- During pregnancy:
  - Follow AED levels as they may drop significantly.
  - Obtain expert obstetrical advice on timing and type of ultrasound to detect fetal malformations.
  - Start oral vitamin K (10 mg/day) in last 4 weeks of pregnancy. This must be prepared by a pharmacy from the parenteral preparation (an oral form of vitamin K is not available in Canada).
- Postpartum:
  - Breastfeeding is generally acceptable. Babies whose mothers are taking barbiturates may be sedated; babies exposed to barbiturates prepartum and not breastfeeding may have barbiturate withdrawal symptoms in the first week after delivery.
  - Follow AED levels as they may rise precipitously in the first weeks post delivery.

### *Status Epilepticus*

- "Convulsive" status epilepticus is recurrent primary or secondarily generalized tonic-clonic seizures with no return to consciousness; secondarily generalized variety is the most common form (>80%).
- Any seizure type can evolve to "nonconvulsive" status epilepticus: (absence, partial complex, simple partial). For example, a patient experiencing continuous or almost continuous absence seizure is in "absence status" but is not convulsing.

- Psychogenic pseudoseizures commonly present as "convulsive" status. Conversely, absence or partial complex status is often misdiagnosed as a psychiatric condition.
- Convulsive status has high morbidity and mortality related to underlying cause and effects on brain caused by the seizures. Brain injury begins at 30 to 45 minutes of status; aggressive treatment of seizures is important to optimize outcome. A suggested treatment protocol is outlined in Table 3.

Table 3: **Initial Management of Convulsive Status Epilepticus**

| Time | Management |
|---|---|
| 0–5 minutes | History, physical examination<br>Oral airway, oxygen<br>Consider intubation<br>Venous blood (glucose, blood counts, electrolytes, calcium, renal function, liver function, antiepileptic blood levels, consider drug screen)<br>Arterial blood gases<br>Monitor ECG, pulse oximetry, blood pressure |
| 5–10 minutes | Start 2 large bore IV saline infusions<br>50 ml 50% dextrose IV<br>Thiamine 50–100 mg IM<br>Lorazepam 0.1 mg/kg IV @ 2 mg/min (usual dose= 4 to 8 mg) **or** diazepam IV 5 mg/min (usual dose=10 to 20 mg) |
| 10–30 minutes | Phenytoin 17–18 mg/kg IV (maximum rate = 50 mg/min) **or** phenobarbital 20 mg/kg IV (50–75 mg/min) |
| 30–60 minutes | If seizures persist after initial phenytoin, start phenobarbital; if seizures persist after initial phenobarbital, use phenytoin<br>Admit to critical care unit, arrange EEG<br>Obtain expert emergency consultation (consider propofol, thiopental) |

***Other General Measures***

- Reduce the risk of burns during seizures: discourage smoking; use microwave ovens and place pots on the rear burners of stoves.
- Showers are preferable to tub baths because of the risks of drowning during an unwitnessed seizure in a bathtub.
- Assess recreational activities, current and planned employment.

- Patients with active epilepsy who are caregivers for young children should not change infants on a table or bathe babies without assistance.
- Assess driving status. Physicians should be aware of their legal obligations to local Departments of Transportation (mandatory vs. discretional reporting).
- Support groups: some patients may benefit from the activities of local and national epilepsy lay organizations.

## Therapeutic Tips

- Obtain a baseline CBC and serum liver transaminases (and repeat in 4 to 6 weeks) if treating with an AED that may cause a hypersensitivity syndrome involving blood and liver. Mild elevations (< 2–3 times normal) of liver enzymes and/or modest reductions in blood counts (e.g., neutropenia with carbamazepine; thrombocytopenia with valproic acid) are relatively common. Neither of these situations requires discontinuation of treatment but the abnormality should be followed with serial studies.
- Do not rely excessively on serum AED levels to guide therapy as their validity for efficacy and toxicity is not established. Some patients will have satisfactory seizure control at low AED levels; some patients have AED dose-related toxicity below the upper end of the quoted "therapeutic range"; some patients tolerate drug levels modestly above the upper end of the therapeutic range. A useful adage is: "treat the patient, not the serum level."
- Drug interactions with many AEDs are potential problems. Drugs with hepatic enzyme enhancing properties (carbamazepine, phenytoin, phenobarbital, primidone) may reduce the levels of concomitant medications. The presence (or absence) of other medications should be considered when selecting an AED.

## *Suggested Reading List*

Brodie MJ, Dichter MA. Antiepileptic drugs. *N Engl J Med* 1996;334:168–175.

Dichter MA, Brodie MJ. New antiepileptic drugs. *N Engl J Med* 1996;334:1583–1590.

Lowenstein DH, Allredge BK. Status epilepticus. *N Engl J Med* 1998;338:970–976.

Report of the Quality Standards Committee of the American Academy of Neurology: Practice parameter. Management issues for women with epilepsy (summary statement). *Neurology* 1998;51:944–948.

CHAPTER 19

# Cataract Surgery Postoperative Care

*Raymond P. LeBlanc, MD, FRCSC*

## Goals of Therapy

- To control inflammation
- To prevent infection
- To maintain eye comfort
- To promote early visual rehabilitation

## Investigations

- Pain: the postoperative eye should be comfortable
  - at worst patient may have a mild foreign-body sensation; more intensive pain suggests increased IOP, increased inflammation and/or infection
- History of recent trauma:
  - any trauma to the eye in the early postoperative phase requires thorough reassessment
- Change in vision: darkened, loss of detail
  - any significant change could indicate a hemorrhage, retinal detachment or other acute intraocular pathology requiring immediate attention
- Visual phenomena: flashing lights or dark shadows
  - requires thorough reassessment
- Itchy, red eye:
  - suggests allergy to medications
- Examination of eye for:
  - swelling of lids and/or conjunctiva suggests drug allergy or infection
  - red reflex (should be confirmed with ophthalmoscope)
  - hyphema/corneal opacity
- Review of ocular medications:
  - reinforce use
  - clarify any confusion
  - discuss with family member
- Verify follow-up visits with surgeon

Figure 1: **Management of Postop Cataract Patient**

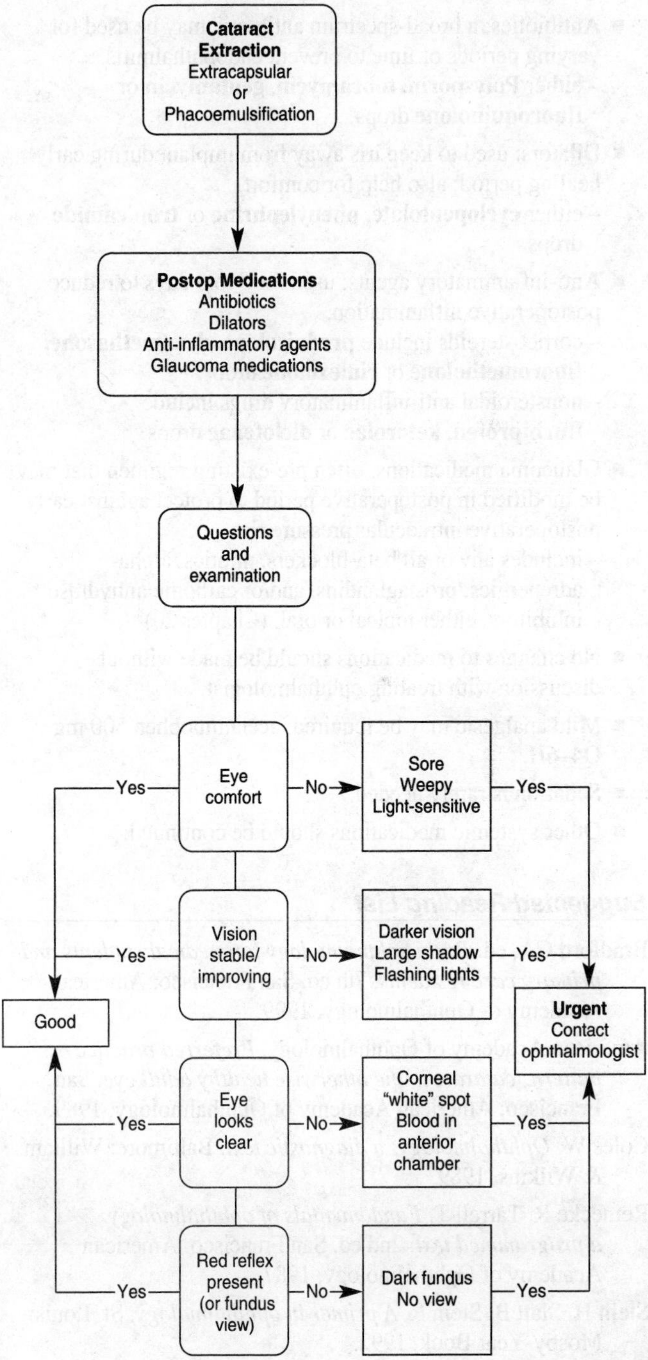
Cataract Extraction
Extracapsular or Phacoemulsification
Postop Medications
Antibiotics
Dilators
Anti-inflammatory agents
Glaucoma medications
Questions and examination
Eye comfort
Yes
No
Sore
Weepy
Light-sensitive
Yes
Vision stable/ improving
Yes
No
Darker vision
Large shadow
Flashing lights
Yes
Good
Urgent
Contact ophthalmologist
Eye looks clear
Yes
No
Corneal "white" spot
Blood in anterior chamber
Yes
Red reflex present (or fundus view)
Yes
No
Dark fundus
No view
Yes

## Therapeutic Choices (Figure 1)

Postoperative medications may include:

- Antibiotics: a broad-spectrum antibiotic may be used for varying periods of time to prevent endophthalmitis.
  - either **Polysporin, tobramycin**, **gentamycin** or **fluoroquinolone** drops.
- Dilators: used to keep iris away from implant during early healing period; also help for comfort.
  - either **cyclopentolate, phenylephrine** or **tropicamide** drops.
- Anti-inflammatory agents: used for 3 to 5 days to reduce postoperative inflammation.
  - corticosteroids include **prednisolone, dexamethasone, fluorometholone** or **rimexolone** drops.
  - nonsteroidal anti-inflammatory drugs include **flurbiprofen, ketorolac** or **diclofenac** drops.
- Glaucoma medications: often pre-existing regimen that may be modified in postoperative period to protect against early postoperative intraocular pressure rise.
  - includes any or all beta-blockers, miotics, alpha-adrenergics, prostaglandins, and/or carbonic anhydrase inhibitors, either topical or oral. (Chapter 20)
- No changes to medications should be made without discussion with treating ophthalmologist.
- Mild analgesic may be required: acetaminophen 500 mg Q4–6H.
- Sedation is rarely needed.
- Other systemic medications should be continued.

## *Suggested Reading List*


Bradford CA, ed. *Basic ophthalmology for medical students and primary care residents*. 7th ed. San Francisco: American Academy of Ophthalmology, 1999.

American Academy of Ophthalmology. *Preferred practice pattern: cataract in the otherwise healthy adult eye*. San Francisco: American Academy of Ophthalmology, 1989.

Coles W. *Ophthalmology: a diagnostic text*. Baltimore: Williams & Wilkins, 1989.

Reinecke R, Tarrell T. *Fundamentals of ophthalmology: a programmed text*. 2nd ed. San Francisco: American Academy of Ophthalmology, 1987.

Stein H, Slatt B, Stein R. *A primer in ophthalmology*. St. Louis: Mosby-Year Book, 1992.

CHAPTER 20

# Glaucoma

*Paul Rafuse, MD, PhD, FRCSC*

## Definition

A group of ocular diseases that have in common an optic neuropathy that causes visual loss. Characteristically, the optic disc is cupped and peripheral field loss precedes deterioration of visual acuity. Elevated intraocular pressure (IOP) is the most important, and only modifiable risk factor for glaucoma. Other risk factors (i.e., vascular diseases) are likely important in the pathogenesis of this neurodegenerative condition.

## Goals of Therapy

- To prevent, halt or slow progressive visual loss
- To preserve the structure and function of the optic nerve
- To eliminate pain and improve vision in acute forms

**NB:** The therapeutic goals are achieved (with medications, laser and/or surgery) by decreasing the IOP.

## Investigations

- Thorough history with special attention to:
  - nature of any ocular disturbances (e.g., loss of peripheral vision, halos around lights, decreased visual acuity)
  - quality of any pain (e.g., deep orbital, brow or headache)
  - associated systemic symptoms (e.g., abdominal pain, nausea and vomiting)

**NB:** The most common varieties are chronic. Generally, only the acute types are accompanied by symptoms.

- Careful assessment of risk factors (Table 1)
- History of drug use that can cause or worsen glaucoma
  - corticosteroids (common)
  - drugs with antimuscarinic activity (e.g., antihistamines, decongestants, antidepressants, antispasmodics, etc.; rare)
- Physical examination
  - positive findings: constricted visual field, optic disc cupping and elevated IOP

**NB:** Screening for elevated IOP *alone* lacks adequate sensitivity and specificity for the detection of glaucoma: many patients with glaucoma do not have high IOPs. Most people with IOPs above the normal range do not have glaucoma.

Table 1: **Risk Factors for the Development of Glaucoma**

| | | |
|---|---|---|
| **Acquired** (Primary) | **Open-angle** | **Closed-angle** |
| | Elevated IOP | Female[1] |
| | Advanced age | Advanced age[1,2] |
| | Black | Black[2] |
| | Positive family history | Positive family history[1,2] |
| | Myopia | Hyperopia[1,2] |
| | Diabetes mellitus | White[1] |
| | Vascular diseases | |
| **Acquired** (Secondary) | Blunt and penetrating trauma | |
| | Previous intraocular surgery | |
| | Previous intraocular inflammation | |
| | Corticosteroid use | |
| **Congenital** | Positive family history | |

*Closed-angle glaucoma can be either acute[1] or chronic.[2]*

- Comprehensive eye examination by an ophthalmologist
- Laboratory tests:
  - automated perimetry
  - optic disc photography

## Therapeutic Choices (Figure 1)

### Nonpharmacologic Choices

- There are no lifestyle modifications proven to alter the outcome of the disease. Aerobic exercise can lower IOP modestly in some patients with glaucoma.
- Surgical or laser procedures are options if drug therapy is unsuccessful (Figure 1).

### Pharmacologic Choices (Table 2)

- Reversible causes of **secondary** and **angle-closure** glaucoma should be treated.
- Excessive IOP, the only modifiable risk factor in chronic primary **open-angle** glaucoma (the most prevalent form), should be treated; all treatment measures in Figure 1 are believed to exert their therapeutic effect by lowering IOP.

#### *Beta-blockers*

Topical **timolol maleate, levobunolol hydrochloride** and **betaxolol hydrochloride** are efficacious ocular hypotensive agents that lack significant ocular side effects. They decrease IOP by inhibiting the formation of aqueous humor. They are contraindicated when some pulmonary and cardiac diseases exist (Table 2). Betaxolol hydrochloride is relatively specific for $beta_1$-receptor blockade and may be used with caution in selected patients with mild obstructive pulmonary disease.

Figure 1: **Management of Open-angle Glaucoma**

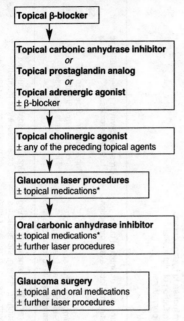

**Treatment is stepped up if optic disc cupping progresses, the visual field deteriorates or IOP control is inadequate.**

**Topical β-blocker**

↓

**Topical carbonic anhydrase inhibitor**
*or*
**Topical prostaglandin analog**
*or*
**Topical adrenergic agonist**
± β-blocker

↓

**Topical cholinergic agonist**
± any of the preceding topical agents

↓

**Glaucoma laser procedures**
± topical medications*

↓

**Oral carbonic anhydrase inhibitor**
± topical medications*
± further laser procedures

↓

**Glaucoma surgery**
± topical and oral medications
± further laser procedures

* *β-blockers, topical carbonic anhydrase inhibitors, prostaglandin analogs, adrenergic agonists and cholinergic agonists.*

**NB:** Systemic absorption of eye drops occurs through the nasal mucosa. This can be reduced by digital occlusion of the nasolacrimal drainage system for several minutes following instillation of the drops.

### *Topical Carbonic Anhydrase Inhibitors*

**Dorzolamide hydrochloride** and **brinzolamide** are two agents available in this class. Like oral carbonic anhydrase inhibitors, they decrease IOP by inhibiting an enzyme involved in the formation of aqueous humor. Both have limited systemic effects when compared to the oral products and have more favorable ocular tolerability than the cholinergic agonists which can cause accommodative spasm and miosis. The newer brinzolamide appears to be equally efficacious to dorzolamide and may be more comfortable on instillation. These drugs are considered in patients with cardiopulmonary contraindications to beta-blockers.

### *Prostaglandin Analogs*

**Latanoprost**, a prostaglandin $F_{2\alpha}$ analog, lowers IOP by increasing uveoscleral outflow. It is highly efficacious and is

Table 2: **Drugs Used in Glaucoma**

| Drug | Dosage | Adverse Effects | Comments | Cost* |
|---|---|---|---|---|
| **Beta-blockers (topical)** | | | | |
| *levobunolol hydrochloride 0.25%, 0.5%* – Betagan, generics | Q12H | Local adverse effects usually minimal – stinging, dry eyes, rarely conjunctivitis. | Avoid in patients with bronchial asthma. Caution in patients with a history of syncope or bradycardia. | $ |
| *betaxolol hydrochloride 0.25%* – Betoptic S | Q12H | Bronchospasm, exacerbation of CHF, bradycardia, syncope, depression, impotence, altered response to hypoglycemia, reduction of high-density lipoproteins. | | $$ |
| *timolol maleate 0.25%, 0.5%* – Timoptic, generics | Q12H | | | $ |
| *timolol maleate gelan 0.25%, 0.5%* – Timoptic-XE | once daily | | | $$ |
| *timolol maleate 0.5% / pilocarpine 2%, 4%* – Timpilo-2, -4 | Q12H | | | $$ |
| **Carbonic Anhydrase Inhibitors (topical)** | | Bitter, sour or unusual taste, stinging, local allergic reaction. | Cross reactivity in patients allergic to sulfonamides. | |
| *dorzolamide hydrochloride 2%* – Trusopt | Q8H | | | $$ |
| *brinzolamide 1% – Azopt* | Q12H | | Brinzolamide: dose can be increased to Q8H after 4 weeks if inadequate response. | $$ |
| *dorzolamide hydrochloride 2% / timolol maleate 0.5%* – Cosopt | Q12H | Combined adverse effects of β-blockers and carbonic anhydrase inhibitors. (see above) | | $$$ |
| **Prostaglandin Analogs (topical)** | | | | |
| *latanoprost 0.005%* – Xalatan | once daily | Foreign body sensation, burning, stinging, itching, increased iris pigmentation, increased eyelash length. | Once daily dosing should not be exceeded. More frequent administration may reduce effectiveness. | $$$ |

| | | | | |
|---|---|---|---|---|
| **Cholinergic Agonists (topical)** | | | | |
| *pilocarpine hydrochloride 0.5%, 1%, 2%, 4%, 6%* – Isopto Carpine, others, Pilopine HS gel | QID (drops)<br>QHS (gel) | Reduced vision in patients with cataracts, blurred vision due to refractive shift, headache, GI upset. | Inhibition of plasma cholinesterase by echothiophate can markedly prolong action of succinylcholine. | $ drops<br>$$ gel |
| *carbachol* – Isopto Carbachol | Q8H | | | $ |
| *echothiophate 0.06%, 0.125%, 0.25%* (irreversible cholinesterase inhibitor) – Phospholine Iodide | Q12H | Iris cysts, cataracts (echothiophate). | | $$–$$$ |
| **Adrenergic Agonists (topical)** | | Local allergic reaction, headache. | | |
| *dipivefrin hydrochloride 0.1%* – Propine, DPE, generics | Q12H | | Dipivefrin is converted by a corneal esterase into the active metabolite epinephrine. | $ |
| *apraclonidine hydrochloride 0.5%* – Iopidine | Q8H | | Controversy exists as to whether the use of apraclonidine and brimonidine is contraindicated in patients taking MAO inhibitors. | $$$ |
| *brimonidine tartrate 0.2%* – Alphagan | Q12H | | Brimonidine: lower incidence of allergy than apraclonidine when used chronically. | $$ |
| **Carbonic Anhydrase Inhibitors (oral)** | | Paresthesias of extremities, metabolic acidosis, hypokalemia, GI upset, urolithiasis, lethargy and depression, aplastic anemia (rare), Stevens-Johnson syndrome (rare). | Cross reactivity in patients allergic to sulfonamides. | |
| *acetazolamide* ❥ – Diamox, Diamox Sequels, generics | 250 mg QID (acetazolamide)<br>500 mg Q12H (Sequels) | | | $4/mo<br>Sequels $45/mo |
| *methazolamide* ❥ – Neptazane | 25–50 mg Q8H | | | $24–35/mo |

❥ *Dosage adjustment may be required in renal impairment – see Appendix I.*

*Legend: $ < $2 $$ $2–4 $$$ > $4*

* *Cost per mL or g – includes drug cost only.*

administered once daily. Clinical experience has not revealed any significant adverse systemic effects, but a few unique (and seemingly innocuous) ocular effects have been noted including darkening of some brown colored irides and lengthening of the eyelashes. Latanoprost may be considered as a first-line agent in individuals with contraindications to the use of beta-blockers.

### *Adrenergic Agonists*

Topical epinephrine, the prototype in this class, is no longer available in Canada. A prodrug, **dipivefrin hydrochloride**, is available and lowers IOP by enhancing aqueous humor outflow. **Apraclonidine hydrochloride** was the first $alpha_2$-specific agonist introduced, but its use has been largely limited to managing acute IOP spikes since chronic use has resulted in an unacceptable rate of ocular allergy. **Brimonidine tartrate** has a higher specificity for the $alpha_2$-receptor and demonstrates a lower allergy rate. It is widely used as an adjuvant agent or primarily when beta-blockers cannot be used.

### *Cholinergic Agonists*

Topical cholinergic agonists may act either directly on the muscarinic receptors activating the ciliary muscle or indirectly through inhibition of ciliary cholinesterase. Both lower IOP by causing an increase in trabecular outflow. Rarely is enough drug absorbed systemically to cause abdominal cramping or diarrhea. **Pilocarpine hydrochloride** and **carbachol** are direct-acting agents. **Echothiophate** is also an irreversible inhibitor of plasma cholinesterase. Because it can markedly prolong the action of succinylcholine, topical echothiophate should be discontinued 2 weeks before elective surgery requiring general anesthesia.

### *Oral Carbonic Anhydrase Inhibitors*

**Acetazolamide** and **methazolamide** lower IOP by decreasing the production of aqueous humor. Their use is normally reserved for advanced chronic cases or acute emergencies because of significant side effects. Approximately 50% of patients are unable to use these drugs. They are more effective IOP-reducing agents than the topical carbonic anhydrase inhibitors. Both oral and topical preparations can show cross reactivity in patients allergic to sulfonamides.

## Therapeutic Tips

- OTC antihistamine products (which carry a caution against use in glaucoma patients due to anticholinergic side effects) will rarely cause a problem in open-angle glaucoma. The caution is made to advise those people without glaucoma but who are at risk for acute angle closure.

### *Suggested Reading List*

Epstein DL, ed. *Chandler and Grant's Glaucoma*. 4th ed. Baltimore: Williams and Wilkins, 1997.

Quigley HA. Medical progress: open-angle glaucoma. *N Engl J Med* 1993;328:1097–1106.

Rafuse PE. Screening those at risk for glaucoma. *Can J Diagn* 1999;16:105–112.

CHAPTER 21

# Red Eye

*Sueda Akkor, MD, FRCSC*

## Definition

Red eye is common in a wide variety of ocular conditions, some with serious consequences that require immediate referral to an ophthalmologist.

## Goals of Therapy

- To preserve eyesight
- To control infection
- To control inflammation
- To provide symptomatic relief

## Etiology

- Infections – conjunctivitis/keratitis: bacterial, viral (herpetic, non-herpetic), other
- Allergy
- Dry eyes: keratoconjunctivitis sicca
- Blepharitis and secondary conjunctivitis/keratitis
- Toxic/chemical/other irritants: topical drugs, contact lens solutions, acids/alkalis, smoke, wind, UV light
- Traumatic injury: corneal abrasions, foreign bodies, hyphema, other
- Ocular inflammation: iritis, episcleritis, scleritis
- Glaucoma: acute angle-closure glaucoma
- Others: lacrimal system infections, pterygium, subconjunctival hemorrhage

## Investigations

The first step is to differentiate the major/serious causes from the minor causes. The following warning signs require referral to an ophthalmologist:

- Limbal/ciliary injection (redness dominant at the corneo-scleral junction)
- Pain **not** relieved by test dose of topical anesthetic drop (proparacaine, tetracaine)
- Pupil abnormalities: miotic or mid-dilated and fixed

Figure 1: **Management of Red Eye**

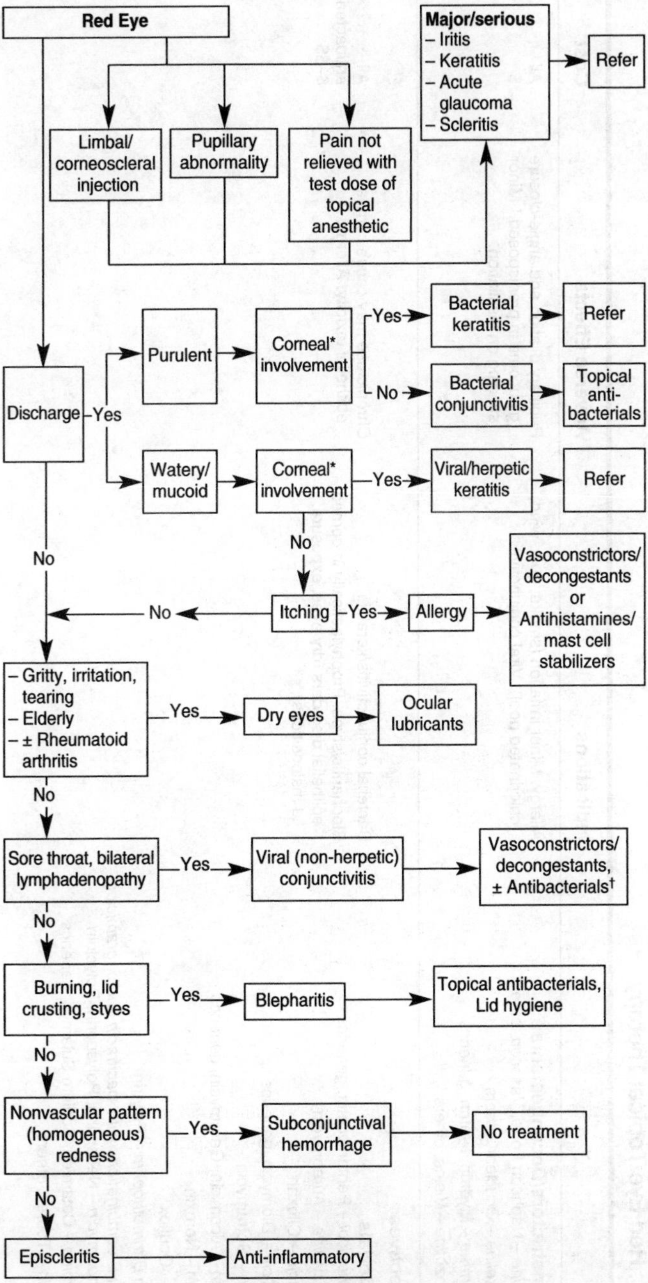
Red Eye
Major/serious
– Iritis
– Keratitis
– Acute glaucoma
– Scleritis
Refer
Limbal/ corneoscleral injection
Pupillary abnormality
Pain not relieved with test dose of topical anesthetic
Discharge
Yes
Purulent
Corneal* involvement
Yes
Bacterial keratitis
Refer
No
Bacterial conjunctivitis
Topical anti-bacterials
Watery/ mucoid
Corneal* involvement
Yes
Viral/herpetic keratitis
Refer
No
No
Itching
Yes
Allergy
Vasoconstrictors/ decongestants or Antihistamines/ mast cell stabilizers
No
– Gritty, irritation, tearing
– Elderly
– ± Rheumatoid arthritis
Yes
Dry eyes
Ocular lubricants
No
Sore throat, bilateral lymphadenopathy
Yes
Viral (non-herpetic) conjunctivitis
Vasoconstrictors/ decongestants, ± Antibacterials†
No
Burning, lid crusting, styes
Yes
Blepharitis
Topical antibacterials, Lid hygiene
No
Nonvascular pattern (homogeneous) redness
Yes
Subconjunctival hemorrhage
No treatment
No
Episcleritis
Anti-inflammatory

* *Corneal staining with fluorescein strip indicates corneal involvement.*

† *Rarely used to prevent secondary bacterial infection.*

Table 1: **Red Eye Topical Therapy**

| Drugs | Indications | Adverse Effects | Cost* |
|---|---|---|---|
| **Vasoconstrictors/Decongestants**<br>*naphazoline* – Naphcon Forte, Vasocon, others<br>*oxymetazoline* – Ocuclear, others<br>*phenylephrine* – Mydfrin, Prefrin, generics<br>*tetrahydrozoline* – Visine, others | Allergy. Minor irritation (smoke, dust, wind, chlorinated pool). Viral conjunctivitis. | Pupillary dilation and angle-closure glaucoma in predisposed.† Minor stinging on instillation. | All<br>$ |
| **Anti-infectives** | | | |
| **Antibacterials**<br>*chloramphenicol* – Pentamycetin, generics<br>*chlortetracycline* – Aureomycin<br>*ciprofloxacin* – Ciloxan<br>*erythromycin* – Diomycin, generics<br>*framycetin* – Soframycin<br>*gentamicin* – Alcomicin, Garamycin, generics<br>*norfloxacin* – Noroxin<br>*ofloxacin* – Ocuflox<br>*polymyxin B/trimethoprim* – Polytrim<br>*polymyxin B combinations with bacitracin and/or gramicidin and/or neomycin* – Neosporin, Polysporin, Polycidin<br>*sulfacetamide* – Cetamide, Sodium Sulamyd, generics<br>*tobramycin* – Tobrex, others | Bacterial conjunctivitis/keratitis.<br>Blepharitis/styes. Prophylactically in corneal epithelial disorders (dry eyes, exposure, lid malpositions). | Chronic use may cause corneal epithelial toxicity. Allergy. | All antibacterials<br>$–$$ |

| | | | |
|---|---|---|---|
| **Antivirals** | Herpes simplex, Herpes zoster (systemic acyclovir or valacyclovir are the only effective antivirals). | Chronic use may cause corneal epithelial toxicity. | |
| *idoxuridine* – Herplex | | | $$ |
| *trifluridine* – Viroptic | | | $$$ |
| Systemic Therapy | | | |
| *acyclovir* – Zovirax, generics ‡ | | | $$$$ |
| *valacyclovir* – Valtrex ‡ | | | $$$$ |
| **Antihistamines/Mast Cell Stabilizers** | Allergies. Sodium cromoglycate in contact lens wear-related giant papillary conjunctivitis.$^{\pi}$ | Minor stinging on instillation. | |
| *sodium cromoglycate* – Opticrom | | | $ |
| *emedastine* – Emadine | | | $$ |
| *lodoxamide tromethamine* – Alomide | | | $$ |
| *levocabastine* – Livostin | | | $$ |
| *nedocromil* – Mireze | | | $$ |
| *olopatadine* – Patanol | | | $$$ |
| *antazoline/naphazoline* – Albalon-A Liquifilm, Vasocon-A | | | $ |
| *antazoline/xylometazoline* – Ophtrivin-A | | | $ |
| *pheniramine maleate/naphazoline* – Naphcon-A, Opcon-A | | | $ |
| **Ocular Lubricants** | Dry eyes, exposure, lid malpositions, blepharitis, minor irritations. | Preservative toxicity, filmy vision. | All $ – $$ (preservative-free unit dose products are more expensive) |
| *carboxymethylcellulose* – Cellufresh, Cellufresh MD, Celluvisc | | | |
| *dextran/polyethylene glycol* – Aquasite | | | |
| *hydroxypropyl methylcellulose* – Genteal, Isopto Tears, Tears Naturale, Tears Naturale II, others | | | |
| *methylcellulose* – Murocel | | | |
| *polysorbate* – Tears Encore | | | |
| *polyvinyl alcohol* – Hypotears, Liquifilm Tears, Refresh, Tears Plus, generics | | | |
| *mineral oil/petrolatum* – Duolube, Hypotears, Lacri-Lube S.O.P., generics | | | |
| *sodium hyaluronate* – Eyestil | | | |
| *sorbitol/carbomer* – Tear-Gel | | | |

(cont'd)

Table 1: **Red Eye Topical Therapy** *(cont'd)*

| Drugs | Indications | Adverse Effects | Cost* |
|---|---|---|---|
| **Anti-inflammatory Agents** | Episcleritis, iritis, scleritis, some keratitis, ocular allergy. | Minor stinging on instillation. | |
| **Steroids** | | Steroids may worsen herpetic/fungal keratitis. | |
| *dexamethasone* – Maxidex, generics | | | $ |
| *fluorometholone* – FML, FML Forte, Flarex | | Long-term steroids may cause glaucoma, cataracts. | $$ |
| *prednisolone* – Inflamase Mild/Forte, Pred Mild/Forte, generics | | | $–$$ |
| *prednisolone/sulfacetamide* – Vasocidin, generics | | | $$ |
| *rimexolone* – Vexol | | | $$ |
| **Nonsteroidals** | | | |
| *diclofenac* – Voltaren Ophtha | | | $$ |
| *flurbiprofen* – Ocufen | | | $$ |
| *ketorolac* – Acular | | | $$ |

* *Cost of smallest unit – includes drug cost only. (For OTC products, add retail mark-up.)*
*Legend: $ < $10 $$ $10–20 $$$ $20–30 $$$$ > $30*
† *See Glaucoma, Chapter 20.*
*Dosage adjustment may be required in renal impairment – see Appendix I.*
‡ *Not available as a topical ophthalmic agent. H. zoster use acyclovir 800 mg 5 times/day for 7 days or valacyclovir 1 g PO TID for 7 days; H. simplex use acyclovir 200 mg QID for 2 weeks.*

π *Giant papillary conjunctivitis is a hypersensitivity disorder seen in patients with contact lenses or artificial eyes. The family practitioner may suspect it in patients complaining of itching and ropy whitish discharge, but diagnosis is made with slit lamp exam by an ophthalmologist.*

- Raised intraocular pressure
- History of iritis/angle-closure glaucoma
- Recent history of trauma

## Therapeutic Choices (Figure 1)

### Nonpharmacologic Choices

- Contact lens wear should be stopped.
- Make-up, smoke, wind, other irritants should be avoided.
- Cold wet compresses should be applied in allergic or viral conjunctivitis.
- Hot wet compresses should be applied in blepharitis/styes.
- Lid hygiene should be used in blepharitis.

### Pharmacologic Choices (Table 1)

Choice depends on underlying cause.

## Therapeutic Tips

- Once the major/serious conditions are ruled out, treatment can be initiated.
- If no improvement is seen after one week, refer.
- Most topically administered eyedrops used in therapy are themselves capable of causing irritation or toxicity.
- Steroids or antibiotic–steroid combinations may worsen herpetic/fungal keratitis and should not be used indiscriminately.
- Long-term use of topical steroids may cause glaucoma and/or cataracts.
- Topical decongestants/vasoconstrictors may provoke angle-closure glaucoma in those predisposed.

## *Suggested Reading List*

Berson FG, ed. *Basic ophthalmology for medical students and primary care residents*. 6th ed. San Francisco: American Academy of Ophthalmology, 1993.

Chawla HB. *Ophthalmology*. 2nd ed. New York: Churchill Livingstone, 1993:89–97.

Vaughan DG, Asbury T, Riordan-Eva P. *General ophthalmology*. 14th ed. Los Altos, CA: Lange, 1995:78–80, 95–136.

CHAPTER 22

# Prevention of Ischemic Stroke

*Robert Côté, MD, FRCPC*

## Goals of Therapy

- To prevent disabling neurologic deficits (stroke) and recurrent transient ischemic attacks (TIA)
- To prevent associated cardiac ischemic events including myocardial infarction (MI)
- To prevent cerebrovascular and cardiovascular-related mortality

## Investigations

- Complete history with attention to:
  - nature, frequency, duration and distribution of symptoms (cerebral localization)
  - identification of vascular risk factors
- Physical examination:
  - complete neurologic assessment
  - visual assessment including eye movements, visual fields, acuity and funduscopy
  - complete vascular examination including auscultation (cranium, cervical, cardiac), palpation (temporal artery, peripheral pulses) and blood pressure in both arms
- Laboratory tests – indicated in patients with TIAs or mild strokes (without disabling deficits):
  - CT brain scan (to rule out hemorrhagic process) and cervical and transcranial ultrasonography
  - CBC, coagulation parameters, blood glucose, renal and hepatic profile
  - in selected cases more specialized blood tests (e.g., ESR, immunologic work-up, testing for hypercoagulable states, antiphospholipid antibodies)
  - baseline ECG (exclude atrial fibrillation)
  - other cardiac tests (e.g., transthoracic or transesophageal echocardiography, Holter monitoring) may be indicated (usually have a higher yield in patients with established cardiac disease or in young stroke patients)
  - cerebral angiography in selected cases to confirm occlusive cerebrovascular disease and to establish appropriateness of endarterectomy. Magnetic resonance imaging (MRI) and/or

Figure 1: **Prevention of Cerebral Ischemia**

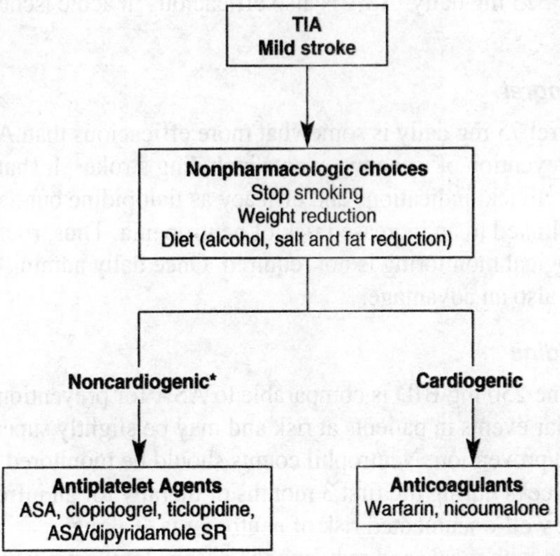
TIA
Mild stroke
Nonpharmacologic choices
Stop smoking
Weight reduction
Diet (alcohol, salt and fat reduction)
Noncardiogenic*
Cardiogenic
Antiplatelet Agents
ASA, clopidogrel, ticlopidine, ASA/dipyridamole SR
Anticoagulants
Warfarin, nicoumalone

** If carotid symptoms and appropriate severe stenosis, consider surgery.*

angiography (MRA) may be required to confirm the diagnosis and/or exclude other neurologic conditions mimicking cerebral ischemia.

## Therapeutic Choices (Figure 1)

### Nonpharmacologic Choices

- Smoking cessation is recommended.
- Vascular risk factors should be controlled through weight reduction and diet modification (reducing alcohol, fat and salt consumption).
- Rehabilitative therapy (physiotherapy, and occupational and speech therapy) should be prescribed if indicated.

### Pharmacologic Choices (Table 1)

#### *Antiplatelet Agents*

Antiplatelet agents are used for long-term prevention of atherothrombotic events (intra-arterial disease with secondary embolic phenomena).

##### ❑ *Acetylsalicylic Acid (ASA)*

The drug of choice for stroke prevention, ASA, reduces vascular events (cardiac and cerebral) by about 25%. It is well-tolerated with few (dose-dependent) side effects. Patient acceptability and low cost are advantages. The optimal dosage (75 to 1300 mg per day) for stroke prevention remains uncertain.[1] The most common dosage is 325 mg daily. ASA is also efficacious in acute ischemic stroke.[2]

#### ❑ *Clopidogrel*

Clopidogrel 75 mg daily is somewhat more efficacious than ASA for the prevention of ischemic events including stroke[3]. It shares the same clinical indications and efficacy as ticlopidine but has not been linked to an increased risk of neutropenia. Thus, routine hematological monitoring is not required. Once daily administration is also an advantage.

#### ❑ *Ticlopidine*

Ticlopidine 250 mg BID is comparable to ASA for prevention of all vascular events in patients at risk and may be slightly superior for stroke prevention. Neutrophil counts should be monitored every 2 weeks during the first 3 months of therapy for an infrequent but well-documented risk of neutropenia. Taking ticlopidine with meals and reducing the dosage temporarily may decrease the incidence of some side effects (e.g., diarrhea which occurs in up to 20% of patients).

#### ❑ *Other Antiplatelet Agents*

**Dipyridamole SR** (400 mg per day) used **in combination with low dose ASA** (50 mg per day) is of benefit for stroke prevention.[4] As well, ASA 100 mg per day combined with an oral anticoagulant appears to provide better protection against cardioembolic events in patients with prosthetic heart valves.[5] Sulfinpyrazone is not effective in stroke prevention.

### *Anticoagulants*

Anticoagulants are used to prevent cerebral ischemic attacks from emboli presumed to be of cardiac origin.

#### ❑ *Heparin*

Heparin is not effective in the management of acute stroke. Available data do not support the routine use of heparin in acute partial atherothrombotic stroke. Its only proven efficacy is in the prevention of deep vein thrombosis in acute ischemic stroke. A risk of bleeding complications is always present, and a CT brain

---

[1] *BMJ 1994;308:81–106.*
[2] *Lancet 1997; 349:1641–1649.*
[3] *Lancet 1996;348:1329–1339.*
[4] *Journal of Neurological Sciences 1996;143:1–13.*
[5] *Chest 1998;114;602S–610S.*

Table 1: **Drugs Used in Prevention of Stroke and Associated Coronary Events**

| Drug | Dosage | Adverse Effects | Drug Interactions | Cost* |
|---|---|---|---|---|
| **Anticoagulants** *heparin* | 80 units/kg. Then 18 units/kg/h adjusted according to APTT (See Chapter 31, Table 4) | Hemorrhagic complications, usually dose-related. Thrombocytopenia (heparin). Skin necrosis (warfarin and heparin). | With heparin, concomitant use of ASA, NSAIDs or other antiplatelets may ↑ hemorrhagic risk. | $† |
| *warfarin* Coumadin, Warfilone | Oral: Dosed to maintain INR between 2.0–3.0 for most cerebrovascular indications; for stroke prevention in patients with **mechanical heart valves**, maintain INR between 2.5–4.5 | Oral anticoagulants are contraindicated in pregnancy. | Effects of oral anticoagulants ↑ by cimetidine, some antibiotics, amiodarone and ↓ by phenytoin, barbiturates, carbamazepine. See Table 3, Chapter 31. | $ |
| *nicoumalone* Sintrom | | | | $ |
| **Antiplatelets** *ASA* Entrophen, generics (coated); Aspirin, generics | 75–1300 mg/d | Bleeding, usually minor (epistaxis, etc.). ASA: gastric intolerance, GI bleeding (gastric ulcers, erosions), nausea, heartburn, constipation, tinnitus usually dose-related. | Hemorrhagic risk ↑ with concomitant use of anticoagulants. | $ |
| *clopidogrel* Plavix | 75 mg daily | Clopidogrel: skin rash (4%); diarrhea (5%) | Clopidogrel: Caution when combined with other hepatically metabolized drugs. Not recommended to combine with ASA 325 mg (↑ antiplatelet effect). | $$$$ |
| *ticlopidine* Ticlid | 250 mg BID | Ticlopidine: diarrhea, skin rash, neutropenia; contraindicated in severe hepatic impairment. | Ticlopidine: ↑ half-life of hepatically metabolized drugs, ↓ digoxin levels, ↑ theophylline levels. Absorption ↓ by antacids. | $$$ |
| *dipyridamole 200 mg sustained-release/ASA 25 mg immediate release* Aggrenox | 1 capsule BID | Headache, diarrhea | | $$$ |

* *Cost of 30-day supply – includes drug cost only.*
*Legend:* *$ < $20* *$$ $20–40* *$$$ $40–60* *$$$$ $60–80*

† *Duration of therapy 5 to 10 days.*

scan is mandatory before initiating IV heparin for acute cerebral ischemia. The dose should be weight based and adjusted according to APTT (Table 1).

### ❑ *Warfarin or Nicoumalone*

Oral anticoagulants are efficacious in preventing cerebral and systemic emboli in acute MI, in valvular and nonvalvular atrial fibrillation and in patients with prosthetic cardiac valves. The risk of bleeding is influenced by many factors (e.g., the intensity of anticoagulation, and concomitant use of high doses of ASA/other drugs with antiplatelet effects).

### ❑ *Low Molecular Weight Heparins (LMWH)*

LMWHs have an antithrombotic effect equivalent to standard heparin but tend to produce less bleeding. Although positive results were reported in acute ischemic stroke with **nadroparin,** a recent randomized trial failed to confirm the initial results.

## Therapeutic Tips

- In most cases antithrombotic treatment should be continued long term, especially in older individuals with atherosclerosis and vascular risk factors.
- If a patient experiences recurrent attacks of cerebral ischemia with a relatively low dose of ASA (i.e., 325 mg per day or less), consideration should be given to using clopidogrel or combination ASA/dipyridamole SR.
- Combination therapy (oral anticoagulant plus ASA 100 mg per day) has been shown to be superior to anticoagulant alone in patients with prosthetic heart valves but with an increased risk of minor bleeding episodes. For patients intolerant of ASA, dipyridamole (225 mg per day) plus an oral anticoagulant may be used.
- Patients with carotid symptoms, ipsilateral to a significant ($\geq$ 70%) carotid stenosis documented by angiography, should be considered for carotid endarterectomy in addition to long-term antiplatelet therapy.

### *Suggested Reading List*

Antiplatelet Trialists' Collaboration. Collaborative overview of randomised trials of antiplatelet therapy–I: Prevention of death, myocardial infarction, and stroke by prolonged antiplatelet therapy in various categories of patients. *BMJ* 1994;308:81–106.

Barnett HJM, Eliasziw M, Meldrum HE. Drugs and surgery in the prevention of ischemic stroke. *N Engl J Med* 1995;332:238–248.

Gorelick PB, Born GVR, D'Agostino RB, et al. Therapeutic benefit. Aspirin revisited in light of the introduction of clopidogrel. *Stroke* 1999;30:1716–1721.

CHAPTER 23

# Hypertension

*S. George Carruthers, MD, FRCP, FACP, FRCPC*

## Goals of Therapy

- To decrease morbidity and mortality attributable to high blood pressure, particularly from stroke, cardiovascular disease, kidney disease
- To provide patients with effective, well-tolerated and convenient treatment that does not diminish quality of life

## Investigations

- Office blood pressure (BP) recordings on at least 3 separate occasions[1]
- Thorough history including: family history of hypertension, heart disease and stroke; personal history of diabetes, cardiovascular disease
- Physical examination focusing on evidence of arterial or arteriolar disease (e.g., diminished pulses, carotid or abdominal bruits, abdominal aneurysm, retinal vascular tortuosity or narrowing)
- Laboratory tests:
  – CBC, urea, creatinine, electrolytes
  – routine urinalysis (in diabetics check for microalbuminuria)
  – total cholesterol, LDL- and HDL-cholesterol
  – ECG

*Note:* Routine echocardiography, carotid ultrasound, ankle to arm index, home BP monitoring or ambulatory BP monitoring is not recommended but may be useful in selected patients.

- Special investigations for secondary hypertension as indicated (e.g., radionuclide renogram, captopril test, digitized renal arteriography for suspected renal artery stenosis; plasma and urinary catecholamines, CT scan, MRI for adrenal medullary and cortical tumors)

[1] *Refer to Can Med Assoc J 1999;161:S1–S22 for detailed description of correct procedure for measuring blood pressure.*

Figure 1: **Pharmacologic Treatment of Hypertension**

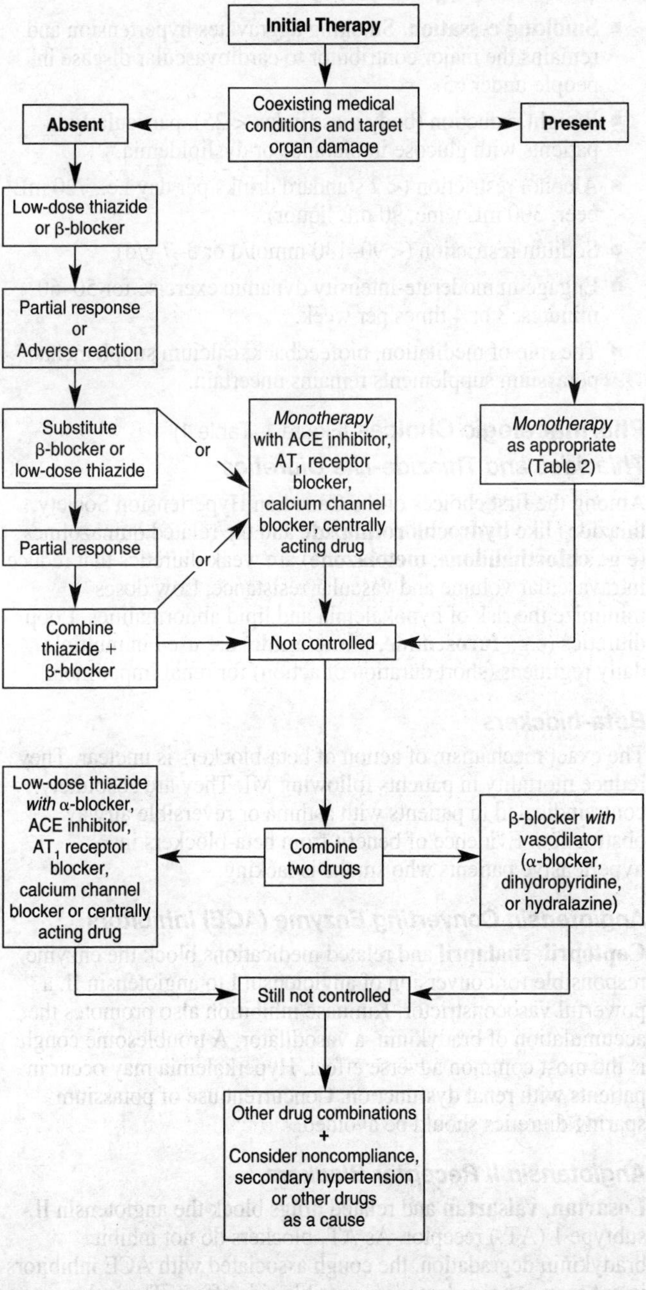
Initial Therapy
Coexisting medical conditions and target organ damage
Absent
Present
Low-dose thiazide or β-blocker
Partial response or Adverse reaction
Substitute β-blocker or low-dose thiazide
or
Monotherapy with ACE inhibitor, AT1 receptor blocker, calcium channel blocker, centrally acting drug
Monotherapy as appropriate (Table 2)
Partial response
or
Combine thiazide + β-blocker
Not controlled
Low-dose thiazide with α-blocker, ACE inhibitor, AT1 receptor blocker, calcium channel blocker or centrally acting drug
Combine two drugs
β-blocker with vasodilator (α-blocker, dihydropyridine, or hydralazine)
Still not controlled
Other drug combinations + Consider noncompliance, secondary hypertension or other drugs as a cause

*Adapted with permission from Ogilvie RI, et al. Report of the Canadian Hypertension Society Consensus Conference: 3. Pharmacologic treatment of essential hypertension. Can Med Assoc J 1993;149:575–584.*

## Therapeutic Choices

### Nonpharmacologic Choices

- **Smoking cessation.** Smoking aggravates hypertension and remains the major contributor to cardiovascular disease in people under 65.
- Weight reduction (body mass index < 25), particularly in patients with glucose intolerance or dyslipidemia.
- Alcohol restriction (< 2 standard drinks per day i.e., 720 mL beer, 300 mL wine, 90 mL liquor).
- Sodium restriction (< 90–130 mmol/d or 3–7 g/d).
- Engage in moderate-intensity dynamic exercise for 50–60 minutes, 3 or 4 times per week.
- The role of meditation, biofeedback, calcium supplements, potassium supplements remains uncertain.

### Pharmacologic Choices (Figure 1, Table 1)

#### *Thiazides and Thiazide-like Diuretics*

Among the first choices of the Canadian Hypertension Society, thiazides like **hydrochlorothiazide** and the related quinazolines (e.g., **chlorthalidone**, **metolazone**) are weak diuretics that reduce intravascular volume and vascular resistance. Low doses minimize the risk of hypokalemia and lipid abnormalities. Loop diuretics (e.g., **furosemide**, **bumetanide**) are used in multiple daily regimens (short duration of action) for renal impairment.

#### *Beta-blockers*

The exact mechanism of action of beta-blockers is unclear. They reduce mortality in patients following MI. They are absolutely contraindicated in patients with asthma or reversible airway obstruction. Evidence of benefit from beta-blockers in hypertensive patients who smoke is lacking.

#### *Angiotensin Converting Enzyme (ACE) Inhibitors*

**Captopril**, **enalapril** and related medications block the enzyme responsible for conversion of angiotensin I to angiotensin II, a powerful vasoconstrictor. Kininase inhibition also promotes the accumulation of bradykinin, a vasodilator. A troublesome cough is the most common adverse effect. Hyperkalemia may occur in patients with renal dysfunction. Concurrent use of potassium-sparing diuretics should be avoided.

#### *Angiotensin II Receptor Blockers*

**Losartan**, **valsartan** and related drugs block the angiotensin II, subtype 1 ($AT_1$) receptor. As $AT_1$ blockers do not inhibit bradykinin degradation, the cough associated with ACE inhibitors is not seen. Angioedema is a possible side effect. These drugs are useful alone or in combination therapy. Long-term effects on morbidity and mortality are unknown.

Table 1: **Commonly Used Antihypertensive Drugs**

| | Daily Dose | | |
|---|---|---|---|
| | **Starting** | **Full** | **Cost*** |
| **Thiazide Diuretics** | | | |
| chlorthalidone (Hygroton, generics) | 12.5 mg | 25 mg | $ |
| hydrochlorothiazide (HydroDiuril, generics) | 12.5 mg | 50 mg | $ |
| indapamide (Lozide, generics) | 2.5 mg | 2.5 mg | $ |
| metolazone (Zaroxolyn) | 2.5 mg | 5 mg | $ |
| **β-blockers** | | | |
| acebutolol (Monitan, Sectral) [ISA] | 200 mg | 800 mg | $$ |
| atenolol (Tenormin, generics) | 25 mg | 100 mg | $ |
| bisoprolol (Monocor) | 2.5 mg | 20 mg | $$ |
| labetalol (Trandate) | 200 mg | 1 200 mg | $$$$ |
| metoprolol (Lopresor, Betaloc, generics) | 50 mg | 200 mg | $ |
| nadolol (Corgard, generics) | 20 mg | 160 mg | $ |
| oxprenolol (Trasicor) [ISA] | 80 mg | 320 mg | $$$ |
| pindolol (Visken, generics) [ISA] | 10 mg | 30 mg | $$ |
| propranolol (Inderal, generics) | 80 mg | 320 mg | $ |
| timolol (Blocadren, generics) | 10 mg | 40 mg | $$ |
| **ACE Inhibitors** | | | |
| benazepril (Lotensin) | 10 mg | 40 mg | $$$ |
| captopril (Capoten, generics) | 25 mg | 100 mg | $$ |
| cilazapril (Inhibace) | 2.5 mg | 10 mg | $$$ |
| enalapril (Vasotec, generics) | 5 mg | 20 mg | $$ |
| fosinopril (Monopril) | 10 mg | 40 mg | $$$ |
| lisinopril (Prinivil, Zestril, generics) | 5 mg | 20 mg | $$ |
| perindopril (Coversyl) | 4 mg | 8 mg | $$$ |
| quinapril (Accupril) | 10 mg | 40 mg | $$ |
| ramipril (Altace) | 2.5 mg | 10 mg | $$ |
| trandolapril (Mavik) | 1 mg | 4 mg | $$$ |
| **Angiotensin II Receptor Blockers** | | | |
| candesartan (Atacand) | 8 mg | 32 mg | $$$$ |
| irbesartan (Avapro) | 150 mg | 300 mg | $$$ |
| losartan (Cozaar) | 25 mg | 50 mg | $$ |
| telmisartan (Micardis) | 40 mg | 80 mg | $$ |
| valsartan (Diovan) | 80 mg | 160 mg | $$ |
| **Calcium Antagonists** | | | |
| amlodipine (Norvasc) [D][V] | 5 mg | 10 mg | $$$ |
| diltiazem (Cardizem, generics) | 120 mg | 360 mg | $$$$ |
| felodipine (Plendil, Renedil) [D][V] | 5 mg | 20 mg | $$$ |
| nicardipine (Cardene) [D][V] | 60 mg | 120 mg | $$$$ |
| nifedipine (Adalat, generics) [D][V] | 20 mg | 80 mg | $$$ |
| verapamil (Isoptin, generics) | 120 mg | 480 mg | $$$ |
| **Centrally Acting Drugs** | | | |
| clonidine (Catapres, generics) | 0.2 mg | 1.2 mg | $$$ |
| methyldopa (Aldomet, generics) | 500 mg | 2 000 mg | $ |
| **Reserpine** (Serpasil) | 0.1 mg | 0.25 mg | $ |
| **α-blockers** | | | |
| doxazosin (Cardura) | 1 mg | 8 mg | $$$ |
| prazosin (Minipress, generics) | 0.5 mg | 20 mg | $$ |
| terazosin (Hytrin, generics) | 1 mg | 10 mg | $$ |
| **Vasodilators** | | | |
| hydralazine (Apresoline, generics) | 50 mg | 200 mg | $$ |
| minoxidil (Loniten, generics) | 5 mg | 20 mg | $$$ |

*[D] Dihydropyridine [ISA] intrinsic sympathomimetic activity [V] vasodilator.*
*Doses in this table are intended only as a guide and may be adjusted according to individual physician and patient requirements.*
*Adapted with permission from Ogilvie RI, et al. Report of the Canadian Hypertension Society Consensus Conference: 3. Pharmacologic treatment of essential hypertension. Can Med Assoc J 1993;149:575–584.*
** Cost of 30-day supply of full dose of antihypertensive – includes drug cost only.*
*Legend: $ < $20 $$ $20–40 $$$ $40–60 $$$$ > $60*

### *Calcium Channel Blockers*

The earliest calcium channel blockers, **verapamil**, **nifedipine** and **diltiazem** are chemically unrelated and exert differing effects on vascular smooth muscle, cardiac myocytes and cardiac conducting tissues. All are effective antihypertensives. Side effects of nifedipine and related dihydropyridines reflect the predominant vasodilation of this group (i.e., flushing, palpitations, pedal edema). Verapamil may impair left ventricular function and cause heart block and should not be used with beta-blockers or negative inotropes (e.g., disopyramide). In larger doses constipation is common. Diltiazem's pharmacologic profile is intermediate to that of verapamil and nifedipine.

### *Centrally Acting Antihypertensives*

**Methyldopa** and **clonidine** exert central $alpha_2$-adrenergic agonist effects that reduce sympathetic drive to the peripheral vasculature. They have a minor role in the treatment of hypertension. Methyldopa is considered safe in pregnancy. The rebound hypertension associated with clonidine withdrawal limits its use, and it must be avoided in patients with poor compliance.

### *Peripheral Sympatholytics*

**Reserpine** appears safe and effective at very low doses but is associated with suicidal depression when used at higher doses.

### *Alpha-blockers*

**Prazosin, doxazosin** and **terazosin** lower BP without the tachycardia associated with the earlier nonselective alpha-blockers. To avoid the first-dose effect of hypotension and occasional syncope, starting doses should be small and given at bedtime. Monotherapy is not recommended.

### *Direct Vasodilators*

**Hydralazine** is out of favor because doses in excess of 200 mg daily are associated with an SLE-like syndrome. Reflex tachycardia and activation of the renin–angiotensin–aldosterone system can be controlled by concurrent beta-blocker or diuretic therapy. **Minoxidil** provokes hirsutism.

### *Combination Products*

Although there are many preparations combining thiazide diuretics with other antihypertensive agents, initiating therapy with these fixed-dose combinations is not recommended. Individual agents should be titrated to effective dosages; once doses have been stabilized, the clinician may then prescribe the combination best suited to the needs of the patient.

## Hypertension with Concurrent Disorders

(Table 2)

Table 2: **Therapeutic Choices for Hypertension with Concurrent Disorders**

| Condition or Risk Factor | Recommended Drugs | Alternative Drugs | Not Recommended |
|---|---|---|---|
| **Ischemic Heart Disease** | | | |
| Angina | β-blockers | Long-acting CCB | Short-acting CCB |
| Recent MI | β-blockers or ACEI or both | CCB (verapamil and diltiazem) if LV function not severely impaired. | Dihydropyridine CCB |
| **Congestive Heart Failure** | ACEI, diuretics | Hydralazine + ISDN.<br>Angiotensin II receptor blocker.<br>Carvedilol or metoprolol<br>Amlodipine or felodipine | |
| **Peripheral Vascular Disease** | | | |
| Raynaud's phenomenon, severe disease | Vasodilators i.e., α-blockers, CCB, ACEI, Angiotensin II receptor antagonists. | | β-blockers in severe disease. |
| Mild disease | Diuretics, ACEI, α-blockers | β-blockers, verapamil | ACEI if underlying renal artery stenosis. |
| **Dyslipidemia** | ACEI, β-blockers with ISA, α-blockers, CCB, centrally acting drugs | Low-dose thiazides. | High-dose thiazides, β-blockers without ISA. |

*(cont'd)*

Table 2: **Therapeutic Choices for Hypertension with Concurrent Disorders** *(cont'd)*

| Condition or Risk Factor | Recommended Drugs | Alternative Drugs | Not Recommended |
|---|---|---|---|
| **Diabetes Mellitus** | ACEI, β-blocker (cardioselective), thiazides | Angiotensin II receptor blockers, long-acting CCBs, centrally acting agents or vasodilators if others contraindicated. | High-dose thiazides. |
| **Asthma** | $K^+$-sparing + thiazide diuretic for patients on salbutamol | | β-blockers. |
| **Gout** | | | Thiazides, but asymptomatic hyperuricemia is not a contraindication. |
| **Pregnancy** | Methyldopa, clonidine, hydralazine, β-blockers | | ACEI, CCB, angiotensin II receptor blockers. |
| **Black Patients** | Low-dose thiazides, CCB | β-blockers, ACEI, angiotensin II receptor antagonists are less effective. | Greater risk of angioedema with ACEI and angiotension II receptor blockers. |

*Abbreviations: + = combined with; ISA = intrinsic sympathomimetic activity; CCB = calcium channel blocker; ACEI = ACE inhibitor; ISDN = isosorbide dinitrate.*

## Managing Severe Hypertension

The most severe forms of hypertension are defined as those in excess of 179 mm Hg systolic and/or 109 mm Hg diastolic.

Hypertension requiring treatment as an urgency or emergency is usually in excess of 200 mm Hg systolic and 120 mm Hg diastolic. The manifestations of these very high pressures may be modified by the age of the patient, the rate of increase of BP, duration of elevated BP and comorbidity such as pre-existent renal disease, abdominal aortic aneurysm, berry aneurysm, coronary artery disease or left ventricular dysfunction.

Many terms have been used to describe extremely high BP. One of the oldest and now least used is the term "malignant" hypertension, reflecting the very poor prognosis associated with papilledema of the ocular fundus (Grade IV, Keith-Wagener-Barker).

Severe hypertension may be triaged into 3 groupings in order of descending severity and risk to the patient, namely *True Emergencies, Urgencies, Pseudo Emergencies* (Figure 2).

*Some "dos" and "don'ts" of managing True Emergencies.*

- Hospitalize, monitor appropriately in ICU, CCU setting
- Choose medications likely to reduce BP, improve hemodynamics and improve or prevent worsening of complications
- Avoid medications likely to aggravate hemodynamics (↑ HR, ↑ pulse pressure, ↑ oxygen consumption, $Na^+/H_2O$ retention). Corollary: if these medications must be used to lower BP, consider using another medication that will blunt or obliterate the undesirable action, e.g., beta-blocker with hydralazine; loop diuretic with minoxidil
- Do not attempt to reduce BP to "normal" and certainly not quickly. Aim instead to lower BP gradually (over 2–6 hrs) to an acceptable level of 160–180 mm Hg systolic or 100–110 mm Hg diastolic. (A figure of ≤25% reduction of mean arterial pressure is often quoted and results in similar numbers, e.g., 230/140 or a mean BP of 170 mm Hg, reduced to mean of about 130 or 170/110 mm Hg)
- Choose treatments over which you have good control, i.e., short acting medications given by the IV route
- During the critical first 4–6 hours, monitor BP and clinical status frequently, in particular CNS, mental status, volume status, renal function, ECG and heart rate
- Start an oral regimen promptly, especially if the patient had previous oral therapy that was discontinued inappropriately e.g., clonidine

Figure 2: **Management of Severe Hypertension**

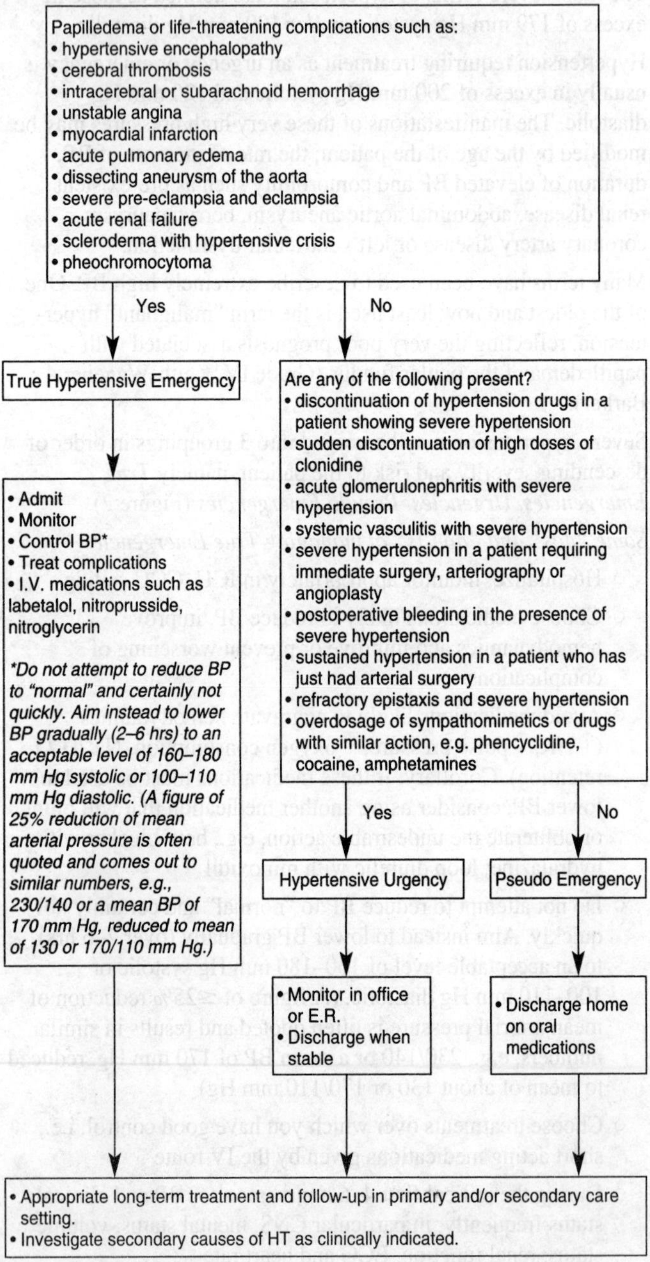
Papilledema or life-threatening complications such as:
• hypertensive encephalopathy
• cerebral thrombosis
• intracerebral or subarachnoid hemorrhage
• unstable angina
• myocardial infarction
• acute pulmonary edema
• dissecting aneurysm of the aorta
• severe pre-eclampsia and eclampsia
• acute renal failure
• scleroderma with hypertensive crisis
• pheochromocytoma
Yes
No
True Hypertensive Emergency
• Admit
• Monitor
• Control BP*
• Treat complications
• I.V. medications such as labetalol, nitroprusside, nitroglycerin
*Do not attempt to reduce BP to "normal" and certainly not quickly. Aim instead to lower BP gradually (2–6 hrs) to an acceptable level of 160–180 mm Hg systolic or 100–110 mm Hg diastolic. (A figure of 25% reduction of mean arterial pressure is often quoted and comes out to similar numbers, e.g., 230/140 or a mean BP of 170 mm Hg, reduced to mean of 130 or 170/110 mm Hg.)
Are any of the following present?
• discontinuation of hypertension drugs in a patient showing severe hypertension
• sudden discontinuation of high doses of clonidine
• acute glomerulonephritis with severe hypertension
• systemic vasculitis with severe hypertension
• severe hypertension in a patient requiring immediate surgery, arteriography or angioplasty
• postoperative bleeding in the presence of severe hypertension
• sustained hypertension in a patient who has just had arterial surgery
• refractory epistaxis and severe hypertension
• overdosage of sympathomimetics or drugs with similar action, e.g. phencyclidine, cocaine, amphetamines
Yes
No
Hypertensive Urgency
Pseudo Emergency
• Monitor in office or E.R.
• Discharge when stable
• Discharge home on oral medications
• Appropriate long-term treatment and follow-up in primary and/or secondary care setting.
• Investigate secondary causes of HT as clinically indicated.

*Adapted from Lebel M. Hypertensive Emergency—or Urgency? Canadian Journal of CME 1998;10(7):73–81.*

- In the case of pre-eclampsia and eclampsia, early delivery must be considered a priority
- Keep an open mind for secondary causes of hypertension such has pheochromocytoma. While the majority of hypertensive crises occur in the much more common primary hypertension, there will be a disproportionate number of secondary forms in this group of patients
- Do *not* use nifedipine liquid capsules to lower BP. You have no control over the outcome of a therapy that can cause precipitous falls in BP and jeopardize cardiac and cerebral blood flows

## Therapeutic Tips

- Consider the patient's age, gender, race, other medical conditions and concurrent medications.
- Start with a low dose of a diuretic or beta-blocker, unless contraindicated.
- Try to achieve BP control with the lowest possible dose of a single medication.
- Consider medications that are of value for other medical conditions (e.g., beta-blockers after MI, ACE inhibitors in symptomatic heart failure).
- Avoid medications likely to aggravate a coexisting disorder (e.g., thiazides with gout, beta-blockers with asthma).
- Unless there are compelling reasons to reduce BP quickly, pressure should be brought to target values (< 140 mm Hg systolic and < 90 mm Hg diastolic) over 3 to 6 months.
- Consider an angiotensin II receptor blocker if ACE inhibitor-induced cough is a problem.
- Combination therapy will be necessary when monotherapy is unsuccessful.
- The patient may assist in BP management by monitoring BP at home and work.
- Consider cost-effectiveness of treatment.
- When treatment is ineffective, consider poor compliance. Consider also excessive salt or alcohol consumption, interfering medications such as NSAIDs and secondary causes of hypertension.
- When BP control is lost in an older patient, consider atherosclerotic renal artery stenosis.
- Consider reducing therapy when BP is controlled and stable for at least 1 year.
- Long-term follow-up is essential, even when therapy is reduced and especially if there is a trial of discontinuation of therapy.

## Pharmacoeconomic Considerations

*Jeffrey A. Johnson, PhD*

Costs of antihypertensive therapy include drug acquisition costs, routine physician visits, care of complications such as stroke and MI and laboratory monitoring. It is important to consider these "downstream" costs for all therapeutic choices. For example, inexpensive diuretics may require more expensive laboratory monitoring. Although drug costs vary considerably, from pennies per day for thiazides to $1-$2 per day for newer agents, the evidence that less expensive medications are more cost-effective is not particularly robust. Because of the limitations to available cost-effectiveness analyses, clinical experience and current treatment guidelines should guide choice of antihypertensive agent in any one patient.

The latest Canadian recommendations for the management of hypertension support the use of newer antihypertensive agents as they have similar overall outcomes compared to older traditional agents. Cost-effectiveness of antihypertensive agents varies according to risk as the benefit of treatment is dependent on severity of hypertension, concurrent risk factors, age and gender. The greatest value will be seen in older patients and those with multiple cardiovascular risk factors. Economic evaluations of the United Kingdom Prospective Diabetes Study have also indicated that intensive intervention for the management of high blood pressure in patients with diabetes is cost-effective.

***Suggested Reading***

*Feldman RD, Campbell N, Larochelle P, et al. 1999 Canadian recommendations for the management of hypertension. CMAJ 1999;161 (12, Suppl.):S1–S17.*

*Pardell H, Tresserras R, Armario P, Hernandez del Rey R. Pharmacoeconomic considerations in the management of hypertension. Drugs 2000;59 (Suppl. 2):13–20.*

*UK Prospective Diabetes Study Group. Cost-effectiveness analysis of improved blood pressure control in hypertensive patients with type 2 diabetes: UKPDS 40, BMJ 1998;317:720–726.*

## Suggested Reading List

1999 Canadian recommendations for the management of hypertension. *Can Med Assoc J* 1999;161:S1–S22.

Chalmers J, World Health Organization—International Society of Hypertension Guidelines Committee. 1999 World Health Organization—International Society of Hypertension Guidelines for the management of hypertension. J Hypertens 1999;17:151–185.

Lifestyle modifications to prevent and control hypertension. *Can Med Assoc J* 1999;160:S1–S50.

The Sixth Report of the Joint National Committee on Detection, Evaluation and Treatment of Hypertension. *Arch Intern Med* 1997;157:2413–2446.

CHAPTER 24

# Dyslipidemias

*Ghislaine O. Roederer, MD, PhD*

## Goals of Therapy

- To reduce cardiovascular disease (CVD)
- To prevent pancreatitis (from severe hypertriglyceridemia)

## Investigations

- Medical history with attention to CVD (past or present), major cardiovascular risk factors (Figure 1 and Table 1) and possible causes of secondary hyperlipidemia (Table 2)
- Family history:
  - premature CVD (before age 45 in males, age 55 in females) in first-degree relatives
  - hyperlipidemia
- Physical examination:
  - weight
  - bilateral brachial blood pressure
  - arcus corneae (especially in the young patient)
  - funduscopy (lipemia retinalis, retinopathies)
  - peripheral pulses
  - cardiac auscultation
  - arterial bruits
  - hepatosplenomegaly
  - lipid deposits (xanthomas)
- Laboratory tests: lipid and lipoprotein levels[1]
  - use the same laboratory for repeated measurements
  - a 12-hour fast is required for triglyceride levels
  - for initial diagnosis of the dyslipidemic phenotype, obtain 2 or 3 measurements at 4- to 6-week intervals to establish a baseline. At least 1 measurement should include a lipoprotein profile (high-density lipoprotein cholesterol [HDL-C], low-density lipoprotein cholesterol [LDL-C])
  - other lab investigations to rule out frequent causes of secondary dyslipidemias (Table 2)

## Classification of Dyslipidemias

*Primary (genetic) vs secondary dyslipidemias:* Possible causes for secondary dyslipidemia must be sought and addressed directly if

[1] ***Note:*** *The Friedwald equation routinely used to calculate LDL-C values (all units mmol/L)* ***LDL-C = TOTAL-C − (HDL-C + TRG/2.2) cannot*** *be used if triglyceride levels > 4.52 mmol/L or if dealing with type III dysbetalipoproteinemia.*

Figure 1: **Management of Dyslipidemia***

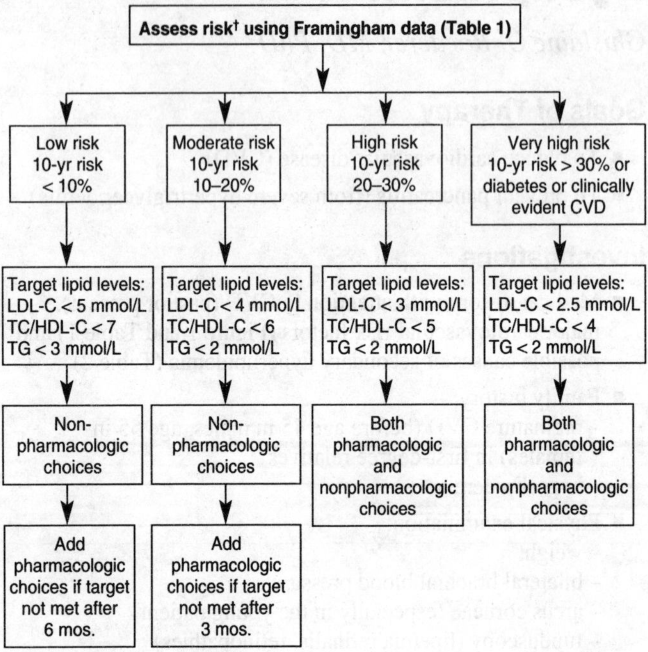
Assess risk† using Framingham data (Table 1)
Low risk 10-yr risk < 10%
Moderate risk 10-yr risk 10–20%
High risk 10-yr risk 20–30%
Very high risk 10-yr risk > 30% or diabetes or clinically evident CVD
Target lipid levels: LDL-C < 5 mmol/L TC/HDL-C < 7 TG < 3 mmol/L
Target lipid levels: LDL-C < 4 mmol/L TC/HDL-C < 6 TG < 2 mmol/L
Target lipid levels: LDL-C < 3 mmol/L TC/HDL-C < 5 TG < 2 mmol/L
Target lipid levels: LDL-C < 2.5 mmol/L TC/HDL-C < 4 TG < 2 mmol/L
Non-pharmacologic choices
Non-pharmacologic choices
Both pharmacologic and nonpharmacologic choices
Both pharmacologic and nonpharmacologic choices
Add pharmacologic choices if target not met after 6 mos.
Add pharmacologic choices if target not met after 3 mos.

* *CMAJ 2000;162:1441–1447.*

† Positive Risk Factors:
*male ≥ 40 yrs, female ≥ 45 yrs; cigarette smoking; systolic blood pressure > 130 mm Hg; diabetes mellitus; low HDL-C (< 0.9 mmol/L). (**Note:** High HDL-C (≥ 1.6 mmol/L) is considered a **negative** (i.e., protective) risk factor for CVD); TC ≥ 5.18 mmol/L*

*Abbreviations: TC = total cholesterol; TG = triglycerides.*

present. If secondary dyslipidemia persists despite proper management of the underlying disease and constitutes an additional risk factor for the condition, then lipid-lowering treatment becomes mandatory (e.g., diabetic dyslipidemia).

- Primary dyslipidemias carrying a *risk for CVD* are (in decreasing order of risk):
  - *heterozygous familial hypercholesterolemia* (hzFH) – associated with severe hypercholesterolemia (LDL-C), premature atherosclerosis and characteristic xanthomas. When diagnosed, family screening (including children) is recommended for early prevention and treatment.
  - *familial combined hyperlipidemia* (FCH) – associated with premature atherosclerosis and characterized by elevated cholesterol and/or triglyceride levels; however, in time, affected persons may display various lipoprotein phenotypes.

– *type III dysbetalipoproteinemia* – associated with coronary and peripheral vascular disease, pathognomonic xanthomas and almost exclusively an E2/E2 phenotype.

- Primary dyslipidemias carrying a *risk for pancreatitis* are (in decreasing order of risk):
  – *familial hyperchylomicronemia* – lipid-lowering drugs are not effective; a strict fat-poor diet (< 10% fat) is the cornerstone of treatment.

Table 1: **Calculation of 10-year risk of Coronary Heart Disease in a Patient Without Diabetes Mellitus or Clinically Evident CVD***

**Part I: Global Risk Assessment Scoring**

| **Risk Factor** | **Men** | **Women** | **Score** |
|---|---|---|---|
| **Age (years)** | | | |
| < 34 | –1 | –9 | |
| 35 – 39 | 0 | –4 | |
| 40 – 44 | 1 | 0 | |
| 45 – 49 | 2 | 3 | |
| 50 – 54 | 3 | 6 | ____ |
| 55 – 59 | 4 | 7 | |
| 60 – 64 | 5 | 8 | |
| 65 – 69 | 6 | 8 | |
| 70 – 74 | 7 | 8 | |
| **Total cholesterol (mmol/L)** | | | |
| < 4.14 | –3 | –2 | |
| 4.15 – 5.17 | 0 | 0 | |
| 5.18 – 6.21 | 1 | 1 | ____ |
| 6.22 – 7.24 | 2 | 2 | |
| ≥ 7.25 | 3 | 3 | |
| **HDL cholesterol (mmol/L)** | | | |
| < 0.90 | 2 | 5 | |
| 0.91 – 1.16 | 1 | 2 | |
| 1.17 – 1.29 | 0 | 1 | ____ |
| 1.30 – 1.55 | 0 | 0 | |
| ≥ 1.56 | –2 | –3 | |
| **Systolic blood pressure (mmHg)** | | | |
| < 120 | 0 | –3 | |
| 120 – 129 | 0 | 0 | |
| 130 – 139 | 1 | 1 | ____ |
| 140 – 159 | 2 | 2 | |
| ≥ 160 | 3 | 3 | |
| **Smoker** | | | |
| No | 0 | 0 | ____ |
| Yes | 2 | 2 | |
| | | **TOTAL RISK POINTS** | ☐ |

**Part II: Calculate 10-year absolute risk for total CVD end points estimated from Framingham data**

| **Risk Points** | | 1 | 2 | 3 | 4 | 5 | 6 | 7 | 8 | 9 | 10 | 11 | 12 | 13 | 14 | 15 | 16 | 17 |
|---|---|---|---|---|---|---|---|---|---|---|---|---|---|---|---|---|---|---|
| **CVD Risk** | Men | 3% | 4% | 5% | 7% | 8% | 10% | 13% | 16% | 20% | 25% | 31% | 37% | 45% | ≥53% | | | |
| | Women | 2% | 3% | 3% | 4% | 4% | 5% | 6% | 7% | 8% | 10% | 11% | 13% | 15% | 18% | 20% | 24% | >27% |

* *CMAJ 2000;162:1441–1447.*

Table 2: **Common Causes of Secondary Hyperlipidemia**

| | |
|---|---|
| Hypothyroidism | Medication: |
| Pregnancy | Thiazide diuretics |
| Excess weight | β-blockers without intrinsic sympathomimetic or alpha blocking activity |
| Alcohol excess | Oral contraceptives |
| Obstructive liver disease | Hormone replacement therapy |
| Nephrotic syndrome | Corticosteroids |

– *familial hypertriglyceridemia* (FHTG) – with a type V phenotype.

*Phenotypic expression* (the description of the lipoprotein anomaly, Table 3) provides no information about the etiology of the disorder. However, proper recognition of the phenotype will provide guidance as to which medication to use.

## Criteria for Intervention

Current recommendations from the Canadian Working Group on Hypercholesterolemia and Other Dyslipidemias[2] include *clinical status* (primary vs secondary prevention), *risk factors* and *HDL-C levels* in the decision tree (Figure 1). Triglycerides may also have an atherogenic role.[3] High triglyceride levels (2.3 to 11.3 mmol/L) are an additional cardiovascular risk factor when associated with atherogenic dyslipidemias (e.g., FCH, insulin resistance, diabetes, renal insufficiency). Individuals with triglycerides in the very high range (> 11.3 mmol/L) are at increased risk for pancreatitis.

Table 3: **Classification of Dyslipidemia Phenotypes***

| | Lipoproteins | | | | Lipids | |
|---|---|---|---|---|---|---|
| **Phenotype** | **Chylomicrons** | **VLDL** | **IDL** | **LDL** | **Cholesterol** | **TG** |
| I | ↑↑ | | | | | ↑↑ |
| IIa | | | | ↑ | ↑ | |
| IIb | | ↑ | | ↑ | ↑ | ↑ |
| III | | | ↑ | | ↑ | ↑ |
| IV | | ↑ | | | | ↑ |
| V | ↑ | ↑ | | | | ↑↑ |

** Fredrickson-Levy classification, based on electrophoretic data.*
*Abbreviations: VLDL = very-low-density lipoproteins; TG = triglycerides; IDL = intermediate-density lipoproteins; LDL = low-density lipoproteins.*

[2] *CMAJ 2000;162:1441–1447.*
[3] *Am J Cardiol 1992;70:19H–25H.*

Table 4: **Dietary Interventions**

| **Step I (Primary Prevention) (patients with no previous CVD)** | **Step II (Secondary Prevention)* (patients with prior CVD/ atherosclerotic disease)** |
|---|---|
| ↓ dietary cholesterol intake to < 300 mg/d | ↓ dietary cholesterol intake to < 200 mg/d |
| Restrict fat intake to 30% of calories | Restrict fat intake to 20% of calories |
| Distribute fat intake equally between saturated, polyunsaturated and monosaturated fats | 7% of daily calories as saturated fat |
| Favor high-fiber intake | |
| Limit simple sugars to 8% of total calories | |
| Limit alcohol consumption to 5% of total calories | |

* *The help of a dietitian is usually required to reach and maintain these goals.*

## Therapeutic Choices (Figure 1)

### Nonpharmacologic Choices

- **Diet**, aimed at reducing blood lipid levels and weight (if needed), should *always* be the first approach to treating all dyslipidemias. A 6-month dietary trial (Table 4) is mandatory before considering medication; during this time, 2 (ideally 3) lipid and lipoprotein measurements should be taken.
- **Increased physical activity** may help decrease cholesterol and triglyceride levels while increasing HDL.
- **Other lifestyle changes** that reduce the risk of CVD (e.g., weight loss, smoking cessation) should be encouraged.

### Pharmacologic Choices (Table 5)

#### *Resins*

The bile-acid-sequestering resins **cholestyramine** and **colestipol** reduce plasma LDL and can slightly increase HDL levels. They have a strong safety record. Resins are the only lipid-lowering agents appropriate for use in children (> 2 years) or in pregnant or lactating women. Some recommend concurrent supplementation with fat soluble vitamins.

#### *HMG CoA Reductase Inhibitors (Statins)*

HMG CoA reductase inhibitors, the most potent LDL-lowering agents, interfere with the atherosclerotic disease process.[4] Significant reductions in CVD morbidity, CVD mortality and

[4] *N Engl J Med 1997;336:153–162.*

Table 5: **Lipid-lowering Agents**

| Drug | Dosage | Effect on Lipoproteins LDL | HDL | TG | Adverse Effects | Comments | Cost* |
|---|---|---|---|---|---|---|---|
| **Resins** | Given daily to TID, AC | ↓↓ | ↑ | ↑ | Constipation, bloating, abdominal fullness, flatulence, ↑ triglycerides, ↑ transaminases (reversible). | Administer 1 h before or 4 h after concurrent medications due to possible adsorption of anionic molecules in the GI tract. Recommend high-fiber diet to ↓ constipation. | |
| *cholestyramine* Questran, Questran Light, generics | 4–24 g/d | | | | | | $–$$$$$ |
| *colestipol* Colestid | 5–30 g/d | | | | | Monitor liver function and triglycerides. Colestipol is available as 5 g powder packets or 1 g caplets. | $$–$$$$$ |
| **HMG CoA Reductase Inhibitors** | Usually given as a single daily dose: | ↓↓↓ | ↑ | ↓↔ | Mild upper GI disturbances, myalgias, sleep disturbances, ↑ CPK, ↑ transaminases (reversible). | All: Monitor liver function and CK at 3, 6, 12 mos then yearly. | |
| *lovastatin* Mevacor, generics | 10–40 mg with evening meal, up to 80 mg/d (40 mg BID) | | | | | Extreme caution if combination therapy with fibrates, erythromycin, cyclosporine or niacin (↑ risk of hepatotoxicity, myopathy/myositis); start with low doses. | $–$$$$$ |
| *simvastatin* Zocor | 5–40 mg with evening meal | | | | | Excellent safety profile. | $$–$$$$ |
| *pravastatin* Pravachol | 10–80 mg QHS | | | | | | $$$–$$$$ |
| *fluvastatin* Lescol | 20–80 mg with evening meal | | | | | | $$–$$$$ |
| *atorvastatin* Lipitor | 10–80 mg at any time | | | (↓↓) | | At doses ≥ 40 mg, atorvastatin has greater TG lowering effect than other statins. | $$–$$$$$ |
| *cerivastatin* Baycol | 0.2–0.3 mg in the evening | | | | | | $$–$$$ |

| | | | | | | | |
|---|---|---|---|---|---|---|---|
| **Niacin (Nicotinic Acid)** generics (regular and slow-release formulations) | Regular: 1.5–6 g/d divided TID, PC<br>Slow release (not recommended): 0.5–2 g/d divided BID, PC | ↓↓ | ↑↑ | ↓↓ | Hot flushes and pruritus (symptoms of vasodilation which abate with time), dry skin, acanthosis nigricans (reversible), reactivation of peptic ulcer, GI disturbances.<br>Severe hepatotoxicity may occur (more frequent with slow-release formulation).<br>↑ blood glucose, uric acid, transaminases. | Greatest HDL-raising effect.<br>Monitor blood glucose, uric acid, transaminases at 3, 6, 12 mos then yearly.<br>Avoid in diabetic patients.<br>Caution if using in combination with statins (potential hepatotoxicity).<br>Reassure and instruct the patient of the following: ↑ medication stepwise (start with 50 mg TID; double dose Q5d to 1.5–2 g/d. If tolerated, max. dose is 6 g/d) after meals. To reduce flushing: avoid hot drinks, hot showers, spicy food, alcohol for 1–2 h after a dose; low-dose ASA daily in the first few weeks of treatment may be helpful. Avoid missing a dose. | $–$$$ |
| **Fibrates** | | ↓↔↑ | ↑↑ | ↓↓↓ | Upper GI disturbances (nausea, abdominal pain, flatulence), myalgias, ↑ bile lithogenicity, ↑ CPK, occasionally ↑ creatinine. | Monitor CK, CBC, liver and renal function at 3, 6 and 12 mos then yearly.<br>May ↑ oral anticoagulant activity.<br>Caution when combining with statins.<br>Very useful in diabetic dyslipidemias. | |
| *clofibrate* Atromid-S, generics | 1–2 g/d divided BID | | | | | | $ |
| *gemfibrozil* Lopid, generics | 600–1200 mg/d divided BID | | | | | | $$$ |
| *fenofibrate* generics | 100 mg BID–QID with meals | | | | | | $$–$$$ |
| *fenofibrate micronized* Lipidil-Micro, generics | 200 mg/d (given once daily with largest meal) | | | | | | $$ |
| *bezafibrate* Bezalip (immediate-release, slow-release [SR] formulations), generics | 200 mg BID–TID<br>SR: 400 mg/d with evening meal | | | | | | $$–$$$ |

* *Cost of 30-day supply – includes drug cost only.*
*Legend: $ < $20 $$ $20–40 $$$ $40–60 $$$$ $60–80 $$$$$ > $80*

*Dosage adjustment may be required in renal impairment – see Appendix I.*

Table 6: **Dose vs Efficacy of HMG CoA Reductase Inhibitors**

| Drug | Dose | Efficacy | | |
|---|---|---|---|---|
| | | LDL | HDL | TG |
| **Lovastatin** | 20 mg | −24% | +7% | −10% |
| | 40 mg | −34% | +7% | −14% |
| | 80 mg | −40% | +9% | −16% |
| **Simvastatin** | 5 mg | −24% | +7% | −10% |
| | 10 mg | −28% | +7% | −10% |
| | 20 mg | −35% | +10% | −17% |
| | 40 mg | −41% | +13% | −19% |
| **Pravastatin** | 10 mg | −22% | | |
| | 20 mg | −32% | | |
| | 40 mg | −34% | +14% | −25% |
| **Fluvastatin** | 20 mg | −20% | +2% | −7% |
| | 40 mg | −25% | +7% | −10% |
| **Atorvastatin** | 10 mg | −39% | +6% | −19% |
| | 20 mg | −43% | +9% | −26% |
| | 40 mg | −50% | +6% | −29% |
| | 80 mg | −60% | +5% | −37% |
| **Cerivastatin** | 0.2 mg | −29% | +6% | −18% |
| | 0.3 mg | −33% | +8% | −25% |

*Abbreviations: LDL = low-density lipoproteins; HDL = high-density lipoproteins; TG = triglycerides.*

total deaths in both primary[5] and secondary[6] prevention have been associated with their use.

Effect on HDL is modest. Within the range of currently recommended dosages, atorvastatin has the greatest triglyceride-lowering effect (Table 6). Statins differ in their structure, pharmacokinetics, in vitro properties and efficacy; no dose-to-dose equivalence can be drawn among them.[7] Increasing the dose may result in further decrease in LDL.

### *Nicotinic Acid (Niacin)*

Niacin is a B vitamin that, at high doses, lowers triglycerides and LDL and raises HDL. The unpleasant side effects of niacin make patient compliance difficult, limiting its usefulness. Slow-release formulations appear to be more hepatotoxic than standard-release products.[8]

5 *N Engl J Med 1995;333:1301–1307.*
6 *Lancet 1994;344:1383–1389.*
7 *Am J Cardiol 1994;73:3D–11D.*
8 *JAMA 1994;271:672–677.*

### *Fibrates*

**Clofibrate, gemfibrozil, fenofibrate** and **bezafibrate** lower triglyceride levels and raise HDL. They are useful in diabetic dyslipidemia. The effect of fibrates on LDL is variable; third generation agents (e.g., bezafibrate, fenofibrate) show a more consistent LDL-lowering effect. The newer fibrates have supplanted clofibrate because of their better safety record and greater potency.

## Therapeutic Tips

- Lipid-lowering drugs must ***always*** be an adjunct, not a substitution, to diet therapy.
- Except for resins, lipid-lowering drugs should be avoided in children and pregnant or lactating women.
- Therapy should be maintained at the lowest dosage required to reach the desired effect.
- Different agents within the same class should be tried in cases of intolerance or lack of efficacy.
- Clinical and laboratory follow-up is essential to monitor lipid-lowering efficacy and adverse effects of therapy.
- Allow 3 months for plasma lipid stabilization after a coronary or other major medical event.
- Because some combination therapies carry an increased risk of drug toxicity, referral should be considered for such patients.

## Pharmacoeconomic Considerations

*Jeffrey A. Johnson, PhD*

A number of cost-effectiveness evaluations of statin medications have been carried out, including both modeling studies and economic evaluations based on clinical trials. Two economic evaluations of simvastatin therapy have been conducted using the results of the 4S study, one of which was specific for the Canadian context. The original cost-effectiveness analysis included both direct and indirect costs (Appendix III), and indicated that in patients with coronary heart disease, simvastatin therapy is cost-effective among both men and women at ages 35 to 70 years with total cholesterol levels prior to treatment of 5.5 to 8.0 mmol per litre. Data for secondary prevention of coronary artery disease in Canada also indicate that simvastatin is a cost-effective approach, with a cost-effectiveness ratio of $6108 to $9876 per year of life gained, depending on the length of time that the clinical benefits were assumed to accumulate.

A recent review of statin therapy from CCOHTA concluded that there is no clear evidence to indicate that one statin is any more or less cost-effective than another. Therefore, it is not clear whether the best strategy is to base treatment choice with cost-minimization (i.e., least expensive drug), or with clinical benefit (i.e., large clinical trial-based evidence) in mind.

It is clear that the greater the base-line risk of experiencing coronary events, the more cost-effective lipid-lowering therapy is. In pharmacoeconomic evaluations of lipid-lowering therapy, it has generally been concluded that secondary prevention is more cost-effective than primary prevention. Baseline risk plays a role in determining cost-effectiveness; as the risk of a coronary event increases (e.g., with higher baseline total cholesterol and LDL and/or lower HDL), the more cost-effective the lipid-lowering therapy will be.

***Suggested Reading***

*Johannesson M, Jonsson B, Kjekshus J, et al. Cost-effectiveness of simvastatin treatment to lower cholesterol levels in patients with coronary heart disease. N Engl J Med 1997;336:332–336.*

*Perras C, Baladi JF. HMG-CoA Reductase Inhibitors: a review of published clinical trials and pharmacoeconomic evaluations. CCOHTA Report 1997: 5E. Ottawa, ON: Canadian Coordinating Office for Health Technology Assessment (CCHOTA); 1997.*

*Riviere M, Wang S, Leclerc C, et al. Cost-effectiveness of simvastatin in the secondary prevention of coronary artery disease in Canada. Can Med Assoc J 1997;156:991–997.*

## *Suggested Reading List*

Expert Panel on Detection, Evaluation, and Treatment of High Blood Cholesterol in Adults. Summary of the Second Report of the National Cholesterol Education Program (NCEP) Expert Panel on Detection, Evaluation, and Treatment of High Blood Cholesterol in Adults (Adult Treatment Panel II). *JAMA* 1993;269:3015–3023.

Fodor JG, Frohlich JJ, Genest JJG, et al. for the Working Group on Hypercholesterolemia and other Dyslipidemias. Recommendations for the management and treatment of dyslipidemia. *CMAJ* 2000;162:1441–1447.

Jialal I. A practical approach to the laboratory diagnosis of dyslipidemia. *Am J Clin Pathol* 1996;106:128–138.

Knopp RH. Drug treatment of lipid disorders. *N Engl J Med* 1999;341:498–511.

Grundy SM. Atherogenic dyslipidemia: lipoprotein abnormalities and implications for therapy. *Am J Cardiol* 1995;75: 45B–52B.

Schectman G, Hiatt J: Dose-response characteristics of cholesterol-lowering drug therapies: Implications for treatment. *Ann Intern Med* 1996;125:990–1000.

CHAPTER 25

# Acute and Postmyocardial Infarction

*Ernest L. Fallen, MD, FRCPC*

## *Acute Myocardial Infarction*

### Goals of Therapy

- To decrease mortality
- To reduce or contain infarct size
- To salvage functioning myocardium/prevent remodeling
- To quickly re-establish patency of infarct related vessel
- To prevent complications

*Note:* IV thrombolytic therapy administered *early* in the course of an evolving acute myocardial infarction (MI) substantially reduces mortality and morbidity.

### Investigations

- 12-lead ECG STAT and at least once daily × 3 days
- Creatine kinase (CK) and CKMB STAT and Q8H × 3 for the first 24 hours, then once daily × 3 *or* total CK plus Troponin T STAT and Q8H × 24 hours, then once daily × 3
- If indicated, an echocardiogram may identify:
  - the site and severity of wall motion abnormalities
  - infarct site in cases of left bundle branch block
  - endocardial thrombus
  - candidates for ACE inhibitor therapy if left ventricular ejection fraction is ≤40%
- Total and LDL cholesterol during the first 24 hours of infarct. The complete lipid profile should be repeated 6 to 8 weeks post-MI. However, it is useful to know the early cholesterol level to initiate lipid lowering therapy as soon as possible when the patient may be most receptive to risk factor modification

### **Therapeutic Choices** (Figure 1, Table 1)

#### Therapeutic Tips

- *Time is of the essence!* It is important to begin thrombolytic treatment as rapidly as possible.

Figure 1: **Treatment of Acute Myocardial Infarction**

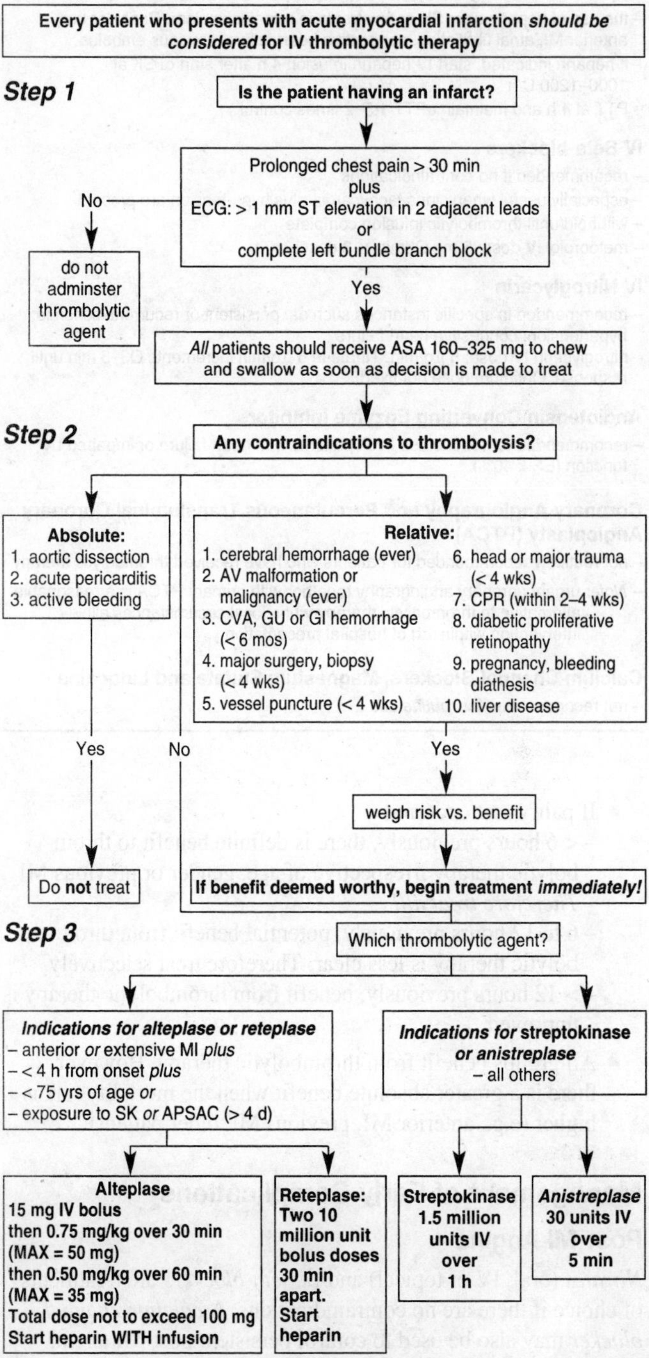
Every patient who presents with acute myocardial infarction should be considered for IV thrombolytic therapy
Step 1
Is the patient having an infarct?
Prolonged chest pain > 30 min
plus
ECG: > 1 mm ST elevation in 2 adjacent leads
or
complete left bundle branch block
No
do not adminster thrombolytic agent
Yes
All patients should receive ASA 160–325 mg to chew and swallow as soon as decision is made to treat
Step 2
Any contraindications to thrombolysis?
Absolute:
1. aortic dissection
2. acute pericarditis
3. active bleeding
Relative:
1. cerebral hemorrhage (ever)
2. AV malformation or malignancy (ever)
3. CVA, GU or GI hemorrhage (< 6 mos)
4. major surgery, biopsy (< 4 wks)
5. vessel puncture (< 4 wks)
6. head or major trauma (< 4 wks)
7. CPR (within 2–4 wks)
8. diabetic proliferative retinopathy
9. pregnancy, bleeding diathesis
10. liver disease
Yes
No
Yes
weigh risk vs. benefit
Do not treat
If benefit deemed worthy, begin treatment immediately!
Step 3
Which thrombolytic agent?
Indications for alteplase or reteplase
– anterior or extensive MI plus
– < 4 h from onset plus
– < 75 yrs of age or
– exposure to SK or APSAC (> 4 d)
Indications for streptokinase or anistreplase
– all others
Alteplase
15 mg IV bolus
then 0.75 mg/kg over 30 min
(MAX = 50 mg)
then 0.50 mg/kg over 60 min
(MAX = 35 mg)
Total dose not to exceed 100 mg
Start heparin WITH infusion
Reteplase:
Two 10 million unit bolus doses 30 min apart.
Start heparin
Streptokinase
1.5 million units IV over 1 h
Anistreplase
30 units IV over 5 min

Table 1: **Adjuvant Therapy for Acute MI**

**Heparin Following Streptokinase (SK) or Anistreplase**
- the use of heparin after SK or anistreplase remains unclear. Consider use in anterior MI, atrial fibrillation, congestive heart failure, previous embolus
- if heparin indicated, start IV heparin infusion 4 h after start of SK at 1000–1200 U/h
- PTT at 4 h and maintain aPTT 1.5–2 times control

**IV Beta-blockers**
- recommended if no contraindications
- especially useful when sinus tachycardia plus hypertension are present
- withhold until thrombolytic infusion complete
- metoprolol IV dose: 5 mg Q2min × 3 doses

**IV Nitroglycerin**
- recommended in specific instances such as: persistent or recurrent ischemia; hypertension; congestive heart failure
- nitroglycerin IV dose: 5 μg/min. Titrate in 5 μg/min increments Q3–5 min until response. Optimum dose not fixed.

**Angiotensin Converting Enzyme Inhibitors**
- recommended for routine use in all patients with heart failure or impaired LV function (EF < 40%)

**Coronary Angiography and Percutaneous Transluminal Coronary Angioplasty (PTCA)**
- not routinely recommended for patients who have received thrombolytic therapy
- *Note*: urgent coronary angiography together with primary PTCA is a reasonable alternative to thrombolytic therapy when local circumstances allow intervention within 1 h of hospital presentation

**Calcium Channel Blockers, Magnesium Sulfate and Lidocaine**
- not recommended for *routine* use

- If pain onset occurred:
  - < 6 hours previously, there is definite benefit to thrombolytic therapy irrespective of age, gender or previous MI. *Therefore treat all!*
  - 6 to 12 hours previously, potential benefit from thrombolytic therapy is less clear. Therefore treat selectively.
  - > 12 hours previously, benefit from thrombolytic therapy is unproven.
- All groups benefit from thrombolytic therapy. However, there is a greater absolute benefit when the mortality risk is higher (e.g., anterior MI, previous MI, older patient).

## Management of Early Complications

### Post-MI Angina

*Nitrates* (oral, IV or topical) and/or *beta-blockers* are treatments of choice if there are no contraindications. A *calcium channel blocker* may also be used to control persistent post-MI angina unresponsive to above agents. Although controversial, there is concern about the safety of short-acting calcium channel blockers in the post-MI patient. If rest angina persists despite treatment, coronary angiography should be considered.

## Dysrhythmias

- Treatment of asymptomatic ventricular ectopy or nonsustained ventricular tachycardia is not warranted.
- For symptomatic ventricular ectopy, *beta-blockers* are sometimes useful. Class IA agents (e.g., quinidine, disopyramide, procainamide) are relatively contraindicated. Class IC agents (flecainide and propafenone) are contra-indicated.
- In the post acute phase of MI, patients with sustained ventricular tachycardia or post cardiac arrest should undergo coronary angiography with or without electrophysiologic studies (Chapter 29).
- Patients with frequent PVCs, complex ventricular ectopy or nonsustained VT plus LV dysfunction may be considered for amiodarone therapy.
- For atrial fibrillation, the ventricular rate can be controlled with a *beta-blocker* or *digoxin*. Verapamil or diltiazem should be avoided in patients with LV dysfunction. (Chapter 28).
- If symptomatic bradycardia occurs, the dose of beta-blocker, calcium channel blocker or digoxin should be reduced or another drug should be substituted. If it persists, consider pacemaker implantation.

## Congestive Heart Failure (See also Chapter 27)

- *ACE inhibitor*, especially if low output syndrome (fatigue, weakness, dyspnea).
- Salt restriction.
- *Diuretic*, especially for cases with dyspnea and pulmonary rales (important to monitor potassium levels).
- *Digoxin* should be considered only if there is:
  – rapid atrial fibrillation
  – dilated left ventricle and S3 gallop rhythm.

## Hypertension

Systemic hypertension increases myocardial oxygen demand and may increase infarct size. An *ACE inhibitor* is the treatment of choice. The addition of a beta-blocker or calcium channel blocker with or without a thiazide diuretic (monitor potassium) should be considered if systolic BP remains > 160 mm Hg or diastolic BP > 95 mm Hg.

### Pericarditis

Pericarditis is common within 72 hours post MI. If symptomatic, **ASA** should be increased to 650 mg QID for 1 to 2 weeks. If pain persists, an NSAID or corticosteroid should be considered. Peri-infarction pericarditis usually resolves spontaneously by the 3rd or 4th day. Discontinuation of anticoagulants is unnecessary if pericarditis presents as part of acute phase MI.

## *Postmyocardial Infarction*

The post-MI phase is defined as the time from transfer to the ward (day 3 to 5) up to 1 year from hospital discharge.

### Goals of Therapy

- To develop a risk stratification profile
- To prevent recurrent ischemic events
- To reduce mortality and morbidity
- To return the patient to an optimum quality of life
- To reduce or reverse modifiable risk factors
- To educate the patient and his/her family

### Investigations

- Symptom-limited exercise test (or submaximal exercise test depending on the risk stratification profile)
- 24-hour Holter recording for patients with suspected ventricular arrhythmias or symptomatic bradyarrhythmias
- A follow-up echocardiogram (2 to 3 weeks post-MI) in patients with a suspected or previously documented endocardial thrombus
- A lipid profile (total cholesterol, LDL, HDL, triglycerides) no sooner than 6 to 8 weeks postdischarge

#### *Risk Stratification Profile* (Figure 2)

The first step in the rehabilitation of the post-MI patient is to assign a risk assessment.

*Note: It is as important to identify the very-low-risk patient, thus sparing him/her unnecessary aggressive investigation and therapy, as it is to identify the high-risk patient for whom aggressive therapy may be life saving.*

A risk stratification profile (Figure 2) should be done three times: on arrival on the ward from the acute coronary unit; at discharge (when patient education ought to be reinforced); following a symptom-limited exercise test 2 to 4 weeks postdischarge. At each stage, the patient may stay within the risk group or be reassigned up or down. Further preventive strategies and treatment decisions rest on the respective risk group, as illustrated in Figure 2.

The intermediate-risk group has the potential for further episodes of ischemia.

## Post-MI Prophylaxis at Time of Hospital Discharge

*All* patients, regardless of risk category or age, should receive **ASA** (160 to 325 mg/d) indefinitely.

*All* patients should be prescribed a **beta-blocker** to be continued indefinitely unless contraindicated as below:

| **Absolute** | **Relative** |
|---|---|
| 1. 2nd or 3rd degree heart block, sick sinus syndrome | 1. Insulin-dependent diabetes with history of hypoglycemic attacks |
| 2. *Overt* CHF | 2. Persistent hypotension (systolic BP < 100 mm Hg) |
| 3. Bronchial asthma | 3. Heart rate persistently < 60 beats/min |
| | 4. COPD, chronic bronchitis |
| | 5. Severe peripheral vascular disease |

**Warfarin** is recommended following acute MI complicated by severe LV dysfunction, CHF, previous emboli, atrial fibrillation or 2D echocardiographic evidence of mural thrombosis. After 1 to 3 months, warfarin should be switched to ASA.

An **ACE inhibitor** is recommended for patients with > Killip Class IIa (see Figure 2 footnote) or LV dysfunction (ejection fraction < 40%).

**Verapamil** or **diltiazem** may be considered in patients *with non–Q wave MI who are free of CHF* if beta-blockers are contraindicated.

**Low molecular weight heparin** combined with **ASA,** the second generation platelet inhibitors (**ticlopidine**, **clopidogrel**) and the glycoprotein IIb/IIIa receptor antagonists **(eptifibatide, tirofiban)** all have proven useful in patients with acute coronary syndromes characterized by either unstable angina or non-Q wave MI.

Evidence to date does not warrant *routine* prophylaxis with organic nitrates, antiarrhythmic agents or calcium channel blockers.

For prescribing information see Table 2.

Figure 2: **Post-MI Risk Stratification**

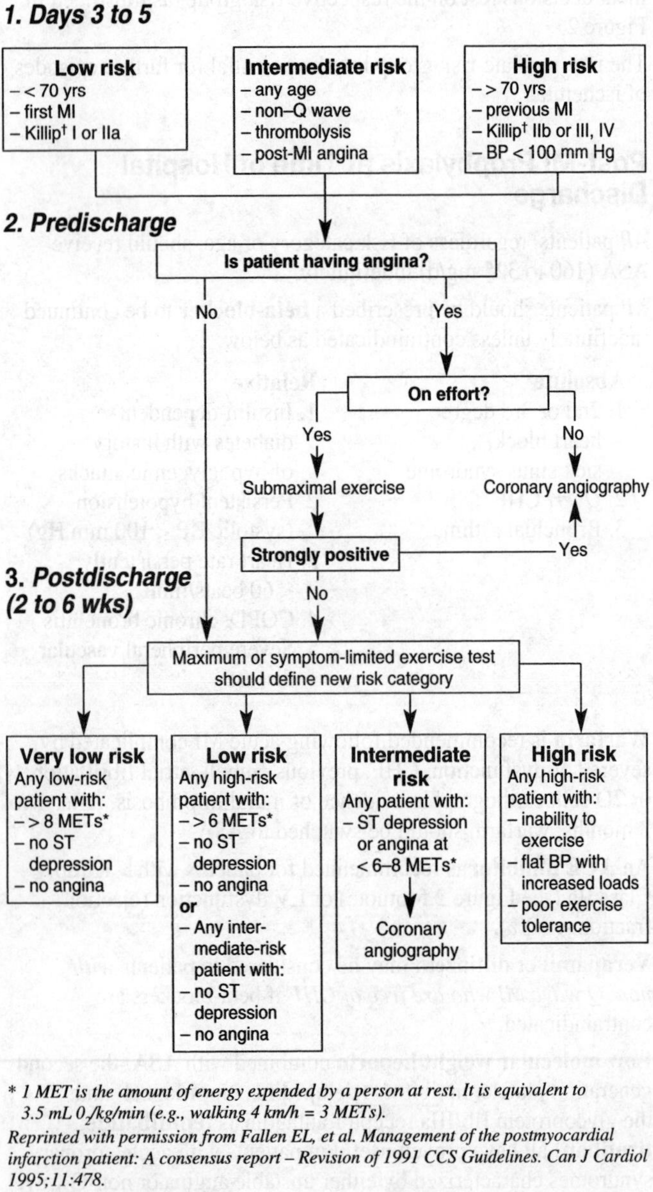
1. Days 3 to 5
Low risk
– < 70 yrs
– first MI
– Killip† I or IIa
Intermediate risk
– any age
– non–Q wave
– thrombolysis
– post-MI angina
High risk
– > 70 yrs
– previous MI
– Killip† IIb or III, IV
BP < 100 mm Hg
2. Predischarge
Is patient having angina?
No
Yes
On effort?
Yes
No
Submaximal exercise
Coronary angiography
Strongly positive
Yes
No
3. Postdischarge (2 to 6 wks)
Maximum or symptom-limited exercise test should define new risk category
Very low risk
Any low-risk patient with:
– > 8 METs*
– no ST depression
– no angina
Low risk
Any high-risk patient with:
– > 6 METs*
– no ST depression
– no angina
or
– Any intermediate-risk patient with:
– no ST depression
– no angina
Intermediate risk
Any patient with:
– ST depression or angina at < 6–8 METs*
Coronary angiography
High risk
Any high-risk patient with:
– inability to exercise
– flat BP with increased loads
– poor exercise tolerance

** 1 MET is the amount of energy expended by a person at rest. It is equivalent to 3.5 mL $O_2$/kg/min (e.g., walking 4 km/h = 3 METs).*

*Reprinted with permission from Fallen EL, et al. Management of the postmyocardial infarction patient: A consensus report – Revision of 1991 CCS Guidelines. Can J Cardiol 1995;11:478.*

*† The Killip classification is a scoring system for heart failure:*

| *Class* | *Clinical Findings* |
|---|---|
| *I* | *No rales, no S3* |
| *IIa* | *Rales < 50% of lungs; no S3* |
| *IIb* | *Rales < 50% of lungs; S3 present* |
| *III* | *Rales > 50%, pulmonary edema* |
| *IV* | *Shock* |

## Rehabilitation

Rehabilitation is the sum of activities required to ensure the best possible physical, psychologic and social conditions so the patient may, by his/her own efforts, regain as normal as possible a place in the community and lead an active, productive life. It includes exercise, risk factor and lifestyle modification, attention to psychosocial factors and management of dyslipidemias (Chapter 24).

### *Exercise*

Guidelines for graduated physical activities post-MI are provided by established cardiac rehabilitation programs in many communities. For general guidelines refer to Figure 3.

Figure 3: **Activities Prescription**

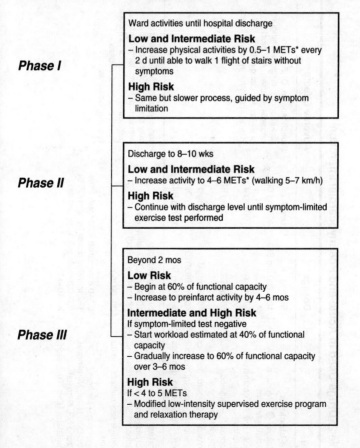

***Phase I***

Ward activities until hospital discharge

**Low and Intermediate Risk**

– Increase physical activities by 0.5–1 METs* every 2 d until able to walk 1 flight of stairs without symptoms

**High Risk**

– Same but slower process, guided by symptom limitation

***Phase II***

Discharge to 8–10 wks

**Low and Intermediate Risk**

– Increase activity to 4–6 METs* (walking 5–7 km/h)

**High Risk**

– Continue with discharge level until symptom-limited exercise test performed

***Phase III***

Beyond 2 mos

**Low Risk**

– Begin at 60% of functional capacity
– Increase to preinfarct activity by 4–6 mos

**Intermediate and High Risk**

If symptom-limited test negative
– Start workload estimated at 40% of functional capacity
– Gradually increase to 60% of functional capacity over 3–6 mos

**High Risk**

If < 4 to 5 METs
– Modified low-intensity supervised exercise program and relaxation therapy

* *1 MET is the amount of energy expended by a person at rest. It is equivalent to 3.5 mL $O_2$/kg/min (e.g., walking 4 km/h = 3 METs).*

Table 2: **Drugs Used in Acute and Postmyocardial Infarction**

| Drug | Dosage | | Adverse Effects | Drug Interactions | Cost* |
|---|---|---|---|---|---|
| **Beta-blockers** | *Starting* | *Usual* | Bronchospasm, CHF, sleep disturbances, dizziness, fatigue, anorexia, nausea, A-V block, bradycardia, claudication, Raynaud's, lethargy, drowsiness. | Enhanced cardiodepressant effect with: calcium channel blockers, antiarrhythmics, anesthetics. | |
| *acebutolol* – Monitan, Sectral, generics | 100–200 mg BID | 400 mg BID | | | $$ |
| *atenolol* † – Tenormin, generics | 50 mg/d | 100 mg/d | | Increased bradycardia with digoxin. | $ |
| | | | | Hypertension with alpha-agonists. | |
| *metoprolol* † – Betaloc, Lopresor, generics | 50 mg BID | 100 mg BID | | Reduced effect with cimetidine. | $ |
| *nadolol* – Corgard, generics | 40–80 mg/d | 120 mg/d | | | $ |
| *propranolol* † – Inderal, generics | 40 mg BID/TID | 40 mg QID | | | $ |
| *timolol* † – Blocadren, generics | 5–10 mg BID | 10 mg BID | | | $ |
| **Nitrates** | *Starting dosages* | | Headache (up to 50%; tolerance may develop), contact dermatitis with topical forms, tachycardia, palpitation, hypotension, syncope (rare), dizziness, nausea, flushing, weakness. | Potential hypotensive effect with vasodilators. | |
| *isosorbide dinitrate* – Isordil, Cedocard SR, generics | 10–30 mg TID (allow a 12H nitrate-free period) | | | | $ |
| *isosorbide mononitrate* – Imdur, Ismo | 30–60 mg/d | | | | $ |
| *nitroglycerin* – Minitran, Nitro-Dur, Nitrol, Nitrolingual, Nitrong SR, Nitrostat, Transderm-Nitro, Trinipatch | 0.3–0.6 mg tablet sublingual PRN<br>1–2 metered doses by spray PRN<br>0.2–0.8 mg/h patch applied daily for 10–12H | | | | SL tablets, spray<br>$<br>Transdermal<br>$$ |

| | | | | | |
|---|---|---|---|---|---|
| **ACE Inhibitors** | *Initial* | *Target* | | | |
| *captopril* – Capoten, generics | 6.25 mg | 37.5 mg Q8h | Proteinuria (1%), neutropenia, rash, hypotension, alterations in taste, nausea, anorexia, dizziness, dry cough. Caution in patients with renovascular hypertension. | ↑ risk of neutropenia with antiarrhythmics, allopurinol, corticosteroids. | $$ |
| *cilazapril* – Inhibace | 0.5 mg | 2.5 mg once daily | | | $ |
| *enalapril* – Vasotec, generics | 2.5 mg | 10 mg BID | | | $$$ |
| *fosinopril* – Monopril | 5 mg | 10 mg once daily | | Hyperkalemia with spironolactone, triamterene, amiloride. | $ |
| *lisinopril* – Zestril, Prinivil, generics | 2.5 mg | 20 mg once daily | | Hypotension with diuretics. | $ |
| *quinapril* – Accupril | 5 mg | 15 mg once daily | | Avoid concurrent therapy with lithium. | $$ |
| *ramipril* – Altace | 2.5 mg | 5 mg BID or 10 mg once daily | | | $$ |
| *trandolapril* – Mavik | 0.5 mg | 2 mg once daily | | | $ |
| **Anticoagulants** | | | | | |
| *warfarin* – Coumadin, Warfilone | Dose PO according to INR (1.5–2 × control) | | | Many drug interactions. See Chapter 29, Table 3. | $ |
| *heparin sodium* – Hepalean | Dose IV according to aPTT | | Hemorrhage, hypersensitivity reactions, thrombocytopenia, alopecia. | | $‡ |
| **low molecular weight heparins:** | | | | | |
| *dalteparin* – Fragmin | 120 IU/kg BID SC | | ↑ risk of bleeding complications if this dose is exceeded. | | $$$$‡ |
| *enoxaparin* – Lovenox | 100 IU/kg Q12H SC | | Hypersensitivity, thrombocytopenia. | | $$$$‡ |
| **Antiplatelet Agents** | | | | | |
| *ASA* – Entrophen, Aspirin, generics | ASA 160–325 mg/d | | Nausea, vomiting, GI hemorrhage, tinnitus, vertigo, hypersensitivity. | | $ |

*(cont'd)*

Table 2: **Drugs Used in Acute and Postmyocardial Infarction** *(cont'd)*

| Drug | Dosage | Adverse Effects | Drug Interactions | Cost* |
|---|---|---|---|---|
| *clopidogrel* – Plavix | 75 mg once daily. | Purpura (5%); rash (4.2%). Similar tolerability to ASA. | Caution with NSAIDs. | $$$$ |
| *ticlopidine* – Ticlid | 250 mg BID. | Diarrhea (12%); rash (5%); neutropenia (2.4%); purpura (2.2%). | Caution with NSAIDs. May ↑ theophylline levels. | $$ |
| **Glycoprotein IIb/IIIa Inhibitors** | | Bleeding, primarily at puncture sites. | Use caution with other drugs that affect hemostasis | |
| *eptifibatide* Integrelin | Bolus 180 μg/kg over 1–2 min, then 2 μg/kg/min. Max: 15 mg/hr | Thrombocytopenia. | | $$$$$ |
| *tirofiban* ❥ Aggrastat | 0.4 μg/kg/min × 30 min, then 0.1 μg/kg/min | | | $$$$$ |
| **Thrombolytics** | (Figure 1) | Bleeding, allergy to streptokinase or anistreplase, hypotension, nausea, fever, reperfusion arrhythmias. | ↑ risk of hemorrhage with oral anticoagulants, heparin and NSAIDs. | |
| *alteplase* – Activase rtPA | | | | $2745/dose |
| *anistreplase* – Eminase | | | | $1700/dose |
| *reteplase* – Retavase | | Cross allergenicity between anistreplase and streptokinase. | | $2700/dose |
| *streptokinase* – Streptase | | | | $375/dose |

❥ *Dosage adjustment may be required in renal impairment – see Appendix I.*
† *Proven efficacy for prophylaxis in post-MI patients.*
‡ *Cost of 3-day supply.*

* *Cost of 30-day supply – includes drug cost only.*
*Legend: $ < $25 $$ $25–50 $$$ $50–75 $$$$ $75–100 $$$$$ > $100*

### Risk Factor and Lifestyle Modification

Compelling evidence shows that modifying risk factors such as hyperlipidemia, smoking and hypertension improves outcome, delays progression of atherosclerosis, reduces mortality and improves functional capacity. For instance, ex-smokers can look forward to a 35 to 50% reduction in mortality whereas the relative risk of sudden cardiac death is 1.6 to 2.2 times in those who continue to smoke. For those willing to comply, psychosocial support, education, exercise programs, relaxation therapy and special teaching programs are helpful as adjunctive measures.

## Pharmacoeconomic Considerations

*Jeffrey A. Johnson, PhD*

Among proven therapies in acute MI, ASA would appear to have a large benefit to cost ratio, given the number of deaths and nonfatal MI that would be prevented in both the short and long term, at a very low cost for the drug itself. Similarly, use of IV beta-blockers in acute MI prevents a significant number of subsequent events at a relatively small cost, as does its continued oral use as post-MI prophylaxis.

Thrombolytic therapy is also cost-effective when compared to other cardiovascular interventions in terms of dollars per years of life saved. Cost-effectiveness studies clearly show that shortening the time to treatment has a critical impact on the cost-effectiveness of thrombolytic therapy, as does the age of the patient. Initiating treatment within 6 hours of AMI is associated with better outcomes, and is therefore more cost-effective. The relative cost-effectiveness of the thrombolytic agents (i.e., streptokinase and alteplase) remains somewhat controversial. The most effective strategy may be one of selective use of the two drugs based on time of presentation, age of the patient and location of the infarction. For the vast majority of patients presenting with AMI with either ST segment elevation or bundle branch block, streptokinase is more cost-effective. The exception would be in younger individuals with a large anteroseptal infarction, who may receive greater benefit from alteplase.

As noted above, continued use of ASA and beta-blockers is economically justified in terms of post-MI prophylaxis. Use of an ACE inhibitor to prevent development of CHF and reduce mortality in MI survivors with low ejection fraction is also associated with a favorable cost-effectiveness ratio when compared to other interventions. Furthermore, participation in cardiac rehabilitation initiated soon after acute MI has shown to be an efficient use of health care resources in terms of the cost per quality-adjusted life years gained.

***Suggested Reading***

*Castillo PA, Palmer CS, Halpern MT, et al. Cost-effectiveness of thrombolytic therapy for acute myocardial infarction. Ann Pharmacother 1997;31:596–603.*

*Collins R, Sleight P, Baigent C, Peto R. Aspirin, heparin, and fibrinolytic therapy in suspected acute myocardial infarction. N Engl J Med 1997;336:847–860.*

*Tsevat J, Duke D, Goldman L, et al. Cost-effectiveness of captopril therapy after myocardial infarction. J Am Coll Cardiol 1995;26:914–919.*

*Oldridge N, Furlong W, Feeny D, et al. Economic evaluation of cardiac rehabilitation soon after acute myocardial infarction. Am J Cardiol 1993;72:154–161.*

## *Suggested Reading List*

Cairns J, Kennedy J, Fuster V. Coronary thrombolysis. Chest 1998;114:6345–6575.

Cairns J, Armstrong P, Belenkie I, et al. Canadian consensus conference on coronary thrombolysis – 1994 update. *Can J Cardiol* 1994;10:517–529.

Fallen EL, Cairns J, Dafoe W, et al. Management of the post-myocardial infarction patient: a consensus report – revision of the 1991 CCS guidelines. *Can J Cardiol* 1995;11:477–486.

The GUSTO Investigators. An international randomized trial comparing four thrombolytic strategies for acute myocardial infarction. *N Engl J Med* 1993;329:673–682.

ISIS-2 Study Group. Randomized trial of intravenous streptokinase, oral aspirin, both or neither among 17,187 cases of suspected acute myocardial infarction. *Lancet* 1988;2:349–360.

Yusuf S, Peto R, Lewis JA, et al. Beta-blockade during and after myocardial infarction: a review of the randomized trials. *Prog Cardiovasc Dis* 1985;27:335–371.

CHAPTER 26

# Angina Pectoris

*John O. Parker, MD, MSc(Med), FACP, FRCPC and*
*John D. Parker, MD, FRCPC*

## *Stable Angina Pectoris*

### Goals of Therapy

- To decrease or abolish symptoms
- To improve exercise tolerance
- To retard disease progression
- To prevent complications

### Investigations

- Thorough history with special attention to:
  - pain: quality, severity, location, radiation, precipitating and relieving factors
  - effect of nitroglycerin
- Physical examination:
  - presence of hypertension, valvular disease, cardiomegaly, heart failure
- Laboratory tests:
  - CBC, blood glucose, creatinine, cholesterol
- Exercise test:
  - not universally required; helps to confirm diagnosis and assess functional status and provides prognostic information

### Therapeutic Choices (Figure 1)

#### Nonpharmacologic Choices

- The patient should be educated to understand the pathophysiology of myocardial ischemia.
- Lifestyle changes should include, when appropriate: dietary modifications to reduce cholesterol, weight reduction, smoking cessation (Chapter 42), avoidance of strenuous exercise (particularly isometric), increased activities (e.g., walking).
- Strenuous activity after meals or in cold weather should be avoided.

Figure 1: **Management of Stable Angina Pectoris**

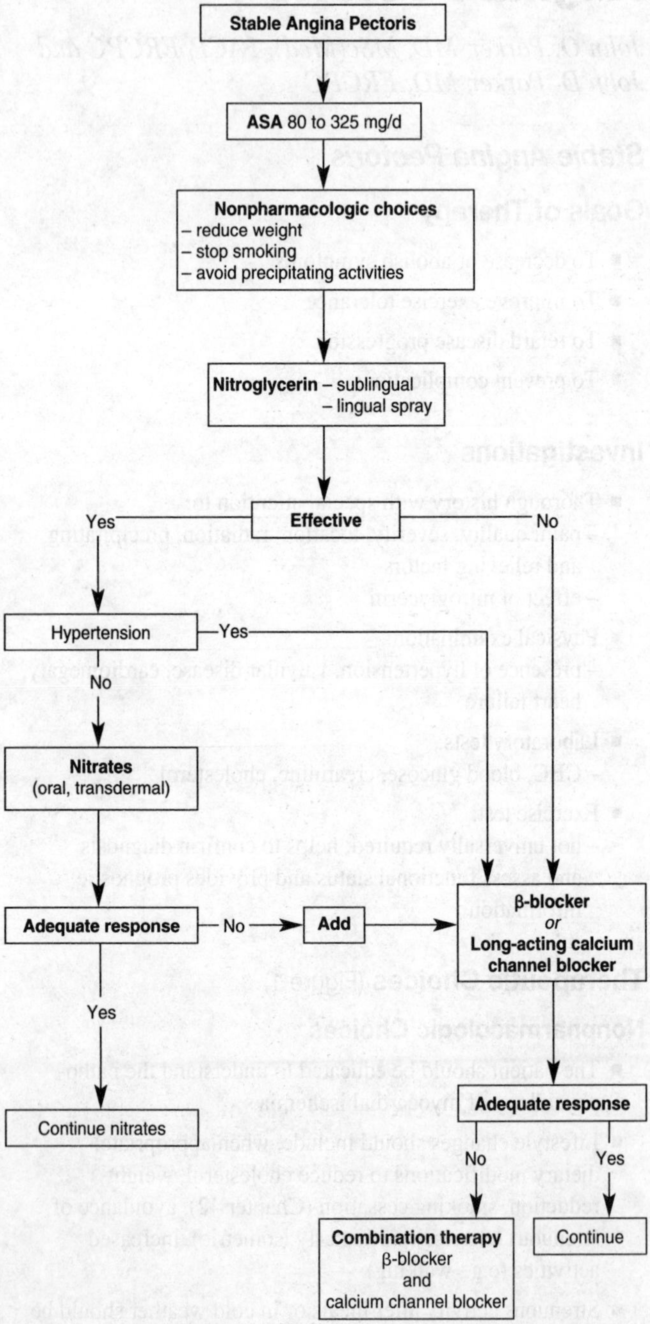
Stable Angina Pectoris
ASA 80 to 325 mg/d
Nonpharmacologic choices
– reduce weight
– stop smoking
– avoid precipitating activities
Nitroglycerin – sublingual
– lingual spray
Effective
Yes
No
Hypertension
Yes
No
Nitrates
(oral, transdermal)
Adequate response
No
Add
β-blocker
or
Long-acting calcium
channel blocker
Yes
Continue nitrates
Adequate response
No
Yes
Combination therapy
β-blocker
and
calcium channel blocker
Continue

## Pharmacologic Choices (Table 1)

All patients should receive **ASA** 80 to 325 mg per day, unless contraindicated. ASA has been shown to reduce the risk of myocardial infarction by one third in patients with stable angina.

### *Treatment of Episodes of Angina*

**Nitroglycerin (GTN)** sublingual tablets (0.3 or 0.6 mg) or lingual spray (0.4 mg) are effective in 95% of patients. A single dose is usually adequate, but 2 or 3 doses over 5 to 10 minutes may be required. **Isosorbide dinitrate (ISDN)** 5 mg, sublingually, is effective but has slower onset than GTN. Each can be used before physical activity for short-term prophylaxis.

### *Long-term Angina Prophylaxis*

The effectiveness of the organic nitrates, beta-blockers and calcium channel blockers varies in subsets of patients and their degree of efficacy is somewhat unpredictable. Nitrates are first-line therapy in patients without hypertension, particularly if the patient responds well to sublingual GTN. Beta-blockers are first choice if the patient has a history of MI. In patients with concomitant hypertension, either a beta-blocker or calcium channel blocker should be considered.

### *Organic Nitrates*

**ISDN** and **isosorbide-5-mononitrate (IS-5-MN)** are available as immediate- and sustained-release tablets. GTN as an ointment and a transdermal patch is effective for angina prophylaxis if administered in a dosing regimen that provides a period of low nitrate exposure of 10 to 12 hours during each 24-hour period. The effects are secondary to the venous and arterial dilating effects that reduce preload and afterload, increase coronary blood flow and improve its distribution. Data are limited concerning the efficacy of GTN oral sustained release.

### *Beta-blockers*

Both selective and nonselective beta-blockers are effective. By lowering heart rate, blood pressure and myocardial contractility, myocardial oxygen requirements are reduced. Beta-blockers are not associated with tolerance during continuous therapy. The intrinsic sympathomimetic activity (ISA) of some agents benefits patients who experience excessive bradycardia with other beta-blockers. Mortality is decreased in patients with previous MI while on beta-blockers.

### *Calcium Channel Blockers*

**Verapamil** and **diltiazem** lower heart rate, whereas the dihydropyridines, including **nifedipine, amlodipine, felodipine** and **nicardipine,** are arteriolar dilators and have a major effect

Table 1: **Drug Therapy for Stable Angina**

| Drug | Dosage | Drug Interactions | Comments | Cost* |
|---|---|---|---|---|
| **Nitrates** | | For all nitrates: Potential hypotensive effect with vasodilators. | For all nitrates: Headache, hypotension, tachycardia, flushing, edema, contact dermatitis with topical forms. | |
| *nitroglycerin* – Nitrolingual Spray, Nitrostat | SL: 0.3–0.6 mg PRN | | | $ |
| | Spray: 0.4 mg PRN | | | $ |
| ointment: Nitrol | Ointment: 1.25–5 cm BID–TID; remove for 12 h per 24 h period | | | $ |
| transdermal: Nitro-Dur, Transderm-Nitro, Minitran | Patch: 0.2–0.8 mg/h for 12 h per 24 h period | | | $$ |
| *isosorbide dinitrate* – Isordil, Cedocard SR, generics | SL: 5 mg PRN | | | $ |
| | Regular: 10–30 mg TID on QID schedule (allow 12 h nitrate-free period) | | | |
| | SR: 20–40 mg BID (7 h apart) | | | $–$$ |
| *isosorbide-5-mononitrate* – Imdur, Ismo | Regular: 20 mg BID (7 h apart) | | | $$ |
| | SR: 30–120 mg once daily | | | $–$$ |
| **Beta-blockers** | | For all β-blockers: With digoxin ↑ bradycardia. Calcium channel blockers and amiodarone may ↑ cardiodepressant effect. | For all β-blockers: Bradycardia, hypotension, fatigue, depression, sleep disorders, dyspnea. Monitor HR, caution in patients with CHF, COPD, diabetes mellitus. | |
| *acebutolol* – Monitan, Sectral, generics | 200–300 mg BID | | | $ |
| *atenolol* – Tenormin, generics | 50–100 mg daily | | | $ |
| *metoprolol* – Betaloc, Lopresor, generics | 50–100 mg BID | | | $ |
| *nadolol* – Corgard, generics | 20–160 mg daily | | | $ |
| *propranolol* – Inderal, generics | 40–60 mg QID | | | $ |

| | | | | |
|---|---|---|---|---|
| **Calcium Channel Blockers** | | Additive myocardial depressant effects with β-blockers, digoxin, amiodarone. Monitor for excessive bradycardia. | | |
| *amlodipine* – Norvasc | 5–10 mg once daily | | Hypotension, flushing, headache, edema. | $$–$$$ |
| *diltiazem* – Cardizem, Cardizem CD, Cardizem SR, generics | Regular: 30–120 mg TID–QID<br>CD: 120–480 mg once daily<br>SR: 60–240 mg BID | | Caution in patients with CHF or bradycardia. | $$–$$$$ |
| *nifedipine* – Adalat PA, Adalat XL, generics | PA: 10–40 mg BID<br>XL: 30–120 mg once daily | | Hypotension, tachycardia, flushing, edema. | $$–$$$$ |
| *verapamil* (renal symbol) – Isoptin, Isoptin SR, generics | Regular: 80–240 mg BID<br>SR: 180–480 mg daily | | Bradycardia, heart block, hypotension, constipation, flushing, edema. | $–$$$ |

(renal symbol) *Dosage adjustment may be required in renal impairment – see Appendix I.*
* *Cost of 30-day supply – includes drug cost only.*
*Legend: $ < $25 $$ $25–50 $$$ $50–75 $$$$ > $75*

on peripheral vascular resistance. The beneficial effects of the calcium channel blockers are secondary to their effect on lowering arterial blood pressure and the reduced heart rate seen with verapamil and diltiazem. They also increase coronary blood flow by dilating conductive arteries. The dihydropyridines also have an effect on coronary resistance vessels, which may be deleterious in some patients by inducing coronary steal with redistribution of flow away from ischemic zones. There is evidence that the use of short-acting calcium channel blockers may be associated with adverse cardiac events. Although no clear data are available concerning the patient with stable angina, it would seem prudent to *avoid the use of short-acting dihydropyridines* in patients with coronary artery disease.

#### Combination Therapy

Nitrates and either beta-blockers or long-acting calcium channel blockers are usually very effective. The increased heart rate seen during nitrate therapy may be blunted by the beta-blocker or rate-limiting calcium channel blocker (i.e., verapamil or diltiazem). Adding a beta-blocker to a rate-limiting calcium channel blocker can be undesirable because excessive bradycardia may occur. Combination therapy allows for titration of doses of individual agents to maximize benefits and to minimize side effects. There are little data to support the use of combination therapy despite the fact that this approach is widely used.

#### Coronary Artery Revascularization

Coronary artery bypass surgery (CABG) or percutaneous transluminal coronary artery (PTCA) angioplasty may be indicated for the patient who is significantly limited by recurrent symptoms despite maximal medical therapy.

## Unstable Angina Pectoris

Patients with unstable angina are a heterogeneous group: those on no medication with new onset exertional angina and those already on maximal antianginal therapy presenting with rest pain and electrocardiographic changes.

### Goals of Therapy

- To reduce episodes of chest pain or other symptoms of myocardial ischemia
- To prevent the onset of MI
- To treat or reverse secondary causes of unstable angina

## Investigations

- Thorough history with special attention to:
  - pain: quality, severity, location, radiation, precipitating and relieving factors
  - effect of nitroglycerin
  - duration of anginal symptoms, previous cardiac events, risk factors
- Physical examination:
  - presence of hypertension, valvular heart disease, heart failure, cardiomegaly
- Laboratory tests:
  - ECG, CBC, electrolytes, creatinine, CPK (MB), troponin levels, blood glucose and cholesterol
- Treadmill exercise test:
  - in patients with atypical pain or no ECG changes to clarify if symptoms are cardiac in origin
  - for predischarge risk stratification
  - to determine severity of underlying coronary artery disease and relative risk of future events

Treadmill exercise testing can be carried out safely in patients with unstable angina who respond well to medical therapy. It is useful in determining whether further invasive diagnostic procedures are required.

### *High-risk Patients*

Certain clinical characteristics at the time of presentation categorize patients into low- and high-risk groups. The following are clinical characteristics of a high-risk patient with unstable angina:

- transient or fixed ST segment depression > 0.5 mm
- transient (< 30 min) but presently *absent* ST segment elevation > 0.5 mm
- new T wave inversion > 1 mm in any 5 leads
- within 4 weeks of myocardial infarction
- drop in BP or CHF with symptoms of ischemia
- clear evidence of ischemia on ASA and heparin

## Therapeutic Choices (Figure 2)

### Nonpharmacologic Choices

- Patients generally should be admitted to hospital for bed rest. A quiet atmosphere, reassurance, explanation of the nature of the problem, analgesia and mild sedation are helpful initial measures.

Figure 2: **Management of Unstable Angina Pectoris**

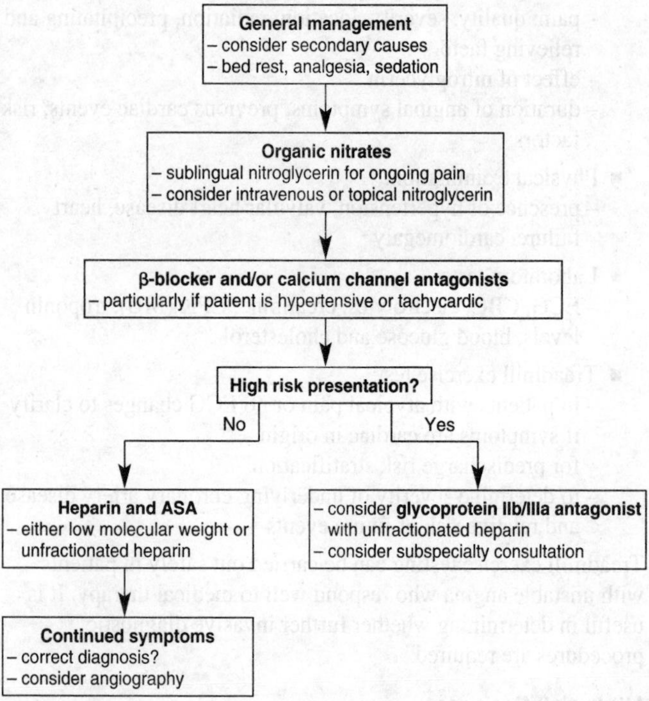
General management
– consider secondary causes
– bed rest, analgesia, sedation
Organic nitrates
– sublingual nitroglycerin for ongoing pain
– consider intravenous or topical nitroglycerin
β-blocker and/or calcium channel antagonists
– particularly if patient is hypertensive or tachycardic
High risk presentation?
No
Yes
Heparin and ASA
– either low molecular weight or unfractionated heparin
– consider glycoprotein IIb/IIIa antagonist with unfractionated heparin
– consider subspecialty consultation
Continued symptoms
– correct diagnosis?
– consider angiography

- Attention to potential secondary causes (i.e., anemia, fever, concurrent infection, congestive heart failure, tachy- or bradyarrhythmias) is mandatory since their management may control the symptoms of unstable angina.

## Pharmacologic Choices (Table 2)

### *Anticoagulant and Antiplatelet Therapy*

Patients presenting with acute coronary syndromes, including unstable angina, have evidence of thrombus formation involving one or more atherosclerotic plaques within their coronary circulation. **ASA** and full-dose **heparin** are effective in reducing the number of episodes of ischemia and the incidence of progression to infarction. During the hospital phase, heparin and ASA are superior to ASA alone in preventing refractory symptoms and the progression to MI. Following discharge from hospital, long-term prophylactic therapy with ASA reduces the incidence of reinfarction and has beneficial effects on mortality.

There is increasing evidence that *glycoprotein IIb/IIIa antagonists* are effective in the therapy of acute ischemic syndromes (both unstable angina and non-Q wave myocardial infarction). It seems

Table 2: **Drug Therapy for Unstable Angina**

| Drug | Dosage | Dosage Adjustment | Adverse Effects | Drug Interactions | Cost* |
|---|---|---|---|---|---|
| **Anticoagulants and Antiplatelet Agents** | | | | | |
| *ASA* Aspirin, Entrophen, generics | 325 mg/d | None. | Gastritis, gastric/duodenal ulceration (rarely bronchospasm). | Heparin/warfarin (bleeding risk with heparin appears to be low); other NSAIDs. | $ |
| *heparin* | 75 U/kg, then 1250 U/h. Adjust dose according to aPTT. | Follow aPTT (should be maintained at 1.5–2 × control). Draw first aPTT 4 h after initial bolus. | Bleeding, thrombocytopenia. | ASA, warfarin (bleeding risk with ASA is low); aPTT response may be blunted with concurrent IV nitroglycerin (controversial). | $† |
| **Low Molecular Weight Heparins** | | | | | |
| *dalteparin* Fragmin | 120 IU/kg SC BID max: 10 000 IU/dose | | Hematoma at injection site, bleeding, thrombocytopenia. | ASA, warfarin (bleeding risk with ASA is low) | $$† |
| *enoxaparin* Lovenox | 100 IU/kg SC BID max: 10 000 IU/dose | | | | $$† |
| **Glycoprotein IIb/IIIa Inhibitors** | | | | | |
| *eptifibatide* Integrilin | Bolus of 180 μg/kg over 1–2 minutes, then 2 μg/kg/min Max: 15 mg/hr | | All: Bleeding (risk of serious bleeding appears to be low). Thrombocytopenia. Allergic reactions. | Extensively tested with unfractionated heparin but safety/efficacy with low molecular weight heparin is unclear. | $$$$† |

*(cont'd)*

Table 2: **Drug Therapy for Unstable Angina** *(cont'd)*

| Drug | Dosage | Dosage Adjustment | Adverse Effects | Drug Interactions | Cost* |
|---|---|---|---|---|---|
| **Glycoprotein IIb/IIIa antagonists** *(cont'd)* | | | | | |
| *tirofiban* ☻ Aggrastat | CrCl ≥ 30 mL/min: bolus dose 0.4 μg/kg/min × 30 min, then maintenance infusion 0.1 μg/kg/min × 72 h. CrCl ≤ 30 mL/min: bolus dose 0.2 μg/kg/min × 30 min, then maintenance infusion 0.05 μg/kg/min × 72 h. | | | ↑ bleeding: ASA, warfarin | $$$$† |
| **Organic Nitrates** | | | | | |
| *IV nitroglycerin* | 10–150 μg/min IV (titrate dose to symptoms and blood pressure) | If symptoms recur ↑ infusion rate by 15–25%. No maximum dosage. | Hemodynamic monitoring is required. For all nitrates: Headache, hypotension, tachycardia, flushing, edema. | For all nitrates: Potential hypotensive effect with vasodilators. See above for interaction with heparin. | $† |
| *nitroglycerin ointment* Nitrol | 2.5–5 cm Q4–6H | | | | $ |
| *nitroglycerin patch* Minitran, Nitro-Dur, Transderm-Nitro, Trinipatch | 0.2–0.8 mg/h | | | | $$ |
| *isosorbide dinitrate* Isordil, generics | 10–30 mg PO TID (on QID schedule) | Often started after stabilization on IV nitroglycerin. | | | $ |

| | | | | | |
|---|---|---|---|---|---|
| **Calcium Channel Blockers** | | | | | |
| **Nondihydropyridines** | | All: Caution in CHF. | | All: additive effect with β-blockers, digoxin, amiodarone. Monitor for excessive bradycardia. | |
| *verapamil* ◗ Isoptin SR, generics | 180–480 mg daily | | Bradycardia, heart block, hypotension, constipation, flushing, edema. | | $$–$$$ |
| *diltiazem* Cardizem CD & SR, generics | 120–360 mg daily | | Bradycardia, hypotension. | | $–$$$ |
| **Dihydropyridines** | | | | | |
| *amlodipine* Norvasc | 5–10 mg daily | | Hypotension, flushing, marked peripheral edema. | | $$–$$$ |
| **Beta-blockers** – See Table 1 | | | | | |

** Cost of 30-day supply – includes drug cost only.*
*† Cost of average 1-day supply.*

*Legend: $ < $25 $$ $25–50 $$$ $50–75 $$$$ > $75*
◗ *Dosage adjustment may be required in renal impairment – see Appendix I.*

that patients with a high-risk clinical presentation (defined above), benefit from therapy with these agents. Agents approved for the therapy of unstable angina are **eptifibatide** and **tirofiban**.

The role of *low molecular weight heparin (LMWH)* in the treatment of unstable angina is controversial. It is possible to conclude from available data that LMWH is at least as effective as unfractionated heparin for unstable angina. LMWH, despite its higher cost, may have economic advantages because it does not require continuous intravenous infusion and monitoring of the partial thromboplastin time (PTT). Most centres presently use glycoprotein IIb/IIIa inhibitors with unfractionated heparin as experience with LMWH is limited.

## Antianginal Therapy

### *Nitrates*

Organic nitrates have potent preload reducing effects and lower myocardial oxygen demand. Their effects on epicardial coronary artery diameter may increase coronary blood supply and myocardial oxygen supply in some patients with severe, epicardial arterial stenoses. There is growing evidence that the nitrates, particularly nitroglycerin, have primary antiplatelet effects. The latter 2 effects may be of particular importance in unstable angina with pain occurring at rest, since these transient episodes of ischemia are probably caused by reductions in coronary blood flow rather than increased cardiac demand.

Organic nitrates are the agent of first choice for therapy of unstable angina. IV nitroglycerin is easily titrated to the patient's symptoms and its effect on systemic arterial blood pressure. Nitroglycerin ointment or an oral formulation may be appropriate in many cases.

### *Beta-blockers*

The role of beta-blockers in the treatment of unstable angina is being re-examined because many ischemic episodes are not preceded by increases in heart rate or blood pressure and appear secondary to a primary decrease in myocardial oxygen supply. When used alone, they may not be effective in preventing ischemic episodes. Patients already on a beta-blocker should continue and their antianginal therapy intensified with another agent. For those not on a beta-blocker, use in combination with nitrates may be appropriate. This is particularly true if the patient is anxious and/or has underlying tachycardia and hypertension. In the patient with refractory symptoms despite treatment with nitrates and heparin, a beta-blocker is appropriate.

### *Calcium Channel Blockers*

Although not first line agents, calcium channel blockers can be effective if the patient continues to have symptoms despite therapy. Diltiazem may be beneficial in the occasional patient with clinical evidence of coronary vasospasm with intermittent episodes of pain accompanied by electrocardiographic evidence of ST segment elevation.

### *Coronary Artery Revascularization*

Coronary artery bypass surgery or percutaneous transluminal coronary artery angioplasty may be indicated in patients with continued symptoms of myocardial ischemia on medical therapy.

## Pharmacoeconomic Considerations

*Jeffrey A. Johnson, PhD*

Available cost-effectiveness data suggest that medical therapy or coronary angioplasty are the preferred initial strategies for low-risk coronary disease, whereas CABG is recommended for many high-risk patients, particularly those with triple-vessel disease and impaired LV function. For patients with milder symptoms and milder coronary disease, revascularization therapy is likely to be less cost-effective. Any assessment of cost of treatment must take into account the cost of investigation, treatment, the morbidity associated with procedures or side effects of drugs, together with that of recurrent hospitalization, prolonged life, and premature death. Taking these factors into account, medical therapy is the least expensive short- and long-term treatment for angina pectoris.

A study commissioned by the Canadian Coordinating Office for Health Technology Assessment focused on the use of nitrates in chronic stable angina. This evaluation indicated that more than $45 million were spent by provincial governments on nitrates. The authors determined that, based on limited evidence available, there were no significant differences in effectiveness of the various products in terms of therapeutic outcomes (e.g. stress test performance, frequency of anginal attacks, use of sublingual nitroglycerin, tolerance and adverse effects). The findings of the review indicated that national savings of $9 million could be achieved if isosorbide dinitrate (ISDN) were to replace other nitrates 50% of the time.

More recently, economic evaluations of the new glycoprotein IIb/IIIa inhibitors in acute coronary syndromes have indicated that costs per death avoided are within reasonable cost-effectiveness ranges ($32,000 to $80,000 per life saved). However, as with revascularization, the use of these drugs in only the highest-risk patients would likely be the most cost-effective therapeutic choice.

***Suggested Reading***

*O'Rourke RA. Cost-effective management of chronic stable angina. Clin Cardiol 1996;19:497–501.*

*Cleland JG. Can improved quality of care reduce the costs of managing angina pectoris? Eur Heart J 1996;17(Suppl A):29–40.*

*Hillegass WB, Newman AR, Raco DL. Economic issues in glycoprotein IIb/IIIa receptor therapy. Am Heart J 1999;138:S24–S32.*

*Holbrook AM, Dolovich L, Grootendorst P, et al. Efficacy, effectiveness and cost analysis of nitrate therapy for the prevention of angina pectoris. Ottawa, ON: Canadian Coordinating Office for Health Technology Assessment, 1996.*

## Suggested Reading List

Braunwald E. Unstable angina: a classification. *Circulation*; 1989;80:410.

Gersh BJ, Braunwald E, Rutherford JD. Chronic coronary artery disease. In: Braunwald E, ed. *Heart disease. A textbook of cardiovascular medicine*. Philadelphia: W.B. Saunders, 1997:1289–1366.

Theroux P, Ouimet H, McCans J, Latour JG, et al. Aspirin, heparin or both to treat acute unstable angina. *N Engl J Med* 1988;319:1105–1111.

Harrington A. Overview of clinical trials of glycoprotein IIb-IIIa inhibitors in acute coronary syndromes. *Am Heart J* 1999;138:276–86.

CHAPTER 27

# Congestive Heart Failure

*Israel Belenkie, MD, FRCPC*

## Goals of Therapy

- To limit factors that precipitate or aggravate heart failure
- To reduce symptoms and improve function
- To improve quality of life
- To prevent progression of the disease
- To reduce morbidity and mortality

## Classification

Of the two broad categories of heart failure, the most common is **systolic failure**, which is due to the impaired pumping ability of the heart. This usually occurs in patients with a left ventricular ejection fraction $\leq 35\%$. Systolic dysfunction may be present without overt heart failure.

In **diastolic heart failure**, systolic function is preserved but diastolic filling is impaired. The left ventricular ejection fraction is $\geq 45\%$. Hypertrophic cardiomyopathy is a unique subgroup of patients in whom diastolic dysfunction is important.

## Investigations (Figure 1)

The history and physical examination are used to assess the severity of congestive heart failure (CHF), to identify precipitating or aggravating causes, and to identify specific causes of heart failure.

- Routine laboratory tests (Figure 1) should be done in all patients and include assessment of cardiac function by echocardiography in most cases.
- Special laboratory tests (Figure 1) are reserved for precipitating causes, complications or for re-evaluation.

## Therapeutic Choices (Figures 2 and 3)

### Nonpharmacologic Choices

Treatment of precipitating or aggravating causes is essential in both systolic or diastolic heart failure.

- Treatment of myocardial ischemia is a priority since these patients may benefit substantially from coronary revascularization by percutaneous transluminal coronary angioplasty (PTCA) or bypass surgery. However, there are

Figure 1: **Investigation of Congestive Heart Failure**

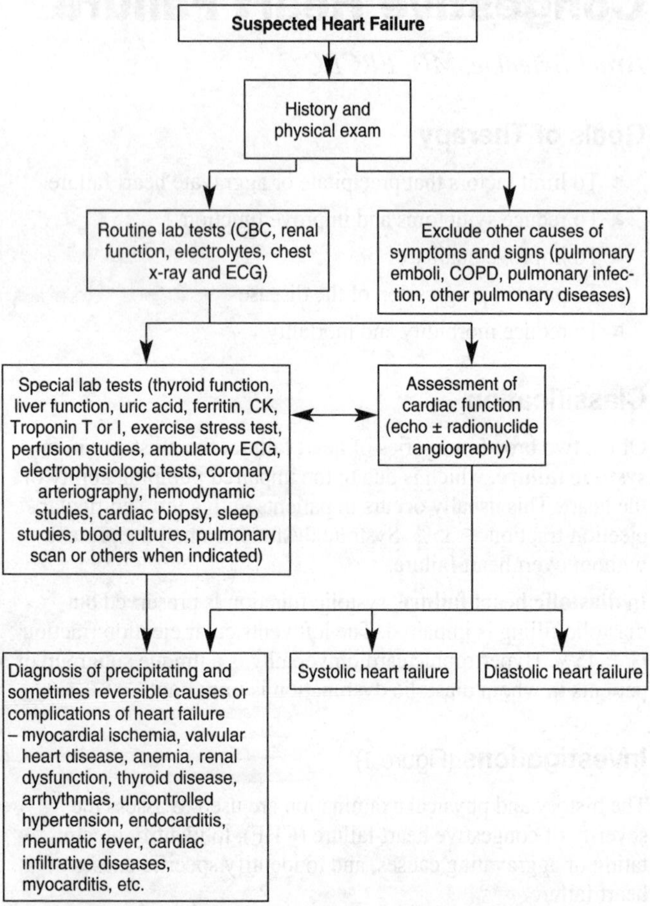
Suspected Heart Failure
History and physical exam
Routine lab tests (CBC, renal function, electrolytes, chest x-ray and ECG)
Exclude other causes of symptoms and signs (pulmonary emboli, COPD, pulmonary infection, other pulmonary diseases)
Special lab tests (thyroid function, liver function, uric acid, ferritin, CK, Troponin T or I, exercise stress test, perfusion studies, ambulatory ECG, electrophysiologic tests, coronary arteriography, hemodynamic studies, cardiac biopsy, sleep studies, blood cultures, pulmonary scan or others when indicated)
Assessment of cardiac function (echo ± radionuclide angiography)
Diagnosis of precipitating and sometimes reversible causes or complications of heart failure – myocardial ischemia, valvular heart disease, anemia, renal dysfunction, thyroid disease, arrhythmias, uncontrolled hypertension, endocarditis, rheumatic fever, cardiac infiltrative diseases, myocarditis, etc.
Systolic heart failure
Diastolic heart failure

limited data on the effects of revascularization on survival in patients with severe heart failure. Current evidence suggests that survival is improved in patients with angina and/or extensive myocardial ischemia. In patients with less severe heart failure, it has been conclusively demonstrated that bypass surgery improves the prognosis of patients with more extensive coronary artery disease. Nevertheless, in patients with severe left ventricular dysfunction and marked left ventricular dilatation or pulmonary hypertension, revascularization is risky and should only be carefully considered; special consideration should be given if reversible mechanical factors are present. In appropriately selected patients, revascularization may result in considerable improvement in cardiac function.

Figure 2: **Management of Systolic Heart Failure**

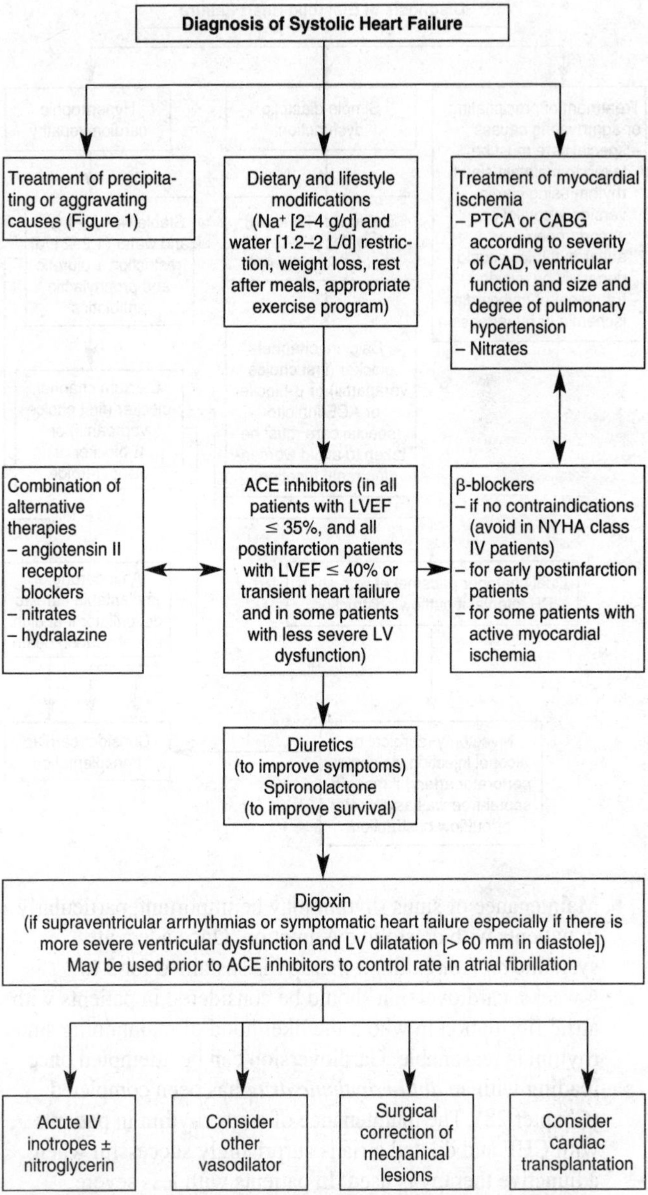
Diagnosis of Systolic Heart Failure
Treatment of precipitating or aggravating causes (Figure 1)
Dietary and lifestyle modifications (Na+ [2–4 g/d] and water [1.2–2 L/d] restriction, weight loss, rest after meals, appropriate exercise program)
Treatment of myocardial ischemia – PTCA or CABG according to severity of CAD, ventricular function and size and degree of pulmonary hypertension – Nitrates
Combination of alternative therapies – angiotensin II receptor blockers – nitrates – hydralazine
ACE inhibitors (in all patients with LVEF ≤ 35%, and all postinfarction patients with LVEF ≤ 40% or transient heart failure and in some patients with less severe LV dysfunction)
β-blockers – if no contraindications (avoid in NYHA class IV patients) – for early postinfarction patients – for some patients with active myocardial ischemia
Diuretics (to improve symptoms) Spironolactone (to improve survival)
Digoxin (if supraventricular arrhythmias or symptomatic heart failure especially if there is more severe ventricular dysfunction and LV dilatation [> 60 mm in diastole]) May be used prior to ACE inhibitors to control rate in atrial fibrillation
Acute IV inotropes ± nitroglycerin
Consider other vasodilator
Surgical correction of mechanical lesions
Consider cardiac transplantation

*Abbreviations: LV = left ventricle; LVEF = left ventricular ejection fraction; PTCA = percutaneous transluminal coronary angioplasty; CAD = coronary artery disease; CABG = coronary artery bypass graft; NYHA = New York Heart Association.*

Figure 3: **Management of Diastolic Heart Failure**

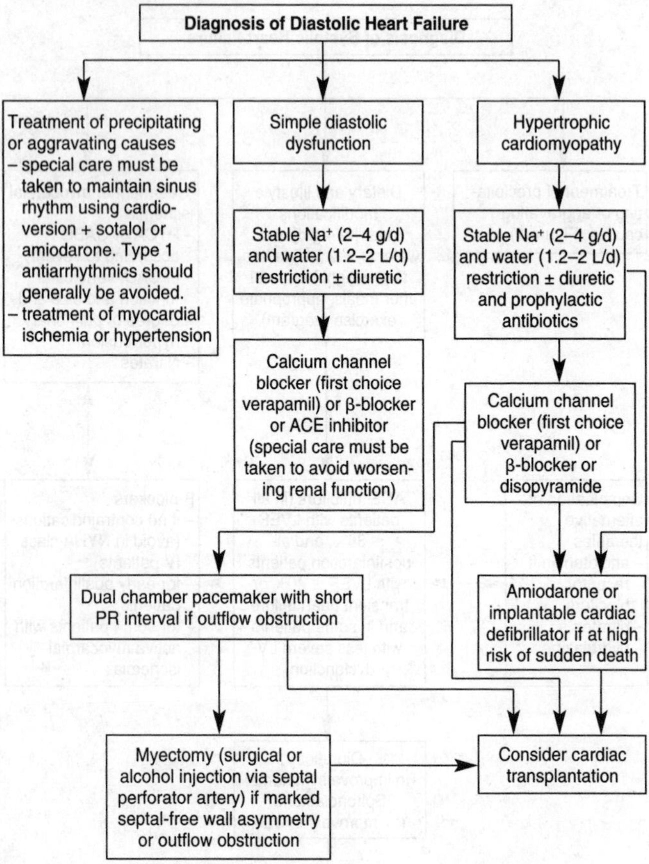
Diagnosis of Diastolic Heart Failure
Treatment of precipitating or aggravating causes
– special care must be taken to maintain sinus rhythm using cardioversion + sotalol or amiodarone. Type 1 antiarrhythmics should generally be avoided.
– treatment of myocardial ischemia or hypertension
Simple diastolic dysfunction
Hypertrophic cardiomyopathy
Stable Na+ (2–4 g/d) and water (1.2–2 L/d) restriction ± diuretic
Stable Na+ (2–4 g/d) and water (1.2–2 L/d) restriction ± diuretic and prophylactic antibiotics
Calcium channel blocker (first choice verapamil) or β-blocker or ACE inhibitor (special care must be taken to avoid worsening renal function)
Calcium channel blocker (first choice verapamil) or β-blocker or disopyramide
Dual chamber pacemaker with short PR interval if outflow obstruction
Amiodarone or implantable cardiac defibrillator if at high risk of sudden death
Myectomy (surgical or alcohol injection via septal perforator artery) if marked septal-free wall asymmetry or outflow obstruction
Consider cardiac transplantation

- Maintenance of sinus rhythm may be important, particularly in patients with diastolic dysfunction. Once adequate systemic *anticoagulation therapy* is sustained for 3 to 4 weeks, cardioversion should be considered in patients with atrial fibrillation in whom the likelihood of maintaining sinus rhythm is reasonable. Cardioversion can be attempted once loading with an *antiarrhythmic drug* has been completed (Chapter 28). The maintenance of sinus rhythm in patients with CHF and dilated atria is surprisingly successful when adjunctive therapy is used. In patients with less severe ventricular dysfunction or idiopathic cardiomyopathy, the use of **sotalol** (160 to 320 mg per day) is recommended; in patients with more severe left ventricular dysfunction or in whom beta-blockers are contraindicated, the use of **amiodarone** (200 mg per day) is recommended. *Because* *of the potential for serious adverse effects, referral to a cardiologist should be made before initiation of amiodarone therapy and sotalol should be initiated under continuous ECG monitoring.*

- Sodium restriction forms the cornerstone of therapy and should be adjusted according to the severity of CHF. Fluid restriction is occasionally necessary. Weight loss, rest after meals and appropriate exercise programs are also important.

## Pharmacologic Choices

### *Angiotensin Converting Enzyme (ACE) Inhibitors* (Table 1)

ACE inhibitors should be given to all patients with symptomatic CHF unless a specific contraindication is present. In asymptomatic patients with moderate left ventricular dysfunction (left ventricular ejection fraction ≤ 35%), they are recommended to prevent deterioration to overt heart failure and to reduce the need for hospitalization. In patients with a recent myocardial infarction and moderate left ventricular dysfunction (left ventricular ejection fraction ≤ 40 %) or in transient heart failure postinfarction, they decrease mortality, prevent progression to overt heart failure and reduce the risk of recurrent myocardial infarction. Therapy should be started as soon as possible postinfarction. In chronic failure, high doses are more effective than lower doses. *It is believed that the benefits are due to a class effect and that ACE inhibitors are largely interchangeable. The major differences are approved indications, dosing schedule and cost* (Table 1). In patients with diastolic heart failure, ACE inhibitors are not first-line drugs but can be used to control arterial hypertension and to help induce regression of left ventricular hypertrophy where this is thought to be a precipitating factor.

### *Angiotensin II Receptor Blockers*

Angiotensin II receptor blockers have hemodynamic effects which are similar to ACE inhibitors, although they do not directly affect the bradykinin pathway. They should be considered in ACE inhibitor-intolerant patients and may be useful in combination with ACE inhibitors in severe failure. It is unknown if different pharmacologic effects between these 2 classes of drugs will translate into different benefits.

### *Nitrates*

Topical or oral nitrates are recommended to improve symptoms and exercise tolerance in patients intolerant of ACE inhibitors or who remain symptomatic despite optimal therapy with ACE inhibitors, diuretics and digoxin or in whom myocardial ischemia is thought to be a factor. Doses of isosorbide dinitrate 30 mg PO TID before meals, or topical preparations 0.4 to 0.6 mg from 8 a.m. to 8 p.m. are recommended. Mononitrate preparations are

Table 1: **ACE Inhibitors Used in Congestive Heart Failure**

| Drug ❥ † | Initial Dose | Targeted Dose | Adverse Effects (common to all ACEIs) | Drug Interactions (common to all ACEIs) | Cost* |
|---|---|---|---|---|---|
| *captopril* Capoten, generics | 6.25–12.5 mg TID | 50 mg TID | Hypotension, hyperkalemia, dry cough, renal insufficiency, angioedema (rare), skin rashes, taste disturbance, proteinuria, neutropenia (rare), headache, dizziness. | Diuretics → hypotension (monitor BP). | $$$ |
| *cilazapril* Inhibace | 0.5 mg once daily | 2.5 mg/d given daily | | Potassium-sparing diuretics → hyperkalemia (monitor $K^+$). | $$ |
| *enalapril* Vasotec | 2.5 mg once daily | 20 mg/d given daily to BID | | Potassium → hyperkalemia (monitor $K^+$). | $$$$ |
| *fosinopril* Monopril | 10 mg once daily | 20 mg/d given daily | | NSAIDs → decreased hypotensive effect (monitor BP). | $$ |
| *lisinopril* Prinivil, Zestril, generics | 2.5–5 mg once daily | 10–20 mg/d given daily | | | $$ |
| *quinapril* Accupril | 5–10 mg once daily | 40 mg/d given daily to BID | | Lithium → lithium toxicity (monitor lithium levels). | $$ |
| *ramipril* Altace | 1.25–2.5 mg BID | 10 mg/d given daily to BID | | | $$ |
| *trandolapril* Mavik | 1 mg | 2–4 mg daily | | | $$–$$$ |

* *Cost of 30-day supply at targeted dosage – includes drug cost only.*
*Legend: $ < $20 $$ $20–40 $$$ $40–60 $$$$ $60–80*

† *Captopril, cilazapril, enalapril, fosinopril, lisinopril, quinapril and ramipril are indicated for heart failure but only captopril, enalapril, lisinopril and ramipril have been shown to reduce morbidity and prolong survival in heart failure.*

❥ *All ACE inhibitors are excreted primarily by the renal route except fosinopril, which is excreted by the renal/hepatic routes. Dosage adjustments may be required in renal impairment for ACEIs excreted primarily by the renal route – see Appendix I; fosinopril does not require dosage adjustment.*

also effective. A nitrate-free period of 10 to 12 hours each day is necessary to prevent loss of nitrate effect.

### *Hydralazine*

Hydralazine combined with nitrates is indicated in patients with symptomatic systolic heart failure who are intolerant of ACE inhibitors and angiotensin II receptor blockers or have refractory CHF despite use of ACE inhibitors, diuretics and digoxin. Although some patients may require lower doses, doses of 75 to 100 mg PO TID were used in studies where hydralazine in combination with nitrates prolonged survival.

### *Diuretics* (Table 2)

Diuretics should be used to control signs and symptoms of CHF. In patients with diastolic dysfunction, they can be a first-line drug; in patients with systolic dysfunction, they are generally reserved for those who are symptomatic despite the use of ACE inhibitors. Low-dose **spironolactone** (12.5 to 50 mg per day) reduces mortality in severe heart failure.

### *Digoxin*

Digoxin should be used to control ventricular response in patients with atrial fibrillation and in patients with symptomatic systolic dysfunction to improve symptoms and exercise tolerance and reduce rehospitalizations. It is particularly effective in those with more severe ventricular dysfunction and ventricular dilatation (diastolic diameter ≥ 60 mm). Maintenance doses should be 0.125 to 0.25 mg PO daily depending on the patient's size and renal function.

### *Beta-blockers* (Table 3)

Beta-blockers should be considered in most patients with chronic heart failure to preserve or improve ventricular function. Started in extremely low doses (i.e., **carvedilol** 3.125 mg PO BID or **metoprolol** 6.25 mg PO BID) after treatment of the failure has been optimized, these *beta-blockers are increased slowly over a period of weeks to months* to maintain doses that average carvedilol 25 mg PO BID or metoprolol 50 mg PO BID. In patients with left ventricular dysfunction postinfarction, they should be started before hospital discharge and continued indefinitely. They can be used to control symptoms of myocardial ischemia in patients with CHF and angina. Although not first-line drugs for diastolic dysfunction, they are beneficial in some patients, controlling heart rate at rest and during exercise and permitting better filling of the ventricle. Beta-blockers can be particularly useful in patients in whom myocardial ischemia is an associated problem. It is uncertain if the benefits of beta-blockers in heart failure are a class effect; important differences may exist as suggested by trial results.

Table 2: **Diuretics Used in Congestive Heart Failure**

| Drug | Dosage | Comments | Adverse Effects | Drug Interactions | Cost* |
|---|---|---|---|---|---|
| **Thiazides and Related Diuretics** | | | **(Common to thiazide and loop diuretics)** | **(Common to thiazide and loop diuretics)** | |
| *chlorthalidone* Hygroton, generics | 50–200 mg/d given daily | Mild diuretic; acts on distal tubule. Use: mild heart failure or with loop diuretic. | Dehydration, hypokalemia, nausea, anorexia, hyperglycemia (more with thiazides), hyperuricemia, weakness, fatigue, rash, increased total cholesterol, ototoxicity (with high doses of loop diuretics). | Lithium → lithium toxicity (monitor lithium levels). Digoxin → digoxin toxicity if $K^+$ depleted (monitor $K^+$). | $ |
| *hydrochlorothiazide* HydroDiuril, generics | 25–200 mg/d given daily to BID | Mild diuretic; acts on distal tubule (+ proximal tubule). Use: mild heart failure or with loop diuretic. | | Antidiabetic agents → increased blood glucose (monitor glucose). Corticosteroids → hypokalemia (monitor $K^+$). | $ |
| *metolazone* Zaroxolyn | 2.5–10 mg/d given daily to BID | Strong diuretic; acts on dilutional distal + proximal tubules. Use: refractory heart failure. | | NSAIDs → decreased diuretic effect; increased renal toxicity (monitor). | $ |
| **Loop Diuretics** | | | | | |
| *bumetanide* Burinex | 1–4 mg/d | Strong diuretic; acts on ascending loop of Henle. Use: alternative to furosemide particularly when renal blood flow is reduced. | See above. | See above. | $–$$$ |
| *ethacrynic acid* Edecrin | 50–400 mg/d given daily to BID | Strong diuretic; acts on ascending loop of Henle (+ other portions of nephron). Use: alternative to furosemide. | | | $–$$$$ |

| | | | | | |
|---|---|---|---|---|---|
| *furosemide*<br>Lasix, generics | 20–500 mg/d given daily to BID | Strong diuretic; acts on ascending loop of Henle (+ proximal + distal tubules).<br>Use: moderate to severe heart failure. | | | \$–\$\$\$\$ |
| **Potassium-sparing Diuretics** | | | **(Common to potassium-sparing diuretics)** | **(Common to potassium-sparing diuretics)** | |
| *amiloride*<br>Midamor | 2.5–10 mg/d given daily to BID | Moderate diuretic; acts on distal tubule.<br>Use: with $K^+$ wasting diuretic. | Hyperkalemia, gynecomastia (with spironolactone). | ACE inhibitors → hyperkalemia (monitor $K^+$).<br>Potassium supplements → hyperkalemia (avoid). | \$ |
| *spironolactone*<br>Aldactone, generics | 12.5–200 mg/d daily to BID<br>12.5–50 mg/d | Mild diuretic; acts on distal tubule.<br>Use: with $K^+$ wasting diuretic.<br>Low dose for mortality benefit. | | | \$ |
| *triamterene*<br>Dyrenium | 50–200 mg/d given daily to BID | Mild diuretic; acts on distal tubule.<br>Use: with $K^+$ wasting diuretic. | | | \$ |

** Cost of 30-day supply – includes drug cost only.*
*Legend: \$ < \$20  \$\$ \$20–40  \$\$\$ \$40–60  \$\$\$\$ \$60–80*

*Dosage adjustment may be required in renal impairment – see Appendix I.*

Table 3: **Beta-blockers Used in Congestive Heart Failure**

| Drug | Dosage | Comments | Adverse Effects | Cost* |
|---|---|---|---|---|
| *carvedilol* Coreg | 3.125–25 mg PO BID | Nonselective, also alpha-blocker resulting in some vasodilating effects. | Orthostatic hypotension, fluid retention. | $$$$ |
| *metoprolol* Betaloc, Lopresor, generics | 6.25–50 mg PO BID | Selective β-blocker. 6.25 mg strength not commercially available. | All beta-blockers: bronchospasm, dyspnea, bradycardia, malaise, fatigue, asthenia, may mask hypoglycemia. | $ |

* *Cost of 30-day supply – includes drug cost only.*
*Legend: $ < $20 $$ $20–40 $$$ $40–60 $$$$ $60–80*

### *Antiarrhythmic Drugs, Pacemakers and Devices*

These should generally be reserved for symptomatic or sustained ventricular arrhythmias or to help maintain sinus rhythm in atrial fibrillation. Class IC agents (flecainide, propafenone) and Class IA agents (quinidine, procainamide) should be avoided. The Class III drug (**sotalol** 160 to 320 mg per day according to severity of heart failure) may be used with caution. **Amiodarone** (200 to 300 mg per day) is effective and usually considered the drug of choice in patients with severe CHF. Serum potassium should be kept ≥ 4 mmol/L in all patients. Antiarrhythmic drug therapy, when indicated, should be started in the hospital setting. Implantable cardiac defibrillators should be used when pharmacologic therapy has failed. A dual chamber (DDD) pacemaker with a short PR interval (0.08 s) may improve symptoms and exercise tolerance in patients with hypertrophic cardiomyopathy and outflow obstruction.

### *Anticoagulation*

The guidelines for systemic anticoagulation therapy in patients with or without CHF are similar. Anticoagulation is strongly recommended in all patients with heart failure and associated atrial fibrillation, demonstrated intraventricular thrombi, acute myocarditis and for the first 3 to 6 months postacute large anterior myocardial infarction. It is not recommended for routine use in sinus rhythm with no other risk factors for emboli. The INR to be achieved is 1.8 to 2.5. In patients at risk from **warfarin** therapy or where warfarin therapy is not indicated, **ASA** 80 mg daily is recommended (Chapter 32).

### *Calcium Channel Blockers*

*In systolic heart failure and in postinfarction patients with left ventricular dysfunction, the use of calcium channel blockers is generally* ***contraindicated.*** In systolic left ventricular dysfunction, the calcium channel blocker, **amlodipine**, may be used in specific cases: hypertension not controlled with ACE inhibitors or with associated angina or where ACE inhibitors are contraindicated and the combination of hydralazine and nitrate is inadequate or not tolerated. In patients with diastolic dysfunction, calcium channel blockers may be used to control arterial hypertension and to help induce regression of myocardial hypertrophy. They also provide symptomatic relief in up to 60% of patients with hypertrophic cardiomyopathy. In diastolic dysfunction, the calcium channel blocker most commonly used is **verapamil** (240 mg per day). **Diltiazem** (180 to 240 mg per day) has also shown benefit. In hypertrophic cardiomyopathy, calcium channel blockers should in some patients be started in hospital as they may cause significant deterioration.

### IV Inotrope or Vasodilator Therapy

**Dobutamine** (5 to 10 μg/kg/min), **milrinone** (0.375 to 0.75 μg/kg/min) or IV **nitroglycerin** (1 to 2 μg/kg/min) ± **dopamine** (5 to 10 μg/kg/min) infusions for 48 to 72 hours can be used to treat patients with acute decompensation of severe systolic heart failure. Special care must be taken to avoid ventricular arrhythmias and hypokalemia.

### Surgical Correction of Mechanical Lesions

Although a number of cardiac reduction and cardiomyoplasty procedures are being offered today, at this time only aneurysm resection and valvular repair are recommended in patients where this is deemed responsible for the progression of heart failure.

### Continuous Positive Airways Pressure (CPAP)

Central sleep apnea is a poor prognostic finding in patients with severe left ventricular dysfunction. Nasal CPAP may reduce apneic periods, improve symptoms and possibly survival. A large trial is now addressing this issue.

## Therapeutic Tips

- ACE inhibitors should be used with care in patients with renal dysfunction, particularly those with a history of hypertension, and are contraindicated in bilateral renal artery stenosis. Although the risks of hyperkalemia and deterioration of renal function are higher in patients with diabetes, the long-term use of ACE inhibitors (when tolerated) has been useful in preserving renal function.
- When ACE inhibitors cause hypotensive symptoms or deterioration of renal function, a reduction in the dosage of diuretics frequently reduces hypotensive symptoms and recuperates lost renal function.

- *Cough* may not be related to the use of ACE inhibitors in some patients with CHF. Whenever possible the ACE inhibitor should be continued despite the cough. Switching to an angiotensin II receptor blocker usually eliminates the cough.
- *NSAIDs* limit the benefits of ACE inhibitors (but not Angiotensin II receptor blockers). ASA can be used without causing this interaction if the dose is 80 mg per day.
- Diastolic heart failure, although due to impaired filling of the left ventricle, is generally associated with hypertension and renal dysfunction and is much more common in older patients. These are all complicating factors that must be considered when choosing one form of therapy over another.
- Patients in periods of acute decompensation of otherwise chronic heart failure should receive **furosemide** IV to assure rapid and complete delivery of the dose as edematous and sluggish bowels may lead to erratic absorption of oral doses.

## *Suggested Reading List*

Consensus recommendations of the management of chronic heart failure. *Am J Cardiol*; 1999;83(2A):1A–38A.

Stauffer JC, Gaasch WH. Recognition and treatment of left ventricular diastolic dysfunction. *Prog Cardiovasc Dis* 1990;32:319–332.

Tardif J-C, Rouleau J-L. Diastolic dysfunction. *Can J Cardiol* 1996;12:389–398.

CHAPTER 28

# Supraventricular Tachycardia

*Anne M. Gillis, MD, FRCPC and*
*D. George Wyse, MD, PhD, FRCPC*

The most common causes of supraventricular tachycardia (SVT) are atrial fibrillation, atrial flutter, atrioventricular node reentrant tachycardia or reciprocating tachycardia utilizing the atrioventricular node and an extra-nodal accessory electrical connection between atria and ventricles (e.g., Wolff-Parkinson-White syndrome). In general, it is safest to assume that patients presenting only with atrial flutter have both atrial flutter and fibrillation, although the atrial fibrillation may not be documented.

## Goals of Therapy

- To convert to sinus rhythm
- To control ventricular rate (chronic atrial fibrillation/flutter)
- To relieve associated symptoms: palpitations, fatigue, dyspnea, presyncope, syncope, angina, heart failure
- To prevent recurrence
- To prevent complications: life-threatening arrhythmia (e.g., Wolff-Parkinson-White syndrome), stroke, other systemic thromboembolism, tachycardia-induced heart failure, myocardial infarction

## Investigations

- Thorough history and physical examination with special attention to detecting underlying structural heart disease
- 12-lead ECG, during SVT and sinus rhythm
- Thorough attempt to document SVT with ECG, including 24-hour ambulatory monitoring and/or event recorders
- Chest x-ray
- 2-D echocardiogram, transesophageal echocardiogram in special circumstances
- TSH, CBC, INR, PTT (for patients with atrial fibrillation/flutter)

Table 1: **Acute Therapy of Persistent Paroxysmal Atrial Fibrillation/Flutter (AF)***

| **Patient Unstable** | **Patient Stable†** | |
|---|---|---|
| | **AF ≥ 48 hours:** | **AF < 48 hours:** |
| Electrical cardioversion 100–400 J → (repeat if necessary) | propranolol 2–10 mg by IV infusion in 1 mg boluses Q1 min<br>or<br>metoprolol 5–15 mg by IV infusion in 5 mg boluses Q5 min<br>or<br>verapamil 5–20 mg IV push in 5 mg boluses Q5 min<br>or<br>diltiazem 0.25 mg/kg IV infusion then 0.35 mg/kg IV 15 min later if necessary<br>or<br>digoxin 0.5–0.75 mg by IV infusion over 30 min, followed by an additional 0.75 mg in divided doses over next 12–24 h | ibutilide‡ 1 mg IV (for patients < 60 kg, 0.01 mg/kg); may repeat × 1 after 10 min<br>or<br>flecainide 200–300 mg po single dose<br>or<br>propafenone 450–600 mg po single dose<br>or<br>electrical cardioversion 100–400 J; repeat if necessary |

* *See Therapeutic Tips and Figure 1 for subsequent cardioversion and antithrombotic therapy.*

† *Procainamide is the drug of choice for Wolff-Parkinson-White-Syndrome.*

‡ *Ibutilide (Corvert) expected to be available from Pharmacia & Upjohn. Torsades de pointes develops in 8% of patients; monitor at least 4 hours after dose.*

## *Paroxysmal Atrial Fibrillation/Flutter*
(Table 1, Figure 1)

### Pharmacologic Choices

Drugs that slow conduction in the AV node are administered to achieve heart rate control (Tables 1 and 2). Beta-blockers and calcium channel blockers are more effective than digoxin but must be used cautiously in patients with heart failure.

#### *Heart Rate Control*

**Digoxin** is effective at rest but is frequently ineffective for heart rate control during exercise.

**Beta-blockers** effectively control heart rate at rest and during exercise but must be prescribed cautiously in patients with heart failure or bronchospastic lung disease.

**Verapamil** effectively controls heart rate at rest and during exercise. **Diltiazem** is less effective, but synergistic effects are observed with digoxin. Nifedipine and other dihydropyridine calcium channel blockers are ineffective as they have no effects on AV node conduction.

#### *Restoration and Maintenance of Sinus Rhythm*

Class I/III antiarrhythmic drugs are effective in converting atrial fibrillation/flutter to sinus rhythm and maintaining it (Table 3).

Figure 1: **Approach to Management of Atrial Fibrillation**

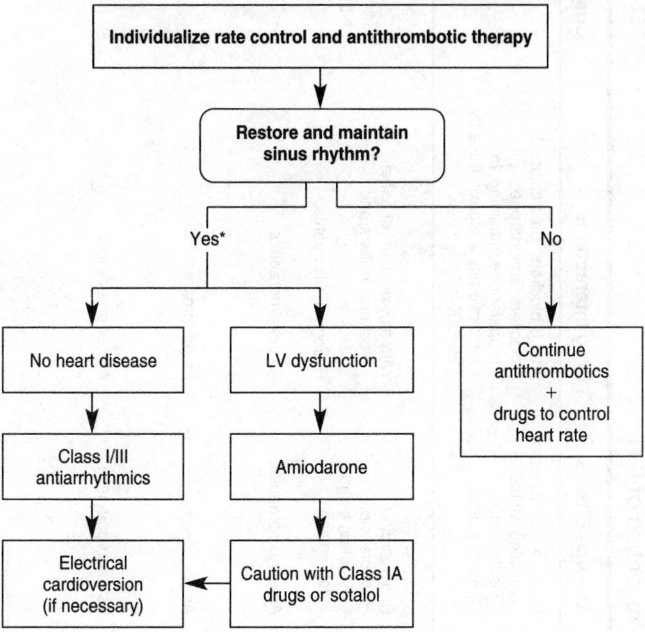
Individualize rate control and antithrombotic therapy
Restore and maintain sinus rhythm?
Yes*
No
No heart disease
LV dysfunction
Continue antithrombotics + drugs to control heart rate
Class I/III antiarrhythmics
Amiodarone
Electrical cardioversion (if necessary)
Caution with Class IA drugs or sotalol

* *See Therapeutic Tips concerning antithrombotic therapy.*

The initial drug of choice remains empiric. A strategy for antithrombotic therapy must be established prior to restoration of sinus rhythm when paroxysmal atrial fibrillation is persistent (i.e., does not stop spontaneously). Atrial fibrillation which is continuous for ≥ 48 hours duration requires specific antithrombotic therapy prior to restoration of sinus rhythm (see Therapeutic Tips). Intermittent, self-administered class I/III therapy at the onset of atrial fibrillation to achieve pharmacologic cardioversion can be used in selected patients.

**Class IA drugs** may cause QRS interval prolongation and QT interval prolongation. Torsades de pointes ventricular tachycardia is the most serious side effect in the setting of marked QT interval prolongation.

**Class IC drugs** cause marked prolongation of conduction velocity that manifests as significant QRS interval prolongation.

**Class III drugs** may cause significant prolongation of the QT interval which may predispose to torsades de pointes ventricular tachycardia.

## Nonpharmacologic Choices

- Direct-current cardioversion is the most rapid method for restoring sinus rhythm in a patient with significant

Table 2: **Heart Rate Control of Fibrillation/Flutter or Termination/Prevention of SVT**

| Drug | Dosage | Dosage Adjustment | Adverse Effects | Drug Interactions | Cost* |
|---|---|---|---|---|---|
| *digoxin* Lanoxin | PO or IV: loading: 1–1.5 mg<br>IV or PO: maintenance 0.125–0.375 mg/d | ↓ maintenance dose in renal insufficiency. | Bradycardia, nausea, vomiting, visual disturbances, proarrhythmia. | With β-blockers, $Ca^{++}$ channel blockers, amiodarone, propafenone, quinidine, in hypokalemia: ↓ digoxin dose by 25–50%. | $ |
| **Beta-blockers** | | | | | |
| *propranolol* Inderal, Inderal-LA, generics | IV: 4–8 mg<br>PO: 80–240 mg/d | Monitor carefully in diabetic patients; caution in patients with CHF or bronchospastic lung disease. | Bradycardia, hypotension, dyspnea, fatigue, depression. | With digoxin, $Ca^{++}$ channel blockers, amiodarone: ↓ dose 25–50%.<br>Hypoglycemic agents. | $<br>LA $–$$ |
| *atenolol* Tenormin, generics | PO: 50–150 mg/d | As per propranolol and ↓ dose in moderate to severe renal insufficiency. | As per propranolol. | As per propranolol. | $ |
| *metoprolol* Betaloc, Lopresor, generics | IV: 5–15 mg<br>PO: 100–400 mg/d | As per propranolol. | As per propranolol. | As per propranolol. | $ |
| *nadolol* Corgard, generics | PO: 20–160 mg/d | As per propranolol and ↓ dose in moderate to severe renal insufficiency. | As per propranolol. | As per propranolol. | $ |

| | | | | | |
|---|---|---|---|---|---|
| **Calcium Channel Blockers** | | | | | |
| *verapamil* Isoptin, Isoptin SR, Verelan, Chronovera, generics | IV: 5–15 mg<br>80 mg PO TID; max. dose 120 mg QID – 240 mg BID | Caution in patients with CHF. | Bradycardia, hypotension, constipation, flushing. | β-blockers, digoxin, amiodarone. | $–$$ |
| *diltiazem* Cardizem, Cardizem CD, Cardizem SR, Tiazac, generics | IV: 0.25–0.35 mg/kg<br>PO: 180–540 mg/d | Caution in patients with CHF. | Bradycardia, hypotension. | As per verapamil. | $$–$$$ |

*Note: The β-blockers suggested are examples only. Atenolol and metoprolol have $\beta_1$ selectivity; both atenolol and nadolol are hydrophilic agents and less likely to cause CNS side effects. Acebutolol, labetolol and timolol would also be effective. Some agents are available as sustained-release preparations.*

** Cost of 30-day supply of oral doses – includes drug cost only.*
*Legend: $ < $30 $$ $30–60 $$$ $60–100*

Table 3: **Drug Therapy for Long-term Prophylaxis of Atrial Fibrillation/SVT**

| Drug | Dosage | Dosage Adjustment | Adverse Effects | Drug Interactions | Cost* |
|---|---|---|---|---|---|
| **Class IA** | | | | | |
| *quinidine* Biquin Durules, generics | 200–250 mg PO Q8H ↑ by 200–250 mg doses if QTc < 460 msec. ↓ dose if QTc ≥ 500 msec. Max. dose 1 g PO Q8H | ↓ initial dose 50% + ↑ dosing interval Q12H in renal failure. Active metabolites accumulate in renal failure but therapeutic blood monitoring of them is not readily available. Careful monitoring of the ECG intervals should guide dosing decisions. | Diarrhea, stomach cramps, tinnitus, fever, rash, thrombocytopenia, torsades de pointes. | ↓ digoxin dose by 50%. | $ Biquin Durules $$–$$$$$ |
| *procainamide SR* Procan SR, Pronestyl SR | 250 mg PO Q6H ↑ by 250 mg increments if QTc < 460 msec. ↓ dose if QTc ≥ 500 msec. Max. dose 1 g PO Q6H | Metabolism depends on rate of acetylation. The active metabolite NAPA accumulates in fast acetylators and in renal failure. Monitor procainamide + NAPA levels and keep sum < 80 μM; monitor ECG intervals. | SLE syndrome, torsades de pointes. | | $–$$$ |
| *disopyramide* Norpace, Norpace CR, Rythmodan, Rythmodan-LA | 100 mg PO Q8H<br>CR and LA: 150–250 mg Q12H<br>↑ by 100 mg increments if QTc < 460 msec. Max. dose 300 mg PO Q8H | ↓ initial dose 50% and ↑ dosing interval Q12H in renal failure. | Urinary retention, constipation, dry mouth, torsades de pointes VT. | | $–$$ |

| | | | | | |
|---|---|---|---|---|---|
| **Class IC** | | | | | |
| *flecainide* Tambocor | 50 mg PO Q12H<br>↑ by 50 mg increments<br>Max. dose 200 mg PO Q12H. ↓ dose if ↑ QRS > 20% from baseline | ↓ initial dose 50% in renal failure; titrate dose based on QRS intervals. | VT proarrhythmia, tremor, blurred vision, CHF. | | $–$$$$ |
| *propafenone* Rythmol | 150 mg PO Q8H<br>Max. dose 300 mg PO Q8H. ↓ dose if QRS prolonged > 20% from baseline | ↓ initial dose 50% in renal and hepatic failure and ↑ dosing interval to Q12H.<br>Active metabolites accumulate in rapid metabolizers. Monitor QRS duration carefully. | Constipation, headache, metallic taste, VT proarrhythmia. | ↓ digoxin dose by 25–50%. | $$$–$$$$ |
| **Class III** | | | | | |
| *sotalol* Sotacor, generics | 80 mg PO Q12H<br>↑ by 80 mg increments if QTc < 460 msec<br>Max. dose 240 mg PO Q12H. ↓ dose if QTc ≥ 500 msec | ↓ initial dose in renal failure.<br>↓ initial dose to 40 mg PO Q12H in the elderly. | Torsades de pointes, hypotension, bradycardia, wheezing. | Digoxin/verapamil/other β-blockers may cause AV block, bradycardia. | $–$$ |
| *amiodarone* Cordarone, generics | 200 mg PO TID × 2 wk then 200 mg daily or accelerated loading dose in hospital | Avoid high loading dose in setting of sinus bradycardia (HR < 50 beats/min). | Pulmonary toxicity, CNS effects, hyper-/hypothyroidism, photosensitivity, corneal deposits, hepatic toxicity. | ↓ quinidine/procainamide dose by 50%.<br>↓ digoxin dose by 50%.<br>↓ β-blockers dose by 50%.<br>↓ warfarin dose by 50%. | $$$ |

* *Cost of 30-day supply – includes drug cost only.*

*Legend:* $ < $30 $$ $30–60 $$$ $60–100 $$$$ $100–140 $$$$$ > $140

hemodynamic compromise, angina or heart failure. Elective cardioversion is effective, particularly after initiation of class I/III drugs to prevent early recurrence and facilitate maintenance of rhythm. These drugs may need to be continued temporarily or permanently.

- When heart rate control cannot be achieved or medications are not well tolerated, catheter ablation of the AV node and implantation of a permanent pacemaker should be considered.
- Catheter ablation techniques may prevent recurrent atrial flutter without inducing complete heart block.
- Antitachycardia pacemakers are effective in terminating some episodes of atrial flutter.
- Some surgical techniques may prevent atrial fibrillation and preserve sinus rhythm; atrial-based pacing prevents atrial fibrillation in the general pacemaker population. The implantable automatic atrial defibrillator is at an early stage of investigation.

## *Chronic Atrial Fibrillation*

### Pharmacologic Choices

- When sinus rhythm cannot be maintained, therapy is aimed at achieving heart rate control (Table 2).
- Chronic anticoagulation is indicated to reduce the risk of systemic thromboembolism (Table 4).

### Nonpharmacologic Choices

- When heart rate control cannot be achieved with drug therapy, catheter ablation of the AV node and implantation of a permanent pacemaker should be considered.

### Therapeutic Tips (Atrial Fibrillation/Flutter)

- If atrial fibrillation has been present for ≥ 48 hours, anticoagulation with **heparin** should be initiated followed by **oral anticoagulation**. Attempts to convert atrial fibrillation should be delayed for at least 3 weeks if present for more than 48 hours before initiation of anticoagulation. Another alternative is anticoagulation with heparin followed by transesophageal echocardiography and then immediate restoration of sinus rhythm if no intracardiac clot is noted on the echo. **Warfarin must be started and continued for 4 weeks after restoration of sinus rhythm (regardless of whether it is done immediately or delayed ≥ 3 weeks).**
- *Antithrombotic therapy* should be considered for all patients with paroxysmal or chronic atrial fibrillation based on risk for systemic thromboembolism (Table 4).

Table 4: **Anticoagulation for Paroxysmal and Chronic Atrial Fibrillation***

| Condition | Drug |
|---|---|
| Patient with no risk factors and Age < 75 yrs | ASA 325 mg/d |
| Patient with any one of the following risk factors: Age < 65 yrs and congestive heart failure, left ventricular dysfunction, mitral valve disease, hypertension, diabetes mellitus, previous stroke or embolism, left atrial enlargement | Warfarin (INR 2.0–3.0) |
| Age ≥ 75 yrs | Individualize therapy: warfarin (INR 1.8–2.5) |

* *See Therapeutic Tips for anticoagulation prior to restoration of sinus rhythm.*

- *Digoxin, beta-blockers and calcium channel blockers are contraindicated for atrial fibrillation in Wolff-Parkinson-White syndrome; these drugs may precipitate ventricular fibrillation.* IV **procainamide** is the drug of choice.
- *The use of Class IC drugs (flecainide and propafenone) for maintenance of sinus rhythm is contraindicated in patients with coronary artery disease and cannot be recommended for patients with significant ventricular dysfunction.* Class III drugs must be used with caution in patients with significant ventricular dysfunction.
- Bradycardia, hypokalemia and hypomagnesemia predispose patients to ventricular proarrhythmia on Class I/III drugs. If patients are taking diuretics, $K^+$ and $Mg^{++}$ levels should be measured before initiation of therapy; regular monitoring during therapy is also required. Twelve-lead ECGs should be performed at each steady-state dose to assess QTc.
- Since antiarrhythmic agents may precipitate bradyarrhythmia, permanent pacemaker implantation may be required in some patients. Twenty-four hour ambulatory ECG monitoring should be performed at each steady-state dose in high-risk patients.
- Because of the toxicity profile, referral to a cardiologist should be made before initiation of **amiodarone** therapy.

## *Supraventricular Tachycardia (SVT)*

The approach to therapy for an acute episode of SVT is illustrated in Table 5.

Table 5: **Acute Therapy for Paroxysmal SVT**

**Termination of Acute Episode**

**A. QRS is ≤ 0.1 s or Patient Known to Have Bundle Branch Block**

1. maneuvers to activate the vagus nerve: Valsalva maneuver, carotid sinus massage, pressure on orbit, diving reflex

↓

2. adenosine 6–12 mg by IV push (max. dose 24 mg)

or

3. verapamil 5–20 mg by IV push in 5 mg boluses Q5 min

↓

4. metoprolol 5–15 mg by IV infusion in 5 mg increments Q5 min

or

5. diltiazem 0.25 mg/kg IV infusion; then 0.35 mg/kg 15 min later

or

6. digoxin 0.5–0.75 mg by IV infusion over 15–30 min, followed by additional 0.75 mg in divided doses over 12–24 h

**B. QRS is > 0.1 s and No Previous ECG or Patient Known to Have QRS ≤ 0.1 s**

1. (Suspect Wolff-Parkinson-White syndrome) procainamide 15 mg/kg given as 25 mg/min infusion if blood pressure stable, then maintenance dose 2–4 mg/min IV

↓

2. electrical cardioversion under anesthesia

The chronic therapy for prevention of paroxysmal SVT is illustrated in Table 6.

## Pharmacologic Choices

- Drugs that slow conduction in the AV node (e.g., adenosine, beta-blockers, calcium channel blockers, digoxin) are effective in terminating and preventing recurrence of *SVT*. Maintenance doses are shown in Table 6.
- Drugs that prolong conduction in atrial muscle effectively terminate and prevent recurrence of SVT in the *Wolff-Parkinson-White syndrome* (Table 3 and 6).

## Nonpharmacologic Choices

- **Catheter ablation is the treatment of choice in patients with Wolff-Parkinson-White syndrome who do not respond to therapy or do not tolerate drug therapy.** AV node ablation of the slow or fast pathway is an effective therapy for AV node reentrant tachycardia. Catheter ablative therapy as a primary alternative to pharmacologic therapy is becoming increasingly popular and is the most cost-effective approach to the management of SVT.
- Antitachycardia pacing is occasionally effective.
- Surgical ablation of the AV node or accessory pathway may be considered when catheter ablation has been unsuccessful.

Table 6: **Chronic Therapy for Paroxysmal SVT**

**A. Recurrences Rare and/or Brief and Hemodynamically Stable; QRS ≤ 0.1 s during PAT or Patient Known to Have Bundle Branch Block**

1. vagal maneuvers

   *or*

2. verapamil PO at onset 80 mg Q2H for up to 3 doses

   *or*

3. metoprolol PO at onset 50–100 mg Q2H for up to 3 doses

   *or*

4. propranolol PO at onset 40–80 mg Q2H for up to 3 doses

**B. Recurrences Frequent and/or Prolonged and Hemodynamically Stable; QRS ≤ 0.1 s during PAT or Patient Known to Have Bundle Branch Block**

1. catheter ablation

   *or* continuous/prophylaxis with:

2. verapamil 160–480 mg/d

   *or*

3. diltiazem 180–540 mg/d

   *or*

4. propranolol 80–240 mg/d

   *or*

5. metoprolol 100–400 mg/d

   *or*

6. atenolol 50–200 mg/d

   *or*

7. equivalent doses of alternative beta-blocker

   *or*

8. digoxin 0.25–0.5 mg/d

   *or*

9. surgical therapy

**C. Recurrences Frequent and/or Prolonged and Hemodynamically Stable; QRS > 0.1 s during PAT in Patient with Known Wolff-Parkinson-White Syndrome**

1. catheter ablation

   *or*

2. continuous prophylaxis with sotalol 160–480 mg/d

   ↓

3. continuous prophylaxis with propafenone 450–900 mg/d plus calcium channel blocker or beta-blocker listed above in B

   ↓

4. continuous prophylaxis with flecainide 100–400 mg/d plus calcium channel blocker or beta-blocker listed above in B

   ↓

5. continuous prophylaxis with amiodarone 200–300 mg/d

**D. Recurrence Hemodynamically Unstable Regardless of Frequency, Duration or QRS Width**

1. catheter ablation or surgical therapy

## Therapeutic Tips (Supraventricular Tachycardia)

- Beta-blockers and calcium channel blockers should be used with caution in patients with congestive heart failure.
- Digoxin and verapamil *as monotherapy* are contraindicated in patients with Wolff-Parkinson-White syndrome.
- Combination calcium channel blockers or beta-blockers with Class I/III antiarrhythmic drugs may be required to prevent SVT in patients with Wolff-Parkinson-White syndrome.

## ***Suggested Reading List***

Murray KT. Ibutilide. *Circulation* 1998;97:493–497.

Sharif MN, Wyse DG. Atrial fibrillation: overview of therapeutic trials. *Can J Cardiol* 1998;14:1241–1254.

Thibault B, Nattel S. Optimal management with class I and class III antiarrythmic drugs should be done in the outpatient setting: protagonist. *J Cardiovasc Electrophysiol* 1999;10:472–481.

CHAPTER 29

# Ventricular Tachyarrhythmias

*Paul Dorian, MD, FRCPC*

## Definitions

**Ventricular tachycardia** (VT) is defined as ≥ 3 consecutive ventricular complexes at a rate > 100 beats/minute on an ECG recording. The clinical and prognostic importance and management of VT depend on whether it is sustained or nonsustained and the presence of associated structural heart disease, particularly LV systolic dysfunction.

**Ventricular fibrillation** (VF) is defined as a rapid, disorganized rhythm without recognizable QRS complexes on the ECG. It is invariably associated with cardiovascular collapse and almost invariably fatal unless the patient is electrically defibrillated. VF frequently results from VT. If VF occurs in the absence of reversible causes, recurrence rates are high.

## Goals of Therapy

- To relieve symptoms, including restoring sinus rhythm as quickly as possible in sustained VT or cardiac arrest
- To prevent the potentially fatal occurrence or recurrence of sustained VT or cardiac arrest

### Classification of VT

- *Asymptomatic:* usually discovered during routine screening ECG or other electrocardiographic monitoring
- *Symptomatic:* may cause palpitations, dyspnea, chest discomfort, presyncope, loss of consciousness, cardiac arrest
- *Sustained:* lasting ≥ 30 seconds or requiring immediate medical intervention; for management decisions, > 15 beats is a reasonable working definition
- *Nonsustained:* < 30 seconds but usually lasting only a few seconds; most commonly < 10 consecutive ventricular complexes
- *In the presence of structural heart disease:* usually coronary, valvular or hypertensive heart disease; left ventricular dysfunction is the most important distinguishing characteristic
- *Unaccompanied by structural heart disease* (in a normal heart)

- *Monomorphic:* all the ventricular (QRS) complexes appear the same
- *Polymorphic:* beat-to-beat variability in the QRS complex morphology

## Investigations

- Careful history with special reference to:
  - syncope or severe presyncope
  - angina, heart failure
  - history suggesting structural heart disease
  - symptom correlation with exercise or stress
- Physical examination:
  - signs of structural heart disease
- 12-lead ECG:
  - signs of MI
  - repolarization abnormalities (prolonged QT interval)

*Note:* A 12-lead ECG documenting ventricular tachycardia is very important. If available, ECG at tachycardia onset (or offset) is very useful.

- Echocardiogram with special reference to:
  - left ventricular size and function
  - right ventricular size
- Holter monitoring with special reference to:
  - presence and morphology of ventricular ectopy and symptom–rhythm correlation
- Treadmill exercise test with special reference to:
  - exercise-induced VT
  - ECG signs and symptoms of myocardial ischemia (or scintigraphic evidence of ischemia if necessary)

**All wide-complex (QRS duration ≥ 0.12 seconds) tachycardias in patients over 50 should be considered VT until proven otherwise.**

**Wide-complex tachycardia in an older patient with a history of heart disease *is almost always* VT, regardless of the morphology of ECG complexes.**

**Most wide-complex tachycardias in any patient of any age group are due to VT.**

## Significance of VT/VF

In the presence of structural heart disease, especially left ventricular dysfunction, asymptomatic VT (usually nonsustained) may indicate a risk of future serious, symptomatic, sustained VT or VF.

**Symptomatic:** The prognostic importance of VT and its management are determined by the underlying cardiac status and the type of VT rather than the severity of symptoms (e.g., even severe symptoms in a patient with nonsustained VT and no structural heart disease are prognostically benign and the patient requires reassurance but not necessarily specific antiarrhythmic therapy).

**Sustained VT** is most often associated with structural heart disease, typically coronary disease with previous MI. It requires investigation and therapy: antiarrhythmic drugs, implanted cardioverter defibrillators or antitachycardia surgery.

**Nonsustained VT** unless symptomatic requires treatment only if likelihood of subsequent sustained VT or cardiac arrest is high.

**VT associated with structural heart disease** is usually symptomatic and associated with a high risk of sudden death or recurrence (if sustained) or asymptomatic but associated with at least a moderate risk of sudden death (if nonsustained).

**VT associated with a structurally normal heart** may be symptomatic but rarely life threatening even if sustained; it requires no therapy if asymptomatic and nonsustained.

**Monomorphic VT** usually implies an abnormal automatic focus in the ventricle or a fixed reentrant pathway associated with a scar. It does not by itself suggest prognosis or therapy.

**Polymorphic VT** usually presents as long runs of nonsustained VT. Myocardial ischemia and abnormalities of repolarization (torsades de pointes VT with QT prolongation) should be considered.

### Significance of VF

VF may complicate acute MI. However, the prognosis for resuscitated patients with VF occurring during the first 48 hours post-MI is similar to that in patients with equivalent severity infarction uncomplicated by VF.

Most out-of-hospital episodes of VF are not caused by acute MI or obvious acute ischemia, although they generally occur in patients with coronary artery disease and prior MI. Most patients with VF are at high risk of recurrence and should be investigated in a similar fashion to patients with sustained VT as well as treated to prevent recurrences.

## Therapeutic Choices (Figures 1 and 2)

### Immediate Therapy for Sustained VT or VF

If the patient is unstable (e.g., has hypotension, angina, heart failure or marked symptoms), **cardioversion** is effective and safe.

A synchronized shock of 50 to 100 J is usually effective for VT. If immediate conversion to sinus rhythm is not considered necessary, antiarrhythmic drug therapy can be given.

For VF, an immediate nonsynchronized shock of 200 to 300 J is required, repeated as necessary at 300 to 360 J until defibrillation is achieved.

**Lidocaine:** 1 to 1.5 mg/kg IV followed by a 1 to 3 mg/minute infusion will occasionally be effective (< 20% of cases of VT) and rarely causes hypotension. If conversion does not occur within 10 to 15 minutes lidocaine will probably be ineffective. There is no good evidence that lidocaine is useful in shock-resistant VF.

**Procainamide:** 10 to 15 mg/kg IV over 30 to 45 minutes will often slow VT and terminate tachycardia. Hypotension may occur, especially at the more rapid infusion rates, and blood pressure should be carefully monitored.

**Bretylium:** 5 to 10 mg/kg IV over 5 to 10 minutes may prevent VF. Data on efficacy in monomorphic VT are limited. It frequently causes severe hypotension and should be used with caution.

**Magnesium:** 2 to 5 g IV over 3 to 5 minutes is the treatment of choice for torsades de pointes VT associated with QT prolongation and a characteristic long–short initiating sequence, and may be useful in the presence of myocardial ischemia. It is of unclear benefit in monoform VT. Magnesium may rarely cause hypotension but is generally safe.

**Amiodarone:** IV amiodarone is effective in terminating VT and especially in preventing early recurrence. The usual dose is 3 to 5 mg/kg IV over 5 to 10 minutes followed by a 0.5 to 1 mg/minute infusion. Hypotension may occur, especially if the drug is administered very rapidly. It is likely the most effective therapy for electrical storm characterized by frequent recurrences of VT/VF and is probably useful in shock-resistant VF.

## Chronic Therapy – Prevention of VT/VF Recurrence

Therapeutic choices for long-term management of sustained VT/VF include both drug therapy (Table 1) and nondrug therapy (implanted cardioverter defibrillators, map guided endocardial resection, catheter ablation).

Sustained monomorphic VT or VF is likely to recur in the absence of treatment. Empiric drug treatment (i.e., without objective documentation of efficacy) is not recommended. Amiodarone therapy is a possible exception.

Indicators of drug efficacy include the inability to deliberately induce VT in the presence of a drug when VT can be induced in its absence, and the marked reduction of the frequency or

Figure 1: **Management of Nonsustained Ventricular Tachycardia (VT) (< 15 beats)**

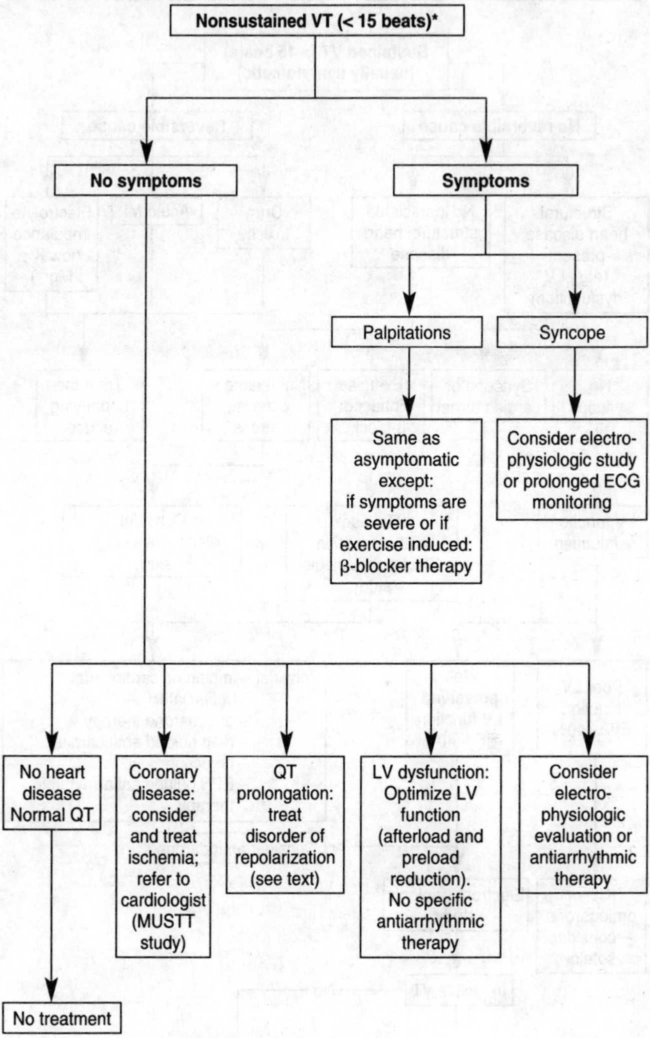
Nonsustained VT (< 15 beats)*
No symptoms
Symptoms
Palpitations
Syncope
Same as asymptomatic except: if symptoms are severe or if exercise induced: β-blocker therapy
Consider electro-physiologic study or prolonged ECG monitoring
No heart disease Normal QT
Coronary disease: consider and treat ischemia; refer to cardiologist (MUSTT study)
QT prolongation: treat disorder of repolarization (see text)
LV dysfunction: Optimize LV function (afterload and preload reduction). No specific antiarrhythmic therapy
Consider electro-physiologic evaluation or antiarrhythmic therapy
No treatment

* *Evidence suggests that patients with nonsustained VT and severe LV dysfunction (ejection fraction < 35%) are at high risk of serious arrhythmias and may profit from electrophysiologic evaluation. (Moss AJ et al, N Engl J Med 1996; 335: 1933–40 and Buxton AE et al, N Engl J Med 1999;341:1882–1890.)*

Figure 2: **Long-term Management of Sustained Ventricular Tachycardia (VT) (> 15 beats) or Ventricular Fibrillation (VF) (after immediate stabilization)**

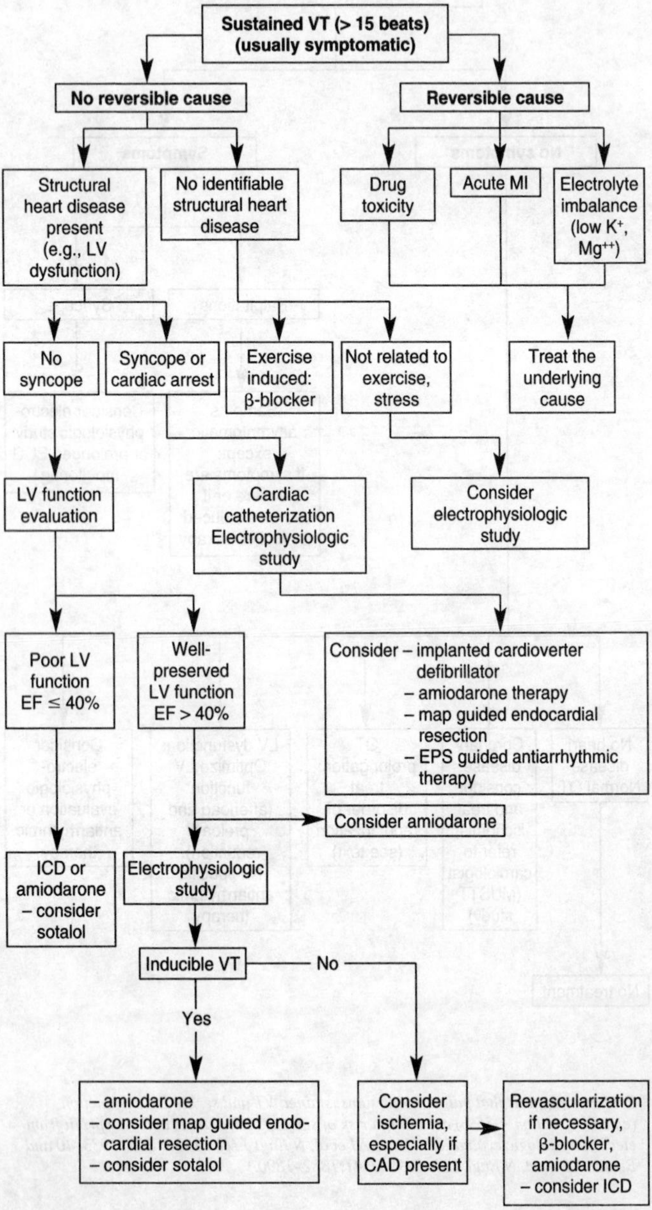
Sustained VT (> 15 beats) (usually symptomatic)
No reversible cause
Reversible cause
Structural heart disease present (e.g., LV dysfunction)
No identifiable structural heart disease
Drug toxicity
Acute MI
Electrolyte imbalance (low K+, Mg++)
No syncope
Syncope or cardiac arrest
Exercise induced: β-blocker
Not related to exercise, stress
Treat the underlying cause
LV function evaluation
Cardiac catheterization Electrophysiologic study
Consider electrophysiologic study
Poor LV function EF ≤ 40%
Well-preserved LV function EF > 40%
Consider – implanted cardioverter defibrillator – amiodarone therapy – map guided endocardial resection – EPS guided antiarrhythmic therapy
Consider amiodarone
ICD or amiodarone – consider sotalol
Electrophysiologic study
Inducible VT
No
Yes
– amiodarone – consider map guided endo-cardial resection – consider sotalol
Consider ischemia, especially if CAD present
Revascularization if necessary, β-blocker, amiodarone – consider ICD

***NB: Implanted cardioverter defibrillator (ICD) therapy may be considered for any patient with sustained VT.***

*Abbreviations: LV = left ventricle; MI = myocardial infarction; VPB = ventricular premature beat; EPS = electrophysiologic study; CAD = coronary artery disease.*

Table 1: **Drug Therapy for VT/VF**

| Drug | Dosage | Dosage Adjustment | Drug Interactions | Comments | Cost* |
|---|---|---|---|---|---|
| **Drugs that slow conduction and prolong repolarization (Class IA)** | | | | | |
| *quinidine* † generics, Biquin Durules | 800–1600 mg/d (sulfate equivalent) | ↓ initial dose by 50% + ↑ dosing interval to Q12H in renal failure. Active metabolites accumulate in renal failure, but therapeutic blood monitoring is not readily available. Careful monitoring of the ECG intervals should guide dosing decisions. | ↓ digoxin dose by 50%. | Long history of use. Frequent GI intolerance. Rare fever, thrombocytopenia. May cause torsades de pointes; (proarrhythmic) VT. | $ Biquin Durules $$–$$$ |
| *procainamide* † Pronestyl, generics, Pronestyl SR, Procan SR | 2–4 g/d | Metabolism depends on rate of acetylation. The active metabolite NAPA accumulates in fast acetylators and in renal failure. Monitor procainamide + NAPA levels; monitor ECG intervals. | | Frequent arthralgias after long term use. May cause SLE syndrome. Rare granulocytopenia. Occasional torsades de pointes. | $$–$$$ |
| *disopyramide* † Norpace, Norpace CR, Rythmodan, Rythmodan-LA | 400–800 mg/d | ↓ initial dose by 50% and ↑ dosing interval to Q12H in renal failure. | | Depresses LV function. Should not be used in patients with LV dysfunction. Dry mouth, urinary retention, blurred vision. May cause torsades de pointes. | $–$$ |

*(cont'd)*

Table 1: **Drug Therapy for VT/VF** *(cont'd)*

| Drug | Dosage | Dosage Adjustment | Drug Interactions | Comments | Cost* |
|---|---|---|---|---|---|
| **Drugs that slow conduction (Class IB and IC)†** | | | | | |
| *mexiletine* Mexitil, generics | 600–900 mg/d | ↓ dose by 50% and ↑ dosing interval to Q12H in renal failure. | Phenytoin and rifampin may ↓ effect. May need to ↑ mexiletine dose. | Frequent CNS side effects. | $$$ |
| *flecainide* Tambocor | 100–200 mg/d | ↓ initial dose by 50% in renal failure. Titrate dose based on QRS intervals. | | Moderately frequent proarrhythmia. Should not be used in patients with LV dysfunction, especially prior MI. Increases mortality compared to placebo in patients who have frequent PVCs following MI. | $$ |
| *propafenone* Rythmol | 600–900 mg/d | ↓ initial dose by 50% in renal and hepatic failure and ↑ dosing interval to Q12H. Active metabolites accumulate in rapid metabolizers. Monitor QRS duration carefully. | ↓ digoxin dose by 25–50%. | Weak β-blocking effect. Depresses LV function. Should be used with great reservation, if at all, in patients with LV dysfunction, especially prior MI. | $$$–$$$$ |
| **Drugs that primarily prolong repolarization (Class III)** | | | | | |
| *sotalol* Sotacor, generics | 160–480 mg/d | ↓ initial dose in renal failure. ↓ initial dose to 40 mg PO Q12H in the elderly. | Digoxin, verapamil, other β-blockers may cause AV block, bradycardia. | Potent β-blocker and bradycardic agent. Often causes fatigue. May cause torsades de pointes, especially at higher doses or with renal dysfunction. May be especially effective in exercise-related arrhythmias. Likely more effective than other drugs in suppressing inducibility of VT. Contraindicated in bronchial asthma. | $–$$ |

| | | | | | |
|---|---|---|---|---|---|
| *amiodarone*<br>Cordarone, generics | Loading dose: 800–1600 mg/d × 7–10 d PO<br>Maintenance dose: 200–400 mg/d PO | Avoid high loading dose in setting of sinus bradycardia (HR < 50 beats/min). | ↓ quinidine/procainamide dose by 50%.<br>↓ digoxin dose by 50%.<br>↓ β-blocker dose by 50%.<br>↓ warfarin dose by 50%. | Very complex drug; also slows conduction, blocks adrenergic activity, blocks $Ca^{++}$ channels. Very long half-life. Frequent adverse effects in many organ systems. Requires close monitoring. Likely the most effective antiarrhythmic drug. Usually used as empiric therapy. | $$$–$$$$ |
| **Other** | | | | | |
| *beta-blockers* | Individualized according to chosen agent | Monitor carefully in diabetic patients.<br>Caution in patients with CHF. | Digoxin.<br>$Ca^{++}$ channel blockers.<br>Amiodarone.<br>↓ dose of hypoglycemic agents by 25–50%. | Especially useful in exercise-induced VT, with ischemia, or VT in the absence of structural heart disease. Of probable but unclear benefit in patients with sustained VT and prior MI. May enhance efficacy of other antiarrhythmic drugs in this setting. Very low proarrhythmic risk. Contraindicated in bronchial asthma. | $ |

*† There is no evidence that any drug with primarily class I activity is of long-term benefit in reducing mortality from VT or VF; in particular, class IB and IC drugs are not recommended in patients with VT or VF and structural heart disease.*

** Cost of 30-day supply – includes drug cost only.*
*Legend: $ < $30   $$ $30–60   $$$ $60–100   $$$$ > $100*

elimination of nonsustained VT episodes or PVCs by the given antiarrhythmic agent. (The latter indicator is unproven and rarely used.)

Patients with a history of VF or cardiac arrest are at risk of recurrence of VF or VT, since their original arrhythmia may have been VT degenerating to VF. Their treatment is similar to that of patients with sustained VT, although markers to judge drug efficacy (inducible VT or VF, PVCs or nonsustained VT on Holter monitoring) are less often present.

### Nonpharmacologic Choices for VT

- Implanted cardioverter defibrillator (ICD):
  - extremely effective in treating VT or VF but requires complex evaluation and follow-up. The AVID trial reported 39% total mortality reduction in ICD-treated patients compared to antiarrhythmic therapy (primarily amiodarone).
- Map guided endocardial surgery:
  - requires careful patient selection, specialized facilities and complex open heart surgery; may be very effective in certain patient subsets.
- Catheter ablation using radiofrequency energy:
  - may be especially effective for VT arising from the right ventricle in patients with apparently normal hearts; experimental for VT following myocardial infarction.

## *Suggested Reading List*

The Antiarrhythmics versus Implantable Defibrillators (AVID) Investigators. A comparison of antiarrhythmic-drug therapy with implantable defibrillators in patients resuscitated from near-fatal ventricular arrhythmias. *N Engl J Med* 1997;337:1576–1583.

Kowey PR, Levine JH, Herre JM, et al. Randomized, double-blind comparison of intravenous amiodarone and bretylium in the treatment of patients with recurrent hemodynamically destabilizing ventricular tachycardia or fibrillation. *Circulation* 1995;92:3255–3263.

Nattel S. Antiarrhythmic drug classifications: a critical appraisal of their history, present status, and clinical relevance. *Drugs* 1991;41:672–701.

Teo KK. Evaluation of therapeutic modalities in patients with life threatening arrhythmias. *Can J Cardiol* 1994;10:333–341.

CHAPTER 30

# Acute Stroke

*Stephen J. Phillips, BSc, MBBS, FRCPC*

Stroke, recognized clinically as the sudden onset of a focal disturbance of central nervous system function, may be caused by cerebral infarction (ischemic stroke; responsible for about 80% of all strokes), intracerebral hemorrhage and subarachnoid hemorrhage.

There is no acute-phase intervention of proven value for intracerebral hemorrhage. Post-acute treatment of primary intracerebral hemorrhage is similar to that of ischemic stroke except that antithrombotic drugs are avoided. Patients with suspected subarachnoid hemorrhage should be referred to a neurosurgical centre. Treatment of subarachnoid hemorrhage is primarily nonpharmacologic, i.e., endovascular and/or surgical ablation of the bleeding source and will not be discussed further.

This chapter focuses on acute-phase medical treatment of ischemic stroke.

## Goals of Therapy

- To minimize brain damage
- To prevent complications
- To reduce risk of recurrence
- To restore function of the individual

## Investigations

- History
  – time of onset, symptoms at onset, course of symptoms since onset
  – antecedent trauma or illness, previous neurovascular events
  – vascular comorbidity (angina, myocardial infarction, heart failure, atrial fibrillation, peripheral and renal vascular disease)
  – vascular disease risk factors (hypertension, smoking, diabetes, cholesterol, alcohol intake, body mass index, exercise, family history of vascular disease or hemostatic disorder)
  – other health problems (particularly peptic ulcer disease and other disorders that predispose to bleeding)
  – pre-stroke cognitive and functional status
  – place of residence and social supports
  – medications (particularly warfarin, ASA and other antiplatelet drugs)

- Physical examination to: localize the lesion by brain region and vascular territory; determine syndromic diagnosis, severity, and cause; and assess comorbid conditions
- Laboratory tests:
  – CBC, INR, PTT, glucose, electrolytes, urea and creatinine
  – ECG
  – Chest x-ray
  – CT brain scan required for almost all patients, immediately for some (Table 1)

Table 1: **Indications for Immediate CT Brain Scan**

| |
|---|
| • Suspected subarachnoid hemorrhage |
| • Patients within 3 hours of stroke onset who are potential candidates for thrombolysis (see Table 2) |
| • Suspected cerebellar stroke (possible need for neurosurgical intervention) |
| • No history available (possibility of subdural hematoma and need for neurosurgical intervention) |
| • Patient on warfarin or heparin (possible need for reversal of anticoagulation) |

  – Carotid Doppler ultrasonography to determine degree of carotid stenosis in patients with non-disabling carotid territory strokes who are fit for surgery. Urgent referral to stroke centre required for carotid stenosis of >50% in men or >69% in women
  – Holter monitor and echocardiography to search for cardiac source of emboli in all patients aged <50, and any patient who has a large-vessel territory (non-lacunar) stroke and neurovascular imaging studies showing no large-vessel disease, provided anticoagulation not contraindicated
  – Other investigations if indicated, e.g., blood cultures if endocarditis suspected; anticardiolipin antibodies, protein C, protein S, and antithrombin III in young patients when other investigations are negative or if indicated by the patient's personal or family history; Factor V Leiden and prothrombin gene mutations in patients with cerebral venous thrombosis

## Therapeutic Choices (Figures 1 and 2)

### I. Minimizing Brain Damage

#### *Restoring Perfusion*

- **Alteplase** administered IV within 3 hours of stroke onset (Tables 2 and 3)

**Dose:** 0.9 mg/kg (max. 90 mg) by IV infusion over 60 minutes with 10% of total dose as bolus at start of infusion.

Figure 1: **Diagnosis and Initial Management of Suspected Acute Stroke**

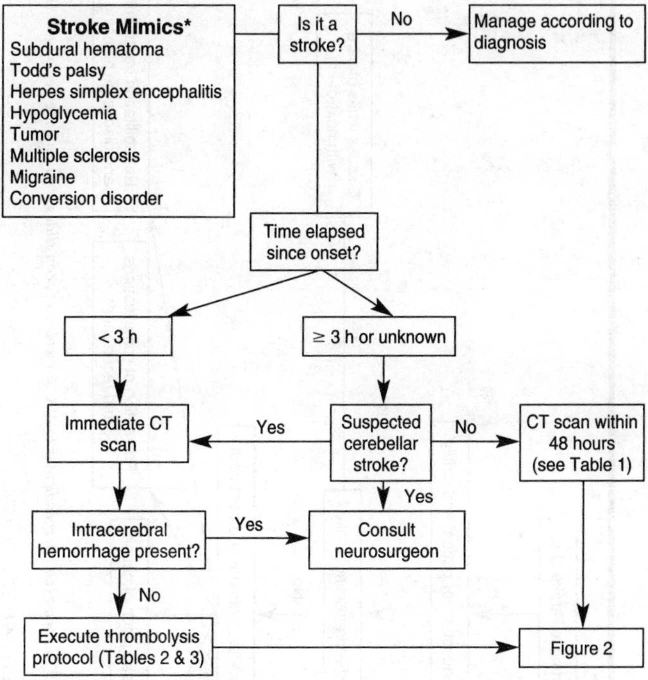
Stroke Mimics*
Subdural hematoma
Todd's palsy
Herpes simplex encephalitis
Hypoglycemia
Tumor
Multiple sclerosis
Migraine
Conversion disorder
Is it a stroke?
No
Manage according to diagnosis
Time elapsed since onset?
< 3 h
≥ 3 h or unknown
Immediate CT scan
Yes
Suspected cerebellar stroke?
No
CT scan within 48 hours (see Table 1)
Yes
Intracerebral hemorrhage present?
Yes
Consult neurosurgeon
No
Execute thrombolysis protocol (Tables 2 & 3)
Figure 2

* *List not exhaustive. Disorders listed are common or require specific treatment or both.*

Intra-arterial administration of thrombolytic agents shows promise but application is likely to be limited.[1] Eligibility criteria and time-window for thrombolysis may be re-defined as more data from randomized trials become available. Nonpharmacologic methods of achieving re-canalization are under investigation.

### *Salvaging Ischemic Brain*

- Oxygen if pulse oximetry shows desaturation.
- Hypothermia is strikingly beneficial in animal models of stroke. Elevated body temperature is associated with poor outcome after stroke. Symptomatic treatment of pyrexia (and investigation of its cause) is recommended.
- Hyperglycemia is associated with poor outcome after stroke, suggesting that blood glucose control may be beneficial[2], but no definitive clinical trial data are available.

[1] *JAMA 1999;282:2003–2011.*
[2] *Stroke 1999;30:793–799.*

Figure 2: **General Management of the Stroke Patient**

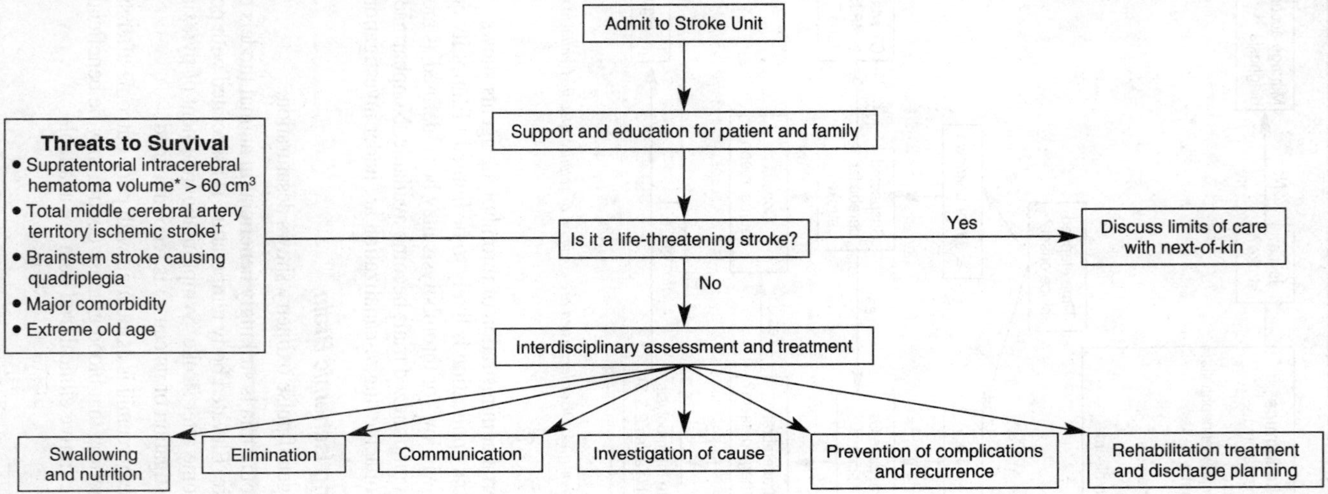
Admit to Stroke Unit
Support and education for patient and family
Threats to Survival
• Supratentorial intracerebral hematoma volume* > 60 cm³
• Total middle cerebral artery territory ischemic stroke†
• Brainstem stroke causing quadriplegia
• Major comorbidity
• Extreme old age
Is it a life-threatening stroke?
Yes
Discuss limits of care with next-of-kin
No
Interdisciplinary assessment and treatment
Swallowing and nutrition
Elimination
Communication
Investigation of cause
Prevention of complications and recurrence
Rehabilitation treatment and discharge planning

* *Hematoma volume (cm3) = A+B+C/2 where A = largest diameter (cm) on CT scan, B = diameter (cm) perpendicular to A, C = number of scan slides (cm) showing hematoma. (Reference: Stroke 1993;24:987–993).*

† *Hemiparesis and hemianopia with either aplasia or visuospatial deficit (Reference: Lancet 1991;337:1521–1526).*

Table 2: **Alteplase in Acute Ischemic Stroke: Eligibility Criteria***

**Inclusion criteria**

- < 3 hours from onset of symptoms
- Disabling neurologic deficit
- Symptoms present ≥ 60 minutes showing no sign of resolution
- Consent of patient or legal next-of-kin (if unavailable, document circumstances in the patient's hospital chart)

**Exclusion criteria†**

- Intracranial hemorrhage on CT
- Suspected subarachnoid hemorrhage
- Previous intracranial hemorrhage
- Cerebral infarct or severe head injury within the past 3 months
- Recent pericarditis
- Major surgery within the past 14 days
- GI or urinary hemorrhage within the past 21 days
- Recent lumbar puncture or arterial puncture at a non-compressible site
- Pregnancy
- BP ≥ 185 mm Hg systolic, or ≥ 110 mm Hg diastolic
- Bleeding diathesis
- Prolonged PTT or INR > 1.2
- Platelet count ≤ 100 × $10^9$ /L
- Blood glucose < 2.8 or > 22 mmol/L

**If patient fulfills all inclusion criteria and no exclusion criteria, alteplase may be given.**

* *Derived from the NINDS t-PA Stroke Study. N Engl J Med 1995;333:1581–1587.*

† *A score >22 on the NIH Stroke Scale, and CT signs of early ischemia are associated with an increased risk of intracerebral hemorrhage but are* ***not*** *absolute contra-indications to alteplase.*

- Acute blood pressure reduction has not been shown to be beneficial, and may be harmful.
- Neuroprotective agents that act at various points in the ischemic cascade are in clinical trials.

### *Neurosurgical Intervention*

- Craniectomy or ventricular shunting is sometimes performed on patients with massive hemispheric or cerebellar infarcts whose level of consciousness is declining. There is no evidence from randomized controlled trials to support this practice but consensus opinion is that patients with cerebellar strokes, in particular, benefit from surgical intervention in this situation.

## II. Preventing Complications

Expert nursing care and early mobilization are the mainstays of treatment.

Table 3: **Alteplase in Acute Ischemic Stroke: Monitoring***

**Vital Signs**
- Baseline, then q15min for 2h after starting alteplase
- Then q30min × 6h
- Then q1h × 4h
- Then q2h × 12h
- Call MD if systolic BP > 180 or if diastolic BP > 110 for two or more readings 5–10 minutes apart

**Neurologic Signs**
- q1h × 12h
- Then q2h × 12h
- Stop infusion and notify MD if there is neurologic deterioration, severe headache, or new nausea or vomiting

**Blood Glucose**
- Call MD if glucose >12 mmol/L

**Medications**
- No ASA, ticlopidine, clopidogrel, heparin or warfarin for 24h.
- Acetaminophen 650mg po or pr q4h if temperature ≥ 38° C or for analgesia.
- $O_2$ via nasal prongs or face mask to keep $O_2$ sat. > 90%.
- After alteplase infusion completed, IV normal saline with KCl

**Investigations**
- CT brain scan after 24 h

* *Derived from the NINDS t-PA Stroke Study protocol (N Engl J Med 1995;333:1581–87).*

### *Aspiration Pneumonia and Malnutrition*

- Screen nutritional status on admission to identify patients who were malnourished pre-stroke.
- Give nothing by mouth if any of the following are present: reduced level of consciousness, severe dysarthria, wet voice, weak cough, impaired palatal sensation, unable to sit, or if aspiration is suspected.
- Monitor recovery of dysphagia using serial bedside swallowing assessments. These are best performed by a dietitian plus a speech-language pathologist or an occupational therapist.
- A videofluoroscopic examination (modified barium swallow) may be required to exclude significant aspiration when the results of the bedside examination are ambiguous.
- Tube feeding may be required if significant aspiration is demonstrated or suspected. Initially, this is usually via nasogastric tube. If swallowing does not recover, gastrostomy tube feeding may be necessary. Parenteral nutrition is required only in exceptional circumstances.
- Give a texture-modified diet for dysphagic patients at lower risk of aspiration. Additional intravenous fluids are often necessary for these patients.

### *Venous thromboembolism*

- Support stockings if mobility limited by leg weakness.
- **ASA** (75–325 mg daily) is protective.
- **Heparin** 5000 U BID SC reduces deep venous thrombosis and pulmonary embolism but carries a small risk of bleeding, does not decrease long-term death or disability, and is not definitely superior to early mobilization, ASA, good hydration and support stockings.
- Low molecular weight heparins and heparinoids have not been adequately tested in stroke patients.

## III. Reducing the Risk of Stroke Recurrence

### *Antithrombotic drug treatment*

#### *Antiplatelet therapy*

- **ASA** 325 mg daily as soon as intracranial hemorrhage excluded by CT scan. Give as a suppository or via nasogastric tube to dysphagic patients. Use enteric coated formulation for patients who can swallow. Use 81 mg enteric coated tablets for patients who cannot tolerate 325 mg daily.
- Platelet **glycoprotein IIb/IIIa inhibitors** are in clinical trial.

#### *Anticoagulant therapy*

- For patients in atrial fibrillation (AF), use **warfarin** at a dose to maintain the INR in the range 2.0 to 3.0, provided there are no contraindications to anticoagulation.
- The best time to initiate anticoagulant therapy is unclear. For patients with minor strokes, warfarin may be started as soon as intracranial hemorrhage has been excluded by CT scan. For patients with major strokes, delay warfarin until a CT scan done about a week after the stroke has excluded hemorrhagic transformation of the infarct.
- Use enteric coated **ASA** 325 mg daily for patients who cannot take warfarin. Other antiplatelet drugs have not been tested adequately in patients with AF.
- Immediate systemic anticoagulation with unfractionated heparin, low molecular weight heparin, heparinoids or specific thrombin inhibitors is *not* recommended in the setting of acute ischemic stroke—not even for patients in atrial fibrillation—because there is no evidence of short- or long-term benefit. Specifically, reduction in early recurrent ischemic stroke is completely offset by an increase in major intracranial and extracranial bleeding.[3]

---

[3] *Anticoagulants for acute ischaemic stroke (Cochrane Review). In: The Cochrane Library, Issue 4, 1999. Oxford: Update Software.*

For post-acute antithrombotic treatment, carotid endarterectomy, and risk-factor modification, see Chapter 22.

## IV. Restoring Function of the Individual

- Rehabilitation should start as soon as the patient is medically stable.
- Optimal rehabilitation is provided by a multidisciplinary team on a stroke unit.
- Family and community supports are important for social reintegration.

## Therapeutic Tips

- In order to administer alteplase *within 3 hours* of stroke onset, patients must be assessed *within 2 hours*. This leaves *1 hour* for clinical assessment, CT scan, blood tests and consent procedures.
- Determining the time of stroke onset is critical in the decision to use alteplase but checking the clock is not a natural reaction in the setting of an acute stroke. Encourage patients and families to think of "time anchors" e.g., what was on the radio or TV at the time or at what point in the patient's daily routine did the symptoms first occur?
- Patients with acute stroke are often unable to communicate. Whenever possible, the next-of-kin should travel with the patient to hospital (or between hospitals, if the patient is transferred to a stroke centre) in order to provide collateral history and consent for treatment before the time-window for intervention closes.
- Any signs of infarction on a CT scan done within 3 hours of stroke onset are usually subtle. If the CT scan of a patient being considered for treatment with alteplase shows a very definite infarct in a location that explains the presenting clinical symptoms and signs, re-check the time of onset.
- Return vials containing unused alteplase to the hospital pharmacy for reimbursement from the manufacturer.
- Treatment of hypertension and hyperlipidemia in patients who have had a stroke should follow the recommendations in Chapters 23 and 24.

## Pharmacoeconomic Considerations

*Jeffrey A. Johnson, PhD*

Based on the results of the large clinical trials, treating acute ischemic stroke patients with alteplase (t-PA) within 3 hours of symptom onset is likely to result in net cost savings to the health care system. The savings would result from reduced lengths of stay for the initial hospitalization, as well as reductions in the need for subsequent inpatient rehabilitation or nursing home admissions. In addition to the positive financial impact, economic modeling predicts a gain of 564 quality-adjusted life years (QALYs) for every 1000 patients treated with t-PA.

Stroke-unit care is likely to be highly cost-effective, and will facilitate the best use of t-PA and other interventions. The development of an organized approach to stroke care must be a major priority for the Canadian health care system.

For the secondary prevention of stroke, the use of ASA is a low-cost and effective strategy that is clearly of benefit. The addition of dipyridamole to ASA may be a cost-effective strategy, but probably only in high-risk patients. Substitution of clopidogrel for ASA is likely not cost-effective in all cases; however, clopidogrel is justified in high-risk patients who are intolerant of ASA.

***Suggested Reading***

*Wein TH, Hickenbottom SL, Alexandrov AV. Thrombolysis, stroke units and other strategies for reducing acute stroke costs. PharmacoEconomics 1998;14: 603–611.*

*Fagan SC, Morgenstern LB, Petitt A, et al. Cost-effectiveness of tissue plasminogen activator for acute ischemic stroke. NINDS rt-PA Stroke Study Group. Neurology 1998;50:883–890.*

*Hankey GJ, Warlow CP. Treatment and secondary prevention of stroke: evidence, costs, and effects on individuals and populations. Lancet 1999;354:1457–63.*

*Wilson E, Taylor G, Phillips S, Stewart PJ, et al, for the Canadian Stroke Systems Coalition. Creating a Canadian Stroke System. CMAJ 2000 in press.*

*Chambers M, Hutton J, Gladman J. Cost-effectiveness analysis of antiplatelet therapy in the prevention of recurrent stroke in the UK. Aspirin, dipyridamole and aspirin-dipyridamole. PharmacoEconomics 1999;16:577–593.*

## *Suggested Reading List*

Gubitz G, Sandercock P, Counsell C. Antiplatelet therapy for acute ischaemic stroke (Cochrane Review). In: *The Cochrane Library,* Issue 3, 1999. Oxford: Update Software.

Gubitz G, Sandercock P, Counsell C, Signorini D. Anticoagulants for acute ischaemic stroke (Cochrane Review). In: *The Cochrane Library,* Issue 4, 1999. Oxford: Update Software.

NINDS rt-PA Stroke Study Group. Tissue plasminogen activator for acute ischemic stroke. *N Engl J Med* 1995;333: 1581–1587.

Stroke Unit Trialists' Collaboration. Organised inpatient (stroke unit) care for stroke (Cochrane Review). In: The Cochrane Library, Issue 3, 1999. Oxford: Update Software.

Wardlaw JM, Yamaguchi T, del Zoppo G. Thrombolytic therapy versus control for acute ischaemic stroke (Cochrane Review). In: The Cochrane Library, Issue 4, 1999. Oxford: Update Software.

CHAPTER 31

# Venous Thromboembolism

*Alexander G.G. Turpie, MD, FRCP(Lond), FRCP(Glas), FACP, FACC, FRCPC*

## *Prophylaxis*

### Goals of Therapy

- To prevent deep vein thrombosis (DVT) and pulmonary embolism (PE)
- To reduce mortality
- To prevent the postphlebitic syndrome

### Clinical Risk Categories

Venous thromboembolism (VTE) is a common cause of morbidity and mortality in hospitalized patients; the frequency varies according to patients' risk category. Consensus conferences have defined these categories based on clinical criteria and made recommendations for thrombosis prophylaxis according to risk group (Table 1). The risk of VTE is also increased in the presence of the following factors related to venous stasis and coagulopathies:

- age
- varicose veins
- immobility (bed rest > 4 days)
- active cancer
- pregnancy
- puerperium
- high-dose estrogen therapy
- previous DVT or PE
- thrombophilia (tendency to thrombosis)
  - antithrombin III deficiency
  - protein C or protein S deficiency
  - activated protein C resistance
  - antiphospholipid antibody
  - lupus anticoagulant
  - factor V Leiden

### Nonpharmacologic Choices

**Caval interruption** by filter is rarely indicated for primary prophylaxis but should be considered in patients in whom anticoagulants have failed or are absolutely contraindicated.

Table 1: **Risk Categories and Thrombosis Prophylaxis**

| Risk Group | Clinical Criteria | Frequency of VTE: Hospitalized Patients (without prophylaxis) | | | Prophylactic Measures (should be continued for a minimum of 5 to 7 d until the patient is fully ambulant) |
|---|---|---|---|---|---|
| | | DVT | Proximal vein thrombosis | Fatal PE | |
| **Low** | Minor surgery (< 30 min); no risk factors other than age.<br>Major surgery (> 30 min); age < 40 yrs, no other risk factors.<br>Minor trauma or medical illness. | 10% | 1% | 0.01% | Mobilize<br>Graduated compression stockings |
| **Moderate** | Major general, urologic, gynecologic, cardiothoracic, vascular or neurologic surgery; age ≥ 40 yrs or other risk factor.<br>Major medical illness: heart or lung disease, cancer, inflammatory bowel disease.<br>Major trauma or burns.<br>Minor surgery, trauma or illness in patients with previous deep vein thrombosis, pulmonary embolism or thrombophilia. | 10–40% | 1–10% | 0.1–1% | Low molecular weight heparin (Table 3)<br>Low-dose heparin (5000 units SC Q12H or Q8H)<br>Graduated compression stockings<br>External pneumatic compression |
| **High** | Fracture or major orthopedic surgery of pelvis, hip or lower limb.<br>Major pelvic or abdominal surgery for cancer.<br>Major surgery, trauma or illness in patients with previous deep vein thrombosis, pulmonary embolism or thrombophilia.<br>Lower limb paralysis (e.g., hemiplegic stroke, paraplegia).<br>Major lower limb amputation. | 40–80% | 10–30% | 1–10% | Low molecular weight heparin (Table 3)<br>Adjusted-dose heparin (aPTT 1.5 × control)<br>Adjusted-dose warfarin (INR 2.0–3.0)<br>External pneumatic compression<br>Combinations |

### Pharmacologic Choices

See Table 1 for prophylactic measures used in different risk categories and Drugs Used in Prophylaxis and Treatment for details on specific drugs.

## *Treatment*

### Goals of Therapy

#### *Deep vein thrombosis (DVT)*

- To prevent major pulmonary embolism
- To prevent thrombus extension
- To enhance thrombolysis
- To prevent postphlebitic syndrome
- To reduce morbidity of acute event

#### *Pulmonary Embolism (PE)*

- To prevent death
- To prevent recurrent thromboembolism
- To prevent chronic thromboembolic pulmonary hypertension

### Investigations

Because the clinical diagnosis of DVT and PE is insensitive and nonspecific, objective diagnosis using specific procedures is important for optimal management.

- **DVT:** Ascending venography, impedance plethysmography, B-mode compression ultrasound (most practical and useful clinically)
- **PE:** Pulmonary angiography, perfusion lung scan, ventilation lung scan, spiral CT, NMRI, DVT tests
- Patients under 40 with recurrent VTE or a family history should be screened for thrombophilia (see Clinical Risk Categories)

### Therapeutic Choices

### General Measures

**Deep Vein Thrombosis**

- Immobilize if symptoms warrant (reduces pain, prevents embolization).
- Elevate limb (reduces edema and pain).
- Avoid pressure on the swollen leg.
- *Analgesics* for pain (NSAIDs are effective but may increase the risk of bleeding, especially when used with anticoagulants).

**Pulmonary Embolism**

- Administer oxygen.
- IV fluids.
- Vasopressor agents.
- Other resuscitory measures (depending on patient's clinical status).

## Pharmacologic Choices

Established DVT and/or PE are initially treated with SC **low molecular weight heparin** or IV **standard heparin** for a minimum of 5 days followed by oral anticoagulation with **warfarin** with at least 2 days of overlap with a therapeutic INR. The duration of oral anticoagulation is dependent on the risk of recurrence of VTE (Table 2).

Table 2: **Duration of Secondary Prophylaxis for Venous Thromboembolism***

| |
|---|
| **3–6 Months** |
| First event with reversible or time-limited risk factor |
| First event with heterozygous activated protein C resistance (APCR) |
| **6 Months Minimum** |
| First idiopathic event |
| **12 Months – Indefinite** |
| Recurrent disease |
| Cancer until resolved |
| Homozygous APCR, antiphospholipid antibody, antithrombin, protein C or S deficiency |

* *Adapted from Myers TM, et al. Antithrombotic therapy for venous thromboembolic disease. Chest 1998;114:561S–578S.*

# *Drugs for Prophylaxis and Treatment of Venous Thromboembolism*

## *Low Molecular Weight Heparins (LMWHs)*

**Enoxaparin**, **dalteparin**, **tinzaparin** and **nadroparin** are approved for both prophylaxis in conjunction with surgery and treatment of VTE (Table 3).

The kinetics of LMWHs are more predictable than those of standard heparin, and their elimination half-life is longer. These properties make weight-adjusted fixed-dose SC dosing of LMWHs an excellent alternative to adjusted-dose IV heparin in the initial treatment of VTE. LMWHs have become the management of choice for initial treatment of DVT for many outpatients. They are also effective in the treatment of PE.

Table 3: **Low Molecular Weight Heparins: Dosage for Prophylaxis and Treatment of Deep Vein Thrombosis***

| | | Prophylaxis | Treatment |
|---|---|---|---|
| *dalteparin* Fragmin | General Surgery:<br>Orthopedics: | 2500 IU/d<br>5000 IU/d | 200 IU/kg once daily<br>max: 18000 IU/d |
| *enoxaparin* Lovenox | General Surgery:<br><br><br>Orthopedics: | 4000 IU (40 mg) Q24H<br><br>3000 IU (30 mg) Q12H | 100 IU or 1 mg/kg BID<br>150 IU or 1.5 mg/kg once daily<br>max: 18000 IU/d |
| *nadroparin* Fraxiparine Fraxiparine Forte | General Surgery:<br>Orthopedics: | 2850 IU/d<br>38 IU/kg Q12H × 3 doses, then 38 IU/kg × 2 d, then 57 IU/kg/d | 171 IU/kg once daily or 86 IU/kg BID<br>max: 17100 IU/d |
| *tinzaparin* Innohep | General Surgery:<br><br>Orthopedics: | 3500 IU once daily<br>50–75 IU/kg once daily | 175 IU/kg once daily<br>max: 18000 IU/d |

* *SC administration*

### *Heparin*

Heparin acts as an anticoagulant by forming a complex with antithrombin III, catalyzing the inhibition of several activated blood coagulation factors. For treatment of VTE, heparin is most commonly given by IV infusion in a dose monitored to prolong the activated partial thromboplastin time (aPTT) to 1.5 to 2.5 times control. It is also effective by SC injection if a sufficiently high dose is given (generally 15 000 to 25 000 units Q12H). An IV bolus (5000 to 10 000 units) should be given with the SC injection in the initial treatment. Monitoring 4 to 6 hours after the SC dose should aim for an aPTT 2.0 to 2.5 times control. A practical weight-based nomogram has been developed for adjusting IV heparin (Table 4).

### *Warfarin*

Warfarin inhibits thrombin formation by interfering with vitamin K metabolism, which is essential in the synthesis of coagulation factors II, VII, IX and X. It is given in a dose adjusted to maintain the INR at 2.0 to 3.0.

#### Monitoring Warfarin Therapy with the INR

A major limitation of the prothrombin time, reported in seconds, is the considerable variability in the results depending on the laboratory technique used. This limitation is largely overcome by the use of the international normalized ratio (INR).

#### Drug Interactions with Warfarin

The most common cause of poor anticoagulant control is drug interactions (Table 5). ASA and NSAIDs contribute to bleeding by inhibiting platelet function.

Table 4: **Body Weight-based Dosing of Intravenous Heparin in Adults*†**

| APTT (seconds) | Dose Change (units/kg/h) | Additional Action | Next APTT (h) |
|---|---|---|---|
| <35 (<1.2×mean normal) | +4 | Rebolus with 80 units/kg | 6 |
| 35–45 (1.2–1.5×mean normal) | +2 | Rebolus with 40 units/kg | 6 |
| 46–70‡ (1.5–2.3×mean normal) | 0 | 0 | 6π |
| 71–90 (2.3–3.0×mean normal) | −2 | 0 | 6 |
| >90 (>3×mean normal) | −3 | Stop infusion for 1 h | 6 |

* *Adapted with permission from: Myers TM, et al. Antithrombotic therapy for venous thromboembolic disease. Chest 1998;114:561S–578S.*

† *Initial dosing: 80 units/kg; maintenance infusion of heparin, at a rate dictated by body weight through an infusion apparatus calibrated for low flow rates: 18 units/kg/h (APTT in 6 hours).*

‡ *The therapeutic range in seconds should correspond to a plasma heparin level of 0.2 to 0.4 units/mL by protamine sulfate titration. When APTT is checked at 6 hours or longer, steady-state kinetics can be assumed.*

π *During the first 24 hours, repeat APTT every 6 hours. Thereafter, monitor APTT once every morning unless it is outside the therapeutic range.*

**Anticoagulation in Pregnancy**

- Heparin is the anticoagulant of choice during pregnancy; SC injections twice daily achieve therapeutic levels.
- Heparin should be stopped at the first sign of labor.
- Warfarin or SC heparin may be used for about 6 weeks after delivery for secondary prevention.
- Women can breast-feed while being treated with warfarin.
- The management of pregnant women with a previous DVT or PE is controversial; heparin, 5000 units SC Q12H throughout pregnancy, is recommended.
- LMWHs do not cross the placental barrier and have been used as alternatives to heparin.

### *Thrombolytic Agents*

Less than 20% of VTE patients are eligible for thrombolytic therapy (i.e., young patients with massive ileofemoral vein thrombosis or patients with major PE). **Streptokinase** (SK), **urokinase** (UK) and **alteplase** are approved for treatment of VTE. The best results are obtained with recent thrombi, but substantial lysis may be obtained in patients with symptoms of up to 14 days' duration.

SK is the least expensive thrombolytic. However, given the prolonged infusions of SK and UK used in VTE, alteplase, with its short infusion, may be more cost effective.

Table 5: **Warfarin Drug Interactions**

| | |
|---|---|
| **Drugs That Increase INR** | |
| *antimicrobials* | *lipid lowering agents* |
| Cefamandole | Bezafibrate |
| Cefotetan | Clofibrate |
| Chloramphenicol | Fenofibrate |
| Ciprofloxacin | Gemfibrozil |
| Co-trimoxazole | Lovastatin |
| Erythromycin | *others* |
| Metronidazole | Alcohol (large amounts) |
| Norfloxacin | Allopurinol |
| *antifungals* | Amiodarone |
| Fluconazole | Cimetidine |
| Itraconazole | Chloral hydrate |
| Ketoconazole | Disulfiram |
| | Paroxetine |
| *hormones* | Phenylbutazone |
| Anabolic steroids | Propafenone |
| Danazol | Sulfinpyrazone |
| Thyroid supplements | Zafirlukast |
| **Drugs That Decrease INR** | |
| Antithyroids | Phenytoin |
| Barbiturates | Primidone |
| Carbamazepine | Rifampin |
| Cholestyramine | Vitamin K |
| Griseofulvin | |
| **Drugs That Increase Hypoprothrombinemia** | |
| ASA | |
| NSAIDs | |

## Pharmacoeconomic Considerations

*Jeffrey A. Johnson, PhD*

A number of recent pharmacoeconomic evaluations have evaluated the use of low molecular weight heparin (LMWH) as a therapeutic choice in the treatment and prevention of venous thromboembolism (VTE). In most analyses of the treatment of VTE, use of LMWH has typically been shown to be more effective and less costly overall, when compared to unfractionated heparin. The cost-effectiveness of LMWH in the treatment of VTE has been demonstrated for in-hospital use, and is even greater when treatment is provided in outpatient settings, leading to potential cost savings of $2000 to $4000 per patient in provincial health system perspectives. There is no evidence however that any one LMWH product is more cost-effective than another in the treatment of VTE.

The most cost-effective therapeutic choice for the prevention of VTE following major surgery or secondary prophylaxis following VTE is less clear. Following major orthopedic surgery, when VTE confirmed by venography is the outcome of interest (i.e., as in clinical trials), LMWH may be more efficacious. When only symptomatic VTE is considered, oral anticoagulation with warfarin is less costly and more effective compared to the use of LMWH. However, in patients for whom monitoring is problematic, or who have a higher risk of bleeding complications, the use of LMWH instead of warfarin could offer specific advantages. Other important considerations that have not yet been resolved are the use in other surgeries and the optimal duration of prophylaxis. External pneumatic compression may be a more cost-effective prophylactic measure than LMWH or warfarin in post-gynecologic surgery.

***Suggested Reading***

*O'Brien B, Levine M, Willan A, Goeree R, Haley S, Blackhouse G. Economic evaluation of outpatient treatment with low-molecular weight heparin for proximal vein thrombosis. Arch Intern Med 1999;159:2298–2304.*

*Rodger. M, Bredeson C, Wells PS, Beck J, Kearns B, Huebsch LB. Cost-effectiveness of low-molecular-weight heparin and unfractionated heparin in treatment of deep vein thrombosis. CMAJ 1998;159:931–938.*

*Schulman S. Long-term prophylaxis in venous thromboembolism. LMWH or oral anticoagulation? Haemostatis 1998;28 (Suppl. 3);17–21,*

*Anderson DR, O'Brien B, Nagpal S, et al. Economic evaluation comparing low molecular weight heparin with other modalities for prevention of deep vein thrombosis and pulmonary embolism following total hip or knee arthroplasty. Ottawa: Canadian Coordinating Office for Health Technology Assessment (CCOHTA); 1998.*

## *Suggested Reading List*

Clagett CG, Anderson FA, Geerts WH, et al. Prevention of venous thromboembolism. *Chest* 1998;114(5 Suppl): 531S–560S.

Haas S, Turpie AG. Building a new era in DVT management. Introduction. *Blood Coagul Fibrinolysis* 1999; Suppl 2: S1–S3.

Hirsh J, Fuster V. Guide to anticoagulant therapy. Part 1: Heparin. *Circulation* 1994;89:1449–1468.

Hirsh J, Fuster V. Guide to anticoagulant therapy. Part 2: Oral anticoagulants. *Circulation* 1994;89:1469–1480.

Thromboembolic Risk Factors (THRIFT) Consensus Group. Risk of and prophylaxis for venous thromboembolism in hospital patients. *BMJ* 1992;305:567–574.

Turpie AGG. Antithrombotic therapy in the new millennium – the role of low molecular weight heparin. *S Afr Med J* 1999;89: Cardiovascular Suppl 3:C151–C155.

CHAPTER 32

# Intermittent Claudication

*Richard I. Ogilvie, MD, FRCPC, FACP*

## Goals of Therapy

- To improve mobility and quality of life
- To increase walking distance and time to claudication
- To increase capacity for regular dynamic leg exercise

## Investigations

- History with special attention to cardiovascular disease risk factors and associated conditions:
  - hypertension
  - diabetes mellitus
  - smoking
  - dyslipidemia
  - angina pectoris/MI
  - congestive heart failure
  - TIA/stroke
- Define walking time to claudication (**severe** < 1/2 city block; **moderate** 1/2 to 1 block; **mild** > 1 block)
- Define duration of symptoms (6 to 12 months are required to develop collateral circulation)
- Physical examination:
  - signs of hypertension, dyslipidemia, diabetes mellitus, atherosclerosis (aortic aneurysm, bruits), heart failure
  - signs of peripheral artery obstruction
  - evidence of acute peripheral artery occlusion (acute onset of continuous pain, pale and cool limb or mottled discoloration, thickened swollen stiff muscles plus pain over the muscle)
  - paresthesia and paralysis require immediate surgical revascularization (fibrinolysis may be considered)
  - resting pain, dependent rubor, cyanosis, muscle atrophy, trophic ulcers suggest severe obstruction
- Laboratory tests:
  - fasting blood sugar and lipid profile
  - hemoglobin, hematocrit, platelet count
  - resting Doppler-derived or sphygmomanometric ankle/arm systolic pressure index (Figure 1)

Figure 1: **Treatment of Intermittent Claudication**

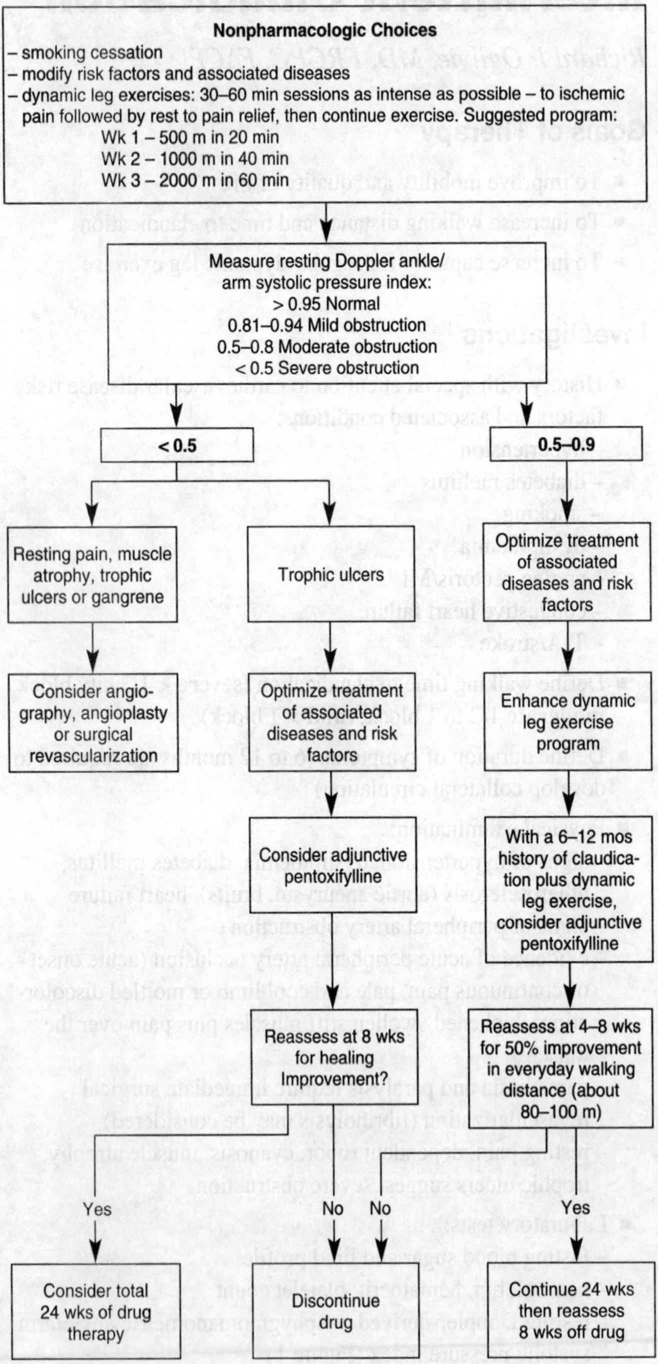
Nonpharmacologic Choices
– smoking cessation
– modify risk factors and associated diseases
– dynamic leg exercises: 30–60 min sessions as intense as possible – to ischemic pain followed by rest to pain relief, then continue exercise. Suggested program:
Wk 1 – 500 m in 20 min
Wk 2 – 1000 m in 40 min
Wk 3 – 2000 m in 60 min
Measure resting Doppler ankle/arm systolic pressure index:
> 0.95 Normal
0.81–0.94 Mild obstruction
0.5–0.8 Moderate obstruction
< 0.5 Severe obstruction
< 0.5
0.5–0.9
Resting pain, muscle atrophy, trophic ulcers or gangrene
Trophic ulcers
Optimize treatment of associated diseases and risk factors
Consider angiography, angioplasty or surgical revascularization
Optimize treatment of associated diseases and risk factors
Enhance dynamic leg exercise program
Consider adjunctive pentoxifylline
With a 6–12 mos history of claudication plus dynamic leg exercise, consider adjunctive pentoxifylline
Reassess at 8 wks for healing Improvement?
Reassess at 4–8 wks for 50% improvement in everyday walking distance (about 80–100 m)
Yes
No
No
Yes
Consider total 24 wks of drug therapy
Discontinue drug
Continue 24 wks then reassess 8 wks off drug

– consider invasive angiography for patients with resting pain, atrophy, cyanosis, nonhealing ischemic ulcers or gangrene for possible revascularization by angioplasty or surgery. The role of angioplasty for patients with chronic intermittent claudication without signs of severe arterial obstruction remains to be defined by clinical trials

## Therapeutic Choices (Figure 1)

### Nonpharmacologic Choices

- Discontinuation of smoking (active and passive) (Chapter 41).
- Time (collateral flow develops over 6 to 12 months).
- Non-drug treatment of obesity, lipid disorders, hypertension, heart failure.
- Regular dynamic leg exercise (5 times per week continuously for an initial period of 8 weeks).

### Pharmacologic Choices

- Optimize control of hypertension, dyslipidemia, diabetes mellitus, angina pectoris and CHF.
- Moderate claudication is not worsened and may be improved during control of hypertension with vasodilators ($alpha_1$-blockers, ACE inhibitors or calcium channel blockers).
- Severe claudication may be worsened by beta-blockers.
- Platelet-active agents (e.g., ASA, clopidogrel) do not improve claudication but may be indicated for the secondary prevention of MI and stroke.
- The role of prostaglandin analogues, L-carnitine or arterial gene therapy has not yet been defined by adequate clinical trials.
- The role of **cilostazol**, a cyclic AMP phosphodiesterase inhibitor selective for phosphodiesterase III is not defined by adequate clinical trials.[1] Long-term safety and drug interactions with other CYP3A4 inhibitors are of concern with this agent.
- Vitamin E or chelation therapy is not effective.
- **Pentoxifylline** alters erythrocyte deformability and reduces blood viscosity, platelet reactivity and plasma hypercoagulability. The controlled-release formulation (400 mg TID) is given with meals to reduce GI upset.

[1] *Cilostazol (Pletal) expected to be available from Pharmacia & Upjohn.*

- Five percent of patients stop therapy due to nausea, vomiting, dyspepsia, belching, bloating or flatulence. Other side effects are dizziness, nervousness, agitation, flushing and palpitations. Adverse effects may ameliorate with dose reduction.
- Pentoxifylline is *contraindicated* in patients with allergy or intolerance to xanthines, during pregnancy or lactation, acute MI, acute hemorrhage or severe hepatic or renal dysfunction. The dose should be reduced in patients with hepatic dysfunction.
- Pentoxifylline probably reduces the efficacy of adenosine in terminating supraventricular arrhythmias. It may enhance effects of theophylline, warfarin, sympathomimetics, antihypertensives and hypoglycemics.
- *Indications*
  - *Mild claudication* is not an indication for pentoxifylline.
  - *Moderate claudication:* cessation of smoking and regular dynamic leg exercise may be more beneficial than pentoxifylline. Dynamic leg exercise for 6 to 12 months after the onset of claudication may allow collaterals to develop. If pentoxifylline is used, a total of 24 weeks of therapy followed by 8 weeks drug-free (as exercise tolerance increases) can decrease or eliminate the need for the drug.
  - Pentoxifylline may be beneficial adjunctive therapy for *trophic ulcers* in diabetic and nondiabetic patients; therapy should be assessed at 4-week intervals with a usual maximum duration of 24 weeks (due to cost – approximately $40 per month, drug cost only).
  - Resting pain, muscle atrophy, trophic ulcers or gangrene should prompt investigation for possible angioplastic or surgical intervention.

## Suggested Reading List


Anon. Cilostazol for intermittent claudication. *Med Lett Drugs Ther* 1999;41:44–46.

Ernst E. Chelation therapy for peripheral arterial occlusive disease. A systematic review. *Circulation* 1997;96: 1031–1033.

Gardner AW, Poehlmann ET. Exercise programs for the treatment of claudication pain. A meta-analysis. *JAMA* 1995;274:975–980.

Hood SC, Moher D, Barber GG. Management of intermittent claudication with pentoxifylline: meta-analysis of randomized controlled trials. *Can Med Assoc J* 1996;15: 1053–1059.

Kleijnen J, MacKerras D. Vitamin E for the treatment of intermittent claudication (Cochrane Review) In: The Cochrane Library, Issue 1, 1998. Oxford: Update Software.

CHAPTER 33

# Raynaud's Phenomenon

*André Roussin, MD, FRCPC*

## Goals of Therapy

- To decrease symptoms (cold-induced blanching of the fingers) in primary (PRP) or secondary Raynaud's phenomenon (SRP)
- To prevent local and systemic deterioration in SRP
- To heal lesions in SRP

## Investigations (Figure 1)

- Thorough history to differentiate between:
  - **PRP** (no associated illness or trauma)
  - **SRP** (secondary to occupational hazards, vascular diseases, connective tissue diseases [CTD], carpal tunnel syndrome, hypothyroidism or other disorders)
  - possible **drug-induced** RP (see Nonpharmacologic Choices)
- Physical examination for:
  - altered pulsations and abnormal Allen's test
  - local signs of CTD (e.g., sclerodactyly) and carpal tunnel syndrome
  - systemic signs of CTD (e.g., telangiectasis, pulmonary fibrosis), vascular diseases and hypothyroidism
- Laboratory tests:
  - nailfold capillary microscopy to detect megacapillaries and other abnormalities suggestive of scleroderma and other CTD
  - ANA (antinuclear antibodies) and ACA (anticentromere antibodies) to detect CTD
  - other tests are less useful as early markers of SRP
  - normal tests suggest PRP

## Therapeutic Choices (Figure 1)

### Nonpharmacologic Choices

- Minimize cold exposure.
- Avoid prescribing medications with vasoconstrictive potential:
  - ergot derivatives including methysergide
  - beta-blockers (unlikely but controversial)
  - bromocriptine.
- Reassure patients that no complications arise from PRP.

Figure 1: **Investigation and Management of Raynaud's Phenomenon**

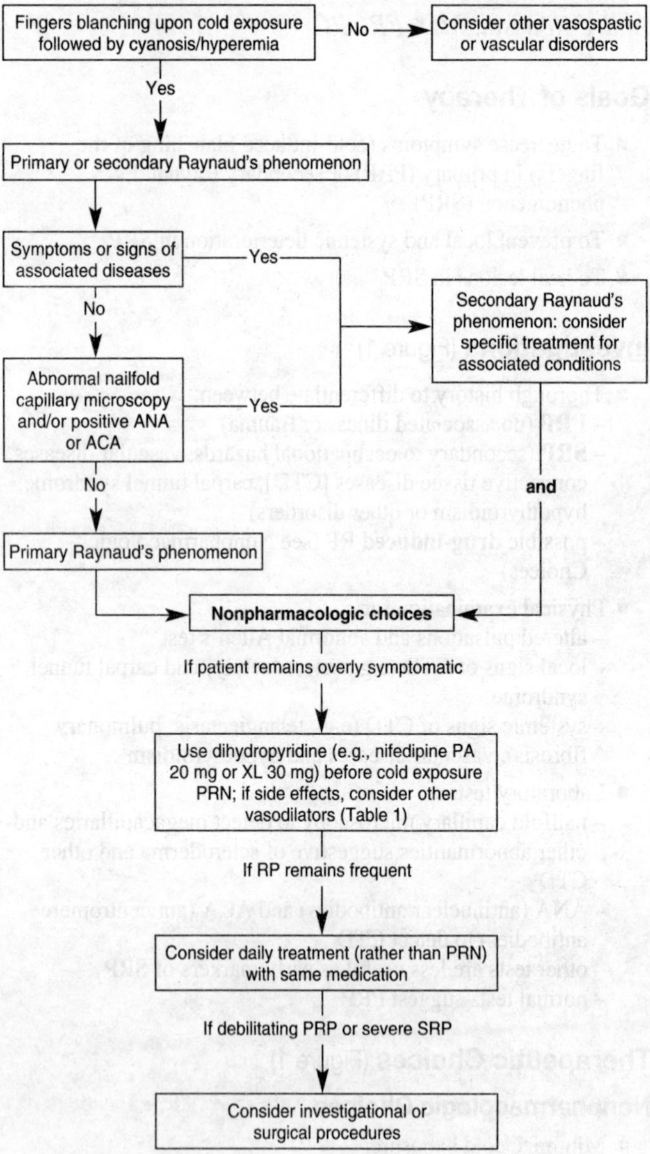
Fingers blanching upon cold exposure followed by cyanosis/hyperemia
No
Consider other vasospastic or vascular disorders
Yes
Primary or secondary Raynaud's phenomenon
Symptoms or signs of associated diseases
Yes
No
Secondary Raynaud's phenomenon: consider specific treatment for associated conditions
Abnormal nailfold capillary microscopy and/or positive ANA or ACA
Yes
No
and
Primary Raynaud's phenomenon
Nonpharmacologic choices
If patient remains overly symptomatic
Use dihydropyridine (e.g., nifedipine PA 20 mg or XL 30 mg) before cold exposure PRN; if side effects, consider other vasodilators (Table 1)
If RP remains frequent
Consider daily treatment (rather than PRN) with same medication
If debilitating PRP or severe SRP
Consider investigational or surgical procedures

- Teach warming exercises such as swinging the arms vigorously (windmill effect).
- Patients should dress warmly (including the head and neck) to avoid a sympathetically mediated vasoconstrictive reflex and use warming devices in mittens or boots if appropriate and affordable.
- Patients should stop smoking and avoid using vibrating tools (grinders, pneumatic hammers, drills, chain saws).

## Pharmacologic Choices (Table 1)

A calcium-blocking agent of the dihydropyridine class (e.g., **nifedipine PA 20 mg or XL 30 mg**) should be used 60 minutes before cold exposure. If side effects limit use, *other calcium channel blockers* may be considered, although they are less effective in RP. Daily administration, at the same or higher dosages, can be used in severe PRP and SRP or in SRP if ulcers are present (e.g., scleroderma).

*Peripheral alpha-blockers* (e.g., **prazosin**) are less effective, and dosage is limited by side effects in nonhypertensive patients. ACE inhibitors are generally not effective.

IV **iloprost** ($PGI_2$ analogue) may be useful for short-term use; however, both IV and oral prostaglandins have not been shown to be effective. Oral **ketanserin** (a serotonin receptor antagonist) reduces frequency of symptoms. Neither drug is commercially available.

## Surgical Choices

- Extremity sympathectomy, particularly by thoracoscopy, in difficult SRP with digital ulcers is not effective in the long term.
- Digital sympathectomy may be more effective.

## Therapeutic Tips

- Since pharmacologic prophylaxis of RP is effective in only 60% of patients at most (usually 40%), it is important to stress nonpharmacologic approaches and reassure patients. Only about 5% of PRP will go on to SRP; it is the underlying disease rather than the RP that will bring complications.
- Medication taken **daily** (as opposed to PRN) during the winter will increase tolerance to side effects (e.g., headaches).
- If dihydropyridines are ineffective (irrespective of side effects), other vasodilators are not likely to be effective.
- Laboratory cold-induced tests do not reliably predict a patient's response to any given drug in RP.
- PRP and SRP respond equally well to medications; frequency of attacks, rather than intensity and duration, is most likely reduced.

Table 1: **Dosages of Drugs Used in Raynaud's Phenomenon**

| Drug | Dosage | Cost* |
|---|---|---|
| **Calcium Channel Blockers** | | |
| **Dihydropyridines** | | |
| *nifedipine*<br>Adalat PA or XL, generics | PA 20 mg or XL 30 mg 30–60 min before cold exposure | $$ |
| *felodipine*<br>Renedil, Plendil | 5–10 mg 60 min before cold exposure | $$ |
| *amlodipine*<br>Norvasc | 5 mg 60 min before cold exposure | $$$ |
| **Others** | | |
| *diltiazem*<br>Cardizem SR or CD, generics | SR 90 mg or CD 180 mg 60–90 min before cold exposure | $$–$$$ |
| **Alpha$_1$ Adrenergic Blockers** | | |
| *prazosin*<br>Minipress, generics | 1–2 mg BID (regular dosage, to avoid risk of syncope with irregular use) | $ |

* *Cost per dose – includes drug cost only.*
*Legend: $ < 0.50 $$ 0.50–1.00 $$$ 1.00–1.50*

## *Suggested Reading List*


Adee AC. Managing Raynaud's phenomenon: a practical approach (review). *Am Fam Physician* 1993;47:823–829.

Coffman JD. Vasospastic diseases. In: Young JR, ed. *Peripheral vascular diseases*. 2nd ed. St. Louis: Mosby, 1996:407–424.

Creager MA, et al. Raynaud's phenomenon and other vascular disorders related to temperature. In: Loscalzo J, ed. *Vascular medicine*. 2nd ed. Boston: Little, Brown and Company, 1996:965–997.

Wigley FM, et al. Intravenous iloprost infusion in patients with Raynaud phenomenon secondary to systemic sclerosis. A multicenter, placebo-controlled, double blind study. *Ann Intern Med* 1994;120:199–206.

Yee AM, Hotchkiss RN, Paget SA. Advential stripping: a digit saving procedure in refractory Raynaud's phenomenon. *J Rheumatol* 1998;25:269–76.

CHAPTER 34

# Syncope

*Robert Sheldon, MD, PhD*

Syncope is defined as a reversible loss of consciousness not requiring specific resuscitative measures, and not associated with generalized seizures. Probably 30–40% of people faint at least once in their life, and about 3–10% of people faint recurrently. Most people who faint have a benign cause, but a few are at risk of death. Common causes of syncope are listed in Table 1.

## Goals of Therapy

- Identify potentially fatal causes of syncope
- Aggressively investigate and treat high-risk patients
- Remove reversible causes of syncope
- Treat patients with therapies appropriate to the degree of their symptoms

Table 1: **Classification of Common Causes of Syncope**

- Obstruction
  - Aortic stenosis
  - Pulmonary emboli
  - Many other rarer causes reported
- Arrhythmias
  - Bradycardias
    - Sinus node disease
    - Complete heart block
  - Tachycardias
    - Supraventricular arrhythmias (uncommon)
    - Ventricular tachycardia
    - Torsades de pointes ventricular tachycardia
- Volume depletion and drugs
  - Volume depletion
    - Diarrhea
    - Diminished oral intake
    - Polyuria
  - Hypotensive drugs
    - Alpha and beta adrenergic blockers
    - Vasodilators
    - Nitrates
- Orthostatic intolerance disorders
  - Reflex syncope syndromes
    - Carotid sinus hypersensitivity
    - Vasovagal syncope syndromes
  - Postural orthostatic tachycardia syndrome
  - Autonomic neuropathies
    - Pure autonomic failure syndromes
    - Multiple system atrophy syndromes

## Investigations

- Complete cardiovascular and neurologic history and physical examination. Determine whether the patient is seizing or fainting, then screen for life-threatening causes such as obstruction, ventricular tachycardia, and asystole or heart block (Figure 1)
- Laboratory investigations should be tailored to the individual patient:
  - ECG
  - Echocardiogram or other noninvasive measure of left ventricular function if structural heart disease suspected
  - Coronary angiography as indicated
  - Patients with structural heart disease should be referred for electrophysiologic assessment
  - Older patients (> 50 years) should have ambulatory ECG monitoring unless the history is strongly persuasive for vasovagal syncope
  - Ambulatory ECGs and stress tests are of limited use in younger patients
  - Implanted, patient-activated loop recorders may be useful in patients with infrequent syncope that eludes conventional attempts at diagnosis
  - Tilt table testing is useful in diagnosing vasovagal syncope

Figure 1: **Diagnostic Approach to the Patient with Syncope**

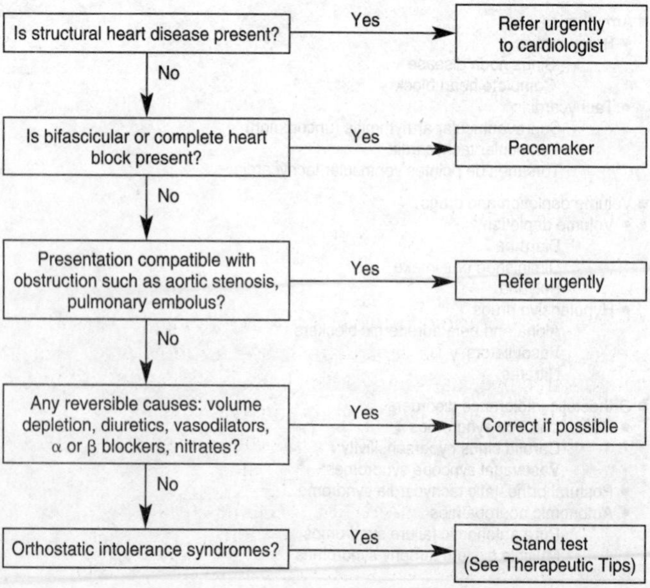
Is structural heart disease present?
Yes
Refer urgently to cardiologist
No
Is bifascicular or complete heart block present?
Yes
Pacemaker
No
Presentation compatible with obstruction such as aortic stenosis, pulmonary embolus?
Yes
Refer urgently
No
Any reversible causes: volume depletion, diuretics, vasodilators, α or β blockers, nitrates?
Yes
Correct if possible
No
Orthostatic intolerance syndromes?
Yes
Stand test (See Therapeutic Tips)

After eliminating potentially fatal causes, and removing reversible causes, most remaining patients will have one of several syndromes of orthostatic intolerance:

- Reflex syncope syndromes
  - Vasovagal syncope
  - Carotid sinus hypersensitivity in the elderly
- Postural orthostatic tachycardia syndrome (POTS)
- Pure autonomic failure syndromes
- Multiple system atrophy syndromes

## Therapeutic Choices

Treatment is directed at the cause of syncope. Treat any reversible causes. Patients with syncope secondary to bradycardia (asystole or complete heart block) should be referred for a permanent pacemaker. Patients with suspected or diagnosed ventricular tachycardia should be referred to a cardiologist, preferably an electrophysiologist. The following addresses treatment of syndromes of orthostatic tolerance.

### *Vasovagal Syncope*

#### Nonpharmacologic Choices

- Reassure the patient that this syndrome is not life-threatening and that it is a physical problem, not a psychiatric disorder. Encourage *increased dietary salt* intake of about 3 to 5 g daily, in the absence of contraindications such as hypertension or heart failure.
- Pacemaker therapy: Dual chamber permanent pacemakers may prevent syncope in patients with highly recurrent syncope in whom drugs are ineffective, contraindicated or not tolerated. Given the invasiveness of this treatment, these rare patients should be assessed at a tertiary referral clinic.

#### Pharmacologic Choices (Table 2)

Drug therapy may be effective in some, although the evidence is mixed.

**Fludrocortisone** should be used if simple salt supplements are ineffective, and may be particularly helpful in adolescents. It is administered once daily and usually has few side effects, the most common being supine hypertension and hypokalemia. Oral potassium supplements are often necessary. The goal is fluid retention, which may precipitate heart failure.

*Alpha agonists* cause venoconstriction and increase venous return, thereby preventing the onset of vasovagal syncope. **Midodrine** is the most useful. Its major side effects are supine

Table 2: **Drugs Used for Treatment of Syndromes of Orthostatic Intolerance**

| Drug† | Initial Dosage | Dose Increments | Adverse Effects | Monitoring | Cost* |
|---|---|---|---|---|---|
| *Sodium chloride* | 3–5 g $Na^+$ daily | | Gastric upset, fluid retention | | $ |
| *Fludrocortisone* Florinef | 0.1 mg daily | 0.1 mg q1–2 weeks to 0.4 mg | Mild edema, supine hypertension, hypokalemia, eczema, thin skin | Check serum $K^+$ and supine BP 1 week after increment | $–$$ |
| *Midodrine* (renal) Amatine | 2.5–5 mg TID ac; none after 5 pm | 2.5 mg TID q1–2 weeks to tolerance, effectiveness, or 15 mg TID | Supine hypertension, headache, shivering, paresthesias, piloerection | Check supine BP 2 h after dose of each increment | $$–$$$$ |
| *Yohimbine* | 4 mg BID | 2 mg BID q1–2 weeks to tolerance, effectiveness, or 8–14 mg BID | Anxiety, tremor, diarrhea | | $ |
| *Metoprolol* Betaloc, Lopresor, generics (other beta-blockers may be used) | 50 mg BID | Up to 100 mg BID | Fatigue, bradycardia, hypotension, depression, bronchospasm | Check HR, BP after each increment | $–$$ |
| *Paroxetine* (renal) Paxil (other serotonin reuptake inhibitors may be used) | 20 mg | 10 mg daily at monthly intervals to 40 mg daily | Headache, nausea, somnolence, agitation, insomnia | | $$–$$$ |

† *See text for specific indications.*
(renal) *Dosage adjustment may be required in renal impairment – see Appendix I.*

* *Cost of 30-day supply – includes drug cost only.*
*Legend: $ < $10 $$ $10–50 $$$ $50–100 $$$$ > $100*

hypertension, headache, shivering, paresthesias, and piloerection. After each dose increment, check for supine hypertension about 2 hours after a dose.

*Beta-blockers* are used to prevent the sympathetic surge that may provoke vasovagal syncope. They should be used cautiously in patients with bronchospastic lung disease and diabetes. There is little evidence that one beta-blocker is better than another.

*Serotonin reuptake inhibitors* prevent syncope in some cases, but may also increase the frequency of fainting.

## Postural Orthostatic Tachycardia Syndrome

Few rigorous clinical trials have been reported. Salt, fludrocortisone, midodrine and beta-blockers are all reasonable empiric treatments.

## Orthostatic Hypotension

The goal of therapy is to relieve symptoms of cerebral hypoperfusion while avoiding treatment side effects. Orthostatic hypotension is often associated with supine hypertension, which complicates its therapy.

### Nonpharmacologic Choices

Remove as many hypotensive and volume-depleting drugs as possible. *Increase dietary salt* intake if not contraindicated. Elevate the head of the bed on blocks or bricks by 15 to 30 cm (this is often not well tolerated). Instruct patients to avoid hemodynamic stress such as getting up quickly, eating large meals, warm environments or hot baths, and heavy exertion.

### Pharmacologic Choices (Table 2)

**Fludrocortisone** increases blood volume and sensitizes peripheral alpha receptors.

**Midodrine** is a pressor amine that causes both venoconstriction (thereby increasing venous return) and arteriolar constriction (to directly increase pressure). Supine hypertension may complicate treatment.

**Yohimbine** is an $alpha_2$ antagonist that stimulates sympathetic outflow. Recent work suggests that many patients have only partial sympathetic denervation and yohimbine stimulates outflow in the remaining nerves. Anxiety, tremor, headache and diarrhea may limit its use.

*NSAIDs* may increase fluid retention and also indirectly cause vasoconstriction. Try **indomethacin** 25 to 50 mg TID or equivalent doses of related drugs.

*Nonselective beta-blockers* (e.g., **propranolol, timolol, nadolol**) block vasodilatory $\beta_2$ receptors.

**Octreotide**, a somatostatin analogue that blocks production of gut vasodilator hormones, may be useful in postprandial hypotension.

### *Driving*

All physicians treating syncope patients should be familiar with their local regulations for the ability of syncope patients to drive. The regulations vary with the cause of syncope and with the therapy, and with the individual province. Know and implement your province's guidelines. The Canadian Cardiovascular Society Conference recommends that the syncope patient:

- *Refrain from driving private or small vehicles*
  - For 1 month after each faint if they faint once/year or less
  - For 3 months after each faint if they faint > once/year
- *Refrain from driving large commercial vehicles*
  - For 3 months after each faint if they faint once/year or less
  - For 12 months after each faint if they faint > once/year

## Therapeutic Tips

- The orthostatic intolerance syndromes can be distinguished based on history and a simple **stand test** in the office. To perform the stand test, first measure blood pressure and heart rate while the patient is supine, then after 2 and 4 minutes of standing. These responses are seen:

  *Normal and vasovagal syncope:* modest rises in heart rate (about 10 bpm) and blood pressure (about 10 mm Hg).

  *Postural orthostatic tachycardia syndrome:* > 30 bpm rise or heart rate > 120 bpm with normal BP or mild orthostatic hypotension.

  *Autonomic failure:* progressive fall in blood pressure of ≥ 20 mm Hg systolic or ≥ 10 mm Hg diastolic with development of presyncope; often no increase in heart rate.

### *Suggested Reading List*

Grubb BP, Karas B. Clinical disorders of the autonomic nervous system associated with orthostatic intolerance: an overview of classification, clinical evaluation, and management. *PACE* 1999;22:798–810.

Atiga WL, Rowe P, Calkins H. Management of vasovagal syncope. *J Cardiovasc Electrophysiol* 1999;10:874–876.

Benditt DG, Fahy GJ, Lurie KG, Sakaguchi S, Fabian W, Samniah N. Pharmacotherapy of neurally mediated syncope. *Circulation* 1999;100:1242–1248.

CHAPTER 35

# Systemic Thromboembolism

*Anne M. Gillis, MD, FRCPC*

Systemic thromboembolism is usually caused by embolism of a clot to a peripheral artery causing acute arterial occlusion. Less frequently tumor, vegetation or a foreign body may cause arterial occlusion. The most common source of clot is the left atrium (atrial fibrillation), left ventricle (prior myocardial infarction or dilated cardiomyopathy), prosthetic valve or ulcerated plaque in the systemic vascular tree. Less frequently, a clot in the venous system may embolize to the systemic system via a patent foramen ovale or atrial/ventricular septal defect. Cerebral embolism is discussed in Chapter 22.

## Goals of Therapy

- To prevent organ damage
- To alleviate pain
- To prevent recurrence

## Investigations

- Complete history with attention to cardiovascular history and identification of cardiovascular risk factors
- Complete physical examination with attention to cardiovascular examination, blood pressure, peripheral pulses and relevant target organs
- Laboratory tests:
  - CBC, coagulation parameters. In selected cases, specialized tests (immunologic work-up, testing for hypercoagulable states, antiphospholipid antibodies, Factor V Leiden)
  - ECG
  - echocardiogram (rule out cardiac souce, consider transesophageal echo)
  - in selected cases, CT angiography, MRI angiography or arterial angiography may be required to identify a vascular source.
  - blood cultures if endocarditis suspected

## Therapeutic Choices

### Acute Therapy

**Heparinize:** 80 units/kg followed by maintenance infusion of 18 units/kg/hour; titrate up or down to maintain PTT 60 to 90 sec (see Chapter 31, Table 4). Follow by **thromboembolectomy** (local thrombolysis, percutaneous catheter aspiration embolectomy or surgical thrombectomy as appropriate). The treatment requires the collaboration of radiologists, vascular surgeons and cardiologists to define the most appropriate intervention.

### Chronic Therapy

Chronic anticoagulation with **warfarin** (maintain INR 2 to 3 for cardiac source; 3 to 4 for prosthetic mechanical valve) if risk of recurrence high, e.g., cardiac source, significant vascular disease or abnormality of coagulation cascade.

## Therapeutic Tips

- Referral to a hematologist for specialized investigations of the coagulation system may be required if the patient has no apparent risk factors.
- Documentation of sinus rhythm at the time of presentation does not exclude atrial fibrillation as a cause of intracardiac thrombus. If the patient has risk factors for atrial fibrillation, continuous ECG monitoring should be performed for at least 48 hrs.
- Local thrombolysis with intra-arterial infusion of **alteplase** (2.5 to 10 mg/hr for 4 to 5 hr) or **urokinase** (4000 IU/min × 4hr, then 2000 IU/min until lysis) may be as effective as catheter or surgical embolectomy although the risk of bleeding complications is higher.
- Prophylactic anticoagulation with warfarin should be considered in high risk patients, e.g., patients with significant left ventricular dysfunction, patients with left ventricular thrombus, high risk patients with atrial fibrillation (Chapter 28).

### Suggested Reading List

Ouriel K, Veith FJ, Sasahara AA. A comparison of recombinant urokinase with vascular surgery as initial treatment for acute arterial occlusion of the legs. Thrombolysis or Peripheral Arterial Surgery (TOPAS) Investigators. *N Engl J Med* 1998;338:1105–1111.

Huettl EA, Soulen MC. Thrombolysis of lower extremity embolic occlusions: a study of the results of the STAR Registry. *Radiology* 1995;197:141–145.

Hess H, Mietaschk A, von Bilderling P, Neller P. Peripheral arterial occlusions: local low-dose thrombolytic therapy with recombinant tissue-type plasminogen activator (rt-PA). *Eur J Vasc Endovasc Surg* 1996;12:97–104.

Reber PU, Patel AG, Stauffer E, Muller MF, Do DD, Kniemeyer HW. Mural aortic thrombi: An important cause of peripheral embolization. *J Vasc Surg* 1999;30:1084–1089.

CHAPTER 36

# Allergic Rhinitis

*D. William Moote, MD, FRCPC*

## Goals of Therapy

- To prevent allergic reaction from occurring, by avoiding exposure
- To suppress and control symptoms produced by the allergic response

## Investigations

- Clinical history and physical examination (Table 1). View nasal mucosa using otoscope
- Skin testing: confirms allergic sensitivity, if present. Little benefit in measuring serum IgE or eosinophilia, which do not correlate well with presence of allergic disease

Table 1: **Differential Diagnosis of Rhinitis**

| Type | Characteristics |
|---|---|
| Seasonal or perennial allergic rhinitis | Nasal obstruction and rhinorrhea are common.<br>Often conjunctival symptoms, sneezing, itching of the nasal mucosa and the oropharynx.<br>Seasonal patterns may be recognized, or perennial symptoms may flare up after exposure to allergens like dust mite or animal danders.<br>Nasal mucosa is swollen, often pale or bluish, and moist. |
| Upper respiratory infections | More episodic, often associated with sore throat or fever and not associated with itch.<br>Nasal mucosa is often red. |
| Vasomotor rhinitis | Obstruction and rhinorrhea are prominent and other symptoms infrequent.<br>May be triggered by irritant exposures such as smoke, temperature changes, strong odors. |
| Nasal polyps | Obstruction is the main complaint.<br>Anosmia is almost always present.<br>Nasal exam will usually detect a polyp. |

## Therapeutic Choices (Figure 1)

### Nonpharmacologic Choices

- Avoidance of allergens allows reduced medication use. Air conditioning reduces pollen exposure. Removing pets from the home will reduce perennial symptoms caused by animal dander. Dust avoidance measures can reduce exposure as much as 60%.

Figure 1: **Management of Allergic Rhinitis**

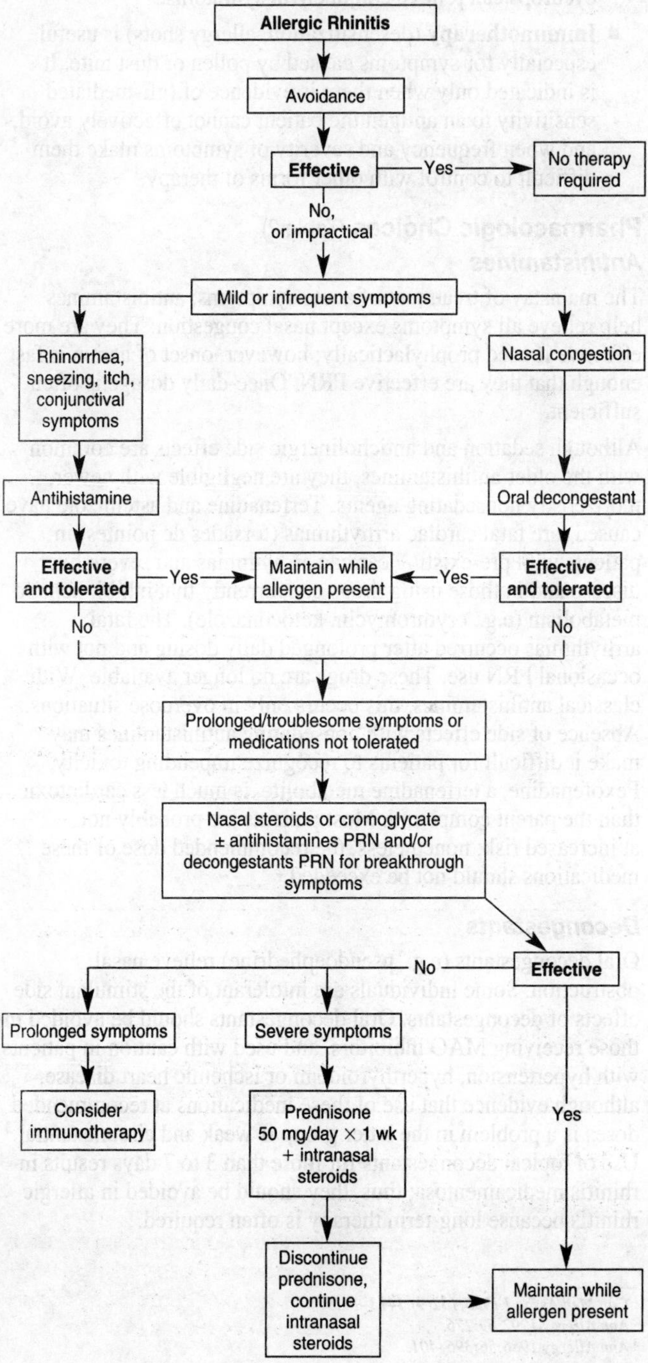

Allergic Rhinitis
Avoidance
Effective
Yes
No therapy required
No, or impractical
Mild or infrequent symptoms
Rhinorrhea, sneezing, itch, conjunctival symptoms
Nasal congestion
Antihistamine
Oral decongestant
Effective and tolerated
Yes
Maintain while allergen present
Yes
Effective and tolerated
No
No
Prolonged/troublesome symptoms or medications not tolerated
Nasal steroids or cromoglycate ± antihistamines PRN and/or decongestants PRN for breakthrough symptoms
No
Effective
Prolonged symptoms
Severe symptoms
Consider immunotherapy
Prednisone 50 mg/day × 1 wk + intranasal steroids
Yes
Discontinue prednisone, continue intranasal steroids
Maintain while allergen present

- Saline nose sprays can help relieve symptoms by washing out mucus and the inhaled allergen. Similarly, lubricant eyedrops can relieve conjunctival symptoms.
- **Immunotherapy** (desensitization, allergy shots) is useful, especially for symptoms caused by pollen or dust mite. It is indicated only when there is evidence of IgE-mediated sensitivity to an antigen the patient cannot effectively avoid, and when frequency and severity of symptoms make them difficult to control with other forms of therapy.[1]

## Pharmacologic Choices (Table 2)

### *Antihistamines*

The mainstay of treatment of acute symptoms, antihistamines help relieve all symptoms except nasal congestion. They are more effective if used prophylactically; however, onset of action is fast enough that they are effective PRN. Once-daily dosage is often sufficient.

Although sedation and anticholinergic side effects are common with the older antihistamines, they are negligible with newer, more costly nonsedating agents. Terfenadine and astemizole have caused rare fatal cardiac arrhythmias (torsades de pointes) in patients with pre-existing cardiac arrhythmias and severe liver disease and in those using drugs concurrently that inhibit hepatic metabolism (e.g., erythromycin, ketoconazole). The fatal arrhythmias occurred after prolonged daily dosing and not with occasional PRN use. These drugs are no longer available. With classical antihistamines, this occurs only in overdose situations. Absence of side effects with nonsedating antihistamines may make it difficult for patients to recognize impending toxicity. Fexofenadine, a terfenadine metabolite, is much less cardiotoxic than the parent compound. Most patients are probably not at increased risk; nonetheless, the recommended dose of these medications should not be exceeded.[2]

### *Decongestants*

Oral decongestants (e.g., pseudoephedrine) relieve nasal obstruction. Some individuals are intolerant of the stimulant side effects of decongestants. Oral decongestants should be avoided in those receiving MAO inhibitors, and used with caution in patients with hypertension, hyperthyroidism or ischemic heart disease, although evidence that use of these medications at recommended doses is a problem in the latter group is weak and circumstantial.[3] Use of topical decongestants for more than 3 to 7 days results in rhinitis medicamentosa; thus, they should be avoided in allergic rhinitis because long-term therapy is often required.

---

[1] *Can Med Assoc J 1995;152(9):1413–1419.*
[2] *Ann Allergy 1992;69:276.*
[3] *Ann Allergy 1986;56:396–401.*

### *Antihistamine–Decongestant Combinations*

Antihistamines and decongestants have complementary effects. Patients taking both drugs may find combination tablets convenient, although many of the combinations include classical antihistamines, which may be sedating. Some combinations (e.g., cold preparations) may also contain analgesics and expectorants, which are not helpful in allergic rhinitis and should be avoided.

### *Topical Therapy*

**Topical corticosteroids** are the mainstay of therapy for chronic rhinitis symptoms. Aqueous preparations generally have better intranasal deposition than pressurized metered-dose inhalers especially when chronic symptoms have caused significant obstruction or there is ciliary dysfunction, as in smokers. Newer preparations have a lower volume spray, which may be preferred by some. Dry powder inhalers are available for some preparations (e.g., budesonide) and offer an alternative for those who dislike aqueous sprays.

Topical steroids act locally and are quickly metabolized once absorbed. Adrenal suppression has not been seen at therapeutic dosages. Data on inhaled steroids in asthma suggest that systemic effects occur at doses in the range of 1000 to 2000 μg of beclomethasone – much higher than those recommended for allergic rhinitis. There are anecdotal reports of nasal septal perforation. No reports in controlled studies confirm this; however, patients should be instructed to aim the spray at the turbinates, not at the septum.

**Topical cromoglycate** sprays have an excellent safety profile but are less effective than the steroids and usually need QID dosing, at least initially.

**Levocabastine** (antihistamine) nasal spray has a rapid onset but is less potent than topical steroids and is not effective for treatment of congestion.

### *Anticipated therapy*

**Leukotriene receptor antagonists** may be of value in the treatment of allergic rhinitis, but their role in routine treatment needs to be further defined. For now, it is helpful to note that in patients using these drugs for asthma, their rhinitis may also improve.[4]

## Pharmacoeconomic Considerations

Topical corticosteroids are the therapy of choice based on cost and effectiveness. Antihistamines are cost effective only for the mildest symptoms.

Quality of life assessments are now being applied in allergic rhinitis. They show a significant impairment in day-to-day

---

[4] *J Allergy Clin Immunol 1998;101(1pt2):S97.*

Table 2: **Drugs Used in Allergic Rhinitis**

| Drug | Dosage | Adverse Effects | Comments | Cost* |
|---|---|---|---|---|
| ***Oral Agents*** | | | | |
| **Antihistamines:** See Chapter 66 (Pruritus). | | | | |
| **Decongestants**<br>*pseudoephedrine*<br>Eltor, Sudafed, others | Adults: 60 mg Q4–6H<br>Sustained release: 120 mg Q12H<br>Children 6–11 yrs: 30 mg Q4–6H (120 mg/d max.)<br>Children 2–5 yrs: 15 mg Q4–6H (60 mg/d max.) | Insomnia, tremor, irritability, headache, nightmares, palpitations. | Rhinitis medicamentosa is not a problem with oral agents but occurs with prolonged use (> 3 days) of topical nasal decongestants. | $† |
| **Antihistamine–Decongestant Combinations**<br>– various combinations and products | In accordance with labelled directions | See Chapter 66, Table 1, for antihistamine adverse effects; as above for decongestants. | Offer convenience to patient requiring an antihistamine and decongestant. | $† |
| ***Topical Agents*** | **Sprays per day in each nostril** | | | |
| *sodium cromoglycate*<br>Cromolyn, others | Adults and children over 5 yrs: 1 QID | Nasal stinging, burning, irritation, sneezing. | Slow onset (significant effects may not be seen for 1 wk in seasonal allergic rhinitis and 2–4 wks in chronic allergic rhinitis), low potency, very safe. | $$ |

| | | | | |
|---|---|---|---|---|
| **Corticosteroids** | | | | |
| *beclomethasone* Vancenase, Beconase AQ, generics | Adults/children ≥ 6 yrs: 1 QID 2 BID | Burning or stinging, nosebleeds. | Slow onset (7–14 d for maximal effect), must be used regularly, long duration, very potent, concern about potential steroid side effects, especially in children. Aiming spray up toward turbinates and away from septum helps avoid septal crusting or irritation. Liquid formats may be more effective than metered-dose inhalers. For once daily dosed medication, administering 1 spray into each nostril BID may be more effective in some situations. | $–$$ |
| *budesonide* Rhinocort Aqua, Rhinocort Turbuhaler, generics | Adults/children ≥ 6 yrs: 2 daily | | | $–$$$ |
| *flunisolide* Rhinalar | Adults: 2 BID Children 6–14 yrs: 1 TID | | | $$ |
| *fluticasone* Flonase | Adults/children ≥ 12 yrs: 2 daily Children 4–11 yrs: 1–2 daily | | | $$$ |
| *mometasone furoate* Nasonex | Adults/children ≥ 12 yrs: 2 daily Children 3–11 yrs: 1 daily | | | $$$ |
| *triamcinolone acetonide* Nasacort, Nasacort AQ | Adults/children > 12 yrs: 2 daily Children 4–12 yrs‡: 1 daily | | | $$$ |
| **Antihistamines** | | | | |
| *levocabastine* Livostin | Adults/children > 12 yrs: 2 BID | Nasal irritation. | Quick onset, short duration, short shelf life. If no improvement in 3 d it should be discontinued. Not effective for congestion. | $$ |

† *Available over the counter – retail mark-up may vary.*
‡ *Only aqueous formulation approved for use in children.*
* *Cost of one unit (spray pump, metered-dose aerosol unit, etc.) or 12 tablets – includes drug cost only.*
*Legend: $ < $10 $$ $10–20 $$$ $20–30*

physical, emotional, occupational, and social functioning.[5] Approximately 15% of the population experiences symptoms of allergic rhinitis, but only 12.3% of these seek medical treatment.[6]

## Therapeutic Tips

- If an antihistamine at recommended dosage does not work, little is gained from changing to a different chemical class. Although older studies of long-term dosing with classical antihistamines have demonstrated loss of effectiveness, they are flawed by lack of evidence of compliance. Newer studies show no loss of effectiveness up to 1 year.
- Most antihistamine preparations are available as syrups for children but are not very convenient for portable PRN dosing. Brompheniramine/phenylpropanolamine (Dimetapp Chewtabs) and loratadine (tasteless) tablets can be chewed.
- Medications are usually started at the maximum dose and then tapered to the minimum required for maintenance.
- Patients with predictable seasonal allergic rhinitis can start medications such as intranasal corticosteroids before the allergen exposure period and take them regularly until the end of the season for maximum effectiveness.
- If desired results are not achieved with once-daily dosing of newer topical steroids, a twice-daily regimen may be more effective, even at the same total daily dose.
- Antihistamines can be used in asthmatic patients; many have a slightly beneficial effect on asthma symptoms.
- For conjunctival symptoms, oral antihistamines are useful. Topical ophthalmic levocabastine provides relief in 10 minutes but is short lasting (12 h). Topical cromoglycate or lodoxamide requires several days for onset. Once opened, levocabastine and cromoglycate should be discarded within a month. In contrast, olopatadine or emedastine eyedrops are both quick in onset and stable once opened.
- In vasomotor rhinitis where watery rhinorrhea is the major problem, ipratropium bromide spray can be helpful. It is quick in onset.
- Topical steroids will shrink nasal polyps, but long-term treatment is required. Anosmia is not usually improved. If surgery is contemplated, the use of topical steroids after surgery may decrease the recurrence rate.

---

[5] *J Allergy Clin Immunol 1997;99(2):S742–S749.*
[6] *J Allergy Clin Immunol 1997;99(1):22–27.*

## *Suggested Reading List*

Anon. Assessing and treating rhinitis: A practical guide for Canadian physicians. Proceedings of the Canadian Rhinitis Symposium. *Can Med Assoc J* 1994;151(4Suppl):1–27.

Dykewicz MS, Fineman S, Skoner DP, et al. Diagnosis and management of rhinitis: complete guidelines on the Joint Task Force on Practice Parameters in Allergy, Asthma, and Immunology. American Academy of Allergy, Asthma, and Immunology. *Ann Allergy Asthma Immunol* 1998;81(5pt2): 478–518.

Milgrom H, Bender B. Adverse effects of medications for rhinitis. *Ann Allergy Asthma Immunol* 1997;78(5):439–444.

CHAPTER 37

# Viral Rhinitis

*Timothy P. Lynch, MD, FRCPC*

## Goals of Therapy

- To lessen interference with activities of daily living
- To improve the discomfort and emotional distress of rhinorrhea
- To improve the discomfort of nasal congestion
- To minimize the potential adverse effects of pharmacologic agents

## Investigations

- The diagnosis of the common cold, which is most commonly due to rhinovirus infections, requires no specific laboratory investigation

## Therapeutic Choices (Figure 1)

Viral rhinitis is not a condition that is life-threatening. Typical symptoms of rhinorrhea and nasal congestion resolve untreated in 7 to 10 days. There is no evidence to support that treatment lessens the risk of developing complications. To improve these symptoms and the patient's quality of life, certain nonpharmacologic and pharmacologic approaches are available. Each pharmacologic agent employed should be directed against a specific symptom.

### Nonpharmacologic Choices

- The avoidance of close contact with someone with a cold is the key to prevention.
- Strict hand-washing techniques limit risk of inoculation and risk of transmission.
- Regular administration of normal saline nose drops may improve nasal congestion in young infants.

### Pharmacologic Choices (Figure 1, Table 1)

#### *Alpha-adrenergic Agents (Decongestants)*

Decongestants are used specifically to relieve nasal congestion and improve rhinorrhea. There is no question that they help most adults by improving nasal air flow. Both short- and long-acting topical agents are available along with long-acting oral formulations.

Figure 1: **Management of Viral Rhinitis**

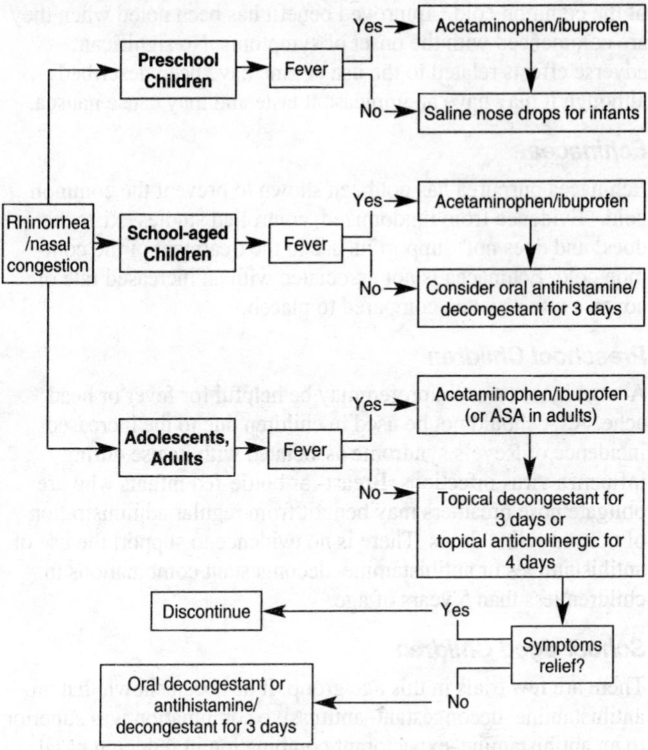
Rhinorrhea /nasal congestion
Preschool Children
Fever
Yes
Acetaminophen/ibuprofen
No
Saline nose drops for infants
School-aged Children
Fever
Yes
Acetaminophen/ibuprofen
No
Consider oral antihistamine/ decongestant for 3 days
Adolescents, Adults
Fever
Yes
Acetaminophen/ibuprofen (or ASA in adults)
No
Topical decongestant for 3 days or topical anticholinergic for 4 days
Symptoms relief?
Yes
Discontinue
No
Oral decongestant or antihistamine/ decongestant for 3 days

### *Anticholinergic Agents*

Aerosolized intranasal atropine derivatives block cholinergic-mediated vasodilatation. They are effective in treating rhinorrhea and provide relief of sneezing but do not improve nasal congestion.

### *Antihistamines*

The anticholinergic effects of some first-generation antihistamines may reduce nasal secretions.

Second-generation or nonsedating antihistamines have no anticholinergic activity. There is no evidence to support their use alone in controlling rhinorrhea or nasal congestion.

### *Vitamin C*

Vitamin C (ascorbic acid) supplementation has not been shown to prevent the common cold. Direct therapeutic benefits in doses of at least 1 g/day remain controversial.[1] It has few adverse effects.

[1] *Nutrition 1996;12(11–12):804–809.*

### *Zinc Lozenges*

Zinc gluconate lozenges may reduce the symptoms and duration of the common cold.[2] Improved benefit has been noted when they are commenced with the onset of symptoms. No significant adverse effects related to the use of zinc have been described although it may have an unpleasant taste and may cause nausea.

### *Echinacea*

Echinacea purpurea has not been shown to prevent the common cold.[3] Evidence from randomized, controlled studies exists that does[3] and does not[4] support its use in the treatment of the common cold. Echinacea is not associated with an increased rate of adverse effects when compared to placebo.

### *Preschool Children*

Acetaminophen or ibuprofen may be helpful for fever or headache. ASA should not be used in children due to the increased incidence of Reye's syndrome associated with its use during influenza virus infections. Breast- or bottle-fed infants who are obligate nose breathers may benefit from regular administration of normal saline drops. There is no evidence to support the use of antihistamines or antihistamine–decongestant combinations in children less than 5 years of age.

### *School-aged Children*

There are few trials in this age group. It has been shown that an antihistamine–decongestant–antitussive combination was superior to an antihistamine–expectorant combination in reducing nasal symptoms.

### *Adolescents and Adults*

Decongestants, either topically or orally, or antihistamine–decongestant combinations have been shown to improve short-term nasal symptoms. Oral decongestants are associated with an increased number of adverse effects. Prolonged use of nasal decongestants is associated with rebound congestion (rhinitis medicamentosa). Anticholinergic agents have also been shown to improve rhinorrhea.

## Therapeutic Tips

- In preschool children
  - combination decongestants–antihistamines have not been shown to be effective
  - accidental ingestion and dosing errors of these products can do much harm

[2] *Can Fam Physician 1998;44:1037–1042.*
[3] *Phytomedicine 1999;6(1):1–6.*
[4] *Am J Med 1999;106(2):138–143.*

Table 1: **Drugs Used in Viral Rhinitis**

| Drug | Dosage | Adverse effects | Drug Interactions | Comments | Cost* |
|---|---|---|---|---|---|
| **Decongestants Systemic** | | | | | |
| *pseudoephedrine* Sudafed, Triaminic Oral Pediatric Drops, others | Adults: 60 mg Q4–6H PRN 120 mg SR Q12H (max. 240 mg/d)<br>Children 6–12 yrs: 30 mg Q4–6H PRN (max. 120 mg/d)<br>Children 2–5 yrs: 15 mg Q4–6H PRN (max. 60 mg/d)‡ | Insomnia, tremor, irritability, headache, night palpitations. | β-blockers: therapeutic effects may be decreased.<br>MAOI's concurrent use contraindicated. | Contraindicated in patients with severe hypertension and coronary artery disease. Use with caution in cardiovascular disease, diabetes, hyperthyroidism, prostatic hypertrophy and angle-closure glaucoma. | $† |
| **Decongestants Topical** | | For all:<br>Burning, stinging and dryness of nasal mucosa.<br>Rebound congestion may occur with > 3–5 days of continuous use.<br>Topical products are associated with fewer systemic adverse effects than oral decongestants. (see above) | | Use with caution in patients with hypertension, cardiovascular disease or hyperthyroidism. | |
| *oxymetazoline* Dristan Long Lasting Nasal Spray, Drixoral Nasal, others | Adults and children ≥ 6 yrs: 0.05% 2 or 3 sprays each nostril Q12H PRN | | | | $† |
| *xylometazoline* Otrivin, Decongest, others | Adults: 0.1% 1–2 sprays or 2–3 drops each nostril Q8–10H PRN<br>Children > 6 yrs: 0.05% 1–2 sprays or 2–3 drops each nostril Q8–10H PRN<br>Children < 6 yrs: 0.05% 1 spray or 1 drop each nostril Q8–10H PRN‡ | | | | $† |

*(cont'd)*

Table 1: **Drugs Used in Viral Rhinitis** *(cont'd)*

| Drug | Dosage | Adverse effects | Drug Interactions | Comments | Cost* |
|---|---|---|---|---|---|
| **Anticholinergic Agents**<br>*ipratropium bromide*<br>Atrovent Nasal Spray | Adults and children ≥ 12 yrs: 0.06% 2 sprays each nostril TID-QID PRN | Nosebleeds, nasal dryness, dry mouth/throat. | | Avoid accidental release of nasal spray into eyes. | $$$ |
| **Antihistamine – Decongestant Combinations**[π]<br>-various combinations and products e.g., | Dosage varies. Refer to specific product information. | Antihistamines: drowsiness, fatigue. Paradoxical stimulatory effects may occur in children and the elderly. Anticholinergic effects: dry eyes, dry mouth, and urinary retention. | Antihistamines: Additive CNS depressive effects with alcohol and other CNS depressants. | As for systemic decongestants (above). | $[†] |
| *brompheniramine/ phenylpropanolamine*<br>Dimetapp Liqui-Gels, others | 4 mg/25 mg | Decongestants: see above. | Decongestants: see above. | | |
| *chlorpheniramine/ phenylpropanolamine*<br>Contac Cold, Ornade, others | 8 mg/75 mg | | | | |
| *chlorpheniramine/ pseudoephedrine*<br>Chlortripolon Decongestant, others | 12 mg/120 mg | | | | |
| *dexbrompheniramine/ pseudoephedrine*<br>Drixoral, others | 2 mg/60 mg | | | | |
| *triprolidine/ pseudoephedrine*<br>Actifed | 2.5 mg/60 mg | | | | |

* *Cost of one unit (spray pump, drops) or 12 tablets — includes drug cost only.*
*Legend: $ < $10 $$ < $10–20 $$$ $20–30*
[†] *Available over the counter — retail mark-up may vary.*
[‡] *There is no evidence to support the use of decongestants in preschool children (JAMA 1993;269:2258–2263).*
[π] *Not inclusive of all available products. Listed products are representative of some available brands; other similar products exist. For a complete listing, see the Compendium of Nonprescription Products 6th ed. Ottawa, ON: Canadian Pharmacists Association, 1999.*

- In school-aged children
  - combination decongestant–antihistamines may be of benefit but risks of treatment should be carefully considered
- In adolescents and adults
  - a short course of topical decongestants or topical anticholinergic agents should be considered first-line therapy

## *Suggested Reading List*

Anderson LD. Anti-histamines and the common cold. A review and critique of the literature. *J Gen Intern Med* 1996;11: 240–244.

Clemens CJ, et al. Is an anti-histamine-decongestant combination effective in temporarily relieving symptoms of the common cold in preschool children? *J Pediatr* 1997;130:463–466.

Hayden FG, et al. Effectiveness and safety of intranasal ipratropium bromide in common colds: A randomized, double blind, placebo-controlled trial. *Ann Intern Med* 1996;125:89–97.

Smith MBH, Feldman W. Over-the-counter cold medications: a critical review of clinical trials between 1950 and 1991. *JAMA* 1993; 269:2258–2263.

CHAPTER 38

# Adult Asthma

*David G. McCormack, MD, FRCPC, FCCP*

## Goals of Therapy

- Maintain normal activity levels
- Prevent symptoms (cough, wheezing, dyspnea)
- Maintain normal (or near normal) spirometry
- Prevent exacerbations
- Avoid side effects of therapy

## Investigations

- Thorough history with particular attention to:
  - pattern of symptoms (seasonal, perennial, etc.)
  - precipitating factors (environmental allergens, occupational exposures, irritants such as smoke, drugs such as ASA, beta-blockers, exercise)
  - previous hospitalizations and intensive care admissions
- Physical examination: wheezing, nasal polyps
- Objective measurements needed to confirm diagnosis and assess severity include:
  - spirometry: reduced expiratory flow rates
  - home peak flow monitoring for patients with severe asthma or poor perception of airway obstruction
  - bronchoprovocation challenge test, using methacholine or histamine, if diagnosis in doubt

## Therapeutic Choices

### Nonpharmacologic Choices

- Known precipitating factors such as environmental allergens and occupational irritants should be avoided.
- Smoking cessation is essential (Chapter 42).
- ASA and other nonsteroidal anti-inflammatory drugs (NSAIDs) should be avoided.
- Hyposensitization therapy to allergens generally is not useful.
- Patient education about asthma symptoms and therapy is essential for optimal management.

Figure 1: **Treatment of Asthma**

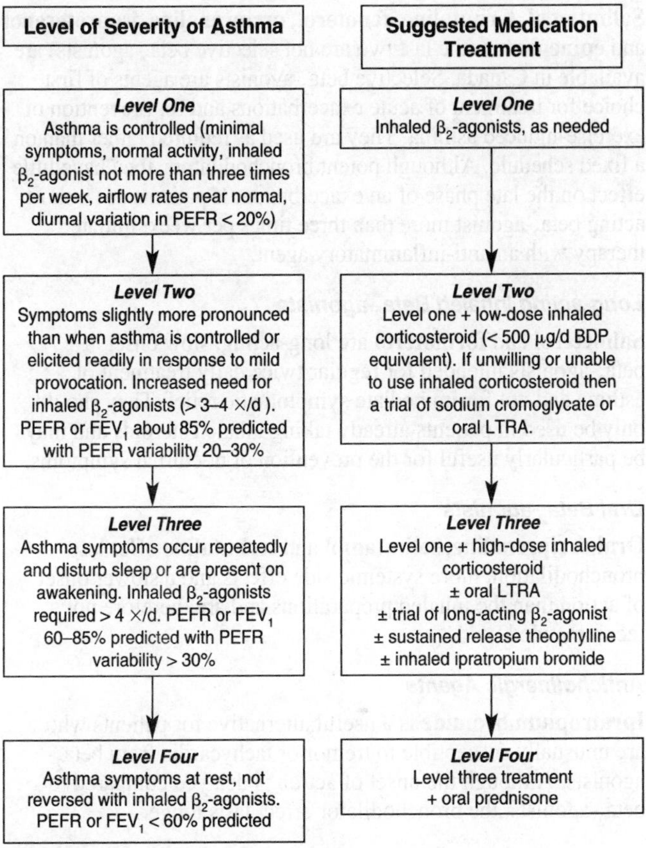
Level of Severity of Asthma
Suggested Medication Treatment
Level One
Asthma is controlled (minimal symptoms, normal activity, inhaled $\beta_2$-agonist not more than three times per week, airflow rates near normal, diurnal variation in PEFR < 20%)
Level One
Inhaled $\beta_2$-agonists, as needed
Level Two
Symptoms slightly more pronounced than when asthma is controlled or elicited readily in response to mild provocation. Increased need for inhaled $\beta_2$-agonists (> 3–4 ×/d ). PEFR or $FEV_1$ about 85% predicted with PEFR variability 20–30%
Level Two
Level one + low-dose inhaled corticosteroid (< 500 µg/d BDP equivalent). If unwilling or unable to use inhaled corticosteroid then a trial of sodium cromoglycate or oral LTRA.
Level Three
Asthma symptoms occur repeatedly and disturb sleep or are present on awakening. Inhaled $\beta_2$-agonists required > 4 ×/d. PEFR or $FEV_1$ 60–85% predicted with PEFR variability > 30%
Level Three
Level one + high-dose inhaled corticosteroid
± oral LTRA
± trial of long-acting $\beta_2$-agonist
± sustained release theophylline
± inhaled ipratropium bromide
Level Four
Asthma symptoms at rest, not reversed with inhaled $\beta_2$-agonists. PEFR or $FEV_1$ < 60% predicted
Level Four
Level three treatment
+ oral prednisone

***Note:** These are not discrete levels of severity and treatment and are best thought of as a continuum to reflect a dynamic therapeutic approach.*

*Abbreviations: BDP = beclomethasone dipropionate, LTRA = leukotriene receptor antagonist*

## Pharmacologic Choices

The initial level of treatment with medication is chosen after an assessment of asthma severity and previous treatment (Figure 1). Treatment should be reviewed every 3 to 6 months, and if control is achieved a stepwise reduction in treatment should be tried.

Inhaled therapy that maximizes delivery of drugs to the respiratory tract and minimizes systemic side effects is the cornerstone of asthma management. The metered dose inhalers (MDI) or dry powder inhalers deliver drugs as effectively as nebulized therapy. Medications include bronchodilators and anti-inflammatory agents (Table 1).

## Bronchodilators

### Short-acting Inhaled Beta$_2$-agonists

**Salbutamol, terbutaline, fenoterol, orciprenaline, isoproterenol** and **epinephrine** (the last two are not selective beta$_2$-agonists) are available in Canada. Selective beta$_2$-agonists are agents of first choice for treatment of acute exacerbations and for prevention of exercise-induced asthma. They are used as required rather than on a fixed schedule. Although potent bronchodilators, they have little effect on the late phase of an exacerbation. If patients use a short-acting beta$_2$-agonist more than three times per week, initiate therapy with an anti-inflammatory agent.

### Long-acting Inhaled Beta$_2$-agonists

**Salmeterol** and **formoterol** are long-acting, slow onset beta$_2$-agonists intended for regular twice daily treatment of asthma and not for immediate symptomatic relief. They should only be used in patients already taking inhaled steroids and may be particularly useful for the prevention of nocturnal symptoms.

### Oral Beta$_2$-agonists

**Oral orciprenaline, salbutamol** and **terbutaline** offer less bronchodilation, more systemic side effects and a slower onset of action than the inhaled preparations and are therefore not recommended.

### Anticholinergic Agents

**Ipratropium bromide** is a useful alternative for patients who are unusually susceptible to tremor or tachycardia from beta$_2$-agonists. Although the onset of action is delayed compared to beta$_2$-agonists, the bronchodilator effect lasts longer.

### Theophylline Products

Oral **theophylline, oxtriphylline** and **aminophylline** are third-line therapy, chiefly due to systemic toxicity and mild bronchodilator activity. They should be administered carefully, according to standard regimens with blood levels monitored. In naive patients titrate the dose slowly to minimize side effects. Cimetidine, erythromycin, quinolones and verapamil may increase theophylline levels. Rifampin, cabamazepine and phenytoin may decrease levels.

## Anti-inflammatory Agents

### Inhaled Corticosteroids

Inhaled **budesonide, beclomethasone dipropionate, fluticasone propionate, flunisolide** and **triamcinolone acetonide** are safe, effective, and cost-effective drugs that block the late phase of asthma. They should be used regularly at the lowest effective dose rather than as needed. They have a higher ratio of topical

Table 1: **Drugs Used in the Treatment of Chronic Asthma in Adults**

| Drugs | Dosage | Adverse Effects | Cost* |
|---|---|---|---|
| **Inhaled $\beta_2$-agonists, Short-acting** | | For all: | |
| *salbutamol*<br>Ventolin, Airomir[†], generics | 100 µg/puff: 1–2 puffs Q4–6H PRN | Nervousness, tremor, tachycardia, palpitations. | MDI $<br>Diskhaler/Rotacaps $$ |
| *terbutaline*<br>Bricanyl | 0.5 mg/puff: 1 puff Q4–6H PRN | | $ |
| *fenoterol*<br>Berotec, Berotec Forte | 100 µg/puff: 1–2 puffs Q6–8H PRN | | $ |
| *orciprenaline*<br>Alupent | 0.75 mg/puff: 1–2 puffs Q4H PRN | | $ |
| **Inhaled $\beta_2$-agonists, Long-acting** | | See above. | |
| *salmeterol*<br>Serevent | 25 µg/puff: 2 puffs BID | | $$$$ |
| *formoterol*<br>Foradil, Oxeze | 12 µg/puff: 1 puff BID or<br>12 µg/cap: 1cap inhaled BID | | $$$ |
| **Theophylline Preparations** | For all: serum levels should be monitored | For all: | |
| *theophylline*<br>Quibron-T/SR, Slo-Bid, Theo-Dur, Uniphyl, generics | 200–300 mg PO Q12H | Nausea, vomiting, abdominal cramps, headache, palpitations. | $–$$ |
| *oxtriphylline*<br>Choledyl, generics | 800–1200 mg/d PO | | $–$$ |
| *aminophylline*<br>Phyllocontin, generics | 225–350 mg PO Q12H | | $ |
| **Anticholinergic Agents** | | | |
| *ipratropium bromide*<br>Atrovent | 20 µg/puff: 2–4 puffs Q6–8H | Dry mouth, metallic taste; mydriasis and glaucoma (if released into eye). | $$ |

*(cont'd)*

Table 1: **Drugs Used in the Treatment of Chronic Asthma in Adults** *(cont'd)*

| Drugs | Dosage | Adverse Effects | Cost* |
|---|---|---|---|
| **Inhaled Corticosteroids** | | For all: | Beclomethasone: |
| *beclomethasone dipropionate*‡<br>Qvar†, Vanceril, generics | 200–2000 µg/d divided BID–QID | Sore mouth, sore throat, dysphonia, oral thrush (can be reduced by rinsing mouth or using spacer). | MDI $–$$$$ |
| *budesonide*<br>Pulmicort | 400–2400 µg/d divided BID–QID | | $$–$$$$ |
| *fluticasone propionate*<br>Flovent | 100–1000 µg/d divided BID–QID | | $$$–$$$$ |
| *triamcinolone acetonide*<br>Azmacort | 1200–3200 µg/d divided BID–QID | | $$ |
| *sodium cromoglycate*<br>Intal | 1 mg/puff: 2 puffs QID<br>20 mg/spincap: 20 mg BID–TID | Rare. | $$–$$$ |
| *nedocromil sodium*<br>Tilade | 2 mg/puff: 4 mg QID | Rare. Unpleasant taste. | $$ |
| **Leukotriene Receptor Antagonists** | | | |
| *zafirlukast*<br>Accolate | 20 mg PO BID<br>1 h before or 2 h after meals | Headache, nausea, diarrhea. | $$$ |
| *montelukast*<br>Singulair | 10 mg PO QHS | Headache, abdominal pain. | $$$$ |

† *Contains non-CFC propellants.*
‡ *Beclovent, Becloforte and Beclodisk were discontinued in March 2000.*

* *Includes drug cost only. Cost of inhaled agents is per unit; cost of oral medications is per 30-day supply.*
*Legend: $ < $15 $$ $15–30 $$$ $30–45 $$$$ > $45*

to systemic activity than do oral steroids. The incidence of pharyngeal candidiasis from deposition of the inhaled corticosteroid in the pharynx can be reduced by mouth rinsing after use and/or using a spacer device.

#### *Sodium Cromoglycate*

This inhaled preparation prevents both the early and late phase of asthma exacerbation although it is used less commonly now because inhaled corticosteroids are more effective. It must be administered regularly to provide significant protection and should not be used to treat exacerbations. It produces few side effects.

#### *Nedocromil Sodium*

This medication has comparable indications to sodium cromoglycate.

#### *Systemic Corticosteroids*

These are useful in both preventing and treating acute exacerbations. The optimal dosage has not been established. The side effects are significant: glucose intolerance, weight gain, mood alterations and hypertension in the short term and osteoporosis, hypertension, cataracts and myopathy in the long term. These can be reduced by treating patients for short periods (1 to 2 weeks) following an acute exacerbation. Side effects with long-term use may be minimized by using alternate-day dosing regimens.

#### *Leukotriene Receptor Antagonists (LTRAs)*

**Zafirlukast** and **montelukast** are the LTRAs currently available. These agents have anti-inflammatory properties and are likely equivalent to low dose (about 200 μg/day BDP equivalent) inhaled corticosteroid therapy. There is no good evidence to suggest that LTRAs should be first-line anti-inflammatory therapy to replace inhaled corticosteroids (unless patients cannot or will not use inhaled corticosteroids).

#### *Other Therapies*

Antihistamines are not useful. The place of **ketotifen** in the treatment of adults has not been established. **Methotrexate** and **gold** have been used in some chronic steroid-dependent asthmatics but should be limited to centers experienced with this therapy.

## Asthma in Pregnancy

The best outcome for pregnancy complicated by asthma occurs with optimal management of asthma. In usual therapeutic doses, the drugs used to treat asthma are nonteratogenic. Information is lacking on the safety of using LTRAs and long-acting beta$_2$-agonists.

## Emergency Treatment

- Priorities include oxygenation, rehydration, bronchodilation and use of anti-inflammatory medications (Figure 2).
- Bronchodilation with metered dose inhalers is equivalent to nebulized therapy.
- Synergistic effects between ipratropium bromide and the beta$_2$-agonists suggest administering these two medications concomitantly.
- Oral or parenteral steroids should be used early in most patients.

Figure 2: **Emergency Treatment of Asthma**

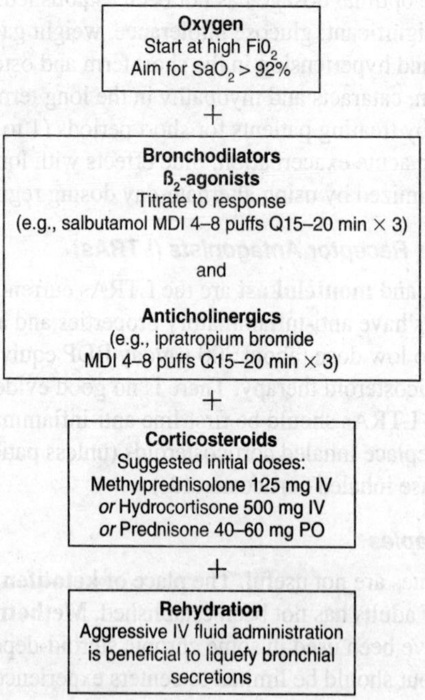
Oxygen
Start at high $FiO_2$
Aim for $SaO_2$ > 92%
+
Bronchodilators
$\beta_2$-agonists
Titrate to response
(e.g., salbutamol MDI 4–8 puffs Q15–20 min × 3)
and
Anticholinergics
(e.g., ipratropium bromide
MDI 4–8 puffs Q15–20 min × 3)
+
Corticosteroids
Suggested initial doses:
Methylprednisolone 125 mg IV
or Hydrocortisone 500 mg IV
or Prednisone 40–60 mg PO
+
Rehydration
Aggressive IV fluid administration
is beneficial to liquefy bronchial
secretions

*Abbreviations: $FiO_2$ = fraction of inspired oxygen; $SaO_2$ = arterial oxygen percent saturation.*

## Pharmacoeconomic Considerations

*Jeffrey A Johnson, PhD*

There is considerable evidence that the prevalence and severity of asthma has increased in the past two decades, leading to increased concern about the growing asthma-related morbidity and mortality, and the associated economic burden. Cost-of-illness analyses for asthma have been carried out for several industrialized nations, principally Australia, United Kingdom, New Zealand, and the US. The costs associated with the management of asthma in the US in 1990 were estimated to be $6.2 billion. Direct medical expenditures accounted for $3.6 billion, or approximately 59% of the total estimate. Canadian estimates for the total direct and indirect costs of asthma were between $504 and $648 million in 1990. Hospital and physician services were found to make up approximately one-third of the total costs.

Published cost-effectiveness evaluations of asthma therapy are limited. The few studies that have been conducted indicate that the additional costs of adding inhaled corticosteroids are almost entirely compensated for by reductions in the costs of other health care services.

***Suggested Reading***

*Weiss KB, Sullivan SD. The economic costs of asthma: a review and conceptual model. PharmacoEconomics 1993;4:14–30.*

*Krahn MD, Berka C, Langlois P, et al. Direct and indirect costs of asthma in Canada, 1990. Can Med Assoc J 1996;154:821–831.*

## *Suggested Reading List*

Barnes PJ. A new approach to the treatment of asthma. *N Engl J Med* 1989;321:1517–1527.

British Asthma Guidelines Coordination Committee. British guidelines on asthma management: 1995 review and position statement. *Thorax* 1997;52:51–524.

Ernst P, Fitzgerald JM, Spier S. Canadian asthma consensus conference summary of recommendations. *Can Respir J* 1996;3:89–100.

Rutten-van Mölken MPMH, Van Doorslaer EKA, Jansen MCC, et al. Cost effectiveness of inhaled corticosteroid plus bronchodilator therapy versus bronchodilator monotherapy in children with asthma. *PharmacoEconomics* 1993;4:257–270.

CHAPTER 39

# Asthma in Infants and Children

*Mark Montgomery, MD, FRCPC*

Asthma is simply airways hyperreactivity (twitchy airways, reactive airways) in the absence of other lung disease. Night cough persisting after a cold, wheeze or shortness of breath limiting activities, all indicate airways hyperreactivity. If there is no evidence of other lung disease such as cystic fibrosis, bronchiolitis, foreign body aspiration or pertussis, the child should be assumed to have asthma and management initiated. If there is little improvement with $beta_2$-agonists or systemic steroids, then the diagnosis of asthma is in doubt. Inadequate response to appropriate therapy mandates reassessment of the patient to establish the appropriate diagnosis or identify concomitant conditions (e.g., gastroesophageal reflux, postnasal drip/sinusitis, vocal cord dysfunction).

## Goals of Therapy

- No cough, wheeze or shortness of breath which interferes with daytime activities, exercise, school attendance or sleep
- $Beta_2$-agonists used for symptom relief less than 3 times/week
- No emergency room visits or hospitalizations
- Normal measures of expiratory airflow, such as peak flows or pulmonary function studies ($FEV_1$)
- No medication side effects

## Therapeutic Choices

### Nonpharmacologic Choices

#### *Environmental Control*

- Avoid exposure to **cigarette smoke.**
- Explore specific allergies to inhalants by history and/or skin testing.
- For those with **house dust mite allergy**:
  - avoid humidifiers, which raise the relative humidity above 40% and promote growth of house dust mite
  - use vinyl mattress and pillow covers
  - avoid down and feather bedding
  - minimize the number of fluffy toys and upholstered furniture in the bedroom
  - remove bedroom carpeting
- For those with **allergy to pets**: avoid exposure.

Figure 1: **Maintenance Therapy of Asthma in Children**

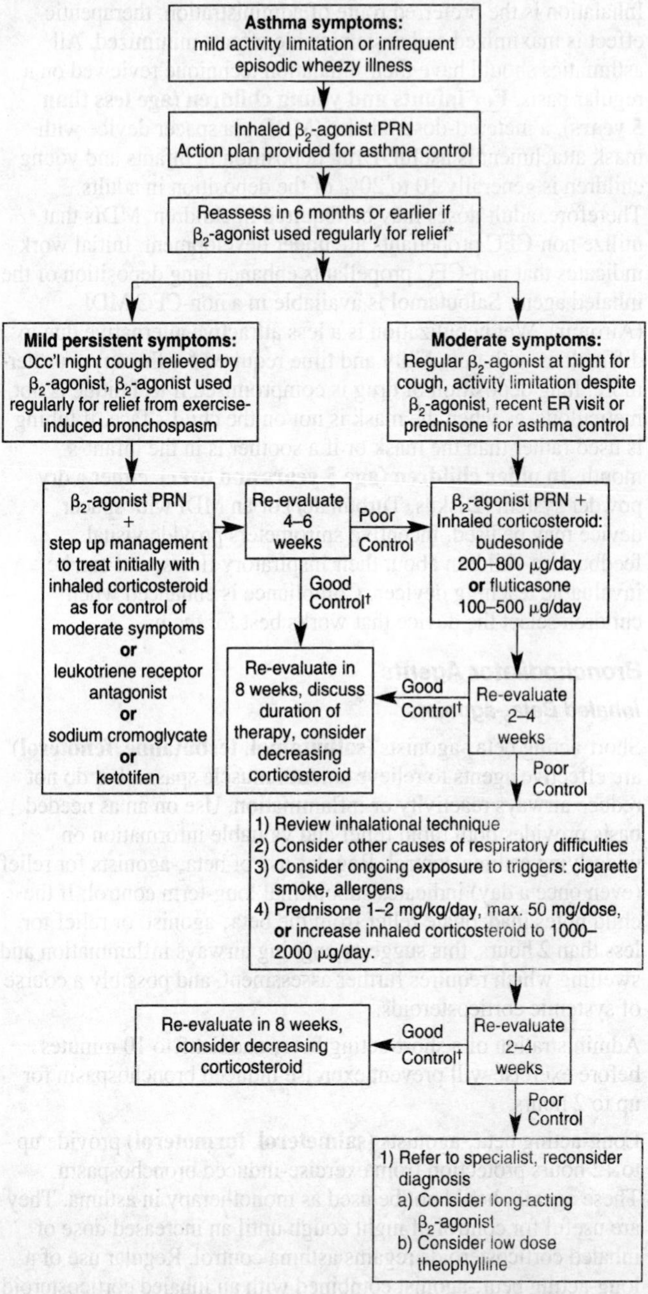
Asthma symptoms:
mild activity limitation or infrequent episodic wheezy illness
Inhaled β2-agonist PRN
Action plan provided for asthma control
Reassess in 6 months or earlier if β2-agonist used regularly for relief*
Mild persistent symptoms:
Occ'l night cough relieved by β2-agonist, β2-agonist used regularly for relief from exercise-induced bronchospasm
Moderate symptoms:
Regular β2-agonist at night for cough, activity limitation despite β2-agonist, recent ER visit or prednisone for asthma control
β2-agonist PRN + step up management to treat initially with inhaled corticosteroid as for control of moderate symptoms or leukotriene receptor antagonist or sodium cromoglycate or ketotifen
Re-evaluate 4–6 weeks
Poor Control
Good Control†
β2-agonist PRN + Inhaled corticosteroid: budesonide 200–800 μg/day or fluticasone 100–500 μg/day
Re-evaluate in 8 weeks, discuss duration of therapy, consider decreasing corticosteroid
Good Control†
Re-evaluate 2–4 weeks
Poor Control
1) Review inhalational technique
2) Consider other causes of respiratory difficulties
3) Consider ongoing exposure to triggers: cigarette smoke, allergens
4) Prednisone 1–2 mg/kg/day, max. 50 mg/dose, or increase inhaled corticosteroid to 1000–2000 μg/day.
Re-evaluate in 8 weeks, consider decreasing corticosteroid
Good Control†
Re-evaluate 2–4 weeks
Poor Control
1) Refer to specialist, reconsider diagnosis
a) Consider long-acting β2-agonist
b) Consider low dose theophylline

* *Regular use $\beta_2$-agonist: use ≥ 3 times/week for relief.*

† *Good asthma control: see Goals of Therapy.*

## Pharmacologic Choices (Figure 1, Table 1)

### *Routes of Administration*

Inhalation is the preferred route of administration: therapeutic effect is maximized and systemic side effects minimized. All asthmatics should have their inhalation technique reviewed on a regular basis. **For infants and young children (age less than 5 years)**, a metered-dose inhaler (MDI) via spacer device with mask attachment is useful. Drug deposition in infants and young children is generally 10 to 20% of the deposition in adults. Therefore, adult doses may be required in children. MDIs that utilize non-CFC propellants are under development. Initial work indicates that non-CFC propellants enhance lung deposition of the inhaled agent. Salbutamol is available in a non-CFC MDI (Airomir). Wet nebulization is a less attractive alternative due to difficulties with portability and time required for therapy. Furthermore, lung deposition of drug is compromised if technique is not meticulous, as when the mask is not on the child's face, if tubing is used rather than the mask or if a soother is in the infant's mouth. **In older children (age 5 years and over)**, either a dry powder system (Diskus, Turbuhaler) or an MDI with spacer device may be used. Incentive spirometers provide visual feedback to children about their inspiratory flows, and can be invaluable teaching devices. Compliance is enhanced when children select the device that works best for them.

### *Bronchodilator Agents*

#### *Inhaled Beta$_2$-agonists*

Short-acting beta$_2$-agonists (**salbutamol**, **terbutaline**, **fenoterol**) are effective agents to relieve smooth muscle spasm, but do not reduce airways reactivity or inflammation. Use on an as needed basis provides both rapid relief and valuable information on underlying asthma control. Regular use of beta$_2$-agonists for relief (even once a day) indicates suboptimal long-term control. If the child notes inadequate relief from the beta$_2$-agonist, or relief for less than 2 hours, this suggests ongoing airways inflammation and swelling which requires further assessment, and possibly a course of systemic corticosteroids.

Administration of a short-acting beta$_2$-agonist 5 to 10 minutes before exercise will prevent exercise induced bronchospasm for up to 2 hours.

Long-acting beta$_2$-agonists (**salmeterol**, **formoterol**) provide up to 12 hours protection from exercise-induced bronchospasm. These agents should not be used as monotherapy in asthma. They are useful for control of night cough until an increased dose of inhaled corticosteroids regains asthma control. Regular use of a long-acting beta$_2$-agonist combined with an inhaled corticosteroid has demonstrated enhanced asthma control over the use of the inhaled corticosteroid alone.

### *Anticholinergic Agents*

Use of **ipratropium bromide** should be restricted to adjunctive therapy in acute severe asthma in children.

#### *Methylxanthines*

**Theophylline** preparations may have an additional anti-inflammatory role in patients already using inhaled corticosteroid therapy. The anti-inflammatory effect of theophylline occurs at serum levels lower than those employed in an attempt to achieve relief of bronchospasm.

### *Agents for Long-term Control*

#### *Inhaled Corticosteroids*

Regular use of inhaled corticosteroids improves pulmonary function and controls symptoms. Although long-term studies have demonstrated safety and efficacy, inhaled corticosteroids do not "cure" asthma. Cessation of regular use may result in return of airways hyperreactivity to the previous status within weeks to months. Regular use reduces the need for oral steroids to treat exacerbations, reduces mortality and may decrease airway remodelling.

**Budesonide** and **fluticasone** possess better benefit/side effect ratios than **beclomethasone**, **flunisolide** and **triamcinolone**.[1] Both budesonide and fluticasone are solely absorbed from the lung and then rapidly cleared from the circulation. Spacer devices are essential for inhaled corticosteroids to improve lung deposition and minimize local side effects. Equivalent doses in terms of asthma control and effects on the HPA-axis are fluticasone 500 μg per day and budesonide 800 μg per day and beclomethasone 1000 μg/day. The effect on asthma control begins to plateau above these levels. Furthermore as these levels are exceeded, the risk of systemic adverse effects such as adrenal suppression, growth suppression and altered bone mineralization are increased. The risk of systemic effects of inhaled corticosteroids depends on inherent individual sensitivity, history of systemic corticosteroid use, compliance with therapy, and adequacy of the inhalation technique.

#### *Sodium Cromoglycate*

Sodium cromoglycate is a safe anti-inflammatory agent. Mild to moderate asthma is controlled in roughly 60% of children. It has also proven useful as an adjunct with beta$_2$-agonists to prevent exercise-induced bronchospasm. Regular use 3 to 4 times per day for 4 weeks is required to determine effect.

---

[1] *Allergy 1997;52 (Suppl 39):1–34.*

Table 1: **Drugs Used for Maintenance Therapy for Asthma in Children**

| Drug | Dosage Chronic Therapy | Adverse Effects | Other | Cost* |
|---|---|---|---|---|
| **Bronchodilator Drugs** | | | | |
| **Short-acting $\beta_2$-agonists** | | | | |
| *salbutamol* Ventodisk, Ventolin, Airomir[†], generics | 2 puffs (100 µg/puff) Q4–6H PRN | For all agents: Tachycardia, palpitations, nervousness, tremor, hypokalemia. | Prevents exercise-induced bronchospasm for up to 2–4 h. Agents provide relief and provide information on asthma control: regular use indicates poor control, use of ≥ 1 canister per month associated with increased risk of asthma mortality. | $-$$ |
| *terbutaline* Bricanyl | 1 puff (0.5 mg/puff) Q4–6H PRN | | | |
| *fenoterol* Berotec | 1–2 puffs (100 µg/puff) Q4–6H PRN | | | |
| **Long-acting $\beta_2$-agonists** | | | | |
| *salmeterol* Serevent | 1–2 puffs (25 µg/puff) OD–BID | As with $\beta_2$-agonists; possibility of tolerance with regular use. | Not to be used as monotherapy, not for immediate relief, provides protection from exercise-induced bronchospasm for 10 h. | $$$$ |
| *formoterol* Foradil, Oxeze | 1 cap or puff (12 µg) inhaled OD–BID | | | $$$ |
| **Anticholinergic Agents** | | | | |
| *ipratropium bromide* Atrovent | 1–2 puffs (20 µg/puff) TID–QID | Dry mouth, metallic taste, mydriasis and glaucoma (if released into eye). | Also available as nebulizer solution. Not used in maintenance therapy. | $$ |

**Prophylactic Drugs**

| | | | | |
|---|---|---|---|---|
| **Inhaled Corticosteroids** | | | | |
| *beclomethasone dipropionate*[‡] Qvar[†], Vanceril, generics | Dose to obtain asthma control 400–1000 μg/d, divided BID–TID. Maintenance dose 200–800 μg/day OD–BID. Regular re-evaluation required to ensure that lowest effective dose of inhaled corticosteroid being used to maintain control. | Oral thrush, dysphonia. Follow linear growth Q3–6 mos with regular asthma reassessments. | Dysphonia and candidiasis can be decreased by use of spacer with MDI and rinsing after use. | MDI $–$$$$ |
| *budesonide* Pulmicort | | | Dose response studies show majority of corticosteroid effect on asthma control is achieved with doses under 800 μg/day; children requiring 800 μg/d or more on a regular basis should be assessed by a specialist. | $$–$$$$ |
| *fluticasone* Flovent | | | | $$$–$$$$ |
| *triamcinolone acetonide* Azmacort | | | | $$ |
| *sodium cromoglycate* Intal | 2 puffs (1 mg/puff) or 1 spincap (20 mg/cap) TID–QID × 4–6 wks, then BID–TID. | Rare. | Used on a regular basis TID–QID Useful for exercise-induced bronchospasm. | $$-$$$ |
| *nedocromil sodium* Tilade | 2 puffs (2 mg/puff) TID–QID | Rare; unpleasant taste. | Useful for exercise-induced bronchospasm. | $$ |
| *ketotifen* Zaditen, generics | Under 3 yrs: 0.5 mg PO BID Older children: 1 mg PO BID | Sedation, weight gain. | May require 8–12 wks for effect. Clinical effectiveness most noted in infants with mild asthma. | $$-$$$ |
| **Leukotriene Receptor Antagonists** | | | | |
| *zafirlukast* Accolate | 12 yrs and older: 20 mg PO BID 1 h before or 2 h after meals. | Headache, nausea. | Zafirlukast: ↑ warfarin serum conc, monitor PT and adjust dose. | $$$ |
| *montelukast* Singulair | 6–14 yrs: 5 mg PO OD ≥ 15 yrs: 10 mg PO OD | Headache, abdominal pain. | | $$$–$$$$ |

*[†] Contains non-CFC propellants.*

*[‡] Beclovent, Becloforte and Beclodisk were discontinued in March 2000.*

** Includes drug cost only. Cost of inhaled agents is per unit; cost of inhalation capsules or oral medications is per 30-day supply.*

*Legend: $ < $15 $$ $15–30 $$$ $30–45 $$$$ > $45*

#### Nedocromil Sodium

Nedocromil sodium is comparable to sodium cromoglycate in anti-inflammatory activity. It prevents antigen-challenge and exercise-induced bronchospasm. Difficulties with taste often limit compliance; a spacer may improve acceptance.

#### Ketotifen

Ketotifen is an oral prophylactic agent with antihistaminic properties. Side effects include sedation and increased appetite. Its clinical effectiveness is most noted in infants with mild persistent asthma.

#### Leukotriene Receptor Antagonists (LTRAs)

Early trials with leukotriene receptor antagonists (**zafirlukast**, **montelukast**) suggest that these oral agents provide broncho-protection in ASA-sensitive asthmatics, and with exercise. Further, these agents may have steroid-sparing properties, allowing improved control of asthma at a reduced dose of inhaled corticosteroid. As monotherapy, these agents exert the equivalent effect of about beclomethasone 200 μg per day on asthma control. The LTRAs have not been associated with any significant side effects. There are reports of development of Churg-Strauss syndrome, an eosinophilic vasculitis, but these most likely represent the unmasking of the vasculitis as systemic corticosteroids are reduced.

### Acute Asthma Management (Figure 2)

An exacerbation of asthma requiring emergency room visit, unscheduled doctor visit or hospitalization is a failure of long-term management. As well as immediate care for respiratory distress, evaluation of the cause of the exacerbation and means of preventing future episodes is essential.

Acute severe asthma should be managed as a pediatric emergency. Initial therapy should be aggressive, and then reduced as the exacerbation settles. Ideally, a child with asthma should not deteriorate once in hospital.

Pulse oximetry or an arterial blood gas should be performed and supplemental oxygen initiated in all asthmatic children with respiratory distress.

The cornerstones of therapy are supplemental oxygen, frequent high dose inhaled beta$_2$-agonist, and systemic corticosteroids. Ipratropium bromide may provide additional bronchodilation. There is no evidence that aminophylline provides additional bronchodilation beyond that produced by frequent high dose beta$_2$-agonist.

Close observation and reassessment of all children with acute severe asthma is mandatory.

Figure 2: **Treatment of Acute Asthma in Children**

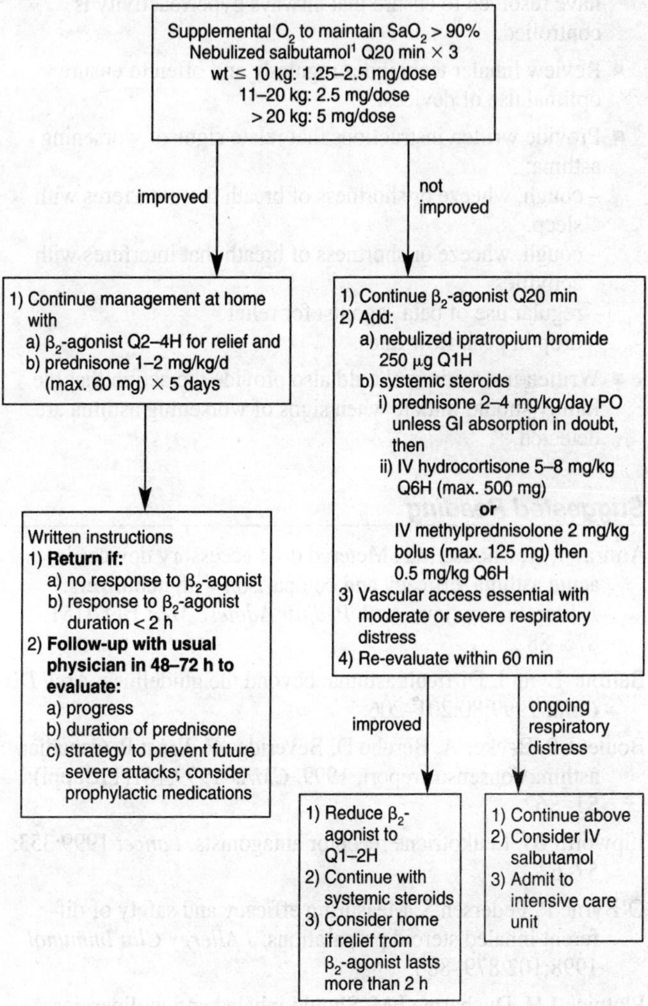
Supplemental $O_2$ to maintain $SaO_2 > 90\%$
Nebulized salbutamol[1] Q20 min × 3
wt ≤ 10 kg: 1.25–2.5 mg/dose
11–20 kg: 2.5 mg/dose
> 20 kg: 5 mg/dose
improved
not improved
1) Continue management at home with
a) $\beta_2$-agonist Q2–4H for relief and
b) prednisone 1–2 mg/kg/d (max. 60 mg) × 5 days
1) Continue $\beta_2$-agonist Q20 min
2) Add:
a) nebulized ipratropium bromide 250 µg Q1H
b) systemic steroids
i) prednisone 2–4 mg/kg/day PO unless GI absorption in doubt, then
ii) IV hydrocortisone 5–8 mg/kg Q6H (max. 500 mg)
or
IV methylprednisolone 2 mg/kg bolus (max. 125 mg) then 0.5 mg/kg Q6H
3) Vascular access essential with moderate or severe respiratory distress
4) Re-evaluate within 60 min
Written instructions
1) Return if:
a) no response to $\beta_2$-agonist
b) response to $\beta_2$-agonist duration < 2 h
2) Follow-up with usual physician in 48–72 h to evaluate:
a) progress
b) duration of prednisone
c) strategy to prevent future severe attacks; consider prophylactic medications
improved
ongoing respiratory distress
1) Reduce $\beta_2$-agonist to Q1–2H
2) Continue with systemic steroids
3) Consider home if relief from $\beta_2$-agonist lasts more than 2 h
1) Continue above
2) Consider IV salbutamol
3) Admit to intensive care unit

[1] *MDIs and dry powder devices (Turbuhaler) have proven as effective as nebulizers in acute severe asthma. Choice of delivery device depends on familiarity with use and availability of health care providers.*

## Therapeutic Tips

- Where possible, agents or situations that worsen asthma should be avoided.
- When triggers cannot be avoided, use medications at an early stage to improve long-term asthma control.

- Use agents for long-term control (i.e., inhaled corticosteroids) for a minimum of several weeks after symptoms have resolved to ensure that airways hyperreactivity is controlled.
- Review inhaler techniques regularly and often to ensure optimal use of devices.
- Provide written instructions that relate signs of worsening asthma:
  - cough, wheeze or shortness of breath that interferes with sleep.
  - cough, wheeze or shortness of breath that interferes with activities.
  - regular use of beta$_2$-agonist for relief.
  - drop in peak flow rates.
- Written instructions should also provide the action that the family should initiate when signs of worsening asthma are detected.

## Suggested Reading

Amirav I, Newhouse MT. Metered dose accessory devices in acute asthma, efficacy and comparison with nebulizers: A literature review. *Arch Pediatr Adolesc Med* 1997;151: 876–882.

Balfour-Lynn I. Difficult asthma: beyond the guidelines. *Arch Dis Child* 1999;80:201–206.

Boulet LP, Becker A, Berube D, Beveridge R, Ernst P. Canadian asthma consensus report, 1999. *CMAJ* 1999;161(11Suppl): S1–S62.

Lipworth BJ. Leukotriene receptor antagonists. *Lancet* 1999;353: 57–62.

O'Byrne P, Pedersen S. Measuring efficacy and safety of different inhaled steroid preparations. *J Allergy Clin Immunol* 1998;102:879–886.

Plotnick LH, Ducharme FM. Should inhaled anticholinergics be added to $\beta_2$-agonists for treating acute childhood and adolescent asthma? A systematic review. *BMJ* 1998;317: 971–977.

CHAPTER 40

# Chronic Obstructive Pulmonary Disease

*Tony R. Bai, MD, FRACP, FRCPC*

## Goals of Therapy

- To decrease or abolish dyspnea
- To decrease sputum production
- To maintain exercise capacity
- To prevent disease progression
- To decrease the frequency of exacerbations
- To maintain arterial blood oxygen saturation above 90%

## Investigations

- A thorough history with special attention to:
  - avoidable environmental factors (e.g., cigarette smoking or occupational exposures)
  - the rate of progression of symptoms
  - the degree of disability
- Physical examination: signs of hyperinflation, airflow obstruction, chronic hypoxemia, pulmonary hypertension
- Laboratory tests:
  - CBC
  - chest radiograph
  - spirometry before and after bronchodilator
  - pulse oximetry ± arterial blood gases if $FEV_1$ < 30% predicted
  - $\alpha_1$ antiprotease level if clinical suspicion of genetic predisposition to emphysema

## Therapeutic Choices (Figure 1)

### Nonpharmacologic Choices

- **Education of patients and their families** through individual and group sessions is essential. Physicians must be aware of patients' expectations and work with them to set realistic goals.
- **Smoking** should be discontinued (Chapter 42).
- **Annual vaccination** against influenza should be given. Pneumococcal vaccination is recommended by some but not all authorities, as no studies specific to COPD have been performed.

Figure 1: **Pharmacologic Management of COPD**

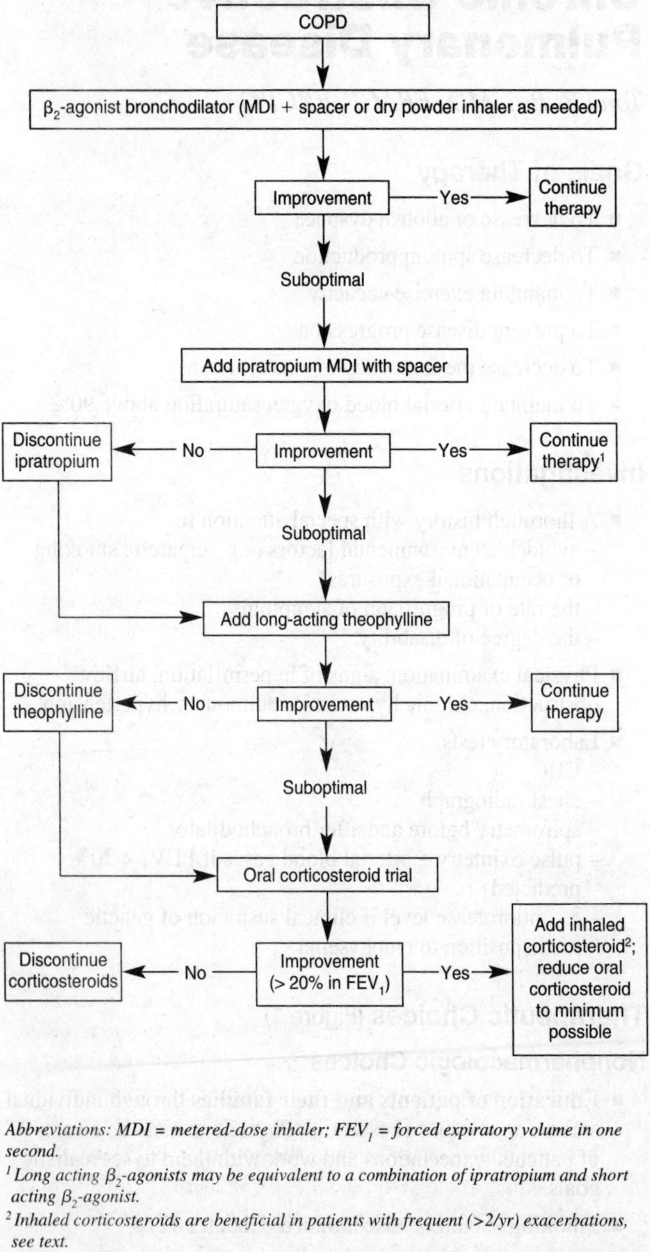
COPD
$\beta_2$-agonist bronchodilator (MDI + spacer or dry powder inhaler as needed)
Improvement
Yes
Continue therapy
Suboptimal
Add ipratropium MDI with spacer
Discontinue ipratropium
No
Improvement
Yes
Continue therapy[1]
Suboptimal
Add long-acting theophylline
Discontinue theophylline
No
Improvement
Yes
Continue therapy
Suboptimal
Oral corticosteroid trial
Discontinue corticosteroids
No
Improvement (> 20% in $FEV_1$)
Yes
Add inhaled corticosteroid[2]; reduce oral corticosteroid to minimum possible

*Abbreviations: MDI = metered-dose inhaler;* $FEV_1$ *= forced expiratory volume in one second.*

[1] *Long acting* $\beta_2$*-agonists may be equivalent to a combination of ipratropium and short acting* $\beta_2$*-agonist.*

[2] *Inhaled corticosteroids are beneficial in patients with frequent (>2/yr) exacerbations, see text.*

- **Rehabilitation programs** providing respiratory, physical and occupational therapy, exercise conditioning, nutritional assistance, and psychosocial and vocational rehabilitation benefit patients regardless of the extent of their disease by reducing symptoms and improving exercise performance and quality of life.

## Pharmacologic Choices (Table 1)

The use of bronchodilators increases airflow and reduces dyspnea in patients with COPD. Inhaled beta$_2$-agonists and anticholinergics are efficacious; some patients who fail to respond to one class may respond to the other.

A small improvement in airflow in COPD patients with severe obstruction may be of significant clinical benefit. There is little evidence that inhaled beta$_2$-agonists or anticholinergic agents potentiate each other when maximal doses are used.

### *Anticholinergic Agents*

**Ipratropium bromide** has a slower onset of action than beta$_2$-agonists, but its duration of action is longer; hence, it is more suitable for regular than intermittent use. It is available as a metered-dose inhaler (MDI) and as a nebulizer solution. The recommended dose (40 μg 3 to 4 times per day) produces less than maximal bronchodilation and may be doubled or tripled without notable side effects. If inhaler technique is inadequate, MDIs should be used with a spacer device (e.g., Aerochamber), which will improve lower respiratory tract deposition. The need for nebulizers in most patients is obviated by the use of a higher dose administered by MDI with a spacer.

### *Beta$_2$-agonists*

**Salbutamol, terbutaline** and **fenoterol** have approximately equal efficacy, side effects, and similar onset and duration of bronchodilator effect. Patients with difficulty coordinating MDIs can benefit from a spacer device or one of the dry powder inhalers (e.g., the Turbuhaler). The Turbuhaler has advantages over other dry powder devices: it is additive-free, contains 200 doses and requires little manipulation. Patient preference will vary for delivery devices. Recommended doses of beta$_2$-agonists result in less than maximal bronchodilation; the dose may be doubled or tripled, although tremor and potential for inducing hypokalemia must be recognized and monitored in patients at risk. Oral beta$_2$-agonists offer few advantages and increase side effects.

Long-acting beta$_2$-agonists (**salmeterol, formoterol**) may be of use in COPD. Published data indicate they are equivalent in efficacy to a combination of short-acting beta$_2$-agonists and ipratropium, yet require less frequent administration.[1,2] In some individuals side effect profiles may be less with an anticholinergic-based regimen, but this requires further study.

### *Theophylline*

The role of theophylline in the treatment of COPD is controversial; it may have little bronchodilator effect beyond that of inhaled agents. The use of long-acting theophylline preparations in the evening has been shown to reduce overnight declines in $FEV_1$ and morning respiratory symptoms. Theophylline may offer added nonbronchodilatory effects such as improved respiratory muscle endurance and ventilatory stimulation. Half of patients with severe COPD can show clinically significant improvements in functional capacity (walking distance, dyspnea) following use of slow-release theophylline despite use of inhaled $beta_2$-agonists and anticholinergics. Theophylline is a third-line drug in the treatment of COPD; if it is used, blood levels in the low therapeutic range (55 to 85 µmol/L) should be the goal to minimize adverse effects. Long-acting preparations (12- or 24-hour) provide stable serum levels and reduce side effects. Theophylline used with an inhaled anticholinergic or adrenergic agent may be more effective than monotherapy, but this varies. The value of adding theophylline is best judged with a 2- to 4-week trial. The outcome should be measured by improvement in expiratory flow rates, 6- or 12-minute walking distance or objectively observed reduction in dyspnea, medication use or nocturnal symptoms.

### *Corticosteroids*

In acute exacerbations of COPD, a 2-week course of corticosteroids is beneficial in hastening recovery and returning lung function to baseline. However, only 10 to 20% of **stable** COPD patients benefit from either systemic or inhaled corticosteroid therapy. In the assessment of a new patient, if airflow obstruction and symptoms persist following smoking cessation and optimal bronchodilator therapy, the patient's corticosteroid response should be assessed by administering **prednisone** (0.6 mg/kg per day) as a single morning dose for 14 days. Objective end points (e.g., spirometry or 6- or 12-minute walking distance) should be evaluated. An improvement in $FEV_1$ of at least 20% and 0.2 L is evidence of significant corticosteroid responsiveness. In these patients, moderate-dose inhaled corticosteroids (e.g., 800 µg per day of **beclomethasone** or **budesonide**, or 400 µg of **fluticasone** in 2 divided doses) should be initiated, and the prednisone dose should be tapered to the minimum needed to maintain major benefits. Recent data suggest that inhaled corticosteroids induce a clinically relevant decrease in the severity and frequency of

[1] *Chest 1999;115:957–965.*
[2] *Am J Resp Crit Care Med 1997;155:1283–1289.*

Table 1: **Medications Used in COPD**

| Drug | Dosage | Adverse Effects | Comments | Cost* |
|---|---|---|---|---|
| **Inhaled Agents** | | | | Cost per unit |
| **$\beta_2$-agonists, short-acting** | | | | |
| *salbutamol* Ventolin, Airomir†, generics | 100 μg/puff: 1–2 puffs Q2–6H PRN not to exceed 8–12 puffs per 24 h | Tremor, nervousness, hypokalemia, tachycardia, palpitations | Usual doses are suboptimal for COPD. | MDI $ Diskhaler/ Rotacaps $$ |
| *fenoterol* Berotec | 100 μg/puff: same as above | | | $ |
| *terbutaline* Bricanyl | 500 μg/puff: same as above | | | $ |
| **$\beta_2$-agonists, long-acting** | | | | |
| *salmeterol* Serevent | MDI 25 μg/puff: 2 puffs BID<br>disk 50 μg/inhalation 1 inhalation BID | As above | | $$$$ |
| *formoterol* Foradil, Oxeze | 12 μg/puff: 1 puff BID may increase to 2 puffs BID, if required | | | $$$ |
| **Anticholinergics** | | | | |
| *ipratropium bromide* Atrovent | 20 μg/puff: 2–4 puffs TID–QID up to 6–8 puffs TID–QID, if tolerated | Dry mouth, metallic taste. | Usual doses are suboptimal for COPD. | $$ |

*(cont'd)*

Table 1: **Medications Used in COPD** *(cont'd)*

| Drug | Dosage | Adverse Effects | Comments | Cost* |
|---|---|---|---|---|
| **Anticholinergic/$\beta_2$-agonist Combinations** | | | | |
| *ipratropium bromide/salbutamol* Combivent | MDI 20 µg/100 µg/puff: 2 puffs Q6H PRN<br>nebulizer: 2.5 mL (0.5 mg/2.5 mg) Q6H PRN | Same as $\beta_2$-agonists and anticholinergics above. | May be used as initial therapy in patients with daily symptoms. Fixed dosage leads to some inflexibility. | MDI $$<br>Inh sol $$$ (20×2.5 mL) |
| *ipratropium bromide/fenoterol* Duovent UDV | nebulizer: 4 mL (0.5 mg/1.25 mg) Q6H PRN | | MDI used with a spacer is preferred for most patients. Consider nebulizers for patients with coordination problems. | $$$$ (20×4 mL) |
| **Corticosteroids** | | | | |
| *beclomethasone*[‡] Qvar[†], Vanceril, generics | 400–800 µg/day divided BID–TID | Oropharyngeal candidiasis, hoarseness (both can be ↓ by using a spacer and rinsing mouth or by using dry powder inhaler). | Poorly absorbed; must be used regularly, not PRN. | MDI $–$$$$ |
| *budesonide* Pulmicort | Same as above | | | $$$–$$$$ |
| *flunisolide* Bronalide | Same as above | | | $$ |
| *fluticasone* Flovent | 200–400 µg/day divided BID | | | $$$ |
| *triamcinolone* Azmacort | Same as beclomethasone | | | $$ |

| Oral Agents | | | | Cost for 30-day supply |
|---|---|---|---|---|
| **Slow-release Theophyllines**<br>Quibron-T/SR, Slo-Bid, Theo-Dur, Uniphyl, generics | 300–900 mg/day | Nausea, vomiting, abdominal cramps, nervousness, tremor, insomnia, tachycardia. | Cimetidine, fluvoxamine, mexiletine, propranolol, quinolones, erythromycin, may ↑ theophylline levels.<br>Rifampin, carbamazepine, phenytoin may ↓ theophylline levels.<br>Lithium levels may be ↓. | $–$$ |
| **Corticosteroids**<br>*prednisone* generics | 0.6 mg/kg/d[π] | Glucose intolerance, weight gain, mood alteration, hypertension, osteoporosis, adrenal suppression, cataracts, myopathy. | Barbiturates, phenytoin, rifampin ↓ steroid effect. | $ |

† *Contains non-CFC propellants.*
‡ *Beclovent, Becloforte and Beclodisk were discontinued in March 2000.*
π *Dosage to optimize airflow obstruction, use for 14 days only as single morning dose; no need to taper medication.*
* *Includes drug cost only. Cost of inhaled agents is per unit; cost of oral medications is per 30-day supply.*
*Legend: $ < $15 $$ $15–30 $$$ $30–45 $$$$ > $45*

exacerbations in severe COPD, and should be prescribed to patients with > 2 exacerbations per year.[3,4] A few severely disabled patients may require maintenance with prednisone 10 mg daily in addition to inhaled steroids.

### *Antibiotics*

The most common infectious agents in exacerbations of COPD are viral. When exacerbations of COPD are accompanied by purulent secretions, broad-spectrum antibiotics directed against typical colonizing bacteria are beneficial. Inexpensive and equally efficacious therapy includes **amoxicillin, co-trimoxazole, erythromycin** or **tetracycline**. The more expensive **quinolones** or newer macrolides may be useful when a resistant gram-negative organism is suspected (e.g., some strains of *Haemophilus influenzae* or *Moraxella catarrhalis*). However, many of the older antibiotics appear as efficacious as the newer, more expensive ones.

### *Oxygen Therapy*

Oxygen therapy reduces the risk of death in selected patients. In COPD patients with significant hypoxemia ($PaO_2 < 55$ mm Hg or $SaO_2 < 90\%$), long-term oxygen therapy may increase the lifespan by 6 to 7 years. Improved survival has only been seen when oxygen is administered for at least 12 hours per day, including nocturnally. The greatest survival benefit is with continuously administered oxygen. Patients whose $PaO_2$ is between 55 and 59 mm Hg may also benefit from supplemental oxygen therapy if there is indirect evidence of hypoxemic end organ damage such as cor pulmonale or polycythemia. Oxygen is usually given through nasal prongs at a flow rate sufficient to produce resting $PaO_2$ between 65 and 80 mm Hg. Flow rates are often increased by 1 or 2 L/min during exercise and sleep. Oxygen therapy may be prescribed with exercise if oxygen desaturation below 88% occurs and there is **objective** evidence of improvement in exercise duration with oxygen administration.

### *Other Therapies*

Mucolytics and ventilatory stimulants have shown little objective benefit in clinical trials and are not recommended in North American consensus guidelines. Noninvasive nasal or face mask ventilatory assistance is useful in acute exacerbations. For patients with emphysema induced by $alpha_1$ antiprotease deficiency, purified $alpha_1$ antitrypsin protein is available for supplemental IV administration. Resection or collapse of large bullae can be helpful, as can lung transplantation.

---
[3] *Thorax 1999;54:287–288.*
[4] *Resp Med 1998;93:161–166.*

## Therapeutic Tips

- The most common mistakes in medical management include inadequate education about medications and techniques for using inhalers, suboptimal dosing, inadequate monitoring and failure to advise the patient to take medication before engaging in physical activity.
- To minimize side effects, long-acting theophyllines should be introduced at 50% of the final dosage for the first week.
- The patient should be encouraged to remain active despite the fact that exercise induces often distressing dyspnea; otherwise a vicious cycle of decreasing mobility can develop.

## *Suggested Reading List*

American Thoracic Society. Standards for the diagnosis and care of patients with chronic obstructive pulmonary disease. *Am J Respir Crit Care Med* 1995;152(Suppl):S77–S120.

British Thoracic Society guidelines for the management of chronic obstructive pulmonary disease. *Thorax* 1997;52 (Suppl 5):S1–S28.

CHAPTER 41

# Croup

*Michael B.H. Smith, MB, BCh, FRCPC*

## Goals of Therapy

- To evaluate and treat the physiological disturbance
- To determine the cause and initiate appropriate therapy
- To provide symptom relief

## Investigations

- Assess degree of airway compromise (Figure 1)
  - **severe obstruction** is likely when there is marked stridor and drooling accompanied by agitation or lethargy. Infants may refuse to feed and children hold their neck extended forward (the sniffing position) in an effort to maximize the diameter of the airway. Cough is often absent or minimal.
  - **mild obstruction** is likely when the child has only mild stridor (obvious only on crying with little or none at rest), is alert and consolable. Usually able to drink fluids. Mild hoarseness without stridor may not require treatment beyond symptomatic modalities.
- Review history to determine the most likely cause for symptoms
  - **acute laryngotracheobronchitis (simple croup)** usually occurs in children aged 6 months to 4 years with preceding viral prodrome, runny nose and mild fever (often < 39°C). The syndrome is characterized by a harsh, barking, seal-like cough, stridor and a hoarse voice peaking on the first day and then resolving over 3 to 5 days. Symptoms are usually most prominent at night. Some authors separate this syndrome from spasmodic croup which is nonfebrile and lasts only 2 to 3 days. In practice it is often not possible to make this distinction and treatment for simple croup is recommended.
  - **acute bacterial tracheitis** occurs at all ages and can be difficult to diagnose because it may resemble croup in the initial stages, then progresses to more severe disease. Often children present with a persistent, painful cough, stridor and progressive toxicity with high fever and increasing respiratory obstruction.
  - **acute supraglottitis (epiglottitis)** occurs most commonly in school age children. It presents in the early stages as above but is rapidly progressive with high fever, drooling

Figure 1: **Assessment of Airway Compromise**

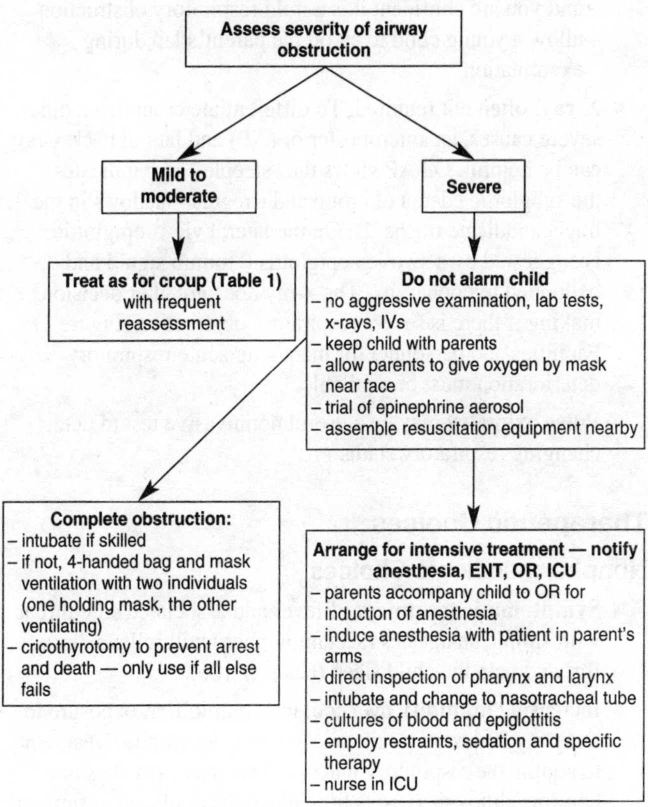
Assess severity of airway obstruction
Mild to moderate
Severe
Treat as for croup (Table 1) with frequent reassessment
Do not alarm child
– no aggressive examination, lab tests, x-rays, IVs
– keep child with parents
– allow parents to give oxygen by mask near face
– trial of epinephrine aerosol
– assemble resuscitation equipment nearby
Complete obstruction:
– intubate if skilled
– if not, 4-handed bag and mask ventilation with two individuals (one holding mask, the other ventilating)
– cricothyrotomy to prevent arrest and death — only use if all else fails
Arrange for intensive treatment — notify anesthesia, ENT, OR, ICU
– parents accompany child to OR for induction of anesthesia
– induce anesthesia with patient in parent's arms
– direct inspection of pharynx and larynx
– intubate and change to nasotracheal tube
– cultures of blood and epiglottitis
– employ restraints, sedation and specific therapy
– nurse in ICU

and stridor. Cough is almost always absent. It is now rare since the introduction of the *Haemophilus influenzae* vaccine.

– other possibilities include **retropharyngeal/peritonsillar abscess** which can cause respiratory obstruction and dysphagia with fever but without stridor, cough and hoarseness. An acute **foreign body obstruction** or **angioneurotic edema** in a child will cause acute respiratory obstruction without fever or other signs of infection.

- Examination:
  – approach the child gently and observe pattern of breathing at rest
  – fatigue, anxiety, restlessness, altered mental status may indicate impending respiratory obstruction
  – hoarse voice, especially on crying, indicates a laryngeal problem (usually croup)

- do not attempt upsetting physical examination (throat inspection, ear examination) unless the child is cooperative and you are confident it is a mild respiratory obstruction
- allow a young child to sit on the parent's lap during examination

- **X-ray**: often not required. To differentiate croup from other severe causes, an anteroposterior (AP) and lateral neck x-ray can be helpful. On AP views the "steeple" sign indicates the subglottic edema of croup and irregular shadows in the trachea indicate tracheitis. On the lateral view, epiglottitis is suggested by a swollen epiglottis ("thumb sign") and ballooned hypopharynx. The x-ray does *not* alter decision making if there is severe respiratory obstruction (Figure 1). Facilities and personnel for managing acute respiratory deterioration must be available.
- **Pulse oximetry** may be a useful noninvasive test to detect changing respiratory status

## Therapeutic Choices

### Nonpharmacologic Choices

- **Symptomatic treatment** of fever and associated sore throat with simple analgesics (acetaminophen) will relieve discomfort and help the child sleep (Chapter 106).
- Increasing **humidity** by a cool mist humidifier, exposure to a steamy bathroom or the outside air is an empiric treatment to soothe the respiratory mucosa. This may provide some comfort although there is little objective evidence to support this practice.
- In rare instances, with severe respiratory obstruction, **IV fluids** and **respiratory support** (oxygen and endotracheal intubation) may be required.

### Pharmacologic Choices (Table 1)

## Therapeutic Tips

- The first priority is assessment of respiratory obstruction, not diagnosis.
- In the majority of patients infectious stridor is simple croup requiring only symptomatic therapy.
- Mild, moderate or severe cases all begin with similar symptoms. While in hospital or the emergency department, frequent reassessment is prudent. On discharge, it is important to inform parents about signs of respiratory compromise and when to return for reassessment.

Table 1: **Drugs Used for Treatment of Croup**

| Drug | Dosage | Adverse Effects | Comments | Cost* |
|---|---|---|---|---|
| **Laryngotracheobronchitis (croup)** | | | Cause: viral, most commonly parainfluenza virus. | |
| *dexamethasone* – Decadron, generics | Initial dose in ER: 0.6 mg/kg[†] PO/IM once<br>If admitted then 0.15 mg/kg/d PO once daily × 3 d while in hospital | Rare with short-term use. | Dexamethasone and budesonide used for mild to moderate obstruction. Currently there is no evidence for repeated doses of steroids. | $ |
| *budesonide* – Pulmicort Nebuamp | By nebulizer:<br>Initial dose in ER: 2 mg once.<br>If admitted then: 2 mg BID × 3 d while in hospital | Rare with short-term use. | | $ |
| *racemic epinephrine 2.25%* – Vaponefrin | By nebulizer:<br>0.5 mL/3 mL NS Q1–3H PRN | Pallor, tachycardia, hypertension. | Epinephrine used for moderate or greater obstruction and requires 3 h period of observation. | $ |
| *l-epinephrine 1:1000* – Adrenalin, generics | By nebulizer:<br>1–3 mL/3 mL NS Q1–3H PRN | | Epinephrine administration is often followed by dexamethasone or budesonide. | $ |
| **Bacterial tracheitis** | | For all: hypersensitivity. | Cause: *S. aureus*, Strep. Group A, *S. pneumoniae*, *H. influenzae*. | |
| *cefuroxime* ❥ – Kefurox, Zinacef, generics<br>**or** | 150 mg/kg/d IV divided Q8H (max. 4.5 g/d) | Eosinophilia, phlebitis. | First-line therapy. | $$ |
| *cloxacillin* – Tegopen, generics<br>**and** | 150 mg/kg/d IV divided Q6H | GI disturbance, interstitial nephritis. | Administer together with cefotaxime. | $ |
| *cefotaxime* ❥ – Claforan | 200 mg/kg/d IV divided Q6–8H | Phlebitis. | Use if unimmunized or suspect co-existing meningitis. | $$ |
| **Supraglottitis (epiglottitis)**<br>same as bacterial tracheitis | | | Cause: *H. influenzae*. | |

** Cost of 1-day supply – includes drug cost only.*
*[†] There is some evidence that doses as low as 0.15 mg/kg may be as effective but this requires further study.*

*Legend:* *$ < $20* *$$ $20–40*
❥ *Dosage adjustment may be required in renal impairment – see Appendix I.*

## *Suggested Reading List*

Ausejo M, Saenz A, Pham B, et al. The effectiveness of glucocorticoids in treating croup: meta-analysis. *BMJ* 1999;319: 595–600.

Custer JR. Croup and related disorders. *Pediatr Rev* 1993;14: 19–28.

Klassen TP. Recent advances in the treatment of bronchiolitis and laryngitis. *Pediatr Clin North Am* 1997;44:249–261.

Cressman WR, Myer CM. Diagnosis and management of croup and epiglottitis. *Pediatr Clin North Am* 1994;41:265.

**CHAPTER 42**

# Smoking Cessation

*Robert P. Nolan, PhD, CPsych*

The efficacy of smoking cessation interventions by health care professionals is well established. Cessation counselling clearly enhances the long-term quit rate (Table 1). Pharmacotherapy in combination with behavioral counselling increases the success rate for sustaining a smoke-free lifestyle at 1 year by approximately five-fold.

Table 1: **Smoking Cessation Treatment and Long-term (6–12 months) Cessation Rates**

| | IHPR[1] | AHCPR[2] | Cochrane Database[3,4] |
|---|---|---|---|
| No Rx | 3% | 7.9% | 4.9% |
| Self-help | 5% | 8.1–11.1% | 4.8% |
| Brief Advice | 10.2% | 10.2% | 5.9% |
| NRT | 14% | 9–20.5% | 14.6–19.4% |
| Behavioral Rx | 24% | 15.1–22.6% | 14.4% |
| NRT + Behavioral Rx | | | 14.8–29.2% |

[1] *Institute of Health Promotion Research, 1998.*
[2] *Agency for Health Care Policy and Research, 1996.*
[3] *The Cochrane Library, 1999.*
[4] *Ibid.*
*See Suggested Reading List for complete citations.*

The *minimum* recommended standard for a smoking cessation interview is to allow for 20 minutes of patient contact, with weekly scheduled patient contacts over at least 4 weeks. Other factors that enhance treatment efficacy include duration of therapy of more than 8 weeks and provision of therapy by multiple providers.

## Goals of Therapy

- **Ask:** assess smoking status and patient readiness to quit
- **Advise:** inform the patient about the importance of quitting, and educate about available pharmacologic and behavioral resources to become smoke-free
- **Assist:** develop a quit plan that specifies a quit date, combines pharmacotherapy and behavioral skills, and provide follow-up support

## Investigations

- Assess smoking status for every patient nine years of age or older, including current status and smoking history, nicotine dependence and motivation to quit.
- If the patient is smoking 20 or more cigarettes per day, and their initial cigarette is consumed within 30 minutes of awakening, it is likely they are significantly nicotine dependent, especially if the patient has experienced symptoms of nicotine withdrawal during a previous quit attempt. Patients who have evidence of nicotine dependence should be considered for nicotine replacement therapy (NRT).
- Assessment of patient motivation to quit provides essential information for tailoring the content and goals of cessation counselling (Figure 1).

Figure 1: **Assessment of Patient Motivation to Quit Smoking**

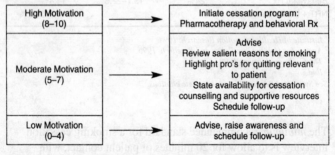

*On a scale from 0 to 10, where 0 is "Not at all," and 10 is "As ready as you can be," how ready are you right now to quit smoking?*

| | | |
|---|---|---|
| High Motivation (8–10) | → | Initiate cessation program: Pharmacotherapy and behavioral Rx |
| Moderate Motivation (5–7) | → | Advise<br>Review salient reasons for smoking<br>Highlight pro's for quitting relevant to patient<br>State availability for cessation counselling and supportive resources<br>Schedule follow-up |
| Low Motivation (0–4) | → | Advise, raise awareness and schedule follow-up |

*A rating in the high range (8 to 10) indicates that the patient is ready to actively participate in developing a quit plan and setting a quit date. A moderate rating (5 to 7) indicates significant ambivalence, which needs to be resolved before developing a quit plan. A low rating (4 or less) indicates the patient is likely to oppose, or not adhere to a quit plan, and more basic intervention is required to help the patient increase their awareness about personal benefits of quitting.*

## Therapeutic Choices

### Nonpharmacologic Choices

#### *Advise*

Advice to patients is to guide behavior change among those already highly motivated, and to stimulate change among those with a low or moderate level of motivation. The challenge is to provide advice that reinforces the patient's motivation and sense of control over their quit plan. This is readily accomplished by suggesting a limited set of cessation aids (vs. a single treatment option) which the patient can choose to include in their quit plan. Constructive delivery of advice is more challenging when patients present with low or moderate motivation to quit. Advice can stimulate awareness of the importance of smoke-free living when motivation for change is low. It can also help patients with only a moderate level of motivation to resolve ambivalence about quitting. The efficacy of providing advice is strengthened when it is linked to information that is personally relevant to the patient (vs. information that is limited to objective facts), and when it is accompanied by a statement that professional support is available. Personally relevant information can be obtained from a collaborative review of current symptomatic complaints, concerns expressed by significant others, effects of smoking on significant others, and changes in the patient's home or work environment that support smoke-free living.

### *Assist – Behavioral Choices*

Best evidence guidelines support a combined behavioral and pharmacologic approach for smoking cessation. The minimum standard for treatment should include giving brief advice with self-help material to educate the patient about:

- Setting a specific quit date within the next 2 weeks, or establishing a schedule to reduce smoking until the patient is smoke-free
- Countering the urge to smoke by distraction, exercise, a relaxation procedure, or a low caloric snack
- Managing "high risk" situations where a lapse to smoking is more likely, through temporary avoidance of that situation or by learning coping skills to manage the specific triggers for smoking in that situation
- Identifying individuals who can provide support and positive modelling of the smoke-free lifestyle
- Establishing feasible goals and rewards that will sustain the patient's motivation to remain smoke-free

Self-help material is widely available to patients. Local group or individual counselling programs are important resources for behavioral skills training and support.

## Pharmacologic Choices

Pharmacotherapies for smoking cessation are designed to manage symptoms of nicotine withdrawal, or symptoms of depressed mood and affect that can become problematic during cessation.

### *Nicotine Replacement Therapy (NRT)* (Table 2)

NRT is the most widely used medication to prevent symptoms of nicotine withdrawal. Symptoms to be monitored include: severe craving, anxiety or irritability, restlessness, nervousness, difficulty with concentration, sleep disturbance, headaches, increased appetite or eating behavior.

In Canada NRT is available in two forms, nicotine polacrilex (gum) and the transdermal nicotine patch. Alternate forms are in a relatively early stage of investigation and include intranasal nicotine spray or nicotine inhaler. Both are not currently available in Canada.

Patients with a high level of motivation to quit, evidence of nicotine dependence, and a current pattern of smoking 10 or more cigarettes per day should be considered for NRT.

To date, available evidence does not support the practice of combining nicotine polacrilex with the transdermal patch as a more effective aid for long-term cessation. Similarly, there are no published controlled clinical trials comparing NRT and bupropion, or the transdermal patch and 4 mg nicotine polacrilex.

#### *Nicotine polacrilex*

Nicotine polacrilex gum is a well-established treatment which enhances the long-term quit rate. The 4-mg dosage demonstrates greater efficacy than the 2-mg dosage. Patients need to be counselled about appropriate use, given that the delivery of nicotine is significantly affected by patient control. Practitioner advice should address chewing technique, pattern of consumption and potential side effects.

Nicotine polacrilex should be used as a substitute for cigarettes, so that the pattern of usage matches the patient's previous pattern of smoking. It is essential for the patient to take intermittent rest periods while chewing each piece. Patients should be directed to regularly "park" the gum on the side of the mouth to avoid rapid absorption of nicotine through the buccal mucosa. They should take from 30 to 45 minutes to consume each piece, and use up to 20 pieces per day. Side effects include gastrointestinal and oral disturbances, jaw discomfort, and hiccoughs. These can usually be avoided through an appropriate method of chewing. Nicotine absorption can be impaired by consuming nicotine polacrilex with acidic beverages, such as coffee or fruit juices, and this combination should be discouraged. The duration of medication usage needs to be monitored, with tapering being initiated at the 12 week interval.

#### *Transdermal nicotine*

The transdermal nicotine patch is well established in facilitating long-term cessation. It does not induce the side effects reported with nicotine polacrilex, as nicotine delivery is regulated at a

Table 2: **Pharmacologic Agents Used for Smoking Cessation**[†]

| Drug | Dosage: Active Treatment | Dosage: Tapering | Adverse Effects | Comments | Cost* |
|---|---|---|---|---|---|
| **Nicotine Replacement Therapy** | | | | NRT manages urge to smoke by preventing symptoms of nicotine withdrawal. | |
| *nicotine polacrilex gum* Nicorette | 2 or 4 mg<br>10–12 pieces/d initially to max. of 20 pieces/d, for 12 wks | 1 piece/d each wk and decrease according to patient's symptoms of withdrawal. | Hiccoughs, GI disturbance, jaw pain and orodental problems. | Use NRT if patient smoking ≥ 10 cigarettes/d, evidence of nicotine dependence, or previous history of nicotine withdrawal and relatively high motivation to quit. | $$ |
| *nicotine transdermal patch* Habitrol | 21 mg/24 h × 3–4 wks | 14 mg/24 h × 3–4 wks, 7 mg/24 h × 3–4 wks | Skin sensitivity and irritation. | | $$$ |
| Nicoderm | 21 mg/24 h × 6 wks | 14 mg/24 h × 2 wks, 7 mg/24 h × 2 wks | | | |
| Nicotrol | 15 mg/16 h × 6 wks | 10 mg/16 h × 2 wks, 5 mg/16 h × 2 wks | | | |
| **Non-nicotine agents** | | | | Manage urge to smoke by preventing disturbed mood/affect. | |
| *bupropion* ● Zyban | 150 mg/d – 300 mg/d divided BID for 7–12 wks. | | Dry mouth and insomnia. ↑ risk of seizures at higher dosage for patients with history of seizures, head injury or bulimia. | Use if patient vulnerable to distressed mood/affect, or history of significant adverse effects or unsuccessful use of NRT. | $$ (300 mg/d × 2 wks) |

* *Cost of 105 pieces of gum or 14 patches – includes drug cost only.*

*Legend: $ < $20 $$ $20–40 $$$ $40–60*

● *Dosage adjustment may be required in renal impairment – see Appendix I.*

† *Adapted from: Bass F. Smoking Cessation: In: Gray J, ed. Therapeutic Choices. Ottawa: Canadian Pharmacists Association, 1998.*

constant rate across a 16- or 24-hour schedule. The major side effect reported is skin irritation or sensitivity, usually mild. It is important to direct patients to rotate the application sites on a daily basis, using the upper arm and upper chest, and ensuring appropriate contact of the patch with the skin surface. Controlled comparisons of the 16- and 24-hour administration formats indicate no significant differences in treatment efficacy. Prolonged use of the patch beyond the standard interval of 8 weeks does not significantly enhance long-term quit rate. There is no demonstrated advantage to tapering the patch dosage following the 8-week course of therapy, or to abruptly end patch usage at this time, so the patient's active participation in making this decision should be encouraged. All trials of the transdermal nicotine patch have included brief advice or counselling, which reinforces the best evidence guideline of a combined therapeutic strategy.

### *Non-nicotine based medications* (Table 2)

Non-nicotine agents designed to decrease emotional distress associated with the urge to smoke are an alternative therapeutic strategy to NRT. Anxiolytics and antidepressants are the principal non-nicotine based medications assessed to date. The following anxiolytics have *not* been found to significantly assist cessation: meprobamate, diazepam, oxprenolol, metoprolol, and buspirone. Antidepressants studied include: imipramine, fluoxetine, doxepin, moclobemide, tryptophan, bupropion and nortriptyline. Some support is reported for the efficacy of fluoxetine, while stronger evidence is available for bupropion. **Bupropion** is currently utilized for smoking cessation in dosages ranging from 150 to 300 mg daily. The relative efficacy of bupropion and NRT has not been determined to guide the selection of either as first-line therapy.

## Therapeutic Tips

- Utilize a structured program for smoking cessation counselling, planned interventions that are brief (e.g., 3-minute contact) or intensive (e.g., 30-minute interview). Programs endorsed by public health care organizations can be readily obtained.
- As smoking is acknowledged as a health problem that is epidemic in nature, a minimum standard of practice should include assessing smoking status in all patient contacts and offering brief advice to smokers about available resources for cessation.
- Patients will likely report previous "failed" attempts to quit smoking. Highlight that previous quit attempts are important learning experiences, which provide information that will

make the current quit plan more likely to succeed. Information to be reviewed that is particularly helpful includes problematic symptoms of withdrawal, or behavioral strategies that were omitted in the previous attempt (see Behavioral Choices).

- The pattern of relapse is rapid. Approximately 66% of self-quitters relapse within the initial 48 hours, and 76% relapse within the initial week. Follow-up should be within the initial week following the quit date, and again within the initial month.

## Suggested Reading List


Bass F. Smoking cessation. In: Gray J, ed. *Therapeutic Choices*. 2nd ed. Ottawa, ON: Canadian Pharmacists Association, 1998.

Canadian Council on Smoking and Health. *Your guide to a smoke free future* (patient booklet). (CCSH, 1000–170 Laurier Ave. W., Ottawa, ON K1P 5V5), 1996.

Fiore MC, Wetter DW, Bailey WC, et al. *Smoking cessation clinical practice guideline*. Rockville, Md: Agency for Health Care Policy and Research, Public Health Service, US Dept of Health and Human Services, 1996. (Summary published in JAMA 1996; 275:1270–1280).

Green LW, Frankisk CJ, eds. *Smoking cessation: A synthesis of the literature of programs*. Institute of Health Promotion Research, University of British Columbia, 1998. (Unpublished Report).

Hughes JR, Stead LF, Lancaster TR. Anxiolytics and antidepressants in smoking cessation. (Cochrane Review). In: *The Cochrane Library*, 2. Oxford: Update Software, 1999.

Silagy C, Mant D, Fowler G, Lancaster T. Nicotine replacement therapy for smoking cessation (Cochrane Review). In: *The Cochrane Library*, 2. Oxford: Update Software, 1999.

CHAPTER 43

# Chronic Liver Diseases

*Mark G. Swain, MD, MSc, FRCPC*

This chapter discusses ascites, spontaneous bacterial peritonitis, hepatic encephalopathy, cholestatic disease (including symptom management), autoimmune chronic hepatitis, alcoholic liver disease (including alcoholic hepatitis), hemochromatosis and Wilson's disease. Esophageal varices are discussed in Chapter 46 and viral hepatitis in Chapter 44.

## Goals of Therapy

- To manage symptoms associated with chronic liver conditions
- To treat complications of chronic disease (e.g., infection)
- To prevent recurrence
- To delay or prevent disease progression
- To decrease mortality from liver-associated causes

## *Ascites (Portal Hypertension)*

### Investigations

- Thorough history with special attention to documented liver disease; other causes of ascites should be ruled out
- Physical examination for features of chronic liver disease (e.g., cutaneous stigmata), hepatosplenomegaly, degree of ascites accumulation (shifting dullness, abdominal protuberance, eversion of umbilicus), signs of portal hypertension (caput medusae, venous hum) or other features of liver failure/complications (GI bleed, asterixis)
- Laboratory tests:
  - ascitic tap (all patients) for neutrophil count, culture, protein/albumin, amylase, lactic dehydrogenase, glucose
  - calculate serum-ascites albumin gradient

### Therapeutic Choices (Figure 1, Table 1)

High plasma aldosterone levels in patients with ascites results in sodium/fluid retention; thus, **spironolactone** (a specific aldosterone antagonist) is the diuretic of choice. **Furosemide** can be added at any time to enhance diuresis and/or control serum potassium levels. **Metolazone** (an extremely potent diuretic) can be added to the spironolactone/furosemide combination if ascites is refractory.

Figure 1: **Management of Ascites Secondary to Portal Hypertension**

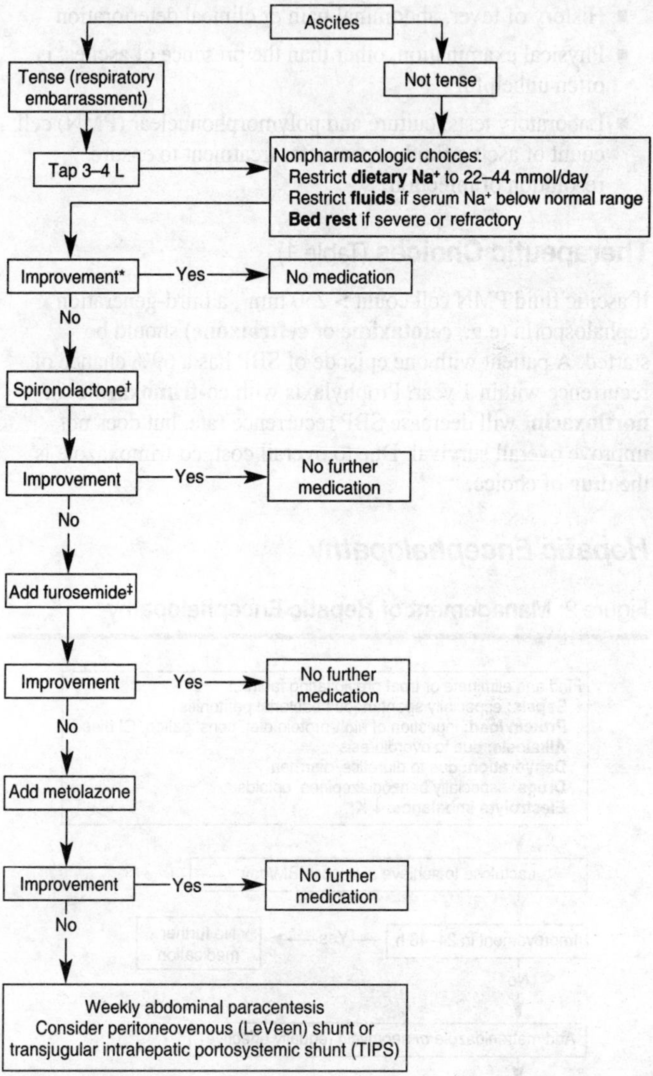
Ascites
Tense (respiratory embarrassment)
Not tense
Tap 3–4 L
Nonpharmacologic choices:
Restrict dietary Na+ to 22–44 mmol/day
Restrict fluids if serum Na+ below normal range
Bed rest if severe or refractory
Improvement*
Yes
No medication
No
Spironolactone†
Improvement
Yes
No further medication
No
Add furosemide‡
Improvement
Yes
No further medication
No
Add metolazone
Improvement
Yes
No further medication
No
Weekly abdominal paracentesis
Consider peritoneovenous (LeVeen) shunt or transjugular intrahepatic portosystemic shunt (TIPS)

** Aim: 1–1.5 kg/day weight loss if peripheral edema, 0.5–1 kg/day if no edema.*

*† Patients developing side effects (e.g., painful gynecomastia) can be switched to another potassium-sparing diuretic (e.g., amiloride).*

*‡ Patients can be started on spironolactone and furosemide simultaneously which often provides a more predictable diuresis with better electrolyte balance.*

***Note:** Diuretics should be given as single doses in the morning. The minimum dose to achieve adequate diuresis should always be used and serum electrolytes, BUN and creatinine monitored before therapy, weekly until stabilized then monthly. Dosage can usually be reduced after diuresis is initiated.*

## *Spontaneous Bacterial Peritonitis (SBP)*

### Investigations

- History of fever, abdominal pain or clinical deterioration
- Physical examination, other than the presence of ascites, is often unhelpful
- Laboratory tests: culture and polymorphonuclear (PMN) cell count of ascitic fluid; repeat after treatment to ensure resolution of infection

### Therapeutic Choices (Table 1)

If ascitic fluid PMN cell count > $250\ mm^3$, a third-generation cephalosporin (e.g., **cefotaxime** or **ceftriaxone**) should be started. A patient with one episode of SBP has a 69% chance of recurrence within 1 year. Prophylaxis with **co-trimoxazole**[1] or **norfloxacin**[2] will decrease SBP recurrence rate, but does not improve overall survival. Due to overall cost, co-trimoxazole is the drug of choice.

## *Hepatic Encephalopathy*

Figure 2: **Management of Hepatic Encephalopathy**

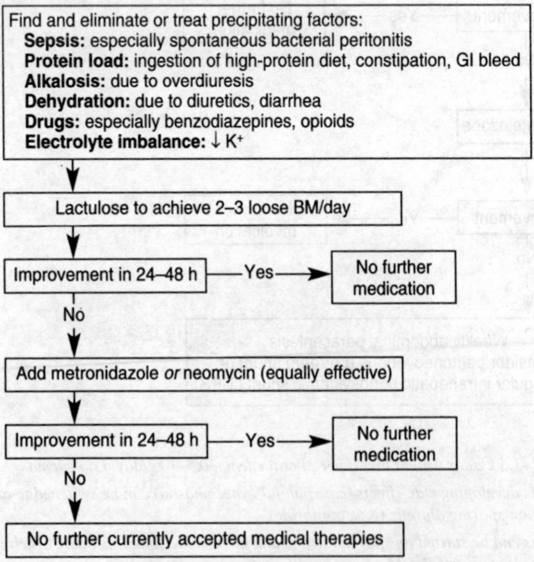
Find and eliminate or treat precipitating factors:
Sepsis: especially spontaneous bacterial peritonitis
Protein load: ingestion of high-protein diet, constipation, GI bleed
Alkalosis: due to overdiuresis
Dehydration: due to diuretics, diarrhea
Drugs: especially benzodiazepines, opioids
Electrolyte imbalance: ↓ K+
Lactulose to achieve 2–3 loose BM/day
Improvement in 24–48 h
Yes
No further medication
No
Add metronidazole or neomycin (equally effective)
Improvement in 24–48 h
Yes
No further medication
No
No further currently accepted medical therapies

[1] *Ann Intern Med 1995;122:595–598.*
[2] *Hepatology 1990;12:716–724.*

## *Cholestatic Disease*

### Goals of Therapy

- To improve or prevent progression of disease
- To improve symptoms (e.g., fatigue, pruritus)
- To improve survival and reduce need for liver transplant
- To adequately manage fat-soluble vitamin deficiencies

### Investigations

- Clinical/biochemical evidence of cholestasis (↑ alkaline phosphatase and later bilirubin) with:
  - for *primary biliary cirrhosis:* positive antimitochondrial antibody (> 95% of cases); confirmed by liver biopsy although not absolutely required if positive antimitochondrial antibody and cholestatic biochemical profile
  - for *primary sclerosing cholangitis:* ductular abnormalities (strictures, beading, etc.) on endoscopic retrograde cholangiopancreatography (ERCP)
- Identify vitamin deficiencies by:
  - prothrombin time (↑ if vitamin K deficient)
  - serum calcium, 25(OH)-vitamin D levels
  - serum vitamin A and/or carotene levels

### Therapeutic Choices (Figure 3, Table 1)

#### *Primary Biliary Cirrhosis (PBC) and Primary Sclerosing Cholangitis (PSC)*

**Ursodeoxycholic acid** (UDCA) has been shown to improve serum liver biochemical tests in PBC[3–5] and PSC. It appears to have limited effect in preventing disease progression in PSC. In PBC a combined analysis of three trials suggested that UDCA significantly reduced the probability of transplantation and/or death after a median of nearly 4 years. It slows disease progression but is not curative.[6] Its effect on symptoms (i.e., fatigue, pruritus) is controversial but likely minimal. **Methotrexate** is experimental for treating PBC or PSC and cannot be recommended for general use. Cholangitis episodes also require treatment with appropriate antibiotics (e.g., ciprofloxacin in outpatients for early mild episodes; ampicillin/gentamicin/metronidazole for hospitalized patients).

---

[3] *N Engl J Med 1991;324:1548–1554.*
[4] *Gastroenterology 1994;106:1284–1290.*
[5] *Hepatology 1994;19:1149–1156.*
[6] *Gastroenterology 1995;108:A1082.*

### *Vitamin Deficiencies*

**Vitamin A, D or K** supplements may be required to treat deficiencies (usually only in chronic cholestasis). The need for **vitamin E** supplements in adults has not been assessed in well designed clinical trials. Vitamin A supplementation is controversial.

### *Management of Pruritus*

Local cutaneous causes of pruritus (e.g., eczema) should be ruled out. **Cholestyramine** will benefit about 90% of patients; it must be continued as long as pruritus is present. **Antihistamines** (e.g., hydroxyzine) are of no proven benefit, but their sedative properties may help. For treatment failures, **rifampin** may be tried. Numerous other therapies have been reported but all are investigational.

# *Autoimmune Chronic Active Hepatitis*

## Investigations

- Marked ↑ in serum transaminases and hypergammaglobulinemia; positive antinuclear antibody (ANA) in about 70% of patients

**Note:** Patient is classically a young woman presenting with either an acute or chronic illness characterized by lethargy, arthralgia, oligomenorrhea, fluctuating jaundice and a cushingoid appearance with striae, hirsutism and acne.

## Therapeutic Choices (Table 1)

Immunosuppression with **glucocorticoids,** with or without **azathioprine,** prolongs life, decreases symptoms, improves serum biochemical abnormalities and diminishes hepatic inflammation on liver biopsy. The goal is to induce remission (decreased serum aminotransferase levels to ≤ twice normal and a follow-up liver biopsy that is normal or shows only chronic persistent hepatitis). Most patients will require therapy for at least 2 to 3 years before attempts to stop prednisone can be made; most will require lifelong therapy. If prednisone cannot be lowered below 10 mg per day, azathioprine may be added to the regimen.

# *Alcoholic Liver Disease*

## Therapeutic Choices

### *Chronic Alcohol-related Liver Disease*

There is no universally accepted medical therapy except **abstention from alcohol**. Some trials suggest potential benefit from long-term propylthiouracil and colchicine, but these therapies are still considered experimental.

Figure 3: **Management of Cholestatic Symptoms**

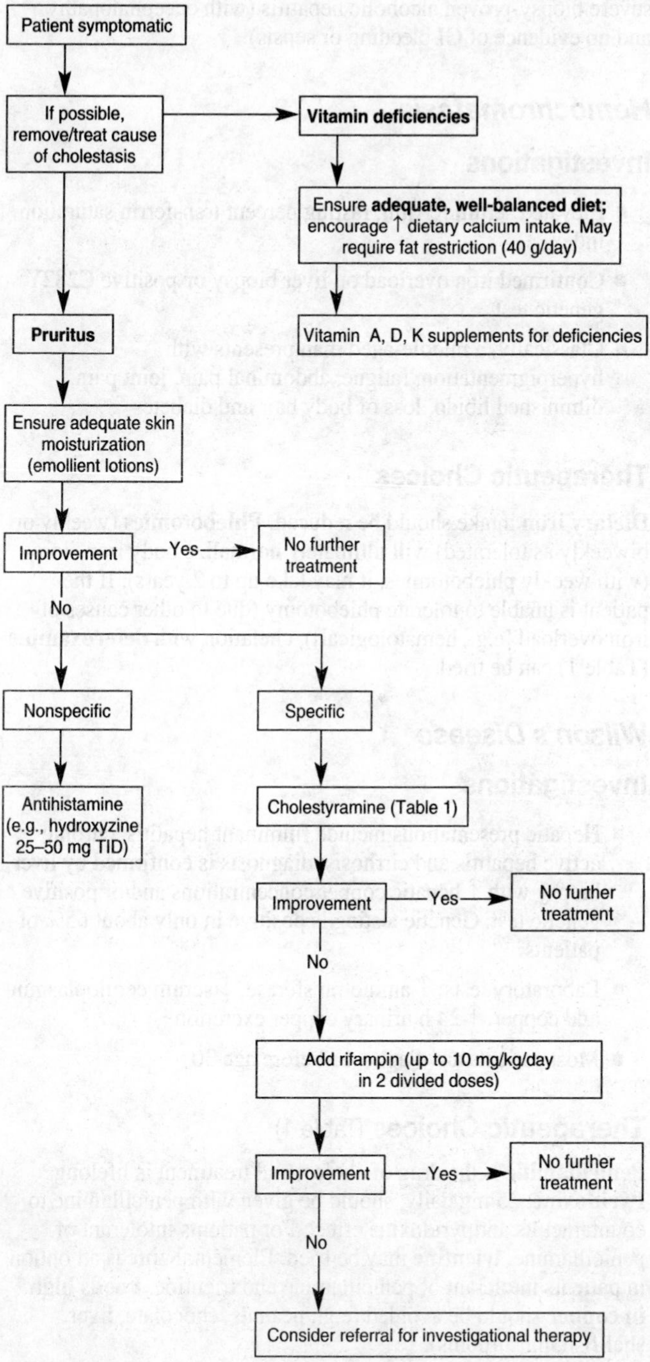
Patient symptomatic
If possible, remove/treat cause of cholestasis
Vitamin deficiencies
Ensure adequate, well-balanced diet; encourage ↑ dietary calcium intake. May require fat restriction (40 g/day)
Pruritus
Vitamin A, D, K supplements for deficiencies
Ensure adequate skin moisturization (emollient lotions)
Improvement
Yes
No further treatment
No
Nonspecific
Specific
Antihistamine (e.g., hydroxyzine 25–50 mg TID)
Cholestyramine (Table 1)
Improvement
Yes
No further treatment
No
Add rifampin (up to 10 mg/kg/day in 2 divided doses)
Improvement
Yes
No further treatment
No
Consider referral for investigational therapy

### *Alcoholic Hepatitis*

**Corticosteroids** improve short-term survival in patients with severe biopsy-proven alcoholic hepatitis (with encephalopathy and no evidence of GI bleeding or sepsis).

## *Hemochromatosis*

### Investigations

- Elevated serum ferritin, fasting percent transferrin saturation index
- Confirmed iron overload on liver biopsy **or** positive C282Y genetic test
- Classically, a middle-aged man presents with hyperpigmentation, fatigue, abdominal pain, joint pain, diminished libido, loss of body hair and diabetes

### Therapeutic Choices

**Dietary iron** intake should be reduced. **Phlebotomies** (weekly or biweekly as tolerated) will ultimately normalize body iron stores (with weekly phlebotomies, it may take up to 2 years). If the patient is unable to tolerate phlebotomy (due to other causes of iron overload [e.g., hematological]), chelation with **deferoxamine** (Table 1) can be tried.

## *Wilson's Disease*

### Investigations

- Hepatic presentations include fulminant hepatitis, chronic active hepatitis and cirrhosis; diagnosis is confirmed by liver biopsy with ↑ hepatic copper concentrations and/or positive genetic test. Genetic testing is positive in only about 65% of patients
- Laboratory tests: ↑ aminotransferase, ↓ serum ceruloplasmin and copper, ↑ 24 h urinary copper excretion
- Most patients are diagnosed before age 30

### Therapeutic Choices (Table 1)

**Penicillamine** is the drug of choice, and treatment is lifelong. **Pyridoxine**, 25 mg daily, should be given with penicillamine to counteract its antipyridoxine effect. For patients intolerant of penicillamine, **trientine** may be tried. Elemental **zinc** is an option in patients intolerant of penicillamine and trientine. **Foods high in copper** should be avoided (e.g., peanuts, chocolate, liver, shellfish, mushrooms).

Table 1: **Drugs Used in Chronic Liver Diseases**

| Drug | Dosage | Adverse Effects | Comments | Cost* |
|---|---|---|---|---|
| **Ascites** | | | | |
| *spironolactone* Aldactone, generics | Starting 100–200 mg/d, ↑ to 400 mg/d with dosage adjustments Q5–7 d | Hyperkalemia, gynecomastia, mastalgia. | If intolerable side effects develop, may switch to amiloride (5 mg/d, can be ↑ to 20 mg/d). | $ |
| *furosemide* Lasix, generics | Starting 40 mg/d, ↑ daily by 20–40 mg until diuresis achieved (up to 160 mg/d) | Common to thiazides/loop diuretics: hyponatremia, hypokalemia, volume depletion, nausea, anorexia, fatigue, hyperuricemia, hyperglycemia with metolazone, ototoxicity with high-dose furosemide, rash, weakness. | | $ |
| *metolazone* Zaroxolyn | Starting 2.5 mg/d, up to 10 mg/d | | | $ |
| **Spontaneous Bacterial Peritonitis** | | | | |
| **Treatment** | | | | |
| *cefotaxime* Claforan | 2 g IV Q8H × 5 d | Hypersensitivity, GI disturbances, pain at injection site, pseudomembranous colitis. | Alternative: other 3rd-generation cephalosporin. | $$$$ |
| *ceftriaxone* Rocephin | 2 g IV Q24H × 5 d | Hypersensitivity, GI disturbances, biliary pseudolithiasis (sludging). | | $$$$ |
| **Prophylaxis** | | | | |
| *co-trimoxazole* Bactrim, Septra, generics | 1 DS tablet 5 ×/week | Hypersensitivity, GI disturbances, blood dyscrasias, skin reactions (rare Stevens-Johnson syndrome). | Prophylaxis to be used only after patient has experienced one confirmed episode of SBP. | $ |
| *norfloxacin* Noroxin, generics | 400 mg/d | GI disturbances, CNS effects, skin rash. | | $$ |

*(cont'd)*

Table 1: **Drugs Used in Chronic Liver Diseases** *(cont'd)*

| Drug | Dosage | Adverse Effects | Comments | Cost* |
|---|---|---|---|---|
| **Hepatic Encephalopathy** | | | | |
| *lactulose*<br>generics | 30 mL BID–QID | Bloating, flatulence, cramps, diarrhea. | Titrate lactulose to produce 2–3 loose BM/d. | \$–\$\$ |
| *metronidazole*<br>Flagyl, generics | 250–500 mg TID | GI disturbances, headache, metallic taste. | Disulfiram-like reaction with alcohol. | \$ |
| *neomycin*<br>Mycifradin | 1 g QID | Malabsorption syndrome, nephrotoxicity, ototoxicity, GI disturbances, rash. | Neomycin and metronidazole are equally effective. | \$\$ |
| **Cholestatic Pruritus** | | | | |
| *cholestyramine*<br>Questran, generics | 4 g before breakfast initially; ↑ in 4 g increments first after breakfast, then at night and then at lunch | Constipation, heartburn, nausea, vomiting. | May bind other drugs given concurrently; separate doses (1 h before or 4–6 h after resin). | \$\$ |
| **Fat-soluble Vitamin Deficiencies** | | | | |
| *vitamin K* | Vitamin K 10 mg IM monthly | | | |
| *vitamin A* | Vitamin A 5 000–10 000 IU/d† PO (aqueous) | | Use of vitamin A is controversial. | \$ |
| *vitamin D* | Vitamin D 1 000 IU Q2 d PO (with 2–3 g elemental calcium/d) | | For examples of calcium products, see Chapter 57. | |

| | | | | |
|---|---|---|---|---|
| **Primary Biliary Cirrhosis** | | | | |
| *ursodeoxycholic acid*<br>Urso | 13–15 mg/kg/d | Diarrhea. | A reasonable treatment for PBC; may be of benefit in PSC but is unproven. | $$$[‡] |
| **Autoimmune Chronic Active Hepatitis** | | | | |
| *prednisone*<br>generics | Sample dosage regimen (e.g., Mayo Clinic) for *autoimmune chronic active hepatitis:*<br>60 mg/d × 1 wk, then 40 mg/d × 1 wk, then 30 mg/d × 2 wks, then 20 mg/d<br>*Alcoholic hepatitis:*<br>40 mg/d for 28 d then taper over 2 wks | Fluid/electrolyte imbalance, suppression of pituitary–adrenal function, hyperglycemia, peptic ulcer, behavioral disturbances, ocular cataracts, glaucoma, cushingoid syndrome, aseptic necrosis of hip. | *Autoimmune chronic active hepatitis:* Gradually taper from 20 mg/d (weeks to months) using serum aminotransferases and clinical status as guides. | $ |
| *azathioprine*<br>Imuran, generics | 50–150 mg/d | ↓ appetite, leukopenia, thrombocytopenia, infection, biliary stasis, hypersensitivity reactions, rash, rare veno-occlusive disease, nausea, vomiting. | Monitor CBC monthly while on azathioprine. | $–$$ |
| **Hemochromatosis** | | | | |
| *deferoxamine*<br>Desferal | 1–4 g by SC minipump over 12 h, adjusted on an individual basis | Allergic reactions, auditory/ocular toxicity, tachycardia, flushing, abdominal discomfort, pain at injection site, hypotension, skin rash, convulsions. | May be beneficial if phlebotomy is not tolerated or contraindicated. | $$$$$ |

*(cont'd)*

Table 1: **Drugs Used in Chronic Liver Diseases** *(cont'd)*

| Drug | Dosage | Adverse Effects | Comments | Cost* |
|---|---|---|---|---|
| **Wilson's Disease** | | | | |
| *penicillamine* Cuprimine, Depen | 1–2 g/d in 4 divided doses, on an empty stomach | Proteinuria, hematologic effects, positive ANA, mouth ulcers, diarrhea, ↓ taste sense, ↓ appetite, nausea, vomiting, hypersensitivity. | Use 24 h urinary copper excretion and serum free copper levels to monitor therapy for adequate removal of copper. | $$–$$$$ |
| *trientine* Syprine[π] | 1–2 g/d in 4 divided doses | Usually well tolerated. Anemia. | | π |
| *zinc* generics | 50 mg (elemental zinc) TID between meals | GI disturbances. | Use in patients intolerant of penicillamine or trientine. | $ |

*† Use minimum effective dose.*
*‡ Based on 750 mg/day × 30 days.*
*π Available through the Special Access Program, Therapeutic Products Directorate, Health Canada.*
*Dosage adjustment may be required in renal impairment – see Appendix I.*
** Cost of 30-day supply unless specified otherwise – includes drug cost only.*
*Legend: $ < $40   $$ $40–80   $$$ $80–125   $$$$ $125–350   $$$$$ > $350*

### *Suggested Reading List*

Autoimmune Hepatitis. In Rothschild MA, Berk PA, Meyer zum Buschenfelde K-H, eds. *Seminars in liver disease*. Vol 11(3). New York: Thieme Medical Publishers, Inc., 1991.

Barton J, McDonnell SM, Adams PC, Brissot P, Powell LW, Edwards CQ, et al. Management of hemochromatosis. *Ann Intern Med* 1998;129:932–939.

Mistry P, Seymour CA. Primary biliary cirrhosis – from Thomas Addison to the 1990's. *Q J Med* 1992;82:185–196.

Runyon BA. Care of patients with ascites. *N Engl J Med* 1994; 330:337–342.

Sternlieb I. Perspectives in Wilson's disease. *Hepatology* 1990;12:1234–1239.

CHAPTER 44

# Viral Hepatitis

*Jenny Heathcote, MB, BS, MD, FRCP, FRCPC*

## Goals of Therapy

- To prevent disease
- To minimize liver damage
- To reduce the spread of infection

# Acute Viral Hepatitis

Acute viral hepatitis is a systemic viral infection that is present for less than 6 months and which causes inflammatory necrosis of the liver.

## Important Features

- Most cases of acute viral hepatitis are asymptomatic.
- A fulminant course occurs in 0.1% (higher rate in pregnant women); immediate referral should be made to a liver transplantation centre because massive necrosis resulting in liver failure can occur.
- Diagnosis must be confirmed serologically.
- Hepatitis B becomes chronic in 1% of healthy adults.
- Hepatitis C becomes chronic in 70% of healthy adults.

### Glossary of Abbreviations

HAV = Hepatitis A virus
HBV = Hepatitis B virus
HCV = Hepatitis C virus
HBsAg = Hepatitis B surface antigen
Anti-HBs = Antibody to HBsAg
HBeAg = Hepatitis Be antigen
Anti-HBe = Antibody to HBeAg
HDV = Hepatitis D (delta) virus
Anti-HCV = Antibody to HCV
HCV RNA = Hepatitis C RNA

## Investigations

The clinical features are nonspecific, regardless of causative virus; viral type is identified by serologic markers.

- Check for parenteral/sexual exposure, medication list, travel/day care exposure, family history of hepatitis B
- Check for persistent nausea and vomiting, drowsiness, bruising (signs of severe disease)
- Check INR; if elevated refer patient to gastroenterologist

Figure 1: **Treatment of Acute Viral Hepatitis**

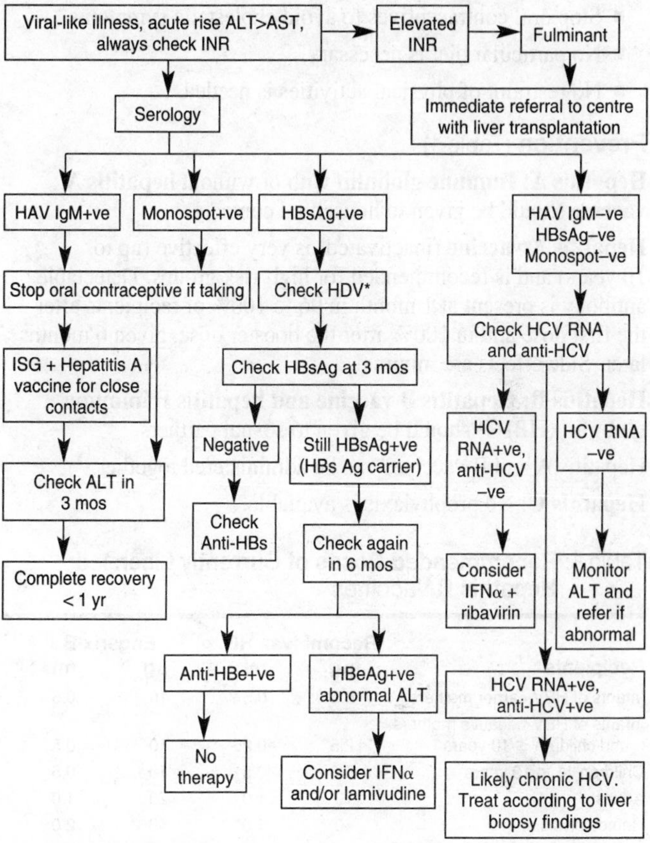
Viral-like illness, acute rise ALT>AST, always check INR
Elevated INR
Fulminant
Immediate referral to centre with liver transplantation
Serology
HAV IgM+ve
Monospot+ve
HBsAg+ve
HAV IgM–ve HBsAg–ve Monospot–ve
Stop oral contraceptive if taking
Check HDV*
Check HCV RNA and anti-HCV
ISG + Hepatitis A vaccine for close contacts
Check HBsAg at 3 mos
HCV RNA+ve, anti-HCV –ve
HCV RNA –ve
Negative
Still HBsAg+ve (HBs Ag carrier)
Check ALT in 3 mos
Check Anti-HBs
Check again in 6 mos
Consider IFNα + ribavirin
Monitor ALT and refer if abnormal
Complete recovery < 1 yr
Anti-HBe+ve
HBeAg+ve abnormal ALT
HCV RNA+ve, anti-HCV+ve
No therapy
Consider IFNα and/or lamivudine
Likely chronic HCV. Treat according to liver biopsy findings

*Abbreviations: HAV IgM = Hepatitis A IgM; HBsAg = Hepatitis B surface antigen; HDV = Hepatitis D (delta) virus; ISG = Immune Serum Globulin; Anti-HCV = Antibody to HCV; IFNα = Interferon alpha.*

** Note: coinfection with HDV does not change treatment course, but is generally more severe.*

- Check serology
  - impossible to distinguish a flare-up of chronic hepatitis B from an acute case; only time will identify the carriers (i.e., all hepatitis B must be followed serologically)
  - acute hepatitis C only HCV RNA+ve first 6 weeks, then anti-HCV becomes positive

## **Therapeutic Choices** (Figure 1)

In most cases no specific therapy is indicated other than supportive care. The majority of patients recover completely without complications or chronic sequelae.

### Nonpharmacologic Choices

- Avoid alcohol for at least 3 months.
- Stop oral contraceptives to avoid cholestatic symptoms.
- No particular diet is necessary.
- No restraint of physical activities is needed.

### Prevention (Table 1)

**Hepatitis A: Immune globulin** with or without **hepatitis A vaccine** should be given to household contacts.

**Hepatitis A vaccine** (inactivated) is very effective (up to 10 years) and is recommended for high-risk groups. Detectable antibody is present at 1 month in 96 to 100% of recipients after the first dose and in 100% after the booster dose, given 6 months later. Side effects are minimal.

**Hepatitis B: Hepatitis B vaccine and hepatitis B immune globulin (HBIG)** should be given to sexual partners.

Hepatitis A and B vaccines can be administered together.

**Hepatitis C:** No prophylaxis is available.

Table 1: **Recommended Doses of Currently Licensed Hepatitis B Vaccines**

| | Recombivax HB | | Engerix-B | |
|---|---|---|---|---|
| **Recipients** | **µg** | **mL** | **µg** | **mL** |
| Infants of HBV-carrier mothers | 5.0 | 0.5 | 10 | 0.5 |
| Infants of HBV-negative mothers and children ≤ 10 years | 2.5 | 0.25 | 10 | 0.5 |
| Children 11 to 19 years | 5.0 | 0.5 | 10 | 0.5 |
| Adults | 10 | 1.0 | 20 | 1.0 |
| Hemodialysis and immunocompromised patients | 40 | 1.0* | 40 | 2.0 |

* *When special formulation is used.*

*From Canadian Immunization Guide, 5th Edition, Health Canada, 1998. Reproduced with permission of the Minister of Public Works and Government Services Canada, 1998.*

# Chronic Viral Hepatitis

Viral hepatitis is chronic when present for 6 months or longer. It can progress to cirrhosis, liver failure and hepatoma. HBV and HCV are the most common causes.

## *Chronic Hepatitis B* (Figure 2)

### Features of Chronic Hepatitis B

**A hepatitis B carrier** is any person who is HBsAg seropositive > 6 months. One percent of HBV carriers per year spontaneously lose HBsAg seropositivity and become immune (i.e, develop anti-HBs).

Figure 2: **Chronic Hepatitis B: Natural History**

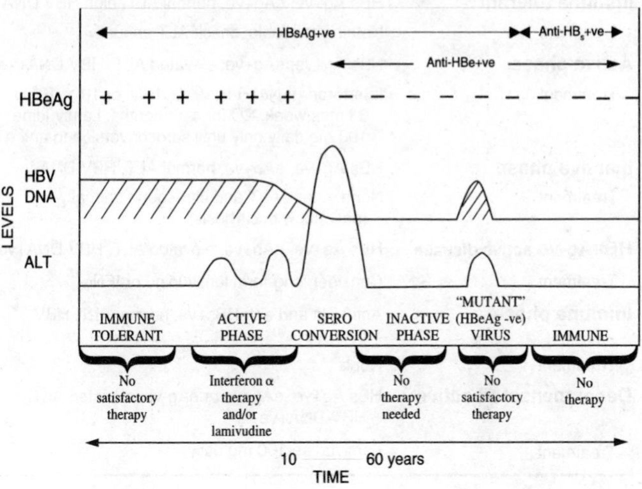
HBsAg+ve
Anti-HBs+ve
Anti-HBe+ve
HBeAg + + + + + + – – – – – – – – – –
HBV DNA
LEVELS
ALT
IMMUNE TOLERANT
ACTIVE PHASE
SERO CONVERSION
INACTIVE PHASE
"MUTANT" (HBeAg -ve) VIRUS
IMMUNE
No satisfactory therapy
Interferon α therapy and/or lamivudine
No therapy needed
No satisfactory therapy
No therapy
10 60 years
TIME

## Investigations

- Check if patient is coinfected with hepatitis D virus
- Check "e" status (HBeAg and anti-HBe) and serum transaminase values

## Therapeutic Choices

### Nonpharmacologic Choices

- Advise against all but modest alcohol consumption (less than 4 drinks weekly).

### Prevention (Table 1)

- All household members and sexual partners require hepatitis B vaccine.
- Hepatitis B vaccine and HBIG should be given at birth to infants of a carrier mother.

### Pharmacologic Choices

Immunosuppressive drugs should be avoided (50% of hepatitis B carriers experience flare-up upon drug withdrawal).

#### *Interferon Alfa (IFNα) (Table 3)*

IFNα is used as an immune stimulant to treat HBsAg carriers who are persistently HBeAg positive with elevated serum transaminase values. It promotes HBeAg+ve to anti-HBe+ve seroconversion which is associated with a fall in serum transaminase to normal.

Table 2: **Therapeutic Options for Chronic Hepatitis B***

| | |
|---|---|
| **Immune tolerant** | HBs Ag+ve, eAg+ve, normal ALT, high HBV DNA |
| Treatment | Nothing available, check ALT annually |
| **Active phase** | HBs Ag+ve, eAg+ve, elevated ALT, HBV DNA+ve |
| Treatment | Interferon (IFNα) 5 × $10^6$ U daily, or 10 × $10^6$ U 3 times/week, SC for 4–6 months. Lamivudine 100 mg daily only until seroconversion to anti-e |
| **Inactive phase** | HBs Ag+ve, eAb+ve, normal ALT, HBV DNA-ve |
| Treatment | None, check ALT and ultrasound annually (patients with cirrhosis) |
| **HBeAg-ve active disease** | HBs Ag+ve, eAb+ve, elevated ALT, HBV DNA+ve |
| Treatment | Consider long-term lamivudine or IFNα |
| **Immune phase** | Anti-HBs and anti-HBc+ve, normal ALT, HBV DNA-ve |
| Treatment | None |
| **Decompensated active** | HBs Ag+ve, eAg+ve or eAg-ve, elevated ALT, HBV DNA+ve |
| Treatment | Lamivudine 100 mg daily |

* *Therapies to be instituted by specialist only.*

All patients with Hepatitis D coinfection relapse after IFNα therapy. HIV and other immunosuppressed patients respond poorly to IFNα.

**Absolute contraindications**: autoimmune disease (SLE, rheumatoid arthritis), severe depression or psychosis, neutropenia (< 1 × $10^9$/L), thrombocytopenia (< 50 × $10^9$/L), cardiac arrhythmias, uncontrolled seizures.

**Relative contraindications**: decompensated liver disease, insulin-dependent diabetes, chronic renal failure, coinfection with HIV, concomitant immunosuppressive therapy, ongoing alcohol or IV drug use.

**Adverse effects:** flu-like symptoms, irritability, depression, hair thinning and diarrhea.

### *Nucleoside Analogue – Lamivudine*

Lamivudine is an oral antiviral agent that effectively inhibits replication of HBV in patients who are both eAg negative or eAb positive with elevated serum HBV DNA values. It should only be given to patients who have an ongoing hepatitis (persistent elevation of ALT and HBV DNA.) It is not yet licensed for use in children.

**Absolute contraindications:** pregnant women or any fertile person not practising effective contraception (i.e., both females and males excluded from treatment).

Note: safer to use in patients with decompensated cirrhosis and in patients on immunosuppressive therapy (than IFNα).

**Relative contraindications:** untreated HIV (promotes viral resistance).

**Adverse Effects:** minimal, but induces mutations which cause resistance to lamivudine in 20% per year in those who do not become HBV DNA negative (by highly sensitive PCR methods).

## *Chronic Hepatitis C* (Figure 3)

### Features of Chronic Hepatitis C

- Anti-HCV is a marker of infection, not immunity.
- Measurement of RNA virus in serum is not routinely available.
- Most acute infections become chronic (in 60 to 70%) whether acquired parenterally or sporadically; up to 40% may later resolve spontaneously likely within the first year of infection.
- 60 to 90% of persons who have ever been IV drug users have chronic hepatitis C.
- Immunosuppressed patients may lose anti-HCV but remain RNA positive.
- Sexual transmission (facilitated by HIV coinfection) rate is 0 to 5%; safe sex is recommended for those with multiple sexual partners.
- Vertical transmission rate is 0 to 5%, depending on titre of RNA in mother (i.e., high titre if coinfected with HIV hence greater transmission rate).

Figure 3: **Chronic Hepatitis C: Natural History**

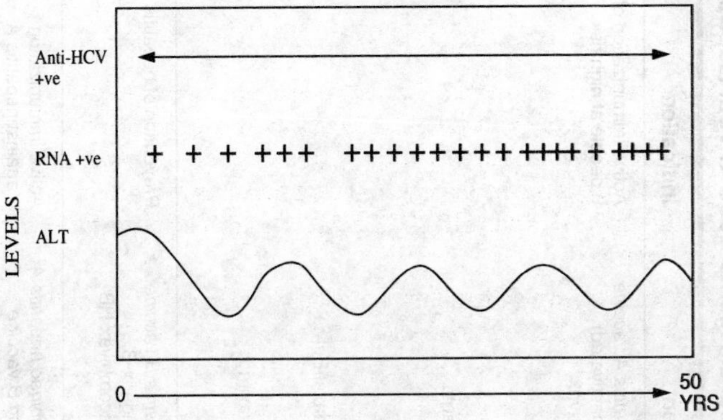
Anti-HCV
+ve
RNA +ve
+ + + +++ ++++++++ ++++ + ++++
LEVELS
ALT
0
50
YRS

*Approximately 1% develop cirrhosis/year*

Table 3: **Agents Used in Viral Hepatitis**

| Agent | Indication | Dosage | Adverse Effects | Comments | Cost* |
|---|---|---|---|---|---|
| *hepatitis A vaccine* (inactivated) | Active immunization of people at high risk | | | | |
| Havrix | | Adults: 1 mL (1440 EL.U) IM at 0 and 6–12 mos | Soreness at site, induration, redness, swelling. | Can be given with immune globulin if person at risk of contacting HAV before adequate anti-HAV antibody titres are achieved. | $$/2 doses |
| | | Children 2–18 yrs: 0.5 mL (720 EL.U) IM at 0 and 6–12 mos | | | $/2 doses |
| Vaqta | | Adults: 1.0 mL (50 U) IM at 0 and 6 mos | | | $$/2 doses |
| | | Children 2–17 yrs: 0.5 mL (25 U) IM at 0, 6 and 18 mos | | | $$/2 doses |
| Epaxal Berna | | Adults and children ≥ 1 yr: 0.5 mL (≥ 500 RU) IM at 0 and 12 mos | | | $$/2 doses |
| Avaxim | | Adults and children ≥ 12 yr: 0.5 mL (160 antigen units) IM at 0 and 6–12 mos | | | $$/2 doses |
| *hepatitis B vaccine* Engerix-B, Recombivax HB | Prevention of hepatitis B | Dose varies with age, product, medical condition (Table 1); 3 doses IM at 0, 1, 6 mos | Soreness and redness at injection site. | Booster not necessary in immunocompetent person. Can be used with HBIG. | $$/3 doses |
| *combined hepatitis A and B vaccine* Twinrex | Active immunization against hepatitis A and B | Adults > 19 yrs: 1 mL IM at 0, 1 and 6 mos. Not yet approved for children. | Soreness at injection site, induration, redness, swelling. | For high-risk occupations and patients with cirrhosis. | $$$/3 doses |

| | | | | | |
|---|---|---|---|---|---|
| *hepatitis B immune globulin (HBIG)* Bayhep B† | Postexposure prophylaxis of hepatitis B | 0.06 mL/kg IM | Can be used with vaccine. | Used to prevent recurrence post liver transplant.<br>It is of no value in treatment of fulminant acute or chronic active hepatitis B. | $$$$/dose |
| *immune globulin* Baygam† | Prophylaxis of hepatitis A; postexposure prophylaxis of hepatitis A if within 2 wks of exposure | Adults: 0.08–0.12 mL/kg IM<br>Children: 0.02–0.04 mL/kg IM<br>If continued exposure, repeat dose in 5 mos | Soreness at injection site, anaphylaxis (rare). | Has no role in prophylaxis of hepatitis B. | $/dose |
| *interferon alfa (IFNα)* Intron A, Roferon-A, Wellferon<br>*interferon alfacon-l* Infergen | Treatment of chronic hepatitis B and C | Hepatitis B: $10 \times 10^6$ U 3×/wk × 16 wks, given SC (or μg equivalent for Infergen)<br>Hepatitis C: $3 \times 10^6$ U (or 9 μg of Infergen) 3×/wk×48 wks | Common: fatigue, fever, muscle aches, asthenia, weight loss, headaches, irritability, hair loss, bone marrow suppression.<br>Less common: pulmonary infiltrates, severe depression. | Intron A, Roferon-A and Infergen are recombinant IFNαs, and Wellferon is a mixture of several IFNαs. No significant differences in efficacy have been shown among the products.<br>For hepatitis C, if HCV RNA still detectable after 12 wks stop treatment. | HBV $5700/course<br>HCV $6000/course |
| *lamivudine* ❸ Heptovir | Treatment of chronic hepatitis B and post liver transplant for chronic hepatitis B | 100 mg/day PO (patients with ↑ ALT,↑ HBV DNA, e/anti-e +ve) | Dizziness, nausea. | 20% of treated patients develop resistant mutants within the first year.<br>Optimum duration of therapy not established. | $140/30 days |

*(cont'd)*

Table 3: **Agents Used in Viral Hepatitis** *(cont'd)*

| Agent | Indication | Dosage | Adverse Effects | Comments | Cost* |
|---|---|---|---|---|---|
| *interferon alpha-2b plus ribavirin* (renal symbol) Rebetron | Treatment of chronic hepatitis C | INF$\alpha$2b $3 \times 10^6$ U 3 ×/wk SC ribavirin 1000–1200 mg/d divided BID PO for 24 wks (genotype 2 and 3), for 48 wks (other genotypes) | INF$\alpha$2b as for INF$\alpha$ above. Ribavirin: hemolytic anemia | Many contraindications (see text). | $9500–10500 /24 wks |

* *Cost of adult therapy, as indicated – includes drug cost only.*
† *Available through Canadian Blood Services.*
(renal symbol) *Dosage adjustment may be required in renal impairment – see Appendix I.*

*Legend: $ < $50 $$ $50–100 $$$ $100–300 $$$$ > $300*
*Abbreviations: EL.U = Elisa units, RU = radioimmunoassay units*

- Risk factors for progressive fibrosis are male gender, age > 40 yrs at acquisition, alcohol consumption > 50 g daily and probably coinfection with HIV/immune suppression.

## Investigations

- Clinical signs of chronic liver disease are infrequent
- ALT > AST and wide fluctuations are observed; levels may be normal for long periods, although liver histology is rarely normal.

Table 4: **Therapy of Chronic Hepatitis C***

| | |
|---|---|
| **Ongoing Hepatitis C** | ALT elevated, HCV RNA+ve, activity ± fibrosis on biopsy |
| Treatment | Interferon alpha-2b plus ribavirin 24 weeks for genotype 2 and 3, 48 weeks for all other genotypes |
| **"Inactive" Hepatitis C** | ALT normal, HCV RNA+ve, therapy not yet proven to be of value, recheck ALT annually (ALT normal, HCV RNA-ve retest in 1 year) |

* *Therapies to be instituted by specialist only.*

## Therapeutic Choices

### Nonpharmacologic Choices

- Any more than modest alcohol use should be avoided (less than 4 drinks weekly).

### Prevention

- No vaccine is available.

### Pharmacologic Choices (Table 3 and 4)

#### *Combination Interferon Alfa-2b Plus Ribavirin*

Combination IFNα2b/ribavirin (Rebetron) is the standard of care.[1] Duration of therapy depends mainly on viral genotype and on viral load; these only need to be tested just prior to starting therapy. When to test for nonresponse and stop therapy is debatable (12 or 24 weeks).

**Expected response to therapy:** genotype 1a, 1b, 4, 5, and 6 – 25 to 29% sustained loss HCV RNA, i.e., 6 months after cessation of 48 weeks treatment.

[1] *CMAJ 2000;162:827–833.*

Genotype 2 and 3 – 67% sustained loss HCV RNA, i.e., after cessation of 24 weeks' treatment.

**Best responders:** low viral load, genotypes 2 and 3, no cirrhosis, females, short duration infection.

Note: if HCV RNA remains negative for more than 6 months after cessation of therapy, likely a 95% chance of remission lasting up to 10 years (data for treatment with IFN alone).

**Absolute contraindications to use of ribavirin:** pregnancy, or any fertile person of either sex not using reliable methods of contraception throughout treatment and for 6 months after cessation of therapy. Renal failure, hemolysis, ischemic vascular disease, or any cardiac problems.

**Relative contraindications:** diabetes, uncontrolled hypertension.

## *Suggested Reading List*

EASL International consensus conference on hepatitis C. Paris 26–28, February 1999, consensus statement. European Association for the study of the liver. *J Hepatol* 1999;30:956–961.

Gutfreud KS, Bain VG. Chronic viral hepatitis C: management update. *CMAJ* 2000;162:827–833.

Hoofnagle JH, Bisceglie AM. The treatment of chronic viral hepatitis. *N Engl J Med* 1997;336:347–356.

Lemon SM, Thomas DL. Vaccines to prevent viral hepatitis. *N Engl J Med* 1997;336:196–204.

CHAPTER 45

# Gastroesophageal Reflux Disease

*Eldon A. Shaffer, MD, DABIM, FACP, FRCPC*

Gastroesophageal reflux disease (GERD) refers to the symptoms (commonly heartburn) resulting when gastric secretions reflux from the stomach to the esophagus. It may lead to inflammatory histopathologic changes (reflux or peptic esophagitis).

## Goals of Therapy

- To relieve symptoms, particularly heartburn
- To promote healing of esophagitis
- To prevent complications (stricture formation, bleeding, progression to Barrett's epithelium)
- To prevent recurrences

### Classification of Symptom Severity*

| Severity of GERD | Criteria |
|---|---|
| Trivial to Mild | Reflux symptoms < 3 times/week<br>Not nocturnal<br>Symptoms do not interfere with daily activity<br>Pain (heartburn) severity rated 1–3 out of 10<br>No major complications |
| Significant | Takes patient to physician<br>Symptoms present for > 6 months<br>Symptoms regularly interfere with daily activity and can awaken patient at night<br>Pain severity rated 7–10 out of 10<br>Complications |

* *Classification does not necessarily correspond to histological severity.*

## Investigations

- History: identify
  - common symptoms of GERD: heartburn, regurgitation of acid or bile, or hypersalivation (water brash)
  - less common features: chest pain, hiccoughs, aspiration (cough, asthma, pneumonia), oropharyngeal symptoms (globus sensation, hoarseness) or ulcers, dental caries, burning mouth syndrome, or rarely odynophagia (pain on swallowing)

- predisposing/associated conditions: pregnancy, obesity, scleroderma

- Indications for diagnostic evaluation include:
  - heartburn refractory to 2 to 4 weeks of therapy with a proton pump inhibitor
  - dysphagia
  - odynophagia
  - atypical chest pain
  - GI bleeding
  - extraesophageal symptoms (respiratory, oropharyngeal)
  - weight loss
- Types of diagnostic evaluation depend on availability and indication:
  - **esophagogastroscopy** is the best test to evaluate mucosal injury: biopsy any suspicious lesion to detect Barrett's epithelium (a premalignant lesion requiring surveillance endoscopy) or carcinoma
  - **barium swallow** assesses peristalsis and detects rings or strictures in patients with dysphagia
  - **esophageal manometry** documents peristalsis and is warranted in patients with atypical chest pain and to eliminate a major motility disorder (e.g., scleroderma) before doing antireflux surgery
  - **24-hour pH monitoring** detects acid reflux into lower esophagus in patients with atypical reflux symptoms, for those who fail standard medical therapy, and as preoperative evaluation before antireflux surgery

## Therapeutic Choices (Figure 1)

### Nonpharmacologic Choices

There is little evidence to support lifestyle changes; however, they are recommended as initial therapy.

- Dietary modifications (avoid chocolate, caffeine, acidic citrus juices, large fatty meals).
- Weight loss if 20% greater than ideal body weight.
- No snacks before bedtime.
- No lying down after meals.
- Reduce alcohol intake.
- Legs under the head of the bed should be elevated on 10- to 15-cm blocks.
- Stop smoking (Chapter 42).
- Avoid tight clothing.

Figure 1: **Management of GERD**

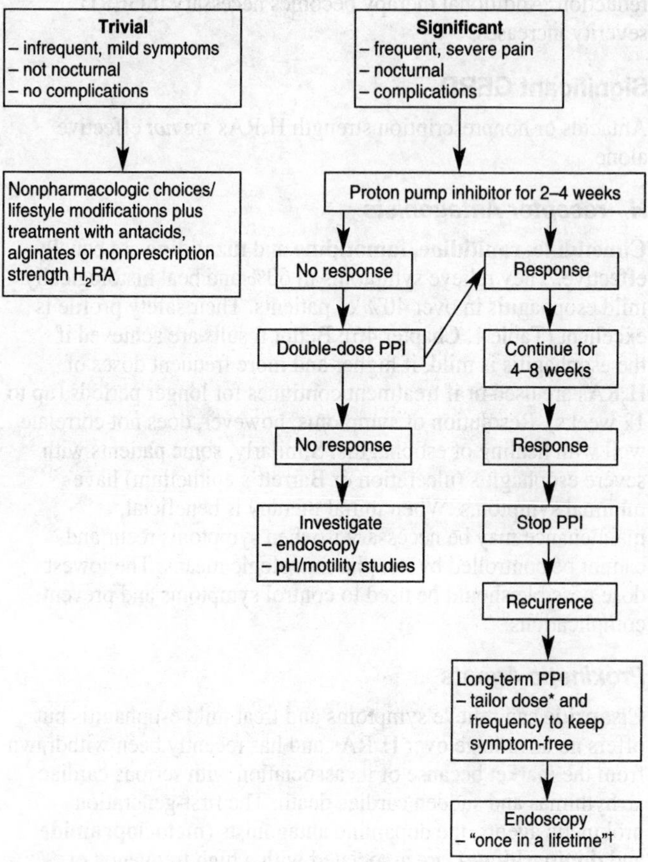
Trivial
– infrequent, mild symptoms
– not nocturnal
– no complications
Significant
– frequent, severe pain
– nocturnal
– complications
Nonpharmacologic choices/ lifestyle modifications plus treatment with antacids, alginates or nonprescription strength $H_2RA$
Proton pump inhibitor for 2–4 weeks
No response
Response
Double-dose PPI
Continue for 4–8 weeks
No response
Response
Investigate
– endoscopy
– pH/motility studies
Stop PPI
Recurrence
Long-term PPI
– tailor dose* and frequency to keep symptom-free
Endoscopy
– "once in a lifetime"†

** May be able to step down to $H_2RA$.*

*† For those on longterm PPI, indicating significant GERD, it is reasonable to evaluate for the presence of Barrett's epithelium (a premalignant lesion) and assess for erosive esophagitis (which requires PPIs) vs a normal esophagus (the "hypersensitive" esophagus which sometimes can be controlled with $H_2RA$).*

## **Pharmacologic Choices** (Tables 1 and 2; refer also to Chapter 46)

### Trivial to Mild GERD

Drugs that impair esophageal motility and lower esophageal sphincter tone should be eliminated when possible (e.g., calcium channel blockers, theophylline, tricyclic antidepressants, beta-blockers, anticholinergic agents).

Most people with mild symptoms frequently do not seek medical attention and will obtain symptomatic relief with **antacids**,

**alginates** or nonprescription strength **$H_2$-receptor antagonists** ($H_2RA$). The latter are expensive and yield relatively little acid reduction. Additional therapy becomes necessary if GERD severity increases.

## Significant GERD

Antacids or nonprescription strength $H_2RAs$ are *not* effective alone.

### *$H_2$-receptor Antagonists*

**Cimetidine, ranitidine, famotidine** and **nizatidine** are equally effective. They relieve symptoms in 60% and heal histologically mild esophagitis in over 40% of patients. Their safety profile is excellent (Table 1, Chapter 46). Better results are achieved if the esophagitis is mild, if higher and more frequent doses of $H_2RAs$ are used or if treatment continues for longer periods (up to 12 weeks). Resolution of symptoms, however, does not correlate well with healing of esophagitis. Similarly, some patients with severe esophagitis (ulceration or Barrett's epithelium) have minimal symptoms. When initial therapy is beneficial, maintenance may be necessary if/when symptoms recur and cannot be controlled by nonpharmacologic means. The lowest dose possible should be used to control symptoms and prevent complications.

### *Prokinetic Agents*

**Cisapride** can relieve symptoms and treat mild esophagitis but offers no advantage over $H_2RAs$ and has recently been withdrawn from the market because of its association with serious cardiac arrhythmias and sudden cardiac death. The first-generation prokinetic agents, the dopamine antagonists (**metoclopramide** and **domperidone**), are associated with a high frequency of adverse effects. The addition of a prokinetic agent to an $H_2RA$ improves the response in those who do not respond to $H_2RA$ therapy alone, but such dual therapy provides no advantage over proton pump inhibitors (PPI) alone.

### *Proton Pump Inhibitors*

Marked suppression of acid secretion eliminates acid reflux episodes and selectively heals all grades of esophagitis in most patients (60% by 4 weeks, 80% by 8 weeks). PPIs are more effective and more cost-effective than $H_2RAs$ for rapid relief of symptoms and healing of esophagitis.[1,2] Occasionally a higher dose (e.g., standard dose twice a day) is necessary in those with continued symptoms. Such high dose PPI use is so effective that it can serve as a diagnostic trial. PPIs can heal ulceration but do

---

[1] *Aliment Pharmacol Ther 1999;13:1003–1013.*
[2] *Am J Gastroenterol 2000;95:395–407.*

Table 1: **Drugs Used in Gastroesophageal Reflux Disease**

| Drug | Dosage | | Adverse Effects | Comments | Cost* |
|---|---|---|---|---|---|
| **Antacids** | | | | | |
| Numerous aluminum hydroxide – magnesium hydroxide combinations | 30 mL (regular strength) 1 h PC and QHS | | Constipation, diarrhea. | ↓ bioavailability of digoxin, tetracycline, quinolone antibiotics; separate dosing by 2 h. | $$ |
| **Alginates** | | | | | |
| Gaviscon, Rafton | 10–20 mL or 2–4 tablets (chewed) PC and QHS, followed by glass of water | | Flatulence, eructation. | Alginates and some antacids contain significant amounts of sodium. Alginates alone have limited value. | $–$$ |
| **$H_2$-antagonists** | | | | | |
| **Nonprescription** | **Treatment** | **Maintenance** | See below. | Comparable in efficacy to antacids. | |
| *famotidine* Pepcid AC, others | 10 mg BID | | | | $ |
| *ranitidine* Zantac-75, others | 75 mg BID | | | | $ |
| **Prescription** | | | | | |
| *cimetidine* Tagamet, generics | 600 mg BID | 600 mg BID | Diarrhea, constipation, headache, fatigue, confusion (most likely in elderly and those with poor renal function), cardiac effects, rash. Cimetidine: gynecomastia, impotence (rare). | Cimetidine ↓ cytochrome P-450 metabolism of several agents (e.g., warfarin, phenytoin, theophylline) – use another $H_2$-antagonist; ranitidine has minor effect. | $ |
| *ranitidine* Zantac, generics | 150 mg BID | 150 mg BID | | | $$ |
| *famotidine* Pepcid, generics | 20 mg BID | 20 mg BID | | | $$ |
| *nizatidine* Axid | 150 mg BID | 150 mg BID | | | $$ |

*(cont'd)*

Table 1: **Drugs Used in Gastroesophageal Reflux Disease** *(cont'd)*

| Drug | Dosage | Adverse Effects | Comments | Cost* |
|---|---|---|---|---|
| **Prokinetic Agents** ‡ | | Diarrhea, abdominal discomfort (cramps, distention), headache. | Anticholinergic drugs may antagonize effects on GI motility. | |
| *metoclopramide* Maxeran, Reglan, generics | 5–10 mg TID AC and QHS | | | $ |
| *domperidone* Motilium, generics | 10 mg TID AC and QHS | Hyperprolactinemia (metoclopramide and domperidone). Drowsiness, fatigue, extrapyramidal reactions (metoclopramide). | | $ |
| **Proton Pump Inhibitors** | | | | |
| *omeprazole* Losec | 20–40 mg/day† | Abdominal pain, nausea, headache. | Omeprazole may interfere with cytochrome P-450 metabolized agents (e.g., diazepam, warfarin, phenytoin). | $$$$–$$$$$ |
| *lansoprazole* Prevacid | 30 mg/day | | | $$$ |
| *pantoprazole* Pantoloc | 40 mg/day | | | $$$ |

† *Not to exceed 20 mg/d in hepatic impairment.*
*Dosage adjustment may be required in renal impairment – see Appendix I.*
‡ *Cisapride (Prepulsid) was withdrawn from the market in August 2000 because of reported association with cardiac arrhythmias and sudden cardiac death.*

* *Cost of 30-day supply – includes drug cost only.*
*Legend: $ < $20 $$ $20–40 $$$ $40–60 $$$$ $60–80 $$$$$ > $80*

Table 2: **Efficacy of Drugs Used to Treat GERD**

| | Acute treatment | | Prevention of |
| --- | --- | --- | --- |
| | **Symptoms** | **Esophagitis** | **recurrences** |
| Antacids | + | – | – |
| Alginates/antacids | + | – | – |
| Metoclopramide, domperidone | + | – | – |
| $H_2$-receptor antagonists | ++ | + | ± |
| Proton pump inhibitors | +++ | +++ | +++ |

*+ Drug of proven value (controlled trials).*
*– Not established (negative trial or not tested).*

not reverse Barrett's epithelium. Their use, short and long term, is safe. Choice between the available proton pump inhibitors should be driven by cost rather than subtle differences in pharmacokinetics.

### *Maintenance Therapy for Significant GERD*

The recurrence rate following successful therapy is extremely high (75 to 90%), particularly for erosive/severe esophagitis. PPIs maintain remission more effectively than $H_2$RAs. Maintenance therapy for such significant disease appears to be long term. Cost and safety are concerns with chronic use of proton pump inhibitors. The dose should be tailored to keep the patient symptom-free. Intermittent courses of therapy are reasonable. Using half the regular dose (e.g., omeprazole 10 mg per day) may have a role but requires individual evaluation for effectiveness. In patients also infected with *Helicobacter pylori*, any relation between prolonged acid suppression during maintenance therapy leading to chronic atrophic gastritis, a potential forerunner of gastric carcinoma, is unclear. Eradication of *H. pylori* in GERD will likely increase the need for PPI.[3] Some patients can be switched to an $H_2$RA in "step down" therapy. The informed patient should be involved in any decision concerning lifelong maintenance therapy.

### *Antireflux Surgery*

Antireflux surgery is effective for reflux control in 80% of well-selected patients. Indications include intractable reflux esophagitis (particularly in a young person) and major complications (aspiration, recurrent stricture or major bleeding).

Laparoscopic approaches may become a reasonable, cost-effective treatment, but will require comparison to outcome analysis of long-term therapy with potent acid-suppressing agents.

[3] *Gut 1995;37:743–748.*

## Pharmacoeconomic Considerations

*Jeffrey A. Johnson, PhD*

A number of pharmacoeconomic evaluations of therapeutic choices for GERD have been conducted. In general, these evaluations indicate that proton-pump inhibitors are more cost-effective than $H_2$-antagonists, for grades II to IV esophagitis. For example, a CCHOTA evaluation indicated that, even though the acquisition cost of an 8-week course of omeprazole was almost three times that of an 8-week course of ranitidine, omeprazole was more cost-effective because downstream costs were avoided due to higher healing rates and lower recurrence rates. The study concluded that substituting maintenance ranitidine therapy with intermittent omeprazole therapy would result in savings of $52,000 and an extra 3,410 weeks of time free from GERD per 1,000 patients treated per year. Maintenance omeprazole would be even more effective, resulting in 6,220 extra weeks free from GERD, but at an additional cost of $348,000 per 1,000 patients treated per year, when compared to maintenance ranitidine therapy.

Recent studies have further supported the economic benefit of using PPIs over other treatment strategies in GERD. Including HRQOL outcomes also indicates that PPI is a cost-effective choice in treating GERD. As might be expected, the cost-effectiveness improves when considering treatment for persons with moderate to severe GERD compared to those with milder symptoms. However, there is also evidence from drug utilization studies to suggest that there may be widespread use of PPIs outside of current prescribing guidelines, which can potentially result in a negative economic impact on drug and total health care budgets.

***Suggested Reading***

*Gerson LB, Robbins AS, Garber A, Hornberger J, Triadafilopoulos G. A cost-effectiveness analysis of prescribing strategies in the management of gastroesophageal disease. Am J Gastroenterol 2000;95:395–407.*

*Pillans PI, Kubler PA, Radford JM, Overland V. Concordance between use of proton pump inhibitors and prescribing guidelines. Med J Aust 2000;172:16–18.*

*Thomson AB, Chiba N, Armstrong D, Tougas G, Hunt RH. The second Canadian gastroesophageal reflux disease consensus: moving forward to new concepts. Can J Gastroenterol 1998;12:551–556.*

### *Suggested Reading List*

Beck IT, Champion MC, Lemire S, Thomson ABR. The second Canadian consensus conference on the treatment of patients with gastroesophageal reflux disease. *Can J Gastroenterol* 1997;11(suppl B).

DeVault KR, Castell DO. Guidelines for the diagnosis and treatment of gastroesophageal reflux disease. *Arch Intern Med* 1995;155:2165–2173.

Moss SJ, Arnold R, Tytgat GNJ, Spechler SJ, Fave GD, Rosin D, Jensen RT. Consensus statement for management of gastroesophageal reflux disease. *J Clin Gastroenterol* 1998;27:6–12.

Sridhar S, Huang J, O'Brien BJ, Hunt RH. Clinical economics review: cost-effectiveness of treatment alternatives for gastroesophageal reflux disease. *Aliment Pharmacol Ther* 1996;10:865–873.

Thomson ABR, Chiba N, Armstrong D, Tougas G, Hunt RN. The second Canadian gastroesophageal reflux disease consensus. Moving forward to new concepts. *Can J Gastroenterol* 1998;12:551–556.

CHAPTER 46

# Peptic Ulcer Disease and Upper Gastrointestinal Bleeding

*A.B.R. Thomson, MD, PhD, FRCPC, FACG*

## *Peptic Ulcer Disease*

Dyspepsia, defined as pain or discomfort in the upper abdomen, is one of the most common complaints bringing patients to consult their family physician. The most common causes of dyspepsia include non-ulcer dyspepsia (NUD), gastroesophageal reflux disease (GERD) (Chapter 45 ), duodenal ulcer (DU) and gastric ulcer (GU). DU and GU are considered to be two of the *Helicobacter pylori*-associated diseases, and both are components of the gastroenteropathy associated with nonsteroidal anti-inflammatory drugs (NSAIDs).

### Goals of Therapy

- To relieve dyspepsia and prevent ulcer disease complications
- To alter the natural history of disease recurrence by curing associated *H. pylori* infection, by eliminating unnecessary use of NSAIDs, or by providing maintenance therapy with potent acid-lowering medications
- To accomplish these goals in a cost-effective manner to optimize the quality of the patient's life

### Investigations

- History and physical examination
  - determine the character of the dyspeptic symptoms (ulcer-like, reflux-like or dysmotility-like)
  - inquire into possible alarm symptoms (dysphagia, anemia, or weight loss)
  - exclude nongastrointestinal sources of pain or discomfort in the upper abdomen (e.g., ischemic heart disease)
  - take a drug history for NSAIDs/ASA use
  - physical examination will usually be normal. Epigastric tenderness is a common but nonspecific finding
- *H. pylori* infection

The only reliable non-endoscopic test for *H. pylori* infection is the $^{14}C$ or $^{13}C$ urea breath test (UBT). The $^{13}C$ (nonradioactive) UBT is recommended for use in children and women of child-bearing years.

Because of the relatively low prevalence of *H. pylori* infection in Canada (about 30% in the adult population), the positive predictive value of serological testing for *H. pylori* is relatively low. On the other hand, a negative serological test for *H. pylori* has a high negative predictive value, confidently indicating that the patient does not have an infection. Under special circumstances it may be necessary to prove *H. pylori* eradication, and this can be accomplished with UBT but not with serology. Where available, the direct cost to the patient of serology is approximately $30 per test, whereas the cost of UBT is about $60.

- Esophagogastroduodenoscopy (EGD)

EGD is the investigation of choice in the patient with ulcer-like dyspepsia, particularly in the patient over the age of 55 with new onset dyspepsia, in any patient with alarm symptoms, when GU is reported on an upper GI series (to obtain biopsies to exclude gastric cancer), or to diagnose an *H. pylori* infection when UBT is not available.

- Upper Gastrointestinal Barium Study

The upper GI series has an approximately 20% false-positive and false-negative rate for ulcer disease, and is generally not recommended. However, barium studies are generally more available than UBT or EGD, and are still used, perhaps falsely, to reassure the physician that nothing serious has been missed. An upper GI series should not be performed in the patient with bleeding from the upper gastrointestinal tract.

## Therapeutic Choices

### Nonpharmacologic Choices

- Bland diets are no longer prescribed. A simple rule of thumb is to use moderation if a food or beverage makes dyspepsia worse. Common offenders are coffee, orange juice, spicy foods, fatty foods, large meals, or eating on the run.
- Smoking – before the importance of *H. pylori* in the etiology of PUD was recognized, patients were advised to stop smoking in order to improve ulcer healing rates and reduce the risk of ulcer recurrence. Now this can be achieved with *H. pylori* eradication. However, the opportunity to recommend to the patient that they stop smoking for general health reasons must not be lost.
- Stress and a type A personality are still considered by many to predispose to ulcer disease. With the discovery that most peptic ulcers are caused by *H. pylori*, the role of stress may be played down, but stress management should be added to the general advice offered about useful lifestyle changes.

## Pharmacologic Choices (Figure 1, Table 1)

### *Approach to the Management*

If the patient is suspected to have an ulcer on the basis of their dyspepsia, there are 3 commonly used approaches:

- *Empirical therapy* – treat with a proton pump inhibitor (PPI) once a day in the morning for 2 to 4 weeks, or an $H_2$-receptor antagonist ($H_2RA$) twice a day for 4 to 6 weeks. See the patient in follow-up and investigate with a UBT for *H. pylori* infection, or with prompt endoscopy for those who do not improve with the initial trial of PPI/$H_2RA$, or those who have frequent recurrences.

  The advantage of empirical therapy is that it is an office-based approach which does not require initial investigations such as UBT or EGD. The disadvantage is that some patients do not lose their dyspepsia, or the symptoms recur and there is no diagnosis.

- *Test-and-treat* – a diagnostic test is performed for *H. pylori*, and a positive test result is treated with triple therapy (Table 2). This approach assumes that if the patient's dyspepsia is caused by DU/GU, then they will be positive for *H. pylori*. About 90% of DU and 70% of GU may be *H. pylori* positive, although the association may be less striking in community practice, or in patients with a past history of an ulcer complicated by bleeding.

  The advantage of this cost-effective approach is that the investigations needed to diagnose *H. pylori*, when available in the community, can be readily used by the family physician and the results are rapidly available. The disadvantage is that serology and UBT are not universally available in all communities in Canada, and the cost of these tests is not usually covered by provincial health care plans.

- *Prompt endoscopy* – the most sensitive and specific means to diagnose the cause of the patient's dyspepsia is EGD, preferably performed within a week of the patient presenting to the medical provider. EGD permits the diagnosis of erosive esophagitis, Barrett's epithelium, gastric or duodenal ulcer, gastric or duodenal erosions, *H. pylori* infection, or gastric cancer. The patient and physician will be reassured, and the patient's future use of medications and health care resources may be lessened.

  The disadvantages of prompt endoscopy are self-evident. In many Canadian communities, the average waiting time to consult a gastroenterologist to arrange for an EGD is at least 6 weeks and may be as long as 4 months. Time is lost from work, the procedure is expensive to the health care system (total cost approximately $400), and there is a very small but real risk of a complication such as aspiration or perforation.

Figure 1: **Management of Suspected Peptic Ulcers**

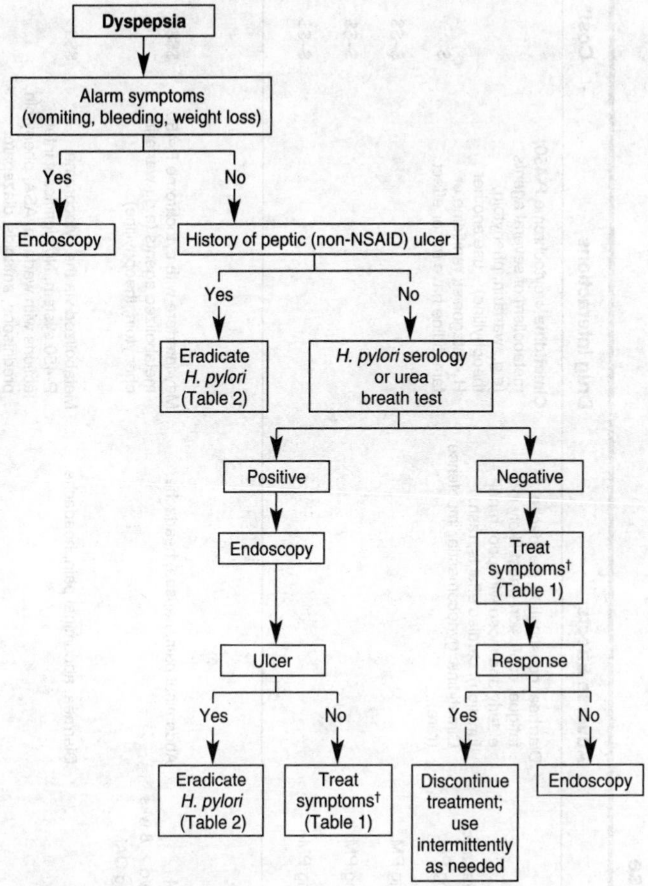
Dyspepsia
Alarm symptoms (vomiting, bleeding, weight loss)
Yes
No
Endoscopy
History of peptic (non-NSAID) ulcer
Yes
No
Eradicate H. pylori (Table 2)
H. pylori serology or urea breath test
Positive
Negative
Endoscopy
Treat symptoms† (Table 1)
Ulcer
Response
Yes
No
Yes
No
Eradicate H. pylori (Table 2)
Treat symptoms† (Table 1)
Discontinue treatment; use intermittently as needed
Endoscopy

† *Treat symptoms; lifestyle changes, diet, short courses (no more than 4 wks) of OTC antacids/$H_2$-receptor antagonist ($H_2RA$) and therapeutic doses of $H_2RA$, proton pump inhibitor.*

*Adapted with permission from Thomson ABR. A suggested approach to patients with dyspepsia. Can J Gastroenterol 1997;11:135–140.*

## *Modest Acid Inhibition*

Over-the-counter (OTC) therapy with antacids or $H_2RAs$ are commonly used by patients before seeking medical advice. They provide moderate benefit for mild symptoms.

Prescription doses of $H_2RAs$ may be used for symptom relief but are much less (30% to 50%) effective for pain relief or ulcer healing than PPIs, and must be used twice a day and for longer periods (4 to 6 weeks for $H_2RAs$ versus 2 to 4 weeks for PPIs).

Table 1: **Drugs Used in Peptic Ulcer Disease**

| Drug | Dosage | | Adverse Effects | Drug Interactions | Cost* |
|---|---|---|---|---|---|
| **$H_2$-antagonists** | **Treatment length:**<br>4–8 wks for DU<br>8–12 wks for GU | | Diarrhea, constipation, headache, fatigue, confusion (most likely in elderly and those with poor renal function), cardiac effects, rash. Cimetidine: gynecomastia, impotence (rare). | **Cimetidine** ↓ cytochrome P-450 metabolism of several agents (e.g., warfarin, phenytoin, theophylline) – use another $H_2$-antagonist; ranitidine or famotidine have minor effect. | |
| | **Treatment** | **Maintenance** | | | |
| *cimetidine*<br>Tagamet, generics | 300 mg BID | 400 mg PM | | | $ |
| *ranitidine*<br>Zantac, generics | 150 mg BID | 150 mg PM | | | $–$$ |
| *famotidine*<br>Pepcid, generics | 20 mg BID | 20 mg PM | | | $–$$ |
| *nizatidine*<br>Axid, generics | 150 mg BID | 150 mg PM | | | $–$$ |
| **Proton Pump Inhibitors** | **Treatment length:**<br>2–4 wks for DU<br>4–8 wks for GU | | | | |
| *omeprazole*<br>Losec | Treatment: 20 mg QAM<br>NSAID-induced: 20 mg/d × 8 wks<br>Maintenance: 10–20 mg QAM | | Abdominal pain, nausea, headache. | May interfere with cytochrome P-450 metabolized agents (e.g., warfarin, phenytoin, theophylline). | $$$$ |
| *lansoprazole*<br>Prevacid | Treatment: 30 mg/d† | | Diarrhea, abdominal pain, headache. | Metabolized via the cytochrome P-450 system. No significant interactions with warfarin, ASA, phenytoin, prednisone, antacids, diazepam. | $$$ |

| | | | | |
|---|---|---|---|---|
| *pantoprazole* Pantoloc | Treatment: 40 mg/d | Diarrhea, headache, dizziness, pruritus. | Metabolized via the cytochrome P-450 system. No interactions with diazepam, phenytoin, nifedipine, theophylline, warfarin, digoxin, oral contraceptives or antacids. | $$$ |
| *misoprostol* Cytotec | Treatment: 200 µg QID | Diarrhea (dose-related), abdominal cramps, flatulence. **Contraindicated in pregnancy** – abortifacient. | | $$$ |
| *sucralfate* ◗ Sulcrate, generics | Treatment: 1 g QID 4–8 wks for DU 8–12 wks for GU Maintenance: 1 g BID | Constipation, aluminum absorption. (Avoid in renal failure.) | Intraluminal drug binding may ↓ absorption of antibiotics, ketoconazole, warfarin, digoxin, NSAIDs, theophylline; separate dosing by 2 h. | $ |

† *Taken 30 min. before breakfast.*

◗ *Dosage adjustment may be required in renal impairment – see Appendix I.*

* *Cost of 30-day (treatment dosages) supply – includes drug cost only.*

*Legend:* $ < $20 $$ $20–40 $$$ $40–60 $$$$ $60–80

Tachyphylaxis (loss of effectiveness over time) may develop quickly, and the $H_2RAs$ have no role to play in the approved regimens used to eradicate *H. pylori*.

### Extensive Acid Inhibition

In order to heal DU with acid-lowering therapy, the intragastric pH must be maintained over 3. The more hours each day that there is a pH >3, the higher the rate of ulcer healing or the shorter the duration of therapy.[1] The duration of use of PPI needed to heal a DU is shortened to one week when triple therapy is used to eradicate an associated *H. pylori* infection. For those individuals with a DU or GU not associated with either *H. pylori* infection or use of NSAIDs, once a day PPI should be used for 2 to 4 weeks, and maintenance therapy must be considered on an individualized basis. The PPIs provide fast symptom relief and high ulcer healing rates: about 80% of DU heal in 2 weeks, 90% in 4 weeks. About 80% of GU heal in 4 weeks, 90% in 8 weeks. Patients with a GU must have a follow-up EGD to prove ulcer healing in order to avoid the rare initial misdiagnosis of a gastric cancer.

### Maintenance Therapy

Continuous use of acid inhibition, preferably with a PPI, may be needed in selected patients with DU/GU not associated with *H. pylori* infection, especially when the ulcer was complicated by bleeding or perforation, or when the patient suffers from frequent recurrences.

Some ulcer patients cured of their *H. pylori* infection may develop *de novo* reflux-like dyspepsia, and require intermittent or continuous PPI. Finally, as discussed later, some high-risk patients requiring continuous use of NSAIDs may need to be maintained on PPIs to reduce the risk of recurrent GU/DU.

### Eradication of H. pylori Infection (Table 2)

Eradication of *H. pylori* infection is more cost-effective than maintenance therapy with acid-lowering medications and reduces the risk of developing gastric cancer or mucosa-associated lymphoid tissue (MALT) lymphoma.

Treatment regimens approved by the Canadian Helicobacter Study Group Consensus and update statements achieve a minimum eradication rate (on an intention-to-treat basis) of at least 80%. First-line therapy includes PPI or ranitidine bismuth citrate (RBC) plus 2 antibiotics (clarithromycin and amoxicillin or metronidazole) twice daily for 1 week (Table 2). Because the prevalence of metronidazole resistance in Canada is about 20% and resistance to amoxicillin is less than 1%, increasing use is made of the amoxicillin-containing regimen.

[1] *Arch Intern Med 1999;159:649–657.*

If the patient fails one triple-therapy regimen, repeat treatment with a different antibiotic combination, or switch RBC for the PPI, or treat for 2 rather than 1 week, or use quadruple therapy (PPI, bismuth, metronidazole plus tetracycline). After successful *H. pylori* eradication, the risk of reinfection is only about 1% per year.

Repeated testing by UBT or endoscopic biopsies to prove eradication is necessary in patients with a complicated ulcer (bleeding or perforation) to ensure healing and prevent recurrence. In the occasional patient who experiences recurrent dyspepsia after the use of an approved eradication regimen, it may be necessary to prove successful eradication before looking for new causes of dyspepsia, such as GERD.

### *NSAID-associated Ulcers*

Unlike *H. pylori*-associated ulcers, GU/DU caused by NSAIDs are more likely to be painless, and patients often present for the first time with a complication such as bleeding or perforation. For *H. pylori*-associated ulcers the ratio of DU:GU is 2:1 to 3:1; the ratio is opposite for NSAID-associated lesions. Over a one year interval, about 3% of NSAID users will develop a GU/DU. This risk is reduced to about 1 to 2%, but not eliminated, by the use of one of the new COX-2 inhibitors.

Table 2: ***H. pylori* Eradication Regimens**

| Regimen | Dosage | Treatment Period | Cost* |
|---|---|---|---|
| **Triple Therapy** | | | |
| PPI† or RBC ❥ | BID | 7 days | $$$$ |
| clarithromycin | 500 mg BID | | |
| amoxicillin | 1 g BID | | |
| PPI‡ or RBC ❥ | BID | 7 days | $$$$ |
| clarithromycin | 250 mg BID | | |
| metronidazole | 500 mg BID | | |
| **Quadruple Therapy** | | | |
| PPI | BID | 7 days | |
| bismuth subsalicylate | 2 tabs QID | | $$$ |
| metronidazole | 250 mg QID | | |
| tetracycline ❥ | 500 mg QID | | |

*Abbreviations: PPI = lansoprazole 30 mg BID or omeprazole 20 mg BID or pantoprazole 40 mg BID. RBC = ranitidine bismuth citrate 400 mg BID.*

*† Available as Hp-Pac (lansoprazole/clarithromycin/amoxicillin). Losec 1-2-3 A refers to an omeprazole/clarithromycin/amoxicillin regimen.*

*‡ Losec 1-2-3 M refers to an omeprazole/clarithromycin/metronidazole regimen.*

** Cost per treatment period – includes drug cost only.*

*Legend: $ < $20 $$ $20–40 $$$ $40–60 $$$$ $60–80*

❥ *Dosage adjustment may be required in renal impairment – see Appendix I.*

The risk of developing an NSAID ulcer is greater in persons over the age of 65, with the use of more than one NSAID, concomitant use of steroids or anticoagulants, a past history of ulcer disease, and coexisting ischemic heart disease. Such an individual should be offered gastric protective therapy with a PPI or misoprostol 200 μg QID. The role of *H. pylori* in the development of NSAID ulcers is unclear. Eradicating *H. pylori* may reduce the risk of developing an ulcer in first-time NSAID users, but there is no need to look for or treat *H. pylori* in chronic NSAID users, since there is a possibility that the infection may reduce the risk of development of NSAID lesions.

## *Upper Gastrointestinal Bleeding* (Figure 2)

Upper gastrointestinal bleeding (UGIB) is a common medical emergency, with a mortality rate of about 7%, especially in older persons with comorbid conditions. Common causes include DU/GU, gastric or esophageal erosions, or esophageal varices. Rarely, there may be massive bleeding from an eroded gastric blood vessel (the Dieulafoy lesion).

### Goals of Therapy

- To resuscitate and save the patient's life
- To prevent hypoxia-related damage to other organs such as kidneys or heart
- To heal the underlying lesion
- To prevent recurrences of UGIB

### Investigations

- History and physical examination:
  - perform quickly and begin appropriate resuscitation to restore circulating blood volume
  - cause of bleeding may be suggested by history: *ulcer disease* – present history of pain, past history of ulcer, use of NSAIDs; *varices* – signs of liver disease in patients at risk e.g., alcohol abuse, infectious hepatitis B or C; retching or vomiting followed by bleeding is suggestive of a Mallory-Weiss tear.
  - prognosis is usually worse if the patient is vomiting fresh blood or passing red blood per rectum.
  - coffee-ground emesis or passage of a melena stool implies slower loss of a smaller volume of blood
- Blood is drawn for "stat" type and cross match (usually 4 units of packed red blood cells or more depending on severity of bleeding), hemoglobin concentration or hematocrit, electrolytes, renal function (creatinine or BUN), and coagulation studies (platelet count, INR and PTT)

Figure 2: **Management of Acute Upper GI Bleeding**

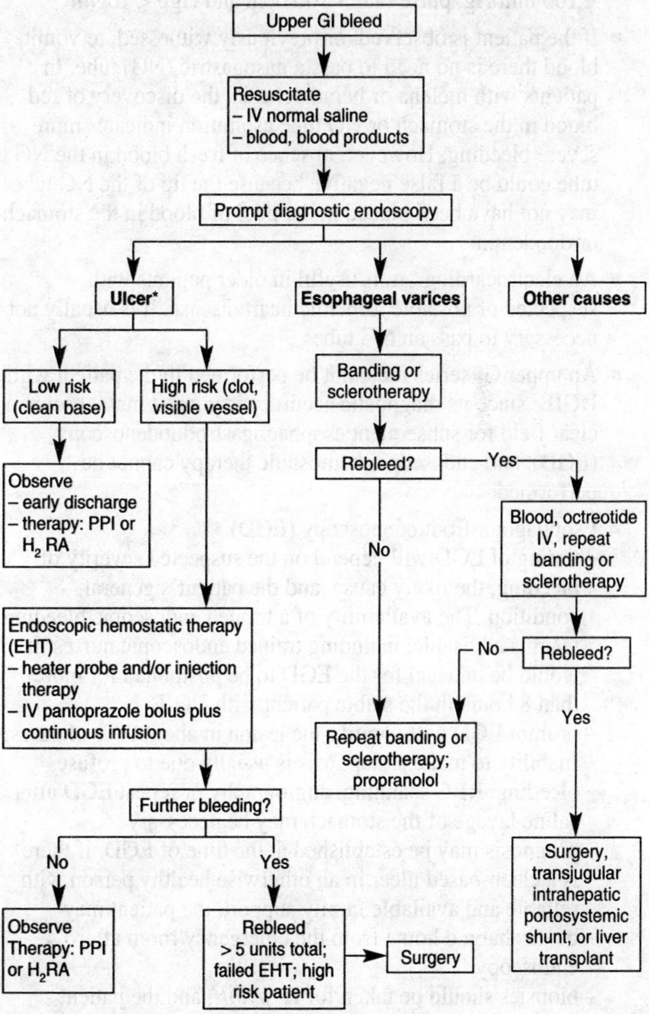
Upper GI bleed
Resuscitate
– IV normal saline
– blood, blood products
Prompt diagnostic endoscopy
Ulcer*
Esophageal varices
Other causes
Low risk (clean base)
High risk (clot, visible vessel)
Observe
– early discharge
– therapy: PPI or $H_2$ RA
Endoscopic hemostatic therapy (EHT)
– heater probe and/or injection therapy
– IV pantoprazole bolus plus continuous infusion
Further bleeding?
No
Yes
Observe
Therapy: PPI or $H_2$RA
Rebleed
> 5 units total; failed EHT; high risk patient
Surgery
Banding or sclerotherapy
Rebleed?
Yes
No
Blood, octreotide IV, repeat banding or sclerotherapy
Rebleed?
No
Yes
Repeat banding or sclerotherapy; propranolol
Surgery, transjugular intrahepatic portosystemic shunt, or liver transplant

** Antral biopsies may be taken at endoscopy to determine H. pylori status.*
*If not done initially, wait 2 weeks after stopping PPI before repeating endoscopy for biopsy or UBT.*
*If H. pylori positive, treat, repeat H. pylori testing and retreat if necessary.*
*If bleeding DU not associated with H. pylori or NSAID use, offer PPI maintenance therapy to minimize risk of recurrent DU and bleeding.*
*Patient with GU, biopsy to rule out gastric cancer.*

- Rapid estimate of blood loss can be made at the bedside: 50% loss of blood volume is suggested by systolic pressure < 100 mm Hg, pulse rate > 100 bpm and Hgb < 10g/dl
- If the patient is observed, or previously witnessed, to vomit blood there is no need to pass a nasogastric (NG) tube. In patients with melena or hematochezia, the discovery of red blood in the stomach or NG tube aspiration indicates more severe bleeding. However, absence of fresh blood in the NG tube could be a false negative because the tip of the NG tube may not have been placed in the pool of blood in the stomach or duodenum
- An electrocardiogram is useful in older patients with suspected or possible ischemic heart disease. It is usually not necessary to pass an NG tube
- An upper GI series must not be performed in the patient with UGIB; since its diagnostic accuracy is poor, it may obscure a clear field for subsequent esophagogastroduodenoscopy (EGD), and endoscopic hemostatic therapy cannot be performed
- Esophagogastroduodenoscopy (EGD)
  - timing of EGD will depend on the suspected severity of bleeding, the likely cause, and the patient's general condition. The availability of a trained endoscopic bleeding team is advisable, including trained endoscopic nurses. It would be unusual for the EGD to be postponed for more than 8 hours in the stable patient with UGIB
  - prompt EGD will identify the lesion in about 90% of cases. Inability to make a diagnosis is usually due to profuse bleeding. RBC scanning, angiography or repeat EGD after saline lavage of the stomach may be necessary
  - prognosis may be established at the time of EGD. If there is a clean-based ulcer in an otherwise healthy person with reliable and available family support, the patient may be discharged home from the emergency room after endoscopy
  - biopsies should be taken for *H. pylori*, and the patient treated appropriately with PPI for 4 weeks if they are *H. pylori* negative, and triple therapy if *H. pylori* positive. In this setting, follow-up testing for *H. pylori* is essential to prove successful eradication and thereby remove the risk of ulcer recurrence and recurrent bleeding

## Therapeutic Choices

### Nonpharmacologic Choices

Efforts are quickly made to ensure protection of the airway, provide supplementary nasal oxygen, and placement of at least two large bore (#18 or larger) IV lines.

### *Endoscopic Treatment*

In the more serious lesions seen in EGD, such as an ulcer with an adherent clot, visible vessel or active bleeding, the bleeding site must be treated endoscopically. This can be achieved with injection of **saline**, **epinephrine** (1:10 000) or a **sclerosant** (e.g., ethanolamine or polidocanol). Alternatively, **thermal techniques** may be used (e.g., heater probe or electrocautery). Recent evidence suggests that a combination of injection plus thermal techniques is preferable. For patients with a high risk of rebleeding, "second look" endoscopy is indicated in 24 to 48 hours.

In **bleeding esophageal varices**, endoscopic sclerotherapy or band ligation may be life saving. Band ligation may be easier to perform in the actively bleeding patient, and multiple bands may be placed at one sitting. The use of an overtube is recommended. Sclerosants include ethanolamine, absolute alcohol, polidocanol, or sodium tetradecyl sulfate. These are of comparable efficacy. For bleeding gastric varices, tissue adhesives (e.g., Krazy Glue®) may be carefully applied. Sclerotherapy is more commonly associated with the complications of esophageal ulceration or stricture than is banding. Either sclerotherapy or banding are useful to stop variceal bleeding, but the patient is just as likely to die from other complications of their underlying liver disease.

For the patient with **portal hypertension** and **varices** that have not yet bled, it remains controversial whether prophylactic therapy is useful to reduce the risk of the first episode of bleeding.

Injection or thermal therapy may be useful for the patient bleeding actively from a **Mallory-Weiss** tear or a **Dieulafoy** lesion.

## Pharmacologic Choices

### *Nonvariceal UGIB*

Meta-analysis has suggested that there is a modest benefit to using IV $H_2$RAs for patients with nonvariceal UGIB, but a single large prospective study has not proven this benefit. Where endoscopic hemostatic therapy (EHT) is not available, **omeprazole** 40 mg BID has been shown to be useful to reduce the risk of rebleeding, the number of units of blood transfused, or the need for surgery. When EHT is available, this may be supplemented with profound acid inhibition using omeprazole or IV **pantoprazole** (see below). Three prospective studies have shown a reduced degree or duration of bleeding, transfusion requirements or need for surgery. Where available, optimal therapy would include early EGD, EHT depending on the nature of the bleeding site, and acid inhibition with IV PPI to stabilize the clot and to reduce ulcer bleeding. Pantoprazole is given IV as an 80 mg bolus over 2 hours followed by 8 mg/hr continuous infusion for 2 to 3 days until the bleeding is stopped, then switch to an oral PPI to heal the associated ulcer. At some stage the patient's *H. pylori* status must be determined, and appropriate eradication therapy offered. Patients whose ulcers are not associated with *H. pylori* infection or NSAID use should be placed and kept on maintenance therapy with a PPI.

### Bleeding Esophageal Varices

For bleeding esophageal varices, sclerotherapy/banding may be supplemented with pharmacologic agents targeted to reduce portal pressure. The long-acting somatostatin analog, **octreotide**, has been shown to improve the prognosis. IV octreotide is given as 100 μg bolus followed by an infusion of 50 μg/hour for up to 2 days after the bleeding stops (mix 500 μg octreotide in 500 mL of 0.9% NaCl and infuse at 50 mL/hr). **Vasopressin** also lowers portal pressure and may be given as a dose of 20 units in 20 mL 5% dextrose over 20 minutes, followed by an infusion of 0.4 units/min for up to 2 days. Caution must be used in the patient with myocardial ischemia or peripheral vascular disease. Where octreotide or banding/sclerotherapy are not available, vasopressin may be given with nitroglycerin in the hope of avoiding ischemic events.

**Beta-blockers** may be used prophylactically in the patient with esophageal varices to prevent the initial bleed, or to reduce the risk of recurrent bleeding.[2] In patients with high-risk (large) esophageal varices, endoscopic ligation of the varices is safe and more effective than propranolol for the primary prevention of variceal bleeding.

## Suggested Reading List


*Peptic Ulcer Disease*

Hawkey CJ, Karrash JA, Szczepanski L. Omeprazole compared with misoprostol for ulcers associated with nonsteroidal anti-inflammatory. *N Engl J Med* 1998;338:727–734.

Hunt RH, Thomson ABR. Canadian *Helicobacter pylori* Consensus Conference. *Can J Gastroenterol* 1998;12:31–41.

Veldhuyzen van Zanten SJO, Flook N, Chiba N, et al. An evidence-based approach to the management of uninvestigated dyspepsia in the era of *Helicobacter pylori*. *Can Med Assoc J* 2000; 162(12 Suppl): S3–S23.


[2] *Hepatology 1997;21:63–70.*

*Upper Gastrointestinal Bleeding*

Khurro M, Yattoo G, Javid G. A comparison of omeprazole and placebo for bleeding peptic ulcer. *N Engl J Med* 1997;336: 1054–1058.

Lai KC, Hui WM, Wong BCY. A retrospective and prospective study on the safety of discharging selected patients with duodenal ulcer bleeding on the same day as endoscopy. *Gastro Endos* 1997;45:26–30.

Lau JYW, Sung SSY, Lan YH. Endoscopic retreatment compared with surgery in patients with recurrent bleeding after initial endoscopic control of bleeding ulcers. *N Engl J Med* 1999;340: 751–756.

CHAPTER 47

# Inflammatory Bowel Disease

*Brian G. Feagan, MD, FRCPC*

The idiopathic inflammatory bowel diseases (IBD) consist of Crohn's disease (CD), ulcerative colitis (UC) and ulcerative proctitis (UP). CD may involve any part of the gastrointestinal tract, while UC is restricted to the colon. UP is a variant of UC, which involves less than 30 cm of the distal colon.

## Investigations

- History:
  - diarrhea, abdominal pain, rectal bleeding and weight loss are the most important symptoms
  - presence of nocturnal diarrhea usually indicates "organic" pathology
  - extraintestinal manifestations (e.g., aphthous ulcers, arthritis, erythema nodosum, iritis, perianal disease, fever)
  - genetics: increased risk with family history, Ashkenazi Jews
  - previous endoscopic/radiologic test results
  - previous medical/surgical treatment
- Physical examination: abdominal tenderness, presence of abdominal mass, malnutrition, perianal disease (fistulae, abscess)
  - growth failure in children (chart height and weight, Tanner stage)
  - extraintestinal manifestations
- Precise diagnosis:
  - biopsy/histopathology, small bowel x-rays
  - presence of small bowel involvement, granulomata is pathognomonic for CD
- 10% of cases cannot be classified and are termed *indeterminate colitis*
- A definitive diagnosis is important since:
  - colectomy cures UC; CD recurs following surgery
  - differential responses to drug therapy (especially aminosalicylates)
- Precise anatomic localization is necessary for selecting drug therapy and planning surgery

- Laboratory tests:
  – measures of inflammation (WBC, Hgb, ESR, albumin)
  – stool cultures

## Goals of Therapy

- To relieve symptoms and improve patients' quality of life
- To improve nutritional status and growth (children/adolescents)
- To prevent disease recurrence
- To prevent development of colon cancer (UC)

## Therapeutic Choices (Table 1)

Therapy is determined by site and extent of disease, and the severity of symptoms.

### Pharmacologic Choices

Management of IBD includes the use of aminosalicylates, corticosteroids, immunosuppressives, antibiotics, antidiarrheals and opioid analgesics.

#### *Aminosalicylates*

Preparations containing **5-aminosalicylic acid** (5-ASA) are formulated to release the drug at specific sites in the GI tract, since efficacy is dependent on luminal concentration. Salofalk, Mesasal and Pentasa release 5-ASA into the small bowel. Sulfasalazine, olsalazine and Asacol release 5-ASA primarily into the colon.

5-ASA has only modest efficacy in active CD (40% efficacy for induction of remission vs 30% with placebo) and is generally used in mild cases. Although clinical trials have evaluated only sulfasalazine and Pentasa for this indication, the other preparations are often used interchangeably.

**Sulfasalazine** has the least favorable adverse effect profile; however, many of these effects are minor and dose-related. The majority of these events (> 90%) are related to the sulfapyridine moiety which is not present in 5-ASA preparations. Oligospermia, reversible on withdrawal of sulfasalazine, has been reported. 5-ASA can be substituted, as male infertility has not been associated with its use.

#### *Corticosteroids*

Patients with a moderately severe exacerbation of CD are treated initially with **prednisone** 40 to 60 mg per day. In those with severe disease, hospitalization and **IV steroids** (e.g., hydrocortisone) may be necessary. Patients who respond to IV therapy are switched to prednisone once stabilized. The prednisone dose is then tapered as improvement occurs (total duration of therapy is 12 to 16 weeks).

Long-term use of corticosteroids is restricted to those unresponsive to other drugs. Patients must be made aware of potential side effects, and informed consent obtained. Osteoporosis is a concern with long-term therapy. Adequate calcium intake, smoking cessation, exercise and, in selected individuals, treatment with vitamin D and bisphosphonates are useful interventions. In addition, use of glucocorticoids is associated with avascular necrosis of the femoral head.

**Budesonide** is rapidly inactivated in the liver resulting in lower systemic bioavailability and a reduced effect on the hypothalamic-pituitary-adrenal axis. It is available as an oral controlled-release capsule for the treatment of terminal ileal/right sided colonic CD, and as an enema for use in UC. In clinical trials, response rates for oral budesonide are marginally less than those observed with prednisone for active CD (50 to 60% vs 70%); Cushing's syndrome occurs less frequently. Budesonide enemas are as effective as other steroid enemas, have a lower incidence of side effects, but are more costly.

### *Immunosuppressives*

**Azathioprine**, **6-mercaptopurine (6-MP)**, or **methotrexate** are used in some refractory patients with CD to control symptoms or reduce the dose of prednisone. All immunosuppressive drugs have important side effects which must be considered (e.g., bone marrow suppression and cytopenias). Hypersensitivity pneumonitis and hepatotoxicity are associated with methotrexate. Pancreatitis occurs in approximately 3% of patients treated with azathioprine or 6-MP.

### *Biologics*

**Infliximab**, a chimeric (murine/human) antibody directed towards tumor necrosis factor alpha (TNFα) has been shown effective for induction of remission[1] and closure of fistulas[2] in patients with active Crohn's disease which is refractory to other forms of treatment. Infusion reactions may be minor (headache, flushing, lightheadedness) or major (manifestations of anaphylaxis). The development of serum sickness, antinuclear antibody formation, rarely a lupus-like syndrome and possibly lymphoma are important concerns.

---

[1] *N Engl J Med 1997;337:1029–1035.*
[2] *N Engl J Med 1999;340:1398–1405.*

Table 1: **Drugs Used in the Treatment of Inflammatory Bowel Disease**

| Drug | Dosage | | Comments | Cost* |
|---|---|---|---|---|
| **Corticosteroids** | | | | |
| Injectable | | | | |
| *hydrocortisone* – Solu-Cortef, generics | 300–400 mg/d IV | | Adverse effects: acne, glucose intolerance, weight gain, hypertension, hypokalemia, osteoporosis, aseptic necrosis of femoral head, adrenal insufficiency with sudden cessation. | $$$ |
| *methylprednisolone* – Solu-Medrol, generics | 40–60 mg/d IV | | No advantage over hydrocortisone. | $$$$$ |
| Oral | | | | |
| *prednisone* – generics | 30–60 mg/d PO (Q am) | | Useful in moderately severe and severe UC and CD. No role in maintenance therapy. | $ |
| *budesonide* – Entocort | 9 mg/d PO (acute exacerbation)<br>3–6 mg/d PO (maintenance) | | Controlled-release capsule for treating CD in the ileum and/or ascending colon. Rapidly metabolized, somewhat fewer adverse effects than conventional corticosteroids. | $–$$ |
| Topical | | | | |
| *hydrocortisone* – Cortenema, Cortifoam, Hycort | 80–100 mg QHS | | Enemas effective in ulcerative proctitis (UP). | $$$ |
| *betamethasone* – Betnesol | 5 mg QHS | | Topical therapy, in general, has less severe adverse effects than systemic therapy. | $$$ |
| *budesonide* – Entocort | 2 mg QHS | | | $$$ |
| **Aminosalicylates** | Active (UC) | Maintenance (UC) | All aminosalicylates are equally effective in UC. | |
| Oral | | | | |
| *sulfasalazine* Salazopyrin, generics | ≥ 4 g/d divided | 2–3 g/d divided | Sulfasalazine 4–8 g/d has shown moderate benefit in CD. Dose-related adverse effects of sulfasalazine: nausea, vomiting, diarrhea, anorexia, headache. Hypersensitivity reactions (rash, fever), aplastic anemia, oligospermia (reversible). | $ |
| *olsalazine* Dipentum | > 1 g/d divided | 1 g/d divided | Olsalazine: ↑ diarrhea, may be minimized by gradually increasing the dose. | $ |

(cont'd)

Table 1: **Drugs Used in the Treatment of Inflammatory Bowel Disease** *(cont'd)*

| Drug | Dosage | | Comments | Cost* |
|---|---|---|---|---|
| *5-aminosalicylic acid* | | | | |
| Asacol, generics | > 1.6 g/d divided | 0.8–1.6 g/d divided | The value of 5-ASA as maintenance therapy in CD is controversial. Best evidence for Asacol 2.4 g/d and Pentasa 3 g/d. | $ |
| Mesasal | > 1.5 g/d divided | 1–1.5 g/d divided | | $ |
| Pentasa | > 2 g/d divided | 1.5–2 g/d divided | Pentasa has shown moderate benefit in active CD. | $-$$ |
| Salofalk | 3–4 g/d divided | 1–2 g/d divided | | $ |
| Topical | | | | |
| Salofalk, Quintasa | Enema: 1–4 g/d<br>Suppositories: 0.5–1 g/d | | Enemas and suppositories effective in UP. | $$–$$$<br>$ |
| **Immunosuppressives** | | | Common adverse effects with all: nausea, stomatitis, GI discomfort, diarrhea, anorexia. | |
| *azathioprine*<br>Imuran, generics | 2.5 mg/kg/d PO | | Major adverse effects with azathioprine and 6-MP: blood dyscrasias and hepatotoxicity. | $ |
| *6-mercaptopurine*<br>Purinethol | 100 mg/d PO | | | $$ |
| *methotrexate*<br>Various | 25 mg IM **Q wk** | | Methotrexate is potentially hepatotoxic.<br>Oral methotrexate has not shown efficacy in controlled trials. | $$$ |
| *cyclosporine*<br>Sandimmune | 4 mg/kg/d IV | | Cyclosporine is nephrotoxic and causes hypertension, seizures. | $$$$$ |
| **Biologics** | | | | |
| *infliximab*<br>Remicade[†] | 5 mg/kg IV × 1, for fistulizing CD<br>5 mg/kg IV × 3 at weeks 0, 2 and 6 | | Adverse effects: nausea, infusion/hypersensitivity reactions. Development of double stranded DNA antibodies and rarely a reversible lupus-like syndrome. Use with antimetabolites may potentiate response and reduce the formation of human anti-chimeric antibodies. | [†] |

*Dosage adjustment may be required in renal impairment – see Appendix I.*

** Cost of 1-day supply – includes drug cost only.*

*[†] Expected to be available in late 2000.*

*Legend: $ < $2   $$ $2–5   $$$ $5–10   $$$$ $10–20   $$$$$ > $20–30*

### *Antibiotics*

Short courses (2 to 4 weeks) of **metronidazole** are useful in treating CD with perianal fistulae. It has a potent disulfiram-like effect if alcohol is ingested and neuropathy may occur with long-term use. The use of metronidazole during pregnancy should be avoided.

### *Antidiarrheals*

Antidiarrheals should be used with caution and avoided in severe disease because of the risk of toxic megacolon. Diphenoxylate with atropine (Lomotil) is a combination of an opiate and an anticholinergic drug which can cause CNS side effects. Loperamide (Imodium) acts on both cholinergic and opiate receptors, but has a lower incidence of adverse effects than diphenoxylate.

### *Opioid Analgesics*

Opioids depress GI motility, and chronic use may lead to narcotic bowel syndrome. The risk for habituation is also high, and in some individuals their use may worsen symptoms.

**Codeine** is useful for pain control and to decrease the number of bowel movements. The use of morphine or meperidine should be avoided; restrict use to severe patients.

## *Crohn's Disease*

## Therapeutic Choices (Figure 1)

### Nonpharmacologic Choices

- Encourage the patient to stop smoking (limited evidence suggests smoking worsens CD).
- Nutritious diet; do not arbitrarily limit food groups. The goal is to ensure an adequate caloric intake. Nutritional supplements or parenteral nutrition may be necessary in selected patients who are malnourished.
- Surgery may be necessary to treat strictures, abscesses, fistulae or for patients refractory to medical management. Recurrence after surgery is almost universal, so conservative surgical management is favored.
- Psychological and social support is important, especially for adolescents.

### Pharmacologic Choices (Table 1)

See previous general discussion of pharmacologic choices in IBD.

- **Corticosteroid** therapy is most effective for the induction of remission (70% response rate). Prednisone (40 to 60 mg/day) is the most commonly used drug.

Figure 1: **Management of Crohn's Disease**

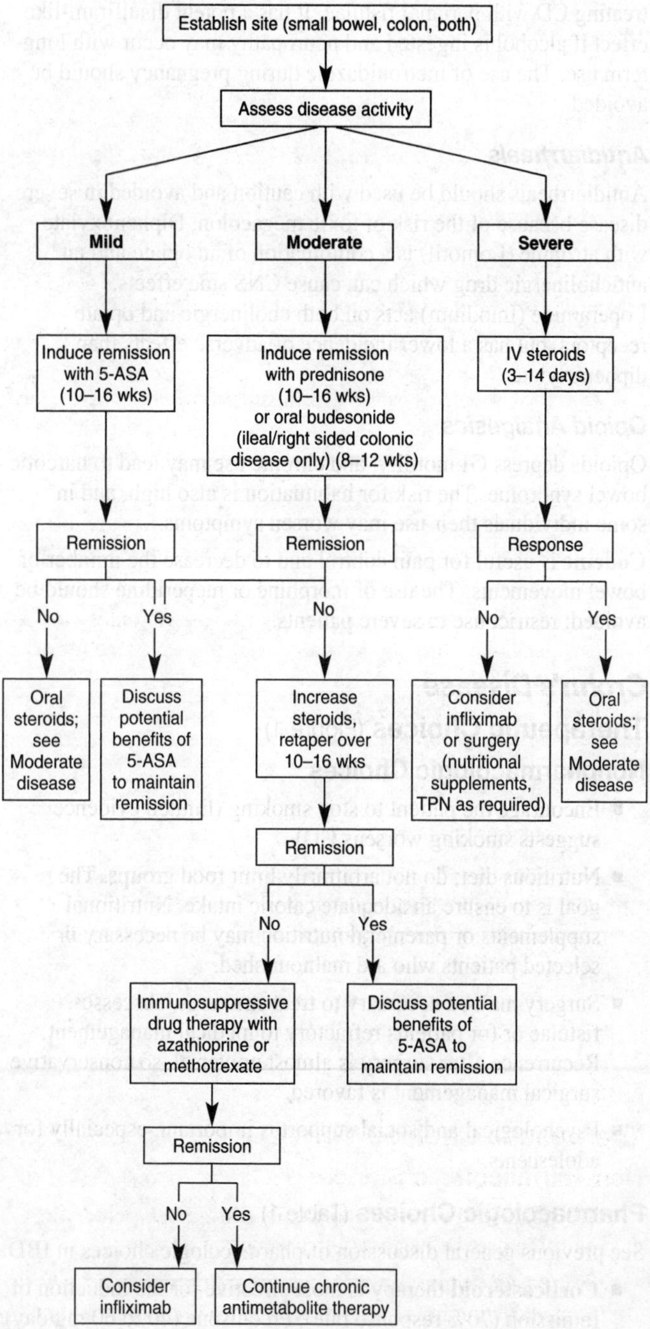
Establish site (small bowel, colon, both)
Assess disease activity
Mild
Moderate
Severe
Induce remission with 5-ASA (10–16 wks)
Induce remission with prednisone (10–16 wks) or oral budesonide (ileal/right sided colonic disease only) (8–12 wks)
IV steroids (3–14 days)
Remission
Remission
Response
No
Yes
No
No
Yes
Oral steroids; see Moderate disease
Discuss potential benefits of 5-ASA to maintain remission
Increase steroids, retaper over 10–16 wks
Consider infliximab or surgery (nutritional supplements, TPN as required)
Oral steroids; see Moderate disease
Remission
No
Yes
Immunosuppressive drug therapy with azathioprine or methotrexate
Discuss potential benefits of 5-ASA to maintain remission
Remission
No
Yes
Consider infliximab
Continue chronic antimetabolite therapy

- Chronic low-dose steroid therapy is *ineffective* for the maintenance of remission. However, some patients experience chronically active disease and may require continuous low-dose prednisone (10 to 15 mg/day) to suppress their symptoms.
- 5-ASA 4 g/day (Pentasa) or 6 to 8 g/day of sulfasalazine is only marginally effective for the induction of remission (approximately 40% response rate vs 30% with placebo) – mild cases only.
- The value of 5-ASA as a maintenance therapy for CD (in distinction to its use in UC) is controversial. Only a modest effect (20% 1-year reduction in relapse rate) is likely. (Consider for patients at high risk for relapse based on previously documented aggressive clinical course and requirement for previous surgery.)
- Patients who receive purine antimetabolites or methotrexate should use effective contraception since these drugs may be teratogenic.
- In pregnancy, methotrexate is absolutely contraindicated and purine antimetabolites are often discontinued (although this is controversial). Aminosalicylates and corticosteroids are safe and their use in pregnancy may continue if indicated.
- **Infliximab** is effective for patients who are refractory to antimetabolite therapy. Consider as primary therapy for patients with moderate to severe disease with fistulae.

## Therapeutic Tips

- 5-ASA preparations rarely worsen symptoms.
- No data support a steroid-sparing effect of 5-ASA.
- Bile salts diarrhea may occur in patients who have had resection of their terminal ileum. This usually responds to cholestyramine or antidiarrheals. $B_{12}$ deficiency may also occur.
- Infusion reactions from infliximab may require treatment with epinephrine, antihistamines and glucocorticoids.

## *Ulcerative Colitis*

## Therapeutic Choices (Figure 2)

### Nonpharmacologic Choices

- Well-balanced diet with supplements or total parenteral nutrition may be necessary in a minority of cases.
- Surgery (colectomy) may be used to treat patients refractory to medical therapy or who have cancerous changes in their colon.

Figure 2: **Management of Ulcerative Colitis**

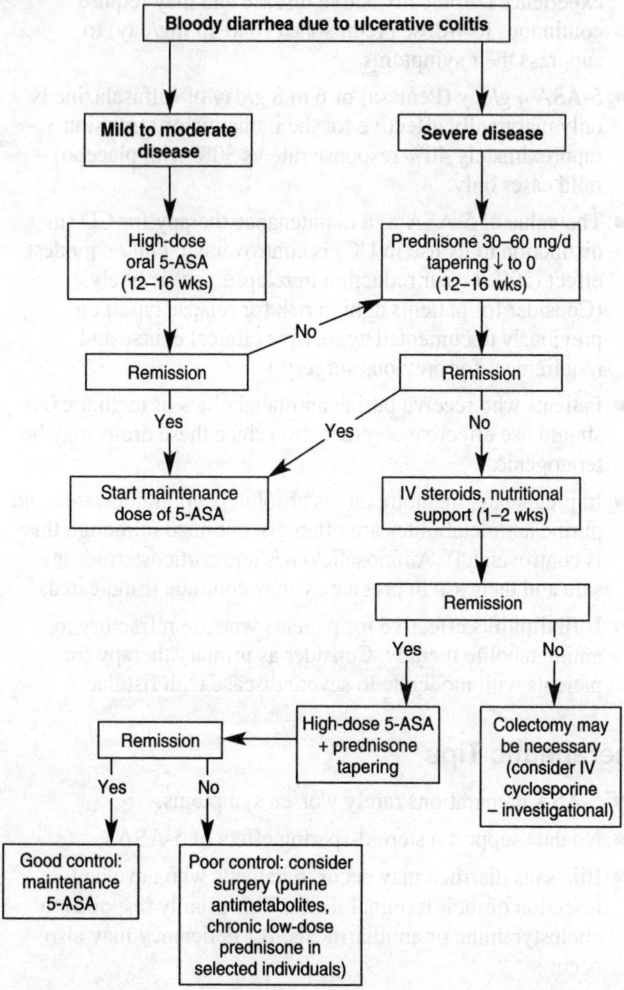
Bloody diarrhea due to ulcerative colitis
Mild to moderate disease
Severe disease
High-dose oral 5-ASA (12–16 wks)
Prednisone 30–60 mg/d tapering ↓ to 0 (12–16 wks)
No
Remission
Remission
Yes
Yes
No
Start maintenance dose of 5-ASA
IV steroids, nutritional support (1–2 wks)
Remission
Yes
No
High-dose 5-ASA + prednisone tapering
Colectomy may be necessary (consider IV cyclosporine – investigational)
Remission
Yes
No
Good control: maintenance 5-ASA
Poor control: consider surgery (purine antimetabolites, chronic low-dose prednisone in selected individuals)

- Colonoscopic surveillance in patients at high risk for cancer (early age of onset, extensive disease, long disease duration) is recommended.
- Although colectomy "cures" UC, pouchitis, a chronic inflammatory condition which occurs after ileal-anal reservoir construction, can be troublesome.

## Pharmacologic Choices (Table 1)

See previous general discussion of pharmacologic choices. **Aminosalicylates** are highly effective (70 to 80%) for the

Figure 3: **Management of Ulcerative Proctitis**

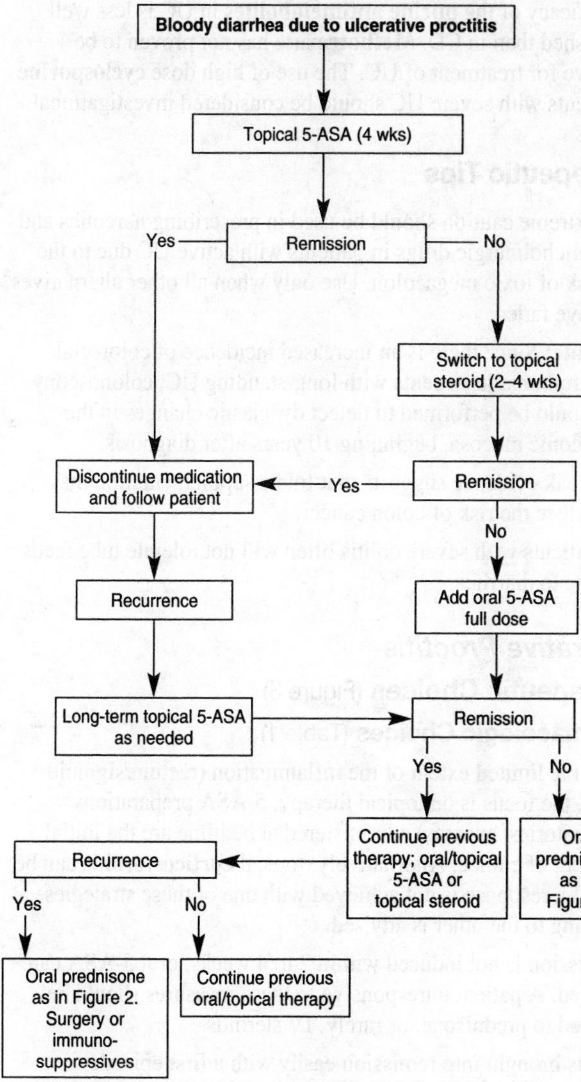
Bloody diarrhea due to ulcerative proctitis
Topical 5-ASA (4 wks)
Yes
Remission
No
Switch to topical steroid (2–4 wks)
Discontinue medication and follow patient
Yes
Remission
No
Recurrence
Add oral 5-ASA full dose
Long-term topical 5-ASA as needed
Remission
Yes
No
Recurrence
Continue previous therapy; oral/topical 5-ASA or topical steroid
Oral prednisone as in Figure 2
Yes
No
Oral prednisone as in Figure 2. Surgery or immuno-suppressives
Continue previous oral/topical therapy

treatment of UC and should be used for both induction (mild to moderate disease) and maintenance of remission (all patients). Sulfasalazine is the least expensive preparation and is well tolerated by most patients. The newer 5-ASA products are useful in patients who are intolerant of sulfasalazine (approximately 20%). Continuous use of **glucocorticoids** or **immuno-suppressives** is reserved for refractory patients who decline surgery. The lowest dose of prednisone found to control disease activity should be used.

The efficacy of the **purine antimetabolites** in UC is less well established than in CD. **Methotrexate** has not proven to be effective for treatment of UC. The use of high dose **cyclosporine** in patients with severe UC should be considered investigational.

### Therapeutic Tips

- Extreme caution should be used in prescribing narcotics and anticholinergic drugs in patients with active UC due to the risk of toxic megacolon. Use only when all other alternatives have failed.
- **Note:** Since there is an increased incidence of colorectal carcinoma in patients with long-standing UC, colonoscopy should be performed to detect dysplastic changes in the colonic mucosa, beginning 10 years after diagnosis.
- Weak evidence suggests that folate supplementation may reduce the risk of colon cancer.
- Patients with severe colitis often will not tolerate tube feeds, due to diarrhea.

## *Ulcerative Proctitis*

### Therapeutic Choices (Figure 3)

#### Pharmacologic Choices (Table 1)

Given the limited extent of the inflammation (rectum/sigmoid colon), the focus is on topical therapy. **5-ASA** preparations (suppositories, enemas) administered at bedtime are the initial treatment of choice. Alternatively, topical **corticosteroids** can be used. If a response is not achieved with one of these strategies, switching to the other is advised.

If remission is not induced within 2 to 4 weeks, oral 5-ASA can be added. A patient unresponsive to these measures should be switched to prednisone, or rarely, IV steroids.

Patients brought into remission easily with a first episode (i.e., within 4 to 8 weeks) may have all medications discontinued. Follow-up is essential; patients with recurring symptoms should receive chronic topical maintenance therapy with 5-ASA.

Patients brought into remission with difficulty should be continued on long-term oral or topical 5-ASA preparations, or steroid enemas, without attempting discontinuation of therapy. Some patients require chronic treatment with low-dose prednisone. Colectomy may be necessary in a few cases, despite the limited extent of the disease.

## Therapeutic Tips

- Topical therapy is preferred.
- A repeat sigmoidoscopy should be performed to ensure that the inflammation has not progressed to more extensive colitis.

### *Suggested Reading List*

Feagan B, McDonald JWD, Rochon J, Fedorak R, Irvine EJ, Sutherland L, et al. Methotrexate for the treatment of Crohn's disease. *N Engl J Med* 1995;332:292–297.

Hanauer SB. Drug therapy: Inflammatory bowel disease. *N Engl J Med* 1996;334:841–848.

Lichtiger S, Present DH, Kornbluth A, Gelernt I, Bauer J, Galler G, et al. Cyclosporine in severe ulcerative colitis refractory to steroid therapy. *N Engl J Med* 1994;330:1841–1845.

Moore TL. Living with inflammatory bowel disease: Can you tell me about medication? *Can J Gastroenterol* 1992;6:235–239.

Pearson DC, May GR, Fick GH, Sutherland LR. Azathioprine and 6-mercaptopurine in Crohn's disease. A meta analysis. *Ann Intern Med* 1995;123(2):132–142.

Sutherland LR, May GR, Shaffer EA. Sulfasalazine revisited: a meta analysis of 5-aminosalicylic acid in the treatment of ulcerative colitis. *Ann Intern Med* 1993;118:540.

CHAPTER 48

# Irritable Bowel Syndrome

*W. Grant Thompson, MD, FRCPC*

The irritable bowel syndrome (IBS) is a collection of symptoms attributed to the intestine (Table 1). Since there is no known pathology or pathophysiology, IBS can only be recognized by its symptoms. The prevalence is about 15% in adults worldwide, and lifetime prevalence is much higher. Most people who have these symptoms do not consult physicians. Nevertheless, IBS accounts for 30% of gut complaints in primary care, and the few that are referred to specialists are a large part of a gastroenterologist's practice. Females with IBS outnumber males 4:1. While the syndrome occurs at all ages, most people see physicians when young. The annual cost of IBS in the US is estimated to be $8 billion.

## Goals of Therapy

- Reassure through a confident diagnosis
- Alleviate symptoms
- Promote coping and normal social and occupational functioning
- Treat psychosocial comorbidity

## Investigations

The history should note the abdominal pain and its relationship with defecation, and altered stool frequency and form (Table 1). Pelvic pain (really lower abdominal pain) may be due to IBS rather than a gynecological cause. Physical findings or 'alarm' symptoms such as rectal bleeding, anemia, fever or profound weight loss are not explained by IBS. The history should also explore the patient's psychosocial circumstances, and the reasons other than the somatic symptoms that he or she has chosen to consult.

In a young person with chronic and typical symptoms (Table 1) and no alarms or family history of colon cancer or inflammatory bowel disease, tests are usually unnecessary. If the patient is over 45, has risk factors for cancer, or atypical and recent onset of symptoms, a barium enema or colonoscopy is wise. The colon disease that must not be missed is cancer. Other tests should be done only as indicated. Difficult, chronic constipation, or persistent diarrhea are not likely due to IBS, and raise different diagnostic and treatment issues.

Table 1: **Rome II Diagnostic Criteria* for IBS**

**Twelve weeks† or more in the past 12 months of abdominal discomfort or pain that has two out of three features:**

- **Relieved with defecation**
- **Onset associated with a change in frequency of stool**
- **Onset associated with a change in form (appearance) of stool**

The following symptoms are not essential for the diagnosis, but one or more are usually present. They add to the physician's confidence that the intestine is the origin of the abdominal pain. The more of these symptoms that are present, the more confident is the diagnosis of IBS:

- Abnormal stool frequency (>3/day or <3/week)
- Abnormal stool form (lumpy/hard or loose/watery stool) >1/4 of defecations
- Abnormal stool passage (straining, urgency, or feeling of incomplete evacuation) >1/4 of defecations
- Passage of mucus >1/4 of defecations
- Bloating or feeling of abdominal distention >1/4 of days

* *In the absence of structural or metabolic abnormalities to explain the symptoms.*
† *The 12 weeks need not be consecutive.*

## Therapeutic Choices (Figure 1)

### Nonpharmacologic Choices

- Diagnosis, explanation, reassurance, prognosis.
- Good doctor–patient relationship — maximizes placebo effect, improves long-term outcome.
- Healthy diet (Canada's Food Guide).
- Avoid food fads, excessive caffeine, alcohol, sorbitol (gums, candies), fructose.
- Many diets proposed by alternative practitioners or over the Internet are nutritionally unsound, and none have proven efficacy.
- Be alert to side effects of drugs and alternative treatments, e.g., senna tea.
- Ensure sufficient dietary fibre (see below).
- Lifestyle adjustment: stress management, relaxation advice, allow quiet time for eating and defecation.
- Treat comorbid conditions: depression, anxiety, panic, life stress.
- Psychological treatments include psychopharmacology; psychotherapy, individual or group; cognitive-behavioral therapy and hypnosis, if available. Benefits in IBS difficult to prove, but may help in difficult cases.
- Avoid inappropriate referral and unnecessary surgery.

## Figure 1: **Management of Irritable Bowel Syndrome**

### Management

**It is essential to make a positive diagnosis, rather than a diagnosis of exclusion, and convincingly convey this to the patient.**

**Education/reassurance — explaining pathophysiology and natural history**

- physiological abnormalities include altered intestinal motility and visceral hypersensitivity
- can be precipitated by previous enteric infection
- diet has no causal role, but may exacerbate IBS
- emotional stress does not cause IBS, but psychosocial factors may exacerbate IBS and/or contribute to the distress it causes
- validate symptoms – i.e., the symptoms are real, not imagined. Gut and brain interact to alter motility (muscle contractions) and/or increase bowel sensation
- **a chronic, relapsing but benign, disorder**

**Healthy lifestyle**

- advise patient regarding balanced diet, exercise, taking time for toilet in morning

**Diet**

- identify excesses, deficiencies (e.g., fad diets)
- diet alone does not cause IBS, but diet modification may alleviate symptoms
- food allergy is rare, and is not part of IBS
- **dietary advice**
  follow Canada's Food Guide;
  limit sorbitol, caffeine, alcohol, fat – they do not cause IBS but may exacerbate symptoms;
  restrict lactose only for proven lactase deficiency;
  refer selected patients to dietitian

**Psychosocial issues**

- important to explore in selected patients
- **"indicators" of difficulty coping with IBS:**
  poor insight; unable to express emotions; comorbid conditions; history of physical or sexual abuse or other major life stress; multiple somatic complaints or abnormal illness behavior; "catastrophizing" symptoms; poor coping mechanisms; inadequate social support

A 2-week symptom diary may assist selected patients to connect diet and stress with aggravation of symptoms. Consider cognitive-behavioral therapy or hypnosis and relaxation therapy in severe cases.

### Drug therapy

- most patients will not require drug therapy
- no single drug has been shown to be beneficial for the IBS symptom complex
- *specific* IBS symptoms ***may*** be amenable to drug therapy – first identify predominant symptom:

**Constipation**

- fibre (or fibre substitute): try wheat bran, up to 20 g/d, as first-line therapy
- Start with 15 or 30 mL of bran daily and titrate dose upward slowly – increase fluid intake
- if fibre supplement shows no benefit (or worsens symptoms) after 4–6 wk, stop or substitute psyllium

**Abdominal pain**

- avoid narcotics
- short-term therapy with antispasmodic agents or peripheral opiate antagonists may be considered, but benefit has not been demonstrated
- tricyclic antidepressants (e.g., amitriptyline) in selected patients with continuous or frequent pain

**Diarrhea**

- loperamide as needed for diarrheal episodes
- prophylactic use of loperamide for predictable episodes of diarrhea (e.g., social events)

**Bloating**

- no medication has been shown to be beneficial
- bloating associated with constipation may respond to treatment of constipation
- consider fibre reduction

**Comorbid conditions**

- treat depression and anxiety if present – IBS may improve as a result

*Adapted with permission from Paterson WG, et al. Recommendations for the management of irritable bowel syndrome in family practice. CMAJ 1999;161:154–160.*

## Pharmacologic Choices (Table 2)

- Very limited. Use only after nonpharmacologic measures fail. It is best to target the most troublesome symptom (see below).
- Predominant diarrhea: loperamide PRN, especially if patient concerned about incontinence.
- Predominant constipation (pellety stools): 2 to 4 table-spoonsful of raw bran or psyllium daily.
- Chronic abdominal pain: low-dose amitriptyline.
- HPB-approved drugs for IBS include dicyclomine, hyoscy-amine, trimebutine and pinaverium. These drugs differ from those approved in other countries, reflecting a lack of agreement about efficacy among regulatory authorities. Only dicyclomine is approved (with caveat) in the US. The efficacy of any of these agents in IBS is unproven[1-3] and this author endorses none of them. If used at all, it should only be for short periods.
- New drugs that may be available in 2000–2001 include:
  - *alosetron* (Lotronex) a 5-$HT_3$ antagonist; Phase III trials suggest efficacy in females with predominant diarrhea.
  - *tegaserod* (Zelmac) a 5-$HT_4$ partial agonist; Phase III trials suggest efficacy in predominant constipation.

### *Prognosis*

- Usually life-long, recurrent.
- Diagnosis is safe when carefully made i.e., the risk of structural disease is low.
- No predilection to structural disease such as diverticular disease, cancer, or IBD.

### *The Difficult-to-Treat Patient*

Difficult-to-treat patients that tend to be referred to specialists often have comorbid conditions such as depression. There may be a history of serious emotional trauma such as sexual abuse. Such patients are best managed with regularly scheduled visits for a sympathetic discussion. Referral to specialists may help as the need arises, and a gastroenterologist can support the primary care physician's diagnosis and management plan. Cure is not a likely long-term result. The emphasis should be on coping, and normal occupational and social functioning.

---

[1] *Gastroenterology 1988;95:232–241.*
[2] *Am J Gastroenterol 1996;91:660–673.*
[3] *Gastroenterol Int 1994;6:189–211.*

Table 2: **Drugs for a Dominant Symptom in Irritable Bowel Syndrome**

| Symptom/Drug | Dose | Adverse Effects | Comments | Cost* |
|---|---|---|---|---|
| **Diarrhea** | | | | |
| *loperamide* – Imodium, generics | 2–4 mg as needed (max. 12 mg/d) | Abdominal cramps, dizziness, dry mouth. | | $$ |
| *cholestyramine* – Questran, generics | 4 g (1 scoop or packet) TID with meals | Constipation, indigestion, nausea and vomiting. | May bind other drugs in GI tract. Do not take 1 hr before or 4 hrs after other medications. | $$ |
| *alosetron – Lotronex*[†] | 1 mg BID | Constipation. Reports of ischemic colitis (causal association not established). | Proven effective only in women with diarrhea-predominant IBS. | † |
| **Constipation** | | | | |
| *psyllium* – Metamucil, Prodiem Plain, others | 4 g BID with meals then adjust (dose varies with product) | Cramps, bloating, flatulence. | Take with fluids. | $ |
| *lactulose* – Duphalac, others | 15–30 mL (10–20 g) BID | Cramps, bloating, flatulence, diarrhea. | | $ |
| **Abdominal Pain** | | | | |
| *dicyclomine* (renal) – Bentylol, generics | 10–20 mg TID-QID then adjust | For all: constipation, drowsiness, dryness of mouth, nose or throat, nausea, headache. | For all: short-term therapy may be considered but **benefit not proven**. | For all: |
| *hyoscyamine sulfate* (renal) – Levsin | 0.125–0.25 mg TID-QID then adjust | | Take before meals if pain occurs after meals. | $–$$ |
| *pinaverium bromide* – Dicetel | 50–100 mg TID | | | |
| *trimebutine maleate* – Modulon | 100–200 mg TID AC | | | |
| Tricyclic antidepressants e.g., *amitriptyline* (renal) – Elavil, generics | 25–100 mg QHS | Drowsiness, dryness of mouth, headache. | For selected patients with intractable pain. See Chapter 5 for drug interactions. | $ |

* *Cost per day – includes drug cost only.*
*Legend: $ < $1 $$ $1–2*

(renal) *Dosage adjustment may be required in renal impairment – see Appendix I.*
† *Expected to be marketed in Canada late 2000.*

### *Suggested Reading List*

Burstall D, Vallis TM, Turnbull GK. *IBS relief*. Minneapolis: Chronimed, 1998.

Paterson WG, Thompson WG, Vanner SJ, Faloon TR, Rosser WW, Birtwhistle RW, Morse JL, Touzel TA, and the IBS consensus conference participants. Recommendations for the management of irritable bowel syndrome in family practice. *CMAJ* 1999;161:154–160.

Thompson WG. *Gut reactions*. New York: Plenum, 1989.

Thompson WG, Heaton KW, Smyth T, Smyth C. Irritable bowel syndrome in general practice: prevalence, management and referral. *Gut* 2000;46:78–82.

Thompson WG, Longstreth GF, Drossman DA, Heaton KW, Irvine EJ, Muller-Lissner SA. Functional bowel disease and functional abdominal pain. *Gut* 1999;45 (Suppl 2):II43–47.

CHAPTER 49

# Lower Urinary Tract Symptoms and Benign Prostatic Hyperplasia

*Richard W. Norman, MD, FRCSC*

## Goals of Therapy

- To improve or abolish lower urinary tract symptoms
- To reduce the risk of surgical intervention
- To prevent the sequelae of long-term bladder outlet obstruction (urinary tract infections, bladder stones, hydronephrosis)

## Investigations

- Thorough history with special attention to:
  - voiding (weak/interrupted stream, dribbling, hesitancy, straining) and storage (nocturia, frequency, urgency) symptoms
  - onset and progression of symptoms and degree of inconvenience
  - details of urethral infection, injury or instrumentation
  - episodes of urinary tract infection, hematuria or urinary retention
- Physical examination:
  - abdomen (bladder distension, flank tenderness)
  - external genitalia (phimosis, meatal stenosis, urethral mass/induration)
  - digital rectal examination (DRE) (documentation of prostate size, consistency, symmetry and tenderness)
- Laboratory tests:
  - urinalysis (and urine culture if pyuria)
  - serum creatinine
  - prostate specific antigen (PSA) (optional and controversial but generally recommended when a diagnosis of prostate cancer would alter treatment in otherwise healthy men between 50 and 70 years of age)
  - symptom score (recommended)
- Other diagnostic tests occasionally required when the history is not clear, there are abnormalities of the physical examination or laboratory tests, or the response to treatment is unsatisfactory:
  - cystoscopy
  - urodynamic studies
  - renal/bladder/transrectal ultrasonography
  - IV pyelography

Figure 1: **Management of Benign Prostatic Hyperplasia**

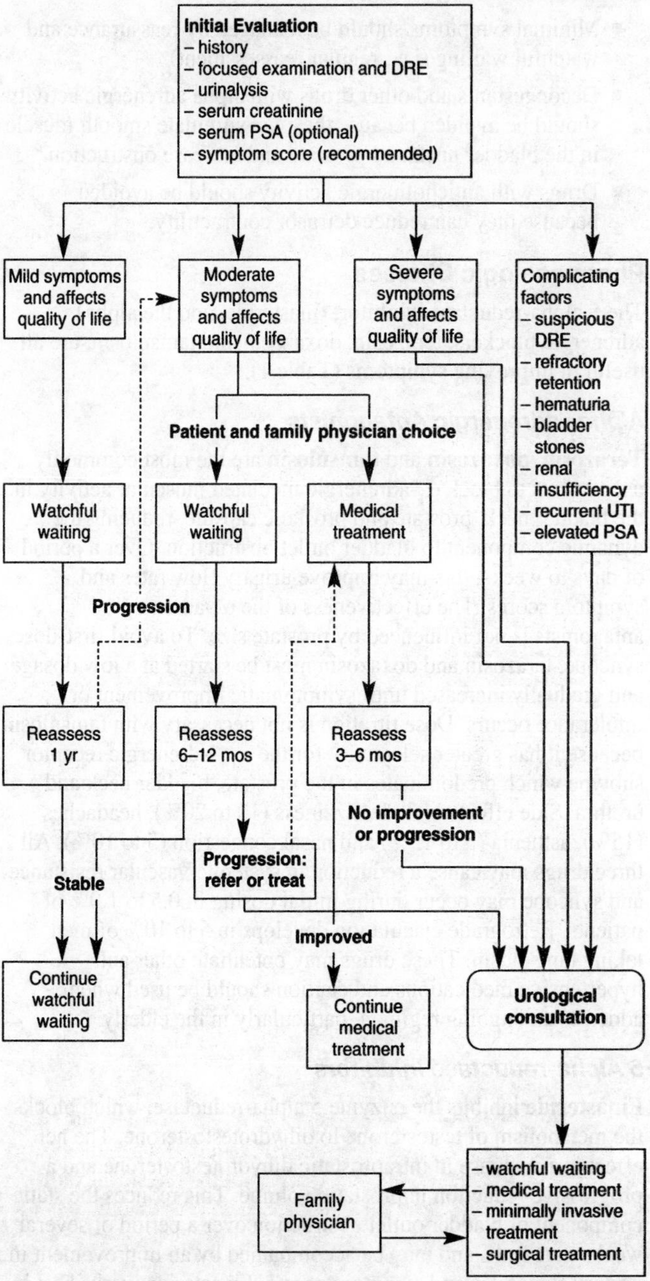
Initial Evaluation
– history
– focused examination and DRE
– urinalysis
– serum creatinine
– serum PSA (optional)
– symptom score (recommended)
Mild symptoms and affects quality of life
Moderate symptoms and affects quality of life
Severe symptoms and affects quality of life
Complicating factors
– suspicious DRE
– refractory retention
– hematuria
– bladder stones
– renal insufficiency
– recurrent UTI
– elevated PSA
Patient and family physician choice
Watchful waiting
Watchful waiting
Medical treatment
Progression
Reassess 1 yr
Reassess 6–12 mos
Reassess 3–6 mos
No improvement or progression
Progression: refer or treat
Stable
Improved
Continue watchful waiting
Continue medical treatment
Urological consultation
Family physician
– watchful waiting
– medical treatment
– minimally invasive treatment
– surgical treatment

*Abbreviations: DRE = digital rectal examination; PSA = prostate specific antigen.*

## Therapeutic Choices (Figure 1)

### Nonpharmacologic Choices

- Minimal symptoms should be managed by reassurance and watchful waiting (i.e., regular reassessment).
- Decongestants and other drugs with alpha adrenergic activity should be avoided because they can stimulate smooth muscle in the bladder neck and prostate and increase obstruction.
- Drugs with anticholinergic activity should be avoided because they can reduce detrusor contractility.

### Pharmacologic Choices

The 5 alpha-reductase inhibitor, finasteride, and the alpha1 adrenergic blockers, terazosin, doxazosin and tamsulosin, are all useful in improving symptoms (Table 1).

#### *Alpha$_1$-adrenergic Antagonists*

**Terazosin, doxazosin** and **tamsulosin** are the most commonly used agents to block $\alpha_1$-adrenergic mediated muscular activity in the bladder neck, prostate and prostatic capsule, reducing the dynamic component to bladder outlet obstruction. Over a period of days to weeks, this may improve urinary flow rates and symptom scores. The effectiveness of the $\alpha_1$-adrenergic antagonists is not influenced by prostate size. To avoid first-dose syncope, terazosin and doxazosin must be started at a low dosage and gradually increased until symptomatic improvement or intolerance occurs. Dose titration is not necessary with tamsulosin because it has greater selectivity for the $\alpha_{1A}$-adrenergic receptor subtype which predominates in the prostate, bladder neck and urethra. Side effects include dizziness (10 to 20%), headaches (15%), asthenia (5 to 15%) and nasal congestion (5 to 10%). All three drugs may cause a reduction in systemic vascular resistance and syncope may occur during initial dosing in 0.5 to 1.0% of patients. Retrograde ejaculation develops in 5 to 10% of men taking tamsulosin. These drugs may potentiate other antihypertensive medications and caution should be used when added to an ongoing regimen, particularly in the elderly.

#### *5 Alpha-reductase Inhibitors*

**Finasteride** inhibits the enzyme 5 alpha-reductase, which blocks the metabolism of testosterone to dihydrotestosterone. The net effect is a decrease in intraprostatic dihydrotestosterone and a progressive reduction in prostatic volume. This reduces the static component of bladder outlet obstruction over a period of several weeks to months and may be accompanied by an improvement in urinary flow rates and symptom scores. Finasteride works best in men with a large prostate. Because of its site specificity, there is a low incidence of side effects (e.g., 3 to 4% sexual dysfunction) and little risk of drug interactions. Finasteride decreases serum PSA levels by approximately 50% in men with BPH and may partially suppress serum PSA in men with prostate cancer.

### *Phytotherapeutic agents*

Saw palmetto (*Serenoa repens*) and African plum tree (*Pygeum africanum*) are examples of plant extracts used by patients to reduce symptoms related to BPH. Some data suggest they may produce a favourable response.[1,2] Identification and pharmacokinetics of active ingredients is often unclear in these mixtures and, until more information regarding their mode of action and long term efficacy and safety becomes available, their role in management will remain unclear.

## Minimally Invasive Approaches

- Long-term catheter drainage is appropriate for patients who are not candidates for any other intervention.

Other options under investigation include:

- Urethral stents
  - both temporary and permanent may be used in patients unable to undergo more definitive surgical treatment.
- Thermotherapy
  - role of intraurethral thermotherapy continues to evolve; results are variable and long-term assessment of effectiveness is lacking.
- Transurethral needle ablation (TUNA) of the prostate
  - intraprostatic placement of needle electrode via urethral route allows heating and necrosis of tissue, but confirmation of long-term benefits is lacking.

## Surgical Approaches

While transurethral resection of the prostate (TURP) and retropubic prostatectomy are traditional means of dealing with an enlarged and obstructing prostate gland, evidence is accumulating that transurethral incision of the prostate and various forms of laser prostatectomy are useful in some patients.

- Transurethral resection
  - most effective treatment for symptomatic BPH and one against which other treatments should be compared.
  - may cause long-term side effects such as impotence, retrograde ejaculation and urethral strictures.

[1] *JAMA 1998;280:1604–1609.*
[2] *Urology 1999;54:473–478.*

Table 1: **Drugs Used in Benign Prostatic Hyperplasia**

| Drug | Dosage | Adverse Effects | Comments | Cost* |
|---|---|---|---|---|
| **$\alpha_1$-Adrenergic Blockers** | | | | |
| *terazosin* Hytrin | 1–10 mg QHS | Dizziness, headaches, asthenia and nasal congestion (5–20%). | Terazosin and doxazosin: dose titrated weekly to desired response. Maximal response seen in 4 weeks. | $$–$$$ |
| *doxazosin* Cardura | 1–12 mg QHS | Syncope (< 1%). Tamsulosin: retrograde ejaculation (5–10%). | Terazosin and doxazosin: may potentiate other antihypertensives. | $$–$$$$ |
| *tamsulosin* Flomax | 0.4–0.8 mg daily 30 min after the same meal | | Start with 0.4 mg/day, if no response in 2–4 weeks increase to 0.8 mg/day. | $$$–$$$$ |
| **5α–Reductase Inhibitors** | | | | |
| *finasteride* Proscar | 5 mg daily | Sexual dysfunction (3–4%). | PSA decreases in patients taking finasteride. Maximal response seen in 6 months. | $$$$ |

** Cost of 30-day supply – includes drug cost only.*
*Legend: $ < $15 $$ $15–30 $$$ $30–45 $$$$ > $45*

- Retropubic prostatectomy
  – required when the prostate is very enlarged or other bladder pathology requires concomitant attention; similar success and side effects to TURP.
- Transurethral incision of the prostate (TUIP)
  – useful for small prostates; associated with a lower incidence of retrograde ejaculation than TURP.
- Laser prostatectomy
  – various forms of this technology allow transurethral coagulation/vaporization/resection of the prostate, often on an outpatient basis with little bleeding; short-term data are encouraging, but long-term data and cost issues require clarification.

## Therapeutic Tips

- Patients with minimum symptoms that do not interfere with their normal activities should be managed by watchful waiting and regular follow-up.
- Patients starting to develop progressive symptoms or moderate inconvenience are candidates for pharmacologic intervention.
- Side effects of terazosin and doxazosin may be reduced by taking at bedtime.
- Terazosin and doxazosin may cause a small decrease in total cholesterol and low-density lipoprotein fraction. The clinical importance of this is unknown.
- Greater selectivity of tamsulosin for the $\alpha_{1A}$-adrenergic receptor subtype, concentrated in the lower urinary tract, and administration with meals, which produces more constant serum drug concentrations, may result in fewer systemic side effects.
- Combination therapy with both classes of drugs shows no additive benefit.
- Drug therapy should be continued indefinitely since symptoms recur when medication is stopped.
- Long-term data are limited to finasteride and show a maintenance of benefit over 5 years and a reduced likelihood of developing urinary retention or requirement for BPH-related surgery.

## Pharmacoeconomic Considerations

*Jeffrey A. Johnson, PhD*

The clinical and economic impact of different treatment options for BPH were recently reviewed and evaluated by the Canadian Coordinating Office for Health Technology Assessment (CCOHTA). The focus of the evaluation was finasteride, compared to TURP and watchful waiting. The results of this review indicated that the relative cost effectiveness of the treatment options is dependent on two main factors: life expectancy and severity of symptoms. For men with mild symptoms, watchful waiting is considered the most cost-effective option. For patients with moderate or severe symptoms, and life expectancy less than 3 years, finasteride is the less expensive option. For patients with life expectancy longer than 4 years, finasteride provides a favorable cost-effectiveness ratio only in patients with moderate symptoms, when compared to surgery or watchful waiting. For patients with severe symptoms, however, using finasteride is likely more expensive than surgery in the long run, and with poorer results.

Unfortunately, no studies are available that evaluate the economic impact of alpha-blockers in the management of BPH. While recent clinical studies suggest that finasteride is most effective in men with large prostates, alpha-blockers work in men with small or large prostates. Alpha-blockers are more effective than finasteride during the first year of treatment, but only finasteride has been shown to induce regression of the gland and offer increased efficacy over time.

Overall, it is likely that the economic cost of BPH treatment will continue to increase due to increased use of both drug therapies. The magnitude of the increase will depend on the degree to which medical therapy substitutes, rather than simply delays, surgical intervention. This will depend on what percentage of men begin long-term therapy, and at what age. At present, the answers to these questions are not available.

---

***Suggested Reading***

*Baladi, J-F Cost-effectiveness and cost-utility analyses of finasteride therapy for the treatment of benign prostatic hyperplasia. Ottawa, ON: Canadian Coordinating Office for Health Technology Assessment, 1995.*

*Eri LM, Tveter KJ. Treatment of benign prostatic hyperplasia. A pharmacoeconomic perspective. Drugs & Aging 1997;10:107–118.*

### *Suggested Reading List*

Boyle P, Gould AL, Roehrborn CG. Prostate volume predicts outcome of treatment of benign prostatic hyperplasia with finasteride: meta-analysis of randomized clinical trials. *Urology* 1996;48:398–405.

Hudson PB, Boake R, Trachtenberg J, Romas NA, Rosenblatt S, Narayan P, et al. Efficacy of finasteride is maintained in patients with benign prostatic hyperplasia treated for 5 years. *Urology* 1999;53:690–695.

Lepor H, Williford WO, Barry MJ, et al. The efficacy of terazosin, finasteride, or both in benign prostatic hyperplasia. *N Engl J Med* 1996;335:533–538.

McConnell JD, Bruskewitz R, Walsh P, Andriole G, Lieber M, Holtgrewe HL, et al. The effect of finasteride on the risk of acute urinary retention and need for surgical treatment among men with benign prostatic hyperplasia. *N Engl J Med* 1998;338:557–563.

Nickel JC, Norman RW. *BPH – A physician's guide to care and counselling*. Montreal: Grosvenor House, 1993.

Norman RW, Nickel JC, Fish D, et al. "Prostate-related symptoms" in Canadian men 50 years of age or older: prevalence and relationship among symptoms. *Br J Urol* 1994;74:542–550.

CHAPTER 50

# Urinary Incontinence and Enuresis

*S.A. Awad, MB, ChB, FRCSC and R.D. Schwarz, MD, FRCSC*

## *Incontinence*

### Goals of Therapy

- To achieve relief of urinary symptoms
- To increase functional capacity of the bladder

### Definitions

**Overflow incontinence** is the leakage of urine due to an overdistended bladder, commonly caused by outlet obstruction (e.g., prostatic hyperplasia) or neurogenic causes (e.g., multiple sclerosis).

**Stress incontinence** is loss of urine due to an increase in intra-abdominal pressure (e.g., cough, exercise). It is more common in women. Weakness in pelvic musculature (e.g., due to childbirth) is the primary cause.

**Urge incontinence** is leakage of moderate to large amounts of urine due to inability to delay voiding when an urge is perceived. Causes include bladder wall hyperactivity or instability and CNS disorders (e.g., parkinsonism, stroke).

**Functional incontinence** is loss of urine because of the inability to get to a toilet. Some causes include physical or cognitive disabilities and environmental barriers. It may also occur in those with a normal neuromuscular anatomy whose mechanism of voiding is functionally disturbed.

**Developmental or maturational incontinence** is the involuntary loss of urine in people with no uropathy or neuropathy whose control has not yet fully developed.

### Investigations

- History and physical examination:
  - to determine type of incontinence
  - to rule out fistula (in women), neurologic lesions, congenital anomalies, bladder infection or other forms of cystitis, bladder cancer, gynecologic disorders, previous pelvic radiation

Figure 1: **Management of Stress Incontinence in Women**

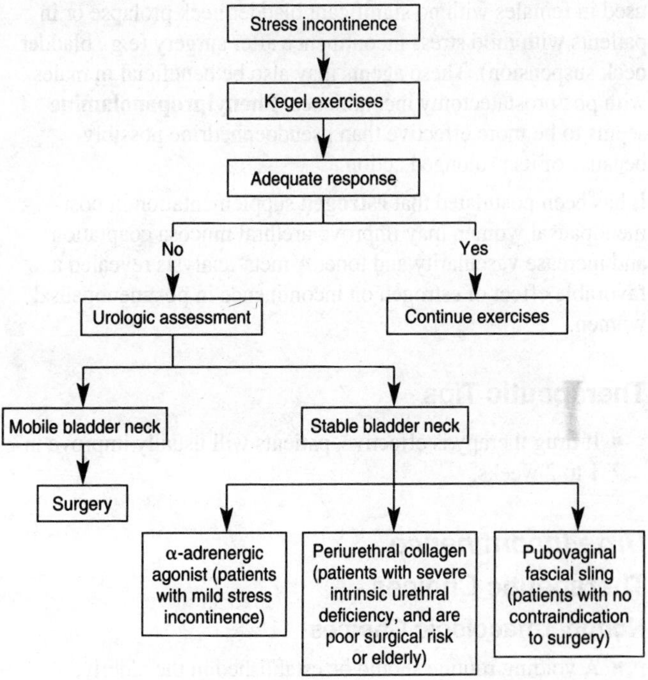
Stress incontinence
Kegel exercises
Adequate response
No
Yes
Urologic assessment
Continue exercises
Mobile bladder neck
Stable bladder neck
Surgery
α-adrenergic agonist (patients with mild stress incontinence)
Periurethral collagen (patients with severe intrinsic urethral deficiency, and are poor surgical risk or elderly)
Pubovaginal fascial sling (patients with no contraindication to surgery)

  – to identify reversible/correctable causes in the elderly (e.g., medications, constipation, inadequate or restricted access to washrooms, delirium, depression)

- Laboratory tests:
  – urinalysis, urine culture and possibly cystoscopy
- A time/volume voiding diary or a cystometrogram helps to demonstrate reduced bladder capacity in urge incontinence. The latter also establishes diminished bladder compliance or instability.

## *Stress Incontinence* (Figure 1)

## Therapeutic Choices

### Nonpharmacologic Choices

- **Kegel exercises** should be the initial therapy. The exercises involve tightening followed by relaxation of pelvic floor (perineal) muscles 10 to 15 times consecutively, 3 to 4 times a day.
- Bladder neck suspension **surgery** to correct bladder neck prolapse may be indicated.

### Pharmacologic Choices (Table 1)

Pharmacotherapy has a limited role. Alpha-adrenergic agents are used in females with no significant bladder neck prolapse or in patients with mild stress incontinence after surgery (e.g., bladder neck suspension). These agents may also be beneficial in males with postprostatectomy incontinence. **Phenylpropanolamine** seems to be more effective than pseudoephedrine possibly because of its prolonged action.

It has been postulated that **estrogen** supplementation in postmenopausal women may improve urethral mucosa coaptation and increase vascularity and tone. A meta-analysis revealed a favorable effect of estrogen on incontinence in postmenopausal women.

### Therapeutic Tips

- If drug therapy is effective, patients will usually improve in 1 to 2 weeks.

## *Urge Incontinence*

## Therapeutic Choices

### Nonpharmacologic Choices

- A voiding routine should be established in the elderly.

### Pharmacologic Choices (Table 1)

Pharmacotherapy is the first-line treatment for urge incontinence with no underlying cause (e.g., in idiopathic detrusor overactivity, more common in females). Drug therapy also seems to be effective in patients with partial neurologic lesions (e.g., multiple sclerosis) but not in complete lesions (e.g., following spinal cord injury); and in chronic cystitis not secondary to bacterial infection. Drugs with **anticholinergic plus smooth muscle relaxant** effects are most effective. They act by increasing the functional capacity of the bladder, partially blocking the detrusor reflex or increasing bladder compliance. Side effects frequently limit treatment.

### Therapeutic Tips

- A satisfactory response is achieved in only about 50 to 60% of patients, even with careful screening and accurate diagnosis.
- Several weeks are required to achieve maximum effect. If no subjective improvement occurs after 4 to 6 weeks, the drug should be discontinued.

# *Enuresis*

## Goals of Therapy

- To manage symptoms
- To reassure the family and to provide advice

## Definitions

**Daytime wetting** in children under 7 years of age is usually related to delayed neurologic maturation of the conscious sensation of bladder fullness and cortical inhibition of detrusor contractions. The episodic wetting is sometimes associated with squatting or urgency.

**Nocturnal enuresis** refers to sleep wetting. The causes are still being debated, and treatments are empirical.

## Investigations

- History and physical examination to exclude:
  - *acute cystitis:* sudden change of voiding pattern, confirmed with urinalysis and culture and sensitivity
  - *posterior urethral valves* in boys: an obstructive voiding pattern
  - *urethral or vaginal ectopic ureter* in girls: void normally but are always damp or wet
  - *occult neuropathy:* usually have bowel dysfunction and show abnormal perineal sensation and/or anal sphincter reflexes
  - *female epispadias or cecoureterocele* (rare): determined by introital exam
  - *stool holders* with urinary symptoms: bladder symptoms improve with proper bowel management (often a "hidden" symptom)
- Diagnostic imaging is **not** indicated in wetters with negative history and physical. Urodynamic evaluation or imaging may be considered in children unresponsive to or intolerant of drug therapy

## Therapeutic Choices (Figure 2)

Treatment, if any, is based on the child's social and developmental indications. Often the knowledge that enuresis is a common problem coupled with an understanding that the child is not "ill" or "at risk" reassures the parent that no treatment is required. Older children may have legitimate psychosocial indications for treatment.

Figure 2: **Management of Daytime and Sleep Wetting in Children**

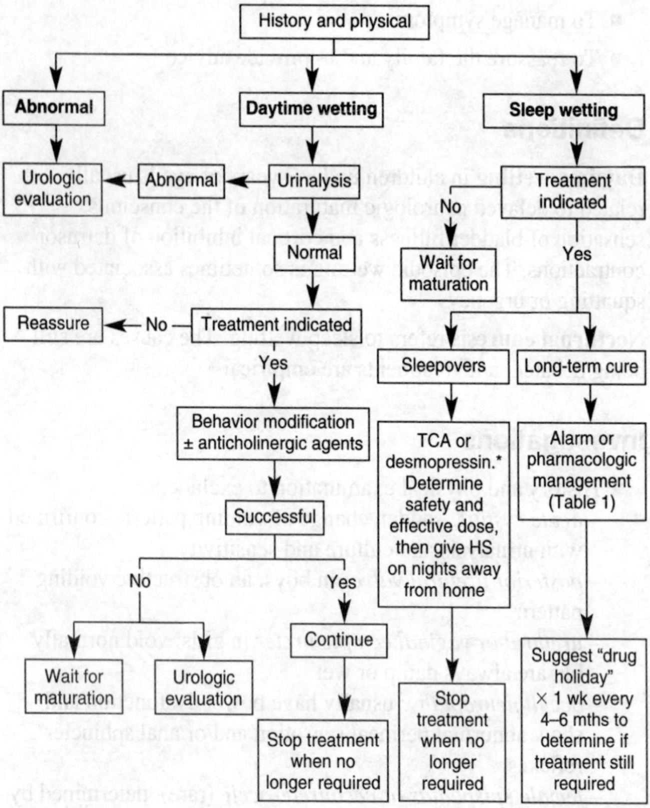
History and physical
Abnormal
Daytime wetting
Sleep wetting
Urologic evaluation
Abnormal
Urinalysis
Treatment indicated
No
Normal
Yes
Wait for maturation
Reassure
No
Treatment indicated
Yes
Sleepovers
Long-term cure
Behavior modification ± anticholinergic agents
TCA or desmopressin.* Determine safety and effective dose, then give HS on nights away from home
Alarm or pharmacologic management (Table 1)
Successful
No
Yes
Continue
Wait for maturation
Urologic evaluation
Suggest "drug holiday" × 1 wk every 4–6 mths to determine if treatment still required
Stop treatment when no longer required
Stop treatment when no longer required

*Abbreviations: TCA = tricyclic antidepressants.*
* *Choice of treatment is empiric and depends on cost, patient choice and response. If unsuccessful with one, can try alternate drug.*

## Nonpharmacologic Choices

- **Behavior modification** using a time-void schedule with rewards for successful toileting may be tried.
- **Alarms** (e.g., Palco or Nitone) serve as a learning tool that, with time and effort, can free the child entirely of symptoms.

## Pharmacologic Choices (Table 1)

If treatment is appropriate for day wetting, a combination of pharmacologic and behavior modification techniques may be used. The anticholinergic/antispasmodic drugs can be tried at very low doses and titrated up to efficacy but avoid side effects.

Table 1: **Drug Therapy of Urinary Incontinence and Enuresis**

| Type of Incontinence | Drug | Dosage | Adverse Effects | Drug Interactions | Cost* |
|---|---|---|---|---|---|
| **Stress** | **Alpha-adrenergic Agonists** | | | | |
| | *phenylpropanolamine* – Entex LA† | 75 mg Q12H | Nervousness, insomnia, dizziness, restlessness. | MAOIs, antihypertensives, neuroleptics; avoid in patients on thyroid medications. | $$ |
| | **Conjugated Estrogens‡** | | | | |
| | Premarin, generics | Vaginal: 1–2 g QHS × 1 wk, then 1–2 ×/wk | Breakthrough bleeding, sodium/water retention, nausea, vomiting, headache, breast tenderness. (See Chapter 72) | Clearance ↑ by rifampin. | $ |
| | | Oral: 0.3–1.25 mg daily | | | $–$$ |
| **Urge** | **Anticholinergic/Antispasmodic$^{\pi}$** | | | | |
| | *oxybutynin* – Ditropan, generics | 2.5–5 mg TID | Dry mouth, flushing, drowsiness, blurred vision, nausea/vomiting, constipation (less frequent with dicyclomine, flavoxate and tolterodine). Experience with tolterodine is, however, limited. | Other drugs with significant anticholinergic side effects (e.g., cyclic antidepressants, neuroleptics). Tolterodine: concurrent use with cytochrome P450–3A4 inhibitors (e.g. macrolides, antifungals) may ↑ serum level; use 1 mg BID. | $–$$ |
| | *tolterodine* – Detrol | 1–2 mg BID | | | $$$ |
| | *dicyclomine* – Bentylol, generics | 10–20 mg TID | | | $# |
| | *flavoxate* – Urispas | 200 mg TID-QID | | | $$$ |
| | **Tricyclic Antidepressants** | | | | |
| | *imipramine* Tofranil, generics | 10–25 mg TID–QID Elderly: 10 mg TID–QID | Drowsiness, insomnia, tremors/paresthesia, dry mouth, blurred vision, orthostatic hypotension, tachycardia, constipation, flushing, perspiration. | MAOIs, barbiturates, carbamazepine, rifampin, cimetidine, fluoxetine, neuroleptics, clonidine, alcohol. | $ |

(cont'd)

Table 1: **Drug Therapy of Urinary Incontinence and Enuresis** *(cont'd)*

| Type of Incontinence | Drug | Dosage | Adverse Effects | Drug Interactions | Cost* |
|---|---|---|---|---|---|
| **Enuresis** | **Anticholinergic/Antispasmodic**[π] | | | | |
| | *oxybutynin* – Ditropan, generics<br>*tolterodine* – Detrol<br>*dicyclomine* – Bentylol, generics<br>*flavoxate* – Urispas | Oxybutynin: 2.5–5 mg BID up to 5 mg TID depending on age, efficacy and side effects; as above for others | See above. | See above. | See above |
| | **Tricyclic Antidepressants** | | | | |
| | *imipramine*<br>Tofranil, generics | 8–12 yrs: 25 mg HS<br>> 12 yrs: 50 mg HS | See above. | See above. | $ |
| | **Antidiuretic** | | | | |
| | *desmopressin*<br>DDAVP | Children ≥ 6 yrs:<br>Nasal spray: 20–40 μg HS<br>Tablets: 0.2–0.4 mg PO HS | Local nasal irritation; (nasal spray); water intoxication, seizures (rare). Restrict fluid intake a few hours before administration. | | $$$$$ |

† *Contains guaifenesin also.*
‡ *In women with an intact uterus: systemic estrogens should be given with a progestin; chronic use of vaginal estrogens may require concurrent progestin use (Chapter 72).*
π *Listed in decreasing order of potency; oxybutynin and tolterodine have comparable efficacy.*
# *Cost of liquid formulation significantly higher than tablets.*
* *Cost of 30-day therapy – includes drug cost only.*
*Legend: $ < $20 $$ $20–40 $$$ $40–60 $$$$ $60–80 $$$$$ > $80*

Occasionally, the child will not respond to this plan or will have unpleasant side effects. Urodynamic evaluation or imaging may be useful in modifying management.

In children with strictly nocturnal enuresis, management options include tricyclic antidepressants (e.g., imipramine), desmopressin or alarm programs. The tricyclic antidepressants or desmopressin can be used to protect the child for sleepovers but neither provide a "cure."

The choice between desmopressin and tricyclic antidepressants is empirical and is usually determined by cost, patient preference and response to therapy. If treatment is unsuccessful with one medication the patient may choose a trial of the other.

## Therapeutic Tips

- If the child is not embarrassed or does not feel social pressure, no treatment may be necessary.
- No single option is best for every child; decision making requires the child's input, interest and commitment.

## *Suggested Reading List*


Appell RA. Clinical safety and efficacy of tolterodine in the treatment of overactive bladder: a pooled analysis. *Urology* 1997;50 (Suppl 6A):90–96.

Fantl JA, Cardozo L, McClish DK, et al. Estrogen therapy in the management of urinary incontinence in postmenopausal women: a meta-analysis. First report of the Hormones and Urogenital Therapy Committee. *Obstet Gynecol* 1994;83: 12–18.

Gajewski JB, Awad SA. Oxybutynin versus propantheline in patients with multiple sclerosis and detrusor hyperreflexia. *J Urol* 1986;135:966–968.

Thruoff JW, Bunke B, Ebner A, et al. Randomized, double-blind, multicenter trial on treatment of frequency, urgency and incontinence related to detrusor hyperactivity: oxybutynin versus propantheline versus placebo. *J Urol* 1991;145: 813–817.

Wein AJ, Barrett D. Physiology of micturition and urodynamics. In: Kelalis PP, King LR and Belman AB, eds. *Clinical pediatric urology*. 3rd ed. Philadelphia: W.B. Saunders, 1992.

CHAPTER 51

# Fibromyalgia

*Andrew Chalmers, MD, FRCPC*

Fibromyalgia is characterized by diffuse musculoskeletal pain accompanied by increased tenderness at specific sites known as "tender points" (Figure 2).

## Goals of Therapy

- To differentiate and treat conditions that also present as diffuse aches and pains but have specific pharmacologic therapies (e.g., polymyalgia rheumatica)
- To reduce pain and fatigue, improve quality of life, educate and promote self-management for conditions that require significant nonpharmacologic therapy and for which drug therapy is of limited benefit

## Investigations (Figure 1)

Figure 1: **Investigation of Diffuse Aches and Pains**

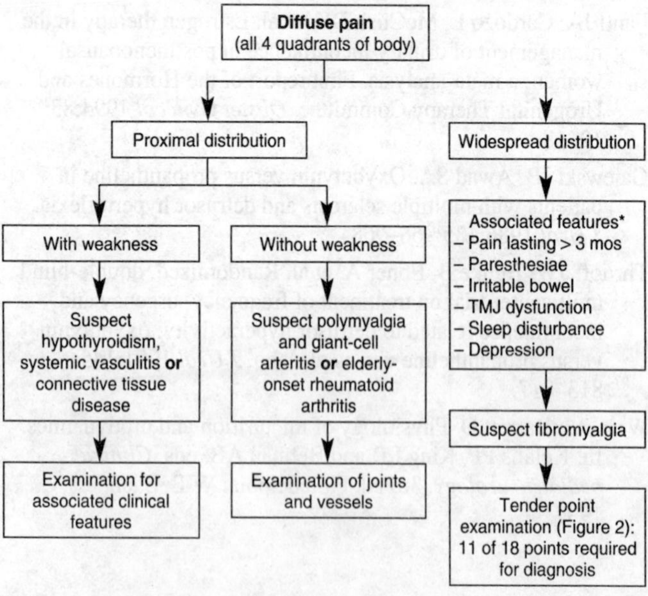
Diffuse pain
(all 4 quadrants of body)
Proximal distribution
Widespread distribution
With weakness
Without weakness
Associated features*
– Pain lasting > 3 mos
– Paresthesiae
– Irritable bowel
– TMJ dysfunction
– Sleep disturbance
– Depression
Suspect hypothyroidism, systemic vasculitis or connective tissue disease
Suspect polymyalgia and giant-cell arteritis or elderly-onset rheumatoid arthritis
Suspect fibromyalgia
Examination for associated clinical features
Examination of joints and vessels
Tender point examination (Figure 2): 11 of 18 points required for diagnosis

* *Note: Lab tests are generally negative (unless fibromyalgia is associated with specific connective tissue diseases).*

Figure 2: **Tender Point Examination**

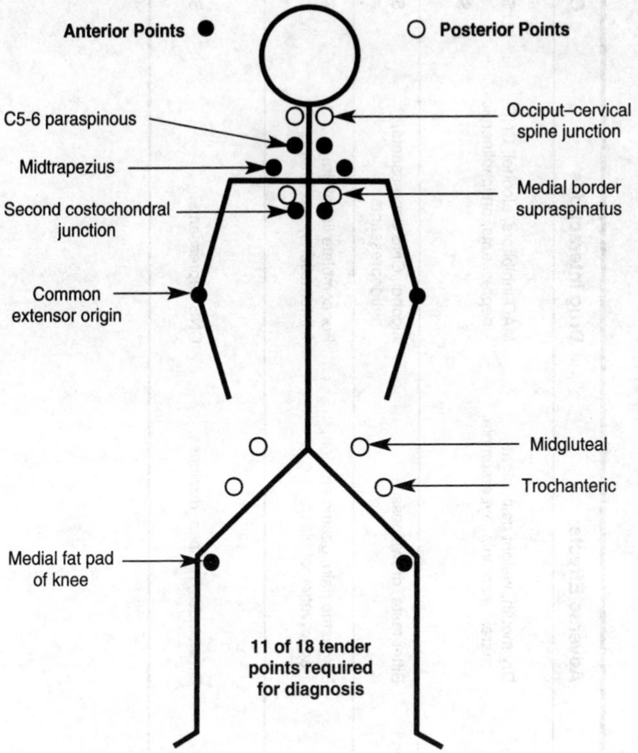
Anterior Points
Posterior Points
C5-6 paraspinous
Midtrapezius
Second costochondral junction
Common extensor origin
Occiput–cervical spine junction
Medial border supraspinatus
Midgluteal
Trochanteric
Medial fat pad of knee
11 of 18 tender points required for diagnosis

*Note: Using thumb pressure sufficient to blanch fingernail.*

# Therapeutic Choices

## Nonpharmacologic Choices

- A comprehensive program of education, nonpharmacologic pain management techniques, graded aerobic exercise and sleep hygiene (Chapter 6) is effective.
- A controlled trial supports the use of biofeedback techniques.[1]
- Multidisciplinary programs focusing on stress management and cardiovascular or aerobic exercise have been found effective.[2]
- Cognitive behavioral therapy is effective in the short term and benefits may persist.

---

[1] *J Rheumatol 1987;14:820–825.*
[2] *Arthritis Care Res 1998;11:397–404.*

Table 1: **Drugs Used in Fibromyalgia**

| Drug | Dosage | Adverse Effects | Drug Interactions | Cost* |
|---|---|---|---|---|
| **Tricyclic Medications** | | | | |
| *amitriptyline* Elavil, generics | 10–20 mg 2–3 h before bedtime | Dry mouth, weight gain, nightmares, insomnia, hypersomnia. | MAO inhibitors, alcohol, CNS depressants, anticholinergics. | $ |
| *cyclobenzaprine* Flexeril, generics | | | | $$–$$$ |
| *zopiclone* Imovane, generics | 7.5 mg QHS (begin with 3.75 mg in the elderly) | Bitter taste, drowsiness. | Alcohol, CNS depressants, antidepressants. | $$ |
| *ibuprofen* Actiprofen, Advil, Motrin, generics | 200 mg QHS | Epigastric pain, gastric erosion, aggravation of ulcer. | For complete list of drug interactions, see Chapter 50. | $ |
| **Muscle Relaxant/Analgesic Combinations** | | | | |
| *methocarbamol* plus *ASA* (Robaxisal) or *acetaminophen* (Robaxacet) | 2 tablets QHS | Drowsiness, nausea, dizziness. | CNS depressants. | $$$ |

** Cost of 30-day supply – includes drug cost only.*
*Legend: $ < $10 $$ $10–20 $$$ > $20*

- Night splints reduce symptoms in patients with temporomandibular joint (TMJ) dysfunction.
- Irritable bowel symptoms may be improved by dietary management.
- Eliminate caffeine-containing products and alcohol.
- Heat, massage and physiotherapy may provide transient benefit during flares. Ultrasound and TENS may help (or occasionally aggravate) symptoms, but should not be used chronically.

### Pharmacologic Choices (Table 1)

- Treat concomitant depression when present.
- Low doses of *tricyclic medications* (e.g., **amitriptyline, cyclobenzaprine**) combined with low doses of **ibuprofen** at bedtime improve sleep disturbance and, in a few patients, reduce pain. Short-term but not long-term efficacy of tricyclics has been demonstrated.[3]
- There is no evidence that the newer antidepressants (serotonin reuptake inhibitors) play a more specific role than treatment of concomitant depression.
- Although **zopiclone** is theoretically of benefit and is used, no evidence has been published as to its efficacy.
- Muscle relaxant/analgesic combinations (e.g., **methocarbamol with ASA or acetaminophen**) are useful, but should **not** be used with other medications.
- Narcotic analgesics or benzodiazepines are not recommended.
- **Human growth hormone** improved symptoms in a placebo-controlled trial, but more evidence is required.[4] Cost and that this treatment could only be performed in tertiary centres are prohibitive factors.

## Therapeutic Tips

- Patients with arthritis may develop concomitant fibromyalgia, which should be treated separately. NSAIDs are usually ineffective for fibromyalgia. Benzodiazepines and corticosteroids should also be avoided.
- Tricyclics should be prescribed 2 to 3 hours before bedtime to minimize hangover effects.
- If tricyclics are not tolerated, zopiclone may be tried.[5]
- Important and sustained clinical improvement occurs only in a minority of patients.

---

[3] *Arthritis Rheum 1994;37:32–40.*

[4] *Am J Med 1998;104:227–231.*

[5] *Scand J Rheumatol 1991;20:288–293.*

### Suggested Reading List

Bennet RM. The fibromyalgia syndrome: myofascial pain and chronic fatigue syndrome. In: Kelly WN, Harris ED, Sledge CB, eds. *Textbook of rheumatology*. Philadelphia: WB Saunders, 1997;511–521.

Leventhal LJ. Management of fibromyalgia. *Ann Intern Med* 1999;131:850–858.

CHAPTER 52

# Chronic Fatigue Syndrome

*Elizabeth Mann, MD, FRCPC*

Fatigue is a common complaint, but chronic fatigue syndrome (CFS) is far less common, occurring in 75 to 450/100,000 people. It is a diagnosis of exclusion. Thorough assessment is required to rule out other potential illnesses, both medical and psychological, and assessment of lifestyle factors (e.g., diet, weight, stress) that reduce one's ability to enjoy life.

## Goals of Therapy

- Make a positive appropriate diagnosis
- Be supportive
- Investigate further complaints as appropriate
- Avoid potentially harmful or unproven therapies
- Treat symptoms

## Investigations

The diagnostic criteria (Table 1) have been revised, simplified and placed in a conceptual framework.

Table 1: **Diagnostic Criteria for Chronic Fatigue Syndrome***

- clinically evaluated fatigue (history, physical, laboratory investigations)
- persistent or relapsing fatigue for ≥ 6 months
- new or definite onset
- not relieved by rest
- substantial, significant reduction in function (occupation, education, social or personal)

PLUS four or more of the following symptoms, concurrent, recurrent or persistent:

- reduced short term memory or concentration
- sore throat
- tender cervical or axillary lymph nodes
- muscle pain
- diffuse arthralgia without arthritis
- new headaches
- unrefreshing sleep
- post-exercise fatigue lasting more than 24 hours

* *Ann Intern Med 1994;121:953–959.*

There must be clinical evaluation to rule out other causes. Other illnesses that are well controlled (e.g., hypothyroidism with replacement L-thyroxine producing a normal TSH) do not preclude a diagnosis of CFS. Well-controlled psychiatric problems also no longer prevent a diagnosis of CFS.

No single factor appears etiologic in this illness. Rather, it is more likely an individual response to a number of potential stimuli including infection, major illness or life stress. Although some patients have psychiatric complaints or prior psychiatric history, many patients do not; it is not felt to be a solely psychologic entity. No consistent biologic markers have been found. No single diagnostic test exists, nor are any tests needed for diagnosis apart from those required to exclude other potential causes (Table 2). Neither viral titres nor neuro-imaging studies are required or helpful in routine clinical practice.

Table 2: **Clinical Evaluation of Prolonged Fatigue***

1. History and physical exam
2. Mental status exam
3. Neurologic and psychiatric exam if indicated
4. Routine laboratory tests
   (CBC with differential, BUN, creatinine, electrolytes, fasting glucose, calcium, phosphorus, ESR or CRP, urinalysis, TSH, liver enzymes, total protein, albumin)
5. Any additional tests as indicated from 1-4 above
6. Label Chronic Fatigue Syndrome if above negative or unhelpful AND all diagnostic criteria are met
7. Label Idiopathic Chronic Fatigue if either duration or severity criteria are not met

* *Ann Intern Med 1994;121:953-959.*

Chronic fatigue syndrome is rare in children younger than 18 years; when it occurs it is more short lived and recovery is good. In population-based US studies CFS occurs predominantly, but not exclusively, in young adult women 30-39, with lower income, who are clerical workers. This contrasts with the reported referral clinic population of affluent well-educated women, probably reflecting sociological factors. It occurs in all races and probably overlaps with fibromyalgia and idiopathic environmental intolerances.

*Recovery* is more often seen in community-based studies and more likely in fatigue of shorter duration. Indeed, fatigue lasting less than 6 months often spontaneously remits, or other causes are found. Recovery is far less likely in patients with CFS for many years, or for those considered severely ill.

## Therapeutic Choices

There are no specific treatments for CFS.

Table 3: **Symptomatic Treatment of Chronic Fatigue Syndrome**

| Drug | Initial Dose | Usual Dose | Comments | Cost* |
|---|---|---|---|---|
| **Antidepressants for Sleep and Mood** | | | See Chapter 5 for more information. | |
| **Tricyclic Antidepressants** | | | All TCAs: No evidence for superiority of any agent. Use side effects (anticholinergic, weight gain) to guide therapy. Useful for nonrestorative sleep. | |
| *amitriptyline* Elavil, generics | 10–25 mg/d | 75–200 mg/d | | $ |
| *desipramine* Norpramin, generics | 10–25 mg/d | 100–200 mg/d | | $$–$$$ |
| **Selective Serotonin Reuptake Inhibitors** | | | All SSRIs: No evidence for superiority of any agent. Can use early in the day for the hypersomnolent. May be better tolerated than TCAs. | |
| *fluoxetine* Prozac, generics | 10–20 mg/d | 20–40 mg/d | | $$–$$$$ |
| *sertraline* Zoloft, generics | 25–50 mg/d | 50–100 mg/d | | $$$ |
| **Other** | | | | |
| *nefazodone* Serzone | 100 mg/d | 300–500 mg/d | | $$$–$$$$$ |
| *trazodone* Desyrel, generics | 50 mg QHS | 50–100 mg QHS | Useful for sleep. May be combined with SSRI. | $ |
| *venlafaxine* Effexor | 37.5 mg/d | 112.5–225 mg/d | | $$$$–$$$$$ |
| **Analgesics for Pain** | | | Other NSAIDs may be used. No evidence for superiority of any agent. | |
| *acetaminophen* Tylenol, generics | | 325–650 mg TID | | $ |
| *ibuprofen* Motrin, Advil, generics | | 200–600 mg TID | | $ |

* *Cost of 30-day supply – includes drug cost only.*
*Legend: $ < $20   $$ $20–40   $$$ $40–60   $$$$ $60–80   $$$$$ >$80*

*Dosage adjustment may be required in renal impairment – see Appendix I.*

### Nonpharmacologic Choices

Nonpharmacologic therapies should be utilized primarily.

- Healthy diet.
- Regular, progressive aerobic exercise.
- Psychologic counselling and lifestyle management.
- *Cognitive behavioral therapy* has resulted in the best outcomes. A randomized trial of 16 sessions which included lifestyle management, gradual and consistent increases in physical activity and counselling regarding belief systems about chronic fatigue and illness, resulted in satisfactory outcome for 73% of the patients randomized to active treatment versus 27% for patients receiving routine care.[1]

### Pharmacologic Choices

- Treat symptoms (Table 3).
  Symptomatic treatment usually includes medication for sleep, most often with low dose antidepressants. There is no convincing evidence that one agent is superior to another. Short trials of 6 to 8 weeks are sufficient to notice benefit.
- There is *no role* for nystatin, intravenous immunoglobulins, fludrocortisone, rigid diets and/or mega vitamin routines.
- Although two small, short-term, clinical trials have been published using *corticosteroids*, there is no convincing evidence that benefit outweighs risk.

## Therapeutic Tips

- Lifestyle issues are major. Minimize the "down" or "couch" time, use graduated progressive exercise and avoid wide swings in activity; it is better to be somewhat (and increasingly) active every day than to do nothing most days and then walk 5 miles.

## *Suggested Reading List*

Fukuda K, Straus SE, Hickie I, et al. The chronic fatigue syndrome: A comprehensive approach to its definition and study. *Ann Intern Med* 1994;121:953–959.

Levine PH. What we know about chronic fatigue syndrome and its relevance to the practising physician. *Am J Med* 1998;105 (3A):100S–103S.

[1] *BMJ 1996;312:22–26.*

CHAPTER 53

# Polymyalgia Rheumatica

*Nikhil Chopra, MD, FRCPC and*
*John G. Hanly, MD, MRCPI, FRCPC*

Polymyalgia rheumatica (PMR) is characterized by aching and stiffness in the muscle groups surrounding the neck, shoulders, pelvic girdle and hips. The etiology is unknown. It rarely affects adults before the age of 50. Pathologically, PMR is characterized by proximal joint synovitis, tenosynovitis and/or bursitis. There is a clear association between PMR and giant cell arteritis (GCA). Approximately 10% of patients with PMR will develop GCA concurrently or subsequent to the diagnosis of PMR; conversely, 50% of patients with GCA will develop symptoms of PMR.

## Goals of Therapy

- To eliminate symptoms of musculoskeletal pain and stiffness and associated malaise
- To restore function
- To minimize the frequency and severity of corticosteroid toxicity

## Investigations

The value of a thorough history and physical examination cannot be overemphasized. PMR is a clinical diagnosis – there are no laboratory tests that are specific for the disease (Figure 1).

- **History:** Patients with PMR complain of significant proximal muscle discomfort, especially around the shoulders, across the neck and in the buttocks and thighs. The pain of PMR is generally severe and usually interferes with activities of daily living. Patients may develop these symptoms insidiously, but many describe an acute onset and can often pinpoint the start of their symptoms to a specific day. Morning stiffness lasting for hours is a prominent feature. Symptoms tend to worsen through the night and movement during sleep causes discomfort which is severe enough to wake the patient. Systemic symptoms such as fever, malaise, anorexia and fatigue may be present. Joint pain and swelling may also occur but is usually confined to the shoulders, hips and knees. Patients should be questioned specifically about symptoms suggestive of associated GCA: temporal headaches, visual disturbances, scalp tenderness and jaw claudication. Untreated, GCA can lead to sudden and irreversible blindness.

- **Physical Examination:** The physical examination is nonspecific but usually reveals a reduction in range of motion of the neck and shoulders. Large and small joint synovitis may be present but is unusual in locations distal to the wrist and ankle. Severe swelling with pitting edema over the dorsum of both hands occurs in 8% of patients. Proximal muscle tenderness may be present but muscle weakness, although difficult to assess due to pain, is not present. Diminished or absent temporal artery pulsation and associated scalp tenderness, coupled with an appropriate history, is suggestive of GCA.
- **Laboratory Tests**
  - A rapid erythrocyte sedimentation rate (ESR) and elevated levels of C-reactive protein (CRP) are usually present.
  - Anemia and/or thrombocytosis may also be found.
  - Temporal artery biopsy is indicated only if there is a clinical suspicion of associated GCA.

The diagnostic approach is outlined in Figure 1 and Table 1.

Figure 1: **Diagnostic Approach in Patients with Suspected Polymyalgia Rheumatica (PMR)**

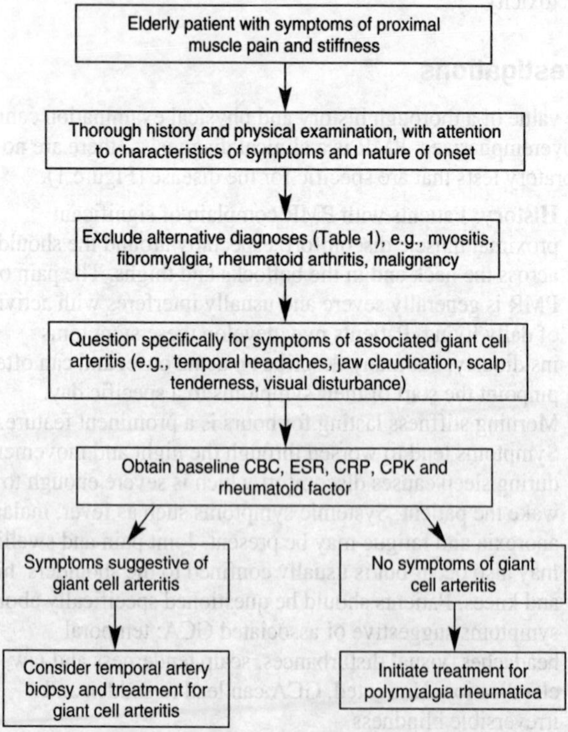
Elderly patient with symptoms of proximal muscle pain and stiffness
Thorough history and physical examination, with attention to characteristics of symptoms and nature of onset
Exclude alternative diagnoses (Table 1), e.g., myositis, fibromyalgia, rheumatoid arthritis, malignancy
Question specifically for symptoms of associated giant cell arteritis (e.g., temporal headaches, jaw claudication, scalp tenderness, visual disturbance)
Obtain baseline CBC, ESR, CRP, CPK and rheumatoid factor
Symptoms suggestive of giant cell arteritis
No symptoms of giant cell arteritis
Consider temporal artery biopsy and treatment for giant cell arteritis
Initiate treatment for polymyalgia rheumatica

Table 1: **Differential Diagnosis of Polymyalgia Rheumatica (PMR)**

| Diagnosis | Distinguishing Features From PMR |
|---|---|
| Myositis | Muscle weakness on physical examination<br>↑ CPK<br>Abnormalities on EMG and muscle biopsy |
| Fibromyalgia | Usually seen in younger patients<br>Widespread pain and tenderness at a significant number of soft tissue sites not limited to the shoulders and hips<br>Normal ESR and CRP |
| Rheumatoid Arthritis | Synovitis distal to the wrist and ankle<br>Seropositivity for rheumatoid factor<br>Inadequate response to low dose prednisone therapy<br>Radiographic erosions |
| Malignancy | As directed by clinical examination, laboratory evaluation (e.g., iron deficiency anemia), and lack of response to conventional therapy. However, the incidence of malignancy is not increased in PMR. |

# Therapeutic Choices

## Pharmacologic Choices

### *Corticosteroids*

Nonsteroidal anti-inflammatory drugs are generally ineffective or provide only partial improvement of symptoms in patients with PMR. Thus, systemic corticosteroids are the cornerstone of therapy. **Prednisone** 10 to 20 mg per day, results in rapid and sustained clinical improvement. Substantial, if not complete, resolution of symptoms occurs within days. In fact, the diagnosis of PMR should be reconsidered if symptoms fail to improve significantly after 1 week of corticosteroid therapy. A diagnosis of GCA necessitates higher doses of corticosteroids.

The dose of corticosteroids is *gradually tapered* once symptoms of PMR have been controlled. Approximately 75% of patients with PMR are able to discontinue steroids completely after 2 years of therapy.[1] A minority of patients may require more prolonged corticosteroid therapy to control their symptoms. Start patients on an initial dose of 15 mg of prednisone daily and

[1] *Ann Rheum Dis 1993;52:847–50.*

reduce by 2.5 mg every 2 weeks until a dose of 10 mg daily is reached. This dose is continued for 4 weeks and, thereafter the daily prednisone dose is tapered by 1 mg every month until completion. Patients should be followed to ensure that symptoms of PMR do not return during the prednisone taper. If symptoms do recur, the dose of prednisone should be increased to the lowest level that was previously effective in controlling symptoms, maintained at that level for 1 month and then tapered as before.

Depot IM **methylprednisolone** (MP) has been compared to oral prednisone in a double-blind study of patients with PMR.[2] Patients on MP received a lower cumulative dose of corticosteroids than patients on oral prednisone; there were also fewer fractures and less weight gain associated with MP. Unfortunately, reduction of pain took longer and fewer patients on MP were able to discontinue corticosteroids completely. Therefore, the role, if any, of IM methylprednisolone in the treatment of PMR is unclear.

*Prevention of Corticosteroid Toxicity*

Corticosteroids are associated with significant side effects, including hypertension, glucose intolerance, cataracts, glaucoma and osteoporosis. The lowest dose of corticosteroid needed to control symptoms should be used for the shortest period of time possible in order to minimize corticosteroid toxicity. Treatment with prednisone doses greater that 7.5 mg daily for greater than 3 months has been associated with significant bone loss. *Bisphosphonates* (**etidronate** 400 mg daily for 2 weeks every 3 months or **alendronate** 5–10 mg daily) have been shown to prevent the bone loss associated with corticosteroid use and should be prescribed in patients with PMR commencing corticosteroid therapy.[3] Exercise, calcium (total daily dose 1500 mg) and vitamin D supplementation (400 to 800 IU daily) also reduce the risk of osteoporosis and should be prescribed in conjunction with bisphosphonates.

### Immunosuppressives

**Methotrexate** and **azathioprine** have been used in the treatment of PMR and GCA primarily to minimize corticosteroid exposure. However, the few studies have yielded conflicting results.[4,5] These drugs should be considered only in those patients with significant corticosteroid toxicity and/or in those unable to wean below 7.5 mg of prednisone daily. Initiation of an immunosuppressive agent should be done in consultation with a rheumatologist.

---

[2] *Br J Rheumatol 1998;37:189–195.*
[3] *N Engl J Med 1997;337:382–387.*
[4] *Ann Rheum Dis 1986;45:136–138.*
[5] *Rheumatol 1996;23:624–628.*

## Therapeutic Tips

- Patients may report a transient increase in musculoskeletal symptoms after each corticosteroid dose reduction. These symptoms usually subside spontaneously over the ensuing week and do not necessarily represent a disease flare.
- The ESR and CRP usually parallel disease activity in patients with PMR. These tests can be used to confirm the clinical suspicion of a disease flare but should not be used in isolation to make treatment decisions.
- Reduction in range of motion of the shoulder may occur in some patients due to a localized rotator cuff tendonitis or capsulitis. This is more likely to occur when there has been a delay in diagnosis and initiation of therapy. A local corticosteroid injection of the subacromial bursa or glenohumeral joint is often helpful.

## *Suggested Reading List*

Evans JM and Hunder GG. Polymyalgia rheumatica and giant cell arteritis. *Clin Ger Med* 1998;14:455–473.

Hazelman BL. Polymyalgia rheumatica and giant cell arteritis. In: Klippel JH and Dieppe PA, eds. *Rheumatology*. 2nd ed. London: Mosby International, 1998. 7:21.1–21.8.

Hunder GG. Giant cell arteritis and polymyalgia rheumatica. *Med Clin North Am* 1997;81:195–219.

Salvarani C, Macchioni P, Boiardi L. Polymyalgia rheumatica. *Lancet* 1997;350:43–44.

CHAPTER 54

# Hyperuricemia and Gout

*Gunnar Kraag, MD, FRCPC*

## Goals of Therapy

- To terminate the acute attack of arthritis
- To prevent recurrence
- To prevent or reverse complications
- To deal with associated disorders

## Stages in Gouty Arthritis

The 4 stages of gouty arthritis are asymptomatic hyperuricemia, acute arthritis, the intercritical period and chronic tophaceous gout.

### *Asymptomatic Hyperuricemia*

Hyperuricemia is not a specific disease nor is it an indication for therapy. It may be secondary to a specific disorder or the ingestion of certain drugs (Table 1). A number of associated conditions (Table 2) deserve treatment. Asymptomatic hyperuricemia ends with the first attack of acute arthritis or nephrolithiasis, usually after more than 25 years of sustained hyperuricemia.

Table 1: **Drugs That May Cause Hyperuricemia**

| | |
|---|---|
| Low-dose salicylates | Phenylbutazone (low dose) |
| Diuretics | Ethambutol |
| Alcohol | Pyrazinamide |
| Cyclosporine | Nicotinic acid |
| Levodopa | IV nitroglycerin |

Table 2: **Conditions Associated With Hyperuricemia**

| | |
|---|---|
| Obesity | Atherosclerosis |
| Hypertension | Ischemic heart disease |
| Hyperlipidemia | Alcohol consumption |
| Myeloproliferative disorders and some cancers | Intrinsic renal disease |
| | Diabetes |

Figure 1: **Treatment of Acute Gout**

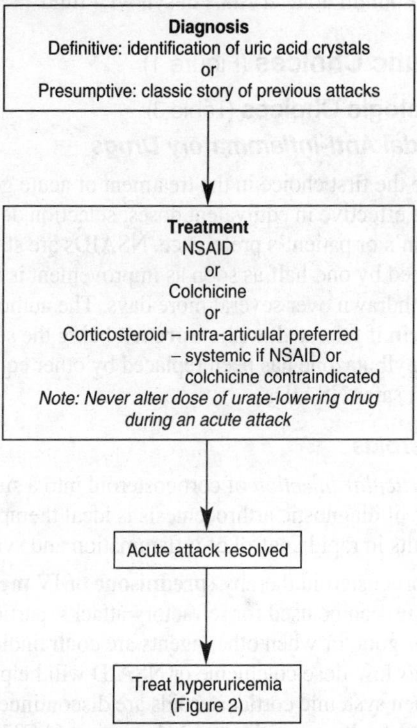

**Diagnosis**
Definitive: identification of uric acid crystals
or
Presumptive: classic story of previous attacks
**Treatment**
NSAID
or
Colchicine
or
Corticosteroid – intra-articular preferred
– systemic if NSAID or colchicine contraindicated
*Note: Never alter dose of urate-lowering drug during an acute attack*
Acute attack resolved
Treat hyperuricemia (Figure 2)


## *Acute Gouty Arthritis*

## Investigations

- History and physical examination:
  - abrupt onset of excruciating joint pain and inflammation of affected joint
  - may be any joint but lower limbs more commonly affected
  - 50% of first attacks occur in the metatarsophalangeal joint of the great toe, which is affected in 90% of patients over time
  - 10% of attacks can be polyarticular
  - mild attacks may resolve over 1–2 days but can take up to several weeks to completely settle
  - precipitants of acute attacks include trauma, acute illness, surgery, alcohol (beer and wine) and drugs (Table 1)
- Laboratory investigations including:
  - serum uric acid may or may not be elevated; several determinations should be made

- 24-hour urine uric acid excretion dictates choice of therapy
- definitive diagnosis by identification of intracellular monosodium urate crystals in synovial fluid

## Therapeutic Choices (Figure 1)

### Pharmacologic Choices (Table 3)

#### *Nonsteroidal Anti-inflammatory Drugs*

NSAIDs are the first choice in the treatment of acute gout. All NSAIDs are effective in equivalent doses; selection depends on the physician's or patient's preference. NSAIDs are started in full doses, reduced by one-half as soon as improvement is noted and then withdrawn over several more days. The author uses **indomethacin** if tolerated, with **naproxen** being the second choice. Phenylbutazone has been replaced by other equally effective but safer NSAIDs.

#### *Corticosteroids*

The *intra-articular injection* of corticosteroid into a single large joint at time of diagnostic arthrocentesis is ideal therapy and usually results in rapid control of inflammation and symptoms.

Systemic corticosteroid therapy (**prednisone** or IV **methylprednisolone**) can be used for refractory attacks, particularly polyarticular gout, or when other agents are contraindicated. *Simultaneous* low-dose colchicine or NSAID will help prevent rebound when systemic corticosteroids are discontinued. A single IM injection of **adrenocorticotropic hormone** (ACTH) can be used as an alternative to corticosteroids.

The side effects of corticosteroids are well known but rarely a problem in the short courses of therapy used in acute gout.

#### *Colchicine*

Colchicine relieves pain within 24 hours in 90% of patients. However, its role is limited due to its toxicity and its questionable value as a diagnostic guide since other conditions including pseudogout, tendonitis and rheumatoid arthritis can also respond to this therapy.

The use of IV colchicine is controversial. It is used when NSAIDs, colchicine or steroids cannot be given by mouth (e.g., postoperatively). Because of severe potential toxicity, IV colchicine should be restricted to hospitalized patients and supervised by physicians experienced in IV use.

## Therapeutic Tips

- The earlier therapy is introduced, the quicker the attack will be resolved.

- Uric acid-lowering agents should never be started or stopped during an acute attack because symptoms may be exacerbated or prolonged.
- The use of colchicine in the treatment of acute gout should generally be discouraged. (Low-dose colchicine is effective for prophylaxis and is not associated with the toxicities of high-dose colchicine used in acute gout.)
- Dietary restriction of purines rarely causes a fall of plasma urate of > 60 μmol/L.
- Avoid use of ASA.

## *Intercritical Period and Prophylaxis*

The intercritical period is asymptomatic. After the initial attack, the interval between subsequent attacks may vary from a few days to many years.

## Therapeutic Choices

### Nonpharmacologic Choices

- Dietary factors can precipitate attacks and include: fasting, overindulgence in purine-rich foods (kidney, liver, anchovies, sardines), pancreatic enzyme therapy in cystic fibrosis and specific foods, beer or wines.
- Reduction in purine intake achieves only modest decreases in serum urate and uric acid excretion. Strict monitoring of purine intake is unnecessary with currently used drugs.
- Weight reduction is important in treating associated conditions (e.g., diabetes, obesity, hyperlipidemia), but strenuous diets may increase uric acid and precipitate an acute gouty attack.
- Alcohol should only be used in moderation. Binge drinking should be avoided.

### Pharmacologic Choices (Figure 2, Table 3)

**Colchicine,** 1 mg per day, is very effective in preventing recurrent attacks. If it cannot be used, a low-dose *NSAID* (e.g., **indomethacin** 25 mg BID or **naproxen** 250 mg BID) may be substituted. If no attacks have occurred for 1 year, the drug can be stopped, but warn the patient about the possibility of an acute attack.

#### *Antihyperuricemic Drugs*

Whether or when to begin long-term antihyperuricemic therapy is controversial. One view is that the first attack is a late event in the gouty diathesis; even if further attacks do not occur, it cannot be

Figure 2: **Treatment of Hyperuricemia**

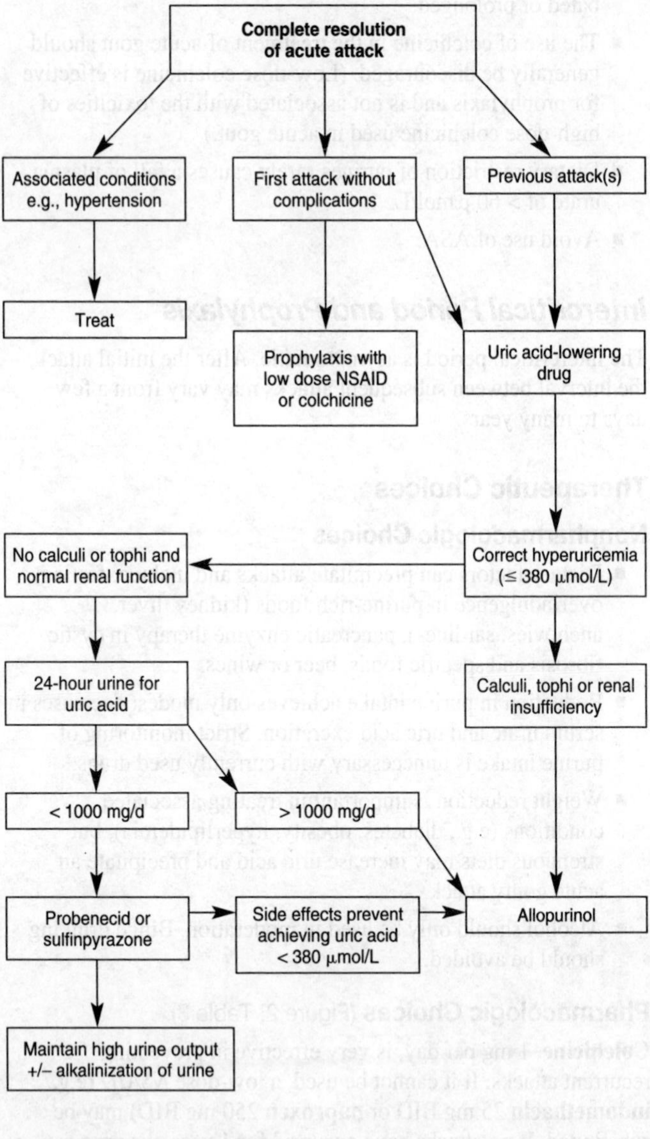
Complete resolution of acute attack
Associated conditions e.g., hypertension
First attack without complications
Previous attack(s)
Treat
Prophylaxis with low dose NSAID or colchicine
Uric acid-lowering drug
No calculi or tophi and normal renal function
Correct hyperuricemia (≤ 380 μmol/L)
24-hour urine for uric acid
Calculi, tophi or renal insufficiency
< 1000 mg/d
> 1000 mg/d
Probenecid or sulfinpyrazone
Side effects prevent achieving uric acid < 380 μmol/L
Allopurinol
Maintain high urine output +/– alkalinization of urine

assumed that renal damage will not. Thus, therapy should be initiated. The other view is that, because recurrence may be delayed for many years and chronic tophaceous gout develops only in a minority, therapy can be delayed until recurrence or detection of tophi. The author treats after the first documented attack of gout.

Table 3: **Drug Therapy of Gout**

| Drug | Dosage | Adverse Effects | Drug Interactions | Comments | Cost* |
|---|---|---|---|---|---|
| **NSAIDs** | | | | | |
| *indomethacin* Indocid, generics | Acute attack: 75 mg STAT, then 50 mg Q6H × 2 d then 50 mg Q8H × 1 d then 25 mg Q8H × 1 d<br>Prophylaxis: 25 mg BID | (For all NSAIDs)<br>GI disturbances; other adverse effects uncommon with short-term therapy.<br>For side effects with long-term use, see Chapter 55. | (For all NSAIDs, see Chapter 55.) | Both agents:<br>Suppositories may be used if oral route inadvisable. | $ |
| *naproxen* Naprosyn, generics | Acute attack: 750 mg STAT, then 500 mg BID × 4–5 d<br>Prophylaxis: 250 mg BID | | | | $ |
| **Colchicine** generics | Acute attack: 0.5–0.6 mg Q1H until relief or side effects occur; max. 10–12 doses<br>Prophylaxis: 0.5–1.8 mg/d; usual: 1 mg/d | Very common: abdominal pain and cramps, diarrhea, nausea and vomiting.<br>Rare: neuropathy, myopathy, bone marrow depression. | | Poor benefit/toxicity ratio.<br>May be given IV: consult specialized references.<br>Dosage should be ↓ in elderly and in renal impairment. | $ |

(cont'd)

Table 3: **Drug Therapy of Gout** *(cont'd)*

| Drug | Dosage | Adverse Effects | Drug Interactions | Comments | Cost* |
|---|---|---|---|---|---|
| **Corticosteroids** | | | | | |
| *triamcinolone hexacetonide* Aristospan | Acute attack: Large joints: 10–20 mg IA Small joints: 2–6 mg IA | Not usually significant after single IA injections. | | | $ |
| *methylprednisolone acetate* Depo-Medrol | Acute attack: Large joints: 20–80 mg IA Medium joints: 10–40 mg IA Small joints: 4–10 mg IA | Not usually significant after single IA injections. | | | $ |
| *methylprednisolone sodium succinate* Solu-Medrol, generics | Acute attack: 50–100 mg IV × 1 dose | Not usually significant after single injection. | | Use when prednisone cannot be used PO. | $$ |
| *prednisone* generics | Acute attack: 30 mg daily × 5 d<br>Effective dose range: 20–50 mg/d | Except for GI disturbances and glucose intolerance, not usually significant in short-term use.<br>Long-term effects are numerous. | Barbiturates, phenytoin and rifampin ↓ steroid effect. | Doses < 20 mg/d tend to be ineffective. Simultaneous low-dose colchicine or NSAID helps prevent rebound when steroid stopped. | $ |
| *ACTH* Acthar | Acute attack: 40 mg IM × 1 dose | Not usually significant after single injection. | | | † |

| | | | | | |
|---|---|---|---|---|---|
| **Uricosurics** | | | | | |
| *probenecid* Benemid, generics | Starting dose: 250 mg BID; titrate gradually; max: 3 g/d | Both agents: May precipitate acute attack during initial phase of therapy; renal calculi, hypersensitivity reactions, GI irritation. | Salicylates ↓ effect of probenecid. Dapsone concentration ↑ by probenecid. Methotrexate plasma levels ↑ by probenecid. Heparin activity ↑ by probenecid. | Both agents: Liberal fluid intake and alkalinizing the urine can help prevent stones. Severe toxicity is rare. | $$–$$$$ |
| *sulfinpyrazone* Anturan, generics | Starting dose: 50 mg BID with meals; titrate gradually; max. 800 mg/d | | Salicylates may ↑ bleeding time, ↓ uricosuric effect of sulfinpyrazone. Action of oral hypoglycemics, insulin and anticoagulants ↑ by sulfinpyrazone. | | $ |
| **Xanthine Oxidase Inhibitors** | | | | | |
| *allopurinol* Zyloprim, generics | Starting dose: 100 mg daily<br>Usual: 300 mg/d titrated to levels: Max. 800 mg/d<br>↓ Maintenance dose in renal impairment:<br>100 mg/d if CrCl 10–20 mL/min;<br>100 mg Q2–3 d if CrCl < 5 mL/min<br>Chemotherapy/irradiation: 600–800 mg/d × 2–3 d before therapy<br>Children with malignancies or enzyme deficiencies: 10 mg/kg/d | Skin rash, GI upset, hepatotoxicity, fever, severe hypersensitivity syndrome, xanthine stones (rare). May precipitate attack during initial phase of therapy. | Half-life of azathioprine and 6-mercaptopurine ↑ by allopurinol.<br>May ↑ toxicity of cyclophosphamide.<br>Allopurinol inhibits hepatic metabolism of warfarin.<br>↑ incidence of rashes when used with ampicillin or amoxicillin. | May need to ↑ dose or combine with uricosuric agents in chronic tophaceous gout.<br>To prevent acute attacks on initiation of therapy, give prophylactic NSAID or colchicine for 2–3 wks.<br>Desensitization to allopurinol can be achieved in some patients, but may recur. | $ |

† *Available through the Special Access Program, Therapeutic Products Directorate, Health Canada.*
*Dosage adjustment may be required in renal impairment – see Appendix I.*

* *Cost of 30-day supply – includes drug cost only.*
*Legend: $ < $10   $$ $10–20   $$$ $20–30   $$$$ > $30*
*Abbreviations: IA = intra-articular.*

The aim of antihyperuricemic therapy is to reduce the serum urate concentration to below 380 μmol/L, the saturation point of monosodium urate in the extracellular fluid.

**Allopurinol**, a xanthine oxidase inhibitor, inhibits the production of uric acid. Clinically very effective, it is one of the most frequently prescribed drugs for hyperuricemia. To avoid unnecessary risks and costs, allopurinol should be reserved for patients with the following indications:

- presence of tophi
- history of renal calculi of any type
- 24-hour urinary uric acid excretion > 1000 mg
- hypoxanthine-guanine phosphoribosyl transferase (HGPRT) deficiency or phosphoribosyl pyrophosphate (PRPP) synthetase overactivity (both ↑ uric acid production)
- renal insufficiency
- uric acid nephropathy
- prophylaxis of hyperuricemia secondary to cytotoxic agents
- allergy to uricosurics

The overall incidence of side effects with allopurinol is about 15 to 20%, but only half of patients with side effects must discontinue therapy. Severe toxicity can occur; the allopurinol hypersensitivity syndrome characterized by fever, rash and severe involvement of the kidney and liver can result in death.

Higher doses of allopurinol and combination with uricosuric agents are occasionally required to speed mobilization of extensive urate deposits in chronic tophaceous gout.

Allopurinol is used before chemotherapy or irradiation and in severe enzyme deficiencies to prevent acute gouty nephropathy.

*Uricosuric agents* (**probenecid** and **sulfinpyrazone**) are effective in 70 to 80% of patients, are safe and do not influence purine metabolism as allopurinol does. They are used in patients < 60 years of age with normal renal function, a 24-hour urine uric acid < 1000 mg and no history of renal calculi. They are ineffective when the glomerular filtration rate is below 30 mL/min. Salicylates at any dose block the uricosuric effect of both drugs and must not be used concomitantly.

Both agents have similar efficacy, but probenecid is better tolerated than sulfinpyrazone.

## Therapeutic Tips

- Asymptomatic hyperuricemia (i.e., before the initial attack of gouty arthritis) should not be treated. A definite diagnosis of gout must be made.

- Patients started on antihyperuricemic therapy should also receive an anti-inflammatory agent for the first 2 to 3 weeks to lower the risk of an acute attack.
- The dose of the antihyperuricemic agent should be titrated against the uric acid levels.
- The dosage of allopurinol should be adjusted according to the creatinine clearance.
- Compliance may be improved by carefully explaining treatment objectives (e.g., allopurinol has no pain-relieving properties and must be used continuously).
- Risk of damage beyond the musculoskeletal system is low: 1% annual incidence of calculi and interstitial renal damage is likely after 10 years of inadequately treated gout.

## Chronic Tophaceous Gout

The best treatment for chronic tophaceous gout is prevention by aggressive management of acute gout and correction of hyperuricemia. Once joint and bone destruction has occurred, it cannot be reversed, and chronic gouty nephropathy often results. The aims of therapy are to control pain and inflammation (usually with NSAIDs) and to decrease serum uric acid levels. The disappearance of tophaceous deposits can be dramatic but may take several years.

### Suggested Reading List

Emmerson BT. The management of gout. *N Engl J Med* 1996; 334:445–451.

Fam AG. Should patients with interval gout be treated with urate lowering drugs? *J Rheumatology* 1995;22:162.

Kelly WN, Harris ED, Ruddy S, et al. *Textbook of rheumatology*. 4th ed. Philadelphia: W.B. Saunders, 1993: Chapters 31, 50 and 76.

Pascual E. The diagnosis of gout and CPPD crystal arthropathy. *Br J Rheumatology* 1996;35:306.

Star VL, Hochberg MC. Prevention and management of gout. *Drugs* 1993;45:212–222.

CHAPTER 55

# Rheumatoid Arthritis

*Marie J. Craig-Chambers BScPhm and*
*J. Carter Thorne, MD, FRCPC*

The "wait and see" approach to rheumatoid arthritis has not been effective. Most patients experienced poor long-term outcomes, including severe functional declines, radiographic progression, economic losses, work disability and premature mortality. Unfavorable outcomes were predicted primarily by more severe disease and only rarely were secondary to medication. Current therapeutic approaches include earlier use of slow-acting and disease modifying antirheumatic medication (DMARD), frequently in combination.

## Goals of Therapy

- To allow the patient to function as normally as possible in the short-term
- To ensure that therapy is as effective as possible in arresting or delaying joint damage and destruction

## Investigations

- A thorough history (subjective)
  – distribution/duration of painful and swollen joints
  – duration of morning stiffness
  – presence or absence of fatigue
  – limitation of function (self-care, productivity, leisure)
- Physical examination (objective). Document:
  – number of painful and swollen joints
  – mechanical joint problems: range of joint motion, crepitus, instability, malalignment and/or deformity
  – extra-articular manifestations (e.g., nodules, sicca syndrome, eye, lung and pericardial involvement, vasculitis, enlarged spleen)
- Baseline laboratory tests for individuals suspected of having a systemic polyarthritis:
  – CBC, platelet count
  – ESR, C-Reactive Protein (CRP)
  – rheumatoid factor titre, antinuclear antibody titre
  – kidney function: creatinine, electrolytes, urinalysis
  – liver function tests: ALT, AST, alkaline phosphatase
  – serum albumin
  – synovial fluid analysis (if crystals/infection suspected)

- X-rays – PA films of the hands and feet (including wrists) as well as other sites affected (x-rays are expected to be normal in early RA but may demonstrate periarticular osteopenia or be used as a baseline for later comparison)

## Therapeutic Choices

### Nonpharmacologic Choices

The arthritis care team (patient, rheumatologist, family practitioner and health professionals including pharmacist, physical therapist, occupational therapist and social worker) can assist with all aspects of care.

- Education (patients and family).
- Balance of rest and activity.
- Joint support and rest (splinting).
- Exercise (e.g., range of motion), aerobic exercise.
- General application of heat (warm water, hot baths, pool therapy) for muscle relaxation and strength building .
- Direct application of ice to inflamed (red, hot, swollen, painful) joints.
- Orthotic supports/supportive footwear.
- Emotional support (patient and family) including use of support organizations (The Arthritis Society, Canada 1–800-848-8384 or website:www.arthritis.ca).
- Importance of proper nutrition to promote wellness.
- Surgery.

### Pharmacologic Choices (Figure 1)

All patients diagnosed with rheumatoid arthritis require referral to a rheumatologist and early introduction of a DMARD in addition to an anti-inflammatory medication. If single DMARD therapy is ineffective or if several severe prognostic factors are present at the start of therapy (severe functional limitations, more than 20 swollen joints, elevated ESR or CRP and elevated rheumatoid factor), combination DMARDs are used increasingly.

#### *Nonsteroidal Anti-Inflammatory Drugs (NSAIDs)* (Table 1)

NSAIDs are used in conjunction with DMARDs to control pain and the local inflammatory reaction. The analgesic effect of salicylates and NSAIDs is prompt but reduction of inflammation may take 2 to 4 weeks. There is no single best NSAID; in general, all are equally effective when used at equivalent dosages (consider cost). There is, however, great variability in patient response to NSAIDs and the ability to tolerate the GI symptoms associated with NSAIDs. Selection should be guided by the prescriber's familiarity with the agent.

Figure 1: **Treatment Strategy for Recent-onset Rheumatoid Arthritis***

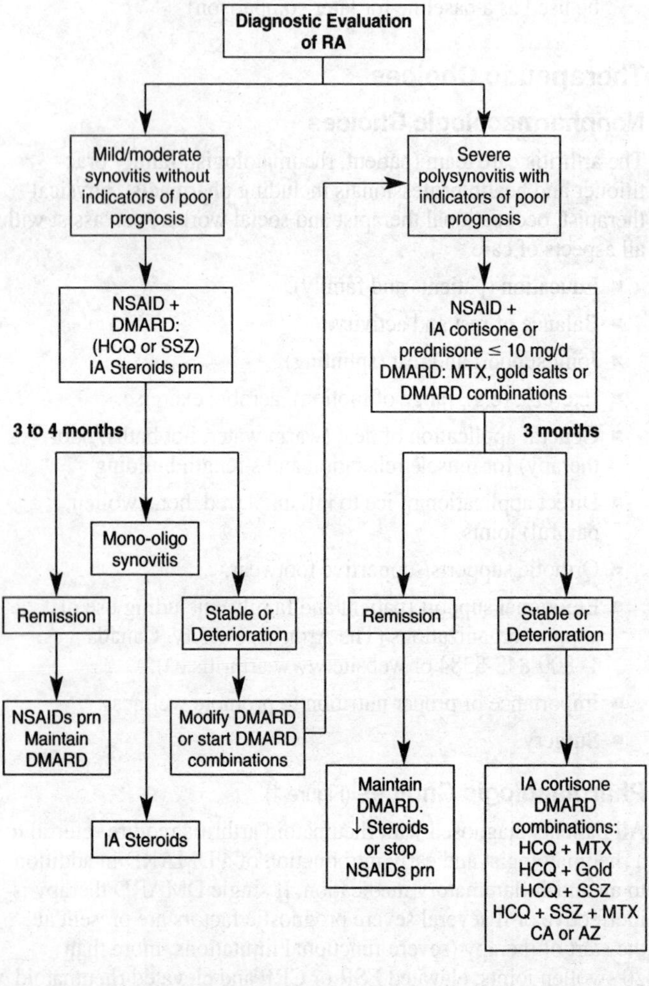
Diagnostic Evaluation of RA
Mild/moderate synovitis without indicators of poor prognosis
Severe polysynovitis with indicators of poor prognosis
NSAID + DMARD: (HCQ or SSZ) IA Steroids prn
NSAID + IA cortisone or prednisone ≤ 10 mg/d DMARD: MTX, gold salts or DMARD combinations
3 to 4 months
3 months
Mono-oligo synovitis
Remission
Stable or Deterioration
Remission
Stable or Deterioration
NSAIDs prn Maintain DMARD
Modify DMARD or start DMARD combinations
Maintain DMARD. ↓ Steroids or stop NSAIDs prn
IA cortisone DMARD combinations: HCQ + MTX HCQ + Gold HCQ + SSZ HCQ + SSZ + MTX CA or AZ
IA Steroids

*Abbreviations: HCQ: hydroxychloroquine; IA = intra-articular; MTX: methotrexate; SSZ: sulfasalazine; CA: cyclosporine A; AZ: azathioprine.*
** Adapted with permission from Can J Diagnosis 1998;Sept(Suppl):4–9.*

None of the traditional NSAIDs is clearly less *gastrotoxic* than another. The use of enteric coated products, suppositories or taking an NSAID with meals may reduce GI symptoms but does not reduce the risk of a major GI bleed. **Misoprostol**, on the other hand, reduces the risk of a bleed in high-risk patients but does not treat stomach symptoms and may need dosage adjustment if GI symptoms (diarrhea, nausea, bloating) occur. GI symptoms do not

Table 1: **NSAIDs Used in Rheumatoid Arthritis**

| NSAID* | Dosage (mg/d) | Adverse Effects | Comments/ Drug Interactions | Cost† |
|---|---|---|---|---|
| **Traditional NSAIDs** | | | | |
| *ASA (enteric coated)*<br>Entrophen, generics | 2600–6000 | **Gastrointestinal**<br>C: Dyspepsia, nausea/vomiting, diarrhea.<br>UC: Gastric and duodenal ulcers.<br>R: Gastric hemorrhage, perforation, small bowel ulceration.<br>**Renal**<br>UC: Fluid retention/edema.<br>R: Renal insufficiency.<br>**Dermatologic**<br>R: Skin rashes.<br>**Central Nervous System**<br>C: Dizziness, headache, tinnitus, loss of hearing (dose related); common with all salicylates, both acetylated and nonacetylated.<br>UC: Tinnitus, loss of hearing with other NSAIDs, disorientation, confusion (tends to occur with indomethacin and tolmetin in younger patients but may occur with all NSAIDs in the elderly).<br>R: Aseptic meningitis (reported with ibuprofen in lupus patients).<br>CNS effects may be dose related and respond to ↓ dosage. | Use one NSAID only. (Exception is cardioprotective doses of ASA.)<br>**Warfarin** – ↑ risk of bleeding due to platelet inhibition and gastric mucosal damage.<br>**Antihypertensives (Diuretics, β-Blockers, ACE Inhibitors; α-Blockers)** – possible reduction in hypertensive effect; may require additional antihypertensive therapy.<br>**Lithium** – may interfere with sodium/water balance. Monitor lithium levels when NSAID added. | $ |
| *choline magnesium trisalicylate*<br>Trilisate | 2000–3000 | | | $$ |
| *diclofenac*<br>Voltaren, generics | 75–200 | | | $–$$$ |
| *diflunisal*<br>Dolobid, generics | 500–1000 | | | $–$$ |
| *etodolac*<br>Ultradol, generics | 400–600 | | | $$$–$$$$ |
| *fenoprofen*<br>Nalfon | 1200–3200 | | | $$–$$$$ |
| *flurbiprofen*<br>Ansaid, Froben, generics | 150–300 | | | $$–$$$ |
| *ibuprofen*<br>Motrin, generics | 1200–3600 | | | $ |
| *indomethacin*<br>Indocid, generics | 50–200 | | | $ |
| *ketoprofen*<br>Orudis, generics | 150–300 | | | $–$$ |
| *nabumetone*<br>Relafen, generics | 1000–2000 | | | $$$–$$$$ |

*(cont'd)*

Table 1: **NSAIDs Used in Rheumatoid Arthritis** *(cont'd)*

| NSAID* | Dosage (mg/d) | Adverse Effects | Comments/ Drug Interactions | Cost† |
|---|---|---|---|---|
| *naproxen* Naprosyn, generics | 500–1500 | **Hepatic** UC: ↑ LFTs. | | $ |
| *oxaprozin* Daypro | 1200–1800 | R: Reye's syndrome in children with chickenpox and flu (primarily ASA), hypersensitivity reaction (hepatitis in adults) with all NSAIDs. | | $$$–$$$$ |
| *piroxicam* Feldene, generics | 10–20 | **Hematologic** | | $ |
| *salsalate* Disalcid | 1500–3000 | C: Antiplatelet effect (not with nonacetylated salicylates). | | $$–$$$ |
| *sulindac* generics | 200–400 | R: Agranulocytosis/aplastic anemia (indomethacin), thrombocytopenia. | | $–$$ |
| *tenoxicam* Mobiflex, generic | 10–20 | **Pulmonary** R: Asthma (patients with ASA hypersensitivity). | | $–$$ |
| *tiaprofenic acid* Surgam, generics | 600 | | | $$ |
| *tolmetin* Tolectin, generics | 1200–2000 | | | $$–$$$ |
| **COX-2 Inhibitors** | | | | |
| *celecoxib* Celebrex | 100–400 | UC: abdominal pain, dyspepsia, diarrhea, skin rash. Renal effects unknown. | Possible cross-sensitivity with sulfa. Incidence unknown. ↓ endoscopic lesions of standard NSAIDs. Unknown if this translates into ↓ GI events. | $–$$$$ |

*Dosage adjustment may be required in renal impairment – see Appendix I.*

** In hepatic disease, reduce dosage.*

*Abbreviations: C (common > 10%); UC (uncommon 1–10%); R (rare < 1%).*

*† Cost of 30-day supply – includes drug cost only.*

*Legend: $ < $ 20 $$ $20–40 $$$ $40–60 $$$$ > $60*

predict GI bleeds and vice versa; in fact, NSAIDs may even result in painless "silent" bleeds because of the analgesic effect of the NSAID.

There is *no added benefit* in combining 2 NSAIDs, but there is increased risk of gastric lesions when NSAIDs are used in combination, including coincidental use of other NSAIDs such as over-the-counter preparations. The only rational risk versus benefit combination of NSAIDs is the addition of low dosage ASA to reduce risk of cardiovascular events. Note that even low dose ASA 325 mg increases the risk of an adverse gastrointestinal event.

Patients at increased risk of a GI bleed (history of recent GI ulcer or bleed, age greater than 65, comorbid diseases) have 2 choices to reduce the risk associated with traditional NSAIDs: cyto-protection with **misoprostol** 200 μg BID or TID or **proton-pump inhibitors**.

A significant reduction in endoscopic lesions was seen in prospective trials of the *COX-2 inhibitor*, **celecoxib**. However, those at most risk of a GI bleed, i.e., the elderly and those with prior GI bleeds, were not included in the COX-2 inhibitor trials. Long term trials to confirm a reduction in serious events including perforation, ulcer, bleeds and death are pending. GI symptoms such as nausea, stomach pain, diarrhea are possible, but less common with the COX-2 inhibitors. As with all NSAIDs, GI symptoms do not predict GI bleeds.

*Non-acetylated salicylates* (**salsalate**, **choline magnesium salicylate**) may be considered in patients with ASA hyper-sensitivity, as the acetyl portion is implicated in allergy.

Evidence does not support the use of one traditional NSAID over another in *renal disease* and it is not yet known what role the COX-2 inhibitors will play.

### ***Disease-Modifying Anti-Rheumatic Medications (DMARDs)*** (Table 2)

These slow-acting agents are recommended for *all patients* diagnosed with active inflammatory disease. It is inappropriate to await the response of anti-inflammatories. DMARD therapy should be initiated in consultation with a rheumatologist. The selection of medication will depend on the intensity of the disease and its stage.

**Methotrexate** (MTX) is the most frequently used DMARD because it is well tolerated, has a low incidence of side effects and a relatively rapid onset of action (8 weeks compared to 3 to 6 months with IM gold and hydroxychloroquine). It is often selected for patients who have more than 5 joint effusions on presentation or who have an incomplete or non-response to hydroxychloroquine plus NSAIDs. It is the agent most frequently used in combination with other medications. Previous concerns regarding liver toxicity have not borne out in clinical practice. Significant reductions in side effects (mouth ulcers, headache, nausea, bone marrow suppression) may be achieved by concomitant **folic acid** 1 mg daily or 5 mg weekly, without adversely impacting efficacy. Methotrexate may be given orally or by IM or SC injection (possibly SC self-injection) always once weekly. The entire dosage must be taken once weekly or if the patient is intolerant of a single dose, divided into 2 or 3 doses 12 hours apart. A response may be seen within 6 to 8 weeks provided the dosage is appropriate for the severity of the arthritis and it is absorbed. If nausea, or lack of benefit occurs with the oral dosage form, consider switching to the injection. Acute pneumonitis, heralded by a sudden onset of shortness of breath and dry cough with or without fever, needs immediate attention and differentiation from rheumatoid lung complications or infection.

Folic acid supplementation is recommended if MTX is combined with other weak folate antagonists (i.e. sulfasalazine).

**Folinic acid** 5–10 mg given 18–24 hours post dose improves severe intolerance without loss of efficacy.

Up to 80% of low dose MTX is excreted in the urine over 24–48 hours. Ten to twenty per cent of patients experience a post-dose effect (nausea, fatigue, headache) within the first 24 to 48 hours, maximally 3 to 4 days post dose. If a single weekly dosage of MTX is missed, loss of benefit may not be felt. However, if 3–4 consecutive weekly doses are missed, a resultant arthritis flare may be seen.

At dosages used in RA, it is difficult to demonstrate an immunosuppressant effect of MTX; it may work more like an anti-inflammatory. However, when considering immunization guidelines, it is classified as an immunosuppressant like azathioprine and cyclosporine.

**Chloroquine** is felt to be more potent than **hydroxychloroquine** (HCQ) but is associated with a significantly higher rate of retinopathy. Risk factors for retinal toxicity are long term use (> 800 g of HCQ) and age > 70 years. If the dosage of HCQ is < 6.0 to 6.5 mg/kg, providing that renal and hepatic function are normal, and there is periodic ophthalmology monitoring, retinopathy occurs very rarely. Both medications have good efficacy, are well tolerated and have few side effects.

**Gold** is not the DMARD of first choice. However, use of IM gold has resulted in a long-lasting remission in some patients, allowing for a once-monthly maintenance dosage or even withdrawal of the medication. With injectable gold, post-injection vasomotor nitritoid reactions, arthralgias, and local pain at the site of injection are possible and are more common with aurothiomalate.

These may be reduced or avoided by switching from the rapidly absorbed aqueous form, **aurothiomalate**, to the oil form, **aurothioglucose**, which is slowly absorbed over 24 hours.

Oral gold, auranofin, is not as effective as IM gold, and diarrhea is common.

**Sulfasalazine** is used in the following situations: in early mild disease as an alternative to hydroxychloroquine, particularly if the patient's concern for ocular toxicity is a barrier; as an alternative to methotrexate if alcohol restriction is not possible; in mild to moderate seronegative RA; in combination therapy with methotrexate and hydroxychloroquine if single DMARD therapy is ineffective (its largest role). GI intolerance can occur and thus a gradually increasing dosage is recommended.

**Azathioprine** and **cyclosporine** are considerations for those who have failed to respond to other DMARDs. They may be used alone but are more often used in combination therapy (e.g., cyclosporine and methotrexate). Use of a gradually increasing dosing regimen is recommended for azathioprine because of GI intolerance . In addition, a small percentage of patients do not have thiopurine methyltransferase, one of the enzymes that metabolizes azathioprine. In these patients, azathioprine has the potential to cause an early, severe reaction with fever, flu-like symptoms, reduced blood cell counts and infection.

Cyclosporine is costly and requires frequent blood pressure and kidney function monitoring. However, at RA dosages, CBC monitoring is required only on a periodic basis and blood level monitoring is not useful in predicting efficacy or toxicity. Use can be limited by headache, occasionally severe and migrainous.

**Penicillamine** has fallen out of favour because it takes a long time for a significant response and because of side effects. **Chlorambucil** and **cyclophosphamide** are not specifically indicated for RA but are sometimes used to treat patients with severe, refractory disease or severe extra-articular complications (e.g., uveitis).

### *Corticosteroids*

Systemic oral corticosteroids are used in RA to *bridge therapy* while awaiting the benefit of slow-acting DMARDs (particularly if the patient is very functionally limited), in systemic extra-articular complications of RA (e.g., pericarditis, pleuritis) and in low doses in the elderly to improve the quality of life. Low dose **prednisone** (10 mg or less) and/or local intra-articular **cortisone** injections are highly effective for relieving symptoms. There is evidence that low dose corticosteroids may slow the rate of joint damage in RA.[1] *Intra-articular injections* are used intermittently

[1] *Arthritis Rheum 1996;39:713–731.*

Table 2: **Disease-modifying Antirheumatic Drugs**

| Drug | Dosage | Adverse Effects | Comments/Drug Interactions | Cost* |
|---|---|---|---|---|
| **Antimalarials**† | | UC: Nausea, abdominal cramps, diarrhea, gas, skin rash.<br>R: Hypopigmentation, hyper-pigmentation, myopathy (avoid in polymyalgia rheumatica, polymyositis). HCQ may exacerbate psoriasis (not a reason to avoid use).<br>Very rare: retinopathy if dose < 6.5 mg/kg and no renal or hepatic impairment. | Avoid concomitant use of related drugs, e.g., quinine. Routine retina protection: sunglasses winter and summer.<br>HCQ dosage may be divided or once daily, with or without food.<br>Time to benefit: 3–6 mos.<br>Ophthalmologic exam Q6–12 mos. | |
| *chloroquine*<br>Aralen | 250 mg/d<br>Maintenance: < 3.5 mg/kg/d | | | $ |
| *hydroxychloroquine (HCQ)*<br>Plaquenil | 200–400 mg/d<br>Maintenance: < 6.5 mg/kg/d | | | $$ |
| *methotrexate*†<br>Rheumatrex, generics | Initial: 7.5 mg once weekly<br>Max.: 25 mg once weekly<br>Give as 1 dose, or at most 2–3 doses 12h apart.<br>PO, IM, SC (self-injection) | C: nausea, flu-like aches, headache 24–48h post dose.<br>R: mouth sores, acute pneumonitis, (may be difficult to distinguish from rheumatoid lung or infection), cytopenia.<br>Very rare: hepatic cirrhosis/fibrosis. | Folic acid supplement 1–5 mg/d ↓ GI effects and mouth sores by 80% without loss of efficacy.<br>Some NSAIDs may ↓ MTX clearance. However, this is not significant with low-dose MTX taken once weekly.<br>Restrict alcohol intake to minimize hepatic injury.<br>Variable oral absorption.<br>Faster onset (6–8 wks) than other DMARDs.<br>Monitor: CBC, liver enzymes, albumin, creatinine Q4–8 wks.<br>Avoid trimethoprim. | $–$$$ |

| | | | | |
|---|---|---|---|---|
| **Gold Salts**[†] <br>**Injectable**<br>*sodium aurothiomalate*<br>Myochrysine (aqueous)<br>*sodium aurothioglucose*<br>Solganal (in oil) | 10 mg and 25 mg test doses 1 wk apart; then 50 mg/wk | C: Post dose reaction: arthralgias, pain at site of injection, vasomotor "nitritoid" reaction (flushing, dizziness, nausea, hypotension).<br>Rash, mouth sores, proteinuria.<br>UC: Pruritus, thrombocytopenia.<br>R: diarrhea, colitis, aplastic anemia, nephrotic syndrome, pulmonary fibrosis (difficult to distinguish from rheumatoid lung). | Post dose reaction more common with aqueous product. Consider switching to oil.<br>Skin rash, mouth sores, proteinuria may be dose related. Consult rheumatologist.<br>Time to benefit: 3–6 mos.<br>Shake multidose vial of Solganal vigorously before use.<br>Monitor: CBC, platelets, urinalysis Q injection. | $$$$<br><br>$$$ |
| *sulfasalazine (enteric coated)*<br>Salazopyrin, generics | 1000–1500 mg BID<br>max: 4 g/d | C: GI intolerance, dizziness, headache, skin rash.<br>R: hypersensitivity: fever, rash, liver enzyme abnormalities.<br>Reversible oligospermia<br>Cytopenias<br>Weak antifolate. Recommend folic acid supplementation if combined with other antifolates (e.g. MTX) or if signs of deficiency. | Better tolerated if start low and go slow (1 tab/day × 1 week, 2 tab/day × 1 week, 3 tab/day × 1 week, then 2 tab BID).<br>Time to benefit: 2–3 months depending how fast the optimal dosage is achieved.<br>May cause sun sensitivity.<br>Do not use if allergic to sulfa medications or G6PD deficiency.<br>May discolor the urine yellow/ orange.<br>Monitor: CBC, liver function tests. | $ |
| *azathioprine* <br>Imuran | 50–150 mg once daily or divided<br>Max: 2.5 mg/kg/day | C: GI distress<br>R: early, severe flu-like illness with fever, infection and cytopenias<br>Myelosuppression<br>Pancreatitis<br>Hepatitis | Long term ↑ risk of malignancy that occurs in renal transplantation patients is not proven in RA.<br>↓ dosage to 1/4 of usual dosage if given with allopurinol.<br>Time to benefit: 2–3 mos depending how fast effective dosage achieved.<br>Monitoring: CBC, LFTs. | $$–$$$$ |

*(cont'd)*

Table 2: **Disease-modifying Antirheumatic Drugs** *(cont'd)*

| Drug | Dosage | Adverse Effects | Comments/Drug Interactions | Cost* |
|---|---|---|---|---|
| *cyclosporine*† <br>Neoral | 2.5 mg–5 mg/kg/d in 2 divided dosages | C: gum hyperplasia, hypertension, hirsutism<br>UC: severe headaches<br>R: nephrotoxicity, cytopenias<br>Side effects such as gum hyperplasia, hypertrichosis, fatigue, GI upset, headache, tremor and paresthesia are generally mild and transient and often resolve spontaneously or with dosage adjustment. | Metabolized by cytochrome P450; many drug interactions. See product monograph.<br>Avoid grapefruit juice totally, not just when taking the medication.<br>Onset of action: 2–3 months after dosage leveling. Start low and go slow.<br>Monitor BP and creatinine Q 2 wks until dose is stable, then monthly. Watch for edema. CBC, $K^+$ and LFT monitoring is recommended only periodically. | $$$$$ |
| *leflunomide*† <br>Arava | Loading: 100 mg/d × 3 d<br>Maintenance: 10–20 mg/d | C: diarrhea<br>U: alopecia, rash, ↑ LFTs<br>R: cytopenia, hepatotoxicity | Time to benefit: 4–12 wks.<br>Avoid alcohol.<br>Potential for teratogenicity; follow elimination procedure pre-pregnancy.<br>Monitor CBC, LFTs Q4–8 wks. | $$$$$ |

*Abbreviations: C (common > 10%); UC (uncommon 1–10%); R (rare < 1%).*
† *Avoid in patients with hepatic impairment.*
*Dosage adjustment may be required in renal impairment – see Appendix I.*

* *Cost of 4-wk supply – includes drug cost only.*
*Legend: $ < $15 $$ $15–30 $$$ $30–45 $$$$ $45–60 $$$$$ > $60*

for isolated joint problems, always ensuring that there is no evidence of local sepsis. *Pulse-dose IV therapy* should be used only under the supervision of a rheumatologist as it does not produce consistent or long-term results. *Prophylactic therapy for corticosteroid-induced osteoporosis* with calcium and Vitamin D supplementation and a bisphosphonate should be considered. If long-term therapy is needed, a medical alert bracelet should be worn.

### Other Agents

The use of new biologic agents, TNF alpha receptor-blockers, **etanercept** (for SC self-injection twice weekly) and **infliximab** (for IV use by protocol) may prove useful in progressive/aggressive disease. **Leflunomide** is an oral disease-modifying agent that inhibits *de novo* pyrimidine synthesis and shows comparable efficacy to methotrexate. Common side effects are diarrhea and alopecia. Skin rash and asymptomatic liver enzyme elevations are uncommon. The cost/benefit profiles for these agents have yet to be determined.

**Minocycline** appears to be moderately effective in early RA; its benefit may be related to its anti-inflammatory effect rather than antibacterial action. There are no comparative trials with other DMARD. GI symptoms and dizziness restricted its use in trials. Like sulfas and penicillamine it has the potential to induce lupus.

In RA, **acetaminophen** may be used on a PRN basis in addition to NSAIDs. Topical heat-producing *rubs* typically contain an "aspirin-like" medication and may provide local, temporary relief to muscle but may actually make a hot, inflamed joint feel worse.

## Therapeutic Tips

- Confirmed diagnosis of RA requires immediate consultation with a rheumatologist who will increasingly choose an aggressive approach using DMARDs.
- RA is a systemic disease with many extra articular features, such as fatigue, fever, chills, alopecia and reduced resistance to infection (in severe disease) due to the overactive yet inefficient immune function. The patient may misinterpret these as MTX side effects when they are more commonly due to the disease itself. Use of low dose MTX has not been noted to cause an increase in infections if the blood work is in the normal range. However, as with all DMARDs, treatment of an active infection should be undertaken prior to the introduction of MTX or other DMARDs.

## *Suggested Reading List*

American College of Rheumatology Ad Hoc Committee on Clinical Guidelines. Guidelines for RA management and monitoring of drug therapy in rheumatoid arthritis. *Arthritis Rheum* 1996;39:713–731.

Pincus TP, O'Dell JR, Kremer JM. Combination therapy with multiple disease-modifying antirheumatic drugs in rheumatoid arthritis: A preventative strategy. *Ann Intern Med* 1999;131:768–773.

Ryan L, Brooks P. Disease-modifying anti-rheumatic drugs. *Curr Opin Rheum* 1999;11:161–166.

West SG. *Rheumatology secrets*. Philadelphia: Hanley & Belfus, 1996.

CHAPTER 56

# Osteoarthritis

*Paul M. Peloso, MD, MSc, FRCPC*

Osteoarthritis (OA), formerly known as degenerative joint disease, encompasses a wide array of rheumatic conditions that share a common final pathway. OA can be generalized (affecting spine, knees, hips, hands or feet), localized (affecting only one joint) or nodal (affecting primarily the hands). It is endemic, increases with age, affects women slightly more often than men and is the leading cause of disability in Canada. Joint pain, crepitus and deformity, with or without swelling, characterize the disease.

## Goals of Therapy

- To reduce or eliminate the joint pain
- To increase patient and joint mobility
- To increase muscle tone around the joint
- To prevent progression and heal the underlying damaged cartilage

## Investigations

- History with attention to:
  - pattern of pain (worse with use and better with rest)
  - duration of stiffness (gelling) – usually < 30 minutes
  - ruling out associated inflammatory conditions although these may coexist
  - identifying predisposing conditions leading to early OA: developmental abnormalities (e.g., slipped capital epiphysis), congenital abnormalities (e.g., benign hypermobility syndrome), occupational factors
  - use of drugs (e.g., prednisone, alcohol) that can lead to avascular necrosis and secondary OA
- Physical examination to confirm deranged joint: active and passive limited range of motion, pain on motion, deformity, bony enlargement, misalignment, crepitus and occasionally swelling
- X-rays to confirm nonuniform joint space narrowing (symmetrical loss suggests an underlying inflammatory condition), osteophytes (new bone), subchondral cyst formation (or geodes) and bony sclerosis; if chondrocalcinosis is suspected on x-ray, diabetes, hemochromatosis, hypophosphatemia and hypothyroidism should be ruled out

- Bone scan – rarely helpful
- CT scan – rarely helpful
- Magnetic resonance imaging – when avascular necrosis is suspected; not routinely indicated
- Joint fluid analysis – high WBC and turbidity suggest other causes

## Therapeutic Choices (Figure 1 and Table 1)

### Prevention

*Primary prevention* is possible through regular physical activity and weight control. *Secondary prevention,* once OA has developed is possible by managing obesity, mechanical stresses and occupational or sports-related trauma. Early and aggressive treatment of inflammatory arthritis, metabolic abnormalities and congenital abnormalities may prevent secondary OA. Adequate intake of **vitamin D** (400 to 800 IU daily) and **calcium** (1000 to 1500 mg daily) and the use of **postmenopausal hormone therapy** delay progression, at least for the knee and hip.

### Nonpharmacologic Choices

The following should be tried prior to most pharmacologic therapies but may be considered at any stage of joint problems. Best results may be obtained using a combined approach (Figure 1).

- *Exercise* (stretching, low-impact aerobics, swimming, stationary cycling or walking) does not cause disease exacerbations and results in improved muscle strength, sense of well-being and functional status. The program should be tailored to the individual and undertaken 3 times a week for at least 20 minutes. Advice from a physiotherapist is helpful for nonadherent or reluctant patients. Many malls are open late evenings and early mornings and are ideal locations for walking.
- *Physical therapies* (i.e., TENS, laser, ultrasound, acupuncture and thermal therapy) may be tried. The most efficacious appear to be TENS and laser.
- Correctly fitted and used *aids* are helpful. A cane reduces forces through a hip or knee by up to 60%. Braces or shoe lifts can help an unstable joint if misalignment or a leg length discrepancy exists. For the neck, a double ruff collar worn at night, and for the back, abdominal and lumbar strengthening, may be helpful.
- *Taping the patella* medially with a broad elasticized tape when the knee is relaxed in slight flexion is beneficial in all patterns of knee OA.

Figure 1: **Approach to Osteoarthritis Treatment**

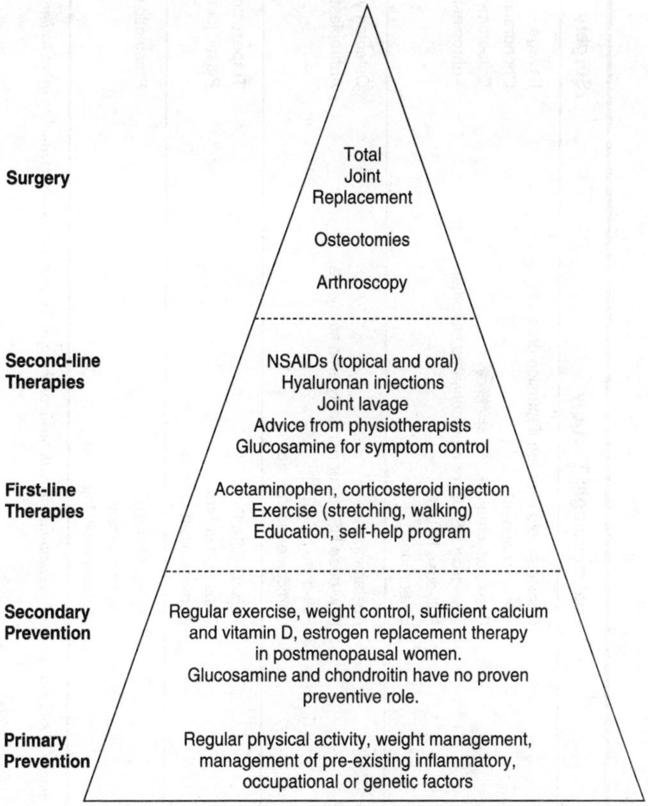
Surgery
Total Joint Replacement
Osteotomies
Arthroscopy
Second-line Therapies
NSAIDs (topical and oral)
Hyaluronan injections
Joint lavage
Advice from physiotherapists
Glucosamine for symptom control
First-line Therapies
Acetaminophen, corticosteroid injection
Exercise (stretching, walking)
Education, self-help program
Secondary Prevention
Regular exercise, weight control, sufficient calcium and vitamin D, estrogen replacement therapy in postmenopausal women.
Glucosamine and chondroitin have no proven preventive role.
Primary Prevention
Regular physical activity, weight management, management of pre-existing inflammatory, occupational or genetic factors

- *Education* (in a group setting), a *positive and supportive attitude* and *regular telephone calls* from nursing staff have been shown to improve pain control. The Arthritis Self Management Program (ASMP) exists in almost all Canadian communities. Trained patient instructors use predesigned teaching modules. Contact the local Arthritis Society or 1–800-321-1433 or http://www.arthritis.ca.

## Pharmacologic Choices (Table 2)

### *Oral and Topical Agents*

**Acetaminophen** is often combined successfully with non-pharmacologic therapies. **Acetaminophen**, **ibuprofen** and **naproxen** have been shown to provide equivalent pain relief. In acute exacerbations, **codeine**, 30 to 60 mg QID, may be necessary for 1 to 2 weeks. Codeine is an alternative in individuals unresponsive to acetaminophen and for whom NSAIDs are contraindicated or not tolerated.

Table 1: **Treatment Choices for Osteoarthritis**

| Joint | Physical Therapy | Pharmacologic Therapy* | Surgery |
|---|---|---|---|
| **Knee** | Quadriceps exercise<br>Walk, swim, bike<br>Weight loss<br>Canes<br>Orthoses for angulation and instability | Corticosteroid injection if effusion present<br>Acetaminophen<br>Capsaicin cream<br>Low-dose NSAID or nonacetylated salicylate<br>Full-dose NSAID<br>Hyaluronan | Lavage<br>Chondral holes<br>Osteotomy<br>Arthroplasty |
| **Hip** | Exercise for range of motion, strength<br>Cane<br>Orthoses for leg length abnormalities | Acetaminophen<br>Low-dose NSAID or nonacetylated salicylate<br>Full-dose NSAID<br>Corticosteroid injection | Osteotomy<br>Arthroplasty |
| **Carpometacarpal** | Ultrasound<br>CMC splints | Topical NSAIDs†<br>Capsaicin cream<br>Corticosteroid injection | Trapezectomy<br>Plastic joint spacer |
| **Distal and Proximal Interphalangeal** | Heat, cold, wax | Topical NSAIDs†<br>Capsaicin cream<br>Corticosteroid injection | Prosthetic surgery |

* *Use in a step-wise approach. Physical therapies should always be recommended and may be used in combination with medical therapy. Surgery is usually tried when other techniques have failed to provide adequate relief. See Table 2 for further information.*

† *Topical NSAIDs are not available in Canada but may be compounded as extemporaneous preparations.*

Topical 0.025% **capsaicin** cream is efficacious in knee OA and possibly other joints. **Topical NSAIDs**, popular in Europe, may be compounded as extemporaneous preparations. About 1 in 3 patients may benefit from this therapy but long-term data are lacking.[1]

The pharmacologic treatment of first choice is **acetaminophen** 500 mg QID; if after 2 to 3 weeks there is little relief, consider a low-dose *NSAID* for 2 weeks and, if unrelieved, a full dose NSAID for 2 weeks. NSAIDs should be avoided in the long term because of concerns about GI problems, particularly in the elderly, those with a history of GI ulcers or with cardiovascular disease. In such patients, continuous use of NSAIDs should be reviewed regularly, conversion back to acetaminophen tried occasionally and either addition of misoprostol or omeprazole or use of a *COX-2 specific NSAID* (**celecoxib**, **rofecoxib**) should be considered. All NSAIDs, including COX-2 inhibitors, may exacerbate hypertension, promote edema and worsen CHF. COX-2 inhibitors clearly show reduced toxicity to the gastrointestinal tract and platelets. In animal studies, some NSAIDs have been shown to retard cartilage formation; although this is controversial, it should caution our use of NSAIDs in OA. NSAIDs may be best used for a 2- to 3- week interval during acute exacerbations of pain or swelling.

The 1995 American College of Rheumatology (ACR) guidelines on the treatment of both hip and knee OA suggest that NSAIDs be considered only when nonpharmacologic treatments and acetaminophen have failed.[2] This was reinforced by the North of England guidelines.[3] Both guidelines favor the use of low dose **ibuprofen** or the *nonacetylated salicylates* such as **salsalate** first. If these are not effective, full dose NSAIDs are indicated.

There is considerable public interest in **glucosamine sulfate** in the treatment of OA. Numerous clinical trials now document its short term efficacy in pain control, compared to ibuprofen and naproxen. **Chondroitin sulfate**, 1200 mg per day, has been shown in several trials to have symptomatic benefit versus placebo; however, only 10% of an oral dose is absorbed. For both these products there is no convincing evidence of disease-modifying properties. Concerns about quality control and minimal knowledge of side effects limit enthusiasm for widespread use.

Clinical trials of *metalloproteinase inhibitors,* which have disease-modifying activity in animals, are underway in Canada.

---

[1] *BMJ 1998;316:333–338.*
[2] *Arthritis Rheum 1995;38:1535–1546.*
[3] *BMJ 1998;317:526–530.*

Table 2: **Pharmacologic Agents Used in Osteoarthritis**

| Drug | Dosage | Comments | Cost* |
|---|---|---|---|
| *acetaminophen* Tylenol, generics | 650 mg Q4H – 1000 mg Q6H | May cause hepatitis if taken in excess or by patients with liver disease. | $ |
| **NSAIDs** (e.g., *ibuprofen* Motrin, generics) | 200 mg TID up to 800 mg TID × 10 d | For comparison of available NSAIDs, see Chapter 55. | $ |
| **Nonacetylated salicylates** | | | |
| *choline magnesium trisalicylate* Trilisate | 1 g BID–TID | Gastrointestinal effects seen in 3% of patients. | $$$ |
| *salsalate* Disalcid | 1 g TID–1.5 g BID | Tinnitus and gastrointestinal effects are common side effects. | $$$ |
| **COX-2 Inhibitors** | | | |
| *celecoxib* Celebrex | 100 mg BID or 200 mg once daily | Edema (4%). Contraindicated in sulfa allergy. | $$$ |
| *rofecoxib* Vioxx | 12.5–25 mg once daily | GI symptoms are common, although less than traditional NSAIDs. | $$$ |
| *capsaicin* Zostrix | Apply to joint area TID–QID<br>May require 14–28 d for optimal effect | Efficacious in knee OA. Continued application necessary for effect; transient burning on application. Avoid contact with eyes, open lesions. | $$$ |

| | | | |
|---|---|---|---|
| *methylprednisolone acetate (intra-articular)*<br>Depo-Medrol | Knee: 40–60 mg<br>Hip: 40–80 mg<br>CMC: 10 mg<br>DIP/PIP: 10 mg | Max: 3 injections/joint/year<br>Joint activity should be minimized for 3 d following injection. Benefits last 4–6 wks. | $$–$$$ |
| *hyaluronans*<br>Neovisc<br>Suplasyn<br>Synvisc | 1 injection/wk × 3–5 wks | Transient pain and swelling on injection. Contains avian protein: avoid in patients with related hypersensitivities. | per 3 injections:<br>$166<br>$199<br>$327 |

*Dosage adjustment may be required in renal impairment – see Appendix I.*
*Abbreviations: CMC = carpometacarpal; DIP = distal interphalangeal; PIP = proximal interphalangeal.*

* *Cost of 1 week's therapy – includes drug cost only.*
*Legend: $ < $2   $$ $2–5   $$$ $5–10*

### *Joint Injection (For Accessible Joints)*

**Corticosteroid** joint injections are used when signs of inflammation exist and may follow or complement oral and topical therapies. They may be most beneficial when crystalline arthritis coexists but may be efficacious even when signs of inflammation are not present. Corticosteroids may act by reducing metalloproteinases that digest cartilage. Benefits can last up to 6 months, but 4 to 6 weeks is about average. No more than 3 to 4 injections of corticosteroid should be given in any one joint per year. Judicious use of rest *postinjection* is advised, but should not exceed 3 days because the loss of muscle bulk and strength is counterproductive. Very rarely, a synovitis is induced within 24 hours following injection.

**Hyaluronan** and its derivatives, proteinaceous derivatives of cartilage, are useful in mild to moderate cases of knee OA, and are indicated prior to NSAIDs. Three injections, separated by 1-week intervals, show benefits lasting up to 6 months. These courses may be repeated. There are no direct comparisons of the different hyaluronan derivatives. About 2% of people injected experience a sterile joint effusion within 1 to 4 days.

Joint lavage with a large-bore needle (14 or 16 gauge) and large volumes of **sterile saline** (500 mL to 2 L) may work by removing joint debris and inflammatory molecules.

**Radioactive yttrium-90**[4] provides a chemical synovectomy; it appears to work best in patients who have responded to intra-articular steroids.

## Surgical Choices

The main indication is pain unresponsive to other measures. The common dictum to be followed is, "can't sleep, can't walk, can't work."

**Arthroscopic techniques** include joint débridement, abrasion arthroplasty to smooth the joint surface, and drilling out portions of osteochondral bone. These loose joint particles may act as a proinflammatory nidus, and burr holes reduce subchondral hypertension. Proper trials are lacking for these approaches, but they continue to have wide support in the surgical community.

Open approaches are **osteotomy** of the distal femur or proximal tibia to redistribute forces through healthier cartilage. This delays the need for total joint replacement but does not provide a permanent solution.

**Total joint replacement** appears to be most appropriate for more sedentary, nonobese, older individuals because subsequent

[4] *May be obtained from Atomic Energy of Canada via your nuclear medicine diagnostic imaging department.*

demands on the prosthesis are lessened. Repeat operations are required in approximately 10 to 15% of patients over a 20-year span, because of either prosthetic loosening or secondary infection.

### Suggested Reading List

Brandt KD. Osteoarthritis. *Rheum Dis Clin North Am* 1999;25(2).

Hochberg MC, Altman RD, Brandt KD, et al. Guidelines for the management of osteoarthritis. *Arthritis Rheum* 1995;38:1535–1546.

CHAPTER 57

# Osteoporosis

*David A. Hanley, MD, FRCPC*

## Goals of Therapy

- Prevention of fractures, disability and loss of independence
- Preservation or enhancement of bone mass

## Investigations

- *History:*
  - height as a young adult (compare with current *measured* height)
  - chronic or acute back pain; development of dorsal kyphosis
  - menstrual history: menarche, occurrence of episodes of oligomenorrhea or amenorrhea (excluding pregnancies), age of menopause (high risk if menopause prior to age 45, or surgical menopause), use of postmenopausal ovarian hormone therapy
  - hypogonadism in males
  - diet: calcium intake, anorexia nervosa, weight loss after age 25, use of calcium or vitamin D supplements, lactose intolerance
  - lifestyle issues: inactivity or prolonged periods of bed rest, smoking history, alcohol intake, excessive caffeine intake
  - medications: glucocorticoids, excessive thyroid hormone replacement, long-term heparin therapy, anticonvulsants, sedatives
  - past medical history: previous fractures; increased propensity to fall; endocrine diseases: hyperthyroidism, hyperparathyroidism, hypogonadism, Cushing's syndrome; renal diseases; organ transplantation; gastrointestinal disease: gastric surgery, malabsorption; chemotherapy for malignancy
  - family history of osteoporotic fracture (particularly hip)
- *Physical examination:*
  - kyphosis
  - muscle weakness (inability to rise from a chair)
  - impaired visual acuity, other disability causing a tendency to fall
- *Laboratory investigations:*
  - all should be normal: complete blood count, calcium, alkaline phosphatase (may be elevated in acute recovery from fracture), creatinine. Consider TSH and serum protein electrophoresis

**Figure 1: Use of Bone Density and Risk Factors in Osteoporosis Management**

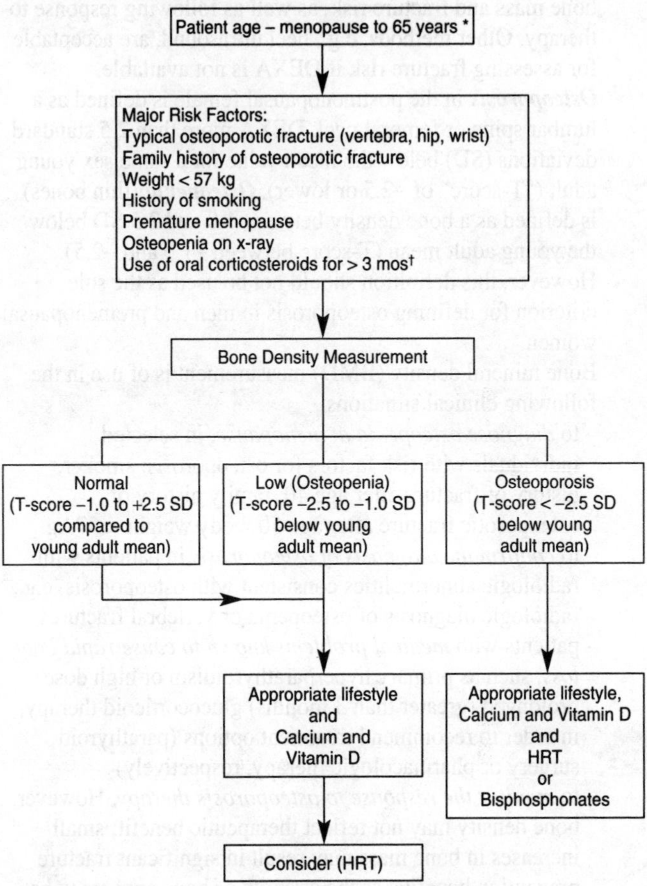
Patient age – menopause to 65 years *
Major Risk Factors:
Typical osteoporotic fracture (vertebra, hip, wrist)
Family history of osteoporotic fracture
Weight < 57 kg
History of smoking
Premature menopause
Osteopenia on x-ray
Use of oral corticosteroids for > 3 mos†
Bone Density Measurement
Normal (T-score −1.0 to +2.5 SD compared to young adult mean)
Low (Osteopenia) (T-score −2.5 to −1.0 SD below young adult mean)
Osteoporosis (T-score < −2.5 SD below young adult mean)
Appropriate lifestyle and Calcium and Vitamin D
Appropriate lifestyle, Calcium and Vitamin D and HRT or Bisphosphonates
Consider (HRT)

* *After age 65, many experts recommend treatment if the patient has had vertebral or hip fracture, regardless of bone density. Bone density measurement is a cost-effective screening tool after age 65.*

† *After menopause or age 50, prolonged (> 3 mos) corticosteroid therapy should be accompanied by bisphosphonate therapy.*

*Abbreviations: SD = standard deviation(s); HRT = hormone replacement therapy.*

– other more specific markers of calcium or bone metabolism are not appropriate routinely

- *Diagnostic imaging:*
  – x-rays are unreliable in diagnosing osteopenia (thin bones) and should only be used for detecting fractures
  – bone scans can be used to identify new fracture activity in patients with back pain and no obvious new fracture on x-ray

- *Bone density measurements* (Figure 1)
Bone density of the spine and hip by Dual Energy X-ray Absorptiometry (DEXA) is the preferred method of assessing bone mass and fracture risk, as well as following response to therapy. Other methods, e.g., heel ultrasound, are acceptable for assessing fracture risk if DEXA is not available.
***Osteoporosis*** in the postmenopausal female is defined as a lumbar spine or femoral neck DEXA more than 2.5 standard deviations (SD) below the mean value for a same sex young adult ("T-score" of –2.5 or lower). ***Osteopenia*** (thin bones) is defined as a bone density between 1.0 and 2.5 SD below the young adult mean (T-score between –1.0 and –2.5). However, this definition should not be used as the sole criterion for defining osteoporosis in men and premenopausal women.
Bone mineral density (BMD) measurement is of use in the following clinical situations:
  - to *diagnose osteopenia at menopause*, in selected individuals with risk factors for osteoporosis: smoker, history of fracture after age 40, family history of osteoporotic fracture after age 50, body weight < 57 kg.
  - to *confirm the diagnosis of osteoporosis* in patients with radiologic abnormalities consistent with osteoporosis, e.g., radiologic diagnosis of osteopenia or vertebral fractures
  - patients with *medical problems known to cause rapid bone loss*, such as primary hyperparathyroidism or high dose prolonged (greater than 3 months) glucocorticoid therapy, in order to recommend treatment options (parathyroid surgery or pharmacologic therapy, respectively)
  - to *monitor the response to osteoporosis therapy*. However, bone density may not reflect therapeutic benefit; small increases in bone mass may result in significant fracture prevention benefits, as the strength of bone appears to be proportional to the square of the density

## Therapeutic Choices

### Nonpharmacologic Choices

- Reduce risk of falling: reduction of hazards for falling in the home, elimination of drugs implicated in falls, e.g., benzodiazepines; exercise to improve strength and coordination.
- Adequate dietary calcium: dairy products; canned fish with bones (sardines, salmon); certain vegetables (broccoli, kale, beans, lentils); almonds.
- Stop smoking, reduce alcohol (< 2 drinks per day) and caffeine (≤ 2 small cups) intake.

## Pharmacologic Choices (Table 1)

Therapies for osteoporosis can be classified as those which prevent bone resorption (antiresorptive) and those which stimulate bone formation. At present, all of the approved drugs (estrogen, alendronate, cyclical etidronate, raloxifene and salmon calcitonin) are *anti-resorptive* in their action. By acting to reduce both the depth and rate of bone resorption, while the mandatory coupled bone formation proceeds normally, these agents cause an initial increase in bone mass. This increase eventually plateaus, as the overall rate of bone turnover is markedly reduced. In contrast, *bone formation agents* like sodium fluoride have been shown to cause a steady gain in bone density for the duration of their use, as much as 30 percent over 4 years.

### *Estrogen (±) Progesterone*

Estrogen, with progesterone (if the patient has not had a hysterectomy), is first choice for *prevention* of osteoporosis in the postmenopause. However, most clinicians rank the bisphosphonates ahead of estrogen for older postmenopausal women with *established* osteoporosis. Some patients cannot tolerate the conventional dose of estrogen. A regime of conjugated estrogen 0.3 mg and medroxyprogesterone acetate 2.5 mg per day combined with a calcium intake over 1000 mg and vitamin D to maintain normal serum 25-OH vitamin D levels, has bone-sparing effects on BMD similar to what might be expected with higher doses of estrogen.[1] The risks and benefits of estrogen therapy are discussed in Chapter 72.

### *Bisphosphonates*

Bisphosphonates are free of significant side effects apart from minor gastrointestinal upset and allergic reactions. An important, although rare side effect of alendronate, is esophageal ulceration.

Cyclical etidronate and alendronate are approved for prevention and treatment of postmenopausal osteoporosis and glucocorticoid-induced osteoporosis. Risedronate is also expected to receive approval for both indications.

**Etidronate** taken for 2 weeks every 3 months increases bone density and prevents vertebral fractures. Safety and efficacy for up to 7 years of cyclical etidronate therapy has been demonstrated.

Didrocal provides 14 days of 400 mg of etidronate followed by 76 days of 500 mg of elemental calcium as calcium carbonate. Calcium supplements are avoided during the 2-week cycle of etidronate.

---

[1] *Ann Intern Med 1999;130:897–904.*

Table 1: **Drugs Used in Management of Osteoporosis**

| Drug | Dosage | Comments | Cost* |
|---|---|---|---|
| **Nutritional Supplements** | | | |
| *calcium* | 1000–1500 mg/d of elemental calcium | Recommend supplements if unable to achieve intake by diet alone. Constipation and nausea are common side effects. | $ |
| *vitamin D*<br>Drisdol, Ostoforte<br>Multivitamins containing vitamin D | 400–1000 IU/d of cholecalciferol (vitamin $D_3$) or ergocalciferol (vitamin $D_2$) | Increases calcium absorption. Higher doses (e.g., 50 000 IU/week) may be needed in some individuals. Possible side effects are hypercalcemia, hypercalciuria, renal calcification and renal stones. Most multivitamin supplements contain 400 IU vitamin D and are the agents most commonly used. | $ |
| **Ovarian Hormone Therapy** | | | |
| **Estrogens** | (Starting dose in brackets) | | |
| *conjugated equine estrogen*<br>Premarin | 0.625 mg/d<br>(0.3 mg × 2–3 mos) | | $ |
| *conjugated estrone sulfate*<br>C.E.S. | 0.625 mg/d<br>(0.3 mg × 2–3 mos) | Synthetic estrogens may be tolerated when equine source estrogens are not. | $ |
| *estrone sulfate* (estropipate)<br>Ogen | 0.625 mg/d<br>(0.3 mg × 2–3 mos) | Modest ↑ risk of venous thromboembolism. | $ |
| *estradiol-17β micronized*<br>Estrace | 1–2 mg/d<br>(0.5 mg × 2–3 mos) | | $ |
| *estradiol-17β transdermal*<br>Estraderm, Vivelle, Climara | 50–100 µg/d<br>(25 µg × 2–3 mos) | Patch is recommended if upper GI disease, liver disease, history of thrombosis or high triglyceride levels. | $$ |

| | | | |
|---|---|---|---|
| **Progestins** | (Dose for 12–14 d/mo) | | |
| *medroxyprogesterone acetate (MPA)*<br>Provera, generics | 2.5, 5 and 10 mg | Start with 10 mg MPA or equivalent if 0–3 yrs postmenopause; 5 mg if 4–10 yrs postmenopause; 2.5 mg if > 10 yrs. Halve dose if taken daily for 30 days. | $ |
| *micronized oral progesterone*<br>Prometrium | 100, 200 and 300 mg HS | More beneficial lipid effects. | $–$$ |
| *norethindrone*<br>Micronor | 0.35 and 0.7 mg | May produce less bleeding and breast stimulation. | $ |
| **Combination estrogen and progestin** | | | |
| *estradiol* 50 μg plus<br>*estradiol* 50 μg/*norethindrone 0.25 μg transdermal*<br>Estracomb | 4 patches over 1st 2 wks, then 4 patches over last 2 wks | | $$ |
| *estradiol* 50 μg/*norethindrone 0.25 μg* or *0.14 μg transdermal*<br>Estalis | 1 patch twice/wk | | $$ |
| **Bisphosphonates** | | | |
| *alendronate*<br>Fosamax | 10 mg/d plus calcium at a different time of day | Best evidence for ↓ fractures.<br>All are poorly absorbed and must be taken on an empty stomach with water only. Side effects are minimal (GI symptoms, altered taste, nighttime leg cramps). Rarely, allergic reactions. Esophageal ulceration is a rare side effect of alendronate; patient must remain upright after taking the pill. Safety in impaired renal function (CrCl < 35 mL/min) is unknown. | $$$$ |
| *etidronate*<br>Didronel, Didrocal | Cyclic: 400 mg/d × 14 d Q 3 mos, then calcium × 76 days | | $$$ |
| *risedronate*<br>Actonel | 5 mg/d plus calcium at a different time of day | Evidence for ↓ fracture rate similar to alendronate. | † |

*(cont'd)*

Table 1: **Drugs Used in Management of Osteoporosis** *(cont'd)*

| Drug | Dosage | Comments | Cost* |
|---|---|---|---|
| **Selective Estrogen Receptor Modulators** | | | |
| *raloxifene* Evista | 60 mg/d | Estrogen–like action on bone and lipid metabolism. Estrogen antagonist in breast and endometrium. Aggravates hot flushes; should not be started until patient is clearly estrogen deficient. Similar risk of venous thromboembolism to HRT. RCT evidence for prevention of bone loss in early postmenopause, vertebral fracture prevention and ↓ incidence of breast cancer. | $$$$ |
| *calcitonin, salmon* Miacalcin | 200 IU/d intranasally | Nasal irritation only notable side effect. | $$$$ |
| Calcimar | 50–100 IU SC/d or Q 2nd day or 5 d/wk | Not approved for osteoporosis: should be restricted to patients who fail conventional therapy. Analgesic effect in addition to antiresorptive effect. Dose is not standardized. Adverse effects: nausea, facial flushing, metallic taste, hypersensitivity (rare). | $$$$$ |

* *Cost of 30-day supply – includes drug cost only.*

*Legend:* $ < $15 $$ $15–30 $$$ $30–45 $$$$ $45–60 $$$$$ >$60

† *5 mg tablet will be available from Procter & Gamble Pharmaceuticals.*

**Alendronate** increases bone mass throughout the skeleton and reduces the risk of all fractures (including hip) by at least 50%.

The dose schedule of etidronate (only 2 weeks every 3 months) and its lower cost are attractive to some patients.

Alendronate, taken continuously, shows more rapid improvement in bone density. The gains in spinal bone density at 3 years with alendronate are marginally greater than those reported with cyclical etidronate (8% vs. 5 to 6%). Alendronate significantly increases bone density at all measured sites including the assessment of total body bone mineral which has not yet been demonstrated with etidronate.

**Risedronate** is also administered continuously. Large, randomized, placebo-controlled trials have shown benefit in prevention of all fractures (including hip), similar to alendronate. A 65% reduction in vertebral fractures compared to placebo was seen in the first year of one clinical trial.[2]

There have been no comparative trials of bisphosphonates; all appear to be effective therapies for osteoporosis. However, only alendronate and risedronate have been clearly shown in randomized controlled trials to prevent all clinical fractures.

### *Selective Estrogen Receptor Modulators*

**Raloxifene** has been shown to prevent postmenopausal bone loss, increasing bone density by approximately 3% and reducing new vertebral fractures by 30–40%. It is an estrogen antagonist in breast and uterine tissue, but has estrogen-like activity in bone and in lipid metabolism. Like estrogen, there is a modest increased risk of deep vein thrombosis and pulmonary embolism in postmenopausal women. It also significantly reduces the risk of diagnosis of estrogen receptor positive breast cancer by 76%.

### *Combination Therapy*

Combining a **bisphosphonate with estrogen or raloxifene** is the subject of several recent or ongoing clinical trials. Estrogen plus a bisphosphonate has additive or synergistic effects on BMD, but no fracture benefit has yet been demonstrated. If a patient continues to lose BMD while taking estrogen, adding a bisphosphonate without stopping estrogen may be considered.

### *Calcitonin*

Calcitonin increases bone mass, particularly in osteoporotic patients with a high rate of bone turnover. It is a very safe agent but is expensive. Salmon calcitonin is longer acting and perhaps more potent than human calcitonin. In addition to its anti-

---

[2] *JAMA 1999;282:1344–1352.*

resorptive effects, calcitonin has demonstrated analgesic properties.

A nasal spray of salmon calcitonin, 200 units once daily, prevents vertebral fractures. The nasal spray is less well absorbed than SC injection. However, the effective treatment dose for injectable calcitonin has not been standardized.

**The following therapies are not recommended unless the above therapies are not tolerated.**

### *Calcitriol*

Calcitriol 0.25 µg BID with calcium 1 g per day showed a fracture prevention benefit compared to patients receiving only calcium supplementation. Serum calcium monitoring is required to avoid hypercalcemia.

### *Androgens*

Hypogonadism is a major diagnostic consideration for males with osteoporosis. Treatment with testosterone is indicated.

Anabolic steroids have been prescribed for women with osteoporosis in selected cases, particularly elderly patients with low muscle mass. Nandrolone decanoate 50 mg IM every 3 to 6 weeks for 1 to 2 years seems to be reasonably well tolerated and moderately effective.

### *Sodium Fluoride*

Fluoride (20 to 40 mg per day) is the most potent stimulator of bone formation currently available, seemingly without stimulating a concomitant increase in bone resorption. A progressive increase in bone mass of 5 to 10 percent is induced per year. There is concern that this increased bone mass seen does not correlate with bone strength, and may be associated with an increased risk of nonvertebral fractures. Therefore, fluoride therapy of osteoporosis should be considered investigational.

## *Conclusion*

Postmenopausal estrogen/progesterone therapy remains the first choice for prevention of osteoporosis for women in the first 10 years postmenopause. Raloxifene has better randomized controlled trial (RCT) evidence for fracture prevention than estrogen and should be considered a solid alternative to estrogen.

After age 60, bisphosphonate therapy should be chosen over ovarian hormone therapy for the treatment of osteoporosis, because of better patient acceptability and better RCT evidence for fracture prevention. Raloxifene and calcitonin are well tolerated alternatives to bisphosphonate therapy in the treatment of established osteoporosis (a fragility fracture and/or bone density in the "osteoporosis" range).

## Therapeutic Tips

- A person over the age of 50 years with a vertebral compression fracture, wrist fracture, or hip fracture should be considered to have osteoporosis until proven otherwise. These individuals should be tested with bone densitometry, if available.
- In all age groups, adequate calcium and vitamin D nutrition preserves or enhances bone mass, and prevents fractures in the elderly.
- For the prevention of osteoporosis in the early postmenopause, estrogen (with progesterone if the woman has not had a hysterectomy) is the treatment of choice. Raloxifene is an alternative, with the potential added benefit of reducing breast cancer risk; the only negative is its lack of effect on menopausal symptoms. Cyclical etidronate and alendronate 5 mg daily, are also approved therapies for the prevention of menopausal bone loss.
- For patients with established osteoporosis (a fragility fracture and bone density in the "osteoporosis" range), bisphosphonate therapy is first line-therapy. Alendronate and risedronate have been clearly shown to prevent all kinds of fractures. Raloxifene and calcitonin have solid evidence for the prevention of vertebral fractures only, and do not seem to increase BMD as much as bisphosphonates. Estrogen does not have comparable RCT evidence for anti-fracture efficacy, but seems to have an effect on BMD similar to bisphosphonates.
- For the prevention and treatment of glucocorticoid-induced osteoporosis, the bisphosphonates are the agents of choice.

## Pharmacoeconomic Considerations

*Jeffrey A. Johnson, PhD*

Hormone replacement therapy (HRT) is considered to be a cost-effective therapeutic choice for the prevention of osteoporosis in postmenopausal women, particularly as it may also decrease the risk of ischemic heart disease.

In women who cannot tolerate HRT, men and in established osteoporosis, etidronate and alendronate are alternative therapeutic choices. While there are no direct comparative trials of bisphosphonates, cyclical etidronate therapy may be more attractive as an initial choice for several reasons. The lower cost and the dosing schedule for etidronate might suggest that it is favorable. Alendronate is, however, the only osteoporosis therapy that has been clearly shown to prevent hip fractures in clinical studies. Alendronate also shows a more rapid improvement in bone density and at all measured sites, not just vertebral bone density. In a recently published economic evaluation of multiple drug treatment strategies, the incremental cost of adding either agent to HRT and calcium therapy remained an attractive investment, ranging from $2331 to $40,965 per vertebral fracture avoided for etidronate and alendronate, respectively.

Salmon calcitonin appears to be as effective as other treatments, but it is considerably more expensive and so should be reserved for situations where both HRT and bisphosphonates are not appropriate. No economic evaluations of raloxifene are available, so specific recommendations cannot be made. Of important consideration for the pharmacoeconomic impact of raloxifene will be the effects on fracture rates, cardiovascular risk, and breast and endometrial cancer, which are not completely known at this time.

***Suggested Reading***

*Rosner AJ, Grima DT, Torrance, GW, Bradley C, Adachi JD, Sebaldt RJ, Willison DJ. Cost effectiveness of multi-therapy treatment strategies in the prevention of vertebral fractures in postmenopausal women with osteoporosis. PharmacoEconomics 1998;14:559–573.*

*Torgerson DJ, Reid DM. The pharmacoeconomics of hormone replacement therapy. PharmacoEconomics 1999;16:9–16.*

## Suggested Reading List

Eddy DM, Johnston CC Jr., Cummings SR, et al, for the National Osteoporosis Foundation. Osteoporosis: review of the evidence for prevention, diagnosis, and treatment and cost-effectiveness analysis. *Osteoporosis Int* 1998; Supplement 4.

Scientific Advisory Board of the Osteoporosis Society of Canada. Prevention and management of osteoporosis: Consensus Statements of the Scientific Advisory Board of the Osteoporosis Society of Canada. *Can Med Assoc J* 1996; 155:921-965.

Scientific Advisory Board of the Osteoporosis Society of Canada. Clinical practice guidelines for the diagnosis and management of osteoporosis. *Can Med Assoc J* 1996;155(8): 1113–1133.

Osteoporosis Society of Canada: Update on diagnostic technologies. Position paper of the Osteoporosis Society of Canada. *Osteoporosis Update* 1999;3(3):2–7.

CHAPTER 58

# Sports Injuries

*James Kissick, MD, CCFP, Dip Sport Med*

The majority of sports injuries encountered by physicians involve the soft tissues: strains, sprains and contusions.

## Goals of Therapy

- To reduce acute symptoms (pain, inflammation) and recurrences
- To correct contributing factors (e.g., malalignment, muscle weakness)
- To return the athlete's weight-bearing capability, flexibility, range of motion, strength and proprioception to normal
- To enable the athlete to participate comfortably and fully in all pre-injury activities

## Therapeutic Choices

For management of specific injuries, see Table 1.

## General Approaches

Acute treatment is best summarized by the RICE protocol:

- **R**est of the injured part.
- **I**ce: Wrap an ice bag, cold pack or package of frozen peas in a damp, thin cloth and apply to the injured area for 15 minutes at a time, at least QID for the first 48 hours (or longer if swelling continues).
- **C**ompression with an elastic bandage if there is swelling such as in an ankle sprain.
- **E**levation: Try to elevate the injured part above the level of the heart.

Initial rehabilitation is directed toward allowing the injured tissues to heal.

Aggravation of the injury must be avoided, but alternative activities should be encouraged (e.g., the runner with a stress fracture of the fibula should not run but can swim or run in deep water).

**NSAIDs** or **ASA** (if not contraindicated) can decrease swelling and discomfort but should be used for short periods only.

The next phase is directed toward restoring and improving flexibility, strength, endurance and proprioception. A progression

Table 1: **Management of Specific Sports Injuries**

| Injury | Investigations | Therapeutic Choices |
|---|---|---|
| **Patellofemoral Syndrome**<br>Anterior knee pain resulting from patellofemoral articulation dysfunction (also known as patellofemoral pain syndrome or anterior knee pain syndrome). | **History** of anterior knee pain, worse with prolonged flexion, running.<br>**Physical examination:** malalignment, pain with patellar pressure, painful quads setting, poor flexibility, medial quadricep (VMO) weakness, lateral patellar tracking.<br>**X-rays** (including skyline view of patella) if trauma or bony pathology is a concern. | **Relief of acute symptoms:** Rest from aggravating activities (emphasize alternative activities); ice, both PRN and postactivity; physiotherapy (ultrasound, etc.), NSAID.<br>**Correction of contributing factors:**<br>*Foot overpronation:* appropriate shoes with straight to slightly curved last, good medial arch and support. If severe, may require custom foot orthotic.<br>*Patellar lateral tracking due to vastus medialis obliquus (VMO) weakness:* VMO strengthening (e.g., closed kinetic chain exercises such as quarter squats, wall sits). Electrical muscle stimulation and/or biofeedback can assist.<br>*Improve flexibility:* quadriceps, hamstrings, gastrocnemius, ilio-tibial band stretches<br>*Taping techniques* (e.g., McConnell[1]) to correct patellar malposition<br>*Correction of training errors:* in runners, more gradual distance increases, fewer hills. Decrease jumping, squats; avoid resisted leg extensions to ≥ 90° flexion.<br>*Patellar stabilizing brace:* with supporting buttress and/or straps. Use with activities or more regularly if subluxation.<br>*Surgery:* e.g., lateral release of tight retinacula, patellar tendon transfer is rarely required and should be a last resort. |
| **Ankle Sprain**<br>Partial or complete tear to ankle-stabilizing ligaments, most commonly lateral (anterior and posterior talofibular, calcaneo-fibular).<br>**Grade I:** No laxity, bears weight without pain, minimal swelling. | **History** of acute inversion (eversion less common).<br>**Physical examination:** tenderness (most marked over injured ligament), swelling, pain with passive inversion and plantar flexion, positive drawer test in Grade III sprains. | **Grade I & II Sprains**<br>Initial RICE protocol.<br>Gradual ↑ weight bearing; may use tape/brace as support. Begin as soon as pain and stability allow (facilitates healing and proprioception).<br>Early range of motion exercises.<br>Stretching in dorsiflexion and plantar flexion.<br>Strengthening: dorsiflexors, plantar flexors, then invertors and evertors. |

| | | |
|---|---|---|
| **Grade II:** Swelling, painful weight bearing, possible slight laxity.<br>**Grade III:** Unstable, significant laxity, complete disruption of at least two ligaments. | **X-rays** PRN[2] | Proprioceptive retraining.<br>Progressive ↑ activities: walk → jog → run → run backward → curves → zig-zags.<br>**Grade III Sprains**<br>Removable cast brace for 3–6 wks (allows icing, physiotherapy); then stirrup-type ankle brace. Once stable, follow protocol for Grudel and Z sprains. Refer for orthopedic consultation if very unstable.<br>Note: Don't forget to check for associated injury more proximally in the leg. |
| **Lower Leg Pain**<br>**"Shin Splints"**<br>Inflammation of the tibialis posterior or anterior at its origin or of the tibial periosteum. | **History** of shin pain, usually in inexperienced and/or inadequately stretched or strengthened athletes.<br>**Physical examination:** tenderness, usually diffuse, at medial border of tibia and adjacent muscle.<br>**X-rays** normal; may need bone scan to differentiate from stress fracture. | Rest from aggravating activities (e.g., running). Alternative activities: cycling, swimming, pool running (running in deep water with flotation belt).<br>Ice.<br>Muscle stretching and strengthening.<br>Correction of predisposing anatomic factors (i.e., with foot orthotics) and training errors.<br>Gradual return to running or activity. |
| **Stress fractures of the tibia/fibula**<br>Failure of bone due to repetitive overload, resulting in microfractures. | **History** of well-localized shin pain with pounding activities.<br>**Physical examination:** localized bony tenderness.<br>**X-rays** usually negative until at least 2 wks after onset; may see periosteal thickening. Bone scan will show discrete increased uptake at stress fracture site. | No pounding activities until pain-free and nontender (usually 6–8 wks).<br>Alternative activities: cycling, swimming, pool running.<br>Flexibility and strength work.<br>Long Air Cast-type brace often provides more comfort and possibly earlier return to pounding activities (if pain-free in Air Cast).<br>Correction of anatomic factors, training errors. |

*(cont'd)*

Table 1: **Management of Specific Sports Injuries** *(cont'd)*

| Injury | Investigations | Therapeutic Choices |
|---|---|---|
| **Stress fractures of the tibia/fibula** *(cont'd)* | Note: Beware of anterior midshaft tibial stress fractures ("the dreaded black line"). On x-ray, appear as a horizontal fissure extending into the cortex of the tibia. These are slow to heal and often go on to nonunion. | Gradual return to running when pain-free and nontender:<br>Wk 1: Run every other d, 1/2 usual distance, 1 min off usual mile pace.<br>Wk 2: Usual run frequency, 3/4 usual distance, 1 min off mile pace.<br>Wk 3: Usual frequency, 3/4 distance, 30 s off mile pace.<br>Wk 4: Usual frequency, full distance, 30 s off mile pace[3].<br>Anterior midshaft tibial stress fractures should be assessed by orthopedic surgeon; may need immobilization. |
| **Lateral Epicondylitis "Tennis Elbow"**<br>Degenerative tears (+/– inflammation) of the common extensor tendon at its origin at the lateral epicondyle of the humerus. | **History** of pain at the lateral elbow, usually due to overuse and/or faulty mechanics.<br>**Physical examination:** tenderness at lateral epicondyle area, painful resisted wrist extension.<br>**X-ray** if any concern (i.e., bony pathology). | Rest from aggravating activities.<br>Tennis elbow "counter-force" brace.<br>Ice, ice massage with "ice cup."<br>Physiotherapy, stretching.<br>Strengthening exercises as improvement occurs.<br>**Correction of faulty mechanics:** *poor strokes, especially backhand (leading with the elbow), correct grip size, string tension to maximum 50–55 lbs, lighter racquet, avoid heavy duty or wet balls.* Suggest consultation with teaching pro.<br>Gradual return to activity.<br>If above unsuccessful, consider corticosteroid injection (e.g., triamcinolone acetonide 20 mg) to common extensor origin area at lateral epicondyle (maximum 3 injections, at least 1 mo apart).<br>If still unsuccessful, consider surgery (usually release of part of common extensor origin and fascia). |

| | | |
|---|---|---|
| **Plantar fasciitis**<br>Microtears of the plantar fascia and inflammation of the periosteum at its calcaneal origin (heel bone). | **History** of pain at plantar aspect of calcaneus, worse upon arising in the morning, getting up after a prolonged sit, and with running or prolonged walking.<br>**Physical examination:** pes planus or cavus, overpronation with walking. Tender at plantar fascial origin at the heel.<br>**X-ray** not usually needed, may show "spur" as a result of more chronic fasciitis. | Limit overpronation, cushion heel. Footwear important; running shoe best. Should wear for all weight bearing. Arch supports, heel pads or cups may be necessary. Custom foot orthotics needed in some cases.<br>Rest from aggravating activities (e.g., bike instead of run).<br>Ice or ice massage.<br>Roll foot on soup can before weight bearing in morning.<br>Stretches: gastrocnemius, soleus, plantar fascia, foot intrinsics.<br>Night splint to prevent ankle plantar flexion while sleeping; decreases fascial shortening and morning pain.[4]<br>Corticosteroid injection if not improving with above (e.g., triamcinolone acetate 20 mg mixed with 0.5 mL xylocaine 1% to tender area).<br>Surgery rarely required. |

[1] *Aust J Phys Ther 1986;32:215.*
[2] *JAMA 1993;269:1127–1132.*
[3] *The team physician's handbook. Philadelphia: Hanley and Belfus, 1990:446.*
[4] *Clin J Sport Med 1996;6:158.*

toward full activity is then undertaken. Before the patient resumes activity, any factors that may have contributed to the injury (improper shoes, poor protective equipment) should be corrected, and sport-specific skills regained.

## *Suggested Reading List*

Hershman EB, Mailly T. Stress fractures. *Clin Sports Med* 1990;9:1.

Kibler WB, Herring SA, Press JM, eds. Functional rehabilitation of sports and musculoskeletal injuries. Gathersburg MO: Aspen, 1998.

Mellion MB, Walsh WM, Shelton Gl, eds. *The team physician's handbook.* 2nd ed. Philadelphia: Hanley and Belfus, 1996.

Reid DC. *Sports injury assessment and rehabilitation.* New York: Churchill Livingstone, 1992.

Stiell IG, Greenberg GH, McKnight RD, et al. Decision rules for the use of radiography in acute injuries: refinement and prospective validation. *JAMA* 1993;269:1127–1132.

Torg JS, Shephard RJ, eds. *Current therapy in sports medicine.* St. Louis: Mosby, 1995.

CHAPTER 59

# Acne

*Rob Miller, MD, FRCPC*

## Definition

A multifactorial disease caused by four factors:

- Increased sebum production
- Comedo formation
- Colonization of the follicle by Propionibacterium, mainly *P. acnes*
- The host's inflammatory response

These four factors are interrelated with increased sebum production being the fundamental factor that causes the subsequent development of the other three.

Acne can be subclassified into different clinical patterns in which one type may predominate:

- Comedogenic acne (closed and open comedones – "whiteheads and blackheads")
- Papulopustular acne (papules and pustules – "pimples")
- Nodulocystic acne (a deeper, more inflammatory form)

Each type can lead to scarring, although it is much more commonly associated with the nodulocystic variety.

## Goals of Therapy

- To minimize the symptoms and cosmetic disfigurement
- To prevent recurrence
- To prevent scarring

## Investigations

- History, including:
  - use/abuse of cosmetic agents including hair gels, mousses, pomades
  - topical (including OTC) and oral medications used in acne treatment and duration of use
  - medications that may positively or negatively affect acne (e.g., oral contraceptives, steroids)
- Laboratory tests: if isotretinoin is to be used, baseline and follow-up pregnancy tests, CBC, liver function tests, fasting serum triglyceride and cholesterol levels

Figure 1: **Management of Acne**

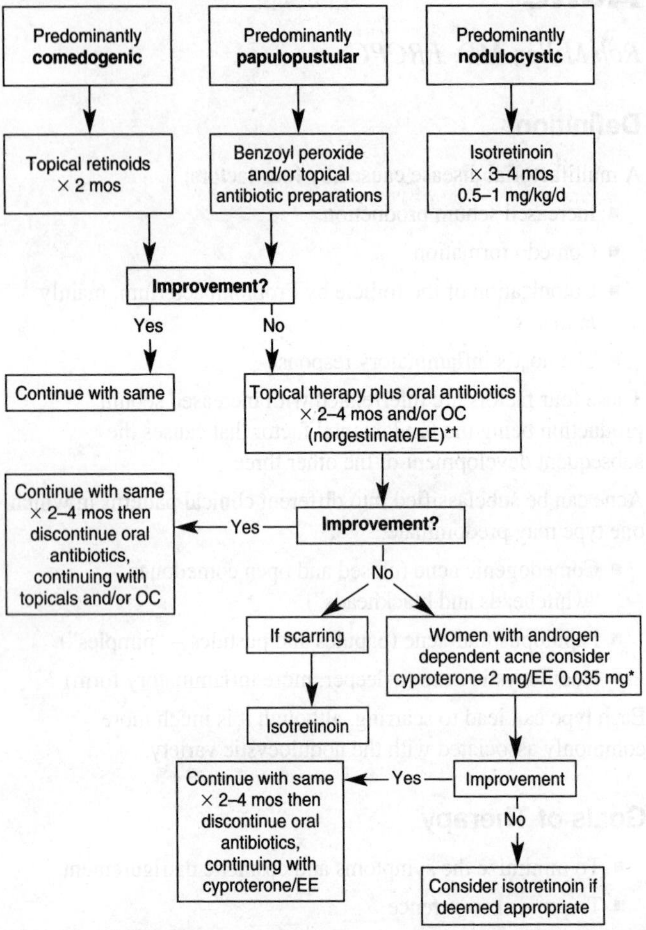
Predominantly comedogenic
Predominantly papulopustular
Predominantly nodulocystic
Topical retinoids × 2 mos
Benzoyl peroxide and/or topical antibiotic preparations
Isotretinoin × 3–4 mos 0.5–1 mg/kg/d
Improvement?
Yes
No
Continue with same
Topical therapy plus oral antibiotics × 2–4 mos and/or OC (norgestimate/EE)*†
Continue with same × 2–4 mos then discontinue oral antibiotics, continuing with topicals and/or OC
Yes
Improvement?
No
If scarring
Women with androgen dependent acne consider cyproterone 2 mg/EE 0.035 mg*
Isotretinoin
Continue with same × 2–4 mos then discontinue oral antibiotics, continuing with cyproterone/EE
Yes
Improvement
No
Consider isotretinoin if deemed appropriate

* *See Table 2.*

† *Consider for women with moderate acne who also require contraception.*

*Abbreviations: OC=oral contraceptives, EE=ethinyl estradiol.*

## Therapeutic Choices

### Nonpharmacologic Choices

- A balanced diet is good for overall health, but there is no evidence that acne is caused by specific foods.
- Squeezing pimples may increase the risk of scarring.
- Avoid excessive cosmetic use and use only non-comedogenic, water-based products.

Table 1: **Topical Acne Preparations**

| Drug | Dose |
|---|---|
| *benzoyl peroxide 2.5%–10%* Acetoxyl, Desquam-X, Panoxyl, others | cream, lotion, gel; apply HS concentrations ≤ 5% available without a prescription |
| **Retinoids** | |
| *tretinoin 0.01%, 0.025%, 0.05%, 0.1%* Retin-A, StieVa-A, Vitamin A Acid, others | cream, gel, solutions; apply HS |
| *isotretinoin 0.05%* Isotrex | gel; apply OD-BID |
| *tazarotene 0.05%, 0.1%* Tazorac | gel; apply HS |
| **Retinoid Analogs** | |
| *adapalene 0.1%* Differin | cream or gel; apply HS |
| **Antibiotics** | |
| *erythromycin 1.5%, 2%* Erysol, Sans-Acne, Staticin, T-Stat | gel, lotion, solution, pads; apply BID |
| *clindamycin 1%* Dalacin T | solution; apply BID |
| **Combinations** | |
| *benzoyl peroxide 5%/erythromycin 3%* Benzamycin | gel; apply BID |
| *tretinoin 0.01%, 0.025% or 0.05%/ erythromycin 4%* Stievamycin | gel; apply HS |
| *neomycin 0.25%/methylprednisolone 0.25%* Neo-Medrol Acne Lotion | lotion; apply OD-BID |
| **Miscellaneous** | |
| *salicylic acid 2%* Acnex, Salac, others | available without prescription |

## Pharmacologic Choices (Figure 1)
## Topical Agents (Table 1)

**Benzoyl peroxide** is a peeling agent that also has some antibacterial action; it is used mainly in papulopustular acne.

**Retinoids (topical isotretinoin, tretinoin tazarotene** and **adapalene)** are used predominantly in comedogenic acne. It is recommended that topical retinoids not be used during pregnancy.

**NB:** Topical tretinoin and benzoyl peroxide have been reported to cause cancer in experimental animal studies. The clinical significance of these reports in humans is unknown.

**Antibiotics (erythromycin, clindamycin)** are used to decrease colonization of skin with *P. acnes*, mainly in papulopustular acne.

Other agents include combinations of topical retinoids and antibiotics, sulfur, salicylic acid, resorcinol and abrasive cleansers (which have largely been displaced by newer topical agents).

## Systemic Agents (Table 2)

### *Antibiotics*

**Tetracycline** is the most commonly prescribed oral agent; 1 g per day reduces the number of *P. acnes* and may exert an anti-inflammatory effect by inhibiting leukocyte chemotaxis. When control is achieved the dosage can often be reduced to 250 to 500 mg per day for maintenance.

Tetracycline during the first trimester of pregnancy is unlikely to cause teeth discoloration or other teratogenic effects, but it is nevertheless contraindicated during all trimesters of pregnancy. It may exacerbate azotemia in patients with pre-existing renal disease.

**Minocycline** has the advantages of once daily dosing and it can be given with food or milk. Information to date on interactions with oral contraceptives is insufficient to conclude whether the risk of pregnancy is increased, decreased or unaffected. Drug-induced lupus and hypersensitivity reactions have become increasingly recognized as a rare complication of minocycline therapy.

**Erythromycin** is an alternative to tetracycline due to its excellent safety profile. Side effects are mainly gastrointestinal (dose related).

### *Hormonal Therapy*

A triphasic oral contraceptive containing norgestimate and ethinyl estradiol (Tri-Cyclen) is approved in Canada for the treatment of women with moderate acne vulgaris who have no contra-indications to oral contraceptive therapy. It must be used for several months in order to see improvement and is usually combined with other systemic therapies (e.g., isotretinoin, tetracycline) and/or topical therapy.

An antiandrogen-estrogen combination containing cyproterone acetate and ethinyl estradiol (Diane-35) is indicated for women with severe acne associated with symptoms of androgenization (seborrhea and mild hirsutism) who have not responded to oral antibiotics and other treatments. When taken as recommended it also provides reliable contraception.

### *Isotretinoin*

Isotretinoin is indicated in the treatment of severe nodulocystic and/or inflammatory acne vulgaris. Patients with other forms of acne for whom the risk of scarring is great and who have not responded to maximal topical and oral antibiotic therapy should be considered for this drug.

Doses of 0.5 to 1 mg/kg/day are prescribed for 16 to 20 weeks in the majority of patients. The medication must be taken with food and can be taken once daily without splitting the dose. Some may

Table 2: **Systemic Drugs Used in Acne Therapy**

| Drug | Dosage | Adverse Effects | Drug Interactions | Cost* |
|---|---|---|---|---|
| **Antibiotics** | | | | |
| *tetracycline* Tetracyn, generics | 500 mg BID initial<br>250–500 mg/d maintenance | GI effects; overgrowth of Candida; photosensitivity; pseudotumor cerebri; may exacerbate azotemia. | GI absorption of tetracycline may be impaired by iron, bismuth, aluminum, calcium, magnesium, in drugs and foods (e.g., dairy products). Separate doses by 2 h. | 1 g/d $ |
| *minocycline* Minocin, generics | 100 mg/d initial<br>50 mg/d maintenance | Dizziness, vertigo, ataxia (dose-related) with minocycline; abnormal cutaneous pigmentation with minocycline. | | 100 mg/d $$ |
| *doxycycline* Vibra-Tabs, generics | 100 mg/d initial and maintenance | Contraindicated in pregnant women, children under 8. | | 100 mg/d $ |
| *erythromycin* Eryc, Erythromid, PCE, others | 500 mg BID initial<br>250–500 mg/d maintenance | GI effects: nausea, vomiting, epigastric distress, diarrhea.<br>Estolate-induced cholestatic jaundice. | May ↑ blood levels of theophylline, cyclosporine, carbamazepine, warfarin, digitalis, ergotamine, methylprednisolone. Concurrent use with astemizole, terfenadine or cisapride is contraindicated. | 1 g/d base $<br>EC caps $$ |
| **Retinoids** | | | | |
| *isotretinoin* Accutane | 0.5–1.0 mg/kg/d for 16–20 wks | Teratogenicity; ocular effects (conjunctivitis, ↓ night vision); bone effects (rarely premature epiphyseal closure); ↑ triglyceride and cholesterol levels (25–50% of patients); ↑ liver function tests in 10% of patients; pseudotumor cerebri; mucocutaneous effects; myalgias (15%); reversible hair loss. | NB: No adverse interaction known between retinoids and oral contraceptives. | 40 mg/d $$$ |

*(cont'd)*

Table 2: **Systemic Drugs Used in Acne Therapy** *(cont'd)*

| Drug | Dosage | Adverse Effects | Drug Interactions | Cost* |
|---|---|---|---|---|
| **Hormonal Therapy** | | | | |
| *EE 0.035 mg/cyproterone 2 mg* Diane-35 | 1 tab/d × 21 days, off for 7 days and repeat cycle | See Chapter 69 | See Chapter 69 | $$ |
| *EE 0.035 mg/norgestimate 0.18 mg × 7 d, 0.255 mg × 7 d, 0.25 mg × 7 d* Tri-Cyclen | 1 tab/d × 21 days, off for 7 days and repeat cycle | See Chapter 69 | See Chapter 69 | $ |

* *Cost of 30-day supply – includes drug cost only.*
*Legend: $ < $20 $$ $20–50 $$$ $50–100*

*Dosage adjustment may be required in renal impairment – see Appendix I.*

require longer treatment times and higher doses. Truncal involvement resolves more slowly than facial. Relapses occur more frequently if lower dosages (e.g., 0.1 mg/kg) are used. If relapses occur, the recommendation is to wait 8 weeks after completion of the first course before reinstituting therapy.

Because of its **teratogenic effects**, use in females of childbearing age requires appropriate contraception as well as baseline and once monthly pregnancy tests. It is appropriate for women to either be abstinent or use two reliable methods of birth control.

If depression, severe headaches, or a decrease in night vision occur, isotretinoin should be discontinued immediately until the etiology of the symptoms can be adequately evaluated.

### *Others*

**Spironolactone**, with its antiandrogen effects, has been used both topically and orally to treat acne although it is not yet approved for this indication. Topical **azelaic acid** is not yet approved for use in Canada. **Zinc** is of unproven value.

### Physical Therapy

- Comedone extraction (care must be taken to avoid unnecessary manipulation).
- Intralesional steroids for inflamed cysts (see Therapeutic Tips).
- Ultraviolet light therapy.
- Chemical peels (of value in treating comedogenic and papulopustular acne not responding to medical therapy).

### *Acne Scars*

It is much easier to prevent acne scars than to treat them. Surgical excision, resurfacing laser, dermabrasion and collagen filling agents are possible treatment options for this complication.

## Therapeutic Tips

- Start with one topical preparation at a time and apply initially only QHS; increase to BID if well tolerated.
- Lower concentrations and cream formulations of benzoyl peroxide and retinoids are, in general, less irritating than the higher concentrations and gels.
- Advise patients to apply preparation over general affected area and not just to individual lesions.
- Warn patients of irritation around mucous membranes and irritation that may be aggravated by sun exposure.
- Advise patients that improvement is slow and may not be seen before 6 to 8 weeks.

- If inflamed cysts are present, do not incise as this causes scarring; they may be managed by intralesional steroid injections after aspiration (0.1 to 0.5 mg triamcinolone acetonide into each cyst).
- If no improvement after 2 months of topical therapy, add oral antibiotic to regimen.
- Patients on long-term antibiotic therapy may develop gram-negative folliculitis (Chapter 68).
- If using isotretinoin, stop all other topical and oral acne therapy (with the exception of OCs if they are being used for contraception and/or being used to treat acne patients with symptoms of androgenization) as they provide no added benefit. Patients should also be advised to stop taking supplements containing vitamin A.

## Suggested Reading List

Leyden JJ. Therapy for acne vulgaris. *N Engl J Med* 1997;336:1156–1162.

Strauss J. Sebaceous glands. In: Fitzpatrick T, Eisen A, Wolff K, et al, eds. *Dermatology in general medicine*. Toronto: McGraw-Hill, 1993:708–726.

White GM. Acne Therapy. *Adv Dermatol*. 1999;14:29–59.

Wolverton S, Wilkin J. *Systemic drugs for skin diseases*. Toronto: W.B. Saunders, 1991.

CHAPTER 60

# Rosacea

*W. Stuart Maddin, MD, FRCPC*

Rosacea is the fifth most common diagnosis made by dermatologists and is estimated to affect 5% of the population. It is a chronic and progressive cutaneous vascular disorder and is often misdiagnosed as adult acne. A high percentage of patients with cutaneous rosacea have some signs or symptoms of ocular involvement (mild conjunctivitis, grittiness, complaint of "dry eyes").

## Goals of Therapy

- Increase awareness of events that can trigger outbreaks of cutaneous rosacea, and how to avoid these triggers
- Make the patient aware of signs and symptoms of ocular rosacea and how they can be managed
- Provide effective topical and systemic agents to reduce the number and severity of recurrences of cutaneous and ocular rosacea
- Provide practical cosmetic suggestions on how to mask rosacea
- Prevent the development of rhinophyma
- Advise the patient on available corrective measures with regard to rhinophyma and telangiectasia

## Investigations

- **Establish the diagnosis:**
  - family history
  - later onset than acne (late 20s to 40s)
  - history of the recurrent bouts of papules and pustules, inappropriate flushing and/or persistent redness of the face
  - history of eye irritation, blepharitis, dry eyes or recurrent styes
  - flare-up of rosacea following sun exposure
- **Physical examination:**
  - presence of papules or pustules along with erythema of the central face; absence of comedones
  - existence of telangiectasia
  - evidence of conjunctivitis, blepharitis, stye formation or complaint of dry eyes
  - nose enlargement (rhinophyma), not common

Figure 1: **Treatment of Rosacea**

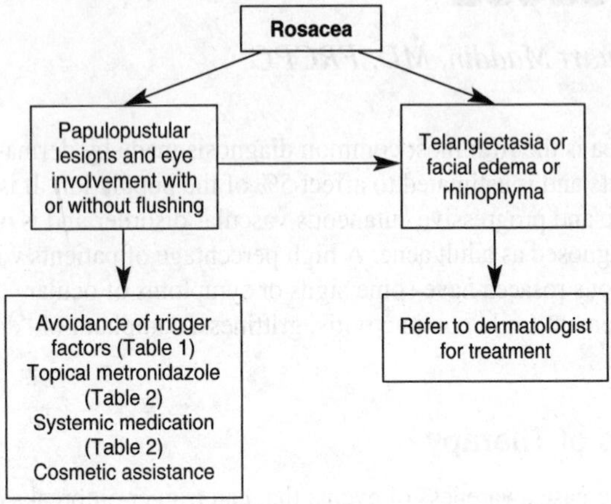
Rosacea
Papulopustular lesions and eye involvement with or without flushing
Telangiectasia or facial edema or rhinophyma
Avoidance of trigger factors (Table 1)
Topical metronidazole (Table 2)
Systemic medication (Table 2)
Cosmetic assistance
Refer to dermatologist for treatment

- **Differential diagnosis:**
  - acne vulgaris, perioral dermatitis, photosensitivity reactions, or discoid lupus erythematosus

## Therapeutic Choices (Figure 1)

### Nonpharmacologic Choices

- Advise patients how to avoid "triggers" that can worsen rosacea (Table 1).
- Protect from the sun with the use of proper clothing, hat and regular use of an effective sunscreen (Chapter 61). The sun and other climatic influences are important in bringing about an exacerbation.
- Avoid hot beverages, soups, spices, vinegar and undiluted alcoholic beverages. Dietary factors are important with regard to flushing.
- Avoid topical corticosteroids – they can precipitate or worsen rosacea by adding to the dermal dystrophy that characterizes the disorder.
- **Scalpel, electrosurgery** or **laser therapy** – telangiectasia and persistent erythema may significantly improve after 1 to 3 laser treatments. In rhinophyma the use of a scalpel to shave the nose or an electric loop or carbon dioxide laser to sculpt the nose to more normal proportions are worthwhile options.

Table 1: **Triggers That can Worsen Rosacea**

| |
|---|
| Sunlight |
| Heat |
| Hot beverages |
| Spicy foods, vinegar |
| Alcohol |
| Application of topical corticosteroids to the face |
| Use of astringents |

### Pharmacologic Choices (Table 2)

## Therapeutic Tips

- Sun protection is very important.
- For female patients, recommend the use of a green tinted foundation which works well at camouflaging the erythema of rosacea.
- When evaluating patients with cutaneous rosacea, inquire about ocular symptoms and examine the eyelids. This is especially important in patients with mild disease who are more likely to be treated with topical treatment alone.
- Start with topical metronidazole. For severe and persistent rosacea, stress avoidance of provocative factors, and use oral antibiotics such as tetracycline, doxycycline, minocycline or erythromycin in full dosage for up to six months.
- Counsel patients with particularly intense erythema, that with successful treatment, posterythema-revealed telangiectasia (PERT) may become apparent. This preempts subsequent worries that the antibiotic therapy "produced" the telangiectasia.
- Pulsed dye laser and other laser systems (e.g., variable pulse width laser) can be very effective for telangiectasia and are being recommended more often as the technology becomes more available.

Table 2: **Drugs Used in Rosacea**

| Drug | Dosage | Adverse Effects | Comments | Cost* |
|---|---|---|---|---|
| **Topical Therapy** | | | | |
| *metronidazole* 0.75% – Metrocream, Metrogel 1% – Noritate | 0.75% gel or cream, or 1% cream applied as thin film BID × 9 weeks, then as needed | Local irritation. | Treatment of choice. If discontinued, relapse can occur. May need up to 12 weeks' therapy to show pronounced improvement. Can be used in combination with oral tetracyclines. | $$ (30 g) |
| **Systemic Therapy** | | | | |
| *tetracycline* ❥ generics | 500 mg BID × 2 wks, then 500 mg OD until rosacea controlled. Then 250 mg OD × 3–4 wks | GI effects; fungal overgrowth; photosensitivity; may ↑ azotemia; pseudotumor cerebri; contraindicated in pregnant women. | Lowest in cost; used in combination with topical metronidazole. Not to be taken with milk or milk products. | $ |
| *minocycline* Minocin, generics | 50–100 mg OD × 6–8 wks | See tetracycline. Also dizziness; vertigo; abnormal cutaneous pigmentation; rarely LE-like syndrome; hepatic dysfunction. | Can be tried if tetracycline fails after compliant 4–6 weeks' trial. No food restriction required. | $$–$$$ |
| *doxycycline* Vibra-Tabs, generics | 100 mg daily × 12 wks | See tetracycline. Photosensitivity may occur. | Given once daily. No food restriction required. Useful for improving ocular rosacea. | $$ |

| | | | | |
|---|---|---|---|---|
| *erythromycin* Eryc, Erythromid, PCE, others | 0.5–1g/day divided × 6–8 wks | GI effects; hepatotoxicity, especially with the estolate; candidiasis. | May be taken with food. FDA Pregnancy Category B – animal studies have failed to show risk to fetus. | $ |
| *isotretinoin* Accutane | 0.5–1mg/kg/day for 4–5 mos | Teratogenicity; cheilitis, dry skin; mucocutaneous effects, myalgia. | For recalcitrant cases.† Provides worthwhile benefit, but not as consistent. Requires at least 2 types of contraception when used in females of childbearing age. | $$$$ (40 mg/d) |

*Dosage adjustment may be required in renal impairment – see Appendix I.*
* *Cost of 30-day supply – includes drug cost only.*

† *Dermatology 1997; 195 (Suppl 1):34–37.*
*Legend: $ < $10  $$ $10–20  $$$ $20–30  $$$$ > $30*

## *Suggested Reading List*

Dahl MV, Katz HI, Krueger GG, et al. Topical metronidazole maintains remissions of rosacea. *Arch Dermatol* 1998;134: 679–683.

Nichols K, Desai N, Lebwohl MG. Effective sunscreen ingredients and cutaneous irritation in patients with rosacea. *Cutis* 1998;61:344–346.

Quarterman MJ, Johnson DW, Abele DC, et al. Ocular rosacea: signs, symptoms, and tear studies before and after treatment with doxycycline. *Arch Dermatol* 1997;133:49–54.

Wilkin J. Rosacea: pathophysiology and treatment. *Arch Dermatol* 1994;130:359–362.

Wilkin J. Use of topical products for maintaining remission in rosacea. *Arch Dermatol* 1999;135:79–80.

## CHAPTER 61

# Sunburn

*Lyn Guenther, MD, FRCPC*

Sunburn is caused by excessive exposure to ultraviolet (UV) radiation. It is characterized by **erythema**, with onset 2 to 6 hours after exposure to a threshold dose of UV radiation; it peaks at 15 to 36 hours and regresses by 72 to 96 hours. **Edema** and **pain** may be present. **Blistering** in severe cases may take a week or more to resolve. Nausea, abdominal cramping, fever, chills and headache may also occur. **Desquamation** with resolution results from cellular injury and death.

Any person, even black, will burn with large doses of UV radiation. Blue- or green-eyed, lighter-skinned individuals who tan poorly and freckle burn more readily. The trunk, neck and head burn at a lower dose of UV radiation than the upper limbs, which burn more readily than the lower limbs.

## Characteristics of Ultraviolet Radiation

UV radiation consists of:

- UVC (200 to 290 nm):
  - filtered by the ozone layer, does not reach the earth
  - emitted by welding arcs, bactericidal and mercury arc lamps
- UVB (290 to 320 nm):
  - the primary cause of sunburn from sunlight
  - 1000 times more erythemogenic than UVA
  - substantially absorbed by the ozone layer
  - does not penetrate glass
- UVA (320 to 400 nm):
  - responsible for most phototoxic reactions to drugs
  - penetrates the skin more deeply than UVB
  - negligibly absorbed by the ozone layer
  - causes 10% of solar erythema
  - can pass through glass

A 1% decrease in ozone results in a 1.5% increase in UVB, leading to a 2 to 6% increase in basal and squamous cell cancers and a 0.3 to 2% increase in melanomas. For every 300 meters above sea level, UV radiation increases by 4%. Radiation effects are enhanced by reflective surfaces (e.g., sand, snow and water). Up to 80% of UV radiation penetrates clouds. Increased humidity decreases the threshold for erythema to UV radiation. In 1992, Environment Canada developed the UV index, which forecasts the intensity of UV rays.

| UV index | Risk | Estimated time for fair-skinned person to burn |
|---|---|---|
| 0–2 | minimal | 1 hour |
| 3–4 | low | <20 min |
| 5–6 | moderate | <15 min |
| 7–9 | high | <10 min |
| ≥10 | extreme | <5 min |

## Prevention of Sunburn

Prevention is critical since repeated sun exposure and sunburns are associated with skin cancer and premature skin aging. One severe sunburn during childhood can double the risk of skin cancer later in life. UV radiation can also suppress the immune system and habitual exposure can cause cataracts.

### Nonpharmacologic Choices

- Cosmetic tanning should be avoided. Pigmentation does not occur without damage and death of epidermal cells.
- Tanning salons should be avoided.
- Outdoor activities at peak UV irradiance times (10:00 a.m. to 4:00 p.m. when your shadow is shorter than you; when the UV index is high or extreme) should be avoided.
- Umbrellas may reduce UV radiation by about 70%; however, they do not protect against reflected radiation.
- Protective clothing (pants, long-sleeved shirts, gloves) and sunglasses should be worn. Loosely woven, white or wet clothing offers less protection. Women's stockings provide minimal protection.
- Wide-brimmed hats (at least 7.5 cm) of tightly woven fabric (not straw) should be worn to protect the face, ears and neck.
- Sun exposure should be minimized while one is taking phototoxic medications or using certain local agents (Table 1), which can interact with UV/visible light to cause a dose-related sunburn.

### Pharmacologic Choices

No sunscreen offers complete protection from the sun. Sunscreens should be adjunctive rather than the primary means of protection.

#### *Topical Sunscreens*

Sunscreens should be used to protect the skin and not to prolong sun exposure. They should provide protection against both UVB

Table 1: **Agents That May Cause Phototoxic Reactions***

| Systemic Drugs | Local Agents |
|---|---|
| Amiodarone | Cadmium sulfide |
| Antibiotics | Yellow pigment in tattoos |
| Ceftazidime | Coal tar derivatives |
| Griseofulvin | Acridine |
| Quinolones | Anthracene |
| Ciprofloxacin | Fluoranthene |
| Nalidixic acid | Naphthalene |
| Norfloxacin | Phenanthrene |
| Ofloxacin | Pyridine |
| Sulfonamides | Thiophene |
| Tetracyclines | Dyes |
| Demeclocycline | Acriflavine |
| Doxycycline | Anthraquinone |
| Tetracycline | Eosin |
| Antineoplastics | Methylene blue |
| Dacarbazine | Rose bengal |
| 5-fluorouracil | Toluidine blue |
| Vinblastine | Furocoumarins |
| Diuretics | Psoralen from plants |
| Furosemide | Leguminoseae family |
| Hydrochlorothiazide | Moraceae family |
| Hematoporphyrin | Figs |
| NSAIDs | Rutaceae family |
| Diclofenac | Bergamot orange |
| Ibuprofen | Gas plant |
| Indomethacin | Lemon |
| Ketoprofen | Lime |
| Naproxen | Umbelliferae family |
| Piroxicam | Angelica |
| Sulindac | Anise |
| Tiaprofenic acid | Bishop's weed |
| Psoralens | Celery |
| Methoxsalen | Cow parsley |
| Trioxsalen | Dill |
| Quinidine | Fennel |
| Quinine | Giant hogweed |
| Retinoids | Wild parsnip |
| Acitretin | Wild carrot |
| Isotretinoin | 5-methoxypsoralen |
| Sulfonylureas | Bergamot oil |
| Tolbutamide | Methoxsalen |
| | Retinoids |
| | Adapalene |
| | Tazarotene |
| | Tretinoin |

* *Radiation in the UVA range causes most drug-related phototoxic reactions.*

and UVA, and have an SPF[1] of at least 30. The FDA rates sunscreens with an SPF of 2–11 as providing minimum protection, 12–29 moderate and ≥ 30 high. The SPF of sunscreens is measured under ideal laboratory conditions and may be considerably less when applied thinly and used outdoors. Topical

[1] $SPF = \frac{\text{least amount of UVB energy to produce erythema with sunscreen}}{\text{least amount of UVB energy to produce erythema without sunscreen}}$

sunscreens should be applied generously (2 mg/cm$^2$) to all exposed surfaces including lips, tops of ears and dorsal aspect of feet. Approximately 30 mL is needed for full coverage. Most people only apply a quarter to half the tested amount, effectively reducing the SPF. Reapplication does not extend the period of protection. A person who burns in 10 minutes will burn in 300 minutes using a sunscreen with an SPF of 30, no matter how many times it is applied. This person will develop erythema in < 300 minutes if the sunscreen is not reapplied after swimming, towelling or sweating. Although sunscreens can prevent sunburn, many biological effects (e.g., immunosuppression, carcinogenicity) can occur before the UV erythema threshold is reached. There is currently no standard assessment of UVA protection.

### *Chemical Sunscreens* (Table 2)

Commercial products usually contain more than one active ingredient. They should be applied 15 to 60 minutes before UV exposure to allow active ingredients to bind to the skin. They can be used in children older than 6 months of age. Chronic sunscreen use has not been associated with vitamin D deficiency. Only a few minutes of sun daily, to the back of one hand, results in sufficient vitamin D production. In addition, adequate amounts of vitamin D can be absorbed from cereal, dairy products and fish.

### *Physical Sunscreens*

**Titanium dioxide, zinc oxide, kaolin, talc (magnesium silicate), ferric chloride, melanin** and **red veterinary petrolatum** protect against UVA and UVB and can be used in people of all ages including infants. They reflect and scatter UV and visible light. Recent data have shown that titanium dioxide and zinc oxide can also absorb UVA wavelengths up to 400 nm. Physical sunscreens are generally thicker, less cosmetically elegant and may rub off easily or melt with the sun's heat. Although they have less risk of sensitization, their occlusive effect may cause miliaria and folliculitis. Micronized titanium dioxide and zinc oxide are relatively transparent to visible light but scatter UV light well.

### *Oral Sunscreens*

There is no effective oral sunscreen. Oral beta-carotene, antimalarials, vitamin A, vitamin E and oral PABA *do not* provide effective protection against sunburn. Combined systemic vitamin C 2 g/day and vitamin E 1000 IU/day provide minimal protection (SPF 1.4). Vitamin C or E in a topical sunscreen may enhance photoprotection.

## Treatment of Sunburn

No effective treatment is available. The following may provide relief if given at the time of sunburn or shortly after.

Table 2: **Chemical Sunscreens**

| Active Ingredient | Comments |
|---|---|
| ***UVB Absorbers*** | |
| **Para-aminobenzoic acid (PABA) esters**<br>Padimate O (octyl dimethyl PABA) | Adhere well to skin.<br>May cause contact/photocontact dermatitis.<br>May cross react with sulfonamides, thiazides, sulfonylurea hypoglycemics, ester anesthetics.<br>PABA may stain fabrics yellow upon sun exposure. |
| **Salicylates**<br>Homosalate (homomenthyl salicylate)<br>Octyl salicylate<br>Triethanolamine salicylate | Rarely cause contact dermatitis.<br>Do not adhere well to skin; easily removed by perspiration or swimming. |
| **Cinnamates**<br>Octyl methoxycinnamate (Parsol MCX)<br>2-ethoxyethyl p-methoxycinnamate (Cinoxate) | Do not adhere well to skin.<br>May cross react with balsam of Peru, coca leaves, benzyl and methyl cinnamate, cinnamic alcohol, cinnamic aldehyde, cinnamon oil. |
| Octocrylene | Photostabilizes dibenzoylmethanes. |
| **Benzylidene camphor derivative**<br>4-methylbenzylidene camphor | Maximum absorption at 300 nm.<br>Photostabilizes dibenzoylmethanes. |
| ***UVA Absorbers*** | |
| **Benzophenones**<br>Oxybenzone (benzophenone-3) | Broad-spectrum UVA/UVB protection.<br>Oxybenzone may cause contact/ photocontact dermatitis. |
| Dioxybenzone (benzophenone-8) | Dioxybenzone may cause contact urticaria/contact dermatitis. |
| **Anthranilates**<br>Menthyl anthranilate | Rarely cause sensitization. |
| **Dibenzoylmethanes**<br>Avobenzone or t-butylmethoxy-dibenzoylmethane (Parsol 1789) | Broad UVA absorption.<br>Better protection against UVA than benzophenones, anthranilates and Mexoryl SX.<br>Photodegradable. |
| **Benzylidene camphor derivative**<br>Terephthalylidene dicamphor sulfonic acid (Mexoryl SX) | Good photostability.<br>Maximum absorption at 345 nm. |

## Nonpharmacologic Choices

**Cool baths** or **wet compresses** for 20 minutes several times a day provide some relief. **Moisturizers** help with dryness and peeling.

## Pharmacologic Choices

**Topical vitamin E (alpha tocopherol)** applied 2 minutes after UV exposure may decrease erythema and edema. The effect is diminished if applied later post-irradiation and is probably insignificant if applied after 5 hours.[1]

**Indomethacin** 25 mg or **ibuprofen** 400 mg Q6H for 4 doses or topical 1% indomethacin, starting at time of insult, may decrease erythema and reduce the degree of epidermal injury.

**Potent topical corticosteroids** transiently decrease erythema by causing vasoconstriction but do not reduce epidermal damage. They may soothe stinging and itching. Their effect is additive when used with indomethacin or ibuprofen.[2]

**Acetaminophen** may relieve pain.

## Therapeutic Tips

- Systemic corticosteroids have little effect in treating sunburn; oral antihistamines have no effect.
- Topical anesthetic sprays are associated with a risk of sensitization and should be avoided.
- After a sunburn, the skin should not be exposed to the sun for at least a week.
- Blistering sunburns may require treatment in a burn unit.
- **Waterproof** sunscreens maintain efficacy after 80 minutes of water immersion.
- **Water-resistant** sunscreens maintain efficacy after 40 minutes of water immersion.
- **Sweat-resistant** sunscreens maintain efficacy after 30 minutes of continuous heavy perspiration.

## *Suggested Reading List*


Buescher LS. Sunscreens and photoprotection. *Otolaryngol Clin North Am* 1993;26(1):13–22.

Dromgoole SH, Maibach HI. Sunscreening agent intolerance: contact and photocontact sensitization and contact urticaria. *J Am Acad Dermatol* 1990;22:1068–1078.

Gonzalez E, Gonzalez S. Drug photosensitivity, idiopathic photodermatoses, and sunscreens. *J Am Acad Dermatol* 1996;35:871–885.

Gould JW, Mercurio MG, Elmets CA. Cutaneous photosensitivity diseases induced by exogenous agents. *J Am Acad Dermatol* 1995;33:551–573.

Lim HW, Cooper K. The health impact of solar radiation and prevention strategies. *J Am Acad Dematol* 1999;41:81–99.

Panthak MA. Sunscreens: topical and systemic approaches for protection of human skin against harmful effects of solar radiation. *J Am Acad Dermatol* 1982;7:285–312.


[1] *Oxidative Stress in Dermatology. New York: Marcel Dekker Inc., 1993:67–80.*

[2] *Dermatology 1992;184:54–58.*

CHAPTER 62

# Burns

*David Warren, MD, FRCPC*

## Goals of Therapy

- Provide early management of serious burns to reduce associated morbidity and mortality
- Triage patients for inpatient, referral and outpatient care
- Optimize cosmetic results and minimize functional morbidity of burns
- Provide appropriate analgesia, burn wound management and follow up

## Investigations

- A thorough history of the burn injury with special attention to:
  - burning agent, its temperature, duration of exposure
  - fire in open or enclosed space, explosion, fall, electrical or chemical exposure
  - past medical history, medications and tetanus status
- Physical examination:
  - general physical examination with attention initially to airway, breathing and circulation
  - head to toe examination to assess for other systemic or musculoskeletal injuries
  - presence of headache, irritability, nausea, confusion, agitation and uncoordination which may indicate **carbon monoxide poisoning**
  - assess for **pulmonary complications**. Upper airway edema may occur from direct thermal injury especially with steam. Smoke inhalation doubles the mortality risk of a burn from systemic and direct toxicant effects to the airway. Indicators would include fire in an enclosed space, inhalation of noxious fumes, facial burns, pharyngeal burns, carbonaceous sputum, hoarseness, elevated carboxyhemoglobin > 5%, abnormal pulmonary function. Pulmonary edema may be an early or late finding
  - assess **depth of wound** (Table 1)
  - assess the **extent of the burn** quantified as the percentage of total body surface area (BSA). The palm size of the victim is approximately 1% BSA, or estimate following the rule of nines (Figure 1)

- some burns due to their extent or potential morbidity should be considered for **referral to a burn centre** or specialized care (Table 2). Transfer should be facilitated by contact between physicians. All pertinent documentation, tests, flow sheets and transfer records should accompany the patient

- Laboratory tests in moderate and severe burns:
  - CBC, electrolytes, glucose, BUN, creatinine, blood type and clotting studies
  - ethanol and drug toxicology if warranted
  - carboxyhemoglobin level and other toxins in suspected inhalation injuries
  - urinalysis and if blood positive or > 30% BSA burn, urine myoglobin
  - arterial blood gas and chest radiograph, often normal early with findings 6 to 24 hours later

Table 1: **Burn Depth Classification**

| Degree | Class | Description | Example | Healing Time |
|---|---|---|---|---|
| 1st | Superficial | involves epidermis: skin red and painful | sunburn | 7 days |
| 2nd | Superficial partial thickness | epidermis and upper dermis: blisters, underlying skin red and moist, very painful | scald with water | 10–21 days |
| | Deep partial thickness | epidermis and deep dermis: some hair follicle and sweat gland damage, blisters to charring | flame, oil | > 14 days, some scarring |
| 3rd | Full thickness | epidermis through dermis to subcutaneous fat: skin pale, painless, leathery | flame, hot metal | scars–will not heal, surgery ± grafts |

## Therapeutic Choices

### Nonpharmacologic Choices

#### *Initial First Aid Management*

- Remove the victim from the source of injury, taking care to limit risk to rescuers in electrical and chemical burn injuries.
- Remove any burning clothing or hot material.
- Assess airway, breathing and circulation (ABC).

## Figure 1: **Rule of Nines Estimation of Body Surface Area for Child and Adult**

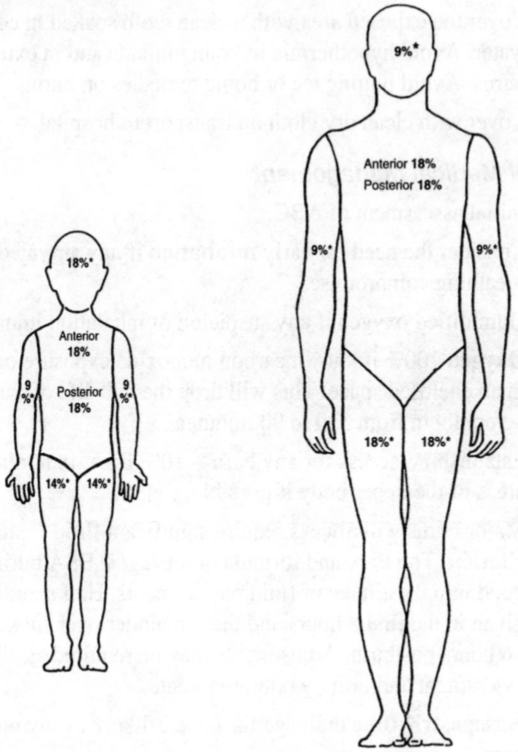
18%*
Anterior
18%
9 %*
Posterior
18%
9 %*
14%*
14%*
9%*
Anterior 18%
Posterior 18%
9%*
9%*
18%*
18%*

** Includes both anterior and posterior aspects.*

## Table 2: **Criteria for Referral or Transfer to a Burn Centre**

- Partial thickness burn > 10% BSA if patient under 10 years or over 50 years of age
- Partial thickness burns > 20% BSA in other age groups
- Partial and full thickness burns involving the face, eyes, ears, hands, feet, perineum, or overlying major joints
- Full thickness burns > 5% BSA
- Significant chemical or electrical burns
- Inhalation injuries
- Patients with pre-existing illness likely to complicate recovery
- Patients with concomitant trauma should be treated initially in an appropriate trauma setting and subsequently transferred to a burn centre
- Children should be treated in facilities with appropriate capabilities and equipment
- Patients with special psycho-social needs and/or rehabilitative support (child abuse, mental health needs, drug addiction)

- In chemical exposures copiously irrigate burn region with lukewarm water until testing demonstrates a normal tissue pH, often prolonged with alkali burns.
- Cover the exposed area with a clean cloth soaked in cool water. Avoid hypothermia in young infants and in extensive burns. Avoid putting ice or home remedies on burn.
- Cover with clean dry cloth on transport to hospital.

### *Initial Medical Management*

- Initial assessment of ABC.
- Consider the need for early **intubation** if any airway or breathing compromise.
- Humidified oxygen if any suspicion of inhalation injury.
- **Oxygen** 100% if known carbon monoxide exposure or fire in an enclosed space. This will drop the half-life of carboxyhemoglobin from 330 to 90 minutes.
- Establish IV access for any burn > 10% BSA, in noninvolved areas of the upper body if possible.
- Major burns will always require significant **fluid resuscitation**. The Parkland formula, 4 mL/kg/% BSA burn, is a good initial estimate of fluid requirements. Half should be given in the first 8 hours and the remainder over subsequent 16 hours postburn. Adjustments may be required as clinical assessment and urinary output indicate.
- **Nasogastric tube** drainage for ileus is likely in any major burn.
- **Bladder catheterization** to monitor appropriate urinary output, minimum 1 mL/kg/h.
- Elevate any encircling limb burn and closely assess for neurovascular status. Chest burns should be assessed for restriction of normal excursion and pulmonary compromise. Surgical escharotomy considered as required.
- Ensure adequate **tetanus prophylaxis**; 0.5 mL tetanus toxoid in previously immunized patient with additional 250 units human immune globulin if previously unimmunized.

### *Burn Wound Management*

- Removal of any attached clothing and loose tissue.
- Gentle washing of the burn surface with sterile water or normal saline.
- Débridement of open blisters and loose tissue.
- Neosporin ointment can be used as an emulsifying agent to remove tar.

- The application of **topical antibiotic** agents will lower the incidence of wound infections. Often not used with superficial burns, they have a more significant role with deeper, more extensive injuries (Table 3).
- Topical antibiotics are applied using sterile technique to approximately 2 mm twice daily or as required if rubbed off. Cleanse the wound prior to reapplication.
- Semi-closed **dressings** permit ambulatory management while maintaining hygiene, limiting mobilization, and preventing tampering with the wound.
  - innermost dressing layer is porous mesh gauze impregnated with nonpetroleum-based water soluble lubricant.
  - second layer is bulky, fluffed coarse mesh gauze to absorb exudate and protect the wound.
  - outer layer of semi-elastic coarse mesh will provide even moderate pressure to keep the dressing in place but should not be constrictive.
  - alternative for superficial partial thickness wounds, semisynthetic occlusive dressings (e.g., Biobrane, DuoDerm, Tegaderm) in flat partial thickness burns.
- Dressing changes:
  - semi-closed dressings; every other day, daily, or twice daily dependent on the wound, antibiotic use and the patient.
  - semisynthetic occlusive dressings; removal, cleansing, and redressing is required if fluid collects beneath, otherwise removal at 7 to 10 days.
- Open therapy is often used on the head, neck and perineum, which are areas difficult to dress and prone to maceration.

## Pharmacologic Choices

- Avoid prophylactic oral and IV antibiotics in all but exceptional circumstances to avoid development of resistant infections.
- **Topical antibiotics** application is discussed above. Various agents have been used with specific indications and limitations (Table 3).

### *Nonsteroidal Anti-inflammatory Drugs (NSAIDs)*

- Have been used to manage pain in minor burns and suppress the inflammatory response in major burns. Standard soft tissue analgesic dosing on a regular basis can be used.

Table 3: **Topical Antibiotics Used in the Treatment of Burns**

| Drug | Application† | Limitations | Comments | Cost* |
|---|---|---|---|---|
| *bacitracin* Baciguent, Bacitin, generics | OD, BID open or semi-closed | Poor eschar penetration, moderate antibacterial spectrum | Transparent, easy to apply, cosmetically acceptable | $ |
| *silver sulfadiazine 1%* Dermazin, Flamazine, SSD | BID–QID open or semi-closed | Only fair penetration, sulfonamide sensitivity (rash), leukopenia | Broad antibacterial spectrum, painless, washable | $–$$ |
| *povidone-iodine 1%* Betadine, Proviodine | BID open or semi-closed | Poor penetration, tissue staining, painful, iodine absorption | Broad antibacterial action | $$ |
| *framycetin sulfate 1%* Sofra-Tulle | OD, semi-closed | Poor penetration, moderate antibacterial action | Easy to use | $ |
| *fusidic acid 2%* Fucidin | OD-QID open or semi-closed | Moderate antibacterial spectrum | Development of resistance | $$–$$$$ |
| *mupirocin 2%* Bactroban | TID, open | Limited antimicrobial coverage | Gram-positive coverage | $$$$ |

*† Approximately 5 g per 1% BSA burn per application.*
** Cost of 7-day supply based on 1% BSA burn – includes drug cost only.*
*Legend: $ < $10   $$ $10–25   $$$ $25–50   $$$$ > $50*

### *Opioid Analgesics*

- In children, potent analgesia with small aliquots of morphine (0.05 to 0.1 mg/kg IV) or fentanyl (1 to 4 μg/kg IV), titrated to effect, are often required initially to manage pain.
- Care should be taken not to suppress the signs of other injuries initially with analgesia.
- Children especially require analgesia to manage their burns.
- Longer term and outpatient analgesia can be achieved with oral codeine.

## Therapeutic Tips

- Avoid contamination of the wound; infection is the major threat to burn outcome.
- Advise patients regarding signs of infection; any evidence of infection should be reviewed quickly and treatment altered as appropriate.
- Outpatient follow-up schedule may be daily initially and extended as dressing requirements and healing progress.
- Electrical burns often have more extensive damage below the surface than is initially identified and should be followed appropriately.

### *Suggested Reading List*

American Burn Association. Guidelines for service standards and severity of classification in the treatment of burn injury. *American College of Surgery Bulletin* 1984;69:24.

American College of Surgeons. Injuries due to burns and cold. In: *Advanced trauma life support*. 6th ed. Chicago: American College of Surgeons, 1997:337–352.

Edlich RF, Moghtader JC. Thermal injury. In: Rosen P, Barkin RM, et al, eds. *Emergency medicine concepts and clinical practice.* 4th ed. St. Louis: CV Mosby, 1997:1573–1584.

Griglak MJ. Thermal injury. *Emerg Med Clin North Am* 1992; 10(2):369.

Schwartz LR. Thermal injury. In: Tintinalli JE, Ruiz E, Krome RL, et al, eds. *Emergency medicine: A comprehensive study guide*. 5th ed. New York: McGraw-Hill, 1999:1281–1286.

CHAPTER 63

# Pressure Ulcers

*Stephen R. Tan, MD*

## Goals of Therapy

- To recognize and modify risk factors for pressure ulcer formation
- To improve existing lesions with the ability to heal
- To recognize and manage the complications of pressure ulcers
- To prevent recurrences in at-risk patients

## Staging of Pressure Ulcers

Table 1: **Staging of Pressure Ulcers**[1]

| | |
|---|---|
| **Stage I** | Non-blanchable erythema of intact skin. In darker skin types, discoloration, warmth, edema, or induration may be indicators. |
| **Stage II** | Partial-thickness skin loss involving the epidermis, dermis, or both. Clinically, this presents as an abrasion, blister, or shallow crater. |
| **Stage III** | Full-thickness skin loss with damage to subcutaneous tissue which extends down to, but not through, underlying fascia. Clinically, this presents as a deep crater that may have undermining of adjacent tissue. |
| **Stage IV** | Full-thickness skin loss with extensive destruction, tissue necrosis, or damage to muscle, bone, or supporting structures such as tendon or joint capsule. Undermining and sinus tracts may be present. |

When eschar is present, a pressure ulcer cannot be accurately assessed until the eschar is removed.

Pressure ulcers do not necessarily progress in order, nor do they heal by reverse staging.

[1] *Agency for Health Care Policy and Research. Treatment of pressure ulcers. Clinical practice guideline #15. Rockville, MD: Department of Health and Human Services, 1994.*

## Investigations

- Complete history, including:
  - risk factors for pressure ulcer formation (Table 2)
  - concurrent medical problems that may impair wound healing, including peripheral vascular disease, diabetes mellitus, immune deficiencies, collagen vascular diseases, malignancy, malnutrition, psychosis, and depression
  - medications, especially steroids or immunosuppressives that impair wound healing

Table 2: **Selected Risk/Causative Factors for Pressure Ulcers**

| Local | Systemic |
|---|---|
| Pressure, especially overlying bony prominences | Malnutrition |
| Shearing forces | Prolonged immobilization (e.g., fractures) |
| Friction | Sensory deficit |
| Excessive moisture | Circulatory disturbance |
| Dry skin | Smoking |

- Physical examination:
  - assess the pressure ulcer for location, depth, size, sinus tracts, undermining, tunneling, exudate, necrotic tissue, and the presence or absence of granulation tissue and epithelialization
- Laboratory tests:
  - albumin

## Therapeutic Choices (Figure 1)

Strategies for the management of pressure ulcers include risk/causative factor modification and local ulcer care.

### Risk/Causative Factor Modification

Healing of pressure ulcers is unlikely unless the underlying causative factors are corrected.

- **Pressure:** External pressure is concentrated over bony prominences and will rapidly lead to tissue necrosis. If pressure is intermittently relieved, minimal skin changes occur. Pressure relief is the cornerstone of both prevention and treatment and may be accomplished by:
  - not placing patients on the pressure ulcer. If possible, raise the ulcer off the support surface. If the ulcer is on a sitting surface, the patient should not be placed in a sitting position.
  - turning bedridden patients every two hours and repositioning sitting individuals every hour.
  - avoiding the placement of patients directly on bony prominences.
  - using soft pillows between bony prominences.
  - using commercially available pressure-reducing surfaces such as air-fluidized, low airloss, alternating air, static flotation, and foam mattresses. There is no compelling evidence that one support surface consistently performs better than all others under all circumstances.

Figure 1: **Pressure Ulcer Therapy**

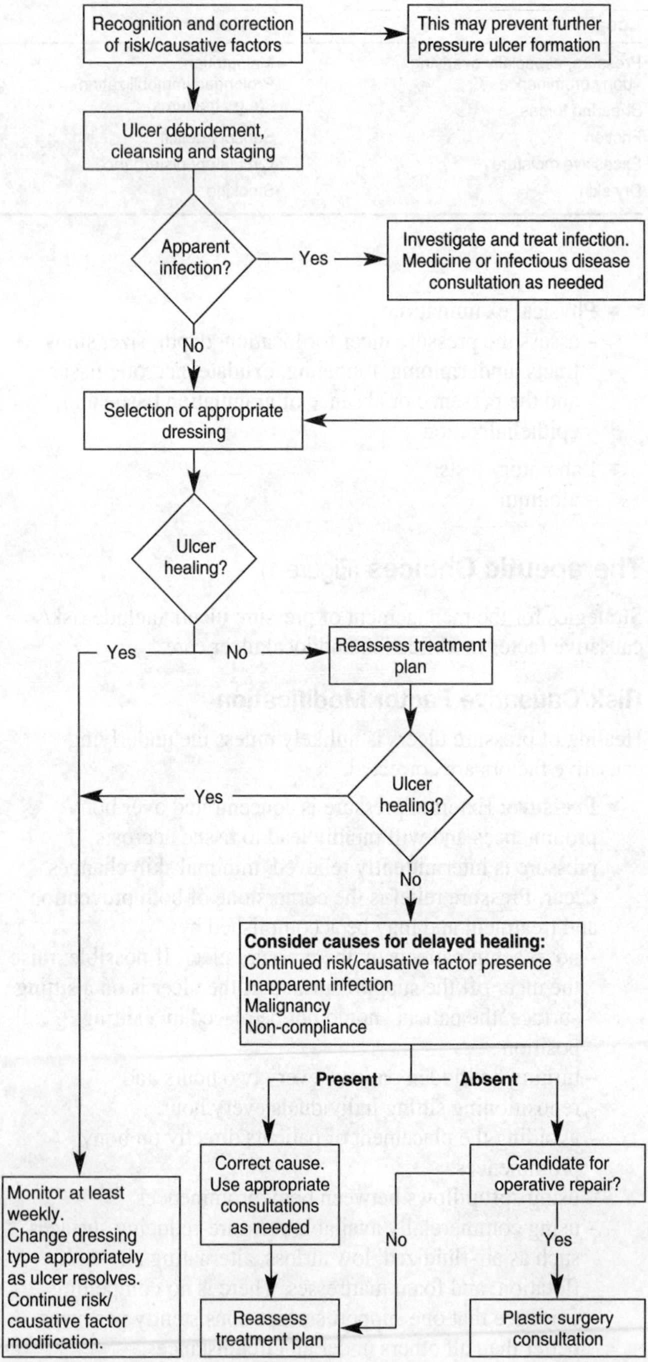
Recognition and correction of risk/causative factors
This may prevent further pressure ulcer formation
Ulcer débridement, cleansing and staging
Apparent infection?
Yes
Investigate and treat infection. Medicine or infectious disease consultation as needed
No
Selection of appropriate dressing
Ulcer healing?
Yes
No
Reassess treatment plan
Ulcer healing?
Yes
No
Consider causes for delayed healing:
Continued risk/causative factor presence
Inapparent infection
Malignancy
Non-compliance
Present
Absent
Correct cause. Use appropriate consultations as needed
Candidate for operative repair?
No
Yes
Monitor at least weekly. Change dressing type appropriately as ulcer resolves. Continue risk/causative factor modification.
Reassess treatment plan
Plastic surgery consultation

- **Shearing forces:** When the head of a supine patient is raised more than 30°, shearing forces occur in the sacral and coccygeal areas. Maintain the head of the bed at the lowest degree of elevation consistent with concurrent medical conditions and other restrictions.
- **Friction:** Friction can be minimized by lifting rather than dragging a bedridden patient across bed sheets, by keeping the bed free of particulate matter such as crumbs, and by keeping sheets loose to avoid restricting movement.
- **Excessive moisture:** A long-term moist environment may result from perspiration or fecal or urinary incontinence. Cleanse the skin and remove moisture at the time of soiling. Moisture barrier creams and incontinence briefs may be used for incontinence. A bowel routine and intermittent or permanent catheterization may be considered.
- **Dry skin:** Well-moisturized skin retains its barrier properties and helps to prevent skin breakdown.
- **Malnutrition:** Encourage dietary intake or supplementation if an individual with a pressure ulcer is malnourished. Give vitamin and mineral supplements if deficiencies are suspected or confirmed. A dietary consultation may be warranted.
- **Immobilization:** Early mobilization is encouraged. A physiotherapy consult may be valuable.
- **Sensory and circulatory compromise:** Optimization of contributing medical problems, such as diabetes, will assist in the healing of existing pressure ulcers and the prevention of new ones.
- **Smoking:** Excessive smoking may cause anorexia, contributing to malnutrition. Smoking also causes vasoconstriction and relative tissue hypoxia, which may impair wound healing.

## Local Ulcer Care

- The ulcer should be monitored at every dressing change and reassessed at least once per week.
- Tracings or color photos may be helpful for record keeping.
- Local ulcer care involves: wound débridement, wound cleansing and appropriate dressing choices.

### *Wound Débridement*

Removal of devitalized tissue and inflammatory agents is necessary to allow granulation tissue formation and subsequent re-epithelialization. Wound débridement may be accomplished in 4 ways:

- *Sharp débridement* with scissors or scalpel is indicated for thick adherent eschars, extensive devitalized tissue, or urgent débridement in infected ulcers. Sterile instruments should be used. If there is bleeding during débridement, pressure should be applied with gauze until the bleeding is controlled. Electrocautery may also be used for hemostasis. A clean, dry dressing may be used for 6 to 24 hours, after which a moist dressing may be reinstated. Algosteril, an absorptive dressing from the xerogels category, also functions as a procoagulant and can be used to obtain hemostasis in oozing wounds.
- *Autolytic débridement* involves synthetic dressings, especially hydrocolloids and hydrogels, to cover a wound and allow devitalized tissue to self-digest with wound fluid enzymes. Autolytic débridement may be appropriate for patients who cannot tolerate other methods and have uninfected wounds. Wounds must be frequently and effectively cleansed to wash out partially degraded tissue fragments at each dressing change.
- *Mechanical débridement* may be performed in several ways, including wet-to-dry dressings, hydrotherapy, or wound irrigation at moderate pressures. Wet-to-dry dressings adhere to eschar and remove the eschar when the dry dressing is removed. They should only be used for débridement and then immediately discontinued. Hydrotherapy and wound irrigation are useful for softening and mechanically removing eschar and debris. Proper irrigation pressure may be obtained using a 35 mL syringe with a 19-gauge angiocatheter.
- *Enzymatic débridement* is performed by applying enzyme-impregnated dressings to wounds.

### Wound Cleansing

- Wounds should be cleansed at initial examination and at each dressing change.
- Irrigation with normal saline may be used to clean most ulcers. Following irrigation, the surrounding skin should be gently patted dry to facilitate optimal adherence of the dressing. Care must be taken to avoid maceration and to avoid the spreading of bacteria to other skin sites.
- To avoid traumatizing the wound, minimal mechanical force should be used when cleansing with gauze, cloth, or sponges. Use the smoothest and softest device possible. Antiseptic agents, hydrogen peroxide, and skin cleansers are toxic to wound tissue and should not be used.
- Whirlpool treatment may be helpful for ulcers with thick exudate, slough, and necrotic tissue, but is inappropriate for clean wounds. Discontinue whirlpool treatment when the ulcer is clean.

### *Choice of Dressings*

The categories of wound dressings are shown in Table 3. Wound dressing choices for ulcer stages are outlined in Figure 2.

- The goals are to choose a dressing that will:
  – keep the ulcer bed continuously moist but not macerated
  – be absorbent enough to control exudate without desiccating the ulcer bed
  – keep the surrounding skin intact and dry
  – protect the wound.
- Studies of different types of moist wound dressings have shown no difference in pressure ulcer healing rates.
- As wounds heal, the dressing needs may change and the wound care plan should be re-evaluated.
- When applying the dressing:
  – dead space should be eliminated by loosely filling all cavities. Tissue must not be overpacked, as this may increase intra-wound pressure and cause additional tissue damage
  – optimal secondary dressings should cover about 3 cm of intact, dry skin around the ulcer
  – dressings should not exert tension on the skin, as the resulting shear forces increase the risk of further tissue breakdown
  – change dressing when drainage has seeped out under the dressing, indicating that the bacterial barrier has been compromised
  – frequency of dressing changes must be individually determined. For uncomplicated wounds, change occlusive dressings every 3 to 7 days, as this minimally disturbs healing tissue between dressing changes. If there are other factors, such as an underlying infection or excessive exudate, the dressing changes should be more frequent.

## Complications

**Infection:** All stage II to IV ulcers are colonized with bacteria. In most cases, adequate cleansing and débridement prevent colonization from progressing to clinical infection, and healing will still occur.

Inapparent infection may occur, with increased bacterial burden and the usual signs of infection absent. Consider a 2-week trial of **topical antibiotics** for clean pressure ulcers that are not healing or are continuing to produce excessive exudate after 2 to 4 weeks of optimal patient care. Contact dermatitis, bacterial resistance, and systemic absorption may occur with topical antibiotics.

Infected pressure ulcers may lead to cellulitis, bacteremia, sepsis, or osteomyelitis. Surrounding erythema or swelling greater than 2 cm may indicate cellulitis. If a sterile probe can be inserted to

Table 3: **Classification of Wound Dressings**

| Dressing | Characteristics | Wound |
|---|---|---|
| **Transparent Films**<br>OpSite<br>TegaDerm<br>Biocclusive | Semi-permeable, highly flexible dressings that reduce evaporative water loss, provide good antibacterial barriers, and reduce shear forces. | Superficial wounds, abrasions, and partial-thickness wounds. |
| **Gauze**<br>*Adherent:*<br>4 × 4 Gauze<br>*Non-adherent:*<br>Telfa<br>N-Terface | Débrides, but painful upon removal unless moistened first. Must be secured in place. | Partial or full-thickness wounds with necrotic debris or covered with antibiotic ointment. |
| **Hydrocolloids**<br>DuoDerm<br>Restore<br>Comfeel | Available as composite sheets with a hydrophilic polymer and a water-impermeable vapor-transmitting backing or in paste form. They are occlusive and provide an excellent barrier. Wound exudate is absorbed and a gel is formed that expands into the wound cavity. Promotes autolytic débridement. Usually requires less frequent changes. | Both partial and full-thickness wounds, especially superficial wounds. |
| **Hydrogels**<br>Intrasite gel<br>Vigilon<br>Nu-Gel<br>Clearsite<br>Duoderm gel | Three-dimensional networks of hydrophilic polymers made from gelatin and polysaccharides. Absorbs exudate with medium capacity and provides cooling and pain relief. Promotes autolytic débridement and granulation. Can both absorb fluid and hydrate desiccated eschars. | Full-thickness wounds with or without undermining. |
| **Xerogels**<br>Kaltostat<br>Algosteril<br>Sorbsan<br>Debrisan<br>Aquacel | Dry dressings with high absorptive capacity that change into a gel-like substance upon contacting wound exudate. After the exudate is absorbed, xerogels act similarly to hydrogels in facilitating moist wound healing. Alginates* are also procoagulants and can be used to obtain hemostasis in oozing wounds. | Full-thickness wounds with slough, with or without undermining. |
| **Foams**<br>Lyofoam<br>Epilock<br>Hydrosorb<br>Allevyn | Polymeric dressings that maximize absorbency and vapor permeability to provide optimal exudate handling. May be combined with a water-impermeable but vapor-transmitting backing to allow vapor loss. When the exudate contacts the backing, evaporative loss facilitates exudate control. Expansion of the foam as it absorbs exudate creates gentle pressure on the wound, possibly reducing wound edema. | Full-thickness wounds with exudate. Can be used around wound drains and tubes or over incisions. |
| **Enzymatic**<br>Collagenase | Enzymatic dressings apply topical débriding agents to devitalized tissue on the wound surface. A clean moist dressing should be applied over the ulcer after enzyme application. | Wounds with eschar. |

** Alginates are xerogels with hemostatic properties.*

## Figure 2: **Dressing Choices for Pressure Ulcers**

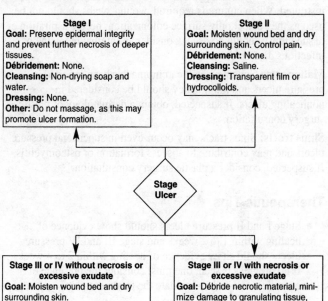

**Stage I**
**Goal:** Preserve epidermal integrity and prevent further necrosis of deeper tissues.
**Débridement:** None.
**Cleansing:** Non-drying soap and water.
**Dressing:** None.
**Other:** Do not massage, as this may promote ulcer formation.

**Stage II**
**Goal:** Moisten wound bed and dry surrounding skin. Control pain.
**Débridement:** None.
**Cleansing:** Saline.
**Dressing:** Transparent film or hydrocolloids.

**Stage Ulcer**

**Stage III or IV without necrosis or excessive exudate**
**Goal:** Moisten wound bed and dry surrounding skin.
**Débridement:**
Autolytic with occlusive dressings.
**Cleansing:** Saline irrigation (35 cc syringe with 19-gauge angiocatheter).
**Dressing:**
1. If very shallow, use hydrocolloids or hydrogel wafers.
2. If dead space present, lightly fill with hydrogels or saline-moistened gauze kept continuously moist.
Remoisten gauze before removal if dried and adherent to tissue.
Apply hydrocolloid dressing over wound filler.

**Stage III or IV with necrosis or excessive exudate**
**Goal:** Débride necrotic material, minimize damage to granulating tissue, keep surrounding skin intact and dry.
**Débridement:**
1. Infection (advancing cellulitis, bacteremia or sepsis) - sharp débridement.
2. Eschars - soften with an occlusive dressing then use sharp débridement.
3. Slough - use mechanical wet-to-dry saline dressings, enzymatic, or autolytic débridement. Switch once slough resolved. Whirlpool baths may be used.
**Cleansing:** Saline irrigation (35 cc syringe with 19-gauge angiocatheter).
**Dressing:**
1. If mechanical débridement is appropriate, use wet-to-dry saline-soaked gauze.
Loosely fill dead space and undermining.
Do not moisten before removal.
2. After sharp débridement with bleeding, dry dressing or alginate for 6-24 hours.
Moisten any dry dressings before removal.
3. If excessive exudate, use xerogels or foams. Protect surrounding skin with barrier ointment.
4. If malodorous or purulent exudate, topical antibacterial agents. If cellulitis, use systemic antibiotics.
5. Once necrosis is no longer present, stop débridement and refer to **Stage III and IV without necrosis or excessive exudate.**

**At all stages: Search for and correct risk/causative factors. Especially relieve local pressure and optimize systemic condition.**

bone, the patient should be considered to have osteomyelitis until proven otherwise, and appropriate **systemic antibiotic therapy** instituted. When culture is required, wound swabs should not be used as they detect only surface colonization; needle aspiration or tissue biopsy should be used. Consider an internal medicine or infectious disease consult.

**Malignancy:** Squamous cell carcinoma has been reported in pressure ulcers and malignancy should be considered in nonhealing ulcers. If suspected, obtain a dermatology or plastic surgery consultation.

**Sinus tracts:** Sinus tracts may occur even in superficial pressure ulcers and may contribute to abscess formation or osteomyelitis. If suspected, consider a plastic surgery consultation.

## Therapeutic Tips

- Stage I and II pressure ulcers should show evidence of healing within 1 to 2 weeks and stage III and IV pressure ulcers should show evidence of healing within 2 to 4 weeks. If no progress is seen, one must consider the presence of complications and re-evaluate the treatment plan.
- In general, stage I, II, and III pressure ulcers are more likely to heal with local therapy. Stage IV pressure ulcers, especially over ischial tuberosities, often require surgical intervention.
- Caregiver time and associated labor costs are often a significant component of the total cost of caring for a pressure ulcer and should be considered when selecting a dressing. Many studies demonstrate that caregiver labor costs can exceed the cost of supplies in wound management. For example, continuously moistened saline gauze is inexpensive, but can consume up to ten times more nursing time than more expensive occlusive dressings such as hydrocolloids or transparent film.
- The early recognition and correction of risk factors will expedite the healing of existing pressure ulcers and may prevent the formation of new pressure ulcers. In a disease associated with such substantial morbidity and mortality, indeed "an ounce of prevention is worth a pound of cure".

## *Suggested Reading List*

Agency for Health Care Policy and Research. *Treatment of pressure ulcers. Clinical practice guideline #15*. Rockville, MD: Department of Health and Human Services, 1994. AHCPR Publication #95–0652. (available at their website http://www.ahcpr.gov)

Bergstrom NI. Strategies for preventing pressure ulcers. *Clin Geriatr Med* 1997;13:437–454.

Goode PS, Thomas DR. Pressure ulcers: local wound care. *Clin Geriatr Med* 1997;13:543–552.

Kanj LF, Wilking SVB, Phillips TJ. Pressure ulcers. *J Am Acad Dermatol* 1998;38:517–536.

van Rijswijk L, Braden B. Pressure ulcer patient and wound assessment: an AHCPR clinical practice guideline update. *Ostomy Wound Manage* 1999;45(suppl 1A):56S–67S.

CHAPTER 64

# Psoriasis

*Jean-Pierre DesGroseilliers, MD, MSc, FRCPC*

Psoriasis is a chronic skin disease with markedly increased epidermal cellular turnover. Many areas of the body are affected and the patient can present to the health care professional in different ways. Before making therapeutic choices, it is essential that other conditions that affect the same areas of the body be ruled out and that the correct diagnosis be established. A regional approach is provided since patients often present with a skin problem affecting their scalp, face, hands and feet, body, fold areas or nails.

## Goals of Therapy

- To improve the physical signs of psoriasis and its secondary psychological effects
- To facilitate the patient's acceptance of this chronic disease coupled with realistic expectations
- To provide psoriasis control for the longest periods possible

## Therapeutic Choices (Figure 1)

### *Scalp*

#### Diagnosis

Seborrheic dermatitis most often mimics psoriasis to the point that some refer to this condition as seborrhiasis. The psoriatic scale is thicker and more adherent. There are often signs of psoriasis on the knees, elbows or sacral area.

#### Pharmacologic Choices

Removal of the scales is essential. This can be done with oil-based products with or without salicylic acid and/or a medium-strength corticosteroid such as betamethasone left on the scalp overnight. Tar-based shampoos can be used in the morning to wash off the oil and scales. It is better to apply this treatment every two to three nights than not at all.

### *Face*

#### Diagnosis

Here, the nature of the scale helps to differentiate:

- Psoriasis – sharply demarcated, silvery scale

Figure 1: **Management of Psoriasis**

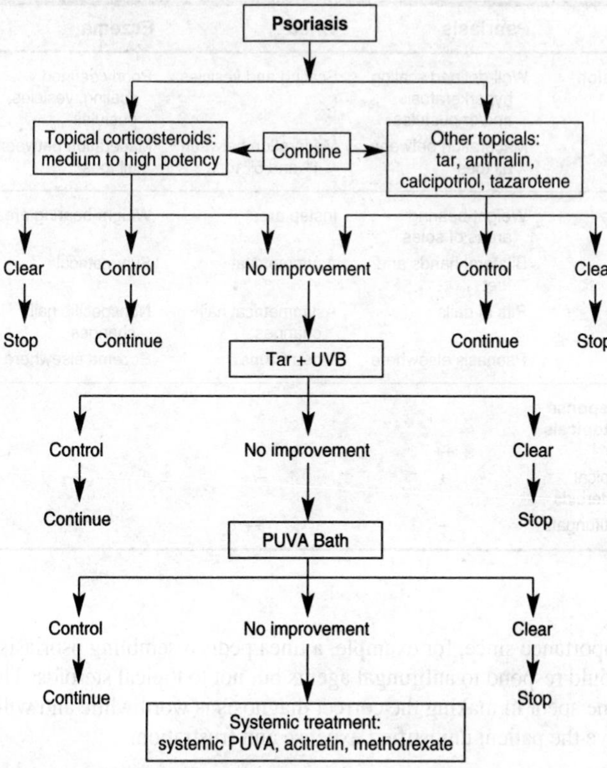
Psoriasis
Topical corticosteroids: medium to high potency
Combine
Other topicals: tar, anthralin, calcipotriol, tazarotene
Clear
Control
No improvement
Control
Clear
Stop
Continue
Continue
Stop
Tar + UVB
Control
No improvement
Clear
Continue
Stop
PUVA Bath
Control
No improvement
Clear
Continue
Stop
Systemic treatment: systemic PUVA, acitretin, methotrexate

- Seborrheic dermatitis - greasy, brownish-yellow scale
- Discoid lupus erythematosus - adherent, carpet-tack scale
- Tinea of face - little or no scale

### Pharmacologic Choices

One percent hydrocortisone cream often is sufficient to control psoriasis of the face as long as it is applied regularly. At first, applications should be in the morning and at bedtime. As improvement occurs, the frequency of application should be decreased to bedtime only and eventually every two to three nights. Avoid using medium strength corticosteroids long term on the face for fear of precipitating rosacea, telangiectasia and ocular changes.

## *Hands and feet*

### Diagnosis (Table 1)

Psoriasis of palms and soles is one of the most difficult dermatologic conditions to treat. The correct diagnosis here is of great

Table 1: **Differential Diagnosis for Psoriasis of the Hands and Feet**

| | Psoriasis | Tinea | Eczema |
|---|---|---|---|
| **Lesion** | Well-defined scaling hyperkeratosis and/or pustules | Scaling and vesicles | Poorly defined scaling, vesicles, pustules |
| | Maceration between all toes | Maceration between 4th and 5th toes | Maceration between all toes |
| **Site** | Weight-bearing areas of soles | Instep area | Weight-bearing area |
| | Bilateral hands and feet | Asymmetrical | Symmetrical |
| | Pits of nails | Asymmetrical nail changes | Nonspecific nail changes |
| | Psoriasis elsewhere | Tinea Cruris | Eczema elsewhere |
| **Response to topicals** | | | |
| Tar | ++ | – | + |
| Topical steroids | + | –/+ | ++ |
| Antifungals | – | ++ | – |

importance since, for example, a tinea pedis resembling psoriasis would respond to antifungal agents but not to topical steroids. The time spent in making the correct diagnosis is worthwhile and will save the patient unjustified expense and frustration.

## **Pharmacologic Choices** (Table 2)

### *Topical Therapy*

Frequent lubrication with vaseline and medium- to high-potency corticosteroid ointment with plastic wrap occlusion.

Newer agents such as calcipotriol (vitamin D derivative) and tazarotene (vitamin A derivative) can be used alone morning and night or with topical corticosteroids or ultraviolet light (UV). Do not use plastic wrap occlusion with calcipotriol or tazarotene as it could result in skin irritation.

### *Phototherapy*

Phototherapy includesUVB with 10% coal tar distillate or UVA with psoralen (PUVA) applied topically as methoxsalen 0.05% in Cetaphil cream. This treatment, as discussed below, is best left to a dermatologist.

### *Systemic Therapy*

Retinoids, such as acitretin 25 to 75 mg daily, give better results than methotrexate 7.5 to 22.5 mg once a week.

Table 2: **Psoriasis Therapies**

| Drug | Dosage | Adverse Effects | Comments | Cost* |
|---|---|---|---|---|
| **Topical Therapy** | | | | |
| Corticosteroids (for a complete listing see Chapter 65 Table 3) | | | | |
| mild potency e.g., *hydrocortisone 1% cream* | Once daily to BID | Few side effects. | Indicated: face and folds<br>Contraindicated: thick plaques | $–$$ |
| mid- to high-potency e.g., *betamethasone, triamcinolone* | Once daily to BID | Local atrophy, tachyphylaxis. Risk of systemic absorption with higher potency agents used over large areas. | Indicated: body<br>Contraindicated: face and folds<br>Effective, not messy. | |
| *coal tar* Alphosyl, Balnetar, Liquor Carbonis Detergens, others | Once daily | Dermatitis, folliculitis, photosensitivity. Malodorous, stains skin and hair. | Indicated: plaques<br>Contraindicated: folds<br>Can be combined with UVB.<br>Effective, economical, longest remission. | $ |
| *anthralin* Anthraforte, Anthranol, Micanol, others | Once daily | Irritating to surrounding normal skin. Stains skin and fabrics. | Indicated: plaques<br>Contraindicated: folds<br>Can be combined with UVB.<br>Effective, economical, longest remission. | $$ |
| *tazarotene 0.05%, 0.1%* Tazorac | Once daily | Skin irritation. | Indicated: body<br>Contraindicated: face and folds<br>Longer remission. | $$$$ |

*(cont'd)*

Table 2: **Psoriasis Therapies** *(cont'd)*

| Drug | Dosage | Adverse Effects | Comments | Cost* |
|---|---|---|---|---|
| *calcipotriol* Dovonex | BID | Skin irritation. | Indicated: body<br>Contraindicated: face and folds<br>Longer remission. | $$$ |
| **Psoralens with UVA (PUVA)** | | | Oral ingestion of, or bathing with a psoralen before exposure to UVA. | |
| *methoxsalen* Oxsoralen, Ultra MOP | Topical: 100 mg/125 mL bath water. Soak in aqueous solution, 15–20 min. before UVA exposure. | Photosensitivity, exaggerated sunburn. | Indicated: total area<br>Use 3 ×/wk<br>Longest remission. | $$$$ |
| | Oral: 0.5–0.8 mg/kg 2 hr before UVA exposure 3 ×/wk. | Nausea, pruritus, cataracts. | Increased risk of skin cancer with long-term PUVA. | $$ (40 mg/dose) |
| **Systemic Therapy** | | | | |
| *methotrexate* ◗ Rheumatrex, generics | 7.5–22.5 mg/wk PO | Bone marrow suppression, hepatotoxicity | Indicated: Total area<br>Contraindicated: liver disease | $$–$$$ |
| *acitretin* Soriatane | 25–75 mg/day PO | Arthralgia, myalgia, alopecia, dry lips and mucosa, hyperlipidemia, hepatotoxicity. | Indicated: hands and feet<br>Teratogen, contraindicated in pregnancy. | $$$$–$$$$$ |

◗ *Dosage adjustment may be required in renal impairment – see Appendix I.*
** Cost of 50 g or 50 mL for topical products or 30-day supply – includes drug cost only.*
*Legend: $ < $10 $$ $10–25 $$$ $25–50 $$$$ $50–100 $$$$$ > $100*

## *Body and extremities*

### Diagnosis

Classical psoriasis with non-pruritic, silvery scaling plaques affecting the elbows, knees and sacral areas is easy to diagnose. Tinea versicolor has a fine orange/brown scale and is limited to the upper thorax. Pityriasis rosea has oval, pink lesions with a fine collarette of central scale, and rarely affects elbows and knees. Eczematous dermatitis is itchy and often crusty, lichenified and excoriated. Tinea corporis has an active periphery with a clear centre and a positive potassium hydroxide (KOH) examination for fungal elements.

### Pharmacologic Choices

The difficulty is to choose the appropriate therapy for the patient from a number of effective topical and systemic pharmacologic agents. The tars used with UVB are either 2% crude coal tar or 10% coal tar distillate. For PUVA bath, 10 tablets of methoxsalen 10 mg are dissolved and added to 125 litres of bath water. For systemic PUVA, the dose of methoxsalen is 0.5 to 0.8 mg/kg body weight given 2 hours prior to UVA radiation.

Usually, PUVA treatments are available only in a dermatologist's office, a psoriasis day-care centre or phototherapy clinic. UVB light sources are at times also available in hospital physiotherapy departments. As a rule, phototherapy is used only if common local treatments with steroids, calcipotriol, tazarotene, tars, or anthralin are ineffective on their own.

If required, it is best to consult a dermatologist who is familiar with phototherapy and the various systemic therapies.

## *Fold areas*

### Diagnosis (Table 3)

In these areas, the diagnosis can be difficult to make, but the treatment is often the same.

### Pharmacologic Choices

In most cases, daily to twice daily applications of a 1% hydrocortisone cream with or without an antimonilial/antifungal agent, such as ketoconazole, will bring about dramatic improvement of the eruption with little or no adverse effects.

## *Nails*

### Diagnosis

Psoriatic nail changes can be hard to differentiate from fungal infection of the nails. Both cause yellowish, white discoloration of the distal nail plate. Only psoriasis, however, produces small "ice pick" pits of the nail.

Table 3: **Differential Diagnosis for Psoriasis in Fold Areas**

| Psoriasis | Tinea | Eczema | Moniliasis |
|---|---|---|---|
| Bright red, well defined | Scaling at edge | Very itchy | Satellite papules and pustules |
| KOH – ve | KOH + ve | KOH – ve | KOH + ve |
| Psoriasis elsewhere | Maceration between 4th and 5th toes | Eczema elsewhere | Affects fold areas mainly |

*Abbreviations: KOH = potassium hydroxide stain which is diagnostic for fungi.*

## Pharmacologic Choices

Most topical therapeutic measures are unsatisfactory and as the overall psoriasis improves the nails often improve. The only treatment that can give satisfactory results in psoriasis of the nails is the use of psoralen topically or systemically with UVA, (PUVA). This treatment can be very prolonged and requires enormous motivation on the part of the patient and the physician.

## Therapeutic Tips

- It is important to customize the treatment to the patient. A number of factors need to be considered when opting for one treatment versus another, and the patient must be an equal partner in the decision process.
  - Can the patient afford the prescribed medication?
  - Is the patient willing to put up with the smell of tar or the stain of anthralin?
  - Can the patient manage to attend phototherapy sessions 5 times per week or only 3 times per week?
  - Does the patient accept the risks of the possible adverse effects of methotrexate, acitretin or PUVA?
- Length of remission is longer with phototherapy but there still is no definitive cure for psoriasis.
- If there is no response to treatment, is the diagnosis the right one?
- The continued care of the patient by the family physician should be the foundation on which occasional evaluations by the dermatologist can be added as needed.

## *Suggested Reading List*

Ashton R, Leppard B. *Differential diagnosis in dermatology*. 2nd ed. Oxford: Radcliffe Medical Press, 1992.

Fitzpatrick TB, et al. *Color atlas and synopsis of clinical dermatology: common and serious diseases.* 3rd ed. New York: McGraw-Hill, 1997.

Jackson R. *Morphological diagnosis of skin disease: a study of the living gross pathology of the skin*. Grimsby, ON: Manticore Publishers, 1998:97–123.

Koo J, Lebwohl M. Duration of remission of psoriasis therapies. *J Am Acad Dermatol* 1999;41:51–59.

Lookingbill DP, Marks JG. *Principles of dermatology*. 2nd ed. Philadelphia: W.B. Saunders 1993:136–142.

CHAPTER 65

# Atopic Dermatitis

*Robert S. Lester, MD, FRCPC*

Atopic dermatitis is an inflammatory skin disease marked by intense pruritus and a tendency to lichenification of the skin. There is a natural tendency in many but not all patients to improve with age.

## Goals of Therapy

- To increase patient/parent understanding of the course of atopic dermatitis and reasonable expectations of management
- To relieve pruritus and decrease or heal lesions
- To minimize and/or manage recurrences

## Investigations

- Complete history with special emphasis on family history of atopic disorders including atopic dermatitis, allergic rhinitis and asthma
- Physical examination: primary sites may vary with age of patients
  - infant stage (birth to 2 years): face and lateral aspects of lower legs
  - childhood phase (2 to 12 years): lichenification in flexural areas
  - adult phase: hand dermatitis; eyelid dermatitis; localized areas of lichenification (e.g., anogenital area)

In all phases, the eruption may become more generalized and inflammation and pruritus may become incapacitating with disturbance of sleep and agitation.

Table 1 lists the associated findings in patients with atopic dermatitis.

## Therapeutic Choices

Refer to Table 2 for general management.

- **Lubrication**
  - attention to dryness of the skin is an important aspect of treatment of atopic dermatitis.

Table 1: **Associated Findings**

| | |
|---|---|
| Dry skin and xerosis | Hyperlinear palmar creases |
| Ichthyosis vulgaris | Dennie-Morgan infraorbital folds |
| Keratosis pilaris | Anterior subcapsular cataracts |
| Pityriasis alba | Keratoconus |

– use agents such as nondrying soaps, nonperfumed oils or oatmeal baths.
– apply lubricating ointments after bathing (e.g., petrolatum)
– encourage use of humidifiers.

- **Antihistamines**
  – primary action of antihistamines may be sedative.
  – sedative antihistamines such as hydroxyzine or diphenhydramine are more effective than the nonsedative types (Chapter 66).
  – topical doxepin may be a useful adjuvant either alone or in combination with topical steroids to control pruritus. Restrict use to smaller areas of involvement as systemic absorption can occur. Advise patients about potential drowsiness.
- **Topical steroids**
  – the mainstay of management is the use of topical steroids twice daily.
  – topical steroids are now available in a wide range of potencies (Table 3). The same drug may show different potency depending on the delivery vehicle used. In general, greater potency occurs when the drug is delivered as an ointment as compared to a cream or lotion.
  – the choice of agent depends on the age, location and extent of skin lesions (Table 4).
  – the lowest potency steroid that is effective should be used. Short courses (1 to 2 weeks) of higher potency topical steroids can be used in all cases of resistant disease.
  – several factors may influence response to topical steroids (Table 5).
  – topical steroids are usually trouble free and highly effective especially when used for brief periods, on limited areas, and without occlusion. More potent topical steroids are associated with increased risks of side effects. Percutaneous absorption varies with the site of application. Least absorption occurs on the palms and soles with maximum absorption occurring in intertriginous areas. Children, as a result of their surface area to weight ratio, absorb relatively more topically applied corticosteroid and are at increased risk for developing systemic adverse effects. Adverse effects attributed to topical steroid use are summarized in Table 6.

Table 2: **General Management of Atopic Dermatitis**

| | |
|---|---|
| Address psychosocial issues | Antihistamines |
| Modify diet (where indicated) | Topical corticosteroids |
| Avoid aggravating factors | Antimicrobials (when indicated) |
| Avoid primary irritants and allergens | Systemic therapy (severe, generalized) |
| Lubrication | |

Table 3: **Potency Classification of Topical Corticosteroids**

| Topical Corticosteroid | Cost* |
|---|---|
| ***Very potent*** † | |
| *betamethasone dipropionate 0.05% in propylene glycol base*<br>Diprolene Glycol, Topilene | $$ |
| *clobetasol propionate 0.05%*<br>Dermasone, Dermovate, others | $$ |
| *halobetasol propionate 0.5%*<br>Ultravate | $$$ |
| ***Potent*** † | |
| *amcinonide 0.1%*<br>Cyclocort | $$ |
| *betamethasone dipropionate 0.05%*<br>Diprosone, Topisone, others | $ |
| *desoximetasone 0.25%*<br>Topicort | $$ |
| *diflorasone acetate 0.05%*<br>Florone | $ |
| *fluocinonide 0.05%*<br>Lidex, Lyderm, Tiamol, others | $ |
| *halcinonide 0.1%*<br>Halog | $$ |
| *triamcinolone acetonide 0.5%*<br>Aristocort C | $$$$ |
| ***Moderately potent*** † | |
| *beclomethasone dipropionate 0.025%*<br>Propaderm | $$ |
| *betamethasone benzoate 0.025%*<br>Beben | $$ |
| *betamethasone valerate 0.05%, 0.1%*<br>Betnovate, Celestoderm V, others | $ |
| *clobetasone butyrate 0.05%*<br>Eumovate | $$ |
| *diflucortolone valerate 0.1%*<br>Nerisone | $$ |
| *fluocinolone acetonide 0.01%, 0.025%*<br>Fluoderm, Synalar | $–$$ |
| *hydrocortisone valerate 0.2%*<br>Westcort | $ |
| *mometasone furoate 0.1%*<br>Elocom | $$ |
| *triamcinolone acetonide 0.1%*<br>Aristocort R, Kenalog, others | $ |
| ***Weak*** † | |
| *desonide 0.05%*<br>Desocort, Tridesilon, others | $ |
| *hydrocortisone 0.5%, 1%, 2.5%*<br>Aquacort, Cortate, others | $ |
| *hydrocortisone acetate 0.1%, 1%*<br>Corticreme, Hyderm, others | $ |
| *methylprednisolone acetate 0.25%*<br>Medrol Veriderm | $ |

† *These classifications are broad guidelines and within any class there may be a range of potencies.*

* *Cost of 15 g – includes drug cost only.*

*Legend: $ < $5 $$ $5–10 $$$ $10–15 $$$$ > $15–20*

- **Antibiotic Therapy**
  - when secondary infection is suspected, bacterial cultures should be taken and the patient treated with appropriate systemic antibiotics.
  - topical combinations of fusidic acid with either betamethasone or hydrocortisone may be used when staphylococcal secondary infection is suspected or in more persistent cases of eczema.
- **Light Therapy**
  - photo (chemo) therapy has been successful in the treatment of severe cases of atopic dermatitis and requires referral to a specialist.
- **Systemic Therapy**
  - short courses of oral corticosteroids or the intermittent use of IM depo-steroids may occasionally be necessary in severe intractable cases.
  - cyclosporine treatment utilized properly may be an effective, safe and well-tolerated treatment for severe atopic dermatitis resistant to conventional therapy.
- **New Approaches to Treatment**
  - immune modulating agents are presently being investigated for the treatment of atopic dermatitis. Topical tacrolimus and topical ascomycin are currently being evaluated in randomized trials.

## Therapeutic Tips

- Do not underestimate the importance of explanation of the natural course and reasonable expectations of therapy to the patient on the first visit.
- Relief of pruritus is essential in the management of atopic dermatitis.

Table 4: **Choice of Topical Corticosteroid**

| Factor | | Choice of Steroid |
|---|---|---|
| Age | Infant | Weak |
| | Child | Weak to moderate |
| | Adult | Moderate to very potent |
| Site | Face | Weak |
| | Intertriginous | Weak |
| | Trunk and extremities | Moderate to potent |
| | Palms and soles | Potent to very potent |
| Extent | Localized | Moderate to very potent |
| | Generalized | Weak to moderate |

Table 5: **Factors Influencing Response to Topical Steroids**

| | |
|---|---|
| Potency of steroid chosen | Frequency of application |
| Concentration of steroid | Occlusion |
| Amount of steroid applied | Vehicle chosen |

Table 6: **Adverse Effects to Topical Corticosteroids**

I. **Systemic**
Hypothalamic-pituitary adrenal axis suppression
Iatrogenic Cushing syndrome
Growth retardation (children)

II. **Local**

A. Catabolic Effects
- Degeneration of dermal collagen
- Epidermal and dermal atrophy
- Telangiectasia
- Purpura and ecchymosis
- Striae
- Disturbances in wound healing
- Steroid acne
- Steroid rosacea
- Steroid perioral dermatitis
- Hypertrichosis
- Infection

B. Modification of Local Response
- Tinea incognito
- Glaucoma and cataracts
- Hypopigmentation

C. Allergic contact dermatitis

- Use the least potent topical steroid which will control symptoms.
- When symptoms are in remission substitute lubrication for medication.
- If unresponsive to therapy, check for occult staphylococcus infection and treat with appropriate antibiotics.
- Do not rely on skin testing. As many as 80% of patients with atopic dermatitis react on skin testing to more than one of a large number of environmental allergens including a multitude of foods. History is more important than testing, and in most patients, dietary manipulation may be unsuitable.

## *Suggested Reading List*

Hanifin JM, Chan S. Biochemical and immunologic mechanisms in atopic dermatitis: new targets for emerging therapies. *J Am Acad Dermatol* 1999; 41(1):72–77.

Krafchik BR. Eczematous Dermatitis. In: Schachner LA, Hansen RC, eds. *Paediatric Dermatology.* 2nd ed. New York: Churchill Livingston, 1995:1(15):685–721.

Lester RS. Atopic Dermatitis. In: Rakel RE, ed. *Conn's Current Therapy.* Toronto: WB Saunders, 1994:803–808.

Lester RS. Corticosteroids. *Clin Dermatol* 1989;7(3):80–97.

CHAPTER 66

# Pruritus

*Laura A. Finlayson, MD, FRCPC*

## Goals of Therapy

- To determine etiology of pruritus in each patient (commonly a skin disease)
- To rule out underlying systemic disease (found in about 20% of pruritic patients without skin disorders)
- To decrease or abolish the itching sensation

## Investigations

- A complete history including:
  - nature, location, duration, severity of pruritus
  - skin rash or dryness
  - past history or symptoms to suggest renal, hepatic, hematopoietic, lymphoreticular or endocrine disease
  - hygiene practices, topical contacts to the skin
  - weight loss or night sweats
  - prescription, over-the-counter and illicit drug use, particularly opiates
- Physical examination with assessment for presence of skin rash or dryness, dermatographism, uremic pigmentation, jaundice, plethora, lymphadenopathy, hepatosplenomegaly
- Laboratory investigations are indicated only if a primary dermatological cause for the pruritus has been excluded and include CBC with differential, fasting serum glucose, liver function tests, renal function tests, chest x-ray
- Depending on the index of suspicion, further investigations may be required to identify underlying systemic disease (Figure 1)

## Therapeutic Choices

Pruritus is a symptom, not a disease. A wide spectrum of cutaneous and systemic conditions can result in the subjective complaint of itching. Once the underlying cause is diagnosed, appropriate management can be prescribed (Figure 1, Table 1).

### Nonpharmacologic Choices

- **Skin hydration:** Dry skin frequently causes or exacerbates pruritus. Overbathing, hot water, harsh soaps and bubble bath preparations dry and irritate the skin and should be avoided.

Figure 1: **Management of Pruritus**

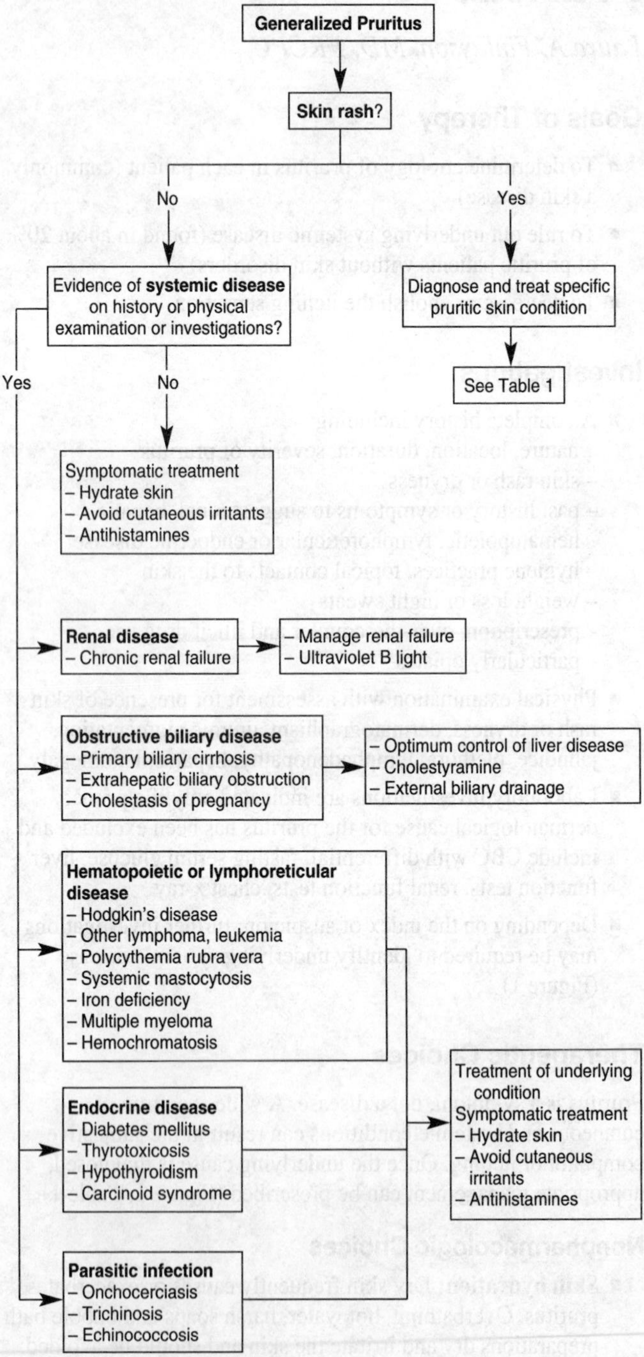
Generalized Pruritus
Skin rash?
No
Yes
Evidence of systemic disease on history or physical examination or investigations?
Diagnose and treat specific pruritic skin condition
See Table 1
Yes
No
Symptomatic treatment
– Hydrate skin
– Avoid cutaneous irritants
– Antihistamines
Renal disease
– Chronic renal failure
– Manage renal failure
– Ultraviolet B light
Obstructive biliary disease
– Primary biliary cirrhosis
– Extrahepatic biliary obstruction
– Cholestasis of pregnancy
– Optimum control of liver disease
– Cholestyramine
– External biliary drainage
Hematopoietic or lymphoreticular disease
– Hodgkin's disease
– Other lymphoma, leukemia
– Polycythemia rubra vera
– Systemic mastocytosis
– Iron deficiency
– Multiple myeloma
– Hemochromatosis
Treatment of underlying condition
Symptomatic treatment
– Hydrate skin
– Avoid cutaneous irritants
– Antihistamines
Endocrine disease
– Diabetes mellitus
– Thyrotoxicosis
– Hypothyroidism
– Carcinoid syndrome
Parasitic infection
– Onchocerciasis
– Trichinosis
– Echinococcosis

Table 1: **Pruritic Skin Diseases**

| Morphology | Skin Disease | Treatment |
|---|---|---|
| Urticarial | Urticaria | Avoid precipitants; antihistamines. |
| | Dermatographism | Avoid precipitants; antihistamines. |
| | Pruritic urticarial papules and plaques of pregnancy | Symptomatic; deliver baby. |
| Dermatitic | Xerosis | Hydrate skin. |
| | Atopic dermatitis | Mild topical corticosteroids. |
| | Contact dermatitis | Avoid precipitants; topical corticosteroids. |
| Dermatitic with burrows | Scabies | Topical permethrin. Treat household contacts. |
| Maculopapular | Drug eruption | Discontinue drug; symptomatic. |
| | Viral exanthem | Symptomatic. |
| Papulosquamous | Lichen planus | Topical or oral corticosteroids. |
| | Lichen simplex chronicus | Cover to prevent scratching; topical corticosteroids. |
| Pustular | Folliculitis | Minimize friction to hair follicles; topical antibiotics. |
| | Miliaria (heat rash) | Keep skin cool; talcum powder. |
| | Insect bites | Prevention; topical antipruritics. |
| Nodular | Nodular scabies | Topical permethrin. |
| | Prurigo nodularis | Cover to prevent scratching; topical corticosteroids. |
| Vesiculobullous | Dermatitis herpetiformis | Dapsone; gluten-free diet. |
| | Bullous pemphigoid | Oral corticosteroids, immunosuppressive agents. |
| | Varicella | Symptomatic; acyclovir. |
| Pigmented macules | Urticaria pigmentosa | Antihistamines; avoid ASA, opiates, rubbing skin. |

However, a daily tepid bath or shower for 5 to 10 minutes, using mild unscented soap mainly on intertriginous areas and feet, can be taken to hydrate skin. Colloidal oatmeal bath preparations or 4 tablespoons of baking soda in the bath can be soothing. An unscented bath oil, baby oil or mineral oil may be applied to the skin shortly before bathing is finished. Skin is then patted with a towel. Unscented moisture cream or white petrolatum should be applied while the skin is still slightly damp to retard water evaporation.

- **Avoid agents that can enhance histamine release** (e.g., ASA, opiates, shellfish, strawberries and red wine).

- **Minimize friction and irritation to the skin.** Clothing should be soft and loose. Wool and synthetic clothing should be avoided. Washing detergent should be well rinsed from clothing, and antistatic agents in the dryer should be avoided. Avoid fragranced products.
- **Minimize scratching.** Generalized pruritus produces a powerful, almost uncontrollable stimulus to scratch the skin. The scratch-itch cycle is self-perpetuating. Fingernails should be kept short. Cool tap water compresses can be applied for acute localized itch.
- **Avoid vasodilatory stimuli** (e.g., excessive exercise, high environmental temperature and humidity, hot showers or baths, spicy foods, caffeine and alcohol).
- **Ensure adequate sleep.** Pruritus is frequently worse at night, mostly because lack of distracting stimuli allows one to focus on the itch. Antipruritic topical lotion, applied just before bedtime, use of light bedclothes, and a sedative or sedating antihistamine may be helpful.

## Pharmacologic Choices

### *Topical Antipruritics*

**Menthol** 0.25 to 0.5%, **camphor** 0.25 to 0.5% in a light nonperfumed lotion (e.g., Sarna lotion), applied TID or PRN, is soothing. **Pramoxine hydrochloride** 1% (e.g., Pramox cream, Sarna P lotion) is a topical anesthetic with low sensitizing potential that may provide short-term relief. Topical benzocaine and other "caine" topical anesthetics and topical diphenhydramine and phenol should be avoided because they can sensitize the skin. Phenol is also contraindicated in pregnancy. **Doxepin** 5% cream (Zonalon) is a topical formulation of a tricyclic antidepressant which relieves pruritus in some patients. Some systemic absorption occurs, therefore it is best used for localized pruritus (less than 10% body surface area) and for a short term (less than 10 days). **Crotamiton** (Eurax), a scabicide, may also be used for its nonspecific antipruritic properties. **Calamine** lotion is helpful for acute conditions such as contact dermatitis but will dry the skin excessively with long-term use.

### *Antihistamines* (Table 2)

Histamine is directly involved in many but not all cases of pruritus; therefore, antihistamines may have a variable effect, providing profound to minimal relief. They are most effective in urticaria. Histamine$_1$ ($H_1$) blockers are the agents of choice because $H_2$ receptors are not directly involved in itch.

First-generation (classical) antihistamines have effects on adrenergic, serotonergic and cholinergic receptors in addition to histamine receptors. They are more likely to cause central

Table 2: **Antihistamines**

| Drug | Dosage (adult) | Sedative Effects | Anticholinergic Effects | Comments | Cost* |
|---|---|---|---|---|---|
| **Alkylamines** | | | | Each of these agents has a longer-acting slow-release form which should not be chewed, crushed or dissolved. | |
| *brompheniramine maleate* Dimetane | 4–8 mg TID–QID | ++ | +++ | | $–$$ |
| *chlorpheniramine maleate*† Chlor-Tripolon, generics | 4 mg Q6H or 8 mg Repetabs Q12H | ++ | +++ | | $–$$ |
| *dexchlorpheniramine maleate* Polaramine | 2 mg TID–QID | ++ | +++ | | $ |
| **Ethanolamines** | | | | This group is particularly useful in acute allergic reactions. High incidence of sedative and anticholinergic effects. Limit long-term use. Diphenhydramine available as an injectable and pediatric liquid. | |
| *clemastine fumarate* Tavist | 2–6 mg/d in divided doses | +++ | ++++ | | $–$$$$ |
| *diphenhydramine HCl* Benadryl, generics | 25–50 mg Q6H | ++++ | ++++ | | $–$$ |
| **Phenothiazines** | | | | Extrapyramidal symptoms, photosensitivity. | |
| *promethazine HCl* Histanil, generics | 12.5 mg QID or 25 mg QHS | ++++ | ++++ | | $ |
| *trimeprazine tartrate* Panectyl | 2.5–5 mg TID | +++ | ++++ | Trimeprazine available as pediatric liquid. | $–$$ |

*(cont'd)*

Table 2: **Antihistamines** *(cont'd)*

| Drug | Dosage (adult) | Sedative Effects | Anticholinergic Effects | Comments | Cost* |
|---|---|---|---|---|---|
| **Piperazines** | | | | | |
| **First generation** | | | | | |
| *hydroxyzine HCl*<br>Atarax, generics | 25–75 mg TID–QID | +++ | ++ | Hydroxyzine: useful in both acute and chronic allergic conditions. Some anxiolytic and antiemetic properties. Occasionally may cause paradoxical excitation in children. | $ |
| **Second generation** | | | | | |
| *cetirizine HCl*[†]<br>Reactine, generics | 10 mg/d | +/0 | +/0 | Cetirizine: long acting and inhibits the late phase reaction of allergy. A metabolite of hydroxyzine. Headache and fatigue in up to 10%. | $$ |
| **Piperidines** | | | | All long acting except cyproheptadine. | |
| **First generation** | | | | | |
| *azatadine maleate*<br>Optimine | 1–2 mg BID | +++ | +++ | Cyproheptadine and azatadine may stimulate appetite and have some antiserotonin effects. | $$–$$$ |
| *cyproheptadine HCl*[π]<br>Periactin, generics | 4–8 mg TID | ++ | +++ | | $$–$$$ |
| **Second generation** | | | | | |
| *loratadine*[†‡π]<br>Claritin | 10 mg/d | +/0 | +/0 | Loratidine available as pediatric liquid. | $$ |
| *fexofenadine*[‡]<br>Allegra | 60 mg BID | +/0 | +/0 | A metabolite of terfenadine lacking the cardiotoxic effects and drug interactions of the parent compound. | $$ |

[†] *Long-acting antihistamines – chlorpheniramine, loratadine, cetirizine, fexofenadine.*
[‡] *Nonsedating antihistamines – loratadine, fexofenadine.*
[π] *Dosage adjustment may be required in hepatic impairment.*

*Dosage adjustment may be required in renal impairment – see Appendix I.*
* *Cost of 7-day supply – includes drug cost only.*
*Legend:* $ < $5 $$ $5–10 $$$ $10–15 $$$$ > $15

sedative and anticholinergic adverse effects. Second-generation antihistamines are less lipid soluble and cross the blood-brain barrier poorly causing fewer CNS effects, and are more selective for the $H_1$ site resulting in fewer anticholinergic effects.

**Choosing an antihistamine:** Patient responses to various agents will vary. The following factors should be considered.

**Precautions and contraindications:** Antihistamines are contraindicated in patients with glaucoma, stenosing peptic ulcer, urinary retention and those taking MAO inhibitors. Antihistamines should be avoided in epileptic or pregnant patients and those with heart disease.

**Drug interactions** (see above): All antihistamines, particularly the sedating ones, should be avoided in patients taking drugs that will depress the central nervous system, including alcohol. Concurrent use with tricyclic antidepressants can cause increased toxicity.

Astemizole and terfenadine have been removed from the Canadian market. Both could cause serious cardiotoxic effects when combined with macrolide antibiotics or systemic antifungals. The remaining second-generation antihistamines (loratadine, cetirizine, fexofenadine) have not been shown to have similar drug interactions.

**Adverse effect profile:** Consider the risk and implications of the various side effects (particularly drowsiness and anticholinergic effects) for each patient (Table 2).

**Individual patient factors:** Antihistamines, particularly the sedating ones, are more likely to cause drowsiness, confusion, hypotension, syncope and dizziness in the **elderly. Children** may show paradoxical excitation rather than sedation.

If a patient is **allergic** to an antihistamine, consider them allergic to other drugs in the same class.

**Occupation:** Working adults and school children can function better and more safely with nonsedating antihistamines (loratadine, fexofenadine) during the day. With cetirizine some drowsiness can occur, however, the incidence and severity of sedation is less than with classical antihistamines. Patients driving or operating heavy machinery should not take sedating antihistamines as up to 40% of subjects have impairment of mental performance equivalent to legal alcohol impairment.

**Underlying condition:** Acute or severe pruritus and skin conditions other than urticaria often respond better to the older antihistamines as the sedative properties may contribute directly to relief of the pruritus. Antihistamines are more effective at preventing histamine release than combating the effects of previously released histamine. Therefore, in chronic pruritic conditions antihistamines should be administered regularly for at least a week rather than intermittently when itch is most severe.

**Response to initial treatment:** Antihistamines are classified by chemical structure (Table 2). If a patient does not respond to an antihistamine from one class, change to an agent from another class. At times, prescribing two antihistamines from different classes at the same time is useful, but it is rarely necessary to prescribe more than two.

### *Other Systemic Pharmacologic Treatments*

**Doxepin,** an antidepressant with potent antihistaminic properties, is useful in some cases of chronic urticaria.[1] It has anticholinergic effects and is contraindicated in patients with congestive heart failure and in those taking MAOIs.

**Ketotifen,** a selective $H_1$ antihistamine that also stabilizes mast cells and inhibits mediator release, is used primarily in asthma prophylaxis but can be useful in urticaria and mastocytosis.

Patients who scratch uncontrollably at night may benefit from a small dose of **diazepam, chlordiazepoxide** or **lorazepam** at bedtime. Large doses of sedating antihistamines, administered at the same time, should be avoided.

**Cholestyramine and colestipol HCl resins** are effective for pruritus related to cholestatic liver disease (Chapter 43). These agents have also been used successfully in uremic pruritus and polycythemia rubra vera.

Future research should clarify whether inhibitors of other inflammatory mediators such as leukotriene antagonists, opiate antagonists, or serotonin antagonists may be effective for some causes of pruritus.

## Phototherapy

**Phototherapy with ultraviolet B (UVB) wavelength** (290–320 nm) is an effective treatment for uremic pruritus. Eight to 10 treatments usually result in symptomatic improvement. Maintenance therapy may be administered as required. UVB phototherapy is often effective for pruritus of other etiology, particularly primary dermatoses.

## Therapeutic Tips

- Histamine$_2$ antagonists (e.g., cimetidine) should not be used unless the $H_1$ receptors are blocked with an $H_1$ antihistamine. $H_2$-antagonists alone can exacerbate pruritus by interfering with a negative feedback mechanism.
- Topical steroids should be avoided in the absence of clinically evident skin disease.

---

[1] *J Am Acad Dermatol 1986;14:375–392.*

- Testing should be done for dermatographism or pressure sensitivity because symptomatic dermatographism or subclinical urticaria is a common cause of pruritus that can be suppressed with antihistamines.
- Even nonsedating antihistamines may have some CNS effects, therefore all patients should be advised to use caution when driving or operating heavy equipment.
- Careful follow-up is required. The itching of scabies, urticaria and drug eruptions may precede onset of skin manifestations. Likewise, symptoms of a systemic disease may eventually develop in a patient with apparent idiopathic pruritus.
- Topical agents may be kept in a refrigerator because the physical cooling enhances their antipruritic effect.
- Antihistamines requiring a single daily dose (e.g., cetirizine or loratadine) are more effective if given in the evening than the morning.
- Sustained-release preparations should be swallowed whole, not crushed or dissolved.

## Suggested Reading List

Du Buske LM. Clinical comparison of histamine $H_1$-receptor antagonist drugs. *J Allergy Clin Immunol* 1996;98(6 Pt 3): S307–S318.

Goldsmith P, Dowd PM. The new $H_1$ antihistamines. *Dermatol Therapy* 1993;11(1):87–95.

Mattila MJ, Paakkari I. Variations among non-sedating antihistamines: are they real differences? *Eur J Clin Pharmacol* 1999;55:85–93.

CHAPTER 67

# Scabies and Pediculosis

*Sandra Knowles, BScPhm and*
*Neil H. Shear, MD, FRCPC*

Scabies and pediculosis are common infestations that cause significant discomfort and are associated with large outbreaks in institutions (e.g., long-term care facilities, schools).

## Goals of Therapy

- To eradicate causative organisms and eggs
- To control symptoms and prevent complications (pruritus, secondary bacterial infection)
- To prevent spread to contacts

## Investigations (Table 1)

- History of exposure and itching
- Physical examination for identification of organism (or evidence of organism such as eggs or nits)

## Therapeutic Choices (Figure 1)

Figure 1: **Management of Scabies or Lice**

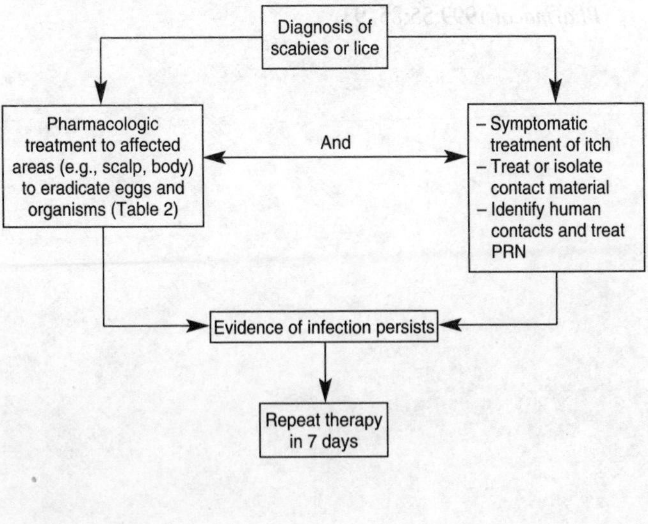
Diagnosis of scabies or lice
Pharmacologic treatment to affected areas (e.g., scalp, body) to eradicate eggs and organisms (Table 2)
And
– Symptomatic treatment of itch
– Treat or isolate contact material
– Identify human contacts and treat PRN
Evidence of infection persists
Repeat therapy in 7 days

Table 1: **Clinical Features of Pediculosis and Scabies**

| Type | Organism | Mode of Transmission | Clinical Features | Diagnosis |
|---|---|---|---|---|
| Pediculosis capitis (head lice) | Pediculus humanus capitis | head-to-head contact | Pruritic scalp with red papules around ears, face and neck. | Detection of lice, eggs or nits close to scalp. |
| Pediculosis corporis (body lice) | Pediculus humanus corporis | via clothing and bedding | Pruritus and skin reactions (usually in the flanks, in the axillae and around the waist and neck); lives in seams of clothing not on the body. | Detection of lice, eggs or nits in the seams of clothing. |
| Pediculosis pubis (pubic lice) | Phthirus pubis | sexual contact; may be associated with other sexually-transmitted diseases | Pruritus in the anogenital area; may also be found on facial hair (including eyelashes) and rarely the scalp. | Detection of lice, eggs or nits in the pubic hair. |
| Scabies | Sarcoptes scabiei | skin-to-skin contact (also via bedding, furniture) | Intense pruritus and an erythematous, papular eruption on skin; lesions most commonly located on finger webs, wrists, waist, areolae and genitals. | Mite visualized as a pinpoint at the end of a burrow; also detection of mites, eggs or feces in skin scrapings. |

### Nonpharmacologic Choices

- Although time-consuming, **lice** and **nits** should be mechanically removed until no eggs or active lice are observed. There are a variety of different louse or nit combs available (e.g., LiceMeister developed by the National Pediculosis Association).
- **Treatment of room:** washing and drying (with heat) pillowcases, sheets, nightclothes, towels, personal articles (e.g., hats, shared helmets, headphones) and stuffed animals is recommended. Alternatively, items which cannot be washed may be dry cleaned or sealed in a plastic bag for two weeks. The patient's room should also be vacuumed. Head lice usually do not exist for more than one day when separated from a person.
- **Combs and brushes:** soak in a disinfectant solution (e.g., 2% Lysol for 1 hour) or in hot water (65°C for 5 to 10 minutes).
- Pediculicide sprays (e.g., R & C II Spray) for inanimate objects are not warranted since head lice generally die within a day when separated from a person.
- Identify and examine **potential human contacts** to prevent a cycle of reinfection. *All* contacts of scabies, even if asymptomatic, require treatment. Pets do not transmit human lice and should not be treated for pediculosis.

### Pharmacologic Choices (Table 2)

## Therapeutic Tips

- Insufficient treatment of itch and fear of infestation may cause patients with scabies to overuse scabicides, resulting in skin irritation and unnecessary repeated therapy.
- Patients should be re-examined 7 days after the first treatment. Evidence of persistent infestation demands a second course of therapy.
- Patients with scabies should be treated from the top of the head **not** the top of the neck.
- In patients with scabies, itching can persist for weeks after mites are eradicated. Medium-potency topical corticosteroids (e.g., betamethasone valerate 0.1% cream) and oral antihistamines (e.g., diphenhydramine) are helpful. (Chapter 66)
- In patients with head lice, treatment may fail if hair is not thoroughly soaked with permethrin. Two bottles are often needed for thick or long hair.
- Crusted scabies in immunocompromised or debilitated patients should be treated with chlorhexidine gluconate wash followed by permethrin 5% cream. Oral **ivermectin**

Table 2: **Drugs Used for Scabies and Pediculosis**

| Drug | Directions | Comments | Cost* |
|---|---|---|---|
| **Pediculicides** | | | |
| *permethrin 1%*<br>Nix Creme Rinse<br>Kwellada-P Creme Rinse | Head lice: Wash hair with conditioner-free shampoo, rinse with water and towel dry. Apply permethrin to saturate the hair and scalp (1/2-1 bottle for adults and children with long hair); leave on for 10 min then rinse.<br>May repeat after 7 d if live lice are observed. | Drug of choice for most patients.<br>May temporarily exacerbate the pruritus, erythema and scalp edema of lice infestation.<br>Burning/stinging, tingling, numbness or scalp discomfort are usually mild and transient.<br>Contraindicated in patients with chrysanthemum allergy. | $ |
| *pyrethrins/piperonyl butoxide*<br>R&C Shampoo/Conditioner, Pronto Lice Killing Shampoo, Licetrol Lice Killing Shampoo<br>*allethrins/piperonyl butoxide*<br>Para Special Shampoo<br>*bioallethrin/piperonyl butoxide*<br>Para Special for Lice & Nits (aerosol) | Shampoo: Apply to thoroughly saturate dry hair and massage scalp; leave on for 10 min. Add a little water; work the shampoo into the hair and skin to form a lather. Rinse thoroughly.<br>Repeat treatment in 7 d.<br>Aerosol: Saturate area (5–10 squirts); wash off after 30 min. | Few adverse effects, although contact dermatitis and eye irritation have been reported.<br>Contraindicated in patients allergic to ragweed, chrysanthemums or other pyrethrin products. | $ |
| *lindane 1% (gamma benzene hexachloride)*<br>Shampoo: generics<br>Lotion (for pubic lice): generics | Shampoo: Apply enough to dry hair to soak hair and skin. Massage for 4 min; add water, a little at a time, to produce lather; massage again for 4 min then rinse.<br>Repeat treatment in 7–10 d.<br>Lotion: Apply to affected area, then dress in clean clothes. Leave on for 8–12 h, then thoroughly wash off. | Avoid contact with eyes, nose, mouth, mucous membranes.<br>Contraindicated in neonates, young children, pregnant women and nursing mothers.<br>Neurotoxicity (e.g., nausea, vomiting, headache, irritability, insomnia, seizures) has been reported after oral ingestion, repeated application, excessive doses or prolonged treatment or in high-risk populations (e.g., young children, elderly, and patients with extensive skin disease). | $ |

(cont'd)

Table 2: **Drugs Used for Scabies and Pediculosis** *(cont'd)*

| Drug | Directions | Comments | Cost* |
|---|---|---|---|
| **Scabicides** | | | |
| *permethrin 5%*† Nix Dermal Cream Kwellada-P Lotion | Massage into all skin areas, from **the top of the head** to the soles of the feet; every bit of skin must be treated, including the fingernails, waist and genitalia; leave on for 8–14 h without interruption, then wash off (shower may be the best way). | Drug of choice for scabies. Pruritus, edema and erythema may temporarily increase after application. Contraindicated in patients allergic to chrysanthemums. | $$ |
| *lindane 1%* (see above) – (lotion recommended; not shampoo) | Apply to all skin areas‡‡ (once); should be left on for 8–12 h and then washed off. | Used when permethrin has been ineffective or is contraindicated. See lindane above. | $ |
| *crotamiton 10%* Eurax cream | Apply to all skin areas‡‡ daily for 2–5 d; wash off 48 h after last application. | Less effective than permethrin. Not recommended for patients with exudative or vesicular dermatitis. | $ |
| *sulfur 5–10%* Sulphur ointment ‡ | Apply to all skin areas‡‡ at bedtime daily for 5–7 d. | Not popular because it is malodorous, requires multiple applications, and stains clothing. Extemporaneously compounded.‡ May be used for small children and pregnant women. | $ |
| *esdepallethrin/piperonyl butoxide* Scabene aerosol | Apply to all skin areas;‡‡ should be left on for 12 h then washed off with soap and water; towels or other protective coverings should be used on floors. To apply to face and scalp, soak cotton with spray and rub on. | A useful therapy for hard to reach places (e.g., mid-scapular). | $$ |

† *Lower strengths are not effective as scabicides.*
‡ *May be commercially available through wholesale distributors in some areas.*
‡‡ *As described for permethrin.*

* *Cost of 1 unit (tube or bottle) of product – includes drug cost only.* ***NB:*** *All products are available without prescription; retail mark-ups may vary.*
*Legend: $ < $10 $$ $10–20*

(available through the Special Access Program, Health Canada) can be used as a single dose therapy (200 µg/kg).

- Various alternative therapies using naturally occurring substances (e.g., tea tree oil, other essential oils [Hair Clean], herbal remedies) have been advocated for the treatment of head lice. However, there is no published evidence to suggest that any of these are consistently effective.
- White petrolatum (e.g., Vaseline) can be applied to eyelashes 2 to 4 times daily for 10 days. Removal of lice and nits with forceps or tweezers prior to application is recommended.

## *Suggested Reading List*


Burkhart CG, Burkhart CN, Burkhart KM. An assessment of topical and oral prescription and over-the-counter treatments for head lice. *J Am Acad Dermatol* 1998;38:979–982.

Downs AM, Stafford KA, Harvey I, Coles GC. Evidence for double resistance to permethrin and malathion in head lice. *Br J Dermatol* 1999;141:508–511.

Elgart ML. A risk-benefit assessment of agents used in the treatment of scabies. *Drug Saf* 1996;14:386–393.

Meinking TL, Taplin D, Hermida JL, et al. The treatment of scabies with ivermectin. *N Engl J Med* 1995;333:26–30.

Pollack RJ. Head lice: Information and frequently asked questions. Laboratory of Public Health Entomology, Harvard School of Public Health. Available from: http://www.hsph.harvard.edu/headlice.html

CHAPTER 68

# Bacterial Skin Infections

*Vincent C. Ho, BSc(Pharm), MD, FRCPC*

## Definitions

**Impetigo:** Superficial skin infection caused mainly by *Staphylococcus aureus*, group A beta-hemolytic streptococci or a combination of both.

**Bullous impetigo:** Bullous form of impetigo caused by *S. aureus* phage group II. The organism elaborates an exfoliating toxin causing superficial skin blistering. In young children, immunocompromised hosts and patients with renal disease, high blood levels of this toxin may lead to generalized skin peeling, the staphylococcal scalded skin syndrome (SSSS).

**Folliculitis:** Superficial infection of the hair follicle most commonly caused by *S. aureus*. *Pseudomonas* folliculitis is associated with hot tub use. Gram-negative folliculitis caused by enterobacteriaceae most often occurs in those on long-term antibiotics for acne. Pseudofolliculitis is inflammation of the hair follicle secondary to friction, irritation or occlusion.

**Furuncle (boil):** Infection of a hair follicle with involvement of subcutaneous tissues, most often caused by *S. aureus*.

**Carbuncle:** Deep-seated infection of several hair follicles by *S. aureus*.

**Erythrasma:** Infection of the stratum corneum with *Corynebacterium minutissimum* that manifests as brown patches in intertriginous areas.

**Erysipelas:** Infection of the superficial subcutaneous tissues caused mainly by group A beta-hemolytic streptococci, but may occasionally be caused by other streptococci or *S. aureus*.

**Cellulitis:** Infection of the deeper subcutaneous tissues caused mainly by group A beta-hemolytic streptococci and occasionally by *S. aureus*. In children (usually < 2 years of age) *Haemophilus influenzae* may be the etiologic agent. Cellulitis associated with diabetic foot is often polymicrobial and broad-spectrum antimicrobial coverage against gram-positive, gram-negative and anaerobic organisms is required.

**Necrotizing fasciitis:** Infection of the superficial layer of the fascia of muscle and may secondarily involve the adjacent muscle and subcutaneous tissues. It is caused by invasive group A streptococci.

## Therapeutic Choices (Figures 1 to 4)

### Nonpharmacologic Choices

- Remove impetigo crusts, which harbor bacteria, by saline compresses or washing with soap and water.
- Occlusion, friction, heat and moisture are predisposing factors for bacterial skin infections. Mild cases may be treated with topical drying agents (e.g., aluminum chloride hexahydrate solution) or topical antiseptics (e.g., chlorhexidine, hexachlorophene, triclosan or povidone-iodine). Occlusive skin care products and clothing should be avoided.
- Incision and drainage of a large and fluctuant furuncle or carbuncle will relieve much of the pressure and pain. With effective antibacterials now available, there is less need for this surgical procedure.

Figure 1: **Management of Impetigo**

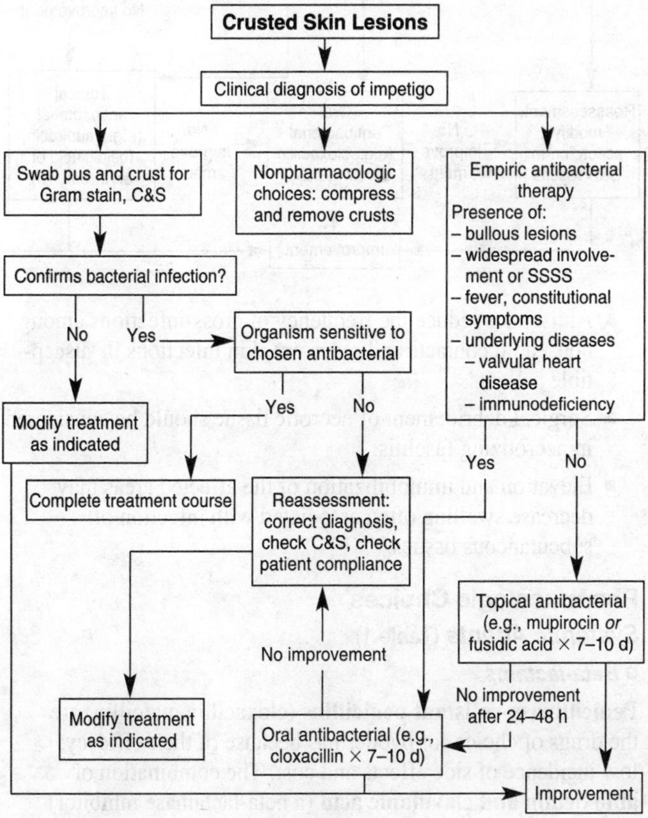
Crusted Skin Lesions
Clinical diagnosis of impetigo
Swab pus and crust for Gram stain, C&S
Nonpharmacologic choices: compress and remove crusts
Empiric antibacterial therapy
Presence of:
– bullous lesions
– widespread involvement or SSSS
– fever, constitutional symptoms
– underlying diseases
– valvular heart disease
– immunodeficiency
Confirms bacterial infection?
No
Yes
Organism sensitive to chosen antibacterial
Yes
No
Modify treatment as indicated
Yes
No
Complete treatment course
Reassessment: correct diagnosis, check C&S, check patient compliance
Topical antibacterial (e.g., mupirocin or fusidic acid × 7–10 d)
No improvement
No improvement after 24–48 h
Modify treatment as indicated
Oral antibacterial (e.g., cloxacillin × 7–10 d)
Improvement

*Abbreviations: SSSS = Staphylococcal scalded skin syndrome.*

Figure 2: **Management of Folliculitis**

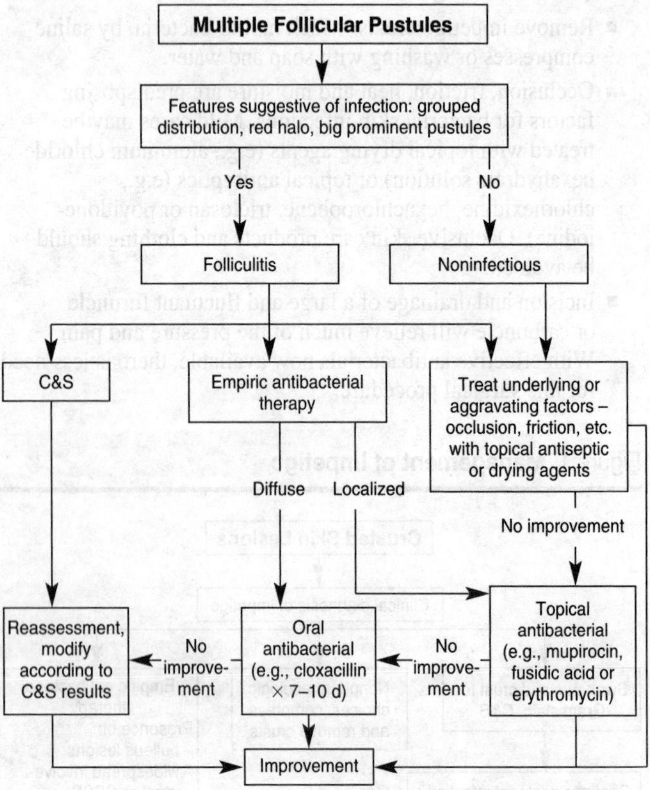
Multiple Follicular Pustules
Features suggestive of infection: grouped distribution, red halo, big prominent pustules
Yes
No
Folliculitis
Noninfectious
C&S
Empiric antibacterial therapy
Treat underlying or aggravating factors – occlusion, friction, etc. with topical antiseptic or drying agents
Diffuse
Localized
No improvement
Reassessment, modify according to C&S results
No improve-ment
Oral antibacterial (e.g., cloxacillin × 7–10 d)
No improve-ment
Topical antibacterial (e.g., mupirocin, fusidic acid or erythromycin)
Improvement

- Antiseptics reduce the frequency of cross-infections among household contacts and recurrent skin infections in susceptible patients.
- Surgical débridement of necrotic tissue should be considered in necrotizing fasciitis.
- Elevation and immobilization of the affected areas may decrease swelling often associated with infection of subcutaneous tissues.

## Pharmacologic Choices

### *Systemic Agents* (Table 1)

#### ▫ *Beta-lactams*

**Penicillinase-resistant penicillins** (cloxacillin, nafcillin) are the drugs of choice for pyodermas because of their efficacy, low incidence of side effects and cost. The combination of **amoxicillin and clavulanic acid** (a beta-lactamase inhibitor) is effective but has no advantage over penicillinase-resistant

Figure 3: **Management of Recurrent Episodes of Folliculitis or Impetigo**

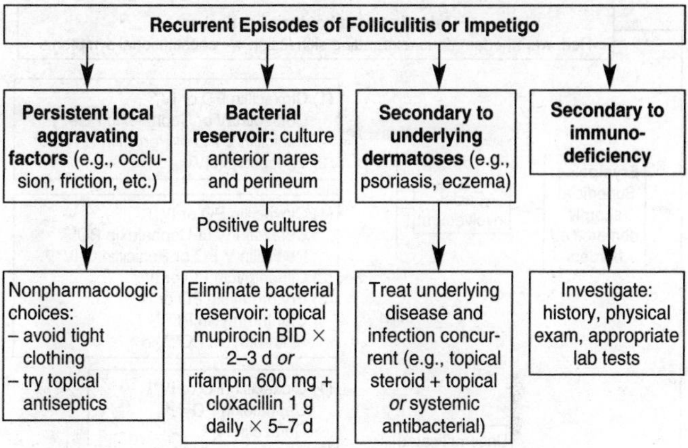
Recurrent Episodes of Folliculitis or Impetigo
Persistent local aggravating factors (e.g., occlusion, friction, etc.)
Bacterial reservoir: culture anterior nares and perineum
Secondary to underlying dermatoses (e.g., psoriasis, eczema)
Secondary to immunodeficiency
Positive cultures
Nonpharmacologic choices:
– avoid tight clothing
– try topical antiseptics
Eliminate bacterial reservoir: topical mupirocin BID × 2–3 d or rifampin 600 mg + cloxacillin 1 g daily × 5–7 d
Treat underlying disease and infection concurrent (e.g., topical steroid + topical or systemic antibacterial)
Investigate: history, physical exam, appropriate lab tests

penicillins for the usual pyodermas. **Cephalosporins** may be used as alternatives in patients with penicillin allergy; however, there is a 10% cross-reactivity between penicillins and cephalosporins. First-generation cephalosporins (cefadroxil, cephalexin) are preferred because they are more active against gram-positive bacteria than second- and third-generation agents.

### ❑ *Macrolides (Erythromycin, Azithromycin, Clarithromycin)*

Erythromycin is a good alternative to penicillin for gram-positive bacterial skin infections in patients allergic to penicillin, and it is also effective against erythrasma. The newer macrolides, clarithromycin and azithromycin, offer once- or twice-daily dosing, shorter treatment duration and better gastrointestinal tolerance but are more expensive.

### ❑ *Clindamycin*

Clindamycin may cause pseudomembranous colitis; it is not indicated for superficial bacterial skin infections except rarely, when first-line therapy is ineffective or not tolerated.

### ❑ *Quinolones*

Quinolones are broad-spectrum antibacterials, but their activity against gram-positive aerobes is relatively weak; ciprofloxacin-resistant strains, including methicillin-resistant *S. aureus*, are emerging. Quinolones should not be used as first-line therapy for superficial bacterial skin infections; they may be indicated for rare cases of *Pseudomonas* folliculitis associated with marked constitutional symptoms.

Figure 4: **Management of Erysipelas, Cellulitis, Necrotizing Fasciitis**

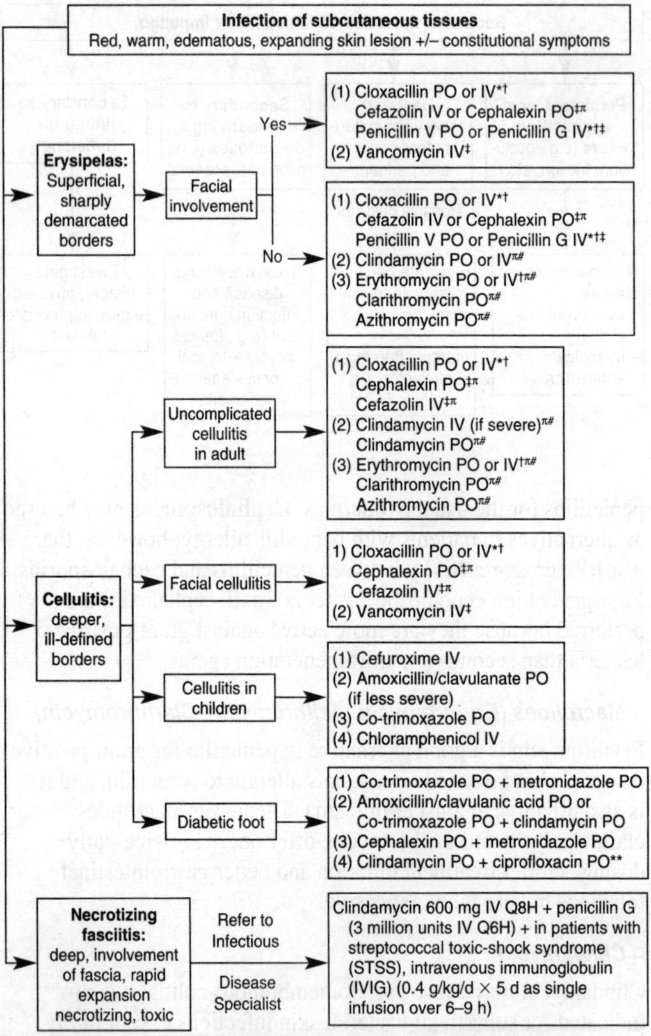
Infection of subcutaneous tissues
Red, warm, edematous, expanding skin lesion +/– constitutional symptoms
Erysipelas: Superficial, sharply demarcated borders
Facial involvement
Yes
No
(1) Cloxacillin PO or IV*†
Cefazolin IV or Cephalexin PO‡π
Penicillin V PO or Penicillin G IV*†‡
(2) Vancomycin IV‡
(1) Cloxacillin PO or IV*†
Cefazolin IV or Cephalexin PO‡π
Penicillin V PO or Penicillin G IV*†‡
(2) Clindamycin PO or IVπ#
(3) Erythromycin PO or IV†π#
Clarithromycin POπ#
Azithromycin POπ#
Cellulitis: deeper, ill-defined borders
Uncomplicated cellulitis in adult
(1) Cloxacillin PO or IV*†
Cephalexin PO‡π
Cefazolin IV‡π
(2) Clindamycin IV (if severe)π#
Clindamycin POπ#
(3) Erythromycin PO or IV†π#
Clarithromycin POπ#
Azithromycin POπ#
Facial cellulitis
1) Cloxacillin PO or IV*†
Cephalexin PO‡π
Cefazolin IV‡π
(2) Vancomycin IV‡
Cellulitis in children
(1) Cefuroxime IV
(2) Amoxicillin/clavulanate PO
(if less severe)
(3) Co-trimoxazole PO
(4) Chloramphenicol IV
Diabetic foot
(1) Co-trimoxazole PO + metronidazole PO
(2) Amoxicillin/clavulanic acid PO or
Co-trimoxazole PO + clindamycin PO
(3) Cephalexin PO + metronidazole PO
(4) Clindamycin PO + ciprofloxacin PO**
Necrotizing fasciitis: deep, involvement of fascia, rapid expansion necrotizing, toxic
Refer to Infectious Disease Specialist
Clindamycin 600 mg IV Q8H + penicillin G
(3 million units IV Q6H) + in patients with
streptococcal toxic-shock syndrome
(STSS), intravenous immunoglobulin
(IVIG) (0.4 g/kg/d × 5 d as single
infusion over 6–9 h)

*Abbreviations: (1) = first line; (2) = second line; (3) = third line (4) = fourth line.*

* *In patients having questionable/minor allergic reactions with penicillin, cephalosporins are an alternative, but they should be avoided in patients describing an anaphylactic reaction to penicillin. Vancomycin, clindamycin, erythromycin, clarithromycin and azithromycin are good alternatives.*

† *IV route is recommended in severe cases.*

‡ *Vancomycin IV is recommended in patients not tolerating or not responding to therapy and in β-lactam-allergic patients (including those with facial involvement of cellulitis/erysipelas).*

π *Avoid in facial cellulitis, since assurance of meningeal penetration is required (in the clinical opinion of the authors).*

\# *Organisms resistant to erythromycin will also be resistant to clindamycin, clarithromycin and azithromycin.*

** *Although this regimen is 4th line for mild diabetic foot infections, it may be considered first line in patients with severe diabetic foot infections when oral therapy is the selected route.*

### *Topical Agents* (Table 2)

**Mupirocin** has a unique mechanism of action and no cross-resistance with other antibacterials; it is as effective as systemic antibacterials for impetigo and superficial folliculitis.

**Fusidic acid** is available in systemic and topical form; its efficacy for superficial pyodermas is similar to mupirocin.

**Bacitracin** and **gramicidin** are active against gram-positive bacteria in vitro, but efficacy for established skin infections is not proven. **Polymyxin B** is active against gram-negative bacteria in vitro; it is often combined with bacitracin or neomycin, but its clinical efficacy is not proven.

The aminoglycosides **neomycin, framycetin** and **gentamicin** are active against gram-negative organisms, staphylococci and streptococci; they are probably less effective than systemic antibiotics for the treatment of established skin infections.

Commonly used for prophylaxis and treatment of infection in serious burn victims, **silver sulfadiazine** is active against staphylococci and gram-negative organisms, including *Pseudomonas*.

## Therapeutic Tips

- **Impetigo** and **folliculitis** may be treated with either topical (mupirocin or fusidic acid) or systemic antibacterials. Systemic antibacterials of choice are the beta-lactams (penicillinase-resistant penicillins or cephalosporins, e.g., cloxacillin or cephalexin). Alternative agents include erythromycin, clarithromycin or clindamycin. Systemic therapy should be used when there is widespread disease, fever or constitutional symptoms or when the patient has valvular heart disease or is immunocompromised.
- **Bullous impetigo**, **furuncles** or **carbuncles** should be treated with systemic antibacterials.
- Systemic antibacterials should be combined with topical measures such as cleaning or compresses to remove crusts that harbor bacteria.
- Avoid topical antibacterials that may cause cross-resistance with systemic antibiotics (e.g., gentamicin).
- Avoid prolonged use of topical antibacterials (> 2 weeks) to prevent development of bacterial resistance.
- Avoid manipulation of furuncles on the central face as this may lead to cavernous sinus thrombosis or brain abscess.
- **Recurrent furunculosis** or **impetigo** may be due to bacterial carriage in the nose or perineum (see Figure 3 for treatment suggestions).

Table 1: **Antibiotics Used to Treat Bacterial Skin Infections**

| Drug | Dosage (A: Adult, C: Children) | Adverse Effects† | Drug Interactions† | Cost* |
|---|---|---|---|---|
| **Penicillins** | | Rash, drug fever. | | |
| *penicillin V* Pen-Vee, PVF K, generics | A: 300 mg PO Q6H<br>C: 25–50 mg/kg/d divided Q6–8H | | | $ |
| *penicillin G* Crystapen, generics | A: 2 million units IV Q4–6H | Electrolyte imbalance possible with high-dose penicillin G $Na^+$ or $K^+$ (> 10 million IU/d). | | $$$$$ |
| **Penicillinase-resistant Penicillins** | | Hypersensitivity reactions (ranging from minor rashes to anaphylactic shock). | | |
| *cloxacillin* Tegopen, generics | A: 250–500 mg PO Q6H<br>C: 25–50 mg/kg PO Q6H | | | $ |
| *amoxicillin/clavulanic acid* Clavulin | A: 250–500 mg PO Q8H<br>C: 40 mg/kg/d of amoxicillin PO divided Q8H | Nausea, vomiting, diarrhea, rash, eosinophilia. | | $$ |
| **Cephalosporins** | | Hypersensitivity reactions (some cross-reactivity with penicillins). | | |
| *cephalexin* Keflex, generics | A: 250–500 mg PO Q6H<br>C: 25–50 mg/kg/d PO divided Q6H | | | $ |
| *cefadroxil* Duricef | A: 1 g PO daily | | | $$ |
| *cefazolin* Ancef, Kefzol, generics | A: 1 g IV Q8H<br>C: 50–100 mg/kg/d divided Q8H | Rash, ↑ AST and ALP, phlebitis. | | $$ |

| | | | | |
|---|---|---|---|---|
| *cefuroxime*<br>Kefurox, Zinacef, generics | C: 100–150 mg/kg/d IV divided Q8H to max. 750 mg IV Q8H | Eosinophilia, anemia, phlebitis, ↑ LFTs. | | $$$$ |
| **Macrolides** | | GI irritation (common), nausea and vomiting.<br>Cholestatic jaundice with erythromycin estolate (rare). | Inhibits cytochrome P-450 enzyme system.‡ | |
| *erythromycin*<br>Erythromid, EES, Eryc, Ilosone, generics | A: 250 mg PO Q6H<br>500 mg IV Q6H<br>C: 30–50 mg/kg/d PO divided Q6H | | | $ |
| *clarithromycin*<br>Biaxin | A: 250–500 mg PO Q12H<br>C: 15 mg/kg/d divided Q12H | | | $$ |
| *azithromycin*<br>Zithromax | A: 500 mg PO on day 1, then 250 mg on days 2–5 (total 1.5 g) | | | $$ |
| *clindamycin*<br>Dalacin-C | A: 150–300 mg PO Q6H<br>450–600 mg IV Q8H<br>C: (> 1 mo) 10–30 mg/kg/d PO divided Q6H | Diarrhea, pseudomembranous colitis.$^{\pi}$ | | $$ |
| *chloramphenicol*<br>Chloromycetin | A: 50–75 mg/kg/d IV divided Q6H | Eosinopenia, aplastic anemia, gray syndrome, fever, rash. | ↑ toxicity of phenytoin<br>↑ INR with warfarin<br>Hypoglycemia with sulfonylureas. | $$$–$$$$ |
| *ciprofloxacin*<br>Cipro | A: 500–750 mg PO BID | Nausea, vomiting, diarrhea, abdominal pain. | Multivalent metallic cations, antacids and sucralfate ↓ absorption of ciprofloxacin.<br>Inhibits cytochrome P-450 enzyme system.‡ | $$ |

*(cont'd)*

Table 1: **Antibiotics Used to Treat Bacterial Skin Infections** *(cont'd)*

| Drug | Dosage (A: Adult, C: Children) | Adverse Effects† | Drug Interactions† | Cost* |
|---|---|---|---|---|
| *co-trimoxazole* ❥ Bactrim, Septra, generics | A: 800 mg/160 mg daily (2 tabs BID or 1 DS tab BID) | Nausea, vomiting, diarrhea, rash, neutropenia, thrombocytopenia, anemia. | ↑ phenytoin levels<br>↑ INR with warfarin<br>Hypoglycemia with sulfonylureas. | $ |
| *metronidazole* Flagyl, generics | A: 500 mg PO BID<br>C: 30–50 mg/kg/d divided TID | Nausea, vomiting, diarrhea, metallic taste, headache, dark urine, neutropenia. | Disulfiram reaction with alcohol.<br>↑ INR with warfarin<br>↓ phenytoin clearance<br>Phenobarb, phenytoin ↓ effectiveness of metronidazole. | $ |

† *Only the most important adverse effects/drug interactions are listed; consult product monograph for complete list.*

‡ *Potential ↑ effect/toxicity of carbamazepine, corticosteroids, cyclosporine, digoxin, theophylline and warfarin.*

π *Commonly associated with clindamycin but any antibiotic may cause this complication.*

❥ *Dosage adjustment may be required in renal impairment – see Appendix I.*

* *Cost per day – includes drug cost only.*

*Legend:* $ < $2 $$ $2–10 $$$ $10–20 $$$$ $20–30 $$$$$ > $30

Table 2: **Topical Antibacterials Used in Superficial Bacterial Skin Infections**

| Drug | Dosage | Antibacterial Spectrum | Adverse Effects | Cost* |
|---|---|---|---|---|
| *mupirocin*<br>Bactroban | BID–TID | Gram-positive | Stinging, allergic contact dermatitis (rare). | $$† |
| *fusidic acid*<br>Fucidin | BID–TID | Gram-positive | Allergic contact dermatitis (rare). | $$ |
| *bacitracin*<br>Baciguent, generics | BID–TID | Gram-positive | Allergic contact dermatitis, anaphylactic reactions following topical application (rare). | $† |
| *polymyxin B*<br>Polysporin cream (with gramicidin), Polysporin ointment (with bacitracin), generics | BID–TID | Gram-negative | Nephrotoxicity when used extensively, allergic contact dermatitis. | $† |
| *neomycin*<br>Neosporin (with polymyxin B and bacitracin) | BID–TID | *S. aureus*, strep, gram-negative | Allergic contact dermatitis, especially when applied to eczematous skin. | $$ |
| *framycetin*<br>Sofra-Tulle dressing | BID–TID | *S. aureus*, strep, gram-negative | Allergic contact dermatitis, cross-reaction with neomycin. | $$ (10×10 cm dressing, 10s) |
| *gentamicin*<br>Garamycin, generics | BID–TID | *S. aureus*, strep, gram-negative | Allergic contact dermatitis. | $$ |
| *silver sulfadiazine*<br>Dermazin, Flamazine, SSD | BID–TID | *S. aureus*, gram-negative, *Pseudomonas* | Allergic contact dermatitis, leukopenia when applied to large area of burned skin. | $ |

*† Available without prescription – retail mark-up not included.*
** Cost of 15g tube – includes drug cost only.*
*Legend: $ < $5 $$ $5–10*

- Recurrent furunculosis in the groin or axillae may be due to hidradenitis suppurativa; dermatologic consultation is suggested.
- **Facial erysipelas** or **cellulitis** may lead to intracranial involvement and cavernous sinus thrombosis; they should be treated with antimicrobials with good CNS penetration e.g., penicillin, cloxacillin or vancomycin.

### *Suggested Reading List*

Danzinger LH, Fish D, Hassan E. Skin and soft tissue infections. In: *Pharmacotherapy, a pathophysiologic approach*. 3rd ed. Connecticut: Appleton and Lange, 1996:2059–2080.

Gentry LO. Therapy with newer oral beta-lactam and quinolone agents for infections of the skin and skin structures: a review. *Clin Infect Dis* 1991;14:285–297.

Gilbert DN, Moellering RC, Sande MA. *The Sanford guide to antimicrobial therapy 2000*. Hyde Park, Vermont: Antimicrobial Therapy Inc., 2000.

Liu C. An overview of antimicrobial therapy. *Comprehen Ther* 1992;18:35–42.

Ontario Anti-infective Review Panel. *Anti-infective guidelines for community-acquired infections*. 2nd ed. Toronto: Queen's Printer for Ontario, 1997:32–35.

Turnidge J, Grayson ML. Optimum treatment of staphylococcal infections. *Drugs* 1993;45:353–366.

CHAPTER 69

# Contraception

*Gillian Graves, MD, FRCSC*

## Goals of Therapy

- To prevent fertilization. Effective contraceptive control and education reduces the rates of maternal and child mortality, as well as population growth
- To tailor the method to an individual's specific needs, lifestyle, age, parity and desire for future fertility

## Therapeutic Choices

### *Assessment of Consumer Needs*

No single method of contraception is ideal for all individuals. The preferred methods in young women are reversible, have high safety profiles and low failure rates. They should not interfere with other physiologic processes, such as vaginal lubrication, spontaneity, or pleasure of either partner. Cost should be affordable.

## Nonpharmacologic Choices (Table 1)

## Pharmacologic Choices (Table 1)

### *Oral Contraceptives* (Table 2)

Oral contraceptives (OCs) have the lowest failure rate outside of surgical sterilization. It is the method of choice for most young couples, especially teens, if combined with condoms (required for STD protection).

OCs containing synthetic estrogen and progestogen have undergone several modifications resulting in dose reduction and the synthesis of newer and more potent steroids. This has been done to increase safety and reliability, and decrease adverse effects that reduce compliance.

"Minipills" (with progestin only) inhibit ovulation and alter cervical mucus and uterine physiology. Triphasic pills claim better cycle control and reduced side effects. Products containing "new progestins" (e.g., desogestrel, gestodene) are less androgenic and may in theory have less atherogenic risk; however, long-term studies are required to quantitate any potential changes in cardiovascular risk profile for users of third-generation OCs compared to older progestins.

**Cardiovascular adverse events** including venous thromboembolism (VTE) and acute myocardial infarction (AMI) are uncommon among OC users. Compared to nonusers, the calculated risk of VTE is 3.5-fold higher with sub-50 μg ethinyl estradiol (EE) OCs. The very low attributable or absolute risks of VTE associated with third-generation OCs (incidence: 2 extra cases per 10 000 or relative risk [RR] 1.3 to 2.4) are of insignificant public health or clinical importance. The VTE risk of 20 μg OCs is equivalent to that of 30–35 μg OCs.[1]

Women with factor V Leiden who use OCs experience a VTE risk 30 times higher than that of OC users.[2] Broad-based screening for this or other thrombophilias (Protein S or C deficiency) is not appropriate (given approximately 5% affected) but should be undertaken with a strong family or personal history of VTE.

The stroke risks are extremely small and do not differ between generations of progestins. Severe hypertension and atypical migraines are risk factors for stroke in women aged less than 45.[3]

AMI risk is decreased with third-generation OCs compared to second generation (RR 0.3). All cardiovascular risks are appreciably higher in pregnancy compared to those on any sub-50 μg EE OC.

In the nonsmoking normotensive woman under the age of 35, the risk of cardiovascular disease is so small that there is no health impact related to the choice of second vs third generation of progestin. Clinicians make thoughtful decisions about which OC to prescribe based on monitoring and controlling an individual's other risk markers for cardiovascular disease, such as obesity (higher risk of VTE: consider second-generation OCs and weight reduction) and smoking (higher risk of AMI and arterial disease: consider third-generation OCs and smoking cessation/reduction).

### Injectable Contraceptives

#### Medroxyprogesterone Acetate (Depo-Provera)

- an injectable contraceptive used worldwide for many years
- extremely safe, effective (99.7%), and private
- dose is 150 mg IM every 3 months
- injection schedule of four times a year facilitates compliance
- produces amenorrhea in the majority of women, but some experience irregular bleeding and progestational side effects such as bloating, weight gain/loss and mood swings
- an excellent product for women who should avoid high estrogen doses, such as migraine sufferers

[1] *Contraception 1998;57:291–301.*
[2] *Lancet 1994;344:1453–1457.*
[3] *BMJ 1999;318:13–18.*

Table 1: **Available Contraceptive Methods**

| Contraceptive Method | Contra-indications | Adverse Effects | Drug Interactions | Comments | Cost* |
|---|---|---|---|---|---|
| **Coital Timing** | Relative: irregular menses | None | None | Requires high motivation; depends on identification of mucous and temperature patterns to identify fertile time; very difficult if there is an irregular cycle or ovulation defects. High pregnancy rates. | |
| **Condom**<br>Various<br>Reality (female condom) | Relative: hypersensitivity to latex | Common: hypersensitivity to latex in either partner | None | Protects against STD including HIV (latex only); best for infrequent intercourse; high failure rate of 10–14%. Use with spermicide. | $0.45–0.70/ condom<br>$2.60/female condom |
| **Diaphragm/Sponge**<br>Ortho Diaphragm Coil<br>Protectaid Sponge | Relative: hypersensitivity, inability to insert<br>Absolute: inability to achieve proper fit, marked uterine prolapse, large cystocele/rectocele, vaginal deformity | Common: hypersensitivity to diaphragm and/or spermicide | None | Best for infrequent intercourse. High failure rate of 10–14%. Use with spermicide. | $40.00/ diaphragm<br>$6.00/4 sponges |
| **Cervical Cap** | Relative: abnormal cervical cytology, chronic cervicitis, recurrent salpingitis<br>Absolute: cervical deformity (i.e., inability to obtain suitable fit) | Common: vaginal discharge, vaginal odor, cervical or fornices ulceration, hypersensitivity (cap or spermicide) | None | Use with spermicide. Protects against STD including HIV. | $35.00/cap |

*(cont'd)*

Table 1: **Available Contraceptive Methods** *(cont'd)*

| Contraceptive Method | Contra-indications | Adverse Effects | Drug Interactions | Comments | Cost* |
|---|---|---|---|---|---|
| **Spermicide**<br>Various | Relative: hypersensitivity | Common: hypersensitivity | None | Use with condom, diaphragm or cervical cap. | \$6.00–\$15.00/unit spermicide |
| **IUD**<br>Gyne-T, Gyne-T 380, Nova-T | Absolute: pregnancy; undiagnosed vaginal bleeding, stenosed cervix, nulliparity, copper allergy | Major: salpingitis, uterine perforation, cervical perforation, endometrial embedding, menorrhagia, pain, infection, ectopic pregnancy | None | Excellent for spacing children in a stable relationship, failure rate 1–5% in 1st yr, risk of PID and tubal infections is too high for nullipara. Immediate risks are insertional infection or perforation. Late risks are infection and ectopic pregnancy. | \$30.00–\$45.00 for copper IUD – lasts 3–5 yrs |
| **Vasectomy** | None | None | None | Method of choice for couples with completed family. Failure rate < 2%. Reversible with more surgery if < 10 yrs since procedure. | Cost-insured service in Canada. Cost of reversal surgery \$3000–\$5000 |
| **Tubal Ligation** | None | Ectopic rates post tubal ligation were 7.3 per 1000. | None | Method of choice for couples with completed family. Low failure rate – 18.5 per 1000 procedures at 10 yrs follow-up. Reversible only if salpingectomy not performed and sufficient length of undamaged tubal remnants remain. | Cost-insured service in Canada. Cost of reversal surgery \$3000–\$5000 |

| | | | | | |
|---|---|---|---|---|---|
| **Oral Contraceptives** (see Table 2) | Relative: estrogen hypersensitivity, classic migraine, gallbladder disease, brittle diabetes<br>Absolute: history of coronary artery disease, hypercholesterolemia, recent history of thromboembolism, recent history of stroke, end-stage renal disease, proliferative retinopathy, symptomatic mitral valve prolapse, estrogen-dependent carcinoma or tumor, smoker > 35 yrs old, current jaundice or pregnancy | Major: rare thromboembolism, stroke, retinal artery thrombosis, myocardial infarction, benign liver tumor, cholelithiasis, hypertension<br>Common: breakthrough bleeding/spotting, amenorrhea, nausea/vomiting, weight gain, bloating, chloasma, breast tenderness, depression, headaches | Antibiotics: reports of failure of OCs in women taking ampicillin, tetracycline, erythromycin, co-trimoxazole or nitrofurantoin. Rifampin is the only antibiotic consistently shown to reduce estrogen levels. Patients with diarrhea or breakthrough bleeding may be at higher risk. There is controversy as to whether barrier is also required at the time of antibiotic use | Lowest failure rate outside of surgical sterilization. Method of choice for most young couples, especially for teens, if combined with condoms. Lower dose estrogen products have increased safety and decreased side effects. Condoms needed for STD protection. | $12.00/mo |
| **Medroxyprogesterone Acetate** Depo-Provera | Thrombophlebitis, thromboembolic disorders, cerebrovascular disease or patients with a past history of these conditions. Known sensitivity to medroxyprogesterone acetate or to the vehicle or vaginal bleeding or urinary tract bleeding. Liver dysfunction or disease. Pregnancy. Undiagnosed breast pathology | Breast tenderness, galactorrhea. Occasionally nervousness, insomnia, somnolence, fatigue, depression, dizziness and headache. Thromboembolic disorders (thrombophlebitis and pulmonary embolism). Skin sensitivity reactions. Hyperpyrexia, change in weight, moon face | Aminoglutethimide may significantly depress the bioavailability of medroxyprogesterone | Injectable contraceptive that is extremely safe and effective (99.7%). Excellent for women who should avoid high estrogen doses, such as migraine sufferers. Condoms needed for STD protection. | $26.00 for 150 mg Q3 mos |

*(cont'd)*

Table 1: **Available Contraceptive Methods** *(cont'd)*

| Contraceptive Method | Contra-indications | Adverse Effects | Drug Interactions | Comments | Cost* |
|---|---|---|---|---|---|
| **Levonorgestrel Implant** Norplant | Active thromboembolic disorders; undiagnosed abnormal genital bleeding; known or suspected pregnancy; acute liver disease; benign or malignant liver tumors; known or suspected carcinoma of the breast | Changes in uterine bleeding or amenorrhea. Pain or itching near the implant site, infection at implant site, removal difficulties. Headache, nervousness, nausea, dizziness, adnexal enlargement, dermatitis, acne, change of appetite, mastalgia, weight gain, hirsutism, hypertrichosis and scalp hair loss | Phenytoin and carbamazepine may reduce efficacy and result in pregnancy. Warn patients of the possibility of decreased efficacy with the use of any related drugs | Efficacy close to that of tubal ligation. Expensive up-front cost. Condoms needed for STD protection. | $475.00/5 yrs |
| **Emergency Postcoital Contraception** | See oral contraceptives | See oral contraceptives | See oral contraceptives | For both regimens the 1st dose should be taken as soon as possible after unprotected intercourse, within 72 hours, followed by a 2nd dose 12 hours later. | |
| *ethinyl estradiol* 50 µg/ *levonorgestrel* 0.25 mg Preven | | | | Preven: 2 tablets initially, then 2 tablets 12 h later. | $5.30/kit |
| *levonorgestrel* 0.75 mg Plan B | | | | Plan B: 1 tablet initially, then 1 tablet 12 h later. | $16.00/kit |

* *Approximate cost per unit (condom, tube, canister, package) – includes drug or contraceptive cost only. Mark-up is not included.*

Table 2: **Oral Contraceptives**

| Composition | Product |
|---|---|
| **50 μg Estrogen** | |
| *EE 50 μg / ethynodiol diacetate 1 mg* | Demulen 50 |
| *EE 50 μg / d-norgestrel 0.25 mg* | Ovral |
| *mestranol 50 μg / norethindrone 1 mg* | Norinyl 1/50, Ortho-Novum 1/50 |
| **Sub-50 μg Estrogen Monophasic** | |
| *EE 35 μg / norethindrone 1 mg* | Brevicon 1/35, Ortho 1/35, Select 1/35 |
| *EE 35 μg / norethindrone 0.5 mg* | Brevicon 0.5/35, Ortho 0.5/35 |
| *EE 35 μg / norgestimate 0.25 mg* | Cyclen |
| *EE 30 μg / desogestrel 0.15 mg* | Marvelon, Ortho-Cept |
| *EE 30 μg / ethynodiol diacetate 2 mg* | Demulen 30 |
| *EE 30 μg / levonorgestrel 0.15 mg* | Min-Ovral |
| *EE 30 μg / norethindrone acetate 1.5 mg* | Loestrin 1.5/30 |
| *EE 20 μg / norethindrone acetate 1 mg* | Minestrin 1/20 |
| *EE 20 μg / levonorgestrel 0.1 mg* | Alesse |
| **Biphasic** | |
| *EE 35 μg × 21 d / norethindrone 0.5 mg × 10 d, 1 mg × 11 d* | Ortho 10/11 |
| **Triphasic** | |
| *EE 35 μg × 21 d / norethindrone 0.5 mg × 7 d, 0.75 mg × 7 d, 1 mg × 7 d* | Ortho 7/7/7 |
| *EE 35 μg × 21 d / norethindrone 0.5 mg × 7 d, 1 mg × 9 d, 0.5 mg × 5 d* | Synphasic |
| *EE 35 μg × 21 d / norgestimate 0.18 mg × 7 d, 0.215 mg × 7 d, 0.25 mg × 7 d* | Tri-Cyclen |
| *EE 30 μg × 6 d, 40 μg × 5 d, 30 μg × 10 d / levonorgestrel 0.05 mg × 6 d, 0.075 mg × 5 d, 0.125 mg × 10 d* | Triphasil, Triquilar |
| **Progestin only** | |
| *norethindrone 0.35 mg* | Micronor |

*Abbreviations: EE = ethinyl estradiol.*

- can be used in the postabortal state (5 days postpartum), or during lactation (6 weeks postpartum)
- duration of action may be up to a year until regular menses returns
- increasing the interval between injections increases the risk of pregnancy
- condoms required for STD protection
- more prospective data needed to document the long-term effect on bone mineral content with prolonged use
- long-term use is not associated with an increase in breast cancer

***Levonorgestrel (Norplant)***

- – efficacy close to tubal ligation
- – progestin-containing rods are implanted in the subcutaneous tissue of the upper, inner arm
- – may cause dysfunctional or breakthrough bleeding
- – occasionally can be difficult to remove the rods
- – similar adverse effects and benefits as injectable medroxyprogesterone acetate
- – expensive up-front costs
- – condoms required for STD protection

## Emergency Postcoital Contraception

- Levonorgestrel (two separate doses of 0.75 mg e.g., 1 tablet of Plan B, taken 12 hours apart) used within 72 hours of unprotected intercourse prevents 85% of expected pregnancies. The Yuzpe method (2 separate doses of ethinyl estradiol 100 μg with levonorgestrel 0.5 mg e.g., 2 tablets of Preven, taken 12 hours apart) prevents 57% of expected pregnancies. The efficacy of both regimens is increased if treatment is provided within 24 hours. Side effects (nausea, vomiting, dizziness and fatigue) with levonorgestrel alone are reduced compared to the Yuzpe method.[4]
- Delaying the first dose of both treatments by 12 hours increases the odds of pregnancy by almost 50%.[5]
- The progestin only method has a good safety record. The combined OC pill method is relatively contraindicated in patients with a history of thromboembolism, and absolutely contraindicated in those with a history of migraine with aura.

## Contraception While Breast-feeding

- Barrier plus spermicides can provide lubrication to the hypoestrogenic vagina but not as effective for contraception as other methods.
- IUD can be inserted 4 to 6 weeks postpartum once involution has occurred and the uterus is firm enough to decrease the risk of insertional perforation. Need to ensure good fundal placement with larger uterine cavity, since efficacy of current copper T devices requires the IUD arms to be near the fundus.
- Progestin-only OCs can be used during lactation, without increasing thromboembolic rates in the puerperium. Must be taken every day at the same time without missing a pill, in order to minimize spotting and maintain contraceptive efficacy.

---
[4] *Lancet 1998;352:428–433.*

[5] *Lancet 1999;353:721.*

- Low-dose combination OCs can be used once the milk supply is well established. There is some decrease in milk quantity; however, no negative effect on the infant has been described.

## Therapeutic Tips

- Age – In the past, OCs were not given to women older than age 35 since earlier publications had indicated an increased rate of myocardial infarction. Recent data have shown that smoking and other cardiovascular risk factors contribute to the myocardial risk in these women. In nonsmoking selected women with no other risk factors, low dose OCs may be considered for contraception or control of dysfunctional uterine bleeding up to the menopause.
- OCs help control anemia and regulate cycles.
- Acne is considered an androgen-dependent condition. OCs with androgenic progestins (e.g., norethindrone acetate) would not be the first choice for individuals with acne vulgaris (theoretical advantage of new progestins). However, OC estrogenicity affects sex hormone binding globulin, which may be more important than the choice of progestin in hirsutism and acne. (See Chapter 59)
- Noncontraceptive health benefits attributed to OC use include a decrease in: the frequency of endometrial cancer, fibroids, endometriosis pain, benign breast disease, functional ovarian cysts, ectopic pregnancy, dysmenorrhea and PID.

## *Suggested Reading List*

Anon. Pill scares and public responsibility. *Lancet* 1996; 347:1707.

Farmer RDT, Lawrenson RA, Thompson CF, Kennedy JG, Hambleton IR. Population-based study of risk of venous thromboembolism associated with various oral contraceptives. *Lancet* 1997;349:83–88.

Lefebvre G, Lea RH, Boroditsky R, Fisher W, Belisle S, Sand M. The benefits of awareness study: an evaluation of a targetted, user-friendly education among oral contraceptive users. *J SOGC* 1996;18:1111–1121.

Peterson HB, Xia Z, Hughes JM, Wilcox LS, Tylor LR, Trussel J. US Collaborative Review of Sterilization Working Group. The risk of ectopic pregnancy after tubal sterilization. *N Engl J Med* 1997;336:762–767.

CHAPTER 70

# Dysmenorrhea

*Glenn H. Gill, MD, CCFP, FRCSC*

## Definition

Dysmenorrhea is menstrual pain, which affects over 50% of menstruating women to some degree, 10% of whom are incapacitated for 1 to 3 days per month. It is most common from age 20 to 25.

## Goals of Therapy

- To decrease or abolish menstrual pain that interferes with everyday activities
- To rule out organic causes of pain that may require alternative therapies

## Investigations

- A thorough history to differentiate primary from secondary dysmenorrhea (Table 1). In primary dysmenorrhea:
  - pain starts within 1 to 4 hours of onset of menses and lasts at most 1 to 3 days
  - pain is described as crampy, located in the lower abdomen and present with each period
  - other symptoms of prostaglandin excess may be present (i.e., nausea, vomiting, diarrhea, backache, thigh pain, headache, dizziness)

Table 1: **Characteristics of Dysmenorrhea**

| Primary | Secondary |
|---|---|
| – absence of identifiable pelvic pathology<br>– occurs in ovulatory cycles<br>– onset within 2 yrs after menarche<br>– pain due to myometrial contractions induced by prostaglandin production in the secretory endometrium | – associated with pelvic pathology (e.g., endometriosis, adenomyosis, uterine myomas, endometrial polyps, intrauterine device, pelvic inflammatory disease, obstructed outflow, congenital mullerian malformations). Diagnostic clues include infertility, dyspareunia, premenstrual or intermenstrual bleeding, pain onset before menses<br>– onset at menarche or after age 25 suggests a possible pelvic abnormality<br>– component of pain may be due to endometrial prostaglandins; therefore partial response to therapy for primary dysmenorrhea may be seen |

Figure 1: **Management of Dysmenorrhea**

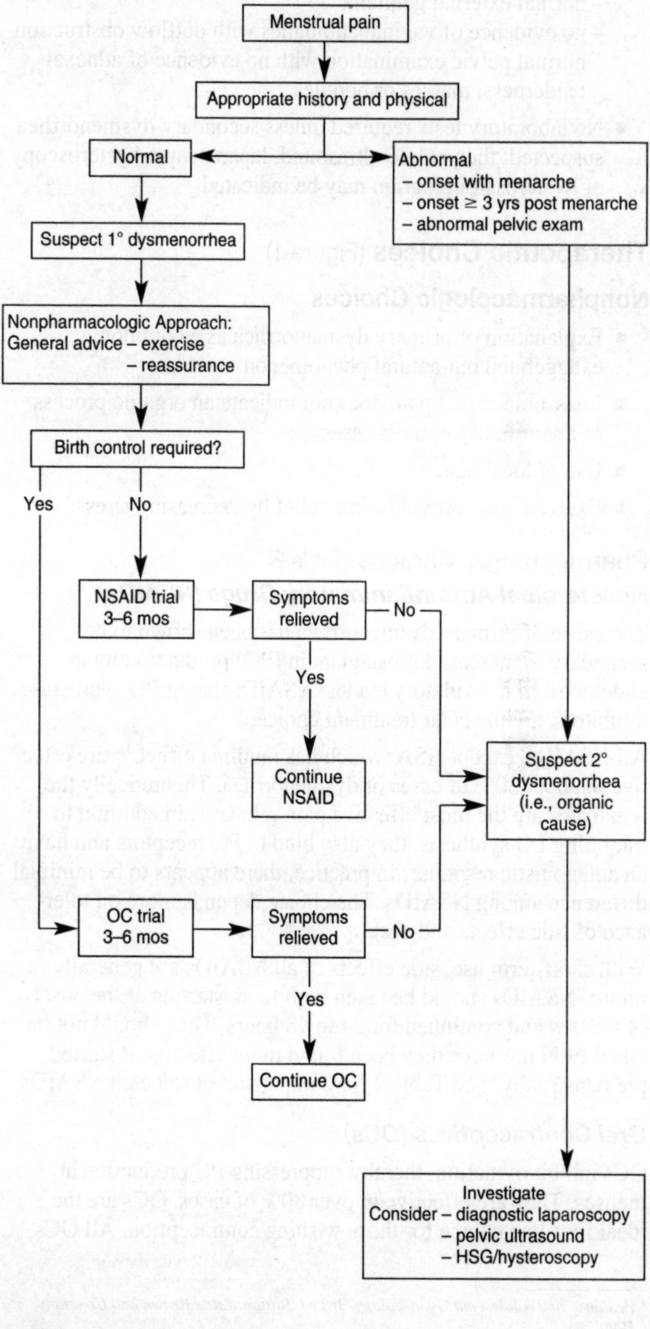
Menstrual pain
Appropriate history and physical
Normal
Abnormal
– onset with menarche
– onset ≥ 3 yrs post menarche
– abnormal pelvic exam
Suspect 1° dysmenorrhea
Nonpharmacologic Approach:
General advice – exercise
– reassurance
Birth control required?
Yes
No
NSAID trial
3–6 mos
Symptoms relieved
No
Yes
Continue NSAID
Suspect 2° dysmenorrhea (i.e., organic cause)
OC trial
3–6 mos
Symptoms relieved
No
Yes
Continue OC
Investigate
Consider – diagnostic laparoscopy
– pelvic ultrasound
– HSG/hysteroscopy

*Abbreviations: OC = oral contraceptive, HSG = hysterosalpingogram.*

- Physical examination for primary dysmenorrhea should reveal:
  - normal external genitalia
  - no evidence of vaginal anomalies with outflow obstruction
  - normal pelvic examination with no evidence of adnexal tenderness, masses or nodules
- No laboratory tests required unless secondary dysmenorrhea suspected; then pelvic ultrasound, laparoscopy, hysteroscopy or hysterosalpingogram may be indicated

## Therapeutic Choices (Figure 1)

### Nonpharmacologic Choices

- Explanation of primary dysmenorrhea as a common, exaggerated but natural phenomenon.
- Reassurance that pain does not indicate an organic process or abnormality in most cases.
- Use of local heat.
- Exercise may provide some relief by decreasing stress.

### Pharmacologic Choices (Table 2)

#### *Nonsteroidal Anti-inflammatory Drugs (NSAIDs)*

The cause of primary dysmenorrhea has been shown to be secondary to increased prostaglandin (PG) production by the endometrium in ovulatory cycles. NSAIDs, being PG synthetase inhibitors, are the clear treatment choice.

All NSAIDs, except ASA, which has minimal effect,[1,2] are effective in about 80% of cases of dysmenorrhea. Theoretically the fenamates are the most effective pain relievers; in addition to inhibiting PG synthesis, they also bind to PG receptors and have an antagonistic response. In practice, there appears to be minimal difference among NSAIDs. The choice depends more on tolerance of side effects and cost.

With short-term use, side effects of all NSAIDs are generally minor. NSAIDs should be taken with food, starting at the onset of menses and continued for 24 to 48 hours. They should not be taken PRN nor have they been found more effective if started premenstrually. See Table 2 for comparison of selected NSAIDs.

#### *Oral Contraceptives (OCs)*

OCs inhibit ovulation, thereby suppressing PG production at menses. They are effective in over 80% of cases. OCs are the ideal first-line choice for those wishing contraception. All OCs

[1] *Pediatric and Adolescent Gynaecology. 3rd ed. Boston: Little Brown and Company, 1990:295.*

[2] *J Pediatr 1981;98:97.*

Table 2: **Drugs Used for Dysmenorrhea**

| Drug | Dosage | Contraindications | Adverse Effects | Efficacy (Clinical Pain Relief) | Cost* |
|---|---|---|---|---|---|
| ***PG Synthetase Inhibitors (NSAIDs)*** (See Chapter 55 for more information on adverse effects and drug interactions of NSAIDs.) | | | | | |
| **Indoleacetic Acid** | | For **all** agents: Hypersensitivity to ASA, active peptic ulcer disease, gastritis, inflammatory bowel disease, existing renal disease, clotting disorders. | For **all** agents: Very common (> 10%): dyspepsia, nausea/ vomiting. Common (5–10%): nonspecific rash/ pruritus, dizziness, headache. | | |
| *indomethacin* Indocid, generics | 25 mg TID to 6×/d | | | 70–80% | $ |
| **Fenamates** | | | | | |
| *mefenamic acid* Ponstan, generics | 250–500 mg QID | | | 86–94% | $$–$$$ |
| **Propionic Acid Derivatives** | | | | 66–90% | |
| *ibuprofen* Motrin, generics | 400 mg QID | | | | $ |
| *naproxen sodium* Anaprox, generics | 275 mg QID | | | | $$ |
| *ketoprofen* Orudis, Rhodis, generics | 50 mg TID | | | | $ |
| *flurbiprofen* Ansaid, Froben, generics | 50 mg QID | | | | $$ |

(cont'd)

Table 2: **Drugs Used for Dysmenorrhea** *(cont'd)*

| Drug | Dosage | Contraindications | Adverse Effects | Efficacy (Clinical Pain Relief) | Cost* |
|---|---|---|---|---|---|
| **Others** ◗ | | | | | |
| *piroxicam* Feldene, generics | 10–40 mg/d | | | ≈ 80% | \$–\$\$ |
| *diclofenac sodium* Voltaren, generics | 50–75 mg/d | | | ≈ 80% | \$ |
| **COX-2 Inhibitors** | | | | | |
| rofecoxib ◗ Vioxx | 25–50 mg/d | | | ≈ 80% | \$\$–\$\$\$ |
| **Oral Contraceptives** Numerous products | According to product monograph | See Chapter 69. | See Chapter 69. | | \$\$\$\$† |

** Cost of 2-day/cycle supply – includes drug cost only.*
*† Cost of one pack of oral contraceptives – includes drug cost only.*
*Legend: \$ < \$2 \$\$ \$2–4 \$\$\$ \$4–10 \$\$\$\$ \$10–15*

◗ *Dosage adjustment may be required in renal impairment – see Appendix I.*

are effective, although in theory monophasic OCs with a more androgenic progestational component are ideal (e.g., levonorgestrel, dl-norgestrel) (Chapter 69).

## Therapeutic Tips

- A therapeutic trial of 3 to 6 months of either an NSAID or OC is usually sufficient to demonstrate effectiveness.
- Pharmacotherapy fails in 20% of patients. These patients usually have secondary dysmenorrhea and require prompt investigation. Diagnostic laparoscopy is the most useful test to differentiate primary from secondary dysmenorrhea. Therapy can then be directed and may involve surgery, such as laser ablation of endometriosis or uterosacral nerve ablation.
- In a small percentage of patients in whom pharmacotherapy fails, extensive investigation will not identify a specific cause. In these patients psychogenic factors should not be overlooked.
- Calcium channel blockers, magnesium, clonidine, transcutaneous electrical nerve stimulation (TENS), acupuncture, omega-3 fatty acids, transdermal nitroglycerin and chiropractor spinal manipulation have been studied. None has shown greater efficacy than NSAIDs or OCs.

## *Suggested Reading List*


Daywood MY. Dysmenorrhea. In: Speroff L, Simpson JL, Sciarra JJ, eds. *Sciarra gynecology and obstetrics.* Vol 5. Philadelphia: JB Lippincott, 1991:1–12.

Emans SJH, Goldstein DP. *Pediatric and adolescent gynecology.* 3rd ed. Boston: Little, Brown, and Company, 1990:291–299.

Fraser IS. Prostaglandins, prostaglandin inhibitors and their roles in gynecological disorders. *Bailliere's Clinical Obstetrics and Gynecology International Practice and Research* 1992;6:829–857.

Rapkin AJ. Pelvic pain and dysmenorrhea. In: Berek JS, Adashi EY, Hillard PA. *Novak's textbook of gynecology.* 12th ed. Baltimore: Williams and Wilkins, 1996:399–428.

Speroff L, Glass RH, Kase NG. *Clinical gynecologic endocrinology and infertility.* 5th ed. Baltimore: Williams and Wilkins, 1994:523–525.

CHAPTER 71

# Endometriosis

*G. Barry Gilliland, MD, FRCSC*

Endometriosis is diagnosed by finding tissue which histologically resembles endometrium at sites outside the uterine cavity. Histological confirmation of a diagnosis of endometriosis requires at least two of the following: endometrial epithelium, endometrial glands, endometrial stroma and hemosiderin-laden macrophages.

## Goals of Therapy

- To treat infertility
- To relieve pain
- To prevent recurrence

## Investigations

- History
  - a history of pelvic pain, dysmenorrhea, dyspareunia, or infertility suggests endometriosis
- Physical examination
  - a pelvic examination that reveals particular tenderness in the uterosacral ligament area (especially around the time of menses) suggests endometriosis
- Laboratory results
  - serum CA 125 (a tumor-associated protein) levels that are significantly elevated (> 35) suggest endometriosis. Endometriosis is, however, only one of many factors that can elevate CA 125 levels. Others include pelvic inflammatory disease, epithelial ovarian cancer and pregnancy. CA 125 levels are more useful for follow-up to determine the effectiveness of some therapies
- Ultrasound
  - can reliably diagnose endometriomas, but its sensitivity is poor for the detection of focal implants
- Laparoscopy and biopsy
  - form the "gold standard" test for endometriosis. Endometriotic tissue may have a typical or atypical appearance. Focal deposits may have the classical blue or black appearance, but they may also appear yellow, brown, white or red (81% of such areas show histological evidence of endometriosis)

## Classification

Although endometriosis is most often classified according to the revised American Fertility Society Classification[†] (r-AFS) there is no direct correlation between the volume of endometriotic tissue and the severity of symptoms.

## Therapeutic Choices

Endometriosis may be treated pharmacologically or surgically, depending on the severity of the disease and the symptoms of the patient. Tables 1 and 2 summarize the nonpharmacologic and pharmacologic choices available. Table 3 summarizes the incidence of the most common clinical adverse effects associated with the hormonal treatment of endometriosis. Individualized therapy is required.

## *Treatment of Endometriosis-associated Infertility*

### *Nonpharmacologic Choices*

#### *Surgery*

- No difference in the success of laparoscopy versus laparotomy in the surgical treatment of endometriosis-associated infertility.
- Laparoscopy offers the advantages of a shorter hospital stay, less pain, and quicker convalescence, but requires surgical expertise and expensive equipment.
- Laparoscopic resection or ablation of minimal or mild endometriosis enhances fecundity in infertile women. Three hundred and forty-eight patients having r-AFS stage I and II disease and no other cause for infertility, who were followed for 36 months after conservative surgery, showed a cumulative probability of pregnancy in the treated group of 30%, compared to 17% in the untreated group. There was no particular advantage to coagulation, laser vaporization, or excision of endometriosis.
- No advantage to using pre- or postoperative medical therapy with surgical therapy.

#### *Assisted Reproductive Technologies*

- The efficacy of IVF- ET (in vitro fertilization – embryo transplant) in treating endometriosis-associated infertility has not been properly evaluated for severity of disease, or for important prognostic variables, including age and duration of infertility.

[†] *Fertil Steril 1985;43:351–352.*

Table 1: **Surgical Approaches to the Treatment of Endometriosis**

| Approach | Comments |
|---|---|
| Conservative surgery – laparoscopy or laparotomy | • Used in endometriosis-associated infertility. Laparoscopy offers advantage of shorter hospital stay, less pain, and quicker convalescence, but requires surgical expertise and expensive equipment.<br>• Used in endometriosis-associated pain. Cytoreductive procedure that is not necessarily curative. |
| LUNA (laparoscopic uterosacral nerve ablation) | • Used with laser ablation in women with dysmenorrhea, dyspareunia, or pelvic pain to relieve endometriosis-associated pain. |
| PSN (presacral neurectomy) | • Used in conjunction with conservative surgery for relieving severe midline dysmenorrhea associated with endometriosis. |
| Hysterectomy | • Definitive therapy for endometriosis-associated pain. Major indication is intractable pain that has not responded to more conservative measures. |
| Hysterectomy plus BSO (bilateral salpingo-oophorectomy) | • Often used as definitive therapy for endometriosis-associated pelvic pain or adnexal masses. |

- With improvements in IVF programs, this form of therapy will likely prove beneficial in milder forms of endometriosis-associated infertility.

## Pharmacologic Choices

### *Ovulation Induction*

- **Clomiphene** 50 mg daily for 5 days (day 3 to 7 of the menstrual cycle), is simple and inexpensive. However, it has only a weak effect. Human chorionic gonadotropin (HCG) is sometimes added in a dose of 5000 to 10 000 units IM at mid-cycle ± intrauterine insemination (IUI).
- **Gonadotropin therapy** (referred to as superovulation or controlled ovarian hyperstimulation [COH]), together with IUI may be used to treat minimal or mild endometriosis-associated infertility. Live birth rates diminish with successive treatments. Because of its expense, this form of therapy should be limited to three cycles.

### *Ovarian Suppression*

- Ovarian suppression is ineffective and is inappropriate to use for endometriosis-associated infertility unless there is severe coexisting endometriosis-associated pain.

## *Treatment of Endometriosis-associated Pain*

Combined medical and surgical treatment may offer the best options to maximize pain relief. As conservative surgery is considered to be cytoreductive in the higher stages of disease, it seems reasonable to use surgery to "reduce" this stage of the disease before initiating medical treatment.

### Nonpharmacologic Choices

#### *Surgery*

The primary goals in the surgical treatment of endometriosis-associated pain include the removal of typical and atypical endometriotic implants and the restoration of pelvic anatomy.

- Definitive therapy of endometriosis-associated pain requires total abdominal hysterectomy and bilateral salpingo-oophorectomy with complete excision or ablation of endometriosis. It is considered 90 to 95% effective pain relief.
  - major indication is intractable pain that has not responded to more conservative measures and in patients who have completed their families.
  - estrogen replacement therapy postoperatively is associated with minimal (1 to 3%) risk of disease recurrence.
- Conservative surgery for endometriosis is a cytoreductive procedure that is not necessarily curative.
  - 60 to 100% of patients experience decreased severity of pain after ablative surgery.
  - recurrence rates range from 13.5 to 40.3% at 5 years.
  - conservative surgery can be performed by laparoscopy or laparotomy and both procedures are equally effective. Potential advantages of laparoscopy include the ability to treat the disease at the time of diagnosis, enhanced removal and ablation of endometriosis, reduced morbidity, shorter hospital stay, rapid recovery and potential decrease in the rate of postoperative adhesion formation.
  - the only prospective, double-blind, randomized, controlled trial to evaluate the effectiveness of laparoscopic surgery on pelvic pain, using both laser ablation and LUNA (laparoscopic uterosacral nerve ablation) in women with dysmenorrhea, dyspareunia or pelvic pain associated with endometriosis, showed 62.5% had pain relief, compared to 22.6% in the untreated control group.
  - two-thirds of women treated with laparoscopy for endometriosis-associated pain will feel improvement for at least one year.
- Presacral neurectomy, in conjunction with conservative surgery for endometriosis, may be effective in relieving severe **midline** dysmenorrhea associated with endometriosis,

Table 2: **Drugs Used to Treat Endometriosis**

| Drug | Dosage | Adverse Effects | Drug Interactions | Comments | Cost* |
|---|---|---|---|---|---|
| *clomiphene* Clomid, Serophene | 25–50 mg/day for 5 days; if ovulation does not occur, a second course of 100 mg/day for 5 days may be given 30 days after the initial course. A maximum of 3 courses may be administered. | Hot flashes, abdominal discomfort (bloating, pain) ovarian enlargement and ovarian cyst formation, visual disturbances (blurring, spots or flashes), dizziness/lightheadedness, breast discomfort. | | Simple and inexpensive. Used to induce ovulation but has only a weak effect in the treatment of endometriosis-associated infertility. Incidence of multiple births is increased. | $ (5 days) |
| **Nonsteroidal Anti-inflammatory Drugs** ➔ various e.g., | | Refer to Table 1, Chapter 55. | Refer to Table 1, Chapter 55. | Contraindicated in patients hypersensitive to ASA, active peptic ulcer disease, gastritis, inflammatory bowel disease, existing renal disease, clotting disorders, asthma. First-line treatment of endometriosis-associated pelvic pain and dysmenorrhea. | All: $ |
| *ibuprofen* Advil, Motrin, generics | 200–400 mg PO QID 100 mg per rectum BID | | | | |
| *naproxen sodium* Anaprox, generics | 275 mg PO QID | | | | |
| *ketoprofen* Orudis, generics | 50 mg PO TID | | | | |
| *flurbiprofen* Ansaid, Froben, generics | 50 mg PO QID | | | | |

| | | | | | |
|---|---|---|---|---|---|
| **Low-dose Oral Contraceptives**<br>various | One tablet daily | Refer to Table 1, Chapter 69. | Refer to Table 1, Chapter 69. | Produce symptomatic pain relief in 75–100% of cases. Used in treating recurrent endometriosis; reduce symptoms in mild disease. | $ |
| **Progestins**<br>*medroxyprogesterone acetate (MPA)* | | Amenorrhea, bloating, edema, weight gain, irritability, mood changes, spotting. | | Used to reduce endometriosis-associated pain. IM MPA significantly delays the resumption of ovulation following the cessation of therapy. Ovulation resumes promptly after stopping oral MPA. | All: $ |
| Depo-Provera (injectable) | 150 mg IM Q6–12 wks | | | | |
| Provera, generics (tablets) | 20–40 mg PO daily | | | | |
| *megestrol*<br>Megace, generics | 40 mg PO daily | | | | |
| *danazol*<br>Cyclomen | 600–800 mg/day in 2 divided doses for up to 6 months. | Edema, acne, oiliness of skin and hair, decreased breast size, amenorrhea, weight gain, hepatic dysfunction, emotional lability (reversible). Voice deepening (2%)(irreversible). | Warfarin, oral hypoglycemic agents, insulin, can have their actions potentiated by danazol.<br>Danazol may increase cyclosporine levels and risk of toxicity. | Highly effective in endometriosis-associated dysmenorrhea, less effective in managing chronic pain. May be used to treat mild recurrent endometriosis pain. | $$$ |

*(cont'd)*

Table 2: **Drugs Used to Treat Endometriosis** *(cont'd)*

| Drug | Dosage | Adverse Effects | Drug Interactions | Comments | Cost* |
|---|---|---|---|---|---|
| **Gonadotropin Releasing Hormone Analogues (GnRH-a)** | | For all: headache, depression/emotional lability, insomnia, vaginal atrophy, hot flushes/sweats, ↓ libido, acne, breast atrophy/tenderness, nausea, edema and weight gain. Bone mineral density ↓ 1–3% with 6 months therapy. | Topical nasal decongestants used concomitantly can reduce absorption of nafarelin (administer decongestants at least 2 hr after nafarelin). | GnRH analogues suppress ovulation. They are used to treat endometriosis-associated pain and recurrent disease pain. Recurrence of endometriosis symptoms may occur within 9–12 months after stopping therapy. Add-back therapy (conjugated estrogen 0.625 mg PO/day plus MPA 2.5 mg PO/day) can improve hypoestrogenic symptoms and control bone mineral density loss. | |
| *nafarelin* Synarel | 200 μg intranasally BID | For nafarelin: nasal irritation. | | | $$$$ |
| *goserelin* Zoladex | 3.6 mg SC monthly | For goserelin and leuprolide: palpitations or cardiac arrhythmias. | | | $$$$$ |
| *leuprolide* Lupron Depot | 3.75 mg IM monthly | | | | $$$$ |

* *Cost of 30-day supply – includes drug cost only.*

*Legend: $ < $50 $$ $50–150 $$$ $150–250 $$$$ $250–350 $$$$$ $350–$450*

*Dosage adjustment required in renal impairment – see Appendix I.*

if the surgeon completely resects the presacral nerve plexus. Results of adding this procedure to conservative surgery are mixed.

## Pharmacologic Choices

### *Nonsteroidal Anti-inflammatory Drugs (NSAIDs)*

- NSAIDs are well tolerated, safe and inexpensive and recommended as a first-line treatment of mild endometriosis-associated pelvic pain and dysmenorrhea.
- These drugs are most effective if started at the onset of symptoms and given continuously thereafter.

### *Oral Contraceptives (OCs)*

- When used continuously, low dose OCs (20 to 35 μg ethinyl estradiol) produce anovulation and amenorrhea.
- Low-dose OCs produce symptomatic pain relief in 75 to 100% of cases of endometriosis-associated pain.
- Women who have used OCs are less likely to develop endometriosis.
- The use of OC, in the usual cyclic fashion may delay the onset or recurrence of disease.

### *Progestins*

- Progestins suppress gonadotropin secretion, thereby inducing a hypoestrogenic acyclic hormonal environment and inhibiting ovulation.
- IM medroxyprogesterone acetate (MPA), 150 mg every 6 to 12 weeks, significantly reduces pain. Treatment delays the resumption of ovulation following cessation of therapy and should not be used in younger women who wish to become pregnant immediately after stopping treatment. IM MPA should be reserved for older patients who do not want to conceive and wish to avoid surgery.
- Continuous oral MPA, 20 to 40 mg per day, also relieves endometriosis-associated pain. Spotting frequently occurs, but ovulation resumes promptly.

### *Danazol*

- Danazol is an androgen agonist that inhibits ovarian estrogen production and causes atrophy of endometrial deposits.
- It is highly effective in the treatment of endometriosis-associated dysmenorrhea but less effective in the management of chronic pelvic pain.
- Endometriomas greater than 1 cm in diameter respond poorly to danazol.

Table 3: **Incidence of the Most Common Adverse Effects Associated with the Hormonal Treatment of Endometriosis**

| Adverse Effect | Oral Contra-ceptives | Medroxy-proges-terone Acetate | Danazol | GnRH analo-gues |
|---|---|---|---|---|
| Weight gain | ++++ | +++ | ++/+++ | + |
| Edema, bloating | ++++ | +++ | ++ | – |
| Breast tenderness | ++++ | – | + | – |
| Acne | – | + | +/++ | + |
| Hirsutism | – | – | + | – |
| Breast reduction | – | – | ++ | + |
| Muscle cramps | – | – | +/++ | – |
| Breakthrough bleeding | ++ | ++ | +/++ | + |
| Headache | + | + | +/++ | +/++ |
| Emotional lability | + | + | +/++ | ++ |
| Hot flushes | – | – | ++/+++ | +++/++++ |
| Vaginal dryness | – | – | ++ | ++/+++ |
| Decreased libido | – | – | +/++ | +/++ |

*Legend: "–" = not reported*

- Doses of 600 to 800 mg per day for 6 months are highly effective in alleviating symptoms of endometriosis, particularly in the early stages of the disease.

## *Gonadotropin Releasing Hormone Analogues (GnRH-a)*

- GnRH analogues (GnRH-a) inhibit the pituitary-gonadal axis, reducing the secretion of LH and FSH required for follicular development. As a result, they produce a markedly hypoestrogenic state, inducing atrophy and regression of endometriotic implants.
- The most common GnRH-a used include:
  – **nafarelin** intranasal, 200 μg twice daily,
  – **goserelin**, 3.6 mg subcutaneously, monthly, and
  – **leuprolide**, 3.75 mg intramuscularly, monthly
- GnRH-a are usually used for 3 to 6 months.
- There appears to be no significant difference in the relief of pain or clinical symptoms between 3 and 6 months of therapy.
- Recurrence of endometriosis symptoms commonly occurs within 9 to 12 months after completion of therapy.
- Adverse effects are common, including: hot flushes, insomnia, mood changes, and vaginal atrophy.
- Bone mineral density decreases about 1 to 3% with 6 months therapy.

- Add-back therapy, consisting of oral conjugated estrogens 0.625 mg daily plus oral MPA 2.5 mg daily, improves the hypoestrogenic symptoms and results in no change of bone density.
- GnRH-a therapy, plus add-back therapy, is as effective as GnRH-a therapy alone in relieving pelvic symptoms of endometriosis.

#### *Antiprogestins*

- Antiprogestins are a group of steroid compounds that bind to progesterone receptors and exert antiprogesterone and antiglucocorticoid activity.
- Mifepristone (RU-486), 100 mg OD, may be effective in the treatment of endometriosis symptoms. This product is not yet on the Canadian market.
- Long-term treatment of endometriosis with RU-486, at a lower dose of 50 mg daily for 6 months, has been reported to be successful. Larger clinical trials are required.

## *Treatment of Recurrent Endometriosis*

### *Nonpharmacologic Choices*

#### *Surgery*

- Conservative surgery may be considered for recurrent disease, if pain relief is required, or a patient declines definitive surgery. Between 20 and 40% of patients suffer recurrence 5 years after conservative surgery. Pregnancy does not influence the average time to recurrence of symptoms.
- Hysterectomy, with or without bilateral oophorectomy, is often used as a definitive therapy for the treatment of endometriosis associated with pelvic pain or adnexal masses. A recent retrospective study of recurrence of symptoms after definitive surgery, with a mean follow-up of 58 months showed that 62% of patients with ovarian conservation had recurrent symptoms and 31% required further surgery. In women with bilateral oophorectomy, 10% had recurrent symptoms and 3.7% required further surgery. The majority of patients who had bilateral oophorectomy had subsequently taken estrogen replacement therapy with no adverse effect on endometriosis. There is no advantage in delaying the introduction of estrogen replacement therapy after surgery.

### Pharmacologic Choices

#### *Treatment of Mild Disease*

- **Low-dose OCs** can reduce symptoms of mild disease (suggested by pelvic tenderness, small nodule). The advantage of low-dose OC therapy is that it can be used for an unlimited time.

- **MPA**, **danazol** or a **GnRH-a** can be used, as previously described, if low-dose OC therapy is ineffective.

### *Treatment of Advanced Disease*

- Medical treatment with **MPA**, **danazol** or a **GnRH** agonist can be used to relieve the pain of advanced disease (suggested by an adnexal mass, a fixed uterus, or obliteration of the cul-de-sac), but this form of therapy may not effectively treat the disease process. Although these drugs may reduce the size of endometriomas, their use is not necessarily associated with a reduction in surgical time or the eventual outcome of surgery.
- Danazol, or a progestin, is an appropriate alternative to a GnRH-a if:
  - GnRH-a treatment has been associated with marked unrecovered bone loss
  - bone density is not being evaluated or
  - the patient has other risk factors for osteoporosis.
- GnRH-a treatment, with an add-back of oral conjugated estrogens 0.625 mg daily plus oral MPA. 2.5-mg daily, can be used as an alternative to repeated treatment with a GnRH-a alone.
- The addition of a bisphosphonate has also been shown to prevent bone loss in a small group of endometriosis patients treated with a GnRH analogue.

## Therapeutic Tips

- Endometriosis must be diagnosed by laparoscopy ± biopsy.
- Chronic pelvic pain is a diagnosis, in itself, and should be treated as such.
- Endometriosis treatment must be individualized. Treatment depends on several factors including: age, reproductive desire, extent of disease, severity of symptoms, response to previous therapies, anticipated side effects and cost (insurance coverage varies considerably).

### *Suggested Reading List*

Schenken RS (guest editor). Endometriosis. *Clin Obstet Gynecol* 1999;42:565–713.

The Canadian consensus conference on endometriosis (Part I). *J Soc Obstet Gynaecol Can* 1999;21:468–498.

The Canadian consensus conference on endometriosis (Part II). *J Soc Obstet Gynaecol Can* 1999;21:574–610.

CHAPTER 72

# Menopause

*John Collins, MD, FRCSC*

## Definition

Menopause is the cessation of menstrual periods and occurs when the ovaries stop producing estrogen. This change takes place naturally when ovarian follicles are depleted at approximately 51 years of age, or following surgical removal of the ovaries, with or without hysterectomy.

## Goals of Therapy

- To reduce symptoms due to estrogen depletion, including hot flushes, sleeplessness, lethargy, depression and symptoms arising from urogenital atrophy
- To prevent disorders that may be less frequent with estrogen therapy, including osteoporotic fractures, myocardial infarction and colonic cancer
- To avoid causing disorders that may be more frequent with estrogen therapy, including endometrial and breast cancer

## Investigations

- Confirm cessation of ovarian activity (Figure 1)
  - if 6 months have elapsed since the last menstrual bleeding, ovarian failure is virtually certain
  - if in doubt, or if symptoms are present while menses continue, two serum FSH values 1 week apart will detect incipient ovarian failure, which is associated with values in excess of 30 IU/L. (An ovulatory rise in FSH lasts only 2 to 3 days and cannot affect both estimates.)
- Health maintenance screening
  - initial examination should include blood pressure measurements, breast examination and cervical cytology
  - mammography is indicated for all women over 50 years of age. It should be considered for younger women who have a higher than average risk
  - lipid screening and bone densitometry may be considered in women with a family history or a strong personal risk profile for heart disease or osteoporosis

## Therapeutic Choices (Figure 1, Tables 1 and 2)

### Nonpharmacologic Choices

Not all women with menopausal symptoms seek medical attention. Many rely on **lifestyle changes**, including exercise and reductions in caffeine and alcohol intake. **Herbal remedies** are also widely used; their effects are unlikely to be due to their minuscule content of estrogen and their beneficial effects remain unproven. Increasing **calcium** intake to 1 g daily and taking **vitamin D** is a useful approach to minimize bone loss.

### Pharmacologic Choices

#### *Preparations* (Table 1)

**Estrogen** preparations are essential to manage symptoms and prevent disease. The efficacy of pharmaceutical estrogen preparations correlates with the amount of estradiol that binds to target organ receptors. Therefore, the therapeutic ratios of benefits and side effects among the various preparations are similar when they are used in pharmacologically equivalent doses.

**Progesterone** preparations (progestins) are necessary among estrogen users who have not had a hysterectomy. Progestins prevent the unrestrained endometrial growth that increases the risk of endometrial cancer.

#### *Dosage Regimens*

**Cyclic administration** emulates estrogen and progesterone secretion in normal menstrual cycles. In this treatment regimen, estrogen is given daily. Progestin is given on the 1st to the 14th days of the calendar month. Most women will have withdrawal bleeding shortly after completing the progesterone phase. The daily estrogen regimen has replaced the regimen in which estrogen is given for the first 21–25 days of the calendar month because some women develop symptoms during the days without estrogen.

**Continuous combined therapy** avoids withdrawal bleeding, but unpredictable spotting or light bleeding occurs in most women during the first year of treatment. Estrogen and progestin are given daily without breaks in the regimen.

#### *Dosage*

Regardless of the product selected, the dose should be the lowest capable of controlling symptoms or known to prevent disease. In the case of conjugated estrogens 0.625 mg per day is a rational starting dose. The starting dose for progestins should be equivalent to 5 mg medroxyprogesterone acetate for cyclic/sequential regimens and 2.5 mg for continuous regimens.

Figure 1: **Treatment of Menopause**

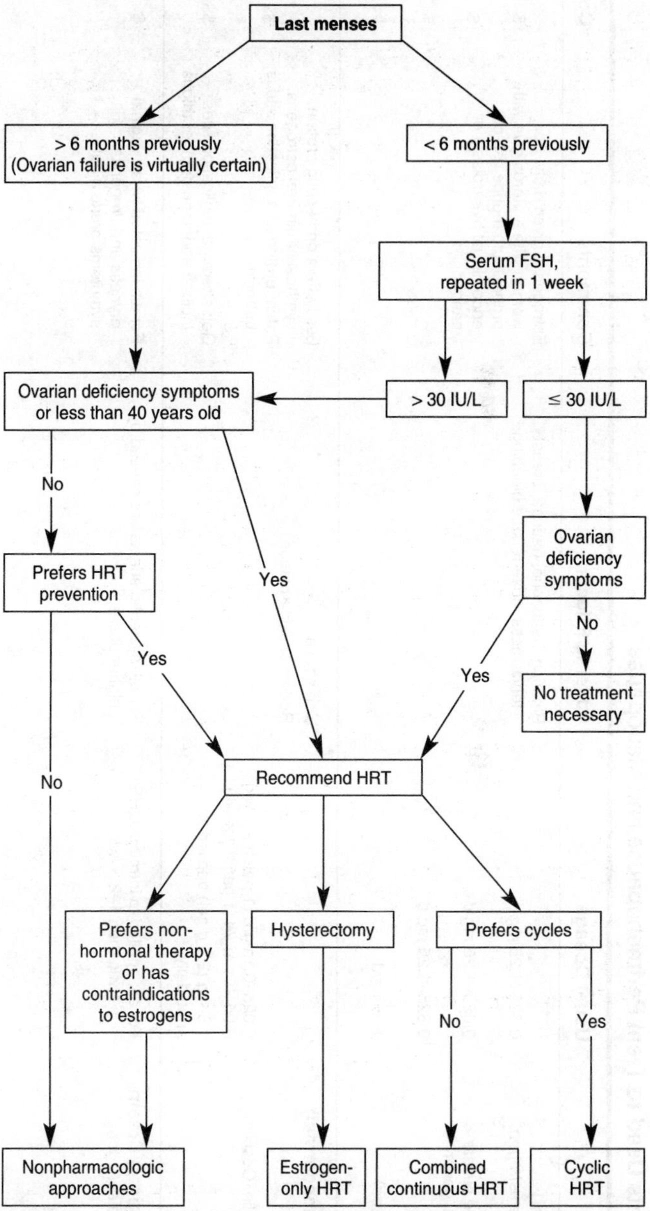
Last menses
> 6 months previously
(Ovarian failure is virtually certain)
< 6 months previously
Serum FSH,
repeated in 1 week
> 30 IU/L
≤ 30 IU/L
Ovarian deficiency symptoms
or less than 40 years old
No
Yes
Prefers HRT
prevention
Yes
No
Ovarian
deficiency
symptoms
No
Yes
No treatment
necessary
Recommend HRT
Prefers non-
hormonal therapy
or has
contraindications
to estrogens
Hysterectomy
Prefers cycles
No
Yes
Nonpharmacologic
approaches
Estrogen-
only HRT
Combined
continuous HRT
Cyclic
HRT

*Abbreviations: HRT = hormone replacement therapy.*

Table 1: **Agents Used to Treat Perimenopause and Menopause**

| Drug | Usual Dosage | Adverse Effects | Comments | Cost* |
|---|---|---|---|---|
| **Estrogens (Oral)** | | Bloating, headache, nausea, breast tenderness, dose-related bleeding. | Estrogen is given daily. For women with a uterus give with progestin to reduce risk of endometrial hyperplasia or cancer. | |
| *conjugated equine estrogen* Premarin | 0.625–1.25 mg/d | | | $ |
| *conjugated estrone sulfate* C.E.S., Congest, generics | 0.625–1.25 mg/d | | | $ |
| *estropipate* Ogen | 0.625–1.25 mg/d | | | $ |
| *estradiol (micronized)* Estrace | 1–2 mg/d | | | $ |
| **Estrogens (Transdermal)** | | See above. | Less effect on hepatic protein synthesis than oral estrogens. | |
| *estradiol-17β* | | | | |
| *Patch* | | Redness, skin irritation. | Patch: preferred application site is buttocks. | $$ |
| Estraderm, Vivelle, Oesclim | 0.025–0.1mg/d (1 patch 2×/wk) | | | |
| Climara | 0.05–0.1 mg/d (1 patch 1×/wk) | | | |
| *Topical gel* Estrogel | 1.5 mg (2.5 g gel) applied to arms daily. | | Gel: alternate application sites include abdomen or inner thighs. | $$ |
| **Estrogens (Vaginal) Cream** | For all: applied to introitus QHS × 1 wk, then 1–2 ×/wk | For all: systemic effects are caused by higher doses. | For all: Indicated when vaginal dryness and urogenital symptoms predominate. | $ |
| *conjugated equine estrogen* Premarin | | | | |
| *dienestrol* Ortho Dienestrol | | | | |
| *estrone* Oestrilin | | | | |

| | | | | |
|---|---|---|---|---|
| **Ring** | | | | |
| *estradiol 2 mg* Estring | 7.5 μg/d continuously | Vaginal discomfort. | Replace ring every 3 months. | $$ |
| **Progestins** | | For all: bloating, irritability, weight gain, mood swings. | Progestin is given on the 1st–14th day of the calendar month for cyclic regimens. Progestins normalize the endometrial response and decrease breakthrough bleeding. When given continuously prevent flow. | |
| *medroxyprogesterone acetate* Provera, generics | 5–10 mg/d cyclically or 2.5–5 mg/d continuously | | | $ |
| *norethindrone* Micronor | 0.35–0.7 mg/d continuously (contraceptive) | | | $ |
| *progesterone (micronized)* Prometrium | 200–300 mg/d QHS cyclically or 100–200 mg/d continuously | | | $$–$$$ |
| **Combination estrogen/progestin (Transdermal)** Estracomb | Estracomb: estradiol 0.05 mg/d (4 patches over 1st 2 wks) estradiol 0.05 mg/d + norethindrone 0.25 mg/d (4 patches over last 2 wks) | As for cyclic estrogens, progestins above. | | $$ |
| Estalis 250/50, 140/50 | Estalis: estradiol 0.05 mg/d + norethindrone 0.25 mg/d or 0.14 mg/d (1 patch 2 ×/wk × 4 wks) | | Can be used as a continuous regimen or in a sequential regimen with an estradiol-only patch. | $$ |

** Cost of 1-month therapy as directed – includes drug cost only.*
*Legend: $ <$15 $$ $15–30 $$$ $30–45*

Table 2: **Contraindications to Estrogen**

| |
|---|
| Recent treatment for breast cancer |
| Abnormal uterine bleeding |
| Active hepatic disease |

## Therapeutic Tips

- **Individual decision-making**
  Although hormone replacement therapy (HRT) appears to provide long-term benefits and increase both life span and quality of life, each woman should make her own decisions concerning HRT. Each woman's health history is singularly unique, and provides a risk profile that leads to more, or less, benefit from HRT. As a result, an unswerving policy applied to all women is unlikely to meet the individual needs of many. Physicians should consider the needs and wants of each patient before recommending a course of therapy for menopause.
- **Premature ovarian failure**
  Less than 1% of North American women experience menopause before age 40. Premature ovarian failure is associated with an early rise in the incidence of cardiovascular disease and osteoporosis. The risk profile of patients who enter menopause prior to age 40 dictates that HRT should be prescribed for all such individuals. Treatment should continue until at least the age of 50, the age when other women are also in or nearing menopause.
- **Route of administration**
  Estrogen preparations may be taken orally, transdermally, vaginally, and parenterally. Although there is some indication that lipid bio-markers may show greater changes with different routes of administration, there is no evidence that route of administration has any bearing on the clinical outcomes of greatest interest, such as fracture.
- **Duration of use**
  Treatment of menopausal symptoms may require several years of hormonal treatment. Prevention of cardiovascular disease and osteoporosis may need much longer use. The rates of myocardial infarction and hip fracture do not reach appreciable levels until women are in their late sixties and seventies. Optimal prevention of these events is seen only among current users of HRT.
- **Unexplained bleeding**
  Estrogen therapy increases the risk of endometrial cancer in postmenopausal women who have a uterus. Therefore, any unexpected bleeding requires investigation. In most cases, a tissue diagnosis may be required.

- **Risk of breast cancer**
  Breast cancer is a serious and common diagnosis in postmenopausal women. Breast cancer incidence is correlated with hormonal events such as pregnancy and age at menopause. The breast cancer risk with HRT mirrors the effect of delayed menopause. The additional risk with each year of HRT is similar to the additional risk with each year of delayed menopause. During the 20 years after age 50, about 45 in every 1000 women will have breast cancer diagnosed. An additional 2 to 6 cases of breast cancer per 1000 women 50 to 70 years of age may be associated with use of HRT for 5 to 10 years.[1]

## *Suggested Reading List*

The Canadian Consensus Conference on Menopause and Osteoporosis. *J SOGC* 1998;20(13 and 14).

Cramer DW, Xu H, Harlow BL. Family history as a predictor of early menopause. *Fertil Steril* 1995;64:740–745.

Limouzin-Lamouthe MA, Mairon N, Joyce CRB, Le Gal M. Quality of life after menopause: influence of hormonal replacement therapy. *Am J Obstet Gynecol* 1994;170: 618–624.

[1] *Lancet 1997;350:1047.*

CHAPTER 73

# Sexual Dysfunction

*Rosemary Basson, MB, BS, MRCP*

## *Erectile Dysfunction*

Erectile dysfunction (ED) is the persistent inability to achieve or maintain an erection sufficiently firm for satisfactory sexual activity.

## Goals of Therapy

- To address underlying conditions that are presenting as ED
- To assess the safety of resuming intercourse and orgasm
- To correct reversible ED
- To safely prescribe medical enhancement for irreversible ED
- To restore sexual intimacy to allow sexual arousal

## Investigations (Figure 1)

- **Sexual history**
  - clarify sexual history and current sexual status (Table 1)
  - identify the presence of reversible ED (Table 2)
  - assess likely efficacy of medical enhancement

Table 1: **Questions to Clarify Sexual History and Current Sexual Status**

1. For how long have you had difficulty getting and keeping erections?
2. On a scale of 1 to 10 where 1 is a flaccid penis, 10 is completely firm and erect and 6 allows (but only just allows) intercourse, how firm are erections when you have sexual play with your partner, when you attempt intercourse, when you waken from sleep, and when you self-stimulate?
3. Despite those changes, are you and your partner still touching each other in sexual ways and being a sexual couple?
4. Your willingness to try and have sex may well be reduced given the disappointments, but do you still have sexual thoughts, sexual fantasies and the desire to self-stimulate, and become aroused mentally if you see or hear something erotic?
5. Your experience of orgasm – has that changed?
6. Are you reaching ejaculation – and has that changed?
7. Does your partner have sexual difficulties? Will I be able to interview your partner? Is your partner in agreement with reinstitution of sexual activity including intercourse?
8. What effects have these difficulties had on you, on your relationship and on your sexual partner?

Figure 1: **Assessment and Management of Acquired Erectile Dysfunction**

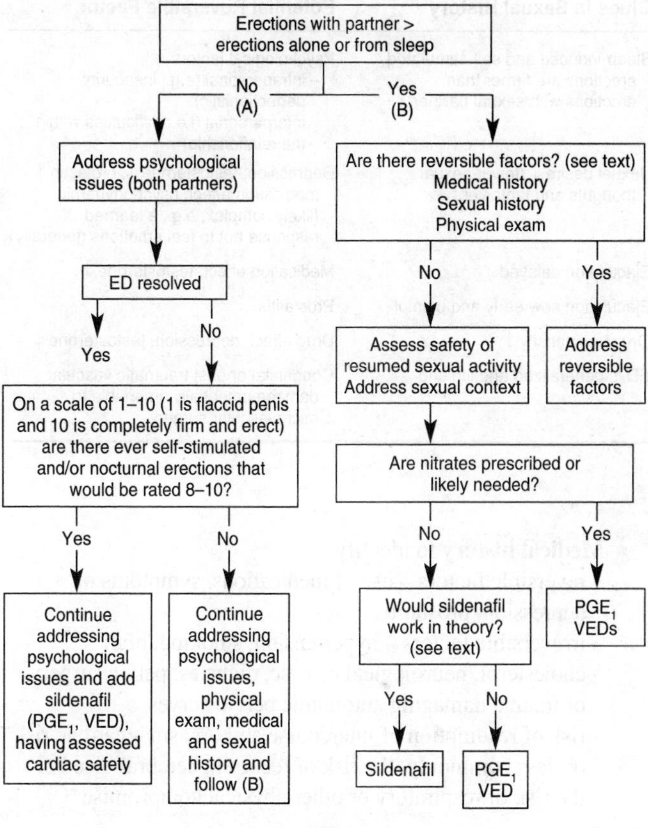
Erections with partner > erections alone or from sleep
No (A)
Yes (B)
Address psychological issues (both partners)
ED resolved
Yes
No
On a scale of 1–10 (1 is flaccid penis and 10 is completely firm and erect) are there ever self-stimulated and/or nocturnal erections that would be rated 8–10?
Yes
No
Continue addressing psychological issues and add sildenafil (PGE1, VED), having assessed cardiac safety
Continue addressing psychological issues, physical exam, medical and sexual history and follow (B)
Are there reversible factors? (see text) Medical history Sexual history Physical exam
No
Yes
Assess safety of resumed sexual activity Address sexual context
Address reversible factors
Are nitrates prescribed or likely needed?
No
Yes
Would sildenafil work in theory? (see text)
PGE1 VEDs
Yes
No
Sildenafil
PGE1 VED

*Abbreviations: $PGE_1$ = alprostadil, VED = vacuum device*

Establish if there is ongoing sexual intimacy with mental sexual arousal. Advise couples who have stopped being sexual together on ways to reinstate sexual intimacy. This is important for drug treatment to be effective. (See Pharmacologic Choices.)

Remind couples, who have deliberately avoided sexual intimacy because of dysfunction, that reinstating sexual intimacy requires effort.

- the first priority is to make time to be together, away from responsibilities.
- reintroducing sexual/sensual/intimate remarks and behaviors throughout the day allows each individual to view the other, once again, as his or her potential sexual partner.

Table 2: **Clues to Potentially Reversible Erectile Dysfunction**

| Clues in Sexual History | Potential Reversible Factor |
|---|---|
| Sleep-induced and self-stimulated erections are firmer than erections with sexual partner. | Psychological factors<br>– intrapersonal (e.g., insecurity, perfectionistic)<br>– interpersonal (i.e., difficulties within the relationship) |
| Sexual desire ↓ (fewer sexual thoughts and fantasies) | Depression, testosterone ↓, prolactin ↑, medication effect, psychodynamic (likely complex, e.g., a learned response not to feel emotions generally) |
| Ejaculation delayed | Medication effect, testosterone ↓ |
| Ejaculation now early and painful | Prostatitis |
| Orgasm intensity ↓ | Drug effect, depression, testosterone ↓ |
| ED is generalized and lifelong | Congenital or past traumatic vascular damage potentially amenable to microvascular surgery |

- **Medical history** to identify:
  - reversible factors – use of medications, symptoms of depression, prostatitis
  - irreversible factors – hypertension, smoking, high cholesterol, neurological disease, diabetes, pelvic surgery or trauma damaging autonomic pelvic nerves
  - risk of resumption of intercourse and orgasm – cardiac risk or, less commonly, the risk of recurrent cerebral bleed or the risk of respiratory or other physical compromise
- **Physical exam**
  - cardiovascular system (CVS) signs may indicate irreversible vascular cause: bruits, hypertension, fundal changes, poor peripheral pulses, cardiac failure

    **Note:** Normal CVS exam does not exclude vascular etiology (endothelial cells lining the corpora cavernosal sinusoids cannot be examined)
  - CNS signs may indicate irreversible neurological damage, including multiple sclerosis, Parkinson's disease, previous Guillain-Barré syndrome, alcoholic neuropathy, spinal cord injury, diabetes

    **Note:** Normal CNS exam does not preclude neurological etiology (the pelvic autonomic nerves cannot be examined)
  - late signs of hypotestosterone state – fine body hair, smooth skin, testicular atrophy, lessening of beard, gynecomastia, hepatomegaly
  - signs of prostatitis from rectal exam

- **Investigation**
  - assess safety of resuming sexual activity – cardiac stress testing to 4 METs is useful to identify silent or symptomatic cardiac ischemia that would also occur with sexual intercourse and orgasm
  - measure free testosterone and prolactin concentrations, as indicated by sexual history
  - determine levels of fasting plasma glucose, lipids and liver function tests as needed – abnormalities in these parameters may clarify the etiology of ED, but correcting them is unlikely to improve the ED

## Therapeutic Choices (Figure 1)

### Nonpharmacologic Choices

#### *Psychological Issues*

Psychological issues may be partly or wholly responsible for ED and:

- may be identified by self-stimulated erections, and erections during sleep that are firmer than those experienced with the sexual partner. In older men, erections during sleep may be absent, and the only evidence of a psychological etiology may be firmer erections during self-stimulation than with the partner.
- require treatment in their own right (e.g., hesitancy on the part of the woman impairs her partner's erection, but her hesitancy may be due to an abusive relationship). Treating psychological issues directly may avoid the need to resort to drugs.
- affect the efficacy of pharmacotherapy. Sildenafil acts via arousal and may not be effective if psychological issues are precluding arousal. $PGE_1$ compliance is likely to be poor if interpersonal issues are not addressed – the flaccid penis was actually an "appropriate" response to the troubled sexual interaction.

#### *Vacuum device (VED)*

Creating a vacuum around the penis can usually draw sufficient venous blood back into the penis. The blood is then trapped by the use of a retaining band around the base of the penis to attain adequate firmness for intercourse. There is a learning curve with the use of VEDs. Warn patients that the tightness of the retention band is critical and the band must be removed by 30 minutes. Some men cannot tolerate the degree of tightness required. Any condition that predisposes to priapism is a relative contraindication to the use of a VED.

## Pharmacologic Choices (Table 3)

### *Sildenafil*

Nitric oxide (NO) is a neurotransmitter that activates cGMP, which, in turn, relaxes sinusoidal smooth muscle to produce erection. Sildenafil selectively inhibits phosphodiesterase type 5, the enzyme responsible for the inactivation of cGMP.

**Note:** Sildenafil can only enhance an erection that is partially developing as a result of effective sexual stimulation and mental sexual arousal.

**Contraindications** to the use of sildenafil include:

- current use of, or likely need to use, any form of nitrate therapy.
- symptomatic hypotension (sildenafil is a mild hypotensive drug).
- previous priapism.
- any condition in which even a slight lowering of systemic pressure would be poorly tolerated, including conditions restricting aortic outflow and volume depletion states.
- conditions predisposing to priapism, e.g., leukemia, polycythemia, myelofibrosis and sickle cell disease.

### *Alprostadil ($PGE_1$) by Intracavernosal Injection*

If sufficient corporal erectile tissue is still present, injected $PGE_1$ will cause erections **even in the absence of mental sexual arousal.** By activating cAMP, $PGE_1$ relaxes sinusoidal smooth muscle to produce an erection. Technique, dose and dilution are critical for efficacy and comfort of erection. ($PGE_1$ directly stimulates nociceptors. Therefore, dilution and dose are critical, particularly in cases of neurogenic ED, which often require only 1 to 3 μg.) Doses up to 40 or 60 μg may be needed for vascular ED.

**Contraindications** to the use of intracavernosal $PGE_1$ include:

- anticoagulation with high INR
- previous priapism
- severe thrombocytopenia
- conditions predisposing to priapism, e.g., leukemia, polycythemia, myelofibrosis and sickle cell disease.

### *Alprostadil$_1$ by Urethral Instillation – MUSE*

Instilling $PGE_1$ into the urethra allows the drug to enter the corpus spongiosum. Retrograde venous passage from spongiosum to cavernosa is unpredictable and depends on the individual's venous anatomy. Thus, a trial of MUSE is necessary to determine efficacy. By entering the communicating veins between the corpora, the drug is introduced into the systemic circulation and systemic side effects are possible.

Table 3: **Drugs for Erectile Dysfunction**†

| Drug | Dosage | Adverse Effects | Drug Interactions | Comments | Cost* |
|---|---|---|---|---|---|
| *sildenafil* ➔ Viagra | 50–100 mg 1 hr before intercourse and not more than once/day. Higher dose may be required for neurogenic or vascular ED. Use only 25 mg in hepatic or renal disease. | Headache: 15%<br>Flushing: 10%<br>Dyspepsia: 5%<br>Nasal congestion: 5%<br>Visual: 2% | Concomitant use of cimetidine, ketoconazole, nefazodone, erythromycin, protease inhibitors inhibit sildenafil metabolism. Use only 25 mg dose.<br>Hypotensive effect of nitrates ↑; concomitant use is contraindicated. | Efficacy dependent on sexual arousal (reflex erections in spinal cord injured men may be enhanced as NO is generated in response to physical stimulation). | $10–11/dose |
| *alprostadil ($PGE_1$) intracavernosal injection* Caverject | **Neurogenic ED:**<br>Begin with 1 μg and titrate (usual dose 2–5 μg).<br>**Vascular ED:**<br>Begin with 4 μg and titrate (usual dose 5–20 μg). 40 μg (occasionally 60 μg) for severe vascular ED.<br>10–30 min before intercourse; not more than once/day and 3 ×/ week (24 hrs between doses). | Penile pain with erection: 10% (dilute reconstituted solution and use minimum dose to avoid).<br>Fibrosis of tunica (rare). | | Caution re: needle stick injury and risk of STD transmission.<br>Caution if known risk of subacute bacterial endocarditis (emphasize strict sterile technique).<br>Stress one time use only of needle and syringe in Caverject kit. Prepared product is stable for 7 days under refrigeration. | $14–21/ 10–20 μg dose |
| *alprostadil ($PGE_1$) intraurethral pellet* MUSE | 250–1000 μg 10–30 min before intercourse; no more than 2 administrations per 24 hrs.<br>Dose is unpredictable from ED etiology; dependent on venous anatomy. | Penile pain: 35%<br>Dizziness: 10%<br>Syncope: rare | Additive to hypotensive agents. | Caution with asymptomatic hypotension – monitor BP during in-office titration. | $21/dose |

* *Cost as indicated – includes drug cost only.*

† ***Note: See contraindications to use of listed drugs in text.***

➔ *Dosage adjustment may be required in renal impairment – see Appendix I.*

**Contraindications** to the use of intraurethral $PGE_1$:
- previous priapism
- symptomatic hypotension
- conditions predisposing to priapism, e.g., leukemia, polycythemia, myelofibrosis and sickle cell disease.

## Therapeutic Tips

- ED is a couple entity. Interview the partner whenever possible – there may be reasons not to intervene.
- Remember that sex is a biopsychosocial entity:
  - if a patient's erections with self-stimulation are more firm and erect than with his partner, addressing the couple's interaction is more relevant than drug therapy. Prescribing $PGE_1$ will fix only the penis. Ordering sildenafil is unlikely to be effective, given the minimal arousal.
- Plan follow-up, since drug failures are usually a result of:
  - lack of sexual arousal,
  - poor technique especially with intracavernosal therapy, or
  - low desire in the partner.
- Reinforce both the contraindication to nitrate use and the assessment of the safety of sex in cardiac patients.

# *Low Sexual Desire in Women*

Hypoactive sexual desire disorder is the persistent or recurrent deficiency or absence of sexual fantasies/thoughts and desire for, or receptivity to, sexual activity, causing personal distress.

## Goals of Therapy

- To address the biological, psychological and interpersonal factors required to nurture a woman's sexual desire
- To construct, with the couple, a model of the female sexual response cycle that clarifies the usual requirement of emotional intimacy (Figure 2)
- To have the couple see the need for referral for relationship counseling, if it becomes clear that interpersonal issues are precluding the intimacy necessary to drive the woman's cycle
- To address a lack of sexual stimuli, or the ineffectiveness of the stimuli to trigger desire
- To clarify the need for psychiatric or psychological referral, when deep-seated intrapsychological issues either prevent a woman from recognizing sexual stimuli, or result in her finding that the effect of arousal is dysphoric

- To address issues such as excessive focus on the act of intercourse, partner sexual dysfunction, lack of sexual skill and knowledge, when these result in an unsatisfactory sexual outcome

## Investigations (Table 4, Figure 2)

- Sexual history including current and past sexual functioning of both partners
- Medical history including medication and mood
- Relationship details, both past and present, focusing on non-sexual intimacy, including trust and respect, safety, birth control, fertility and stressors
- Lab investigations, only if indicated by medical or sexual history

## Therapeutic Choices

### Nonpharmacologic Choices

- Counsel or refer the couple when their emotional intimacy is insufficient to drive the cycle.
- Address the lack of stimuli when this is evident.
- Clarify psychological factors when these are inhibiting the effectiveness of sexual stimulation. If necessary, refer the patient.

Table 4: **Sexual Concerns**

1. How long have you had concerns with respect to your sexual desire?
2. Do you sometimes have sexual thoughts, sexual daydreams and fantasies (even though you may not act on them)?
3. Currently, would you have sexual feelings, arousal from something that could be erotic, e.g., a picture, a book, a movie, music, dancing.
4. Many women self-stimulate – is that something you still do from time to time?
5. What would have been your answers to the above questions previously?
6. A large proportion of women's sexual desire, especially in longer-term relationships is "receptive" or responsive. Women can go happily through their day not really sensing any sexual need. However, if they are not too distracted or depressed or feeling distanced from their partner, they can respond to their partner or to other sexual stimuli. What are the circumstances when you would expect your desire to be there and find that it isn't?
7. For many women, feeling emotionally close and able to trust their partner is as important to them as sensing their partner is physically sexually attractive. How is the emotional intimacy with your partner?
8. Can you slowly respond to your partner's sexual touch – even if initially you have no sexual need? Does the touching gradually become more pleasant and arousing? Does anything negative happen (the stimulation is not what you want, or intercourse is attempted too soon, or there is some pain, e.g., with penetration). Can you stay focused on the experience? Are you able to guide your partner as to what pleases you? Is there anything being done to you that is discomforting?

Figure 2: **Model of Female Sexual Response Cycle**

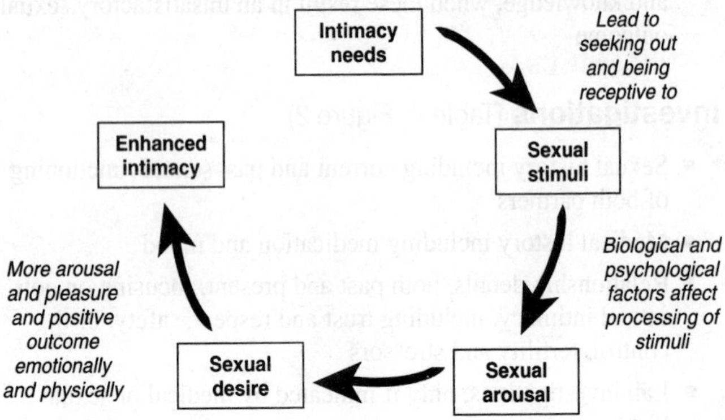
Intimacy needs
Lead to seeking out and being receptive to
Sexual stimuli
Biological and psychological factors affect processing of stimuli
Sexual arousal
Sexual desire
More arousal and pleasure and positive outcome emotionally and physically
Enhanced intimacy

- Common psychological factors include:
  - distractions
  - "dysphoric arousal" – often previous abuse
  - constant self-monitoring – these women are often perfectionists, with generally high self-imposed standards and low self-esteem
  - expectation of pain – a past history of dyspareunia can interfere with the processing of sexual stimuli, even if pain is currently absent
  - diminished motivation to be sexual, together with decreased sexual thinking and sexual expectation, which occur when the outcome is negative, e.g., dyspareunia or partner's sexual dysfunction. In this situation, address the primary problem.

## Pharmacologic Choices (Table 5)

- **Androgen replacement therapy** may be considered for women who, coincident with surgical, chemotherapeutic or, occasionally, natural menopause, no longer respond mentally or physically to previously effective stimuli. Measure free (bioavailable) serum testosterone, because androgen therapy may be effective in these women if they have low, or immeasurable, free testosterone levels. Estrogen replacement therapy can exacerbate the lack of testosterone due to an increase in sex hormone-binding globulin, decreasing free and bioavailable testosterone.

Table 5: **Androgen Replacement in Women**

| Drug | Dose | Comments | Cost* |
|---|---|---|---|
| *testosterone undecanoate* Andriol | 40 mg PO Q2 days | Adverse effects not seen at this dose. Higher doses risk adverse androgen effects. Warn patient she should not experience acne worse than any previously with her menses. | $$ |
| *testosterone cypionate* Depo-Testosterone | 25 mg IM monthly | As for testosterone undecanoate. | $ |
| *tibolone*† Livial | 2.5 mg PO daily | Synthetic steroid with estrogenic, progesterogenic and mild androgenic activity | † |

** Cost of 30-day supply – includes drug cost only.*
*Legend: $ < $10 $$ $10–20*
*† Available through the Special Access Program, Health Canada.*

## *Suggested Reading List*

*Erectile Dysfunction*

Chapters 1–5, *Can J Human Sexuality* 1998;7(3) published by Sex Information and Education Council of Canada (SIECCAN).

Drory Y, Shapira I, Fisman E, Pines A. Myocardial ischemia during sexual activity in patients with coronary artery disease. *Am J Cardiology* 1995;75:835–837.

Muller J, Mittleman M, MacClure M, Sherwood J, Tofler G. Triggering myocardial infarction by sexual activity. Low absolute risk and prevention by regular physical exertion. *JAMA* 1996;275(18):1405–140.

*Low Sexual Desire in Women*

Basson R. The female sex response: a different model. *J Sex Marital Ther* 2000;26:51–65.

Basson R. Androgen replacement in women. *Can Fam Physician* 1999;45:2100–2107.

CHAPTER 74

# Diabetes Mellitus

*M.A. Boctor, MD, DMSc, FRCP(C)*

Diabetes mellitus is defined as a chronic metabolic disturbance that is characterized by fasting or postprandial hyperglycemia. Diabetes mellitus is not a single disease entity. Rather, it is a heterogeneous syndrome that is caused by an absolute or relative lack of insulin, or resistance to the action of insulin, or both. When severe, diabetes mellitus affects carbohydrate, lipid, and protein metabolism. Severe long-term diabetes mellitus may lead to complications involving small blood vessels (microangiopathy), large blood vessels (macroangiopathy) and nerve damage (neuropathy) that affect multiple organs and systems.

## Goals of Therapy

To maintain the long term health of the person affected with diabetes, therapy should:

- Control symptoms
- Establish and maintain optimum metabolic control, while avoiding hypoglycemia
- Prevent, or minimize the risk of, complications
- Achieve optimum control of comorbidities such as hypertension and dyslipidemia

## Diagnostic Approach and Criteria (Figure 1)

The diagnosis of diabetes mellitus is established by:

- The presence of symptoms of diabetes plus a casual (random) plasma glucose ≥ 11.1 mmol/L,

  or
- A fasting plasma glucose (FBG) ≥ 7.0 mmol/L. This must be confirmed by a second test done on a subsequent day

  or
- A plasma glucose level ≥ 11.1 mmol/L at 2 hours after a 75 g oral glucose tolerance test.

## Screening

A fasting plasma glucose level should be measured every three years in individuals over 45 years of age. Earlier and more frequent testing should be considered in individuals at a higher risk of diabetes.

Figure 1: Diagnosis of Diabetes

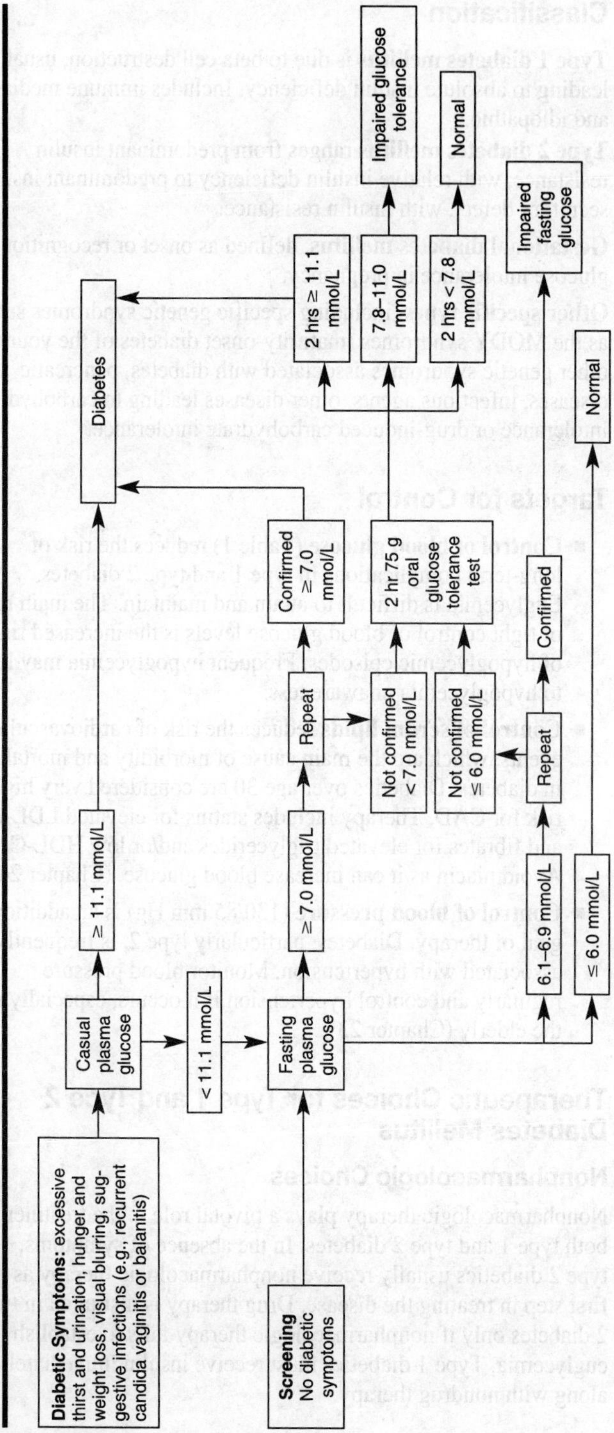
Diabetic Symptoms: excessive thirst and urination, hunger and weight loss, visual blurring, suggestive infections (e.g. recurrent candida vaginitis or balanitis)
Casual plasma glucose
< 11.1 mmol/L
≥ 11.1 mmol/L
Diabetes
Screening No diabetic symptoms
Fasting plasma glucose
≥ 7.0 mmol/L
Repeat
Confirmed ≥ 7.0 mmol/L
Not confirmed < 7.0 mmol/L
2 hr 75 g oral glucose tolerance test
2 hrs ≥ 11.1 mmol/L
7.8–11.0 mmol/L
Impaired glucose tolerance
2 hrs < 7.8 mmol/L
Normal
6.1–6.9 mmol/L
Repeat
Not confirmed ≤ 6.0 mmol/L
Confirmed
Impaired fasting glucose
≤ 6.0 mmol/L
Normal

## Classification

**Type 1 diabetes mellitus** is due to beta cell destruction, usually leading to absolute insulin deficiency. Includes immune mediated and idiopathic.

**Type 2 diabetes mellitus** ranges from predominant insulin resistance, with relative insulin deficiency to predominant insulin secretory defect, with insulin resistance.

**Gestational diabetes mellitus**, defined as onset or recognition of glucose intolerance in pregnancy.

**Other specific types**, including specific genetic syndromes such as the MODY syndromes (maturity-onset diabetes of the young), other genetic syndromes associated with diabetes, pancreatic diseases, infectious agents, other diseases leading to carbohydrate intolerance or drug-induced carbohydrate intolerance.

## Targets for Control

- **Control of blood glucose** (Table 1) reduces the risk of long-term complications in type 1 and type 2 diabetes. Euglycemia is difficult to attain and maintain. The main risk of tight control of blood glucose levels is the increased risk of hypoglycemic episodes. Frequent hypoglycemia may lead to hypoglycemia unawareness.
- **Control of serum lipids** reduces the risk of cardiovascular events, which are the main cause of morbidity and mortality in diabetes. Diabetics over age 30 are considered very high risk for CAD. Therapy includes statins for elevated LDL-C and fibrates for elevated triglycerides and/or low HDL-C. Avoid niacin as it can increase blood glucose. (Chapter 24)
- **Control of blood pressure** (130/85 mm Hg) is an additional goal of therapy. Diabetes, particularly type 2, is frequently associated with hypertension. Monitor blood pressure regularly and control hypertension if it occurs, especially in the elderly (Chapter 23).

## Therapeutic Choices for Type 1 and Type 2 Diabetes Mellitus

### Nonpharmacologic Choices

Nonpharmacologic therapy plays a pivotal role in the treatment of both type 1 and type 2 diabetes. In the absence of symptoms, type 2 diabetics usually receive nonpharmacologic therapy as the first step in treating the disease. Drug therapy is instituted in type 2 diabetes only if nonpharmacologic therapy fails to establish euglycemia. Type 1 diabetics must receive insulin immediately, along with nondrug therapy.

Table 1: **Levels of Glucose Control and Their Importance**

| | Ideal Non-diabetic | Optimal Target Goal | Suboptimal, Action May be Required | Inadequate, Action Required |
|---|---|---|---|---|
| Glycated Hb (%) Upper limit of assay | ≤ 100 | ≤ 115 | 116–140 | > 140 |
| Fasting or pre-meal glucose (mmol/L) | 3.8–6.1 | 4–7 | 7.1–10 | >10 |
| 1–2 hrs post-meal glucose (mmol/L) | 4.4–7 | 5.0–11 | 11.1–14 | >14 |
| Attainability | Difficult | Difficult | Attainable in most diabetics | |
| Risk of long-term complications | Very low | Very low | Moderate | High |

Nonpharmacologic therapy involves:

- **Education** to make the patient a full participant in the diabetes health care delivery team and ensure that he or she can effectively and safely manage the disease. A well-structured educational program should include:
  - a basic understanding of diabetes
  - the role of diet, exercise and medications in its control
  - a recognition of when, how and why self-monitoring of blood glucose is necessary
  - the management of sick days
  - the recognition and treatment of hypoglycemia
  - a knowledge of the major side effects of medications and how to adjust drugs in response to changes in diet and activity
  - care of the feet.
- **Nutritional management** designed to individualize the diet. Counseling should be provided by a registered dietician and include instruction on nutrients from all the basic food groups. Total caloric consumption in type 2 diabetics should be reduced to decrease weight and improve metabolic control. For patients on insulin, tailor the distribution of food intake into meals and snacks according to the individual's preference, lifestyle and medications taken. In type 1 diabetics, the amount and type of carbohydrate have the most immediate impact on the level of blood glucose. Patients are advised to fix carbohydrate consumption or count the amount of carbohydrate ingested.

- **Self-monitoring of blood glucose levels** usually results in improved diabetic control, allows appropriate recognition of low blood glucose levels and provides immediate feedback as to the effects of therapy. Monitoring before each meal and before bedtime is an absolute minimum in individuals on intensive therapy. Self-monitoring is an integral component of therapeutic plans in type 1 and type 2 diabetics treated with insulin and oral hypoglycemic agents. It is also useful in diabetics treated with diet only.
- **Physical activity and exercise** should form an integral part of the management of type 2 diabetes. In these patients, physical activity and exercise improve cardiovascular function, enhance insulin sensitivity, lower blood pressure and lipid levels, and improve glycemic control. Educate type 1 and type 2 diabetics treated with insulin about the effect of exercise on blood glucose and how to adjust insulin dosage. As well, teach these patients how to time their meals and/or regulate food consumption to ensure the safety of the prescribed exercise regimen.
- **Periodic reassessments**, including directed histories and physical examinations. Physical examinations are intended to detect comorbidities and complications. Periodic reassessments should include:
  - blood pressure measurements
  - foot examinations
  - tests of long-term control such as glycated hemoglobin
  - assuring the accuracy of blood glucose measurements made by the patient
  - reinforcement of skills learned in education and dietary counseling.

Periodic reassessments should be based on an each individual's needs. Glycated hemoglobin is generally indicated every 3 to 4 months for patients on insulin and at least every 6 months for individuals on nutritional therapy or oral hypoglycemics.

## Pharmacologic Choices for Type 1 Diabetes

Start all type 1 diabetics on human insulin at the time of diagnosis. Human insulin is less immunogenic, has an earlier onset and peak of action, and a shorter duration of action than animal preparations. Commonly used insulin preparations are shown in Table 2. Beef/pork insulin preparations are no longer produced in North America. Pure pork preparations are still available.

### *Insulin Regimens for Type I Diabetics* (Table 3)

Intensive treatment regimens control blood glucose more effectively than conventional regimens and reduce the risk of

Table 2: **Human Insulin and Analogues**

| Type of Insulin* | Onset (h) | Peak (h) | Duration (h) |
|---|---|---|---|
| **Rapid-acting**<br>*Insulin lispro*<br>Humalog | 0.5–0.75 | 0.75–2.5 | 3.5–4.75 |
| **Short-acting**<br>*Regular Insulin*<br>Humulin R<br>Novolin ge Toronto | 0.5–1 | 0.75–4.5 | 5.0–7.5 |
| **Intermediate-acting**<br>*NPH*<br>Humulin N<br>Novolin ge NPH | 1–2 | 4–12 | 12–24 |
| **Intermediate-acting**<br>*Lente*<br>Humulin L<br>Novolin ge Lente | 2–4 | 7–15 | 12–24 |
| **Long-acting**<br>*Ultra lente*<br>Humulin U<br>Novolin ge Ultralente | 3–4 | 8–16 | 24–28 |

* *Premixed preparations contain specified proportions of Regular and NPH insulin (Novolin and Humulin mixtures) or lispro and lispro NPH (Humalog mixtures). Cost of insulins (drug cost only) ranges $11–23/10 mL vial.*

long-term diabetic complications. Newly diagnosed type 1 diabetics, as well as type 1 diabetics who have not achieved control on conventional therapy, should be offered the option of an intensive diabetes management regimen.

Most type 1 diabetic patients require approximately 0.5 U of insulin per kg of lean body mass. To avoid hypoglycemia, initiate therapy with a lower dose and subsequently adjust the dosage of insulin according to blood glucose monitoring. Regular home monitoring allows patients to correct for abnormal blood glucose levels, adjust the dosage more accurately for diet and exercise, and readjust the amount of insulin injected based on the blood glucose. For optimum control, regular insulin should be administered 20 to 30 minutes before meals. Rapid-acting insulin may be more conveniently administered shortly before eating.

Continuous subcutaneous insulin infusions (CSII), using insulin pumps, can achieve an even tighter and more reproducible degree of control but at a significantly increased cost to the patient.

The use of rapid-acting insulin in multidose insulin regimens, or CSII, improves postprandial glucose and may also diminish hypoglycemia, especially early nocturnal hypoglycemia.

Table 3: **Insulin Regimens**

| | Rapid or Short-acting | Intermediate or Long-acting | Remarks |
|---|---|---|---|
| **Conventional** | None | Once daily N or L before breakfast | Unlikely to achieve control |
| | None | Twice daily breakfast and supper N or L | Improved morning levels |
| | Breakfast and supper R or H | Breakfast and supper N or L | Most widely used regimen; better meal control |
| | Breakfast and supper R or H | N or L breakfast U supper | U more likely to last until next morning |
| | Breakfast and supper R or H | N or L breakfast N or L bedtime | More likely to last until next morning |
| **Intensive MDI** | R or H before each meal | N, L or U supper or bedtime | Usually good control, flexible |
| | R or H before each meal | Twice daily breakfast and supper or bedtime N, L, or U | Better suited for people with varying schedules |
| **Intensive CSII** | R or H basal and boluses as per program | None | Most flexible, can achieve even better control than MDI. Most expensive. Diabetic ketoacidosis may occur quickly with discontinuation |

*Abbreviations: N = NPH insulin; L = Lente insulin; U = Ultralente insulin; R = Regular insulin; H = Insulin lispro; MDI = multidose insulin regimen; CSII = Continuous subcutaneous insulin infusion.*

### *Adverse Effects of Insulin Therapy*

- **Hypoglycemia** is the most common side effect of insulin therapy and occurs more frequently in patients on tight diabetic control. The only way to avoid hypoglycemia is through unacceptably loose control.
  - hypoglycemia is most commonly the result of either a missed meal or an unusual amount of exercise.
  - frequent hypoglycemic events may lead to hypoglycemia unawareness.
  - patients should be taught to account for diet and physical activity when planning insulin treatment regimens.

- **Mild hypoglycemia** is manifested by adrenergic symptoms, such as sweating, tremors, tachycardia, hunger and a general sensation of weakness. It can easily be treated by the patient with an oral source of sugar. A small glass of unsweetened juice will usually raise the blood glucose approximately 2 mmol/L.
- **Severe hypoglycemia** requires assistance in its recognition and/or treatment. Neuroglycopenic symptoms, including confusion, altered behavior and disorientation, can progress to seizures and coma and prevent the patient from appropriately treating the hypoglycemic episode. If the patient is conscious, an oral glucose preparation should be used. Unsweetened juice, Lifesavers or sugar cubes may be useful. Oral glucose and dextrose do not require digestion. In **unconscious patients**, 1 mg of glucagon IM or SC temporarily increases blood glucose, allowing for the intake of oral carbohydrate. Glucagon is not effective in malnourished patients, or alcohol-induced hypoglycemia. IV administration of 50 mL of 50 percent dextrose in water is the treatment of choice under these circumstances.
- **Localized fat hypertrophy** is most often the result of frequent reutilization of the same injection site.
- **Allergic reactions**, such as urticaria, angioedema rashes and local erythema, are rare with human insulin.
- Immune-mediated **insulin resistance**, due to the production of anti-insulin antibodies, is rare with human insulin. Patients who have developed immune-mediated resistance to animal insulins should be switched to human insulin. The dose should be reduced substantially at the initiation of the switch. Concentrated regular insulin, 500 U/mL, may be useful in the treatment of patients requiring very large doses of insulin.

## Pharmacologic Choices for Type 2 Diabetes

Pharmacologic therapy for type 2 diabetes is indicated if control is not achieved within 2 to 4 months following the initiation of nonpharmacologic therapy. Drug treatment is warranted initially in symptomatic type 2 patients.

### *Oral Antidiabetic Agents* (Table 4)

#### *Insulin Secretagogues*

- **Sulfonylureas**
  - stimulate basal insulin secretion and increase meal-stimulated insulin release.
  - do not correct the impaired early phase insulin response.
  - can produce hypoglycemia.
  - may result in weight gain.
  - differ from each other in dose, rate of absorption, duration of action, and route of elimination.

Table 4: **Oral Antidiabetic Agents**

| Drugs | Dosage/Comments | Peak/ Duration (h) | Adverse Effects | Drug Interactions | Contraindications | Cost* |
|---|---|---|---|---|---|---|
| **Sulfonylureas** | | | | | | |
| *tolbutamide* generics | 500 mg BID–TID max. 3 g/d | 2–4/2–12 | Hypoglycemia, weight gain, nausea, abdominal pain, heartburn, fullness, jaundice (cholestatic and/or mixed) skin rashes, bone marrow suppression, hemolytic anemia, headaches. | Hypoglycemic effect potentiated by salicylates, sulfonamides and monoamine oxidase inhibitors. Beta blockers may mask hypoglycemic symptoms. Alcohol and rifampin may accelerate clearance. | Allergy to sulfonylureas, type 1 diabetes, pregnancy. | $ |
| *chlorpropamide* Diabinese, generics | 100–500 mg daily in one dose | 2–6/24–72 | Prolonged hypoglycemia. | | Alcohol-associated flushing, hyponatremia. | $ |
| *glyburide* Diaβetic, Euglucon, generics | 2.5–20 mg/d BID if >10 mg | 2–4/18–24 | Prolonged hypoglycemia. | | | $ |
| *gliclazide* Diamicron, generics | 40–320 mg/d divided does if ≥ 160 mg | 4–6/12–24 | | | Antiplatelet effect. | $ |
| **Carbamoyl Benzoic Acid Derivatives** | | | Hypoglycemia, esp. if meal not taken, weight gain. | Clearance inhibited by ketoconazole, miconazole and erythromycin. | Allergy to repaglinide, type 1 diabetes, pregnancy. | |
| *repaglinide* GlucoNorm | 0.5–4 mg 0–3 min before meals | 1/3 | | Enhanced clearance with barbiturates, rifampin and carbamazepine. | | $$$ |

| | | | | | | |
|---|---|---|---|---|---|---|
| **Biguanides**<br>*metformin* ◗<br>Glucophage, generics | 500–2500 mg/day start low and go slow to minimize GI side effects<br>Little additional benefit at doses >1500 mg<br>No weight gain<br>Lower triglycerides | 3/8–12<br>Max. effect in 1 month | Nausea, diarrhea, abdominal discomfort, anorexia, metallic taste, lactic acidosis if hepatic or renal disease. | Potentiates other oral agents, alcohol potentiates effect. | Hepatic impairment, renal impairment, previous lactic acidosis. | $–$$ |
| **Alpha-glucosidase Inhibitors**<br>*acarbose* ◗<br>Prandase | 50–100 mg TID with each meal<br>Start low and go slow<br>No weight gain. Insignificant systemic absorption | Covers meals | Flatulence, diarrhea, abdominal pain, cramps, nausea. | Potentiates other hypoglycemic agents.<br>May ↓ metformin bioavailability. | Allergy to acarbose, inflammatory bowel disease. | $$ |
| **Thiazolidinediones** | Resumed ovulation in previously anovulatory women (e.g., polycystic ovarian syndrome). ↑ risk of pregnancy if adequate contraception not used | Slow onset. Max. effect in 1 month | Weight gain, fluid retention and hemodilution.<br>Idiosyncratic, hepatitis with troglitazone.†<br>Varying effects on lipids; ↑ HDL, ↑ LDL, ↓ triglycerides (pioglitazone). | Potentiates other oral hypoglycemic agents. | Hypersensitivity to thiazolidinediones. | |
| *rosiglitazone*<br>Avandia | 4–8 mg daily in 1–2 doses | | | | | $$$$ |
| *pioglitazone*‡<br>Actos | 15–45 mg once daily | | | | | ‡ |

◗ *Dosage adjustment may be required in renal impairment – see Appendix I.*
* *Cost of 30-day supply – includes drug cost only.*
*Legend: $ < $10 $$ $10–25 $$$ $25–50 $$$$ > $50*
† *Troglitazone (Rezulin) was never marketed in Canada.*
‡ *Expected to be marketed in Canada late 2000.*

***Combinations***
***Well studied:*** *sulfonylureas + metformin; acarbose + sulfonylureas; acarbose + metformin; thiazolidinediones + sulfonylureas; thiazolidinediones + metformin. Triple Therapy: sulfonylureas with metformin + thiazolidinedione or repaglinide + metformin or repaglinide + thiazolidinedione. Insulin + sulfonylureas; insulin + metformin; insulin + sulfonylurea–metformin combination, insulin + thiazolidinediones.*
***Not well studied:*** *acarbose + insulin; repaglinide + sulfonylureas; acarbose + sulfonylureas + metformin.*

- **Repaglinide**
  - a newly introduced carbamoyl benzoic acid derivative which produces an earlier insulin response to meals, thus lowering postprandial glucose levels.
  - short acting, and should only be taken with meals.
  - fasting glucose usually drops after about a month of regular use.

### *Drugs That Increase Tissue Sensitivity to Insulin*

- **Biguanides**
  - **metformin** is the only available biguanide. Its main action is to decrease hepatic glucose production.
  - metformin may also lower glucose absorption and enhance insulin-mediated glucose uptake.
  - metformin does not lead to weight gain.
  - used alone, metformin does not cause hypoglycemia, but it can potentiate the hypoglycemic effects of insulin and sulfonylureas.
- **Thiazolidinediones**
  - **troglitazone** was never marketed in Canada. **Rosiglitazone** has been recently marketed and **pioglitazone** is under review.
  - thiazolidinediones enhance insulin sensitivity, lowering both blood glucose and circulating insulin levels.
  - these drugs increase peripheral glucose uptake, enhance fat cell sensitivity to insulin and lower hepatic glucose output.
  - thiazolidinediones are associated with some weight gain due to subcutaneous fat increases, and occasionally water retention. They do not produce hypoglycemia although they may enhance the hypoglycemic effects of insulin and sulfonylureas.

### *Drugs That Delay the Digestion of Complex Carbohydrates*

- **Alpha-glucosidase inhibitors**
  - **acarbose** is the only alpha-glucosidase inhibitor on the Canadian market.
  - acarbose inhibits intestinal alpha-glucosidases, thus delaying the digestion of starches and disaccharides, thereby reducing postprandial glucose levels. Acarbose does not significantly inhibit intestinal lactase.
  - hypoglycemia in patients treated with an alpha-glucosidase inhibitor should be treated only with glucose.

### *Insulin*

In type 2 diabetics, insulin may be used singly or in combination with an oral agent in a nighttime insulin, daytime pill regimen. Because of their underlying resistance to insulin, many type 2 diabetics require higher doses of insulin.

### ***Stepwise Approach to the Pharmacologic Treatment of Type 2 Diabetes*** (Figure 2)

The choice of therapeutic agent should be tailored to the patient's needs, the desired therapeutic effect and the presence of contraindications. Patients are usually started on one oral drug. If adequate control is not achieved with monotherapy, a second oral agent, from a different therapeutic class, may be added. If patients are not controlled on combination oral therapy, insulin therapy may be instituted. The United Kingdom Prospective Diabetes Study suggests that obese patients who were controlled on metformin therapy may have had better outcomes than those treated with insulin or sulfonylureas. The addition of a thiazolidinedione or metformin to diabetics not well controlled on insulin may improve control in some patients and lower insulin requirements.

## Diabetic Ketoacidosis (Table 5)

- Diabetic ketoacidosis is characterized by severe hyperglycemia, volume depletion, acidosis, depressed levels of consciousness and marked ketonemia.
- Patients are depleted in sodium, potassium, chloride and water. Despite potassium depletion, serum potassium is frequently elevated at the time of presentation.
- Prerenal azotemia may be present. Hyperglycemia, as well as high triglycerides and free fatty acids, may result in pseudohyponatremia.
- Diabetic ketoacidosis may be seen at first presentation in patients with type 1 diabetes and may also occur when insulin is discontinued.
- Diabetic ketoacidosis often occurs in patients with established diabetes who have a severe stressful illness, such as a severe infection, surgery, trauma or myocardial infarction.
- Patients with diabetic ketoacidosis should be hospitalized for therapy.

## Diabetes in Pregnancy

Carbohydrate intolerance during pregnancy can occur in patients who are either diabetic prior to pregnancy or become diabetic during pregnancy.

### Pre-existing Diabetes in Pregnancy

Poor diabetic control at the time of conception increases the risk of spontaneous abortion, prenatal mortality and morbidity and congenital malformations. Both retinal and renal disease may

Figure 2: **Stepwise Approach to Type 2 Diabetes**

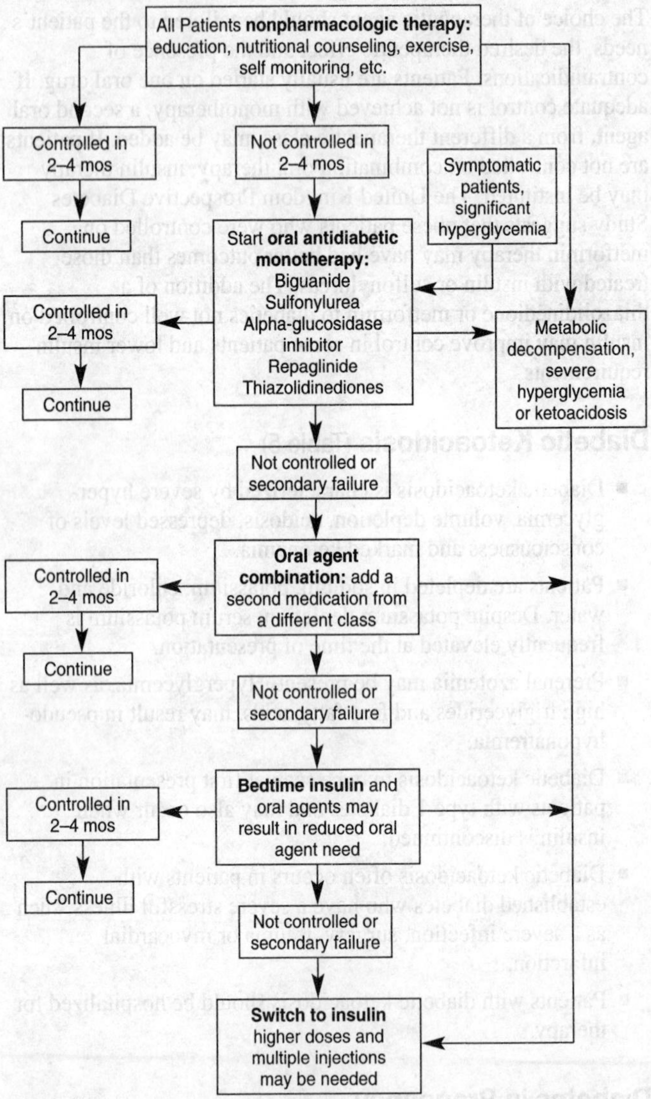
All Patients nonpharmacologic therapy: education, nutritional counseling, exercise, self monitoring, etc.
Controlled in 2–4 mos
Not controlled in 2–4 mos
Symptomatic patients, significant hyperglycemia
Continue
Start oral antidiabetic monotherapy: Biguanide Sulfonylurea Alpha-glucosidase inhibitor Repaglinide Thiazolidinediones
Controlled in 2–4 mos
Metabolic decompensation, severe hyperglycemia or ketoacidosis
Continue
Not controlled or secondary failure
Oral agent combination: add a second medication from a different class
Controlled in 2–4 mos
Continue
Not controlled or secondary failure
Bedtime insulin and oral agents may result in reduced oral agent need
Controlled in 2–4 mos
Continue
Not controlled or secondary failure
Switch to insulin higher doses and multiple injections may be needed

worsen significantly in the mother during pregnancy. Pregnancy should therefore be planned carefully. Patients are best followed by specialized diabetes health care teams with experience in the management of diabetic pregnancy. Diabetic control should be optimized prior to pregnancy and the patient carefully screened for microvascular complications. Oral hypoglycemic agents should be discontinued prior to conception, with control

Table 5: **Management of Diabetic Ketoacidosis**

| | |
|---|---|
| **Fluids**: Patient is always volume depleted (average 7 L). Normal saline (0.9% NaCl) 2 L in the first 2 hrs then individualize. A good urinary output is reassuring. May use 0.45% NaCl (½ NS) initially if serum glucose > 50 mmol/L. Change to IV 5% dextrose in water (D5W) when blood glucose drops to 14 mmol/L or less. | |
| **Insulin:** 10 units regular insulin as IV bolus followed by 0.1 U/kg/hr (5–10 U/hr). Best to mix 50 U in 500 mL NS and piggy back into main IV. | |
| **Potassium:** Potassium chloride is the preparation of choice. If serum $K^+$ < 3.5 mmol/L, add 40 mmol to each L of fluid; 3.5–5.5 mmol/L, add 20 mmol to each L of fluid; > 5.5 mmol/L, no added potassium especially if anuric. | |
| **Bicarbonate:** Sodium bicarbonate should be given if acidosis is severe (e.g., pH < 7.0) but only for partial correction (e.g., 10 mL 8.4% NaHCO3), then reassess. | |
| **Laboratory tests:** Initial CBC, glucose, electrolytes, urea, creatinine and ABG. Cultures as indicated. Radiology as indicated. Repeat electrolyte and glucose hourly, ABG only if continuing severe acidosis. | |
| **Supportive care:** Keep warm and rested. Nasogastric tube if vomiting, urinary catheter if anuric (may have significant retention). | |
| **Pitfalls:** Acetone smell may be absent, undetected or unrecognized by some.<br>Temperature may be low initially – absence of fever does not rule out infection.<br>Leukocytosis is usually present and does not necessarily mean infection.<br>Low serum sodium may be due to pseudohyponatremia.<br>High serum potassium is caused by acidosis and may be seen in spite of severe total body potassium depletion.<br>Ketostix detect aceto-acetate but not hydroxybutyrate.<br>Dehydration may mask a respiratory infection; reassess after rehydration and stabilization.<br>Severe abdominal pain or signs of an acute abdomen need to be reassessed after stabilization – they often disappear.<br>Premature switching to subcutaneous insulin and/or discharge result in high recurrence and readmission rates. | |

optimized either with diet or, if necessary, diet and insulin. If conception occurs in a patient treated with oral medications, these drugs should be stopped as soon as pregnancy is diagnosed and the patient switched to insulin for control of blood glucose.

## Gestational Diabetes (Figure 3)

Gestational diabetes is carbohydrate intolerance of varying severity detected, or first recognized, during pregnancy. It is associated with increased risk of macrosomia, neonatal hypoglycemia, hyperbilirubinemia, hypocalcemia and polycythemia. It may result in an increased risk of childhood obesity and diabetes in the offspring. Gestational diabetes indicates an increased risk for future diabetes in the mother.

Figure 3: **Diagnosis of Gestational Diabetes**

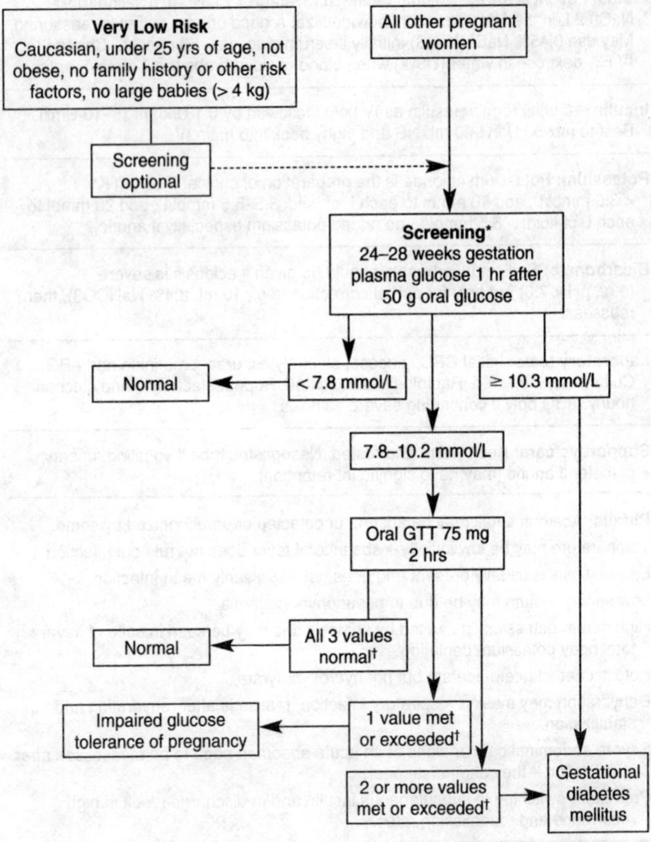
Very Low Risk
Caucasian, under 25 yrs of age, not obese, no family history or other risk factors, no large babies (> 4 kg)
All other pregnant women
Screening optional
Screening*
24–28 weeks gestation
plasma glucose 1 hr after 50 g oral glucose
Normal
< 7.8 mmol/L
≥ 10.3 mmol/L
7.8–10.2 mmol/L
Oral GTT 75 mg
2 hrs
Normal
All 3 values normal†
Impaired glucose tolerance of pregnancy
1 value met or exceeded†
2 or more values met or exceeded†
Gestational diabetes mellitus

* *Screening may be done earlier if very high risk or previous gestational diabetes mellitus.*

† *Abnormal values: Fasting > 5.3 mmol/L*
*1 hr > 10.6 mmol/L*
*2 hr > 8.9 mmol/L*

## Therapeutic Choices for Diabetes in Pregnancy

### Nonpharmacologic Choices

- **Dietary counseling** by a registered dietician is essential. Diet is best divided into meals and snacks. Diet should aim at providing the needs for the pregnant woman and the conceptus while avoiding starvation and ketosis.
- **Patient monitoring of pre-meal and post-meal blood glucose levels**. Targets for control are a fasting plasma glucose level of less than 5.3 mmol/L, and 1 and 2 hour postprandial glucose levels less than 7.8 mmol/L and

6.7 mmol/L, respectively. Elevated postprandial glucoses are more predictive of macrosomia than is the fasting plasma glucose.

- **Aerobic exercise**, particularly use of the upper body, should be encouraged.

## Pharmacologic Choices

**Insulin** is the only approved pharmacologic therapy for hyperglycemia in pregnant women. Its use should be tailored to achieve the targets outlined above. Such tight control frequently necessitates multidose insulin regimens. Women who have had gestational diabetes should have an oral glucose tolerance (75 g 2 hour) performed 6 weeks to 6 months postpartum to rule out the presence of ongoing glucose intolerance.

## Therapeutic Tips

- All diabetics should be assessed every 3 to 6 months. Their home monitoring records should be studied and the occurrence and frequency of hypoglycemia should be noted. Parameters to be followed include diabetic control, blood pressure levels, body weight changes and presence of complications. Foot examination is an integral part of such an examination.
- Inadequate control is frequently related to inadequate dietary compliance or poor adherence to medications.
- The use of snacks is important in diabetics on conventional insulin therapy and may be important in diabetics on sulfonylureas. Diabetics treated with acarbose, metformin, repaglinide, rapid-acting insulin-based multidose insulin regimens may not necessarily require snacks.
- All diabetics should be encouraged to wear a medi-alert bracelet or equivalent.

## Pharmacoeconomic Considerations

*Jeffrey A. Johnson, PhD*

The lifetime costs and benefits of intensive insulin therapy as practiced in the DCCT have been examined in only one study. For approximately 120 000 persons in the US who would meet the eligibility criteria for the DCCT, implementing intensive rather than conventional therapy would result in 611 000 years of life gained at an additional cost of $4.0 billion over the lifetime of the population. The incremental cost per year of life gained was $28 661, i.e., intensive therapy would cost $28 661 more than conventional therapy to gain one additional year of life. Such cost-effectiveness is considered to be a good value when compared to other health care interventions. This value, however, may not be completely applicable to the entire population of diabetic patients because of the strict criteria used in the DCCT. Economic evaluations of the United Kingdom Prospective Diabetes Study have also indicated that intensive policies are cost-effective, including the management of high blood pressure.

The use of ACE inhibitors in the prevention of diabetic nephropathy has also been evaluated from a pharmacoeconomic perspective. A cost-effectiveness analysis of three strategies in type 2 diabetes, either screening for gross proteinuria, screening for microalbuminuria, or treatment of all patients 50 years and older was recently published. The results suggest that treating all middle-aged diabetic patients with ACE inhibitors provided additional benefit at modest cost, with an incremental cost-utility ratio of $7500 (US) per QALY-gained.

***Suggested Reading***

*The DCCT Research Group. Lifetime benefits and costs of intensive therapy as practiced in the Diabetes Control and Complications Trial. JAMA 1996;276:1409–1415.*

*UK Prospective Diabetes Study Group. Cost-effectiveness analysis of improved blood pressure control in hypertensive patients with type 2 diabetes: UKPDS 40. BMJ 1998;317:720–726.*

*Golan L, Birkmeyer JD, Welch HG. The cost-effectiveness of treating all patients with type 2 diabetes with angiotensin-converting enzyme inhibitors. Ann Intern Med 1999;131:660–667.*

## Suggested Reading List

Canadian Diabetes Association: Clinical practice guidelines for the management of diabetes in Canada. *Can Med Assoc J* 1998;159 (suppl. 8) S1–S29.

DCCT Research Group: The effect of intensive treatment of diabetes on the development and progression of long term complications in insulin dependent diabetes mellitus. *N Engl J Med* 1993;329:977–986.

UKPDS Study Group: Intensive blood-glucose control with sulfonylureas or insulin compared with conventional treatment and risk of complications in patients with type 2 diabetes, (UKPDS 33). *Lancet* 1998;352:837–853.

American Diabetes Association: clinical practice recommendations 2000. *Diabetes Care* 2000;23:(suppl. 1).

Lebovitz HE, ed. *Therapy for diabetes and related disorders*. 3rd ed. Virginia: American Diabetes Association, 1999.

CHAPTER 75

# Thyroid Disorders

*Jay Silverberg, MD, FRCPC, FACP*

## Goals of Therapy

- To evaluate and manage patients with hyperthyroidism
- To diagnose and treat patients with hypothyroidism
- To differentiate between the various causes of thyroid enlargement and treat patients with goitres, particularly individuals with a solid nodule

## *Hyperthyroidism*

Hyperthyroidism is a syndrome characterized by excessive production and release of thyroid hormones (thyroxine [$T_4$] and triiodothyronine [$T_3$]). The more common causes of hyperthyroidism are:

- **Graves' disease** (the most common cause of hyperthyroidism) – caused by the production of an antibody capable of stimulating the thyrotrophin (TSH) receptor on the surface of thyroid cells.
- **Toxic adenoma** – a benign tumor of the thyroid capable of producing excessive amounts of thyroid hormones.
- **Toxic multinodular goitre** (found primarily in the elderly) – a condition in which thyroid follicles autonomously produce excess quantities of thyroid hormones.
- **Subacute thyroiditis** (and its variants) – results from the excessive release of thyroid hormone from an inflamed thyroid gland.
  - *classical subacute thyroiditis* – characterized by hyperthyroidism, as well as pain in the thyroid and malaise
  - *silent subacute thyroiditis* – associated only with hyperthyroidism (no pain in the thyroid or malaise)
  - *postpartum thyroiditis* – similar to silent subacute thyroiditis, but occurs in the postpartum period

Other rare causes of hyperthyroidism include:

- Iatrogenic hyperthyroidism
- Factitious hyperthyroidism, characterized by hyperthyroidism in a patient who has a small atrophic gland and a low 24-hour $^{131}I$ uptake
- Hyperthyroidism produced by extrathyroidal sources of thyroid hormone (certain teratomas of the ovary [struma ovarii] and rarely, metastatic follicular carcinoma of the thyroid)

- Hyperthyroidism caused by excessive TSH production (TSH-producing pituitary tumors [thyrotrophomas] or rarely, selective pituitary resistance to thyroid hormone)
- Hyperthyroidism resulting from the excessive production of the placental hormone human chorionic gonadotropin (hydatidiform mole or hyperemesis gravidarum)
- Hyperthyroidism caused by excessive administration of iodine (iod-Basedow's disease).

## Investigations

- A thorough history, with attention to weight loss, heat intolerance, excessive sweating, palpitation, increased frequency of bowel habits and tremulousness
- Physical findings, which may include tachycardia, goitre, warm moist skin and tremor. Patients with Graves' disease may also have eye findings (Graves' orbitopathy), skin changes (pretibial myxedema), and finger and joint changes (Graves' acropachy)
- Laboratory tests, including:
  - *TSH levels* – a key measurement. Except for TSH-dependent causes of hyperthyroidism, the serum TSH is undetectable. Keep in mind that pituitary and hypothalamic hypothyroidism, as well as the non-thyroidal illness syndrome, can be associated with a depressed TSH
  - *free thyroxine ($FT_4$)* and *free triiodothyronine ($FT_3$)* – elevated in all but the most subtle forms of hyperthyroidism
  - *anti-thyroperoxidase (anti-TPO)* and *anti-thyroglobulin (anti-Tg) antibodies* – usually elevated in Graves' disease and occasionally in subacute thyroiditis
  - *$^{131}I$ uptake and pertechnetate scan of the thyroid* – important investigations to differentiate among the 4 common causes of hyperthyroidism previously described

## Therapeutic Choices

### Nonpharmacologic Choices

- Adequate nutrition, hydration and rest (especially in the elderly) – because all hyperthyroid patients are hypermetabolic
- Radioactive iodine ($^{131}I$) – can be used to treat most forms of hyperthyroidism, except subacute thyroiditis. May be used in children, but never in pregnancy. Main drawbacks are post-ablative hypothyroidism and occasional exacerbation of Graves' orbitopathy (this usually occurs in patients with orbitopathy already present before treatment).

- Subtotal thyroidectomy in patients with Graves' disease, a toxic adenoma or a toxic multinodular goitre – restores patients to euthyroidism faster than any other form of treatment. Main concerns are damage to the recurrent laryngeal nerve, which may result in hoarseness, or damage to the parathyroid glands. In the hands of a skilled surgeon, these complications are rare.

**Pharmacologic Choices** (Table 1)

- The thionamide drugs **propylthiouracil** (PTU) and **methimazole** (MMI) are important in the management of hyperthyroid patients, with the exception of patients with subacute thyroiditis.
  – both drugs decrease the thyroid production of $T_4$ and $T_3$
  – PTU also reduces the conversion of $T_4$ to $T_3$
  – several weeks to months of treatment with PTU or MMI restores euthyroidism in Graves' patients
  – PTU and MMI should be given for 1 to 2 years; at the end of this time, 17 to 50% of patients will be in remission. Generally, women with small goitres and mild hyperthyroidism are most likely to go into remission after a course of PTU or MMI treatment
  – important adverse effects include gastrointestinal upset, mild elevation in liver enzymes and rash. Rarer, but more serious, adverse effects include liver toxicity and agranulocytosis.
  – care must be taken in prescribing PTU or MMI during pregnancy because these drugs cross the placenta and can cause fetal goitre and hypothyroidism. Many clinicians use only PTU in pregnancy because of the unresolved contention that MMI may cause the rare congenital complication, aplasia cutis, in offspring.
  – daily dose of PTU in pregnancy should never be higher than 200 mg during the third trimester of pregnancy.
  – PTU is the drug recommended for women who wish to nurse.
- **Iodine**, given orally or intravenously as a saturated solution of potassium iodide or as Lugol's solution to patients with Graves' disease scheduled for surgery, lowers thyroid hormone production and decreases the vascularity of the gland.
- **Lithium**, **glucocorticoids**, and **sodium ipodate** have occasionally been used as second-line drugs in unusual circumstances.
- **Beta-blockers** are important adjuvant drugs because they reduce hyperthyroid symptoms caused by excessive beta adrenergic stimulation (e.g., palpitations, tremor and sweating). Beta-blockers generally do not alter circulating $T_4$ levels. However, nonselective beta-blockers, such as propranolol, may decrease circulating $T_3$ levels.

### Thyroid Storm

Thyroid storm is a rare medical emergency and is characterized by thyrotoxicosis, with fever, and tachycardia or tachyarrhythmias, and altered mental status. It occurs more often in the elderly, when an untreated, or under-treated, hyperthyroid patient suffers a concurrent stress (e.g., pneumonia). Thyroid storm must be treated aggressively because its mortality is high. Treatment includes:

- high doses of **PTU** (up to 1200 mg per day) or **MMI** (up to 80 mg per day), as well as IV sodium iodide (0.5 to 1 g every 12 hours) or Lugol's solution (8 drops PO every 6 hours)
- **beta-blockers** (e.g., propranolol 40 to 120 mg every 6 hours orally or 0.5 to 2 mg IV over 15 minutes every 6 hours) with cardiac monitoring and **glucocorticoids** (e.g., hydrocortisone 300 mg IV followed by 100 mg IV every 8 hours)
- ensuring that hyperpyrexia, congestive heart failure, cardiac arrhythmias and dehydration are properly managed.

### Hypothyroidism

Hypothyroidism is a syndrome characterized by low circulating levels of $T_4$ and $T_3$, or rarely, tissue resistance to the thyroid hormones. Hypothyroidism can result from pathology in:

- the thyroid (primary hypothyroidism)
- the pituitary (secondary hypothyroidism)
- the hypothalamus (tertiary hypothyroidism)
- the peripheral tissues (generalized resistance to thyroid hormones, usually caused by a defect in the beta receptor for $T_4$ and $T_3$)

Some important causes of primary hypothyroidism include:

- Hashimoto's thyroiditis, an autoimmune form of hypothyroidism
- post-ablative hypothyroidism, usually resulting from the use of $^{131}$I for Graves' disease
- the hypothyroid phase of subacute thyroiditis
- infiltrative diseases, such as amyloidosis
- congenital causes, such as aplasia of the thyroid or dyshormonogenesis
- drugs (e.g., lithium)
- ingestion of goitrogens (e.g., cassava)
- iodine deficiency (rare in North America)

## Investigations

- A thorough history, with attention to weight gain, fatigue, cold intolerance, slow pulse, dry hair and skin, and cognitive and mood changes

- Physical findings, which include goitre, bradycardia, coarse hair, dry skin, facial puffiness, slowing of thought processes, depressed mood and delayed deep tendon reflexes
- Laboratory tests, including:
  - *TSH measurement* – probably the most important laboratory investigation. The TSH is elevated in primary hypothyroidism and low or low-normal in secondary or tertiary hypothyroidism. In generalized resistance to thyroid hormones, the TSH is in the high normal range, or elevated
  - *free $T_4$ and free $T_3$ levels* – decreased or low-normal in primary, secondary and tertiary hypothyroidism; increased in generalized resistance to thyroid hormones
  - *anti-thyroperoxidase (anti-TPO) and anti-thyroglobulin (anti-Tg)* – elevated in Hashimoto's thyroiditis and occasionally in subacute thyroiditis

## Therapeutic Choices

### Pharmacologic Choices (Table 1)

- **Sodium levothyroxine** is the currently accepted treatment for all types of hypothyroidism (iodine may be used to treat iodine deficiency and certain congenital types of hypothyroidism, but this is not usually an issue in clinical practice)
  - usual initial dosage is 6 to 10 μg/kg/day for newborns, and 1.6 μg/kg once daily for adults. Adjust dosage until serum TSH is within the normal range.
  - changes in dosage should not take place more frequently than every 4 to 6 weeks
  - levothyroxine is usually well tolerated, and generally without adverse effects when used in the appropriate dosage.
  - individuals with coronary heart disease may experience an exacerbation of angina if they are placed on a full therapeutic dose of levothyroxine immediately. In these patients, treatment is usually initiated at a very low dose (12.5 μg/day) and slowly titrated upwards every 4 weeks until the TSH is normalized
  - patients with elevated TSH levels, but normal concentrations of circulating thyroid hormones, have a condition known as compensated hypothyroidism; this condition is particularly common in elderly patients. Treatment of compensated hypothyroidism is controversial. Generally, treatment with levothyroxine is instituted if the TSH is greater than 10 mU/L, if positive titres of anti-TPO and anti-Tg antibodies are present, or if the patient has suggestive symptoms.

Table 1: **Drugs Used in Thyroid Disorders**

| Drug | Dosage | Adverse Drug Reactions | Drug Interactions | Comments | Cost* |
|---|---|---|---|---|---|
| *radioactive iodine* ($^{131}I$) | Hyperthyroidism: 5–10 mCi in Graves' disease, 15–29 mCi in toxic adenoma and toxic multinodular goitre | Hypothyroidism. Usually none; new patients may suffer some thyroiditis, occasionally with mild pain. Nausea may occur. Occasional exacerbation of Graves' orbitopathy. | | A single dose usually cures patients with Graves' disease. | $$$$$ per dose |
| *propylthiouracil* ‡ Propyl-Thyracil | Hyperthyroidism: 50–100 mg PO BID–QID. Thyroid storm: Up to 1200 mg/day divided Q4–6H | GI upset, rash, elevated liver function tests (not common), neutropenia (rare, but most serious of side effects; usually reversible with discontinuation of the drug, but may present with serious bacterial sepsis). | Oral anticoagulants – altered hypothrombinemic response; monitor prothrombin time. | Patients started on either drug should be counseled regarding side effects. Methimazole should not be used in pregnancy or lactation. | $–$$$ |
| *methimazole* ‡ Tapazole | Hyperthyroidism: 5–10 mg PO BID–QID. Thyroid storm: Up to 80 mg/day divided Q4–6H | | | | $–$$$ |
| *iodine* Lugol's solution (Strong Iodine Solution) | Before thyroidectomy: 2–6 drops Lugol's sol'n TID for 10 days before surgery. Thyroid storm: 8 drops of Lugol's sol'n Q6H for 2–3 days or sodium iodide 0.5–1 g IV Q12H, given after PTU or MMI has been started. | Hypersensitivity reactions: skin rashes, mucous membrane ulcers, anaphylaxis, metallic taste, rhinorrhea, parotid and submaxillary swelling. | | Must not be used before PTU or MMI for thyrotoxic crisis. If used, $^{131}I$ therapy cannot be used in the short term. | $† |

| | | | | | |
|---|---|---|---|---|---|
| *propranolol*<br>Inderal, generics | Hyperthyroidism: 20–40 mg PO BID<br>Painless (silent) thyroiditis: 10–20 mg PO BID<br>Thyroid storm: 40–120 mg PO Q6H or 0.5–2 mg IV over 15 min Q6H with cardiac monitoring. Titrate dose cautiously based on cardiac status. | Bradycardia, hypotension, dyspnea, fatigue, depression. | With digoxin, $Ca^{++}$ channel blockers, amiodarone, additive bradycardia. | Contraindicated in patients with asthma or congestive heart failure. | $ |
| *dexamethasone*<br>Decadron, generics<br>*hydrocortisone*<br>A-Hydrocort, Solu-Cortef, generics | Thyroid storm: dexamethasone 2 mg PO Q6H or hydrocortisone 300 mg IV followed by 100 mg Q8H (for 2–3 days or until stable)<br>Myxedema coma: hydrocortisone 100 mg IV Q8–12H until patient is stable | Glucose intolerance, weight gain, mood alteration, hypertension, osteoporosis, adrenal suppression, cataracts, myopathy. | With barbiturates, phenytoin, and rifampin (may ↓ steroid effect). | | $[π]<br>$$$–$$$$[π] |
| *levothyroxine ($L\text{-}T_4$)*<br>Eltroxin, Synthroid, generics | Hypothyroidism: Initially, 1.6 µg/kg/day PO, titrated with serum TSH Q6–12 wks until TSH normalizes. Newborns – 6–10 µg/kg/day<br>Myxedema coma: Initially, 300–500 µg IV, followed by 100 µg daily, given IV or PO | Due to overdosage and induced hyperthyroidism (e.g., heat intolerance, weakness, fatigue, nervousness, insomnia, tachycardia). | Cholestyramine, colestipol, ferrous sulfate and sucralfate decrease thyroxine absorption.<br>Anticonvulsants and rifampin accelerate thyroxine metabolism.<br>Effects of oral anticoagulants are ↑ by $T_4$; monitor for excessive hypoprothrombinemia.<br>Dose of antidiabetic agent may need to be ↑; monitor blood glucose. | Sensitive TSH assays allow dosing to be individualized.<br>When stable, TSH levels should only be performed at intervals of 6–12 mos. | $ |

† *Extemporaneously compounded.*

‡ *Initial doses are arbitrary. Patients with larger goitres and more active disease may require larger initial doses.*

π *Cost of 3 days of therapy.*

* *Cost of 30-day supply – includes drug cost only.*

*Legend:* $ < $10  $$ $10–20  $$$ $20–30  $$$$ $30–60  $$$$$ > $60

**Myxedema coma** is a rare condition with a high mortality. It is characterized by profound hypothyroidism manifested by hypothermia, bradycardia, hypotension, hypoventilation and coma. Myxedema coma is usually present in elderly patients with neglected or severe undiagnosed hypothyroidism. These patients often have a major concurrent illness.
Therapy should be directed towards:
- correcting hypothermia
- addressing acid-base and electrolyte abnormalities
- managing respiratory and cardiovascular problems
- administering thyroid hormone replacement. High doses of **levothyroxine** (e.g., 300 to 500 μg IV followed by 100 μg per day) are often required. Glucocorticoids are often given but their use remains unproven.

## *Thyroid Enlargement (Goitre)*

Any enlargement of the thyroid gland is termed a goitre. Goitres are often classified as nodular or diffuse. Many of the conditions noted under the above sections on hyperthyroidism and hypothyroidism are associated with goitre. Many goitres are also associated with euthyroidism and are frequently found in middle-aged and elderly individuals. The cause of these goitres is not known.

### Investigations

- A thorough history, addressing dysphagia, stridor, voice changes, neck pain and any symptoms of hyperthyroidism or hypothyroidism
- Physical examination, documenting the size of the goitre, its texture and nodularity and whether it moves with swallowing, as well as any signs of hyperthyroidism or hypothyroidism
- Laboratory tests, including:
  - *TSH levels* – will determine if the goitre is associated with hyper- or hypothyroidism
  - *anti-TPO and anti-Tg antibodies* – will determine if the goitre is the result of an autoimmune process
  - *thyroid ultrasound* – will give an objective measurement of the goitre size or any nodule contained therein
  - *thyroid pertechnetate scan* – will provide information on whether any nodules contained in the goitre are "cold, warm, or hot"

## Therapeutic Choices

### Nonpharmacologic Choices

Any large goitre that causes compressive symptoms or raises malignancy concerns requires surgery.

### Pharmacologic Choices

Some goitres will shrink with **levothyroxine** therapy. When using levothyroxine in this context, titrate the dosage until the TSH level is in the low-normal or slightly depressed range.

## *Single Thyroid Nodule*

A single thyroid nodule, or a dominant thyroid nodule in a multinodular goitre, is an important problem because this type of nodule may be malignant. However, most of these nodules are benign.

## Investigations

- A thorough history, focusing on factors that may raise suspicion that a thyroid nodule may be malignant, including:
  - male sex
  - a nodule that appears for the first time in a young or elderly individual
  - a nodule that rapidly increases in size
  - a history of irradiation to the neck
- Physical examination frequently cannot distinguish a benign from a malignant nodule. Any nodule that does not move with swallowing should be viewed with suspicion
- Laboratory tests may help identify the nature of a thyroid nodule. These include:
  - *TSH level* – will assist in determining whether the nodule is a toxic nodule. Toxic nodules are associated with a decreased TSH level and are seldom malignant
  - *thyroid ultrasound* – will reveal if the nodule is solid or cystic. It will not, however, determine if a nodule is benign or malignant
  - *thyroid pertechnetate scan* – frequently done to determine if the nodule is "cold". Generally, most malignant nodules are cold on scanning. However, the majority of cold nodules are benign. Thus, this test has only limited value
  - *fine needle aspiration biopsy of the nodule* – by far the most useful test to determine the nature of the thyroid nodule. This test usually provides enough information to decide whether a nodule is likely benign and can be followed conservatively, or whether the nodule is likely malignant and requires surgery

## Therapeutic Choices

### Nonpharmacologic Choices

- **Surgery** – remove any nodule that is suspicious for a thyroid malignancy, on the basis of a cytological examination. If surgery confirms a malignancy, perform a total thyroidectomy, except for the smallest of thyroid cancers.
- **Radioactive iodine ($^{131}I$)** – administer several weeks after surgery, once hypothyroidism is established, to patients with well-differentiated thyroid cancer.

### Pharmacologic Choices

- **Levothyroxine**, in suppressive doses, is sometimes used to treat benign thyroid nodules in an attempt to shrink the nodule. This therapy is often unsuccessful. Patients who have undergone total thyroidectomy and $^{131}I$ therapy for a well-differentiated thyroid cancer are kept on levothyroxine in doses sufficient to keep the TSH at an undetectable level.

## *Suggested Reading List*


Arem R, Escalante D. Subclinical hypothyroidism: epidemiology, diagnosis, and significance. *Adv Intern Med* 1996;213–250.

Dabon-Almirante CL, Surks MI. Clinical and laboratory diagnosis of thyrotoxicosis. In: *Endocrinology and metabolism clinics of North America*. Vol. 27. Philadelphia: W.B. Saunders, 1998:25–35.

Hefland M, Redfern CC. Screening for thyroid disease: an update. *Ann Intern Med* 1998;129:144–158.

Mckenzie JM, Zakarija M. Hyperthyroidism. In: DeGroot LJ, ed. *Endocrinology*. 3rd ed. Philadelphia: W.B. Saunders, 1995:676–711.

Surks MI, Chopra IJ, Mariash CN, et al. American Thyroid Association guidelines for use of laboratory test in thyroid disorders. *JAMA* 1990;263:1529–1532.

CHAPTER 76

# Common Anemias

*N. Blair Whittemore, MD, FRCPC*

The treatments of **iron deficiency anemia, megaloblastic anemia** and **anemias which respond to erythropoietin** are discussed in this chapter.

## Definition

- In general, patients with hemoglobin (Hgb) values 2 standard deviations below the mean should be considered anemic and require investigation.
- Normal mean Hgb for men is 155 ± 20 g/L; for women, 140 ± 20 g/L

*Note:* Occasionally patients may be "normal" with Hgb values below 2 standard deviations of the mean, but one must exclude occult disease. Previous hemogram values are valuable in determining the significance of the current result.

## Goals of Therapy

- To determine the etiology of the anemia and replace any identified deficiencies

## Investigations

- History and physical examination including:
  - medication intake: antineoplastic and zidovudine therapy will usually cause macrocytosis; several drugs are associated with altered folate metabolism and macrocytosis including anticonvulsants (phenytoin, primidone), triamterene, trimethoprim and oral contraceptives
  - alcohol intake
  - dietary history (strict vegetarians are at risk of vitamin $B_{12}$ deficiency)
  - gastric or small bowel surgery (terminal ileal resection) may predispose to $B_{12}$ deficiency
  - chronic blood loss and other potential causes of iron deficiency
  - chronic inflammatory or malignant disease
  - diminished hepatic, renal or thyroid function
- Laboratory tests:
  - RBC indices, Hgb, hematocrit, white blood cell (WBC) count with differential, peripheral blood smear

- serum iron, total iron-binding capacity (TIBC), serum ferritin
- stool for occult blood
- other tests may include liver function tests, *red cell* folate rather than serum folate (the former is a better reflection of folate stores), serum $B_{12}$; with low serum $B_{12}$ levels, a Schilling test with and without intrinsic factor, plus serum antibody to intrinsic factor should be done to clarify etiology
- urine for RBC, hemoglobinuria

## Morphologic Classification of Anemia

- **microcytic:** low mean corpuscular volume (MCV) (Table 1)
- **normocytic:** normal MCV
- **macrocytic:** high MCV (Table 2). A falsely elevated MCV may be caused by cold agglutinins or marked leukocytosis, readily seen on a peripheral blood smear

Table 1: **Laboratory Evaluation of Microcytosis**

| Cause | Serum Fe | TIBC | % saturation | Ferritin | Bone marrow Fe stores | Hgb $A_2$ and Hgb F |
|---|---|---|---|---|---|---|
| Iron deficiency (Table 2) | ↓ | ↑ | ↓ | ↓ | 0 | N |
| Anemia of chronic disease | ↓ | N or ↓ | N or ↓ | N or ↑ | N or ↑ | N |
| Thalassemia trait | N | N | N | N or ↑ | N | ↑ β thal, N α thal |
| Sideroblastic anemia | N or ↑ | N or ↑ | N or ↑ | N or ↑ | ↑ | N |

*Abbreviations:* ↑ *= increased;* ↓ *= decreased; N = normal; 0 = none; TIBC = total iron-binding capacity; Hgb $A_2$ = $A_2$ hemoglobin; Hgb F = fetal hemoglobin; β thal = β thalassemia; α thal = α thalassemia.*

Table 2: **Appearance on Peripheral Smear of Some Causes of Macrocytosis**

| Appearance on Smear | Causes |
|---|---|
| Round macrocytes with target cells | Alcoholism or liver disease |
| Oval macrocytes with hypersegmented neutrophils | $B_{12}$ or folate deficiency (megaloblastic anemia) |
| Dimorphic red cell picture with or without hyposegmented neutrophils | Myelodysplasia |

## Iron Deficiency Anemia

### Table 3: Potential Causes of Iron Deficiency Anemia

Inadequate ingestion (dietary deficiency or increased requirements)
- Growth spurts in infants, young children, adolescents
- Pregnancy
- Elderly "tea and toaster" (investigate other causes first)

Impaired absorption
- Partial gastrectomy
- Malabsorption syndromes

Blood loss (most important cause)
- Genitourinary
  - Menstruation (most likely in women 15–45 yrs)
- Gastrointestinal (most likely in men and postmenopausal women)
  - Peptic ulcer
  - Hiatus hernia
  - Cancer
  - Telangiectasia
  - Jogger's anemia
- Phlebotomy
  - Polycythemia
  - Blood donor
  - Diagnostic phlebotomy
- Trauma/surgery

## Therapeutic Choices

### Pharmacologic Choices (Table 4)

#### *Iron Supplements*

Various oral iron salts are available; they differ in their elemental iron content (see below).

| Salt | mg/tablet | mg elemental Fe/tablet |
|---|---|---|
| Ferrous sulfate | 300 | 60 |
| Ferrous gluconate | 300 | 35 |
| Ferrous fumarate | 200 | 66 |
| Ferrous ascorbate | 275 | 33 |

With the diagnosis of iron deficiency anemia established, **oral iron replacement therapy** may be started immediately while the underlying cause is sought. Approximately 30 mg of elemental iron is absorbed from a dose of 180 mg of elemental iron per day. The Hgb should rise 10 g/L every 7 to 10 days if there are no complicating features (e.g., continued blood loss or impaired marrow production).

Upon restoration of the Hgb, iron stores begin to be replenished. This may take a further 6 to 9 months and can be monitored by measuring serum ferritin. Replenishing iron stores may be very difficult or only transient if menstruation causes the deficiency. In such cases it may be necessary to continue iron therapy (30 to 60 mg elemental iron per day) until menopause.

If there is a benign cause of recurrent bleeding for which surgery is not indicated, oral iron therapy may be continued indefinitely. **Parenteral iron therapy** is required infrequently. Indications for its use are malabsorption/intolerance to oral iron preparations and iron losses exceeding maximal oral replacement. *Note:* Response to oral and parenteral iron occurs at the same rate in normal circumstances.

## Therapeutic Tips

- The cause of anemia should be established; iron deficiency is only a sign.
- Failure to respond to therapy may reflect:
  - continued bleeding, but there should be a good reticulocyte response indicating active red cell production
  - inadequate dose or duration of therapy
  - poor compliance
  - associated disease (e.g., inflammatory states, neoplastic disease) or concomitant deficiency (vitamin $B_{12}$, folic acid, thyroid)
  - incorrect diagnosis, for which a bone marrow aspirate is probably required
- Oral iron therapy is preferred.
- If GI side effects occur with oral iron, stopping therapy for 3 to 4 days and resuming at a lower dose may be helpful as this effect appears to be related to the amount of elemental iron. Switching to a liquid preparation to regulate dosage more precisely may also help.
- Nonenteric-coated iron salts should be used. Enteric-coated and time-released iron preparations are intended to reduce side effects but may be ineffective because of failure to release iron in the gastric environment.
- There is little evidence to support the therapeutic advantage of preparations of iron combined with substances to enhance iron absorption (e.g., ascorbic acid) and they are considerably more expensive.
- Treatment should continue long enough to replenish iron stores.

## *Megaloblastic Anemia*

Megaloblastic anemia (MCV > 100 fL) occurs due to a deficiency of vitamin $B_{12}$ or folate. Paresthesias with or without ataxia are the most common neurologic manifestations and may be present before anemia or macrocytosis.

Evaluation of macrocytosis should include serum folate, red cell folate and serum $B_{12}$ to differentiate single deficiency of $B_{12}$ or folate from combined deficiency.

Major causes of macrocytic anemia include alcoholism, folate/vitamin $B_{12}$ deficiency and chemotherapy.

## Therapeutic Choices

### Nonpharmacologic Choices

For those with alcoholism, *abstinence* is necessary to reverse the macrocytosis.

### Pharmacologic Choices (Table 4)

#### *Vitamin $B_{12}$*

Vitamin $B_{12}$ (cyanocobalamin or hydroxocobalamin) is given in amounts sufficient to meet the daily needs of 2 to 3 μg and replenish tissue stores of 1 to 2 mg.

Parenteral therapy is necessary in $B_{12}$ deficiency secondary to *lack of intrinsic factor or malabsorption*. Hydroxocobalamin has some advantage theoretically, but from a practical point of view cyanocobalamin is satisfactory and more readily available. Doses greater than 100 μg per day exceed available binding sites; the excess is renally excreted. Oral therapy with large daily doses (1000 μg) of vitamin $B_{12}$ has been used, but unpredictable absorption, cost and compliance make it of questionable value.

In those with *dietary* deficiency, oral therapy with 200 to 500 μg per day is satisfactory; parenteral administration to replenish $B_{12}$ stores may be considered to ensure compliance and correction of the deficiency. Lower doses prevent dietary deficiency. This may be provided via a multivitamin tablet containing at least 15 μg of vitamin $B_{12}$.

#### *Folic Acid*

Inadvertent administration of pharmacologic doses of folic acid may aggravate the neurologic deficit seen in patients with neurologic manifestations secondary to vitamin $B_{12}$ deficiency. Thus, folic acid should be administered **only** for folic acid deficiency or prophylactically where there is increased demand (e.g., pregnancy[1] or hemolysis).

Although a parenteral preparation is available, folic acid deficiency is generally treated orally; even in patients with malabsorption, the relatively large doses (usually 1 mg per day with the daily requirement being 100 to 400 μg) permit sufficient absorption to correct the deficiency.

---

[1] *For recommended intake in pregnant women at high risk of having a pregnancy affected with a neural tube defect, see Chapter 98.*

Table 4: **Drugs Used to Treat Anemia**

| Drug | Dosage | Adverse Effects | Comments | Cost* |
|---|---|---|---|---|
| **Iron Deficiency Anemia** | | | | |
| **Oral Ferrous Salts†** | 100–195 mg elemental Fe/d<br>Usual: 180 mg elemental Fe/d divided TID | GI (nausea, epigastric distress, constipation and/or diarrhea). | Preferred replacement therapy (safe, inexpensive, generally well tolerated). Optimal absorption occurs on an empty stomach, but frequency of GI side effects may ↑ (dose-related). Starting treatment with 1 tablet daily after a meal × 7–10 d and ↑ step-wise to 1 tablet after each meal often prevents side effects.<br>No iron salt has a particular advantage over another.<br>Iron ↓ absorption of etidronate, tetracycline, levodopa, penicillamine, fluoroquinolones, methyldopa, levothyroxine (separate administration by 2 h).<br>↓ hematological response to iron with concomitant vitamin E, chloramphenicol.<br>↓ absorption of iron with concomitant use of cholestyramine, antacids containing aluminum/magnesium salts, sodium bicarbonate, calcium carbonate. | |
| *ferrous sulfate*<br>many | | | | $ |
| *ferrous gluconate*<br>many | | | | $ |
| *ferrous fumarate*<br>Palafer, generics | | | | $ |
| *polysaccharide-iron complex*<br>Niferex-150 | 150 mg elemental Fe/d | Well-absorbed, excellent GI tolerance (indicated for patients who cannot tolerate other oral iron salts). | | $ |
| **Parenteral Iron** | Total dose = Hgb iron deficit + amount needed to replenish iron stores (refer to manufacturers' information for details) | IM: Discomfort and temporary discoloration at injection site, localized/generalized urticaria, transient metallic taste (common) rarely accompanied by loss of taste, nausea, vomiting, headache, dizziness, flushing of face, palpitations and sensations of pressure in the chest (occasional). | Iron sorbitol: given deep IM into upper outer quadrant of buttock by Z-track technique (↓ or prevents tracking to SC tissues and resultant discoloration, which may persist for years). | |
| *iron sorbitol*<br>Jectofer (IM) | | | | $2.70/100 mg |
| *iron dextran*<br>Dexiron (IV) | | | | $26.20/100 mg |
| Infufer (IV) | | | | $28.60/100 mg |

| | | | |
|---|---|---|---|
| **Parenteral iron** *(cont'd)* | | Systemic adverse effects occur more commonly with larger than normal doses, especially in underweight people.<br>IV: Anaphylaxis (< 1%), arthralgia, fever, myalgia, headache, GI distress, urticaria, exacerbation of arthritic symptoms in those with rheumatoid arthritis (may be managed with acetaminophen). | |
| **Megaloblastic Anemia** | | | |
| **Parenteral Vitamin $B_{12}$**<br>*cyanocobalamin*<br>Rubramin, generics<br>*hydroxocobalamin*<br>generics | Suggested approach:<br>100 µg cyanocobalamin SC/IM daily × 1 wk, then 200 µg SC/IM weekly × 8–10 wks, then 200 µg SC/IM monthly for life | Usually nontoxic. However, mild transient diarrhea, peripheral vascular thrombosis, itching, transitory exanthema, feeling of swelling of entire body, pulmonary edema and congestive heart failure early in treatment and anaphylactic shock have been reported. | <br><br>$<br><br>$ |
| **Folic Acid**<br>generics | 1 mg/d | Allergic reactions including erythema, pruritus and/or urticaria. | $ |

† *Liquid preparations are more expensive.*

* *Cost of 30-day supply – includes drug cost only.*
*Legend: $ < $10*

### Therapeutic Tips

- Serum potassium should be monitored carefully in patients with severe pernicious anemia complicated by heart failure. Administration of diuretics and the intracellular shift of potassium associated with rapid reticulocytosis may cause hypokalemia and its complications unless supplementary potassium is given. Serum $K^+$ should be monitored daily for the first 3 to 5 days of diuretic treatment.
- As Hgb rises in response to vitamin $B_{12}$, the MCV gradually decreases and the patient may become microcytic, with Hgb plateauing below normal. If this occurs, oral iron should be added to therapy to achieve the maximum Hgb response.

## *Anemias Treated with Erythropoietin*

Erythropoietin is a glycoprotein produced primarily by the peritubular capillary adventitial cells of the kidney and, to a lesser extent, by the Kupffer cells of the liver. It is essential for the synthesis of hemoglobin.

**Recombinant erythropoietin** has been approved for the treatment of anemia caused by *chronic renal failure*, *cancer* or *cancer therapy in non-myeloid malignancies*, in *patients infected with the HIV virus who are undergoing zidovudine therapy*, in *patients undergoing elective surgery* with hematocrits less than 39% with an estimated blood loss of 1000 to 3000 mL and in *those donating autologous blood before surgery* (Table 5).

Maintenance doses for each indication must be individualized and should be the lowest possible to maintain the desired hemoglobin level, decreasing by 25 to 50 IU/kg/dose Q 4 to 8 weeks.

Adverse effects are not common but may include headache, nausea, diarrhea, arthralgia, hypertension and allergic reactions. Uncontrolled hypertension is a contraindication to initiation of erythropoietin therapy. In patients with chronic renal failure, blood pressure must be closely monitored and well controlled. If the hematocrit rise exceeds 4% in any two week period, erythropoietin should be reduced or withheld as this may aggravate hypertension or seizures.

Serum $B_{12}$, red cell folate and serum ferritin levels should be assesssed with the latter being at least 100 ng/mL.

**Iron supplements** should be given to patients with lower values throughout erythropoietin therapy.

Erythropoietin is expensive (possibly more than $400/week) and coverage by provincial and private insurance plans varies from province to province; thus, one should inform the patient and check their plan before initiating therapy.

Table 5: **Dosage of Erythropoietin**

| Condition | Erythropoietin Dose | |
|---|---|---|
| | **Initial** | **Increments** |
| ***Chronic Renal Failure*** | 50–100 IU/kg SC 3 ×/wk × 8 wks | 25–50 IU/kg SC 3 ×/wk Q 8 wks to maximum of 300 IU/kg<br>When Hgb approaches 120 g/L, ↓ dosage by 25 IU/kg/dose |
| ***Cancer or Cancer Therapy (erythropoietin level ≤ 500 mu/mL)*** | 150 IU/kg SC 3 ×/wk | 50 IU/kg/dose SC 3 ×/wk Q 8 wks to a maximum of 300 IU/kg<br>If Hgb increases by more than 20 g/L/month, ↓ dose by 25%; if no ↑ with maximum dose, therapy should be discontinued. |
| ***Zidovudine-treated HIV patient (erythropoietin level ≤ 500 mu/mL)*** | 100 IU/kg SC 3 ×/wk | 50 IU/kg/dose Q 8 wks to a maximum of 300 IU/kg |
| ***Pre-operative*** | 600 IU/kg SC on days -21, -14, -7 and day of surgery | |

## *Suggested Reading List*


Brown RG. Determining the cause of anemia. *Postgrad Med* 1991;89:161–170.

Massey AC. Microcytic anemia. Differential diagnosis and management of iron deficiency anemia. *Med Clin North Am* 1992;76:549–566.

Schilling RF. Anemia of chronic disease: a misnomer. *Ann Intern Med* 1991;115:572–573.

Wymer A, Becker DM. Recognition and evaluation of red blood cell macrocytosis in the primary care setting. *J Gen Intern Med* 1990;5:192–197.

CHAPTER 77

# Dehydration in Children

*Gary I. Joubert, MD, FRCPC*

## Goals of Therapy

- To treat shock/impending shock
- To treat dehydration using an appropriate fluid and route
- To treat electrolyte imbalances
- To prevent complications (seizures or edema)

## Fluids in Infants and Children

Newborn and young children have a much higher water content than adolescents and adults (Table 1) and are more prone to both water and salt (sodium [$Na^+$], potassium [$K^+$]) loss during illness.

Table 1: **Age vs Percentage of Body Water**

| Age | % Body Water |
|---|---|
| Newborn | 75–80 |
| Child ≤ 1 yr | 70–75 |
| Child 1–12 yrs | 60-70 |
| Adolescent/adult | 55–60 |

## Investigations

- Thorough history with attention to:
  – underlying cause(s): vomiting and/or diarrhea or other excessive fluid loss
  – frequency and amount of loss
  – frequency and amount of urinary output
- Physical examination to assess clinical manifestations and degree of dehydration
- Laboratory tests: electrolytes, BUN, creatinine, glucose, urinalysis as indicated clinically

The **assessment of dehydration** in infants and children is challenging (Table 2). This difficulty is related to a child's ability to maintain adequate blood pressure in the face of moderate to severe dehydration.

Table 2: **Estimation of Dehydration**

| Extent of Dehydration | Mild | Moderate | Severe |
|---|---|---|---|
| **Weight loss – Infants** (under 1 yr) | 5% | 10% | 15% |
| **Weight loss – Children** (over 1 yr) | 3–4% | 6–8% | 10% |
| **History** | decreased intake<br>duration of illness<br>decreased urine output<br>activity<br>frequency of vomiting<br>diarrhea | decreased intake<br>duration<br>frequency of vomiting and diarrhea<br>marked decreased urine<br>listless, weight loss | very decreased intake<br>longer duration<br>frequency of vomiting and diarrhea<br>anuria<br>obtunded |
| **Pulse** | normal | slightly increased | rapid |
| **Blood pressure** | normal | normal to orthostatic, > 10 mm Hg change | orthostatic to shock |
| **Behavior** | normal | irritable | hyperirritable to lethargic |
| **Thirst** | slight | moderate | intense |
| **Mucous membranes*** | normal | dry | parched |
| **Tears** | present | decreased | absent, sunken eyes |
| **Anterior fontanelle** | normal | normal to sunken | sunken |
| **External jugular vein** | visible when supine | not visible except with supra-clavicular pressure | not visible even with supra-clavicular pressure |
| **Skin*** (less useful in children > 2 yrs) | capillary refill < 2 sec | slowed capillary refill (2–4 sec), decreased turgor | significant delayed capillary refill (> 4 sec) and tenting; skin cool, acrocyanotic, or mottled* |
| **Urine specific gravity** (SG) | > 1.020 | > 1.020, oliguria | oliguria or anuria |
| **Lab values** | normal BUN/creatinine | increased BUN/creatinine | increased+++ BUN/creatinine, increased Hgb, low glucose |

** These signs are less prominent in patients who have hypernatremia.*

Figure 1: **Management of Isonatremic Dehydration**

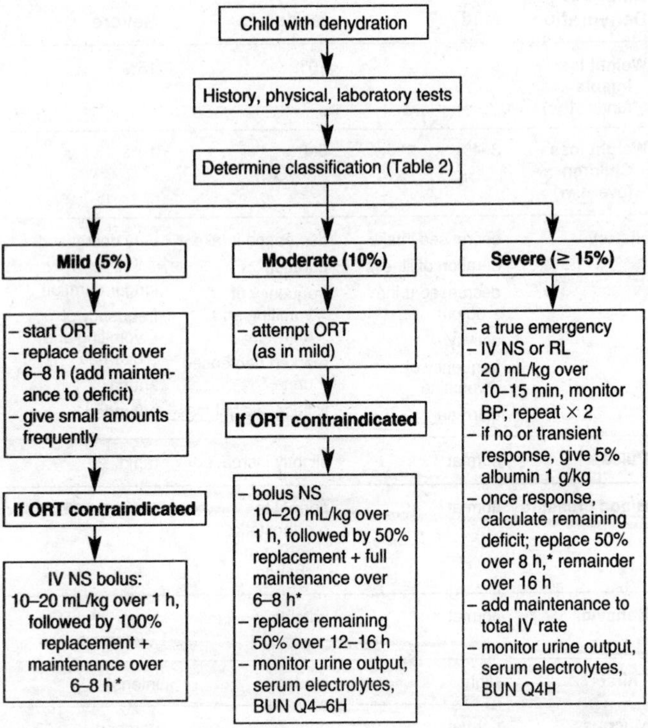
Child with dehydration
History, physical, laboratory tests
Determine classification (Table 2)
Mild (5%)
Moderate (10%)
Severe (≥ 15%)
– start ORT
– replace deficit over 6–8 h (add maintenance to deficit)
– give small amounts frequently
If ORT contraindicated
IV NS bolus: 10–20 mL/kg over 1 h, followed by 100% replacement + maintenance over 6–8 h*
– attempt ORT (as in mild)
If ORT contraindicated
– bolus NS 10–20 mL/kg over 1 h, followed by 50% replacement + full maintenance over 6–8 h*
– replace remaining 50% over 12–16 h
– monitor urine output, serum electrolytes, BUN Q4–6H
– a true emergency
– IV NS or RL 20 mL/kg over 10–15 min, monitor BP; repeat × 2
– if no or transient response, give 5% albumin 1 g/kg
– once response, calculate remaining deficit; replace 50% over 8 h,* remainder over 16 h
– add maintenance to total IV rate
– monitor urine output, serum electrolytes, BUN Q4H

* *Replacement therapy after bolus should contain 50–60 mmol/L $Na^+$ plus a source of glucose (e.g., D5W) plus appropriate $K^+$. An ideal solution is 0.33% NaCl ($Na^+$ 51.3 mmol/L) + D3.3W (3.3 g glucose/100 mL) + appropriate $K^+$. $K^+$ should not exceed 4 mmol/kg/d and replenishment should be done gradually over 2 d.* ***No urine output, no $K^+$.***

*Abbreviations: NS = 0.9% NaCl; ORT = oral replacement therapy; RL = Ringer's lactate.*

## Therapeutic Choices

Treatment of dehydration involves replacing fluid deficits, then maintaining normal hydration.

The calculation of the **fluid deficit** for a given degree of dehydration can be based on historical or objective information (e.g., predehydrational and present dehydrated weight). When the predehydrational weight is known:

*Deficit liters (L) = predehydrational weight (kg) – present weight (kg).*

Predehydrational body weight can be estimated by:

*Body weight (kg) = (age × 2) + 10.* This gives an estimated weight at or about the 50th percentile for age and can be used for children up to 10 years of age.

**Maintenance fluid** (Table 3) is the amount of fluid required to maintain normal hydration. Maintenance fluids are linked to caloric requirements and take into account insensible losses.

Dehydrational illnesses are classified into 3 types depending on serum $Na^+$ concentration (Table 4).

**Isonatremic dehydration** (Figure 1) is the most common form of dehydration, with loss of both $K^+$ and $Na^+$. $K^+$ can be added to the IV mixture following establishment of urinary output. $K^+$ administration should not exceed 4 mmol/kg/d. Higher $K^+$ concentrations can be used in life-threatening hypokalemia.

**Hypernatremic dehydration** usually develops slowly and is corrected slowly to prevent cerebral edema and seizures. Shock is treated aggressively by using 0.9% NaCl until urinary output is re-established, then 0.45% NaCl + D5W is used to correct dehydration states and restore $Na^+$ to normal levels.

The goal of therapy is to reduce serum $Na^+$ by 10 to 15 mmol/ L/day and to restore hydration to normal in no less than 48 hours. If the serum concentration drops rapidly (i.e., > 10 to 15 mmol/ day or > 1 mmol every 2 hours), the IV solution should be changed to 0.9% NaCl + D5W.

Table 3: **Maintenance Fluid and Electrolyte Requirements in Children**

**Fluids**

| Weight (kg) | Daily Fluid Requirement | Hourly Rate |
|---|---|---|
| 0–10 | 100 mL/kg | 4 mL/kg |
| 11–20 | 1000 mL + (50 mL/kg × each kg > 10) | 40 mL/h + (2 mL/kg × each kg > 10) |
| > 20 | 1500 mL + (20 mL/kg × each kg > 20) | 60 mL/h + (1 mL/kg × each kg > 20) |

| | | |
|---|---|---|
| **Daily Electrolytes** | $Na^+$ | 2.5–3 mmol/kg |
| | $K^+$ | 2–2.5 mmol/kg |

**Calculation of Maintenance Fluid Requirements (using information from Table 3)**

*Example:* For a 15-kg child use information for 11–20 kg

| **Fluids:** | Daily fluid | Hourly fluid rate (quick calculation) |
|---|---|---|
| For the first 10 kg | 10 kg × 100 mL/kg = 1000 mL | 10 kg × 4 mL/kg = 40 mL |
| For the next 5 kg | 5 kg × 50 mL/kg = 250 mL | 5 kg × 2 mL/kg = 10 mL |
| | **Total 1250 mL or 52 mL/h** | **Total 50 mL/h** |

**Electrolytes:**

| | |
|---|---|
| $Na^+$ | 15 kg × 3 mmol/kg/d = 45 mmol/d (45 mmol/1250 mL or 36 mmol/L) |
| $K^+$ | 15 kg × 2 mmol/kg/d = 30 mmol/d (30 mmol/1250 mL or 24 mmol/L) |

*Suggested commercially available solution best meeting the needs would be 0.2% NaCl/D5W + 20 mmol KCl/L.*

Table 4: **Types of Dehydration**

| Type of Dehydration (frequency) | Serum $Na^+$ (mmol/L) | Serum Osmolality (mOsm/kg) |
|---|---|---|
| Isonatremic (80%) | 130–150 | Normal: 280–295 mOsm/kg<br>Equal water and salt loss |
| Hypernatremic (15%) | > 150 | Elevated: 295 mOsm/kg<br>Water loss > salt loss |
| Hyponatremic (5%) | < 130 | ↓ or normal or ↑<br>Must determine subgroup |

**Hyponatremic dehydration** is classified into 3 subgroups:

- excessive water.
- $Na^+$ depletion.
- fictitious lowering of serum $Na^+$ concentration due to increased glucose, electrolytes, lipids and proteins.

Shock must be treated aggressively using isotonic saline (0.9% NaCl).

Symptomatic hyponatremia is usually related to the degree of serum $Na^+$ depletion. Children with serum $Na^+ > 120$ mmol/L rarely demonstrate any clinical manifestations; when serum $Na^+$ drops below 120 mmol/L, neurologic manifestations (e.g., seizures) are common. Children who are symptomatic require aggressive replacement using hypertonic saline (3% NaCl) to achieve a serum $Na^+ > 125$ mmol/L.

Serum $Na^+$ deficit can be calculated as follows:

*$[Na^+]$ deficit = ($[Na^+]$ desired − $[Na^+]$ actual) × body weight (kg) × total body water (L/kg).*

After initial elevation of $Na^+$ to > 125 mmol/L, the remaining deficit can be replaced over 24 to 48 hours.

**Calculation of Fluid Deficit and Replacement for Isonatremic Dehydration**

*Example:* For a 15-kg child who is 10% isonatremic dehydrated

*Fluids:* Total fluid replacement equals *deficit* replacement plus *maintenance.* Fluid deficit in 10% dehydration is 100 mL/kg; in 5% dehydration 50 mL/kg

(i) Deficit replacement calculation = 15 kg × 10% (100 mL/kg)
= 1.5 L or 1500 mL
Need to replace 50% or 750 mL over first 8 h at a rate of 94 mL/h

(ii) Maintenance = 52 mL/h (from Table 3 calculation)

(iii) Total = 146 mL/h (94 mL/h + 52 mL/h) for first 8 h, then reduce to 100 mL/h for next 16 h (replacing remaining 750 mL over 16 h + maintenance [47 mL/h + 52 mL/h ≈ 100 mL/h])

*Electrolytes:*

$Na^+$ loss would be approximately 120 mmol (8–10 mmol/kg/d) and $K^+$ loss would be approximately 120 mmol (8–10 mmol/kg/d).

*Using a rehydration solution of 0.45% NaCl + D5W at the above rate will replace 115 mmol of $Na^+$. $K^+$ 40 mmol/L (not to exceed 4 mmol/kg/d) will replace 60 mmol of total loss. Replacement of $K^+$ will make up losses over the next 2 d.*

It is important to remember that dehydrated children with **ongoing fluid losses** need those losses replaced *in addition to* their estimated deficit plus maintenance fluids. Usually fluid losses are replaced on a ratio of 1cc to 1cc. Fluid loss replacement such as those above the usual sensible and insensible losses (i.e., high urine output in a diabetic, nasogastric replacement loss, excessive, ongoing vomiting and diarrhea) also need to be adjusted for electrolyte loss.

## Oral Rehydration Therapy (ORT)

ORT is the treatment of choice in children with mild to moderate dehydration. It can be used in all types of dehydration provided that hypo- and hypernatremic dehydration are not at the extreme of the spectrum.

The fluid deficit is calculated and replaced over 6 to 8 hours using frequent small amounts of fluids. The fluid should be a balanced electrolyte solution acceptable to the GI tract and should facilitate $Na^+$ transport. Solutions ideal for ORT contain $Na^+$ 45 to 75 mmol/L, $K^+$ 20 mmol/L and glucose 20 to 24 g/L; 100 to 150 mL/kg/day is given to the child.

Table 5: **Oral Replacement Solutions**

| **Product** | **Composition** | | | | **Cost*** |
|---|---|---|---|---|---|
| | **Dextrose g/L** | **$K^+$ mmol/L** | **$Na^+$ mmol/L** | **$Cl^-$ mmol/L** | |
| Enfalac Lytren | 20 | 25 | 50 | 45 | $$$$ |
| Gastrolyte | 17.8 | 20 | 60 | 60 | $ |
| Pedialyte | 25 | 20 | 45 | 35 | $$ |
| Pediatric Electrolyte | 20 | 20 | 45 | 35 | $$ |

** Cost per liter – includes drug cost only (retail mark-up not included).*
*Legend: $ < $5  $$ $5–10  $$$ $10–15  $$$$ $15–20*

Commercially available preparations (Table 5) may be used to rehydrate the child with observation in an ambulatory/emergency room setting or at home.

Children who have been started on IV replacement therapy can be switched to ORT at any point. It is important to ensure that no contraindications (shock or impending shock, high diarrheal purge rates, intractable vomiting, altered sensorium) are present.

### *Suggested Reading List*


Boineau FG, Lewy JE. Estimation of parenteral fluid requirements. *Pediatr Clin North Am* 1990;37:257.

Castell HB, Fidorick SC. Oral rehydration therapy, fluid and electrolyte therapy. *Pediatr Clin North Am* 1990;37:295.

Jospe N, Gorbes G. Fluids and electrolytes – clinical aspects. *Pediatr Rev* 1996;17(11):395–403.

Kallen RJ. The management of diarrheal dehydration in infants using parenteral fluids. *Pediatr Clin North Am* 1990;37:265.

CHAPTER 78

# Hypovolemia

*Peter J. McLeod, MD, FRCPC, FACP*

Dehydration in children is discussed in Chapter 77.

Hypovolemia is a generic term encompassing volume depletion and dehydration. Volume depletion, or loss of salt and water from the intravascular space, is more frequently associated with hypotension and tachycardia than is dehydration. Dehydration, such as from excess sweating, implies loss of water from both extracellular (intravascular and interstitial) and intracellular spaces.

## Goals of Therapy

- Restoration of normal volume to relieve symptoms and prevent organ damage

## Investigations

- History:
  - symptoms of hypovolemia include thirst, fatigue and postural lightheadedness
  - causes of hypovolemia include hemorrhage; volume losses from GI tract, kidneys, skin, respiratory tract; fluid sequestration or third-space losses
- Physical exam:
  - determine the presence and severity of hypovolemia
  - pulse: heart rate (HR) increase of more than 30 beats/min on standing from recumbent position is the most accurate sign of volume depletion. Supine tachycardia is insensitive
  - blood pressure: postural decline of systolic pressure of more than 20 mm Hg suggests volume depletion
  - low jugular venous pressure (JVP) is suggestive of volume depletion but skin turgor, capillary refill time and eyeball tension are insensitive. Moist mucous membranes and axillae argue against hypovolemia
- Laboratory tests:
  - blood: in hypovolemia, hematocrit and albumin concentrations increase and urea increases disproportionately to creatinine. Sodium concentration may be normal, low or high
  - urine: hypovolemia is suggested if urine volume is < 20 mL/hr; $Na^+$ is < 20 mmol/L; osmolality is > 450 m0sm/kg

## Therapeutic Choices (Figure 1 and Table 2)

Therapy is designed to restore volume while replacing ongoing losses.

- **Hypovolemia suspected but uncertain:** consider an IV fluid challenge of 500 mL of normal saline over 30 minutes. Closely monitor HR and BP to determine if low cardiac output is due to hypovolemia.
- **Mild hypovolemia:** oral therapy is usually adequate. Water, juices, soft drinks or soup broth with extra salt or a commercially-available electrolyte solution (Chapter 77) may be used. Rice-based oral solutions have proven effective for diarrheal conditions in developing countries.
- **Moderate or severe hypovolemia** or inability to ingest oral fluids: IV therapy is required and 3 types of solutions are used:
  – *dextrose 5% in water* (D5W) distributes throughout total body water and is useful for true dehydration. It is a poor plasma volume expander as very little remains in the intravascular space.

Figure 1: **Management of Suspected Hypovolemia**

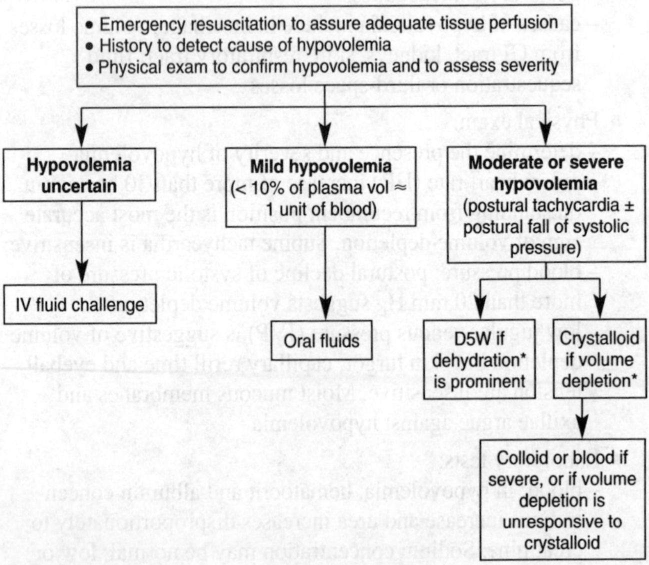
• Emergency resuscitation to assure adequate tissue perfusion
• History to detect cause of hypovolemia
• Physical exam to confirm hypovolemia and to assess severity
Hypovolemia uncertain
Mild hypovolemia (< 10% of plasma vol ≈ 1 unit of blood)
Moderate or severe hypovolemia (postural tachycardia ± postural fall of systolic pressure)
IV fluid challenge
Oral fluids
D5W if dehydration* is prominent
Crystalloid if volume depletion*
Colloid or blood if severe, or if volume depletion is unresponsive to crystalloid

* *Dehydration refers to loss of intracellular water leading to elevated plasma sodium and osmolality. Patients with dehydration may or may not have hypotension and tachycardia. Volume depletion results from loss of salt and water from the extracellular space. Volume depleted patients exhibit circulatory instability.*

Table 1: **Intravenous Solutions for Hypovolemia**

| Crystalloids | Na+ concentration mmol/L | Use |
|---|---|---|
| 0.9% sodium chloride (normal saline [NS]) | 154 | initial treatment of hypovolemia |
| 5% dextrose with 0.9% sodium chloride (D5WNS) | 154 | hypovolemia and dehydration |
| 5% dextrose in water (D5W) | 0 | dehydration; poor plasma volume expander |
| 0.45% sodium chloride (half-normal saline [½ NS]) | 77 | hypovolemia with hypernatremia |
| 3.3% dextrose with 0.3% sodium chloride (2/3–1/3) | 51 | maintenance fluids |
| 5% dextrose with 0.45% sodium chloride (D5–½ NS) | 77 | maintenance fluids |
| **Colloids** | | **Use** |
| Albumin | | volume expander, useful for hypoproteinemic hypovolemia |
| Pentastarch | | volume expander, alternative to blood |
| Blood | | packed cells with saline indicated for hemorrhage |

- *sodium chloride 0.9%* (normal saline [NS]) is the fluid of choice for initial treatment of volume depletion. Like other crystalloid solutions, it distributes to extracellular fluid. For every liter infused, 300 mL remains in the intravascular space and the remainder goes to the interstitial space.
- *colloid solutions*, including albumin, pentastarch and blood, are better intravascular volume expanders than NS. Their cost is high and the duration of benefit is relatively short; use is not justified in most hypovolemic states. Blood is an excellent intravascular volume expander. Packed red blood cells with normal saline is indicated for hemorrhagic hypovolemia.

## Determining Fluid Requirements

There is no precise formula since disease, age, source and rate of fluid loss influence needs. In severe hypovolemia, with obvious hemodynamic compromise, give at least 1 liter of NS over 30 minutes and a second liter over the next hour. Closely monitor HR, BP and JVP, watching for improvement or fluid overload. In less severe hypovolemia, give 250 to 500 mL/h of NS. Colloid solutions may be needed if NS is ineffective. Maintenance fluids must be added to those given to correct the deficit. In adults, maintenance is possible with approximately 30 mL/kg/day or 2000 to 2500 mL/day containing 75 mmol of $Na^+$ and 50 mmol of $K^+$.

Other commercially available crystalloid solutions are more costly and, aside from dextrose 3.3% with sodium chloride 0.3% (2/3–1/3) or dextrose 5% with sodium chloride 0.45% (D5–1/2 NS), they play very little role. Users of other crystalloids must be aware of their contents, e.g., Ringer's lactate contains calcium, potassium and lactate in addition to sodium, and may not be suitable for some patients.

## Therapeutic Tips

- If presence of hypovolemia is uncertain, consider a fluid challenge.
- Dextrose in water is a poor plasma volume expander; normal saline is the fluid of first choice.
- Additional potassium may be required for fluid loss associated with diarrhea, vomiting or over-diuresis with diuretics.
- Colloid solutions are usually reserved as second-line plasma volume expanders; burns and other volume losses containing protein may require additional colloid.
- Bicarbonate may be required in severe metabolic acidosis.

## *Suggested Reading List*

Brown GR. Hypovolemia. In: Gray J, ed. *Therapeutic Choices*. 2nd ed. Ottawa, ON: Canadian Pharmacists Association, 1998:598–603.

McGee S, Abernethy WB, Simel D. Is this patient hypovolemic? *JAMA* 1999;281:1022–1029.

Rose RB, Hypovolemic states. In: *Clinical physiology of acid-base and electrolyte disorders*. New York: McGraw Hill, 1994.

CHAPTER 79

# Edema

*David J. Hirsch, MD, FRCPC*

Edema is a sign, not a specific illness. Therapy is inappropriate until the underlying cause is defined.

**Unilateral dependent edema** should prompt an assessment of local venous and lymphatic drainage and a search for local infection. **Bilateral dependent edema** or anasarca is usually seen in patients with pregnancy, nephrotic syndrome, renal insufficiency, liver disease, heart failure or pericardial disease. Because of the wide range of serious illnesses causing edema, the approach outlined here must be general, and should be individualized for every patient.

## Goals of Therapy

- To define the cause
- To reduce swelling if it causes reduced mobility, skin breakdown or infection, or discomfort
- To avoid elimination of all edema
- To avoid electrolyte disturbances

## Investigations

- History with attention to:
  - salt intake
  - location of edema (peripheral, facial, ascites)
  - evidence of pregnancy, heart disease, renal disease, liver disease
  - previous diuretic use
- Physical examination:
  - weight, postural BP and pulse
  - severity of edema and its location (unilateral vs. bilateral)
  - evidence of cardiac failure, pleural effusion, ascites, hepatic enlargement or stigmata of hepatic failure
- Laboratory tests:
  - urinalysis
  - serum electrolytes and creatinine
  - liver function tests
  - chest x-ray

Figure 1: **Management of Edema**

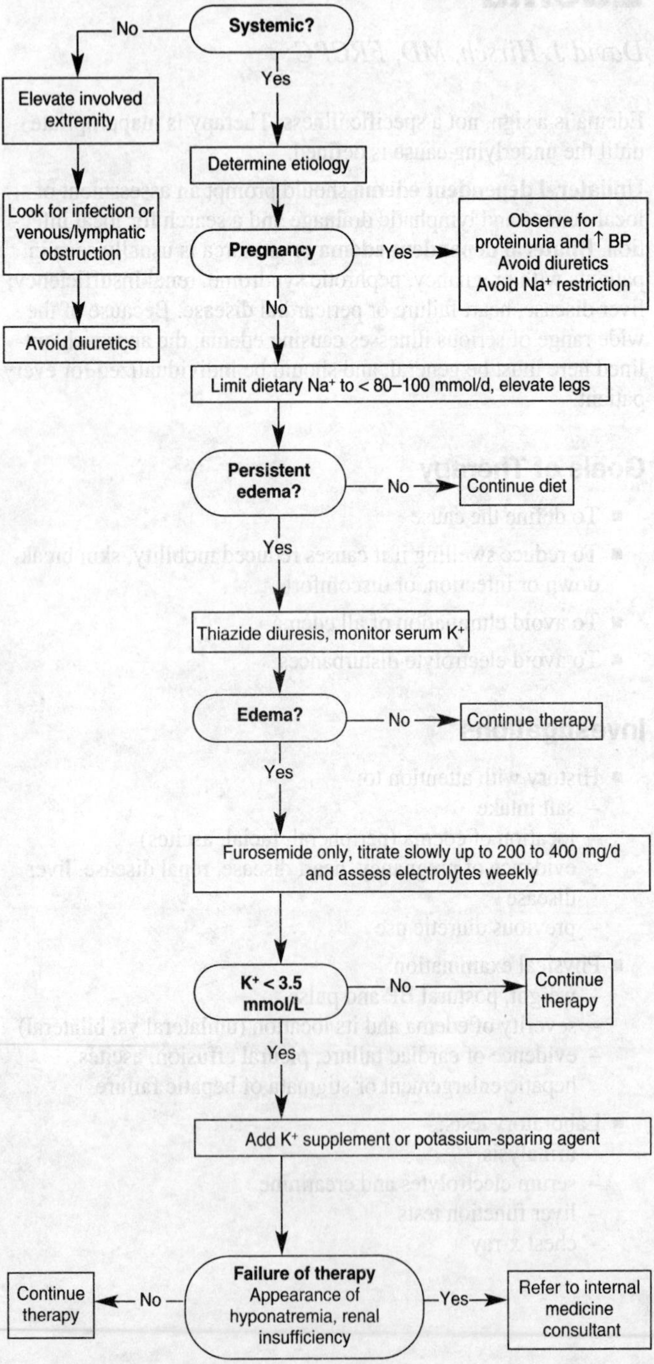
Systemic?
No
Yes
Elevate involved extremity
Determine etiology
Look for infection or venous/lymphatic obstruction
Pregnancy
Yes
Observe for proteinuria and ↑ BP
Avoid diuretics
Avoid Na+ restriction
No
Avoid diuretics
Limit dietary Na+ to < 80–100 mmol/d, elevate legs
Persistent edema?
No
Continue diet
Yes
Thiazide diuresis, monitor serum K+
Edema?
No
Continue therapy
Yes
Furosemide only, titrate slowly up to 200 to 400 mg/d and assess electrolytes weekly
K+ < 3.5 mmol/L
No
Continue therapy
Yes
Add K+ supplement or potassium-sparing agent
Failure of therapy
Appearance of hyponatremia, renal insufficiency
No
Continue therapy
Yes
Refer to internal medicine consultant

## Therapeutic Choices (Figure 1)

### Nonpharmacologic Choices

- Restriction of dietary sodium intake to < 80 mmol/day.
- Rest and elevation of the legs.
- Addition of supportive hose (if possible).

### Pharmacologic Choices

Medications should only be used if nonpharmacologic measures have failed to control edema after attempted treatment of any underlying specific disease process.

### Diuretic Therapy (Table 1)

- Indications:
  - if edema cannot be reduced to the point where shoes can be worn.
  - presence of skin breakdown in the lower limbs.
  - scrotal or vulvar edema.
  - pitting edema extending to the thighs or anterior abdominal wall.
- Pregnant women should **not** receive diuretics for edema without advice from a consultant.

#### *Thiazides*

Mild edema in the absence of renal insufficiency can be treated with a thiazide diuretic, using up to 100 mg of **hydrochlorothiazide** per day if nonpharmacologic measures fail. Serum potassium should be monitored.

#### *Loop Diuretics*

Failure of a thiazide response usually indicates a need for a loop diuretic, e.g., **furosemide**. Dosage starts at 20 to 40 mg per day as a single dose, and is doubled every 2 days until the patient notes the onset of diuresis. The effective dose should then be used as a single daily dose until sufficient edema reduction improves the patient's symptoms. The patient should monitor daily weight and avoid a reduction of more than 1 kg per day. Serum electrolytes and creatinine should be carefully followed.

In some patients a single daily dose of loop diuretic, even if titrated to the effective level, does not produce sufficient diuresis to control edema. If so, it may be reasonable to add a second dose of the loop diuretic at the dosage level previously found to be effective. In some patients this approach may be more effective than simply increasing the single daily dose of diuretic.

#### *Potassium-sparing Therapy*

Hypokalemia (< 3.5 mmol/L) indicates a probable need for potassium supplements or the use of $K^+$-sparing agents, e.g.,

Table 1: **Diuretic Agents**

| Drug | Daily Dose | Adverse Effects | Drug Interactions | Comments | Cost* |
|---|---|---|---|---|---|
| **Thiazide Diuretics** | | | For all thiazides: | | |
| *hydrochlorothiazide* HydroDiuril, generics | 25–100 mg | Hypokalemia, hyponatremia, hypovolemia, hyperuricemia, hyperglycemia, impotence, rash. | Lithium: lithium toxicity (monitor $Li^+$ levels). Digoxin: digoxin toxicity if ↓ $K^+$ (monitor $K^+$). Antidiabetic agents: ↑ blood glucose (monitor). Corticosteroids: hypokalemia. NSAIDs: ↓ diuretic effect, ↑ renal toxicity. | Good initial agent, often ineffective if renal insufficiency present. | $ |
| **Others:** | | | | | |
| *metolazone* Zaroxolyn | 2.5–10 mg | | | No advantage over hydrochlorothiazide, generally more expensive. | $ |
| *chlorthalidone* generics | 25–100 mg | | | | $ |
| *indapamide* Lozide, generics | 1.25–2.5 mg | | | | $ |
| **Loop Diuretics** | | | As for thiazides. | | |
| *furosemide* Lasix, generics | 20–500 mg | As for thiazides; ototoxicity if rapidly injected. | | Effective in refractory edema, useful in renal insufficiency. | $–$$$ |
| *ethacrynic acid* Edecrin | 25–200 mg | As for furosemide. | | No advantage over furosemide clinically, more ototoxic. | $–$$ |
| *bumetanide* Burinex | 0.5–10 mg | As for furosemide. | | No advantage over furosemide. | $–$$$ |

| | | | | | |
|---|---|---|---|---|---|
| **Potassium-sparing** ❥ **Agents** | | | Avoid NSAIDs, ACE inhibitors, potassium supplements: may cause severe hyperkalemia. | | All: $–$$ |
| *spironolactone* Aldactone, generics | 25–300 mg | Hyperkalemia, gynecomastia, GI upset, headache. | | Gynecomastia is common. | |
| *triamterene* Dyrenium | 100–300 mg | Hyperkalemia, acute renal failure (esp. with NSAIDs). | | Occasional reports of renal stones or acute renal failure. | |
| *amiloride* Midamor | 5–20 mg | Hyperkalemia. | | Probably fewest side effects clinically. | |

❥ *Dosage adjustments may be required in renal failure – see Appendix I.*

* *Cost of 30-day supply – includes drug cost only.*
*Legend: $ < $20  $$ $20–40  $$$ > $40*

**spironolactone, triamterene** or **amiloride**. Although all are effective, amiloride has the least number of long-term side effects. Triamterene can occasionally result in decreased renal function and spironolactone can cause gynecomastia, if taken for long periods of time. All $K^+$-sparing agents may increase diuresis, so that volume depletion must be constantly monitored. Hyperkalemia in diabetics or those patients taking NSAIDs or ACE inhibitors is common.

### *Combination Diuretic Therapy*

If furosemide alone fails to induce a diuresis after doses of up to 400 mg per day, combination diuretic therapy may be required; the combination of **furosemide with a potassium-sparing agent** may be effective. However, on many occasions the use of a combination of **thiazide and furosemide** is required to cause diuresis in refractory patients. There is no evidence that metolazone is preferable to other thiazide diuretics. This type of therapy should be monitored closely, preferably in a hospital, because of the risk of complications including sudden massive diuresis, hypokalemia, hypomagnesemia, hyponatremia and acute hypotension with volume depletion. A combination of 25 mg hydrochlorothiazide with 80 to 200 mg of furosemide is often effective, but diuresis may be delayed for a few days following initiation of treatment.

### *Idiopathic Edema*

Commonly seen in young to middle-aged females, particularly those very concerned with their appearance or weight. In some patients, there will be considerable complaint about edema not apparent to physicians. In other cases, patients have been able to document sudden shifts in weight of 3 or 4 kg from one day to another, often with the appearance of mild ankle edema. Thorough investigation in these cases fails to identify the usual causes of edema listed above, and the pathophysiology of this syndrome is not clear. The use of diuretics in these patients is best avoided: many do not respond to thiazide diuretics and require slow tapering of the dosage to avoid rebound edema on discontinuation of the diuretic. This group of patients reinforces the point that edema should not be treated pharmacologically unless there are clear indications to do so. **Diuretics should not be used for cosmetic purposes alone.**

## Therapeutic Tips

- The goal of therapy is to reduce edema to the point of comfort, not to abolish it: pre-renal azotemia and volume depletion can result if edema is completely removed.

- The appearance of refractory hypokalemia, elevated serum creatinine or hyponatremia usually indicates overdiuresis and/or progression of the underlying problem to a more complicated state; consultation and reduction of medication is appropriate.
- $K^+$-sparing agents should be avoided in patients with diabetes or reduced renal function. Dosage reductions of diuretics are not generally needed in liver or renal disease.
- Combination diuretic preparations (e.g., thiazide plus $K^+$-sparing agent) should be avoided due to inflexibility in dosage adjustment.
- In patients where a target weight can be set, thiazides or loop diuretics can be given intermittently. Once an effective dose has been found by titration, that dose can be given only on days when the target weight is exceeded. This will reduce the risks of volume depletion, hyperuricemia and electrolyte disturbance.

## *Suggested Reading List*

Brater DC. Diuretic therapy. *N Engl J Med 1998;339:387–395.*

Schrier RW. Pathogenesis of sodium and water retention in high-output and low-output cardiac failure, nephrotic syndrome, cirrhosis, and pregnancy. *N Engl J Med* 1988;319: 1065–1072, 1127–1134.

Streeten DH. Idiopathic edema: pathogenesis, clinical features and treatment. *Endocrinol Metab Clin North Am* 1995;24: 531–547.

CHAPTER 80

# Hypercalcemia

*Donna M.M. Woloschuk, PharmD, CACE, FCSHP*

## Goals of Therapy

- To correct dehydration
- To enhance renal excretion of calcium
- To inhibit accelerated bone resorption
- To treat the underlying disorder

## Investigations

- Initiating treatment (general measures) immediately will not interfere with diagnostic tests
- History and physical examination, with special attention to:
  - duration of symptoms if symptomatic (anorexia, nausea, vomiting, constipation, malaise, drowsiness, polydipsia, polyuria), or of hypercalcemia if asymptomatic
  - history of, or physical findings consistent with, familial hypocalciuric hypercalcemia, primary hyperparathyroidism, granulomatous diseases, malignancy, nonparathyroid endocrine disorders, immobilization, acute/chronic renal insufficiency or milk-alkali syndrome
  - medications that cause or aggravate hypercalcemia (thiazide diuretics, lithium, excess vitamin A or D, estrogens, antiestrogens, progestins, androgens, parenteral nutrition, ingestion of > 3 g elemental calcium per day)
- Laboratory evaluation:
  - serum calcium and albumin (see Table 1 to calculate correction) *or* ionized calcium
  - serum phosphate, serum creatinine, BUN, 24-hour urine creatinine and calcium
  - alkaline phosphatase (fractionated for bony source, if available)
  - serum parathyroid hormone
  - other tests based on history or physical findings of hypercalcemia-associated conditions, as required

## Therapeutic Choices (Figure 1)

- Aggressiveness of initial interventions depends on the magnitude of hypercalcemia.
- Definitive therapy for long-term control of hypercalcemia requires diagnosis of the underlying condition.

Figure 1: **Management of Hypercalcemia**

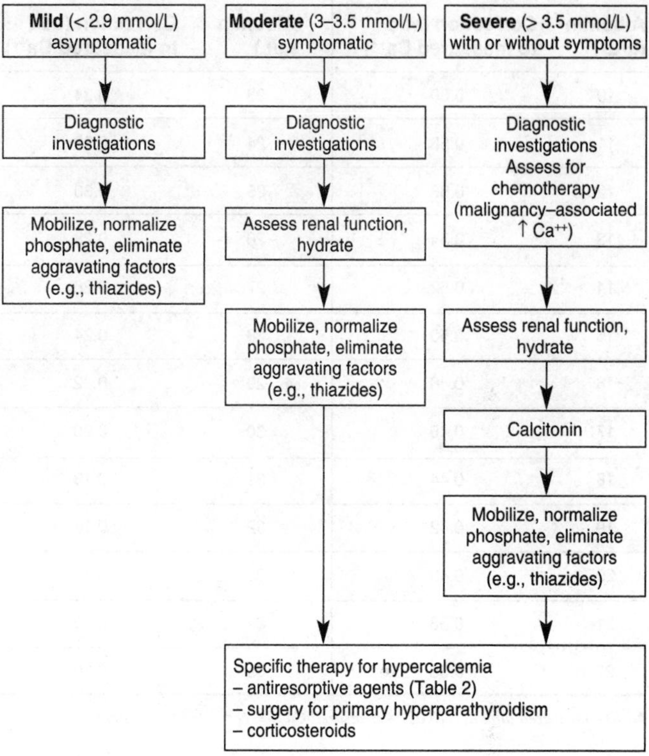
**Mild** (< 2.9 mmol/L) asymptomatic
**Moderate** (3–3.5 mmol/L) symptomatic
**Severe** (> 3.5 mmol/L) with or without symptoms
Diagnostic investigations
Diagnostic investigations
Diagnostic investigations Assess for chemotherapy (malignancy–associated ↑ Ca++)
Mobilize, normalize phosphate, eliminate aggravating factors (e.g., thiazides)
Assess renal function, hydrate
Mobilize, normalize phosphate, eliminate aggravating factors (e.g., thiazides)
Assess renal function, hydrate
Calcitonin
Mobilize, normalize phosphate, eliminate aggravating factors (e.g., thiazides)
Specific therapy for hypercalcemia
– antiresorptive agents (Table 2)
– surgery for primary hyperparathyroidism
– corticosteroids

## Nonpharmacologic Choices

### *Mobilize*

Hypercalcemia is exacerbated by immobilization. Ambulation helps to reduce bone resorption and normalize serum calcium.

### *Diet*

Dietary changes rarely correct hypercalcemia. Patients with vitamin D-mediated hypercalcemia may benefit from dietary calcium restriction. Excessive use of calcium supplements or calcium-containing antacids should be curtailed in all patients.

## Pharmacologic Choices

## General Measures

### *Stop Offending Agents*

If possible, offending agents should be discontinued and replaced with agents that do not exacerbate hypercalcemia.

Table 1: **Serum Calcium Correction (mmol/L) for Low Serum Albumin***

| Albumin (g/L) | Correction (add to measured $Ca^{++}$) | Albumin (g/L) | Correction (add to measured $Ca^{++}$) |
|---|---|---|---|
| 10 | 0.60 | 23 | 0.34 |
| 11 | 0.58 | 24 | 0.32 |
| 12 | 0.56 | 25 | 0.30 |
| 13 | 0.54 | 26 | 0.28 |
| 14 | 0.52 | 27 | 0.26 |
| 15 | 0.50 | 28 | 0.24 |
| 16 | 0.48 | 29 | 0.22 |
| 17 | 0.46 | 30 | 0.20 |
| 18 | 0.44 | 31 | 0.18 |
| 19 | 0.42 | 32 | 0.16 |
| 20 | 0.40 | 33 | 0.14 |
| 21 | 0.38 | 34 | 0.12 |
| 22 | 0.36 | 35 | 0.10 |

* *(40 – measured albumin) (0.02) + measured $Ca^{++}$ = corrected $Ca^{++}$ value.*

### *Hydrate*

Expansion of intravascular volume enhances renal calcium clearance. Hydration alone usually reduces serum calcium by ≤ 0.6 mmol/L. This effect is present only during hydration. Serum magnesium and potassium may also decrease and should be monitored and replaced as needed.

Patients with mild to moderate asymptomatic hypercalcemia should drink 3 L per day of noncaffeinated beverages to achieve and maintain euvolemia. Patients with moderate to severe symptomatic hypercalcemia should receive 0.9% NaCl injection until euvolemic, then the infusion rate should be reduced to maintain normal hydration. Volume correction may require 2 to 3 L of fluid within the first 8 hours. Patients with a significant volume deficit may need 3 to 5 L of fluid therapy in the first 24 hours. Renal dysfunction, a result of volume loss or permanent renal damage, is common among hypercalcemic patients. Careful monitoring of hydration is essential, especially in elderly patients and those with permanent renal damage.

A loop diuretic (e.g., furosemide) should be used to prevent fluid overload and heart failure, as needed, but only after dehydration is corrected. Thiazide diuretics are contraindicated because they impair calcium excretion.

### *Normalize Serum Phosphate*

Hypophosphatemia (seen mostly in primary hypoparathyroidism and malignancy-associated hypercalcemia) exacerbates hypercalcemia by increasing renal synthesis of 1,25–dihydroxy-vitamin D, reducing bone formation and increasing bone resorption. Oral phosphates (1 to 2 g elemental phosphate per day) can be given safely in all patients except those with renal insufficiency, to increase serum phosphate into the low normal range (0.8 to 1 mmol/L). Calcium phosphate can precipitate and cause serious organ damage (heart, kidney, lungs, blood vessels) if phosphate levels are increased to > 1 mmol/L or if IV phosphate is administered.

## Specific Measures (Table 2)

### *Primary Hyperparathyroidism*

**Surgery** is the first-line measure for control of primary hyperparathyroidism. In the < 10% of patients for whom surgery is not an option, pharmacologic therapy may be required. **Estrogen** therapy (conjugated estrogens 0.625 to 2.5 mg per day) lowers serum calcium concentrations (0.25 to 0.5 mmol/L) without affecting parathyroid hormone levels in postmenopausal women. This may be useful for women with mild to moderate hyperparathyroidism. Oral **phosphate** therapy can also be used if the dose is titrated to normalize serum calcium, and appropriate monitoring is provided.

### *Granulomatous Diseases*

Excess production of 1,25–dihydroxyvitamin D is characteristic of granulomatous diseases. Specific therapy includes restriction of vitamin D and calcium intake, and avoiding excessive exposure to sunlight. **Corticosteroids** counteract the effects of vitamin D. Hydrocortisone 200 to 300 mg IV is given every 3 to 5 days in acutely ill patients. Ambulatory patients may benefit from prednisone (or equivalent) 25 mg per day. The dose should be tapered when calcium control is achieved.

### *Malignancy*

**Antineoplastic therapy** aimed at the underlying malignancy is the key to long-term calcium control. Not all patients are candidates for this therapy. **Bisphosphonates** are first-line drugs if effective antineoplastic therapy is not available or appropriate,

Table 2: **Antiresorptive Agents for Treatment of Hypercalcemia**

| Drug | Dosage | Adverse Effects | Comments | Cost* |
|---|---|---|---|---|
| *calcitonin salmon*<br>Calcimar, Caltine | 3–8 IU/kg Q12H SC<br>max. 8 IU/kg Q6H | Nausea, vomiting (dose dependent), hypersensitivity reactions. | Inhibits release of $Ca^{++}$ from bone and stimulates urinary $Ca^{++}$ excretion.<br>Used for rapid early effect (within 6 h).<br>Tachyphylaxis develops in 2–7 d; combining with glucocorticoids may ↑ efficacy and ↓ tachyphylaxis.<br>Use with bisphosphonate for long-term control.<br>Extent of $Ca^{++}$ lowering ≤ 0.8 mmol/L.<br>Skin test before therapy if suspected sensitivity. | \$–\$\$/d |
| *clodronate disodium*<br>Bonefos, Ostac | 600–1500 mg IV single dose over 2 h or<br>300 mg/d IV over 2 h (usually × 5 d) | Uncommon. | **Dilute in 0.5–1 L saline or dextrose before infusion;** fatal acute renal failure reported from infusion < 2 h.<br>Onset – 2 d; maximal effect – 6 d; duration – variable (2–3 wks in hypercalcemia of malignancy). | \$–\$\$\$/single dose<br>\$\$/5 d |
| | 800–1600 mg PO BID (2 h AC or 2 h PC) | GI upset, diarrhea, muscle cramps. | Significant drug interactions with PO iron, calcium, magnesium, aluminum (e.g., antacids). | \$\$–\$\$\$\$/30 d |
| *etidronate disodium*<br>Didronel | 7.5 mg/kg/d IV over 2 h × 3 d | Febrile reaction within 24–48 h, interferes with normal bone mineralization and increases risk of fractures with long-term exposure. | **Dilute in ≥ 250 mL saline or dextrose before infusion**; acute renal failure reported with infusions ≤ 2 h.<br>Onset – 24 h; maximal effect – 72 h after first dose. | \$\$\$/3 d |
| *pamidronate disodium*<br>Aredia | 30–90 mg IV over 2 h single dose (based on serum $Ca^{++}$ result prior to hydration) | Febrile reaction within 24–48 h of infusion. | Same as clodronate. Case reports of safe and effective use (without dosage modification) in patients on hemodialysis. | \$–\$\$\$\$/single dose |

| | | | | |
|---|---|---|---|---|
| *plicamycin* † (renal-dosing symbol) (*mithramycin*) Mithracin | 12.5–25 μg/kg IV over 4–12 h | Nausea, vomiting (worse with rapid infusion), renal tubular necrosis, thrombocytopenia, hepatotoxicity. | Very effective, potent agent.<br>Onset 6–12 h; maximal effect – 10 d; duration up to 6 wks.<br>Risk of bone marrow toxicity ↑ if dose is repeated.<br>Rarely used – safer alternatives available.<br>May be given in smaller fluid volume; therefore, an alternative agent in heart failure or fluid overload. | † |

(renal-dosing symbol) *Dosage adjustment may be required in renal impairment — see Appendix I.*

† *Available through the Special Access Program, Therapeutic Products Directorate, Health Canada.*

* *Cost of supply for specified treatment period – drug cost only.*

*Legend: $ < $200   $$ $200–300   $$$ $300–400   $$$$ $400–500*

if the patient has severe hypercalcemia (> 3.5 mmol/L, with or without symptoms), or if the patient has multiple myeloma. For acute management, parenteral **pamidronate** or **clodronate** are drugs of choice. Rapid infusion of pamidronate and clodronate is safer than once thought, making outpatient therapy convenient. In patients who respond, prolonged treatment with clodronate or pamidronate can maintain calcium at acceptable levels. Patients with multiple myeloma or selected solid tumors also benefit from reduced bone pain, decreased skeletal morbidity and prevention of hypercalcemia recurrence if prolonged therapy is used. Parenteral **etidronate** is also effective for acute management, but requires repeated daily doses, has a higher risk of renal toxicity, and is more likely to interfere with normal bone mineralization than other bisphosphonates. Information about the use of other bisphosphonates (e.g., alendronate) for serum calcium control is limited to case reports. There are no controlled clinical trials that investigate their use in hypercalcemic states. **Calcitonin** is effective to rapidly reduce serum calcium levels in severe hypercalcemia. **Mithramycin** is also effective for this indication; however, its significant adverse effects make it an unsuitable choice for all but the most severe or resistant cases of hypercalcemia.

## Therapeutic Tips

- Overly aggressive use of loop diuretics can aggravate hypercalcemia by depleting extracellular fluid volume; routine use with hydration therapy is discouraged.
- To reduce serum calcium rapidly (within 6 to 12 hours) in severe hypercalcemia of malignancy, use calcitonin plus hydration. Serum calcium usually declines ≤ 0.8 mmol/L at 12 to 24 hours following combined therapy. To augment and prolong serum calcium control, use definitive therapy (e.g., chemotherapy) for the underlying cause. If chemotherapy is not an option, use a bisphosphonate when dehydration is corrected and adequate urine output is achieved (preferably within 24 hours of hypercalcemia diagnosis).
- Premedication with acetaminophen 650 mg can prevent bisphosphonate-induced fever in patients with hypercalcemia of malignancy.
- Adjunctive glucocorticoid therapy (e.g., prednisone 40 to 100 mg per day for up to 1 week) is particularly useful in patients with lymphoma, myeloma, lymphoid leukemia and breast cancer (if hypercalcemic flare is caused by hormonal treatment).

### *Suggested Reading List*

Allerheiligen DA, Schoeber J, Houston RE, Mohl VK, Wildman KM. Hyperparathyroidism. *Am Fam Physician* 1998; 57:1795–1802.

Body JJ, Bartl R, Burckhardt P, et al. Current use of bisphosphonates in oncology. *J Clin Oncol* 1998;16: 3890–3899.

Bushinsky DA, Monk RD. Calcium. *Lancet* 1998;352:306–311.

Kaye TB. Hypercalcemia: how to pinpoint the cause and customize treatment. *Postgrad Med J* 1995;97:153–156, 159–160.

CHAPTER 81

# Potassium Disturbances

*Jean Ethier, MD, FRCPC*

## Goals of Therapy

- To restore the ratio of intracellular to extracellular potassium to prevent life-threatening cardiac arrhythmias and improve neuromuscular conductivity
- To re-establish normal body stores of potassium ($K^+$) and prevent undue losses or accumulations

## Investigations

- History with attention to possible etiology (Table 1)
- Physical examination to assess cardiac rhythm, paresis, muscle weakness, paresthesias, blood pressure (in suspected hypokalemia)
- Laboratory tests:
  - urea, creatinine, $Na^+$, $K^+$, $Cl^-$, glucose
  - arterial or venous gases or total $CO_2$
  - spot urine for $Na^+$, $K^+$, $Cl^-$ and osmolality to calculate the transtubular $K^+$ concentration gradient (TTKG); 24-hour urine collection for $Na^+$, $K^+$ and creatinine
  - renin, aldosterone, cortisol in selected cases
  - magnesium in refractory hypokalemia, especially when patient is at risk for hypomagnesemia (e.g., taking diuretics, cisplatinum)

Table 1: **Common Causes of Potassium Disturbances**

| Hyperkalemia | Hypokalemia |
|---|---|
| Drug-induced: $K^+$ supplements, NSAIDs, ACE inhibitors, $K^+$-sparing diuretics, digoxin overdose, cyclosporine, trimethoprim or co-trimoxazole (high-dose or in susceptible patients, i.e., elderly, renal failure), heparin, beta-blockers, pentamidine | Diarrhea, vomiting |
| Digoxin use (potentiates risk of arrhythmia) | Inadequate dietary intake |
| Renal failure, diabetes, adrenal insufficiency | Drug-induced: diuretics, laxatives, amphotericin B, aminoglycosides, long-term corticosteroid therapy, antipseudomonal penicillins |
| Familial history of hyperkalemia | Digoxin use (potentiates risk of arrhythmia) |
| Acidosis | Familial history (Bartter's syndrome) |
| Crush injury, trauma, hemolysis, tumor lysis | Mineralocorticoid excess (hypertension) |
| | Metabolic alkalosis |
| | Osmotic diuresis (diabetes) |

Figure 1: **Management of Hyperkalemia**

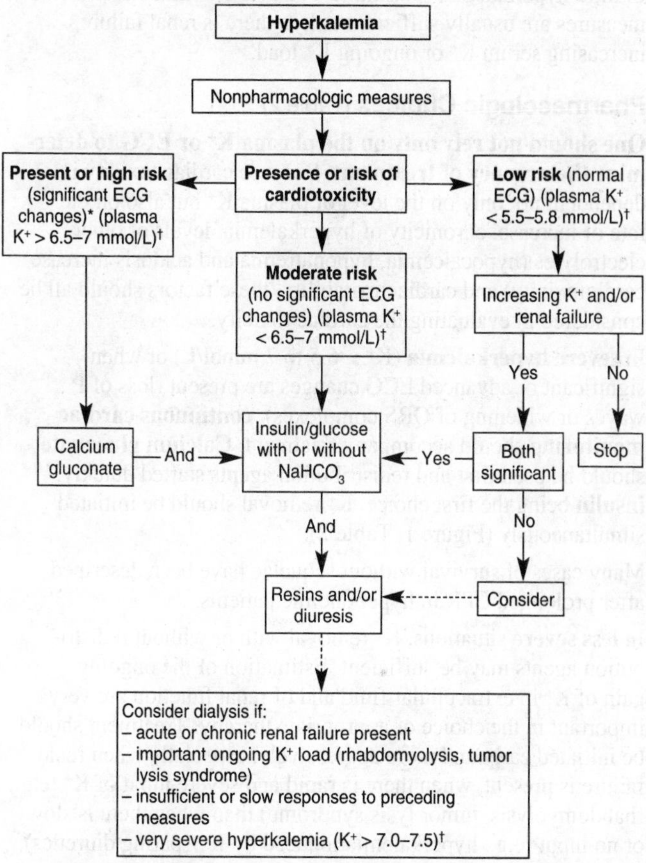
Hyperkalemia
Nonpharmacologic measures
Present or high risk (significant ECG changes)* (plasma K+ > 6.5–7 mmol/L)†
Presence or risk of cardiotoxicity
Low risk (normal ECG) (plasma K+ < 5.5–5.8 mmol/L)†
Moderate risk (no significant ECG changes) (plasma K+ < 6.5–7 mmol/L)†
Increasing K+ and/or renal failure
Yes
No
Calcium gluconate
And
Insulin/glucose with or without NaHCO3
Yes
Both significant
Stop
No
And
Resins and/or diuresis
Consider
Consider dialysis if:
– acute or chronic renal failure present
– important ongoing K+ load (rhabdomyolysis, tumor lysis syndrome)
– insufficient or slow responses to preceding measures
– very severe hyperkalemia (K+ > 7.0–7.5)†

* *Loss of P waves or widening of QRS complexes or more severe changes are considered significant but not isolated peaked T waves.*

† *Plasma potassium level is given only as indicative;* ***therapy should not rely only on the plasma level.***

- rule out pseudohyperkalemia (possible with thrombocytosis, severe leukocytosis, in vitro hemolysis or forearm contraction)
- ECG

## *Hyperkalemia*

## Therapeutic Choices (Figure 1)

### Nonpharmacologic Choices

- $K^+$ supplements and drugs inducing hyperkalemia should be stopped (Table 1).

- Dietary $K^+$ intake should be reduced to ≤ 60 mmol/day.

In mild hyperkalemia (plasma $K^+$ < 5.5 to 6.0 mmol/L) these measures are usually sufficient unless there is renal failure, increasing serum $K^+$ or ongoing $K^+$ load.

## Pharmacologic Choices (Table 2)

**One should not rely only on the plasma $K^+$ or ECG to determine the urgency of treatment.** Because cardiac toxicity is dependent not only on the level of plasma $K^+$ but also on the rate of increase, chronicity of hyperkalemia, levels of other electrolytes (hypocalcemia, hyponatremia and acidosis increase cardiotoxicity) and cardiac irritability, these factors should all be considered in evaluating the cardiac toxicity.

In **severe hyperkalemia** ($K^+$ > 6.5 to 7 mmol/L) or when significant or advanced ECG changes are present (loss of P waves or widening of QRS complexes), **continuous cardiac monitoring** should accompany treatment. **Calcium gluconate** should be used first and redistribution agents started quickly, **insulin** being the first choice. $K^+$ removal should be initiated simultaneously (Figure 1, Table 2).

Many cases of survival without sequelae have been described after prolonged CPR in hyperkalemic patients.

In **less severe** situations, $K^+$ removal with or without redistribution agents may be sufficient. Estimation of the ongoing gain of $K^+$ in extracellular fluid and of renal function are very important in the choice of appropriate therapy. Treatment should be initiated early and more aggressively, especially when renal failure is present, when there is rapid and severe input of $K^+$ (e.g., rhabdomyolysis, tumor lysis syndrome) than when there is slow or no input (e.g., hyperkalemia induced by $K^+$-sparing diuretics).

### *Membrane Antagonists*

Hyperkalemia reduces the magnitude of the resting potential (RP) (less negative) that approaches the threshold potential (TP), leading to an increased risk of arrhythmia and conduction defects. Membrane antagonists correct the difference between RP and TP in excitable tissues. They have a rapid onset but a relatively short duration of action.

IV infusion of **calcium gluconate** raises the TP, restoring the difference between the TP and the RP. **Note:** Calcium should be infused more slowly in patients receiving digoxin because of the risk of hypercalcemia-induced digoxin toxicity.

### *Redistribution Agents*

Redistribution agents promote an intracellular shift of $K^+$ and increase $[K^+_{intracellular}]/[K^+_{extracellular}]$ or RP. These agents act quickly and for a longer period than membrane antagonists.

Table 2: **Treatment of Hyperkalemia**

| Therapy | Dose | Onset (O), Duration (D) of Action | Comments |
|---|---|---|---|
| *calcium gluconate 10%* | 10–20 mL IV over 2–5 min; may repeat once after 5 min (depending on ECG) | O: 1–3 min<br>D: 30–60 min | Continuous ECG monitoring required; ↑ digoxin toxicity; incompatible with $NaHCO_3$-containing solutions (precipitation). |
| *hypertonic saline (NaCl 3%)* | 50–100 mmol IV | O: 5–10 min<br>D: 2 h | Risk of hypertonicity. |
| *sodium bicarbonate ($NaHCO_3$)* | 50–100 mmol IV over 5 min; repeat Q10–15 min (depending on ECG) | O: variable, within 1 h<br>D: 2 h | Variable response; risk of tetany if hypocalcemia present (give calcium first); watch for $Na^+$ overload. |
| *insulin with glucose* | Bolus: 5–10 units IV with 25–50 g of glucose over 5 min. If less urgent, infuse 10 units insulin in 500 mL of 10% dextrose | O: 30 min<br>D: 4–6 h | Risk of hypoglycemia. |
| *salbutamol*<br>Ventolin, generics | 10–20 mg by nebulizer | O: 30 min<br>D: 2–4 h | Reserved for life-threatening cases when other treatments have failed; risk of arrhythmia or angina; variable response. |
| *sodium polystyrene sulfonate resin*<br>Kayexalate, generics | PO: 20–30 g in 50–100 mL of 20% sorbitol Q4–6H PRN<br>PR: 30–50 g in 100–200 mL of water or 10% dextrose Q4–6H PRN; retain at least 30–60 min | O: 1–2 h PO<br>30–60 min PR<br>D: 4–6 h | Constipating; watch for $Na^+$ overload; risk of colonic ulceration or necrosis with hypertonic enema. Cleansing enema before PR use recommended. Cleansing enema after PR use is to be given after evacuation of the resins or after retention for 1–6 h. |
| *furosemide* ➊<br>Lasix, generics | 40–250 mg PO/IV depending on renal function | O: 30–60 min<br>D: to end of increased diuresis (about 4–6 h) | Risk of volume depletion; transient ototoxicity with high-dose furosemide. |

➊ *Dosage adjustment may be required in renal impairment – see Appendix I.*

**Insulin** increases the cellular uptake of $K^+$ independent of glucose uptake. This effect is proportional to insulinemia; to achieve the expected result, insulin must be administered IV. **Glucose** (40 to 50 g per 10 units insulin) is given to avoid hypoglycemia. Bolus administration of glucose should be avoided because the acute increase in plasma tonicity can induce a rise in plasma $K^+$.

The correction of metabolic acidosis with **sodium bicarbonate ($NaHCO_3$)** induces an intracellular shift of $K^+$. $NaHCO_3$ administration in the absence of a low serum bicarbonate concentration or pH has a similar effect but to a much smaller degree. $NaHCO_3$ administration also can induce bicarbonaturia with an increase in renal $K^+$ excretion. The increased $Na^+$ concentration has a membrane antagonist effect. To avoid an acute increase in $K^+$, hypertonic $NaHCO_3$ solutions should not be used.

Insulin administration may be faster, more reliable and more effective than $NaHCO_3$. $NaHCO_3$ may not be useful as the sole initial treatment of hyperkalemia, especially if there is no, or only mild, acidosis present. It has, however, a synergistic effect with insulin in the presence of mild metabolic acidosis. $NaHCO_3$ is still recommended when severe acidosis is present. **Note:** The correction of acidosis in hypocalcemic patients may induce tetany.

The beta$_2$-agonist, **salbutamol**, is effective in lowering plasma $K^+$. Its effect is similar to insulin, but the mechanism is different; concurrent administration of insulin and salbutamol has a synergistic effect. High doses of nebulized salbutamol have a similar effect to IV salbutamol; however, up to 50% of renal failure patients are resistant to this therapy. Salbutamol should be reserved for young patients or life-threatening situations when other therapies have failed, because it is arrhythmogenic and has the potential to exacerbate angina.

### *Potassium Removal*

**Cation-exchange resins** (e.g., sodium polystyrene sulfonate) promote the exchange of $Na^+$ for $K^+$ in the bowel; they also bind calcium and magnesium. **Note:** The $Na^+$ released in exchange for $K^+$ (2 mmol of $Na^+$ per mmol of $K^+$) may lead to volume overload. Because they are constipating, they must be given with a laxative, usually sorbitol. Sorbitol-induced diarrhea can enhance $K^+$ loss. Oral administration is more effective but is much slower than the rectal route.

Rectal ulceration or colonic necrosis has been described when sodium polystyrene sulfonate mixed in sorbitol is given orally or by enema postoperatively. Necrosis may be caused by sorbitol rather than by resins. The duration of drug contact with the mucosa may be a risk factor. A cleansing enema (sodium-free) is recommended to reduce the risk. Use of sorbitol should be avoided when the resin is administered by enema, especially in postoperative patients.

Despite the widespread clinical use of resins and their apparent efficacy, a recent study has questioned the $K^+$-lowering effect of single-dose resin-cathartic therapy.[1]

The administration of **loop diuretics** in patients with sufficient renal function can significantly increase renal $K^+$ excretion.

### Dialysis

If large amounts of $K^+$ need to be removed rapidly, **hemodialysis** is the technique of choice. Because time is required to prepare the equipment and to insert a catheter, other treatments must be initiated while preparing for dialysis. Continuous hemodialysis may also be useful. Peritoneal dialysis is far less efficient in acutely reducing plasma $K^+$.

### Therapeutic Tips

- The treatment of chronic hyperkalemia should focus on the cause or pathophysiological mechanism (Table 1). The modalities are similar to the ones used in acute hyperkalemia ($NaHCO_3$, diuretics, resins).
- Mineralocorticoids (9-alpha-fludrocortisone) may be used in patients with hypoaldosteronism.

## *Hypokalemia*

### Therapeutic Choices

#### Nonpharmacologic Choices

- Reduce or stop medication leading to $K^+$ loss if clinically appropriate.
- Determine and treat the etiology (Table 1).
- If the deficit is slight (plasma $K^+$ = 3.0 to 3.5 mmol/L) and there are no ongoing losses or clinical conditions warranting prompt treatment, dietary intake of potassium-rich foods should be adequate. If there are still unusual losses, $K^+$ supplements will be needed.

#### Pharmacologic Choices

The appropriate pharmacologic approach is determined by:

- **Relative urgency for treatment** (Table 3).

---

[1] *J Am Soc Nephrol 1998;9:1924–1930.*

Table 3: **Management of Hypokalemia**

| Urgency to Treat | Clinical Status | Rate of $K^+$ Administration |
|---|---|---|
| **Urgent** (immediate treatment required) | Severe hypokalemia (plasma $K^+ < 2.5$ mmol/L)<br>Symptomatic hypokalemia (respiratory muscle weakness or paresis, paralysis)<br>Cardiac arrhythmia or conduction disturbances | 20–40 mmol* in the first hour with continuous ECG monitoring and frequent serum $K^+$ measurements to adjust further rate of administration. When plasma $K^+ = 3.0$ mmol/L, remaining deficit should be corrected more slowly. |
| **Less urgent** (prompt treatment required) | Plasma $K^+ = 2.5–3.0$ mmol/L<br>Hypokalemia with digitalis toxicity, myocardial infarction or ischemia<br>Hypokalemia with diabetic ketoacidosis (risk of insulin-induced life-threatening hypokalemia)<br>Hypokalemia with hepatic insufficiency (risk of hepatic encephalopathy) | 10–20 mmol over one hour (↑ serum $K^+$ by 0.25–0.5 mmol/L) with ECG monitoring if > 10 mmol/h. Should be repeated according to control value of serum $K^+$. The remaining deficit should be corrected more slowly. |
| **Not urgent** | Plasma $K^+ > 3.0–3.5$ mmol/L | Initially, 40–60 mmol/d (divided doses), preferably PO (or IV), is usually sufficient. |

* *Larger quantities have been given in extreme life-threatening hypokalemia.*

- The **estimated deficit** for an adult with plasma $K^+ = 3.0$ mmol/L is approximately 200 to 400 mmol and for plasma $K^+ = 2.0$ mmol/L, approximately 500 to 700 mmol.
  **Note:** The true deficit will be *smaller* with an intracellular shift of potassium (e.g., periodic paralysis or hyperadrenergic state) and *larger* with an extracellular shift of potassium (e.g., acidosis or insulin deficit).
- **Ongoing losses** must be added to the deficit when replacement therapy is planned. Renal losses can be estimated based on urine $K^+$ levels and the volume excreted per hour.
- In the presence of renal failure the treatment should be more cautious.

### *Potassium Salts* (Table 4)

In most cases **potassium chloride** (KCl) is the salt of choice, and **oral administration** is the preferred route. If there is no paralytic ileus or suspected absorption problem, oral administration of KCl can rapidly increase plasma $K^+$ (40 to 60 mmol of a liquid preparation will increase plasma $K^+$ by 1.0 to 1.5 mmol/L).

**Potassium bicarbonate** or **potassium citrate** should be reserved for hypokalemic patients with metabolic acidosis (e.g., renal

Table 4: **Oral Potassium Salts**†

| Salt | Dosage Form | Adverse Effects | Comments | Cost* |
|---|---|---|---|---|
| *potassium chloride* | Liquid or powder:‡ K-10, Kaochlor, K-Lyte/Cl, K-Lor, Roychlor, generics | Unpleasant taste, aftertaste, nausea, heartburn. | Rapid absorption, good bioavailability. Salt of choice, especially in alkalotic patients. Inconvenient for transport. | $–$$ |
| | Wax matrix: Slow-K, generics | GI symptoms (less frequent than with liquid), GI ulceration (rare). | Avoid in patients with delayed GI transit or impaired esophageal or intestinal motility. Empty wax matrix may appear in stool. | $ |
| | Micro-encapsulated: K-Dur, Micro-K | May be less ulceration than with wax matrix. | | $ |
| *potassium citrate* (bicarbonate/citric acid) | Effervescent tablets: K-Lyte | Same as potassium chloride. | Useful for patients with metabolic acidosis. More convenient for transport. Useful for hypokalemia secondary to thiazides given for kidney stones. ↑ urinary citrate excretion. | $$ |
| | Crystals or liquid: Polycitra-K | | | $–$$ |
| *potassium gluconate* | Liquid: Kaon, generics | | Useful in patients with acidosis. | $–$$ |

† *Potassium chloride and potassium phosphate are available in parenteral form.*
‡ *Salt substitutes also contain potassium chloride.*

* *Cost of 30-day supply of a 20 mmol/d dose – includes drug cost only.*
*Legend: $ < $10 $$ $10–20*

tubular acidosis, diarrhea). **Potassium phosphate** is used when severe hypophosphatemia is present.

**IV administration** of potassium should be reserved for patients requiring urgent treatment or those unable to take oral supplements (e.g., postsurgery, paralytic ileus). IV potassium should be administered via a large peripheral vein at a maximum concentration of 40 to 60 mmol/L to avoid sclerosis. Higher concentrations should be administered via a central line with the catheter positioned away from the right atrium or ventricle. In patients with severe hypokalemia, $K^+$ should be administered in a dextrose-free solution to avoid stimulating insulin secretion and subsequent intracellular $K^+$ shift.

The **rate of administration** depends on the urgency to treat (Table 3).

### *Potassium-sparing Diuretics* (Table 5)

If renal $K^+$ losses are involved in the pathogenesis of hypokalemia (e.g., hyperaldosteronism, concomitant use of other diuretics), $K^+$-sparing diuretics may be used to decrease these losses; they also prevent or decrease magnesium losses. **Triamterene, amiloride and spironolactone** are equally effective but differ in side effects. The most frequent and serious side effect is hyperkalemia.

$K^+$-sparing diuretics should be avoided in patients with renal or adrenal insufficiency, the elderly, patients with diabetes, and patients taking other drugs that may increase plasma $K^+$ (Table 1).

Table 5: **Potassium-sparing Diuretics***

| Drug | Dosage | Adverse Effects |
|---|---|---|
| *spironolactone* ➔<br>Aldactone, generics | 25–200 mg/d (in single or divided doses); up to 400 mg/d in patients with hyperaldosteronism | Hyperkalemia, gynecomastia, androgen-like side effects, GI symptoms |
| *triamterene* ➔<br>Dyrenium | 50–300 mg/d (in single or divided doses) | Hyperkalemia, muscle cramps, GI symptoms, triamterene renal stones (1 in 1500), acute renal failure (especially with NSAIDs) |
| *amiloride* ➔<br>Midamor | 5–20 mg/d | Hyperkalemia, muscle cramps, headaches, GI symptoms (rare) |

* *For information on drug interactions and cost, see Chapter 79.*

➔ *Dosage adjustment may be required in renal impairment – see Appendix I.*

## Therapeutic Tips

- Using $K^+$ supplements and $K^+$-sparing diuretics together greatly increases the risk of hyperkalemia and should be avoided. Combined use may be required temporarily at the beginning of replacement therapy if renal $K^+$ losses are very high; however, frequent monitoring of plasma $K^+$ is mandatory, and one of the drugs should be stopped when plasma $K^+$ reaches 3.0 to 3.5 mmol/L.

## *Suggested Reading List*


Allon M. Treatment and prevention of hyperkalemia in end-stage renal disease. *Kidney Int* 1993;43:1197–1209.

DeFronzo RA, Smith JD. Clinical disorders of hyperkalemia. In: Narins RG, ed. *Clinical disorders of fluid and electrolyte metabolism.* 5th ed. New York: McGraw-Hill, 1994:697–754.

Kamel SK, Halperin ML. Treatment of hypokalemia and hyperkalemia. In: Brady HR, Wilcox CS, eds. *Therapy in nephrology and hypertension.* 1st ed. Philadelphia: W.B. Saunders, 1999:270–278.

Krishna GG, Steigerwalt SP, Pikus R, et al. Hypokalemic states. In: Narins RG, ed. *Clinical disorders of fluid and electrolyte metabolism.* 5th ed. New York: McGraw-Hill, 1994:659–696.

Rose BD. *Clinical physiology of acid-base and electrolyte disorders.* 4th ed. New York: McGraw-Hill, 1994:776–799.

CHAPTER 82

# Acute Otitis Media in Childhood

*Ross A. Pennie, MD, FRCPC*

## Definition

Acute otitis media (AOM) is a suppurative infection of the middle ear cavity occurring most commonly in preschool children. Affected children usually have earache and fever. Two-thirds of cases are due to bacteria; most of the remaining third are probably due to viruses. Most patients recover without antibiotics; antibiotic therapy hastens the resolution of pain in only 1 out of every 12 children treated. Whether antibiotic therapy decreases the incidence of acute mastoiditis remains unclear.

## Goals of Therapy

- To control pain
- To eradicate infection
- To prevent complications
- To avoid unnecessary antibiotics

## Investigations

- Presenting signs of earache in children:
  - children will usually describe an earache
  - infants react by crying, sleeplessness, irritability
- Inspection of the eardrum (otoscopy):
  - wax and debris should be removed from the ear canal to obtain a clear view
  - the eardrum should be examined for loss of mobility, opacity, bulging, loss of ossicular landmarks and redness

*Note:* The following also cause redness of the eardrum in children **without** AOM:

- crying and agitation
- the common cold
- chronic otitis media with effusion
- aggressive examination or manipulation of the external ear canal

- If the diagnosis of AOM is uncertain, the presence of fluid/pus behind the eardrum should be determined by looking for one of the following:
  - decreased drum mobility on pneumatic otoscopy
  - abnormal profile on tympanometry
  - abnormal reading with acoustic otoscope
- Examination for other causes of apparent earache:
  - pharyngitis, tonsillitis
  - tooth abscess
  - foreign body in the ear canal
- Examination for complications of AOM:
  - ruptured eardrum (perforation visible, pus oozing)
  - mastoiditis (tender, boggy, swollen mastoid region)
  - intracranial infection (lethargy, confusion, stiff neck, vomiting, focal neurologic signs)

## Therapeutic Choices (Figure 1)

### Nonpharmacologic Choices

- Heat applied to the painful ear may provide comfort to an older child.
- Aspiration of pus from the middle ear cavity (tympanocentesis or myringotomy) may relieve the infection when earache and fever do not resolve after 3 days of antibiotics.

### Pharmacologic Choices

- Acetaminophen is indicated for pain relief.
- Oral antihistamines and decongestants do **not** improve outcome.
- Antibiotic therapy (Tables 1 and 2).
- Antibiotics speed the resolution of symptoms of AOM in only a minority of children (1 out of every 12 treated).
- Children who receive repeated courses of antibiotics are at increased risk of developing infections caused by antibiotic-resistant bacteria.
- There should be decreased emphasis on antibiotic therapy in the management of most children with AOM.
- In deciding whether or not to prescribe antibiotics for AOM, the practitioner must balance the potential risks and benefits involved. The following recommendations have been made:[1]
  - The high spontaneous recovery rate of AOM may warrant watchful waiting for 48–72 hours before initiating antibiotic therapy in children over 2 years of age, if appropriate follow-up can be assured.

[1] *The Antibiotic Resistance Education Project. Protecting patients from antimicrobial resistance: the role of the family physician. University of British Columbia, Dept. of Pediatrics. Vancouver, 1999.*

Figure 1: **Management of Acute Otitis Media**

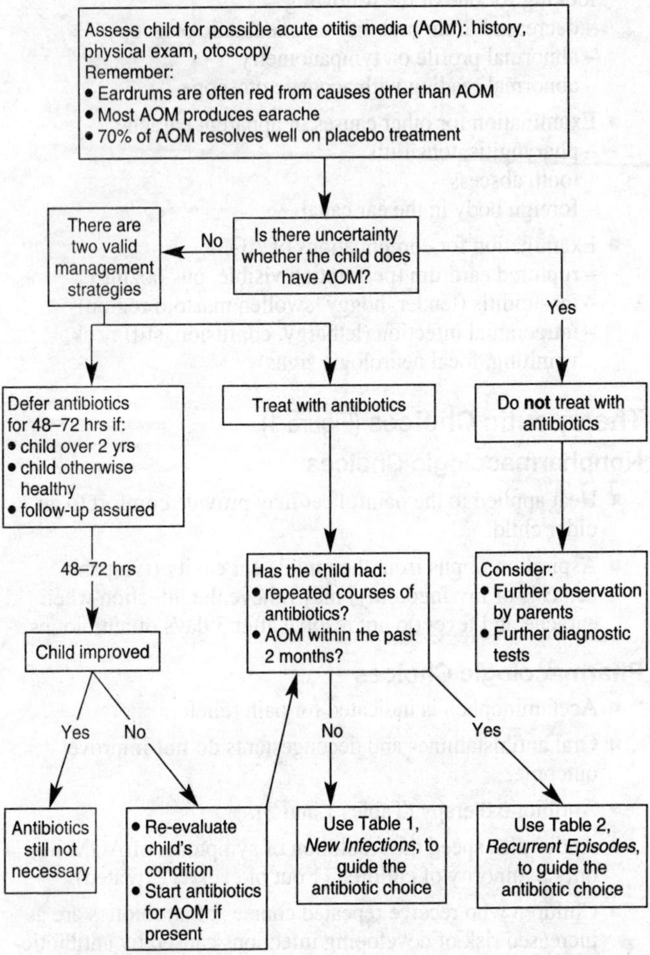
Assess child for possible acute otitis media (AOM): history, physical exam, otoscopy
Remember:
• Eardrums are often red from causes other than AOM
• Most AOM produces earache
• 70% of AOM resolves well on placebo treatment
Is there uncertainty whether the child does have AOM?
No
Yes
There are two valid management strategies
Defer antibiotics for 48–72 hrs if:
• child over 2 yrs
• child otherwise healthy
• follow-up assured
Treat with antibiotics
Do **not** treat with antibiotics
48–72 hrs
Child improved
Yes
No
Antibiotics still not necessary
• Re-evaluate child's condition
• Start antibiotics for AOM if present
Has the child had:
• repeated courses of antibiotics?
• AOM within the past 2 months?
No
Yes
Use Table 1, *New Infections*, to guide the antibiotic choice
Use Table 2, *Recurrent Episodes*, to guide the antibiotic choice
Consider:
• Further observation by parents
• Further diagnostic tests

- Antibiotic therapy for AOM should be initiated when middle ear effusion, ear pain, fever and irritability have not improved after 48–72 hours.
- Amoxicillin remains the treatment of choice for AOM requiring antimicrobial therapy.
- For children under age 2 years, a 10-day course is recommended. For older children, a 5-day course is as effective as 10 days.
- Persistent middle ear effusion (OME) following successful therapy for AOM is to be expected and does not require specific therapy (Figure 2).

The choice of antibiotic rests mainly on which one of the following three scenarios best represents the episode of AOM:

**New Infections** (Table 1):
- no episodes of AOM have occurred in previous 2 months
- most bacterial causes are susceptible to amoxicillin
- consider using high-dose amoxicillin (80 to 90 mg/kg/day) because lower doses cannot achieve bactericidal levels against drug-resistant strains of pneumococcus

**Failure of current treatment or recurrence within 2 months after an episode of AOM** (Table 2). Such infections may be due to:
- beta-lactamase-producing bacteria resistant to amoxicillin or pivampicillin
- pneumococci with reduced susceptibility to penicillins and cephalosporins (higher dose is needed). Such strains may be resistant to macrolides
- organisms resistant to co-trimoxazole

**Infection in a newborn less than 1 month of age:**
- gram-negative enteric bacteria frequently cause AOM in this age group
- hospital admission to rule out bacterial sepsis and initial treatment with IV ampicillin and cefotaxime are recommended

## Therapeutic Tips

- Two weeks after the start of successful antibiotic therapy, 80% of children with AOM may have middle ear effusions (and thus abnormal-looking eardrums). Do not prescribe antibiotics for a child who looks and feels better but has abnormal-appearing eardrums on follow-up.
- For children under age 2 years, a 10-day antibiotic course is recommended. For older children, a 5-day course is equally effective, less costly and shortens the time interval during which the child is exposed to the risks of antibiotic therapy.
- No matter what the age group, azithromycin should be given only for 5 days because it has an unusually prolonged elimination half-life.

## Prevention of Recurrent Acute Otitis Media

- Because of the concern about inducing bacterial resistance, prophylactic antibiotics for recurrent AOM are no longer recommended.
- Pneumococcal vaccine is **ineffective** in preventing AOM.
- The incidence of AOM has not fallen since the introduction of universal immunization against *Haemophilus influenzae* type b.

Table 1: **Antibiotics for *New Episodes* of Acute Otitis Media***

| Antibiotic | Pediatric Dosage† | Advantages | Disadvantages | Cost‡ |
|---|---|---|---|---|
| *amoxicillin* ➜ Amoxil, generics | 40–60 mg/kg/d divided TID or 80–90 mg/kg/d divided TID | Effective against 85–90% of bacteria that cause AOM.<br>Most active agent vs. pneumococci with ↓ susceptibility to penicillins and cephalosporins.<br>Excellent safety profile.<br>Better oral absorption than ampicillin. | Occasionally causes mild diarrhea.<br>Maculopapular skin rash occurs uncommonly but is difficult to distinguish from a concomitant viral exanthem. | Chewable tabs $$<br>Liquid $<br>Caps $ |
| *co-trimoxazole* ➜ Bactrim, Septra, generics | 8–10 mg/kg/d trimethoprim divided BID | BID dosing.<br>Liquid formulation has a long shelf-life at room temperature, making the drug suitable for travelers. | Not active against group A *Streptococcus*.<br>Resistance is increasing among strains of Pneumococci and *H. influenzae*.<br>Probably causes rash more commonly than amoxicillin.<br>May cause leukopenia if taken for several weeks. | $ |
| *pivampicillin* ➜ Pondocillin | 60–80 mg/kg/d divided BID | Better absorbed than ampicillin; therefore, higher blood levels can be achieved, permitting BID dosing.<br>Same excellent safety profile as amoxicillin. | No improvement in antibacterial spectrum or side effect profile compared to amoxicillin, despite ↑ cost. | $$$ |

* *The child has had no episodes of AOM within the preceding 2 mos.*
† *Duration of treatment: 5 days for children over 2 yrs; 10 days if under 2 yrs.*
➜ *Dosage adjustment may be required in renal impairment – see Appendix I. In acute otitis media the recommended dosages are moderate and thus adjustments are not usually necessary.*

‡ *Cost of 10-day supply – includes drug cost only.*
*Legend:* $ < $10   $$ $10–20   $$$ $20–30

Table 2: **Antibiotics for *Recurrent Episodes* of Acute Otitis Media***

| Antibiotic | Pediatric Dosage† | Advantages | Disadvantages | Cost‡ |
|---|---|---|---|---|
| *amoxicillin* Amoxil, generics | 80–90 mg/kg/d (high dose only) | Effective against 85–90% of bacteria that cause AOM. Most active agent vs. pneumococci with ↓ susceptibility to penicillins and cephalosporins.<br>Excellent safety profile.<br>Better oral absorption than ampicillin. | Occasionally causes mild diarrhea.<br>Maculopapular skin rash occurs uncommonly but is difficult to distinguish from a concomitant viral exanthem. | \$–\$\$ |
| *amoxicillin/ clavulanic acid* Clavulin | 40–60 mg/kg/d amoxicillin divided TID | Excellent safety profile of amoxicillin.<br>Active against most bacteria likely to cause AOM. | Diarrhea occurs in about 50% of patients but does not necessarily lead to discontinuing the drug. | \$\$\$\$ |
| *cefaclor* Ceclor, generics | 40 mg/kg/d divided BID or TID | Active against most bacteria likely to cause AOM. | Antimicrobial activity in vitro not as great as with other similar drugs.<br>Serum-sickness reaction in about 1% of children. | \$\$\$ |
| *cefixime* Suprax | 8 mg/kg/d given once daily | Active against amoxicillin-resistant strains of *H. influenzae* and *M. catarrhalis.*<br>Once daily dosing. | Not active against *S. aureus.*<br>Poor in vitro activity vs pneumococci exhibiting reduced susceptibility to penicillins and cephalosporins.<br>Diarrhea occurs in about 10% of patients. | \$\$\$ |

*(cont'd)*

Table 2: **Antibiotics for *Recurrent Episodes* of Acute Otitis Media*** *(cont'd)*

| Antibiotic | Pediatric Dosage[†] | Advantages | Disadvantages | Cost[‡] |
|---|---|---|---|---|
| *cefprozil* Cefzil | 30 mg/kg/d divided BID | Active against most bacteria likely to cause AOM.<br>Good-tasting liquid formulation is well absorbed.<br>Low incidence of diarrhea or gastro-intestinal upset. | | $$$$ |
| *cefuroxime axetil* Ceftin | 30–40 mg/kg/d divided BID | Active against most bacteria likely to cause AOM.<br>Pediatric suspension is available as single-dose sachets suitable for travelers. | Diarrhea occurs more frequently when higher doses are used.<br>Because of the potential to cause bitter after-taste, Ceftin suspension should be taken with food and/or juice. | $$$$ |
| *azithromycin* Zithromax | First day: 10 mg/kg<br>Days 2–5: 5 mg/kg<br>Administer once daily at bedtime | Active against most bacteria likely to cause AOM.<br>Good-tasting liquid formulation.<br>Low incidence of diarrhea or gastrointestinal upset.<br>Convenient once daily dosing and short 5-day course. | Pneumococci exhibiting reduced susceptibility to penicillins and cephalosporins are sometimes resistant to azithromycin. | $$$ |

| | | | | |
|---|---|---|---|---|
| *clarithromycin* ❥<br>Biaxin | 15 mg/kg/d divided BID | Active against most bacteria likely to cause AOM.<br>Better tolerated than erythromycin. | Pneumococci exhibiting reduced susceptibility to penicillins and cephalosporins are sometimes resistant to clarithromycin.<br>Diarrhea or vomiting occur in 15% of patients.<br>Because of the potential to cause bitter aftertaste, Biaxin suspension should be taken with food and/or juice. | $$$$ |
| *erythromycin/sulfisoxazole* ❥<br>Pediazole | 40 mg/kg/d erythromycin divided TID or QID | Active against most bacteria likely to cause AOM. | About 40% of patients experience abdominal pain, nausea or vomiting because of the erythromycin component.<br>Rashes are probably more common with sulfonamides than other antibiotics. | $$ |

* *Failure of current treatment or recurrence within 2 mos after an episode of AOM.*
† *Duration of treatment: 5 days for children over 2 yrs; 10 days if under 2 yrs.*
❥ *Dosage adjustment may be required in renal impairment – see Appendix I. In acute otitis media the recommended dosages are moderate and thus adjustments are not usually necessary.*
‡ *Cost of 10-day supply except 5-day supply for azithromycin – includes drug cost only.*
*Legend: $ < $10 $$ $10–20 $$$ $20–30 $$$$ $30–40*

Figure 2: **Management of Serous Otitis Media (SOM)**

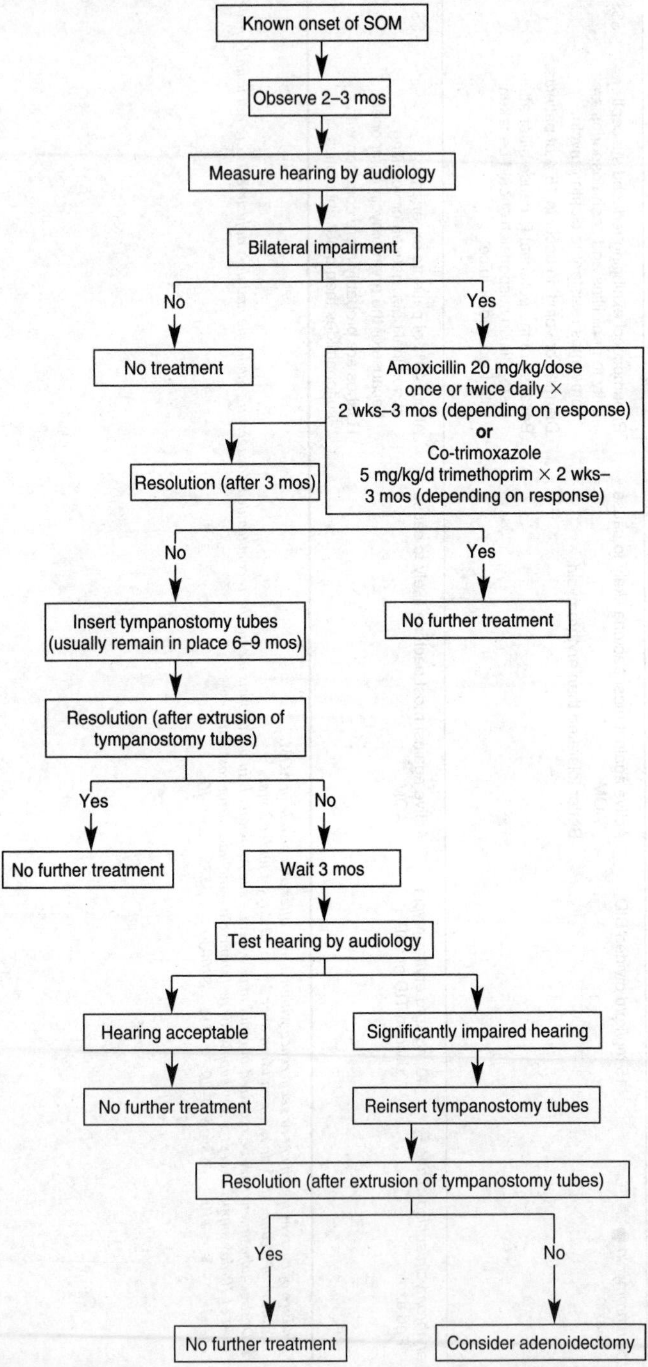
Known onset of SOM
Observe 2–3 mos
Measure hearing by audiology
Bilateral impairment
No
Yes
No treatment
Amoxicillin 20 mg/kg/dose once or twice daily × 2 wks–3 mos (depending on response)
or
Co-trimoxazole 5 mg/kg/d trimethoprim × 2 wks–3 mos (depending on response)
Resolution (after 3 mos)
No
Yes
Insert tympanostomy tubes (usually remain in place 6–9 mos)
No further treatment
Resolution (after extrusion of tympanostomy tubes)
Yes
No
No further treatment
Wait 3 mos
Test hearing by audiology
Hearing acceptable
Significantly impaired hearing
No further treatment
Reinsert tympanostomy tubes
Resolution (after extrusion of tympanostomy tubes)
Yes
No
No further treatment
Consider adenoidectomy

## **Management of Serous Otitis Media** (Figure 2)

Serous otitis media, also known as otitis media with effusion (OME), is fluid in the middle ear cavity without associated earache or fever. This condition often follows episodes of acute otitis media and is only significant when it causes hearing loss.

### ***Suggested Reading List***


Cogeni BL. Therapy of acute otitis media in an era of antibiotic resistance. *Pediatr Infect Dis J* 1999;18:371–372.

Dowell SF, Butler JC, Giebink GS, et al. Acute otitis media: management and surveillance in an era of pneumococcal resistance — a report from the Drug-resistant *Streptococcus pneumoniae* Therapeutic Working Group. *Pediatr Infect Dis J* 1999;18:1–9.

Kaleida PH, Casselbrant ML, Rockette HE, et al. Amoxicillin or myringotomy or both for acute otitis media: results of a randomized clinical trial. *Pediatrics* 1991;87:466–474.

Kozyrskyi AL, Hildes-Ripstein GE, Longstaffe SE, et al. Treatment of acute otitis media with a shortened course of antibiotics. A meta-analysis. *JAMA* 1998;279:1736–1742.

Marchant CD, Carlin SA, Johnson CE, Shurin PA. Measuring the comparative efficacy of antibacterial agents for acute otitis media: the "Pollyanna Phenomenon." *J Pediatrics* 1992;120:72–77.

Paradise JL. Managing otitis media; a time for change. *Pediatrics* 1995;96:712–713.

CHAPTER 83

# Streptococcal Sore Throat

*David P. Speert, MD, FRCPC*

## Goals of Therapy

- To provide symptomatic relief
- To prevent suppurative complications
- To prevent nonsuppurative complications, i.e., acute rheumatic fever
- To prevent spread of group A streptococci to contacts

## Investigations

The probability of culturing group A streptococci is greatest in a child with an acute sore throat who is > 3 years, lacks signs of a viral upper respiratory infection and has signs and symptoms as listed below. However, the diagnosis of streptococcal pharyngitis (strep throat) should be considered seriously in any child presenting with an acute sore throat, with or without "classical" signs and symptoms.

- Differential diagnosis: a partial list of etiologic agents for acute sore throat includes:

| | |
|---|---|
| *Streptococcus*, group A | *Mycoplasma pneumoniae** |
| *Streptococcus*, groups C and G | *Chlamydia trachomatis** |
| *Neisseria gonorrhoeae* (Consider sexual abuse if recovered from child's throat) | *Arcanobacterium hemolyticum** |
| *Corynebacterium diphtheriae* | *Chlamydia pneumoniae** |
| Viruses (adenoviruses, enteroviruses, cytomegalovirus, Epstein-Barr, influenza and parainfluenza viruses) | |

*role in acute pharyngitis is controversial

- Clinical diagnosis of streptococcal infection: adenitis and positive throat cultures are the only predictive features. Although not diagnostic, signs and symptoms include:
  - signs: tender cervical adenopathy, erythematous pharynx and tonsils, pharyngeal exudate, excoriated nares, scarlatiniform rash
  - symptoms: sore throat, headache, abdominal pain, nausea, vomiting, fever (Chapter 106)

Figure 1: **Management of Acute Sore Throat**

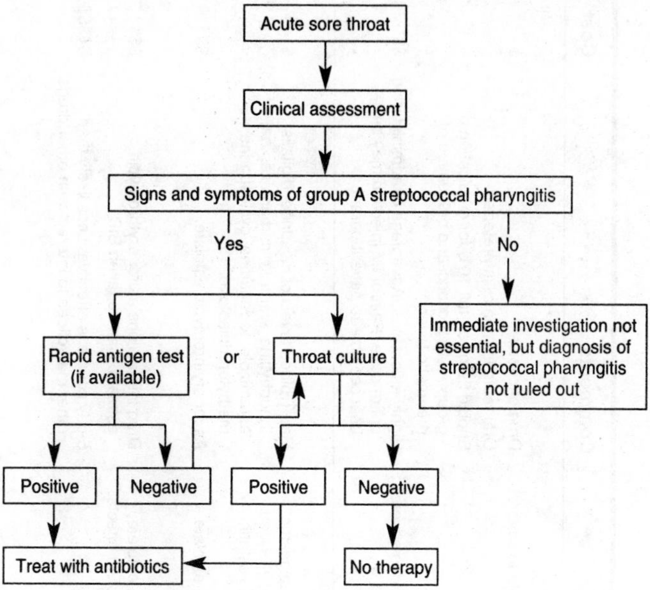
Acute sore throat
Clinical assessment
Signs and symptoms of group A streptococcal pharyngitis
Yes
No
Rapid antigen test (if available)
or
Throat culture
Immediate investigation not essential, but diagnosis of streptococcal pharyngitis not ruled out
Positive
Negative
Positive
Negative
Treat with antibiotics
No therapy

- Laboratory diagnosis:
  - throat culture is "gold standard" (results available in 24 to 48 hours). Viral throat culture rarely affects therapy (results available in days to weeks)
  - antigen screen of throat secretions (rapid test): results available in 7 to 70 minutes but only 50 to 70% sensitive
  - streptococcal serology (antistreptolysin O [ASO] and others): useful retrospectively in patients who have possible complications of streptococcal infection (e.g., rheumatic fever)

## Therapeutic Choices (Figure 1)

### Pharmacologic Choices (Table 1)

Antibiotic therapy for group A streptococcal pharyngitis can shorten the course of the acute illness and prevent both suppurative and nonsuppurative complications.

**Penicillin** is the drug of choice. **Erythromycin** is the preferred alternative in patients allergic to penicillin. Although **cephalosporins** are effective, they should *not* replace penicillin as the drug of choice.

Acetaminophen may be given for fever and pain. Lozenges and gargles may be indicated for symptomatic treatment of sore throat.

Table 1: **Drugs for Treatment of Group A Streptococcal Pharyngitis**

| Drug | Dosage | Adverse Effects | Comments | Cost* |
|---|---|---|---|---|
| **Penicillins** | | | | |
| *penicillin V* PVF K, V-Cillin, generics | < 27 kg: 125 mg PO TID × 10 d<br>≥ 27 kg: 250 mg PO TID × 10 d | Hypersensitivity (mild to severe). | Drug of choice.<br>Oral route for penicillin preferred.<br>Should be given full 10 d for eradication of group A streptococci and prevention of rheumatic fever. | $<br>$$ |
| *benzathine penicillin G* Bicillin L-A | < 27 kg: 600 000 units IM, single dose<br>> 27 kg: 1 200 000 units IM, single dose | Hypersensitivity (mild to severe). | Highly efficacious. Advantage of administering entire dose. Pain of IM injection may be unacceptable to patient/parent. | $$† |
| **Macrolides** | | | | |
| *erythromycin estolate* Ilosone, generics | 20–30 mg/kg/d in 2 to 4 divided doses × 10 d<br>Max.: 1 g/d | Nausea, vomiting, epigastric distress, diarrhea, elevated liver enzymes, cholestatic jaundice. | May ↑ blood levels of cisapride, digitalis, theophylline, warfarin, carbamazepine, astemizole, terfenadine, cyclosporine, methylprednisolone. | $ |
| *erythromycin ethylsuccinate* EES, generics | 40–50 mg/kg/d in 2 to 4 divided doses × 10 d<br>Max.: 1 g/d | As for erythromycin estolate. | As for erythromycin estolate. | $$ |
| *clarithromycin* Biaxin | Adult: 250 mg PO BID × 10 d<br>Children: 125 mg PO BID × 10 d | As for erythromycin estolate; lower frequency of GI effects. | Drug interactions as for erythromycin estolate. Can be taken BID. | $$$ |
| *azithromycin* Zithromax | > 16 yrs: 500 mg × 1 d, then 250 mg/d × 4 d | | 5-day course is effective. Less likely than other macrolides to interact with other drugs. | $$$$$ |

| | | | | |
|---|---|---|---|---|
| **Cephalosporins** | | | | |
| *cephalexin* (kidney symbol) Keflex, generics | 25–50 mg/kg/d in 2 to 4 divided doses × 10 d<br>Max.: 1 g/d | Hypersensitivity. Cross-allergenicity with penicillins. | Use if treatment failure with penicillin. | \$\$–\$\$\$ |

*† Cost of single dose.*

** Cost of 10-day supply of suspension based on 20 kg weight for pediatric dosage except azithromycin 5-day supply of tablets for adult dosage – includes drug cost only.*

*Legend: \$ < \$5   \$\$ \$5–10   \$\$\$ \$10–15   \$\$\$\$ \$15–25   \$\$\$\$\$ > \$25*

(kidney symbol) *Dosage adjustment may be required in renal impairment – see Appendix I.*

## Therapeutic Tips

- If the antigen detection test is unavailable or is negative, a culture should be obtained and antibiotics may be withheld until the results are available in 24 to 48 hours. This approach does not increase the risk of acute rheumatic fever but avoids the unnecessary use of antibiotics. Patients with positive cultures for group A streptococci should be recalled and treated with antibiotics.
- Since there is no efficient way to differentiate between the acutely infected child and the carrier of group A streptococci, all symptomatic patients with positive cultures should receive antistreptococcal therapy. A large percentage of cases of acute rheumatic fever develop after mild or subclinical streptococcal infections.
- The early institution of antibiotic therapy shortens the duration of fever, cervical adenitis and pharyngeal injection and hastens the overall clinical improvement. Early treatment can hasten the return of children to school or to daycare and minimize work time lost by their parents.
- Repeat cultures are not necessary at the end of therapy, and cultures need not be obtained from asymptomatic family contacts.
- It is impossible to reliably differentiate between acute streptococcal infection and chronic carriage; a means of eradicating chronic carriage is therefore desirable. Unfortunately, penicillin, the drug of choice for treating acute streptococcal sore throat, often fails to eradicate *pharyngeal streptococcal carriage*. Some advocate the use of **clindamycin** (20 mg/kg/day divided TID for 10 days) or the addition of **rifampin** (20 mg/kg/day; maximum = 600 mg) for the final 4 days of penicillin therapy to attempt to interrupt chronic pharyngeal carriage of group A streptococci.

## Suggested Reading List

Dajani A, Taubert K, Ferrieri P, Peter G, Shulman S. Treatment of acute streptococcal pharyngitis and prevention of rheumatic fever: a statement for health professionals. *Pediatrics* 1995;96:758–764.

Gerber MA. Treatment failures and carriers: perception or problems? *Pediatr Infect Dis J* 1994;13:576–579.

Markowitz M, Gerber MA, Kaplan EL, et al. Treatment of streptococcal pharyngotonsillitis: Reports of penicillin's demise are premature. *J Pediatr* 1993;123:679–685.

Shulman ST. Evaluation of penicillins, cephalosporins and macrolides for therapy of streptococcal pharyngitis. *Pediatrics* 1996;97:955–959.

CHAPTER 84

# Bacterial Meningitis

*Ari Bitnun, MD, Upton Allen, MBBS, MSc, FAAP, FRCPC and Ronald Gold, MD, MPH, FRCPC*

## Goals of Therapy

- To eradicate bacteria
- To manage acute complications (increased intracranial pressure, dehydration, seizures, subdural effusion)
- To minimize or prevent permanent neurologic damage

## Investigations

- Signs and symptoms. Meningitis should be suspected in the following:
  - *Infants less than 24 months of age:* any infant with fever and significant alteration in consciousness (irritability and/or lethargy); signs of meningeal irritation (neck stiffness, Brudzinski and Kernig signs) are often lacking, especially in infants less than 6 months of age
  - *Children and adults:* any person with sudden onset of fever, neck stiffness, severe headache, alteration in level of consciousness (occasionally agitation or combativeness rather than more usual lethargy or stupor)
  - In addition, pain on movement, vomiting and seizures may be present in *all ages*
- Lumbar puncture (LP)
  - indicated in any person suspected of bacterial meningitis. The procedure is contraindicated only in the presence of *definite* signs of marked increase in intracranial pressure (coma, decerebrate posture, hypertension, bradycardia, irregular respiration)
  - if performance of LP must be delayed, empiric antibiotic therapy should be started after blood culture obtained
- Examination of cerebrospinal fluid (CSF)
  - CSF in bacterial meningitis usually shows pleocytosis ($> 1\times10^9$/L WBC, mainly neutrophils), glucose $\leq 2$ mmol/L and protein $\geq 0.4$ g/L. However, initial CSF may have $< 1\times10^9$/L WBC in 33% and normal protein in 20% of cases
  - Gram's stain is positive in 80% of cases not previously treated with antibiotics
  - detection of bacterial antigens with latex agglutination correlates highly with Gram's stain and is most useful in cases treated with antibiotics before lumbar puncture.

Table 1: **Bacterial Meningitis: Risk Factors, Pathogens and Empiric Treatment**

| **Age Group/Risk Factor (Mechanism)** | **Pathogens** | **Initial Antibiotics*** |
|---|---|---|
| Infants < 6 wks of age | *E. coli*<br>Group B *streptococcus*<br>*Listeria monocytogenes*<br>*S. pneumoniae**<br>*N. meningitidis* | Ampicillin + gentamicin<br>or<br>Ampicillin + cefotaxime |
| Infants 6 wks-3 mos of age<br>(Lack of natural antibody; impaired host defenses in premature infants) | as above +<br>*H. influenzae* (rare) | Ampicillin + cefotaxime |
| Otherwise normal infants ≥ 3 mos of age, children and adults<br>(Lack of natural antibody up to 24 mos) | *S. pneumoniae**<br>*N. meningitidis*<br>*H. influenzae (rare)* | Ceftriaxone<br>or<br>Cefotaxime |
| Elderly<br>(Impaired host defenses) | *E. coli*<br>*S. pneumoniae**<br>*Listeria monocytogenes* | Ampicillin + ceftriaxone |
| CNS malformation<br>(Direct access of bacteria from skin) | *S. epidermidis*<br>*S. aureus*<br>*S. pneumoniae* | Vancomycin + cefotaxime |
| Head trauma<br>(Direct access of bacteria from skin or nasal mucosa) | *S. aureus*<br>*S. pneumoniae** | Cloxacillin |
| Neurosurgery<br>(Foreign body impairs host defenses) | *S. aureus*<br>*S. epidermidis* | Vancomycin |
| Chronic middle ear infection<br>(Direct extension through petrous bone) | *P. aeruginosa* | Ceftazidime<br>+/– tobramycin or amikacin |
| Asplenia, sickle cell disease<br>(Impaired clearance of bacteremia; impaired IgM synthesis) | *S. pneumoniae**<br>*N. meningitidis*<br>*H. influenzae (rare)* | Ceftriaxone<br>or<br>Cefotaxime |
| Agammaglobulinemia<br>(Lack of IgG) | *S. pneumoniae**<br>*N. meningitidis*<br>*H. influenzae (rare)* | Ceftriaxone<br>or<br>Cefotaxime |
| Terminal complement component deficiency (C5–8)<br>(Lack of bactericidal activity against *Neisseria*) | *N. meningitidis* | Ceftriaxone<br>or<br>Cefotaxime |
| Cancer chemotherapy<br>(Impaired cellular immunity) | *S. pneumoniae**<br>*N. meningitidis*<br>*Listeria monocytogenes*<br>*H. influenzae (rare)* | Ampicillin + ceftriaxone<br>or<br>Ampicillin + cefotaxime |

*** Initial regimen should include vancomycin if S. pneumoniae is a likely possibility.***

Latex agglutination is reliable in detecting antigens in CSF of group A and C meningococci (*Neisseria meningitidis*), most pneumococci (*Streptococcus pneumoniae*), *Haemophilus influenzae* type b and group B streptococci. It is much less reliable in detecting group B meningococcal antigen

- Blood and CSF should be obtained for culture to maximize the probability of identifying the infective cause
- CT scan[1] or other imaging studies are indicated in the presence of definite signs of impending herniation due to increased intracranial pressure

## Pharmacologic Choices

### *Antibiotic Therapy*

Initial parenteral antibiotic choice should be based on age and risk factors so as to cover the most likely pathogens (Table 1). Meningitis due to *H. influenzae* type b has virtually disappeared in Canada. Because of concerns regarding penicillin-nonsusceptible strains of meningococci and pneumococci, penicillin G should not be used until antibiotic susceptibilities have been determined. Once the pathogen and its antibiotic susceptibilities are known, therapy should be changed, if possible, to a drug of first choice that is less expensive and/or less toxic (Tables 2 and 3).

It is currently recommended that **vancomycin** be used in addition to **ceftriaxone** or **cefotaxime** as empiric therapy for presumed pneumococcal meningitis in *children older than 3 months of age,* because of the problem of *penicillin- and cephalosporin-resistant pneumococci.* This combination should be used to treat *children 1 to 3 months of age* if *S. pneumoniae* is suspected.

*Children with immediate hypersensitivity to β-lactam antibiotics* may be treated empirically with **vancomycin** and **rifampin** if they are presumed to have pneumococcal meningitis. Treatment failures have occurred with **chloramphenicol**, which should not be used unless the organism is known to have a minimal bactericidal concentration (MBC) value of 4 μg/mL or less for this drug.[2] Since at least 3 days are required to obtain this information, the use of chloramphenicol in combination with vancomycin is not a practical option for the child with presumed pneumococcal meningitis.

Due to the fact that *infants under 1 month of age* may have pneumococcal meningitis, **vancomycin** should be added to the usual antibiotic combination for neonatal sepsis if the CSF shows characteristic gram-positive diplococci *or* bacterial antigen testing suggests pneumococcal meningitis.

---

[1] *J Pediatr 1987;111:201–205.*

[2] *Pediatrics 1997;99:289–299.*

Table 2: **Antibiotic Therapy for Bacterial Meningitis**

| Pathogen | Drug of First Choice | Alternative | Days of Treatment* |
|---|---|---|---|
| *S. pneumoniae* | Penicillin G† | Cefotaxime or ceftriaxone ± vancomycin | 7–10 |
| *N. meningitidis* | Penicillin G | Ceftriaxone, Cefotaxime | 5–7 |
| *H. influenzae* type b | Ceftriaxone, Cefotaxime | Ampicillin (if β-lactamase negative) | 7–10 |
| Group B *Streptococcus* | Ampicillin | Penicillin | 14–21 |
| *E. coli* | Cefotaxime, Ceftriaxone | Gentamicin | 21 |
| *Listeria monocytogenes* | Ampicillin | Co-trimoxazole, vancomycin | 21 |

* *Duration of therapy in uncomplicated cases.*
† *Vancomycin with cefotaxime or ceftriaxone should be the initial regimen if S. pneumoniae is suspected.*

### Response Monitoring

The most important criterion for assessing response to therapy is improved brain function (i.e., improvement in level of consciousness and normalization of behavior and responsiveness). Approximately 10% of patients will have persistent or recurrent fever that is rarely caused by failure of eradication of bacteria from the CSF.

In cases of pneumococcal meningitis, a repeat lumbar puncture should be considered after 24 to 48 hours if the organism is penicillin- or cephalosporin-nonsusceptible and the patient's condition has not improved or has worsened.

Given the emergence of penicillin- and cephalosporin-nonsusceptible pneumococci, an infectious disease expert should be consulted if the patient with presumed pneumococcal meningitis does not appear to be responding to the appropriate empiric therapy (e.g., vancomycin and cefotaxime or ceftriaxone) after 24 to 48 hours.

### Anti-inflammatory Therapy

The use of adjunctive **dexamethasone** in children over 6 weeks of age with bacterial meningitis may be considered after weighing potential benefits and risks. Intravenous dexamethasone therapy reduces the incidence of severe deafness due to *H. influenzae* type b meningitis. The effectiveness of dexamethasone in meningitis caused by other bacteria and its safety and efficacy in neonatal or adult meningitis are unknown.

Table 3: **Intravenous Antibiotics for Treatment of Bacterial Meningitis**

| Antibiotic | Dose (Maximum) | Frequency | Adverse Effects | Drug Interactions | Cost* |
|---|---|---|---|---|---|
| *penicillin G* | 70 000 units/kg/dose (2–4 million units/dose) | Q4–6H | Hypersensitivity, rash, drug fever, positive Coombs' test. | Tetracycline may ↓ effect. | $ |
| *ampicillin* Ampicin, generics | 75 mg/kg/dose (2.5 g/dose) | Q6H | Hypersensitivity, GI effects, rash, seizures with excessively rapid IV. | ↑ incidence of rash with concurrent use of allopurinol. | $$ |
| *cloxacillin* Tegopen, generics | 50 mg/kg/dose (3 g/dose) | Q6H | Hypersensitivity, rash, eosinophilia. | | $ |
| *ceftriaxone* Rocephin | 80 mg/kg/dose (2 g/dose, 4 g/d) | Q12H × 48 h, then once daily | Phlebitis, hypersensitivity, ↑ AST, superinfection. | | $$$$$ |
| *cefotaxime* Claforan | 50 mg/kg/dose (2 g/dose) | Q6H | Phlebitis, hypersensitivity, positive Coombs' test. | | $$$$ |
| *ceftazidime* Ceptaz, Fortaz, Tazidime | 50 mg/kg/dose (2 g/dose) | Q8H | Phlebitis, hypersensitivity, positive Coombs' test, ↑ AST. | | $$$$$ |

*(cont'd)*

Table 3: **Intravenous Antibiotics for Treatment of Bacterial Meningitis** *(cont'd)*

| Antibiotic | Dose (Maximum) | Frequency | Adverse Effects | Drug Interactions | Cost* |
|---|---|---|---|---|---|
| *gentamicin* ❥ † Cidomycin, Garamycin, generics | 2.5 mg/kg/dose | Q8H | Nephrotoxicity – usually reversible, ↑ risk with dose, duration; ototoxicity (often reversible). | ↑ ototoxicity with loop diuretics. ↑ nephrotoxicity with nephrotoxic drugs. Can be inactivated if mixed with some penicillins. | $$ |
| *vancomycin* ❥ Vancocin | 10–15 mg/kg/dose (1 g/dose) | Q6H | Phlebitis, hypotension, flushing with rapid IV. | ↑ toxicity with other ototoxic or nephrotoxic drugs. | $$$$$ |

❥ *Dosage adjustment may be required in renal impairment – see Appendix I.*
* *Cost per 70 kg per day – includes drug cost only.*
*Legend: $ < $25 $$ $25–50 $$$ $50–75 $$$$ $75–100 $$$$$ > $100*

† *Other aminoglycosides may be indicated, depending upon antibiotic susceptibilities.*

Table 4: **Use of Dexamethasone in Children With Bacterial Meningitis**

| | |
|---|---|
| Age | Consider in children ≥ 6 wk of age.<br>Do **not** use in infants < 1 mo of age. |
| Dose | 0.6 mg/kg/d, IV divided Q6H × 4 d. |
| Timing | IV push before or concurrently with first dose of antibiotics.<br>Do **not** start dexamethasone more than 4 h after first dose of antibiotics. |
| Viral meningitis | Discontinue if bacterial meningitis unlikely. |
| Precautions | Measure hemoglobin and stool for occult blood daily.<br>Discontinue if gross blood in stool or melena occurs. |

In addition, dexamethasone may potentially reduce the penetration of antimicrobial agents into the CSF. This is of particular concern with regard to use of vancomycin in meningitis due to penicillin-nonsusceptible *S. pneumoniae*. Dexamethasone is recommended for the treatment of *H. influenzae* type b meningitis and should be considered for *S. pneumoniae* and *N. meningitidis* meningitis (Table 4).

Significant bleeding from the gastrointestinal tract, such as perforated duodenal ulcer or hemorrhage requiring transfusion, has been observed in approximately 0.8% of dexamethasone-treated children.

## Prevention of Meningitis

The virtual disappearance of meningitis due to *H. influenzae* type b (Hib) is due to the efficacy of the vaccine. Vaccines are available against the A, C, Y and W135 serogroups of *N. meningitidis* but not against serogroup B; these are recommended only for outbreak control and for some high-risk patients. Pneumococcal conjugate vaccines have been shown to reduce the incidence of pneumococcal bacteremia and meningitis and are likely to play a major role in prevention of pneumococcal meningitis in the future.

Household and close contacts of patients with meningitis due to *H. influenzae* and *N. meningitidis* should be given antibiotic prophylaxis with **rifampin** (10 mg/kg/dose, maximum 600 mg/dose, Q12H for 4 doses) or **ceftriaxone** (125 mg for children < 12 years, 250 mg for persons > 12 years, single dose IM) or **ciprofloxacin** (500 mg PO single dose for adults and postpubertal children). The 4-day regimen of rifampin used to treat *H. influenzae* type b disease (20 mg/kg, 600 mg maximum, once daily for 4 days) is also effective for meningococcal prophylaxis. The index case should receive chemoprophylactic antibiotics (in addition to the antibiotics used to treat the meningitis) before discharge from hospital unless the infection was treated with ceftriaxone or cefotaxime.

## Suggested Reading List

American Academy of Pediatrics. Committee on Infectious Diseases. Therapy for children with invasive pneumococcal infections. *Pediatrics* 1997;99:289–299.

American Academy of Pediatrics. Dexamethasone therapy for bacterial meningitis in infants and children. In: Peter G, ed. *1997 Red Book: Report of the Committee on Infectious Diseases*. 24th ed. Elk Grove Village, IL: American Academy of Pediatrics, 1997:620–622.

American Academy of Pediatrics. Pneumococcal Infections. In: Peter G, ed. *2000 Red Book: Report of the Committee on Infectious Diseases*. 25th ed. Elk Grove Village, IL: American Academy of Pediatrics, 2000:452–460.

Kaplan SL. Clinical presentations, diagnosis, and prognostic factors of bacterial meningitis. *Infect Dis Clin North Am* 1999;13:579–594.

Klugman KP, Madhi SA. Emergence of drug resistance: impact on bacterial meningitis. *Infect Dis Clin North Am* 1999;13:637–646.

Saez-Llorens X, McCracKen GH. Antimicrobial and anti-inflammatory treatment of bacterial meningitis. *Infect Dis Clin North Am* 1999;13:619–636.

## CHAPTER 85

# Prevention of Bacterial Endocarditis

*Hillar Vellend, MD, FRCPC*

## Principles

- Systemic antibiotics should be administered to patients with types of valvular heart disease or cardiac history known to be associated with significant risk of endocarditis at the time of procedures associated with a high probability of transient bacteremia (Table 1). Most cases of endocarditis cannot be attributed to such invasive procedures.
- The prophylaxis for dental, oral, respiratory tract or esophageal procedures is directed against α-hemolytic (viridans) streptococci (Table 2).
- The prophylaxis for genitourinary or GI (excluding esophageal) procedures is directed against *Enterococcus faecalis* (enterococci) (Table 2).
- The antibiotic(s) should be administered to provide effective serum concentrations at the time of the anticipated bacteremia and for a few hours thereafter. How antibiotics interfere with bacteria during development of endocarditis is unknown.

Table 1: **Conditions and Procedures Recommended for Endocarditis Prophylaxis**

| Cardiac Conditions Associated with Risk of Endocarditis | Dental or Surgical Procedures for Which Endocarditis Prophylaxis is Recommended |
|---|---|
| *High Risk*<br>Prosthetic cardiac valves<br>Previous bacterial endocarditis<br>Complex cyanotic congenital heart disease<br>Surgically constructed systemic-pulmonary shunts or conduits<br>*Moderate Risk*<br>Most congenital cardiac malformations<br>Rheumatic valvular heart disease<br>Hypertrophic cardiomyopathy<br>Mitral valve prolapse with valvular regurgitation (murmur and/or ECHO/Doppler demonstration) | All dental procedures likely to induce bleeding, including professional cleaning<br>Tonsillectomy and/or adenoidectomy<br>All operations that involve oral, respiratory or intestinal mucosa<br>Sclerotherapy for esophageal varices<br>Esophageal dilatation<br>ERCP with biliary obstruction<br>Biliary tract surgery<br>Cystoscopy<br>Urethral dilatation<br>Prostatic surgery<br>Any surgery or drainage procedure involving an abscess, infected tissue or body fluid (urine, bile, amniotic fluid, peritoneal fluid, etc.) if patient is not already receiving appropriate antibiotics |

Prophylaxis is **NOT** recommended for flexible bronchoscopy or GI endoscopy with or without biopsy, transesophageal echocardiography, vaginal delivery, cesarean section, vaginal hysterectomy, therapeutic abortion, cardiac catheterization, transvenous pacemaker insertion.

Table 2: **Antibiotic Prophylaxis for Bacterial Endocarditis**

| **Dental, Oral, Respiratory Tract or Esophageal Procedures**<br>**Drug** | **Adult Dosing** | **Pediatric Dosing** |
|---|---|---|
| **Standard Regimen** | | |
| *amoxicillin* | 2 g PO 1 h before procedure | 50 mg/kg PO 1 h before procedure |
| **Unable to Take Oral Medications** | | |
| *ampicillin* | 2 g IV 30 min before procedure | 50 mg/kg IV 30 min before procedure |
| **Allergic to Penicillin** | | |
| *clindamycin* | 600 mg PO 1 h before procedure | 20 mg/kg PO 1 h before procedure |
| *or cephalexin** | 2 g PO 1 h before procedure | 50 mg/kg PO 1 h before procedure |
| *or cefadroxil** | 2 g PO 1 h before procedure | 50 mg/kg PO 1 h before procedure |
| *or clarithromycin* | 500 mg PO 1 h before procedure | 15 mg/kg PO 1 h before procedure |
| *or azithromycin* | 500 mg PO 1 h before procedure | 15 mg/kg PO 1 h before procedure |
| **Allergic to Penicillin and Unable to Take Oral Medications** | | |
| *clindamycin* | 600 mg IV 30 min before procedure | 20 mg/kg IV 30 min before procedure |
| *or cefazolin** | 1 g IV 30 min before procedure | 25 mg/kg IV 30 min before procedure |

| | | |
|---|---|---|
| ***High-risk patient*** | | |
| **Standard Regimen** | | |
| *ampicillin* plus<br>*gentamicin* | 2 g IV plus<br>1.5 mg/kg (max: 120 mg) IV 30 min before procedure | 50 mg/kg IV plus<br>1.5 mg/kg IV 30 min before procedure |
| then *amoxicillin*<br>or *ampicillin* | 1.5 g PO 6 h later<br>1 g IV 6 h later | *then* 25 mg/kg PO 6 h later<br>25 mg/kg IV 6 h later |
| **Allergic to Penicillin** | | |
| *vancomycin* plus<br>*gentamicin* | 1 g IV infused over 1–2 h plus<br>1.5 mg/kg (max: 120 mg) IV 30 min before procedure | 20 mg/kg IV infused over 1–2 h plus<br>1.5 mg/kg IV 30 min before procedure |
| ***Moderate-risk patient*** | | |
| **Standard Regimen** | | |
| *amoxicillin* | 2 g PO 1 h before procedure | 50 mg/kg PO 1 h before procedure |
| or a*mpicillin* | 2 g IV 30 min before procedure | 50 mg/kg IV 30 min before procedure |
| **Allergic to Penicillin** | | |
| *vancomycin* | 1 g IV over 1–2 h 30 min before procedure | 20 mg/kg IV over 1–2 h 30 min before procedure |

* *Cephalosporins should not be used in individuals with immediate-type hypersensitivity reaction (urticaria, angioedema or anaphylaxis) to penicillins.*

## Therapeutic Tips

- It is important to recognize the limitations of evidence on which current recommendations are based. No adequate clinical trials have been done to establish the efficacy of the recommended drug regimens. Well-documented cases of infective endocarditis have occurred in spite of appropriate prophylaxis. The results of a recent population-based case-control study of dental and cardiac risk factors further question the value of the well-entrenched practice of antibiotic prophylaxis for bacterial endocarditis.

## *Suggested Reading List*


Dajani AS, Taubert KA, Wilson W, et al. Prevention of bacterial endocarditis. Recommendations by the American Heart Association. *JAMA* 1997;277:1794–1801.

Durack DT. Antibiotics for prevention of endocarditis during dentistry: time to scale back? *Ann Intern Med* 1998;129:829–831.

Hall G, Heimdahl A, Nord CE. Bacteremia after oral surgery and antibiotic prophylaxis for endocarditis. *Clin Infect Dis* 1999;29:1–10.

Strom BL, Abrutyn E, Berlin JA, et al. Dental and cardiac risk factors for infective endocarditis. A population-based, case-control study. *Ann Intern Med* 1998;129:761–769.

CHAPTER 86

# Community-acquired Pneumonia

*Thomas J. Marrie, MD, FRCPC*

Community acquired-pneumonia (CAP) is characterized by:

- at least one respiratory symptom (cough, shortness of breath, pleuritic chest pain, hemoptysis, sputum production);
- one or more of: fever, chills, myalgia, headache, arthralgia;
- a new opacity on chest radiograph.

Any of the following physical findings may be present (rarely none are present): crackles, wheezes, findings of consolidation of pulmonary tissue (dullness to percussion, increased tactile and vocal fremitus, bronchial breathing, whispered pectoriloquy), pleural friction rub.

## Goals of Therapy

- To assess the severity of the pneumonia as a guide to deciding on the appropriate location for treatment, i.e., home, hospital ward or intensive care unit
- To relieve symptoms (fever, cough, pleuritic chest pain, sputum production, dyspnea)
- To promptly recognize and minimize complications: metastatic infection (meningitis, purulent pericarditis, endocarditis, osteomyelitis); empyema; cavitation; pneumothorax; septic shock; respiratory failure; adverse drug reactions; worsening of comorbid conditions (e.g., ischemic heart disease, diabetes mellitus)
- To provide compassionate end of life care if this scenario emerges

### *Points to remember when approaching a patient with CAP*

- Many microbial agents can cause pneumonia but the clinical presentation in general does not allow an etiological diagnosis. However, *Streptococcus pneumoniae* accounts for about 50% of all cases of CAP that require hospital admission (Table 1).
- Each microbe can result in an illness that spans the spectrum from mild to life threatening.
- Noninfectious illnesses may mimic pneumonia, e.g., postobstructive pneumonia secondary to cancer of the lung, vasculitis involving the pulmonary vessels, pulmonary embolism with infarction.

Table 1: **Most Common Pathogens in Community-acquired Pneumonia***

| | |
|---|---|
| Pneumonia treated on an ambulatory basis | |
| *Mycoplasma pneumoniae* | 24% |
| *Streptococcus pneumoniae* | 5% |
| *Chlamydia pneumoniae* | 5% |
| *Haemophilus influenzae* | 2% |
| *Legionella pneumophila* | 1% |
| *Miscellaneous* | 11% |
| *Unknown* | 48% |
| Pneumonia requiring admission to hospital | |
| *Streptococcus pneumoniae* | 17%† |
| *Haemophilus influenzae* | 7% |
| *Staphylococcus aureus* | 3% |
| *Legionella pneumophila* | 1% |
| *Mycoplasma pneumoniae* | 14% |
| *Chlamydia pneumoniae* | 10% |
| *Aerobic gram-negative bacilli (Escherichia coli; Klebsiella species; Enterobacter species; Serratia species; Pseudomonas aeruginosa, etc.)* | 4% |
| *Pneumocystis carinii* | 2%‡ |
| *Mycobacterium tuberculosis* | 2% |
| *Fungi* | 1% |
| *Anaerobes* | 5% |
| *Unknown* | 34% |

* *Up to 10% of patients with CAP have more than one pathogen identified.*

† *Studies that have used serological methods in addition to blood and sputum culture to diagnose pneumococcal pneumonia have found that 32–55% of patients with CAP have this infection.*

‡ *This can be up to 12% of all cases of CAP in cities with large populations of HIV-infected individuals.*

- Knowledge of local susceptibility patterns of *S. pneumoniae*; *Haemophilus influenzae* and *Branhamella catarrhalis* is useful. In 1996 in Canada, 8.9% of *S. pneumoniae* isolates showed intermediate resistance to pencillin; 4.4% showed high level resistance. High dose penicillin can be used to treat these patients provided they do not have meningitis. Isolates that are resistant to penicillin are often multidrug resistant (e.g., 96 to 99% of isolates with high level penicillin resistance are resistant to cefaclor, cefixime, cefuroxime and cefpodoxime; almost 50% to macrolides; 70% to co-trimoxazole; 35% to tetracycline; 24% to cefotaxime.)
- Be aware of local epidemiological patterns such as outbreaks or endemic foci of *Legionella* species; *Coxiella burnetii* or Hantavirus

## Investigations

- A detailed history and physical examination with special reference to:

- vital signs – a respiratory rate > 30 in an adult is the single most sensitive and specific sign of severe pneumonia
- oxygenation status – oxygen saturation should be measured in all patients with CAP presenting to an emergency room; an arterial blood gas should be done on those with an oxygen saturation of < 92%, and those with chronic obstructive lung disease.
- chest radiographs – posterior-anterior and lateral views
- laboratory tests for those presenting to an emergency room with CAP
  – assessment of oxygenation status as above
  – CBC and differential white blood cell count
  – electrolytes, glucose, urea nitrogen and creatinine
  – blood cultures: two aerobic bottles drawn at separate site
  – sputum for Gram's stain and culture if available. Special requests such as culture for *Mycobacterium tuberculosis*; *Legionella* species; fungi (*Blastomyces dermatiditis*, *Cryptococcus* species, etc) are dictated by the clinical setting
  – urine for *Legionella* antigen (if the clinical suspicion of Legionnaires' disease is high) will only detect serogroup 1 infections. Patients who require intensive care admission because of progressive pneumonia should have this test
  – serological studies as dictated by the clinical setting, e.g., suspected *Mycoplasma pneumoniae* pneumonia. An acute and 10- to14-day convalescent phase serum sample is usually required. In patients with suspected Legionnaires' disease, a convalescent sample should be collected 6 weeks following the acute phase sample

## Therapeutic Choices

The successful management of pneumonia (Figure 1) includes an accurate assessment of the severity of the illness (Table 2) and selection of the most appropriate site for treatment. Initial antibiotic therapy often must be empiric. Once an etiological diagnosis has been established, therapy can be selected (Table 3). Antibiotics and dosages used in the treatment of CAP are listed in Table 4.

## Therapeutic Tips

- Patients presenting to an emergency room with pneumonia should receive antimicrobial therapy *as soon as possible* after diagnosis.
- The *change from an IV to an oral antibiotic* can be made when the following criteria are met: two normal temperature readings (< 37.5° C orally) over 16 hours in previously

Figure 1: **Initial Management of Community-acquired Pneumonia (CAP)**

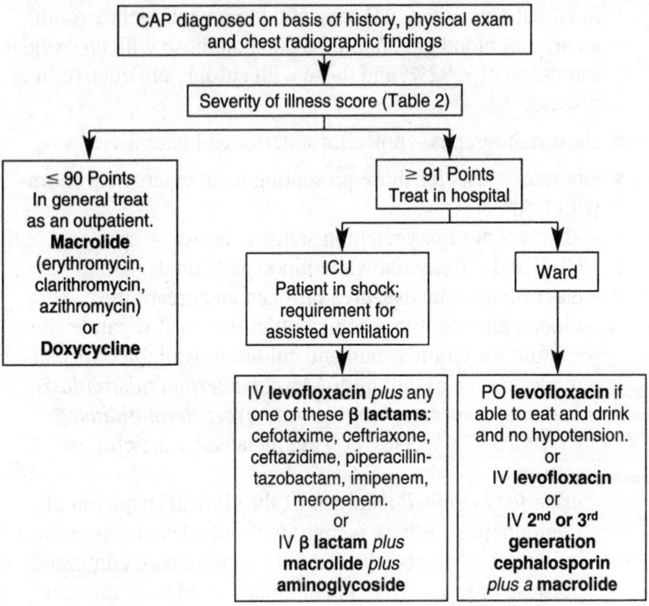
CAP diagnosed on basis of history, physical exam and chest radiographic findings
Severity of illness score (Table 2)
≤ 90 Points In general treat as an outpatient. Macrolide (erythromycin, clarithromycin, azithromycin) or Doxycycline
≥ 91 Points Treat in hospital
ICU Patient in shock; requirement for assisted ventilation
Ward
IV levofloxacin plus any one of these β lactams: cefotaxime, ceftriaxone, ceftazidime, piperacillin-tazobactam, imipenem, meropenem. or IV β lactam plus macrolide plus aminoglycoside
PO levofloxacin if able to eat and drink and no hypotension. or IV levofloxacin or IV 2nd or 3rd generation cephalosporin plus a macrolide

Table 2: **Pneumonia-specific Severity of Illness Score***

| **Patient characteristic** | **Points assigned** |
|---|---|
| Males | age (years) |
| Females | age (years) minus 10 |
| Nursing home residence | +30 |
| **Comorbid illness** | |
| Neoplastic disease | +30 |
| Liver disease | +20 |
| Congestive heart failure | +10 |
| Cerebrovascular disease | +10 |
| Renal disease | +10 |
| **Physical examination findings** | |
| Altered mental status | +20 |
| Respiratory rate > 30/min | +20 |
| Systolic BP < 90 mm Hg | +20 |
| Temperature < 35° C or > 40° C | +15 |
| **Laboratory findings** | |
| Pulse > 125/min | +10 |
| pH < 7.35 | +30 |
| BUN > 10.7 mmol/L | +20 |
| Sodium <130 mmol/L | +20 |
| Glucose > 13.9 mmol/L | +10 |
| Hematocrit < 30% | +10 |
| pO2 < 60 mm Hg | +10 |
| Pleural effusion | +10 |

* *Adapted with permission from Fine MJ, Auble TE, Yealy DM, et al. A prediction rule to identify low-risk patients with community-acquired pneumonia. N Engl J Med 1997;336:243–50.*

Table 3: **Antimicrobial Therapy for Community-acquired Pneumonia Caused by Specific Pathogens**

***Streptococcus pneumoniae***
Penicillin susceptible (MIC <0.1 mg/L) – penicillin G, amoxicillin, a macrolide
Intermediate resistance (MIC 0.1 – 1 mg/L ) – amoxicillin-clavulanate
High-level resistance (MIC > 4 mg/L) – penicillin G 2 MU q4h IV; cefotaxime 1 g q8h IV; ceftriaxone 1 g q24h IV or levofloxacin. If there is concomitant meningitis use vancomycin plus ceftriaxone.

***Moraxella catarrhalis or Haemophilus influenzae***
2nd or 3rd generation cephalosporin or amoxicillin clavulanate

***Staphylococcus aureus***
Methicillin susceptible – cloxacillin
Methicillin resistant – vancomycin

***Legionella* species**
Fluoroquinolone or macrolide plus rifampin.

***Mycoplasma pneumoniae, Chlamydia pneumoniae***
Doxycycline or macrolide

***Coxiella burnetii***
Doxycycline or fluoroquinolone.

**Aerobic gram-negative bacilli** (*Escherichia coli, Enterobacter* spp, *Serratia* spp, *Proteus* spp, etc.) 2nd or 3rd generation cephalosporin

febrile patients; white blood cell count returning towards normal; subjective improvement in cough; subjective improvement in shortness of breath; negative blood cultures for a respiratory pathogen (if done). If blood cultures are positive, the duration of IV therapy should be dictated by the organism recovered from the blood.

- When the following criteria are met in addition to those above, the patient should be ready for *discharge*: absence of complications from the pneumonia (e.g., empyema); absence of complications from comorbid illnesses (e.g., myocardial infarction); absence of complications from treatment (e.g., severe adverse drug reactions); physiological stability as indicated by an oxygen saturation of 92% or greater while breathing room air at sea level for those who do not have chronic obstructive lung disease (for patients with chronic obstructive lung disease, a return to baseline status is desirable); pulse rate of < 100 beats per minute and respiratory rate of 24 or less.
- Check patients with *ongoing fever* (> 37.5° C PO) for empyema: if a pleural effusion is greater than 1 cm on a chest film with the affected side down, the effusion should be aspirated and sent for culture (aerobes, anaerobes and *M. tuberculosis*), white cell count, LDH, protein. Drug fever, which may mimic pneumonia, should be kept in mind and the diagnosis reconsidered.

Table 4: **Antibiotics Used to Treat Pneumonia**

| Drug | Dosage | Adverse Effects/Comments | Cost* |
|---|---|---|---|
| **Beta-lactams** | | | |
| **Penicillins** | | | |
| *penicillin V* – Pen-Vee, PVF K, generics | 300 mg TID PO | ***Penicillins:*** hypersensitivity reactions, rash, nausea, vomiting, pseudomembranous colitis, interstitial nephritis. | $ |
| *amoxicillin* – Amoxil, generics | 500 mg TID PO | | $ |
| *amoxicillin/clavulanate* – Clavulin | 500 mg TID PO | | $$ |
| *cloxacillin* – Tegopen, generics | 500 mg QID PO | | $ |
| *piperacillin* – Pipracil | 3 g Q4H IV | | $$$$ |
| *piperacillin/tazobactam* – Tazocin | 3.375 g Q6H IV | | $$$$ |
| **First-generation Cephalosporins** | | | |
| *cefazolin* – Ancef, Kefzol, generics | 2 g Q8H IV | ***Cephalosporins:*** hypersensitivity reactions, rash, nausea, vomiting, pseudomembranous colitis, renal and hepatic dysfunction, phlebitis and pain at site of IM injection. Cefotaxime is safe in hepatobiliary disease. | $$$ |
| **Second-generation Cephalosporins** | | | |
| *cefaclor* – Ceclor, generics | 250 mg TID PO | | $$ |
| *cefprozil* – Cefzil | 500 mg Q24h | | $$ |
| *cefuroxime axetil* – Ceftin | 500 mg BID–TID PO | | $$ |
| *cefuroxime sodium* – Kefurox, Zinacef | 750 mg Q8H IV | | $$$ |
| **Third-generation Cephalosporins** | | | |
| *cefixime* – Suprax | 400 mg daily PO | | $$ |
| *ceftriaxone* – Rocephin | 1–2 g Q24H IV | | $$$–$$$$ |
| *cefotaxime* – Claforan | 1–2 g Q6–8H IV | | $$$–$$$$ |
| *ceftazidime* – Ceptaz, Fortaz, Tazidime | 1–2 g Q8H IV | | $$$$ |
| **Penems** | | | |
| *imipenem/cilastatin* – Primaxin | 500 mg Q6H IV | ***Imipenem:*** hypotension, nausea with rapid infusion; seizure activity with high levels. | $$$$ |
| *meropenem* – Merrem | 0.5–1 g Q8H IV | ***Meropenem:*** less likely to cause seizures. | $$–$$$ |

| | | | |
|---|---|---|---|
| **Macrolides** | | | |
| *erythromycin* – Erybid, Eryc, Erythromid, PCE, Ilosone, generics | 500 mg QID PO | Abdominal cramping, nausea, vomiting, diarrhea, rash, cholestatic hepatitis. (Fewer side effects with azithromycin and clarithromycin.) | $ |
| *clarithromycin* ❥ – Biaxin | 500 mg BID PO | | $$ |
| *azithromycin* – Zithromax | 500 mg 1st d, 250 mg × 4 d PO | Azithromycin given daily × 5 d is equivalent to erythromycin QID × 10 d. | $$ |
| **Fluoroquinolones** | | *Ciprofloxacin is not a first-line agent for CAP.* | |
| *ciprofloxacin* ❥ – Cipro | 500–750 mg BID PO<br>400 mg Q12H IV | Abdominal pain, photosensitivity, hepatitis, pseudomembranous colitis. Cartilage toxicity – avoid in children. | PO: $$<br>IV: $$$$ |
| *levofloxacin* ❥ – Levaquin | 250–500 mg Q24H PO or IV | *Drug interactions:* Ciprofloxacin may ↓ theophylline elimination; concomitant antacids, sucralfate ↓ absorption of quinolones; ciprofloxacin may prolong INR if given with warfarin. | PO: $$<br>IV: $$$ |
| **Aminoglycosides** | | | |
| *gentamicin* ❥ – Garamycin, Cidomycin, generics | 1.5 mg/kg Q8H IV<br>or | Nephrotoxicity, ototoxicity. | $$$ |
| *tobramycin* ❥ – Nebcin, generics | 5–7 mg/kg once daily | | $$$ |
| **Other** | | ***Co-trimoxazole:*** hypersensitivity reactions, nausea, vomiting, diarrhea, rash, false ↑ serum creatinine, renal impairment, neutropenia, thrombocytopenia, anemia, agranulocytosis. | |
| *co-trimoxazole* ❥ – Bactrim, Septra, generics | 160/800 mg BID PO | | $ |
| *tetracycline* ❥ – generics | 500 mg QID PO | | $ |
| *doxycycline* – Vibramycin, Vibra-tabs, generics | 100 mg BID PO | *Drug interactions:* ↑ phenytoin levels, ↑ INR with warfarin, hypoglycemia with sulfonylureas, ↑ nephrotoxicity with cyclosporine. | $$ |
| *rifampin* – Rifadin, Rofact | 300 mg BID PO | ***Tetracycline, doxycycline:*** nausea, vomiting, photosensitivity, candidiasis, pseudotumor cerebri.<br>*Drug interactions:* calcium, aluminum, magnesium, iron ↓ absorption.<br>***Rifampin** should never be used as a single agent for CAP.* | $$ |

❥ *Dosage adjustment may be required in renal impairment – see Appendix I.*
* *Cost of 1-day supply – includes drug costs only.*

*Legend:* $ < $1 $$ $1–10 $$$ $10–50 $$$$ > $50

- Follow-up chest radiographs should be done for *all tobacco smokers over age 35* and for *all patients over age 50.* Two percent of all patients with CAP will have cancer of the lung and, in 1% of the total, the cancer is not diagnosed on the initial radiographs.
- For those 65 years of age and older as well as for patients with recurrent pneumonia, the goal is to *prevent another episode.* A checklist is useful and should include a search for causes of aspiration and measures to prevent recurrent aspiration.
- Pneumococcal and influenza *vaccine status* should be reviewed and the patient immunized if indicated.

## Suggested Reading List

Berntsson E, Lagergard T, Strannegard O et al. Etiology of community-acquired pneumonia in outpatients. *Eur J Clin Microbiol* 1986;5:446–447.

Davidson R, Canadian Bacterial Surveillance Network, Low DE. A cross Canada surveillance of antimicrobial resistance in respiratory tract pathogens. *Can J Infect Dis* 1999;10: 128–133.

Doern GV, Pfaller MA, Kugler K, Freeman J, Jones RN. Prevalence of antimicrobial resistance among respiratory tract isolates of Streptococcus pneumoniae in North America: 1977 results from the SENTRY Antimicrobial Surveillance Program. *Clin Infect Dis* 1998;27:764–770.

Fine MJ, Auble TE, Yealy DM, et al. A prediction rule to identify low-risk patients with community-acquired pneumonia. *N Engl J Med* 1997;336:243–250.

Marrie TJ, Peeling RW, Fine MJ, et al. Ambulatory patients with community-acquired pneumonia: The frequency of atypical agents and clinical course. *Am J Med* 1996;101:508–515.

CHAPTER 87

# Tuberculosis

*J. Mark FitzGerald, MD, FRCPI, FRCPC and Thomas J. Marrie, MD, FRCPC*

## Goals of Therapy

- To prevent latent infection from progressing to clinically active disease
- To treat active disease (by eradicating *Mycobacterium tuberculosis* from the affected organ) and relieve symptoms (fever, sweats, weight loss, cough)
- To prevent person-to-person spread

## Investigations

- Thorough history with special attention to:
  - risk factors for acquisition of tuberculosis (TB) (e.g., exposure, travel, occupation)
  - risk factors for reactivation of dormant infection (e.g., HIV, recent contact, predisposing medical conditions, ethnicity)
  - history of TB contact, skin test information and details of treatment
- Physical examination (often unrewarding especially for pulmonary TB):
  - nutrition status, fever, choroid tubercles, rales, rhonchi, meningitis
  - concomitant diseases that may affect treatment (e.g., HIV)
- Laboratory tests:
  - chest x-ray
  - urinalysis
  - sputum smear and culture for acid-fast bacilli (AFB)
  - urine smear and culture for AFB if renal TB suspected
  - lumbar puncture with smear and culture of spinal fluid for AFB, plus sugar, protein and cell count if meningitis suspected
  - CBC, creatinine, ALT, AST, alkaline phosphatase, bilirubin
  - HIV serology strongly recommended for all patients
  - in HIV positive persons, blood cultures and stool samples for mycobacteriology
- Special procedures:
  - sputum induction in an appropriately ventilated room has a high yield
  - bronchoscopy with transbronchial biopsy in some cases. A rapid diagnosis is possible by demonstrating caseating granulomata on biopsy

  - aspiration of pleural effusions with culture, chemical and cytological analysis, and pleural biopsy for culture and histology (positive 60%) may be useful
- Polymerase chain reaction (PCR) for detection of mycobacterial antigens in body fluids is used in some laboratories
  - major advantage is rapid diagnosis, generally < 48 h
  - most useful in diagnosing meningeal TB
- Tuberculin skin (Mantoux) testing has 3 indications: *diagnosis of infection*, *diagnosis of disease* and as an *epidemiologic tool* (Figure 1). It should not be performed on persons with previous severe blistering tuberculin reactions, documented active TB, extensive burns or eczema, infections or vaccinations with live virus vaccines in the past month (e.g., mumps or measles)
  - *false negative* tests occur especially in the seriously ill who are often anergic. Patients' recall of test results cannot be relied upon. Test results may vary by 15% between arms and between different observers
  - the Mantoux test is read at 48 to 72 hours following intradermal inoculation, by measuring the widest diameter of *induration* (not erythema)
  - in general, a positive Mantoux > 15 years after BCG vaccination should not be attributed to the vaccine, especially if given in infancy
  - reactivity to tuberculin antigen can diminish to non-reactivity with age. However, repeat TB skin testing may boost reactivity. Thus it is important in populations who are going to have serial testing (e.g., nursing home residents, health care workers) to determine those whose response has waned over time by using the *two step test*. A second test dose is administered 2 to 3 weeks after the first
  - a negative PPD should not preclude consideration of the diagnosis

*Note:* Maintain a high index of suspicion for TB in immunocompromised patients; manifestations are atypical. Miliary disease is common and sputum smears are often negative.

## Therapeutic Choices

### Nonpharmacologic Choices

- All patients with known or suspected tuberculosis disease (usually pulmonary) should be hospitalized in a single negative pressure room and placed on respiratory precautions. Isolation may be discontinued when consecutive sputum smears are negative for AFB on 3 separate days or there is evidence of adherence to an appropriate treatment regimen for a minimum of 2 weeks in those who are AFB

## Figure 1: **Diagnosis and Management of Latent *M. tuberculosis* Infection**

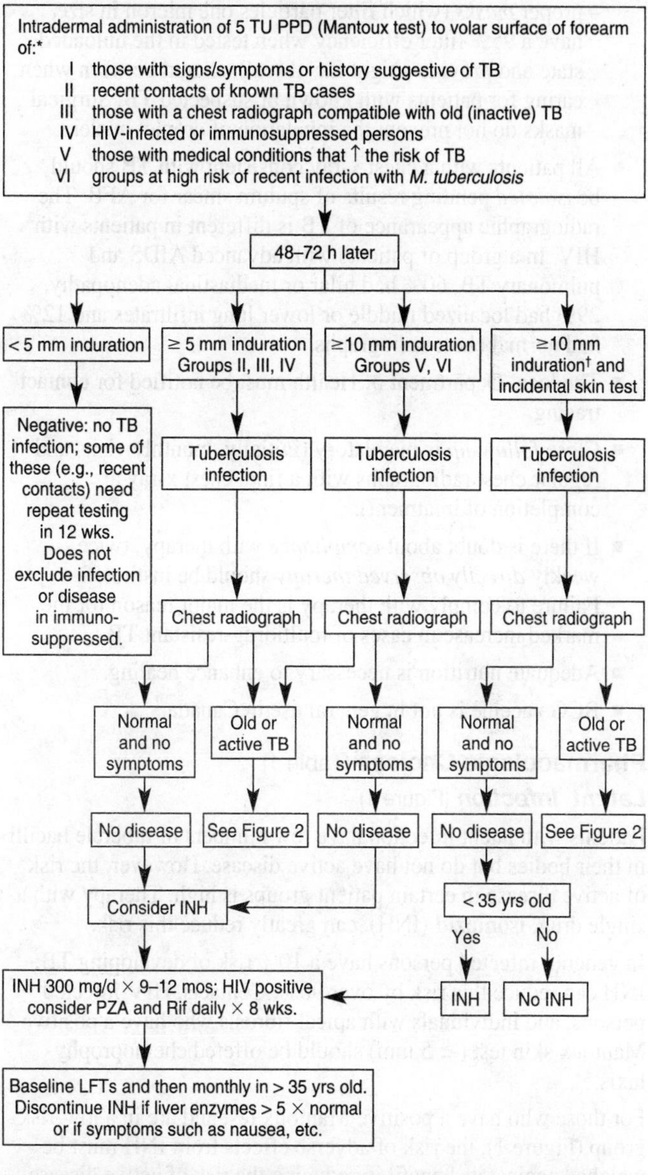
Intradermal administration of 5 TU PPD (Mantoux test) to volar surface of forearm of:*
I those with signs/symptoms or history suggestive of TB
II recent contacts of known TB cases
III those with a chest radiograph compatible with old (inactive) TB
IV HIV-infected or immunosuppressed persons
V those with medical conditions that ↑ the risk of TB
VI groups at high risk of recent infection with M. tuberculosis
48–72 h later
< 5 mm induration
≥ 5 mm induration Groups II, III, IV
≥10 mm induration Groups V, VI
≥10 mm induration† and incidental skin test
Negative: no TB infection; some of these (e.g., recent contacts) need repeat testing in 12 wks. Does not exclude infection or disease in immuno-suppressed.
Tuberculosis infection
Tuberculosis infection
Tuberculosis infection
Chest radiograph
Chest radiograph
Chest radiograph
Normal and no symptoms
Old or active TB
Normal and no symptoms
Normal and no symptoms
Old or active TB
No disease
See Figure 2
No disease
No disease
See Figure 2
Consider INH
< 35 yrs old
Yes
No
INH 300 mg/d × 9–12 mos; HIV positive consider PZA and Rif daily × 8 wks.
INH
No INH
Baseline LFTs and then monthly in > 35 yrs old. Discontinue INH if liver enzymes > 5 × normal or if symptoms such as nausea, etc.

* *Several other antigens (e.g., CMI Multitest) should be inoculated onto the other arm. There are issues re: false positive and negative reactions as well as cost for these antigens. If there is no reaction to these antigens the patient is anergic, and a negative Mantoux is meaningless.*

† *In the US, a 15 mm cut-off is used but this is based on the relatively high prevalence of atypical mycobacterial infection there.*

*Abbreviations: LFTs = liver function tests; INH = isoniazid; PZA = pyrazinamide Rif = rifampin.*

positive. Continue isolation for duration of hospital stay or until cultures are negative in patients with pulmonary or laryngeal multiple drug resistant TB.

- proper *masks* (which filter particles one micron in size, have a 95% filter efficiency when tested in the unloaded state and provide a tight facial seal), should be worn when caring for patients with known or suspected TB. Surgical masks do not prevent the inhalation of droplet nuclei.

- All patients with a chest x-ray consistent with TB should be *isolated* pending results of sputum smear for AFB. The radiographic appearance of TB is different in patients with HIV. In a group of patients with advanced AIDS and pulmonary TB, 60% had hilar or mediastinal adenopathy, 29% had localized middle or lower lung infiltrates and 12% had normal chest radiographs.
- The local Department of Health must be notified for contact tracing.
- Close *follow-up* is mandatory (initially, monthly visits and regular chest radiographs with a final chest x-ray at completion of treatment).
- If there is doubt about *compliance* with therapy, twice weekly *directly observed therapy* should be instituted. Failure to comply with therapy is the major reason for the marked increase in cases of multidrug-resistant TB.
- Adequate nutrition is necessary to enhance healing.
- BCG vaccine is not in general use in Canada.[1]

## Pharmacologic Choices (Table 1)

### *Latent Infection* (Figure 1)

Patients with latent infection have low numbers of tubercle bacilli in their bodies but do not have active disease. However, the risk of active disease in certain patient groups is high. Therapy with a single drug, **isoniazid** (INH), can greatly reduce this risk.

In general, infected persons have a 10% risk of developing TB; INH can reduce this risk by over 90%. Contacts, HIV-infected persons, and individuals with apical fibrosis who have a positive Mantoux skin test (≥ 5 mm) should be offered chemoprophylaxis.

For those who have a positive Mantoux test and are in a low-risk group (Figure 1), the risk of adverse effects from INH must be weighed against its benefit in reducing the risk of active disease. In patients with no risk factors, the risk of adverse effects from INH is low for those < 35 years of age. This group should be

[1] *JAMA 1994;172:698–702.*

Figure 2: **Management of Pulmonary *M. tuberculosis* Disease**

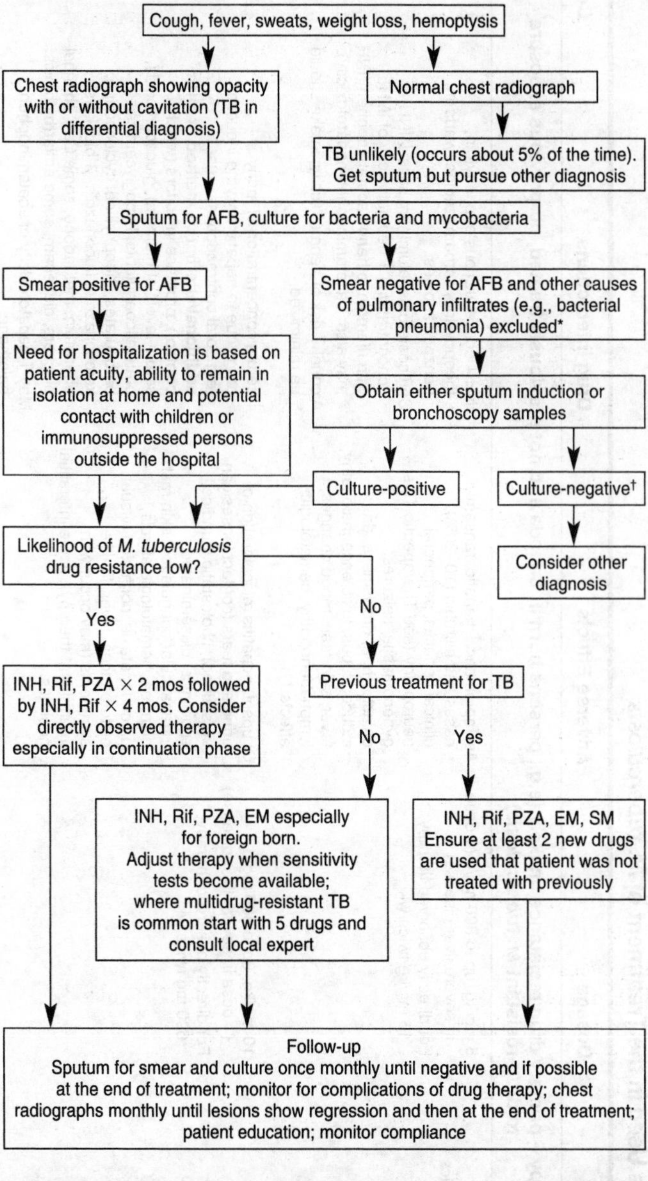
Cough, fever, sweats, weight loss, hemoptysis
Chest radiograph showing opacity with or without cavitation (TB in differential diagnosis)
Normal chest radiograph
TB unlikely (occurs about 5% of the time). Get sputum but pursue other diagnosis
Sputum for AFB, culture for bacteria and mycobacteria
Smear positive for AFB
Smear negative for AFB and other causes of pulmonary infiltrates (e.g., bacterial pneumonia) excluded*
Need for hospitalization is based on patient acuity, ability to remain in isolation at home and potential contact with children or immunosuppressed persons outside the hospital
Obtain either sputum induction or bronchoscopy samples
Culture-positive
Culture-negative†
Likelihood of M. tuberculosis drug resistance low?
Consider other diagnosis
Yes
No
INH, Rif, PZA × 2 mos followed by INH, Rif × 4 mos. Consider directly observed therapy especially in continuation phase
Previous treatment for TB
No
Yes
INH, Rif, PZA, EM especially for foreign born. Adjust therapy when sensitivity tests become available; where multidrug-resistant TB is common start with 5 drugs and consult local expert
INH, Rif, PZA, EM, SM Ensure at least 2 new drugs are used that patient was not treated with previously
Follow-up
Sputum for smear and culture once monthly until negative and if possible at the end of treatment; monitor for complications of drug therapy; chest radiographs monthly until lesions show regression and then at the end of treatment; patient education; monitor compliance

** 50% of pulmonary TB cases will be smear negative. Therefore, with suspicious chest x-ray and clinical scenario, initiate empiric antituberculosis therapy.*

*† 15% of pulmonary TB cases will be culture negative but diagnosis is based on response to therapy in the appropriate clinical setting.*

*Abbreviations: INH = isoniazid; Rif = rifampin; SM = streptomycin; PZA = pyrazinamide; EM = ethambutol.*

Table 1: **Drugs Used in the Treatment of *M. tuberculosis***

| Drug | Dosage | Adverse Effects | Drug Interactions | Cost* |
|---|---|---|---|---|
| **First-line Therapy – primary drug resistance unlikely (e.g., persons born in Canada and not previously treated, no previous exposure to drug-resistant *M. tuberculosis*)** | | | | |
| *isoniazid*<br>Isotamine, generics | 5 mg/kg, up to 300 mg/d (↓ dose in severe liver disease)<br>For directly observed therapy, 15 mg/kg twice/wk | Asymptomatic ↑ hepatic transaminases and bilirubin (10–20%), clinical hepatitis, peripheral neuropathy (see Therapeutic Tips), gynecomastia, seizures, galactorrhea, drowsiness, drug-induced lupus, toxic encephalopathy, fever, skin rash, mood changes, lymphadenopathy, hematologic effects.† | INH ↑ concentrations of phenytoin, theophylline, carbamazepine, warfarin, benzodiazepines.<br>Corticosteroids, aluminum salts ↓ INH concentrations. ↑ hepatotoxicity of INH‡ with rifampin, ethanol, acetaminophen (INH may also ↑ acetaminophen hepatotoxicity).<br>Alcohol ↑ risk of hepatotoxicity; intake should be minimized. | $ |
| *rifampin*<br>Rifadin, generics | 10 mg/kg, up to 600 mg/d (↓ dose in severe liver disease)<br>For directly observed therapy, 600 mg twice/wk | GI upset, hepatitis, discoloration of urine and tears (contact lenses can be stained), cholestatic jaundice, subclinical disseminated intravascular coagulation, skin rash, diarrhea, hematologic effects,† urticaria, ataxia, confusion, visual disturbances, fever, flu-like symptoms (may occur with intermittent therapy), acute interstitial nephritis. | ↓ serum concentration of many drugs due to hepatic enzyme induction (e.g., oral contraceptives – use **additional/alternative method of birth control**), protease inhibitors (which ↑ serum levels of rifampin), glucocorticoids, oral anticoagulants, hypoglycemics, barbiturates, theophylline, cyclosporine, ketoconazole, fluconazole, β-blockers, phenytoin, methadone, some $Ca^{++}$ channel blockers, diazepam, some antiarrhythmics.<br>May ↑ hepatotoxicity of acetaminophen, halothane. | $–$$$ |

| | | | | |
|---|---|---|---|---|
| *pyrazinamide* Tebrazid, generics | 15–25 mg/kg, up to 2 g/d (divided doses). Usual dose: 1.5 g/d For directly observed therapy, 2500 mg twice/wk | Hepatotoxicity (rare with 2-mo therapy), rash, arthralgia, ↑ uric acid (acute gout rarely seen), drug fever, hematologic effects,† GI upset. | ↓ levels of INH. | $$$ |
| *ethambutol* Myambutol, Etibi | 15–25 mg/kg/d For directly observed therapy, 2400 mg twice/wk. | Ocular toxicity (↓ visual acuity, central scotomata, red–green color blindness due to retrobulbar neuritis [rare at 15 mg/kg/d]) (see Therapeutic Tips), GI upset, rash, Stevens-Johnson syndrome (rare), toxic epidermal necrolysis, hematologic effects,† headache, dizziness, confusion, hallucinations. | ↓ cyclosporine blood levels. | $–$$ |
| *streptomycin* | 15 mg/kg/d, up to 1 g IM or 15–25 mg/kg IM twice/wk Not to exceed total of 120 g | Vestibular/cochlear toxicity, ataxia (may be permanent), nystagmus, proteinuria, hypersensitivity with fever, rash, hematologic effects.† | Additive toxicity with other neurotoxic, ototoxic or nephrotoxic drugs. | $$$–$$$$$ |
| **Second-line Therapy** | | | | |
| *cycloserine* Seromycin$^{\pi}$ | 15 mg/kg/d, up to 500 mg/d | Headache, irritability, behavior abnormalities, psychosis, seizures, aggravation of pre-existing psychiatric condition; peripheral neuropathy (especially when used with INH); rarely, may cause megaloblastic or sideroblastic anemia. | Ethionamide and alcohol may potentiate CNS toxicity of cycloserine. | $$$$$ |

*(cont'd)*

Table 1: **Drugs Used in the Treatment of *M. tuberculosis*** *(cont'd)*

| Drug | Dosage | Adverse Effects | Drug Interactions | Cost* |
|---|---|---|---|---|
| *ethionamide* Trecator$^{\pi}$ | 15–20 mg/kg/d, up to 750 mg/d given in divided doses. | Hepatitis, arthralgia, GI disturbances, altered taste, peripheral neuritis, possible antithyroid effects (has produced clinical hypothyroidism); fatigue, depression, frozen shoulder syndrome, galactorrhea, ↑ salivation. | May ↑ CNS toxicity of cycloserine. | π |
| **Aminoglycosides** | | Vestibular/cochlear toxicity, nephrotoxicity. | Other oto- or nephrotoxic drugs may potentiate aminoglycoside toxicities. | |
| *kanamycin* – Kantrex$^{\pi}$ | 15 mg/kg/d IM | | | π |
| *amikacin* – Amikin | 15 mg/kg/d IM | | | $$$$$ |
| *capreomycin* Capastat Sulfate$^{\pi}$ | 15 mg/kg/d IM Max: 1 g/d for all aminoglycosides | | | π |

* *Cost of 30-day supply – includes drug cost only.*
*Legend: $ < 25 $$ $25–50 $$$ $50–75 $$$$ $75–100 $$$$$ > $100*
† *May include any of eosinophilia, thrombocytopenia, transient leukopenia, hemolytic anemia, agranulocytosis, or sideroblastic or aplastic anemia.*
‡ *Cross-hepatotoxicity may occur between drugs that are chemically related (e.g., INH, pyrazinamide and ethionamide). All of these agents should be avoided if a reaction to one of them occurs.*
*Dosage adjustment may be required in renal impairment – see Appendix I.*
π *Available through Special Access Program, Therapeutic Products Directorate, Health Canada.*

offered INH prophylaxis. For those with risk factors for reactivating dormant infection, age should not preclude offering chemoprophylaxis. **Isoniazid** for 9 months is an acceptable regimen. If the source case may have been INH resistant, **rifampin** for 6 months may be substituted. Short course daily prophylaxis with **rifampin and pyrazinamide** for 8 weeks is comparable to 6 months of INH in HIV-positive patients.

### *Active Tuberculosis* (Figure 2)

Treatment should always be with multiple drugs. Directly observed therapy is encouraged although its use in all cases of TB is debated. Knowledge of the local epidemiology of resistance is essential to appropriate treatment. A four-drug regimen (**INH, rifampin, pyrazinamide** and **streptomycin** or **ethambutol**) is preferred for *initial empiric therapy*. Adjust therapy when susceptibility results are available (usually 2 months after initiation of therapy). This is also a good opportunity to consider twice weekly supervised therapy. Suspect resistance when disease is contracted in Africa, Asia, Central or South America, New York,

Table 2: **Suggested Regimens for Multidrug-resistant *M. tuberculosis*—Initiate in Consultation with a Local Expert**

| Resistance Pattern | Treatment | Duration |
|---|---|---|
| INH, SM, PZA | Rif, PZA, EM, amikacin* | 12–18 mos |
| INH, EM (± SM) | Rif, PZA, oflox/cipro, amikacin* | 12–18 mos |
| INH, Rif (± SM) | PZA, EM, oflox/cipro, amikacin* | 18–24 mos Consider surgery† |
| INH, Rif, EM (± SM) | PZA, oflox/cipro, amikacin* plus 2 others‡ | 24 mos after conversion π Consider surgery† |
| INH, Rif, PZA (± SM) | EM, oflox/cipro, amikacin* plus 2 others‡ | 24 mos after conversion π Consider surgery† |
| INH, Rif, PZA, EM (± SM) | Oflox/cipro, amikacin* plus 3 others‡ | 24 mos after conversion π Consider surgery† |

* *Capreomycin may be used if there is resistance to amikacin.*
† *Surgery may be required to resect nonhealing cavitary lesions.*
‡ *May choose from ethionamide, cycloserine, para-aminosalicylic acid.*
π *Refers to conversion from positive to negative sputum smear and culture.*

*Abbreviations: INH = isoniazid; SM = streptomycin; PZA = pyrazinamide; EM = ethambutol; Rif = rifampin; Oflox = ofloxacin; Cipro = ciprofloxacin.*
*Data from a murine model indicate that ethionamide, sparfloxacin, ofloxacin, capreomycin, clarithromycin and clofazimine are active against a multidrug-resistant tuberculous isolate. In this model, despite in vitro resistance, INH had moderate activity. (J Antimicrob Agent Chemother 1993;37:2344–2347).*
*Sparfloxacin, ciprofloxacin and ofloxacin have activity against M. tuberculosis. Ciprofloxacin and ofloxacin are synergistic when combined with rifampin or INH. The role of these agents in the treatment of TB awaits further study. (J Antimicrob Agent Chemother 1993;32:797–808).*

Miami or following exposure to a patient with known drug resistant disease. For susceptible organisms **INH, rifampin and pyrazinamide** should be given for 2 months followed by **INH and rifampin** for 4 months. This regimen can be used for empiric therapy in areas where there is no INH resistance. For regimens to treat multidrug-resistant TB, see Table 2. Re-infection has occasionally been reported, especially in the presence of HIV infection.

### Treatment During Pregnancy

The preferred initial treatment regimen is **INH, rifampin** and **ethambutol**. The risk of teratogenicity with **pyrazinamide** has not been determined but it is unlikely to be teratogenic. Its use should therefore be considered if resistance to one of the initial choices is suspected and susceptibility to pyrazinamide is likely. Therapy for 9 months with **INH and rifampin** should be adequate if **ethambutol** is substituted for pyrazinamide for the first 2 months and the organism is fully sensitive. Breast-feeding need not be discouraged since only small concentrations of anti-TB drugs appear in breast milk, and they do not produce toxicity in the newborn.

## Therapeutic Tips

- All patients given INH should receive **pyridoxine** 25 to 50 mg per day to prevent peripheral neuropathy.
- Color vision should be assessed at baseline and monitored every 2 months in patients receiving ethambutol.
- Consider initiating directly observed therapy which is rapidly becoming the accepted standard of care.

### Suggested Reading List


Belusa MLF, Cocchiarella L, Conly J, et al. Guidelines for preventing the transmission of tuberculosis in Canadian health care facilities and other institutional settings. *Can Commun Dis Rep* 1996;2251:1–50.

Canadian Thoracic Society, Standards Committee (Tuberculosis). *Canadian Tuberculosis Standards*. 5th ed. Ottawa: Canadian Lung Association, 2000.

FitzGerald JM, Houston S. Tuberculosis: The disease in association with HIV infection. *Can Med Assoc J* 1999;161:47–51.

Menzies D, Tannenbaum TN, FitzGerald JM. Tuberculosis: Prevention. *Can Med Assoc J* 1999;161:717–724.

Schluger NW, Rom WN. Current approaches to the diagnosis of active pulmonary tuberculosis. *Am J Respir Crit Care Med* 1994;149:264–267.

CHAPTER 88

# Acute Osteomyelitis

*Simon Dobson, MD, FRCPC*

## Goals of Therapy

- To cure the acute infection
- To minimize morbidity (e.g., loss of limb function)
- To prevent recurrence and progression to chronic osteomyelitis

## Investigations

- History:
  - duration of symptoms: fever, pain, redness, swelling, limp or other loss of function or movement
  - any penetrating wound
  - vascular insufficiency
  - neuropathic ulcer of the diabetic foot
- Examination:
  - tenderness over affected bone (often exquisite). No pain is elicited if advanced neuropathy of diabetic foot
  - range of movement in affected limb (any suggestion of septic arthritis)
- Laboratory tests:
  - CBC and acute-phase reactants (erythrocyte sedimentation rate, C-reactive protein) as baseline
  - blood culture (positive in 30 to 60%)
  - culture of diabetic ulcer unreliable as colonizers will be present. Best to culture bone obtained surgically through intact skin
- Imaging:
  - x-ray – may be normal initially; changes (e.g., periosteal reaction) are not evident for at least 10 days after onset
  - rarefaction of bone visible only when 50% loss of bone density (early in neonates, later in older children)
  - x-ray does not rule out diagnosis in diabetic foot. Chronic osteopathy may be present
- Bone scan: imaging using technetium $99^{m}$-labeled methylene diphosphonate has improved early diagnosis. Early "blood pool images" should be taken as well as later bone uptake images to help differentiate cellulitis from bone infection. A negative bone scan does not rule out osteomyelitis. In neonates an x-ray may be more reliable. Other causes of enhanced bone turnover (e.g., fracture or tumor) will also give a positive result

**Note:** If the clinical findings suggest osteomyelitis, management should not be delayed until a bone scan is obtained.

- Probe diabetic ulcer with sterile instrument. If bone can be reached, this has high specificity and positive predictive value for osteomyelitis (89%) but low sensitivity. Best initial evaluation is x-ray plus a probe for bone. If both negative, treat for soft tissue infection but repeat x-ray in 2 weeks (Figure 2)

Table 1: **Initial Empiric Therapy of Acute Osteomyelitis***

| Characteristics | Causative Organisms | Empiric IV Antibiotic |
|---|---|---|
| **Hematogenous Osteomyelitis** | | |
| Most common type.<br>Predominantly in children.<br>Blood-borne bacteria lodge in bone as nidus of infection.<br>Possible in any bone but usually in long bones: femur 36%, tibia 33%, humerus 10%.<br>Vertebral osteomyelitis not uncommon in adults. Predisposing factors are IV drug abuse, trauma, other source of infection (e.g., urinary tract).<br>In neonates, septic arthritis often coexists. | **Children:** *S. aureus*, group A streptococci Rare: *H. influenzae*,† *S. pneumoniae*, gram-negative enterics<br>**Neonates:** group B streptococci, gram-negative enterics, *S. aureus*<br>**Adults:** *S. aureus*, gram-negative enterics | **Children:** cloxacillin‡ + cefotaxime (if *H. influenzae* suspected)<br>**Neonates:** cloxacillin‡ + cefotaxime (to cover gram-negative enterics)<br>**Adults:** cloxacillin‡ |
| **Spread from Contiguous Sites** | | |
| Common in elderly.<br>Predisposing factors include surgery, soft tissue infection.<br>e.g., mandible, skull. | *S. aureus*, anaerobes, gram-negative organisms, mixed infection | Clindamycin ± gentamicin |
| **Penetrating Trauma** | | |
| All ages.<br>e.g., puncture wound of foot. | *P. aeruginosa*, *S. aureus* | Cloxacillin‡ and ticarcillin (or ceftazidime) + gentamicin |
| **Vascular Insufficiency** | | |
| Diabetic foot. | *S. aureus*, streptococci, gram-negative bacilli, anaerobes | Imipenem-cilastatin or ciprofloxacin + clindamycin |

* *The site and origin of infection and organism responsible are largely related to age.*
† *H. influenzae is of decreasing importance due to success of immunization.*
‡ *A semisynthetic, penicillinase-resistant penicillin (e.g., cloxacillin) provides coverage against S. aureus and streptococci.*

- Aspiration: A bacteriologic diagnosis of aspirate from the subperiosteum or bone greatly aids further management. An organism can be obtained in up to 80% of cases. Early consultation with an orthopedic surgeon is recommended.

Figure 1: **Management of Acute Osteomyelitis**

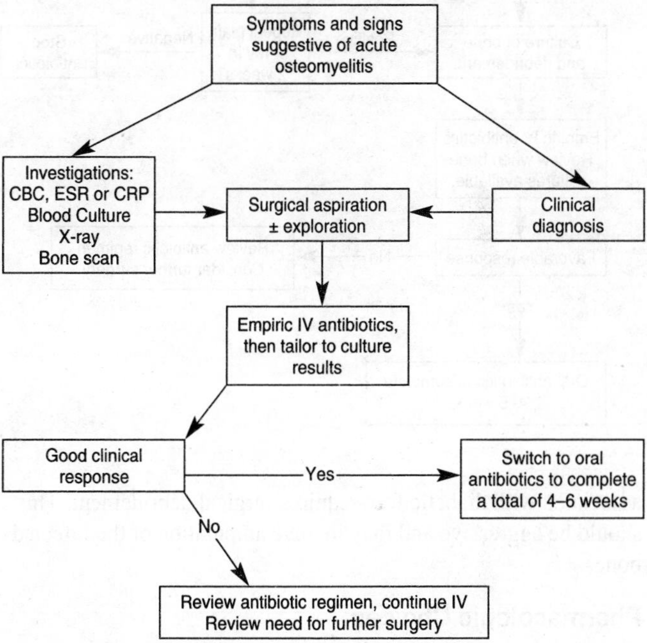
Symptoms and signs suggestive of acute osteomyelitis
Investigations: CBC, ESR or CRP Blood Culture X-ray Bone scan
Surgical aspiration ± exploration
Clinical diagnosis
Empiric IV antibiotics, then tailor to culture results
Good clinical response
Yes
Switch to oral antibiotics to complete a total of 4–6 weeks
No
Review antibiotic regimen, continue IV Review need for further surgery

*Abbreviations: ESR = erythrocyte sedimentation rate; CRP = C-reactive protein.*

## Therapeutic Choices (Figure 1)

### Surgical Drainage

Antibiotics do not penetrate well into collections of pus or into bone in which blood supply is compromised by infection. Surgical decompression and exploration are necessary when there has been a delay in presentation or diagnosis, when pus has been found on aspiration or when there is x-ray evidence of bone destruction. For early disease the role of immediate surgery has been controversial. However, if swelling, pain, tenderness and fever do not resolve within days after starting antibiotics, surgical exploration should be considered. Suspicion of osteomyelitis secondary to a penetrating injury (e.g., to the calcaneus) requires bone exploration, débridement and culture. Osteomyelitis

Figure 2: **Management of Diabetic Foot Osteomyelitis**

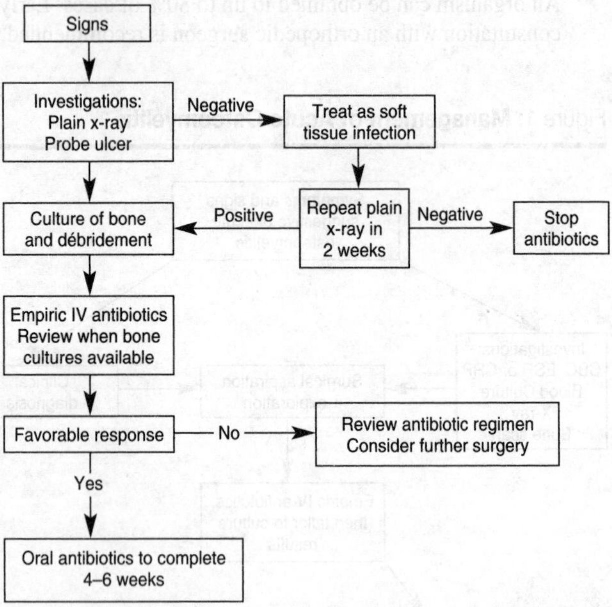
Signs
Investigations:
Plain x-ray
Probe ulcer
Negative
Treat as soft tissue infection
Culture of bone and débridement
Positive
Repeat plain x-ray in 2 weeks
Negative
Stop antibiotics
Empiric IV antibiotics
Review when bone cultures available
Favorable response
No
Review antibiotic regimen
Consider further surgery
Yes
Oral antibiotics to complete 4–6 weeks

associated with diabetic foot requires surgical débridement. This should be aggressive and may involve amputation of the infected bone.

## Pharmacologic Choices

### *Antibiotics*

While cultures are pending, empiric IV antibiotic therapy, based on the most likely infecting organism, should be started (Table 1). A definitive choice can be made once the organism and sensitivities are identified (Table 2). The role of adjunctive antibiotics such as fusidic acid or rifampin has not been studied systematically. They cannot be used alone for staphylococcal infections because resistance develops rapidly.

Mild diabetic foot infection may be treated with an oral regimen of amoxicillin/clavulanic acid or ciprofloxacin plus clindamycin.

**Duration of antibiotic therapy** should be a minimum of 4 weeks; many authorities recommend 6 weeks. More severe initial presentation, extensive bone involvement, and slow resolution of systemic and local signs indicate a 6-week course. In osteomyelitis following penetrating injury, 10 to 14 days of treatment is sufficient if adequate débridement has been performed.

Table 2: **Choice of Antibiotics for Acute Osteomyelitis**

| Organism | Initial IV Antibiotic | Oral Antibiotics (for completion of course) |
|---|---|---|
| *S. aureus* | Cloxacillin or Clindamycin | Cloxacillin or Cephalexin or Clindamycin |
| *Streptococcus* group A | Penicillin | Penicillin or Amoxicillin or Clindamycin |
| *Streptococcus* group B | Penicillin | In neonates oral antibiotics not appropriate |
| *H. influenzae* | Cefotaxime or Cefuroxime | Amoxicillin or Cefixime (if ampicillin-resistant) |
| Coliforms | Cefotaxime | In neonates oral antibiotics not appropriate |
| *P. aeruginosa* | (Ceftazidime or Ticarcillin) + Gentamicin | No suitable oral preparation available for children. Ciprofloxacin for adults |
| Mixed aerobic/ anaerobic | Imipenem-cilastatin | Ciprofloxacin+ clindamycin or amoxicillin-clavulanate |

In diabetic foot, 4 to 6 weeks of therapy is required. If no débridement of bone occurs, a 10- to 12-week course has been curative. If all infected bone has been completely removed, 2 to 3 weeks may be sufficient.

## *Sequential Intravenous–Oral Antibiotic Therapy*

Since a long course is required, a switch from the IV to oral route has many advantages, particularly shortened hospital stay and reduced complications from IV cannulae. This has been the subject of a position paper by the Canadian Paediatric Society.[1] IV antibiotics should be continued until the patient is systemically better, the temperature is normal and local signs of inflammation and tenderness are improved. This may take several days. The same high concentrations of antibiotic can be achieved with the oral route but with certain provisos:

- Compliance is vital. For children, the taste of the oral antibiotic is the most important factor. Cloxacillin liquid preparations are unpalatable; cephalexin has a more acceptable taste.

[1] *Can J Infect Dis 1994;4:10–12.*

Table 3: **Antibiotics Used in Treatment of Acute Osteomyelitis***

| Antibiotic | Dosage Pediatric (P)/Adult (A) | Adverse Effects | Comments | Cost† |
|---|---|---|---|---|
| *amoxicillin*<br>Amoxil, generics | (P) 100 mg/kg/d divided Q8H PO<br>(A) 0.5–1 g Q8H | GI effects, rash, eosinophilia. | Can be taken with food. | $<br>$ |
| *amoxicillin-clavulanate*<br>Clavulin | (P) 100 mg of amoxicillin/kg/d divided Q8H PO<br>(A) 0.5–1 g of amoxicillin Q8H PO | | | $<br>$ |
| *cefazolin*<br>Ancef, Kefzol, generics | (P) 100 mg/kg/d divided Q8H IV<br>(A) 2 g Q8H IV | | | $<br>$$ |
| *cefixime*<br>Suprax | (P) 8 mg/kg/d given Q24H PO | GI effects, especially diarrhea; hypersensitivity. | Can be taken with food. | $ |
| *cefotaxime*<br>Claforan | (P) 150 mg/kg/d divided Q8H IV<br>(A) 2 g Q8H IV | Phlebitis, hypersensitivity, positive Coombs' test. | | $$<br>$$$ |
| *cefuroxime*<br>Kefurox, Zinacef, generics | (P) 150 mg/kg/d divided Q8H IV<br>(A) 1.5 g Q8H IV | Phlebitis, eosinophilia, ↓ hematocrit, positive Coombs' test, neutropenia. | | $$<br>$$ |
| *ceftazidime*<br>Ceptaz, Fortaz, Tazidime | (P) 150 mg/kg/d divided Q8H IV<br>(A) 2 g Q8H IV | Phlebitis, eosinophilia, positive Coombs' test, ↑ AST, superinfections. | | $$$<br>$$$ |
| *cephalexin*<br>Keflex, generics | (P) 100–150 mg/kg/d divided Q6H<br>(A) 0.5–1 g Q6H | GI effects, rash, eosinophilia, leukopenia, positive Coombs' test, ↑ AST. | Oral liquid preparations more palatable than cloxacillin and flucloxacillin. | $ |
| *ciprofloxacin*<br>Cipro | (A) 400 mg Q12H IV or 750 mg Q12H PO | | Not recommended in pediatric patients unless exceptional circumstances | $$$<br>$ |
| *clindamycin*<br>Dalacin C | (P) 40 mg/kg/d divided Q6H IV or 30 mg/kg/d divided Q8H PO<br>(A) 450–600 mg Q8H IV or PO | Rash, neutropenia, ↑ AST and alkaline phosphatase, pseudomembranous colitis. | May need to ↓ dosage in hepatic failure. | IV<br>$$<br>PO<br>$ |

| | | | | |
|---|---|---|---|---|
| *cloxacillin*<br>Tegopen, generics | (P) 200 mg/kg/d IV or<br>150–200 mg/kg/d PO divided Q6H<br>(A) 2 g Q4H IV or<br>1 g Q6H PO | Rash, eosinophilia, GI effects. | May alter INR with warfarin. Oral liquid preparations unpalatable. Should be taken on empty stomach. | $<br>$<br>$$<br>$ |
| *gentamicin* [renal]<br>Cidomycin, Garamycin, generics | (P) 6 mg/kg/d divided Q8H<br>(A) 5–7 mg/kg/d divided Q8H or once daily if renal function permits | Nephrotoxicity usually reversible, ↑ risk with dose, duration. Ototoxicity often reversible. | ↑ toxicity with other nephrotoxic or ototoxic drugs. | $$<br>$$ |
| *imipenem-cilastatin* [renal]<br>Primaxin | (A) 500 mg Q6H IV | Caution in beta-lactam sensitivity. Risk of seizures if dose exceeded in renal failure. | | $$$$ |
| *penicillin G (IV)* [renal]<br>generics | (P) 200 000 units/kg/d divided Q4–6H<br>(A) 4 million units Q6H | GI effects, hypersensitivity, rash, drug fever, positive Coombs' test. Monitor $K^+$ and $Na^+$ when using high-dose parenteral penicillin G. | | $<br>$$ |
| *penicillin V (PO)* [renal]<br>Pen-Vee, PVF K, generics | (P) 100 mg/kg/d divided Q6H PO<br>(A) 600 mg Q6H PO | | | $<br>$ |
| *ticarcillin* [renal]<br>Ticar | (P) 300 mg/kg/d divided Q6H IV<br>(A) 3 g Q6H IV | Hypersensitivity, inhibition of platelet function, hypokalemia. | Contains 5.2 mmol of sodium/g. Can inactivate aminoglycosides if mixed. | $$<br>$$$ |

* *Therapy is initiated with IV antibiotics. When the patient is systemically better, a switch can be made to oral antibiotics under certain conditions – see Pharmacologic Choices.*

[renal] *Dosage adjustment may be required in renal impairment – see Appendix I.*

† *Cost per day (pediatric dosage based on 20 kg) – includes drug cost only.*

*Legend: $ < $10 $$ $10–50 $$$ $50–100 $$$$ $100–150*

- No underlying immunocompromise is present.
- Patient is beyond neonatal age group.
- The dose of oral antibiotic is larger than that usually used for minor infections (Table 3).
- Patient will attend for regular review.
- Adequacy of antibiotic concentrations is measured. The most practical method is to measure the serum bactericidal titre (SBT) against the organism, using a blood sample drawn 45 to 90 minutes after an oral dose is given. The desired titre is ≥ 1:8. An inadequate dose of antibiotic, refusal to take all the dose or poor absorption may lead to failure in reaching the desired level. Inability to achieve this target or failure to improve clinically should lead to resumption of IV antibiotics. If no organism was isolated but the patient has recovered well on the empiric antibiotic regimen, a switch to a comparable oral antibiotic can still be made.

### Follow-up

Success of treatment is judged by careful follow-up of systemic signs (i.e., fever and well-being, local signs of decreasing inflammation and tenderness and return of full function). ESR gradually returns to normal over several weeks. The C-reactive protein returns to normal in a matter of days.

## Suggested Reading List

Canadian Paediatric Society, Infectious Diseases and Immunization Committee. The use of antibiotic therapy as an adjunct in treatment of bone and joint infections. *Can J Infect Dis* 1994;4:10–12.

Caputo GM, Cavanagh PR, Ulbrecht JS, et al. Assessment and management of foot disease in patients with diabetes. *N Engl J Med* 1994;331:854–860.

Eckman MH, Greenfield S, MacKey WC, et al. Foot infections in diabetic patients: decision and cost-effectiveness analyses. *JAMA* 1995;273:712–720.

Grayson MC, Gibbons GW, Balogh K, et al. Probing to bone in infected pedal ulcers. *JAMA* 1995;273:721–723.

Lew DP, Waldvogel FA. Osteomyelitis. *N Engl J Med* 1997;336: 999–1007.

Nade S. Acute haematogenous osteomyelitis in infancy and childhood. *J Bone Joint Surg Br* 1983;65:109–119.

Unkila-Kallio L, Kallio M, Eshola J, et al. Serum C-reactive protein, erythrocyte sedimentation rate and white blood cell count in acute haematogenous osteomyelitis of children. *Pediatrics* 1994;93:59–62.

CHAPTER 89

# Septic Shock

*Anthony W. Chow, MD, FRCPC, FACP*

## Goals of Therapy

- To restore fluid volume
- To improve tissue perfusion and oxygen delivery
- To correct metabolic acidosis and coagulation defects
- To reduce oxygen demand
- To eradicate causative pathogens
- To neutralize the biologic effects of exotoxins and/or endotoxins
- To manage complications (e.g., acute renal failure, acute respiratory distress syndrome [ARDS], disseminated intravascular coagulation [DIC], multiple organ dysfunction syndrome [MODS])
- To prevent nosocomial infections
- To prevent progression from sepsis syndrome to full septic shock

## Classification of Sepsis and Septic Shock

Patients should be categorized into 1 of 3 syndromes (Table 1).

Table 1: **Classification of Sepsis and Septic Shock**

| Clinical Staging | Diagnostic Criteria |
|---|---|
| Sepsis syndrome without shock (incipient septic shock) | Clinical evidence suggestive of infection plus:<br>Signs of a systemic inflammatory response to infection (all of the following):<br>Tachypnea: > 20 breaths/min or > 10 L/min if mechanically ventilated.<br>Tachycardia: > 90 beats/min.<br>Hyperthermia or hypothermia > 38.4°C or < 35.6°C.<br>Evidence of altered organ perfusion (one or more of the following):<br>Hypoxia: $PaO_2/FIO_2 < 280$ (in the absence of other pulmonary or cardiovascular disease).<br>Oliguria: < 0.5 mL/kg for at least 1 h in patients with urinary catheters.<br>↑ plasma lactate (> normal upper limit).<br>Altered mental status. |
| Septic shock<br>Early<br><br>Refractory | Clinical diagnosis of sepsis syndrome as outlined above plus:<br>Early: Hypotension* lasting < 2 h, responsive to conventional therapy.<br>Refractory: Hypotension* lasting > 2 h despite conventional therapy. |

** < 90 mm Hg or a 40 mm Hg decrease below baseline.*

Figure 1: **Early Management of Septic Shock (First 4 Hours)**

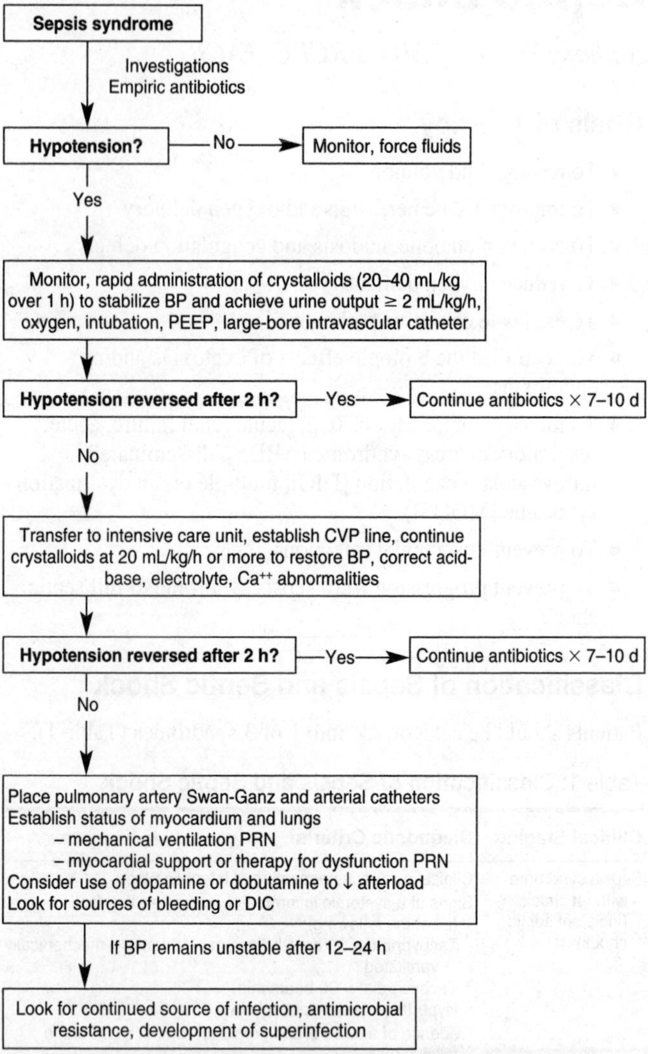
Sepsis syndrome
Investigations
Empiric antibiotics
Hypotension?
No
Monitor, force fluids
Yes
Monitor, rapid administration of crystalloids (20–40 mL/kg over 1 h) to stabilize BP and achieve urine output ≥ 2 mL/kg/h, oxygen, intubation, PEEP, large-bore intravascular catheter
Hypotension reversed after 2 h?
Yes
Continue antibiotics × 7–10 d
No
Transfer to intensive care unit, establish CVP line, continue crystalloids at 20 mL/kg/h or more to restore BP, correct acid-base, electrolyte, Ca++ abnormalities
Hypotension reversed after 2 h?
Yes
Continue antibiotics × 7–10 d
No
Place pulmonary artery Swan-Ganz and arterial catheters
Establish status of myocardium and lungs
– mechanical ventilation PRN
– myocardial support or therapy for dysfunction PRN
Consider use of dopamine or dobutamine to ↓ afterload
Look for sources of bleeding or DIC
If BP remains unstable after 12–24 h
Look for continued source of infection, antimicrobial resistance, development of superinfection

*Abbreviations: PEEP = positive end-expiratory pressure; CVP = central venous pressure; DIC = disseminated intravascular coagulation.*

## Investigations

- Thorough history with special attention to underlying disease, precipitating event and possible sites of infection
- Physical examination to localize the site and extent of infection, assess end organ dysfunction and ascertain

evidence of DIC or disseminated infection (e.g., skin rash, purpura, ecthyma gangrenosum, subcutaneous nodules)

- Clinical monitoring of vital signs, urine output, weight, level of consciousness
- Laboratory monitoring:
  - arterial blood gases
  - electrolytes, plasma lactate, acid-base status
  - BUN or serum creatinine
  - liver function tests
  - serum calcium and phosphate
  - chest x-ray, ECG
  - coagulation status
  - stool for occult blood
  - Gram's stain and cultures from blood, urine, sputum, other body sites
  - imaging studies to search for loculated infection
- Additional investigations may be necessary to monitor cardiopulmonary status and to localize the site of infection

## Therapeutic Choices (Figure 1)

### *Resuscitation and Monitoring*

Meticulous monitoring of the patient's circulating volume and ventilatory status and immediate resuscitation if required, is essential. If simple measures do not quickly restore hemodynamic stability, intensive care should be considered with invasive hemodynamic monitoring and aggressive cardiovascular support.

Early institution of **mechanical ventilation** and **sedation** and the judicious use of **muscle relaxants** or **neuromuscular blockade** may help to reduce oxygen demand and improve oxygen delivery and extraction at the tissue level. **Adequate caloric intake** with trace element and vitamin supplements is important to retard intense catabolism in patients with significant protein–calorie malnutrition.

### *Localization and Evacuation of Loculated Infections*

In addition to plain radiographs and tomograms, ultrasonography and computed tomography are invaluable for localizing nidus of infection in the thorax, abdomen, pelvis or the central nervous system. Loculated abscesses should be drained, and necrotic tissues must be adequately débrided. Infected foreign bodies should be removed.

### *Anticipation and Prevention of Complications*

*Acute respiratory distress syndrome (ARDS):* Anticipate and treat supportively, i.e., ventilatory support, **inhaled beta$_2$-agonists**.

The value of corticosteroids, ibuprofen, prostaglandin $E_1$, pentoxifylline or antioxidants is unproven.

*Electrolyte and acid-base status:* Correct initial hyponatremia and acidosis; anticipate and correct hypocalcemia and tetany.

*Edema, pericardial and pleural effusions:* Maintain adequate intravascular volume before using diuretic to mobilize extravascular fluid.

*Acute renal failure:* Avoid nephrotoxic drugs; monitor and dialyze PRN.

*Thrombocytopenia and DIC:* Administer fresh frozen plasma and platelets PRN. Heparin reduces thrombin generation, interrupts formation of fibrin microthrombi and reduces fibrinolysis but has not been shown to affect survival.

*Deep Venous Thrombosis*: Prevention of deep venous thrombosis may be accomplished by use of **unfractionated heparin**, **low molecular weight heparins** or venous compression devices (Chapter 31).

*Impaired gastrointestinal motility and stress ulcers:* Impaired motility may manifest as abnormal gastric emptying or as adynamic ileus. Stress ulceration is another common complication in the acutely ill. The judicious use of a gastrointestinal prokinetic agent and agents to prevent stress ulcers (e.g., **histamine $H_2$-receptor antagonists**, **proton pump inhibitors**, **sucralfate**) may be beneficial.

*Hepatic dysfunction:* Avoid drugs requiring biotransformation in the liver.

*Central nervous system dysfunction:* Anticipate irrational behavior; manage seizures with anticonvulsants.

*Nosocomial infections:* Strict adherence to aseptic technique and infection control principles are required to minimize the development of nosocomial infections. Every effort should be made to reduce the number of invasive intravascular catheters. Peripheral venous catheters should be changed routinely every 48 to 72 hours; when such catheters are inserted emergently, they should be replaced within 24 hours. Nasogastric and nasotracheal intubation should be avoided to prevent nosocomial sinusitis. The value of selected digestive tract decontamination in reducing the incidence of nosocomial pneumonia remains controversial.

## Pharmacologic Choices

### *Empiric Antimicrobial Therapy*

Antimicrobial therapy remains the cornerstone of treatment for sepsis syndrome and septic shock. However, the underlying disease, comorbid conditions and development of complications (e.g., ARDS, MODS) often dictate the eventual outcome of therapy.

Table 2: **Common Pathogens in Patients with Sepsis Syndrome or Septic Shock**

| Source of Infection | Common Pathogens | Initial Antibiotic Regimen |
|---|---|---|
| Oral cavity, lower respiratory tract | *Streptococcus viridans, Streptococcus pyogenes, Streptococcus pneumoniae, Haemophilus influenzae, Klebsiella pneumoniae, Peptostreptococcus* spp., *Bacteroides* spp., *Fusobacterium* spp., *Legionella pneumophila.* | Third-generation cephalosporin *or* Extended spectrum penicillin |
| Gastrointestinal tract, female pelvis | Enteric gram-negative bacilli, *Bacteroides fragilis, Peptostreptococcus* spp., *Clostridia* spp., *Enterococcus* spp. | Extended spectrum penicillin +/− aminoglycoside *or* Ciprofloxacin + metronidazole |
| Urinary tract | *Escherichia coli, Pseudomonas aeruginosa*, other enteric gram-negative bacilli, *Staphylococcus saprophyticus, Enterococcus* spp. | Ciprofloxacin *or* Aminoglycoside |
| Cardiac valves | *Staphylococcus aureus, Streptococcus viridans, Enterococcus* spp., *Corynebacterium* spp., *Coxiella burnetii*, HACEK group (*Haemophilus aphrophilus, Actinobacillus actinomycetemcomitans, Cardiobacterium hominis, Eikenella corrodens, Kingella* spp.). | Penicillin +/− vancomycin |
| Central nervous system | *Neisseria meningitidis, H. influenzae, S. pneumoniae, S. aureus*, enteric gram-negative bacilli, *Bacteroides* spp., *Nocardia asteroides, Peptostreptococcus* spp. | Extended spectrum penicillin |
| Necrotizing skin and soft tissues | *S. aureus*, enteric gram-negative bacilli, *B. fragilis, Clostridia* spp., *Peptostreptococcus* spp., *Enterococcus* spp. | Extended spectrum penicillin +/− aminoglycoside |
| Intravascular devices-associated | *S. aureus, Staphylococcus epidermidis, Staphylococcus haemolyticus*, enteric gram-negative bacilli, *Candida* spp. | Vancomycin |

Initial antimicrobial therapy is empiric because gram-positive and gram-negative infections as well as mycobacterial, fungal and viral infections can present as sepsis syndrome or septic shock, which are clinically indistinguishable. Antibiotic selection is based on the most likely source/site of infection and hence the most likely causative microorganisms and their anticipated susceptibility profiles (Tables 2 and 3). The choice of antimicrobial agents (Table 4) may also be influenced by the presence of acute renal or hepatic failure, hypersensitivity reactions, need for fluid restriction, local antimicrobial susceptibility patterns, emergence of resistance and drug interactions.

Table 3: **Spectrum of Antibiotics Used in Sepsis Syndrome and Septic Shock**

| Pathogen | β-lactams | Aminoglycosides | Fluoroquinolones | Glycopeptides |
|---|---|---|---|---|
| Staphylococci | ++ I/C, MER, P/T + others | ± | ++ | +++ (incl. MRSA) |
| Streptococci | ++ ctaz ++ + others | – | + | ++ + |
| Enterococci | ++ I/C ++ + P/T ± others | ++ | + | +++ |
| *Haemophilus* | +++ | – | ++ | – |
| Enteric gram-negative bacilli | ++ ctrx, cfax, ctiz +++ others | +++ | +++ | – |
| *Pseudomonas,* resistant gram-negative bacilli | ++ ctrx, cfax, ctiz +++ others | ++ | +++ | – |
| Anaerobes | +++ I/C, MER, P/T (incl. *B. fragilis*) + ctaz, ctrx ++ ctiz | – | – | – |

*MRSA = methicillin-resistant S. aureus.*
***Activity:*** *– none; ± negligible; + some; ++ moderate; +++ excellent.*
***β-lactams:*** *imipenem/cilastatin (I/C), meropenem (MER), piperacillin/tazobactam (P/T), ceftazidime (ctaz), ceftriaxone (ctrx), ceftizoxime (ctiz), cefotaxime (cfax).*
***Aminoglycosides:*** *gentamicin, tobramycin, amikacin.* ***Fluoroquinolones:*** *ciprofloxacin, levofloxacin.*
***Glycopeptides:*** *vancomycin, teicoplanin.*

Antibiotics should be administered IV in critically ill patients and be reassessed within 3 to 5 days. Adjustments are guided by culture results, in vitro susceptibility patterns and clinical response.

### *Vasoactive Agents for Cardiovascular Support*

Although rapid fluid administration alone may be sufficient to restore hemodynamic stability, vasopressors are often necessary to restore minimal tissue perfusion pressure and enhance myocardial contractility.

**Dopamine** (2 to 25 µg/kg/min) is usually selected first because it more effectively maintains organ blood flow. The dose is titrated until systolic BP is maintained at > 90 mm Hg and urine output at > 30 mL/h. Renal and mesenteric circulations may be selectively preserved. **Dobutamine** (2 to 25 µg/kg/min, titrated as with dopamine) is similar to dopamine but has little chronotropic activity. **Isoproterenol** (5 µg/mL/min) increases the cardiac

Table 4: **Intravenous Antimicrobial Drugs Used in Sepsis Syndrome and Septic Shock**

| Drug | IV Dosage | Adverse Effects | Comments | Cost* |
|---|---|---|---|---|
| **Extended Spectrum β-lactams** | | Hypersensitivity, hepatitis, interstitial nephritis, neutropenia, hypoprothrombinemia, eosinophilia, positive Coombs' test, pseudomembranous colitis, seizures. | Have become mainstay of treatment due to lack of nephrotoxicity and broad-spectrum activity vs gram-negative organisms.<br>No drug interactions; serum concentration monitoring not required.<br>Imipenem, ceftazidime may be used with caution in patients allergic to penicillin.<br>Ceftizoxime is often chosen to cover anaerobes in head/neck, intra-abdominal, female pelvic or necrotizing skin infections. | |
| *imipenem/cilastatin*<br>Primaxin | 1 g Q6H | | | $$$$$ |
| *meropenem*<br>Merrem | 0.5–1 g Q8H | | | $$$–$$$$ |
| *piperacillin/tazobactam*<br>Tazocin | 2 g Q4H | | | $$ |
| *ticarcillin/clavulanate*<br>Timentin | 3 g Q4H | | | $$ |
| *ceftazidime*<br>Ceptaz, Fortaz, Tazidime | 2 g Q6H | | | $$$$$ |
| *ceftriaxone*<br>Rocephin | 1–2 g Q24H | | | $$ |
| *ceftizoxime*<br>Cefizox | 1–2 g Q8H | | | $ |
| *cefotaxime*<br>Claforan | 2 g Q6-8H | | | $$–$$$ |
| **Aminoglycosides** | | Nephrotoxicity, ototoxicity, neuromuscular blockade. | May be required as combination therapy with β-lactams for *Pseudomonas* or multiresistant gram-negative bacilli.<br>Often avoided in septic shock due to nephrotoxicity and ototoxicity; serum drug levels monitored to guide dosing and avoid toxicity.<br>Desired levels (μg/mL):<br>*Peak*: *Gentamicin* 10, *Tobramycin* 10, *Amikacin* 40<br>*Trough*: *Gentamicin* < 2, *Tobramycin* < 2, *Amikacin* < 10<br>↑ nephrotoxicity when used with vancomycin. | |
| *gentamicin*<br>Garamycin, Cidomycin, generics | 1.5 mg/kg Q8H or 4–7 mg/kg once daily | | | $ |
| *tobramycin*<br>Nebcin, generics | 1.5 mg/kg Q8H or 4–7 mg/kg once daily | | | $ |
| *amikacin*<br>Amikin | 7.5 mg/kg Q12H or 15–20 mg/kg once daily | | | $$ |

*(cont'd)*

Table 4: **Intravenous Antimicrobial Drugs Used in Sepsis Syndrome and Septic Shock** *(cont'd)*

| Drug | IV Dosage | Adverse Effects | Comments | Cost* |
|---|---|---|---|---|
| **Fluoroquinolones** | | GI upset, insomnia, headache, cartilage damage, rash, seizures (rare). | Oral formulations available for step-down therapy. Serum levels not monitored. Ciprofloxacin: ↑ theophylline (toxicity), ↑ caffeine levels; may cause nephrotoxicity with cyclosporine; may ↑ INR with warfarin. | |
| *ciprofloxacin* Cipro | 400 mg Q8–12H | | | $$–$$$ |
| *levofloxacin* Levaquin | 250–500 mg Q24H | | | $–$$ |
| **Glycopeptides** | | Nephrotoxicity, ototoxicity, phlebitis; "red man syndrome" (flushing/rash, hypotension) if vancomycin infused too rapidly (< 1 h). | Enhanced nephrotoxicity when vancomycin used with aminoglycosides. Teicoplanin has longer half-life. Desired serum levels: *peak* 40 μg/mL, *trough* < 10 μg/mL. Useful if serious infection with coagulase-negative staphylococci or enterococci or if methicillin-resistant *S. aureus* present. | |
| *vancomycin* Vancocin | 1 g Q12H | | | $$$$ |
| *teicoplanin* ‡ | 10 mg/kg/d | | | ‡ |
| **Others** | | Rash, thrombophlebitis, GI effects, pseudomembranous colitis, blood dyscrasias, ↑ liver function tests (clindamycin), metallic taste (metronidazole). | Often chosen to cover anaerobes in head/neck, intra-abdominal, female pelvic or necrotizing skin infections, but lack coverage against facultative gram-negative organisms (most often used with aminoglycosides or fluoroquinolones). Clindamycin: may ↑ neuromuscular blocking action of other agents; may require dosage adjustment in hepatic failure. Metronidazole: ↑ lithium levels; ↑ INR with warfarin; disulfiram-like reaction with alcohol; acute psychosis and confusion with disulfiram. | |
| *clindamycin* Dalacin C | 600 mg Q6H | | | $$ |
| *metronidazole* Flagyl, generics | 500 mg Q8H | | | $$ |

| | | | | |
|---|---|---|---|---|
| *erythromycin*<br>Erythrocin | 15–20 mg/kg/d, divided Q6H | Venous irritation/ thrombophlebitis; rarely prolongation of QT interval, ventricular arrhythmias, ototoxicity.<br>Caution if hepatic dysfunction. | Often included in initial empiric therapy if *Legionella* is suspected.<br>Erythromycin: ↑ theophylline, carbamazepine, cyclosporine levels; ↑ INR with warfarin; ↑ risk of ventricular arrhythmias with astemizole and terfenadine. | $ |

*‡ Available through Special Access Program, Therapeutic Products Directorate, Health Canada.*

*Dosage adjustment required in renal impairment – see Appendix I.*

** Cost of 7-day supply – includes drug cost only.*

*Legend: $ < $200 $$ $200–500 $$$ $500–750 $$$$ $750–1000 $$$$$ > $1000*

index but has little effect on mean arterial pressure. Its marked effect on increasing heart rate in some patients limits its usefulness. **Norepinephrine** (0.1 to 0.2 μg/kg test dose, then 0.5 μg/kg/min) has intense peripheral vasoconstricting activity but can be used effectively to restore arterial pressure in patients with severe cardiovascular collapse. It may be administered as an adjunct to dopamine if hypotension persists but should be tapered down and discontinued in favor of dopamine infusion as soon as the clinical situation has improved.

### *Other Therapies*

Short-term administration of **corticosteroids** at replacement or physiologic stress doses (e.g., hydrocortisone 100 mg IV TID daily for 5 days) was beneficial in achieving 7-day shock reversal in a prospective, randomized, double-blind placebo-controlled study.[1] In contrast, controlled trials of pharmacologic doses of corticosteroids have not demonstrated benefit.[2]

**Immunotherapy** to neutralize or remove specific exotoxins may be worthwhile if etiologic agents are identified (e.g., diphtheria, botulism, anthrax, clostridial septicotoxemia, toxic shock syndrome); however, as specific antisera are seldom available, **immunoglobulins** pooled from healthy donors are often used empirically.

**Antiendotoxin therapy** with a human monoclonal antibody (HA-1A) initially yielded encouraging results. However, subsequent multicentre trials failed to demonstrate benefit when administered to patients within six hours of the onset of septic shock or among children with meningococcal septic shock.

**IV immune globulins (IVIG)** (0.4 g/kg/day for 5 to 7 days) have been used as empiric adjunctive therapy for fulminant *Haemophilus*, pneumococcal, group A and group B streptococcal and *Pseudomonas* sepsis, and sepsis associated with staphylococcal toxic shock syndrome and streptococcal superantigens. Their efficacy in sepsis syndrome remains unproven except in hereditary or acquired immunodeficiency. Evidence suggests that IVIG can at least neutralize staphylococcal and streptococcal superantigen activity in vitro.

**Naloxone, ibuprofen, indomethacin** and **pentoxifylline** have been or are being investigated as adjunctive therapies in septic shock, but definitive studies showing sustained improvements in haemodynamics or survival are lacking. **Anticytokine therapy** with **antibodies to tumor necrosis factor, soluble tumor necrosis factor receptors** and **interleukin-1 receptor antagonists** were investigated but not found to be effective adjunctive therapies in septic shock.

---

[1] *Crit Care Med 1999;27:723–732.*
[2] *Crit Care Med 1995;23:1294–1303.*

## Therapeutic Tips

- Empiric broad-spectrum antibiotic therapy primarily directed at enteric gram-negative bacilli must be initiated early in *neutropenic* patients (Chapter 97). The classic symptoms and signs of infection, other than fever, are often absent, making it much more difficult to localize the primary source of infection. Infections (especially gram-negative) in these patients tend to disseminate rapidly and widely and are associated with a high mortality rate. The clinical response and eventual outcome is often dictated by the speed of bone marrow recovery and successful avoidance of complications (e.g., superinfections).
- *Persistent bacteremia,* despite appropriate antimicrobial therapy, suggests a valvular or endovascular infection, a loculated abscess with dissemination or the emergence of resistant microorganisms.
- *Culture-negative infections* are particularly common among patients who have received partial antimicrobial therapy before cultures are obtained and in immunocompromised patients undergoing bone marrow or solid organ transplants. The possibility of fastidious or culture-negative organisms, particularly *Legionella* spp., rickettsia, invasive fungi and viruses, should be seriously considered and appropriate investigations implemented.

## *Suggested Reading List*

Baumgartner JD, Calandra T. Treatment of sepsis: past and future avenues. *Drugs* 1999;57:127–132.

Bone RC. Managing sepsis: what treatments can we use today? *J Crit Illness* 1997;12:15–24.

Briegel J, Forst H, Haller M, et al. Stress doses of hydrocortisone reverse hyperdynamic septic shock: a prospective, randomized, double-blind, single center study. *Crit Care Med* 1999;27:723–732.

Task Force of the American College of Critical Care Medicine, Society of Critical Care Medicine. Practice parameters for hemodynamic support of sepsis in adult patients in sepsis. *Crit Care Med* 1999;27:639–660.

Wheeler AP, Bernard GR. Treating patients with severe sepsis. *N Engl J Med* 1999;340:207.

Zeni F, Freeman B, Natanson C. Anti-inflammatory therapies to treat sepsis and septic shock: a reassessment. *Crit Care Med* 1997;25:1095–1100.

CHAPTER 90

# Sexually Transmitted Diseases

*John W. Sellors, BSc, MSc, MD, CCFP, FCFP*

## Goals of Therapy

- To abolish symptoms of the infection, if any
- To prevent recurrence
- To prevent the spread of infection to sexual partners
- To decrease the probability of complications (which may be life-threatening or disabling) or permanent damage to reproductive and other systems
- To eliminate genital warts with as little pain and residual damage as possible

## Investigations

- History for:
  - duration of symptoms, if any
  - duration of specific risk factors
  - specific complaints of sexual partner (e.g., anogenital sores, discharge)
  - previous therapy and response
  - recent childbirth, urinary tract surgery or intrauterine contraceptive device (IUCD) insertion (for pelvic inflammatory disease)
- Physical examination:
  - inspection of affected areas for lesions; genital herpes lesions/crusts are usually on an erythematous base
  - anoscopy (if perianal warts are present)
  - in women: speculum examination for signs of infection, using water as a lubricant
  - in men: signs of urethral discharge; palpation for inguinal lymphadenopathy or abnormalities of the testes/epididymides
  - systemic signs of syphilis
- Laboratory tests and other investigations:
  - swabs from affected areas and smears for Gram's stain
  - urine specimen microscopic examination and culture
  - for chlamydia, nucleic acid amplification testing, i.e., polymerase chain reaction (PCR) or ligase chain reaction (LCR) of the first 10 to 15 mL of voided urine is accurate in males. It is also an option for females when a vaginal examination is not possible

- scrotal ultrasound if available and epididymo-orchitis suspected
- CBC, ESR, C-reactive protein, urine and serum β-HCG, VDRL, transvaginal pelvic ultrasonography (preferable to transabdominal) if PID suspected[1]
- darkfield microscopy examination of specimen and VDRL

Table 1: **Differential Diagnosis of Vaginitis/Vaginosis**

| | Candidiasis | Trichomoniasis | Bacterial Vaginosis |
|---|---|---|---|
| ***Signs/symptoms*** | | | |
| Pruritus | + | + | − |
| Odor | − | + | + |
| Discharge | cheesy | purulent | grey/milky |
| Inflammation | + | + | − |
| ***Simple tests*** | | | |
| pH | ≤ 4.5 | > 4.5 | > 4.5 |
| "Whiff" test | − | ± | + |
| ***Microscopic findings*** | | | |
| Specific | mycelia | trichomonads | clue cells |
| PMNs | ++ | +++ | − |
| Lactobacilli | + | − | − |

## Therapeutic Choices

### *Vaginitis* (Table 1)

For management, see Figure 1; for treatment, see Table 2.

Patients should be instructed to complete the full, continuous course of therapy, even during menstruation.

Recurrent vulvovaginal candidiasis (at least 4 proven episodes per year) requires investigation and possibly referral. Predisposing causes, if present, should be addressed (e.g., use of systemic antibiotics, poorly controlled diabetes, consideration of HIV testing and counseling).

Nonsexually transmitted causes of vaginitis are numerous (e.g., tampons/other foreign bodies, douches, deodorant sprays, lubricants, perfumes, contraceptive chemicals, dyes in colored toilet tissue, scented napkins, bubble bath, detergents, seasonal allergy, allergy to latex condoms/semen).

### *Cervicitis and Urethritis due to Chlamydia Trachomatis or Neisseria Gonorrhoeae* (Figures 1 and 2)

Azithromycin or doxycycline are the drugs of choice for chlamydial infection (Table 3).

[1] *Because the accuracy of clinical and laboratory diagnosis for PID is not good, clinicians must follow women carefully and judge when to refer them for more definitive tests (e.g., laparoscopy).*

Selective screening of high-risk women (shaded box, below) is important for detection of sexually transmitted (chlamydial) cervicitis because symptoms are often minor and unlikely to result in health-care-seeking behavior.

**Indications for Chlamydial Screening**[2]

Intermenstrual bleeding

Frequent urination (on enquiry, not a presenting complaint)

New sexual partner in previous year

Mucopurulent (opaque or yellow) endocervical discharge

Easily induced mucosal bleeding of cervix

Test of cure is not recommended unless symptoms persist or recur after treatment, possibly due to poor compliance or reinfection, or when amoxicillin or erythromycin is used to treat chlamydia in pregnancy.

### *Epididymo-orchitis*

Epididymo-orchitis is treated the same way as urethritis (Table 3, Figure 2), but the antichlamydial regimen should be given for at least 10 days and until resolution occurs. Scrotal elevation and bed rest are advisable.

In men over 35 years of age, urethral cultures may be negative but urine cultures suggestive of infection; in this case, treat for urinary tract infection (Chapter 91).

### *Pelvic Inflammatory Disease (PID)*

For management, see Figure 3; for outpatient treatment, see Table 4.

### *Syphilis*

For management, see Figure 4; for treatment, see Table 5. Individuals with HIV infection and syphilis and those with suspected or proven tertiary syphilis should be referred.

### *Genital Herpes (Chapter 94)*

### *Genital Warts* (Figure 5)

There is no specific laboratory test commonly available to detect human papillomavirus (HPV). Examination (3 minutes after applying 3 to 5% acetic acid) using a magnification device may

---

[2] *Arch Intern Med 1992;152:1837–1844.*

Figure 1: **Management of Vaginitis and Cervicitis**

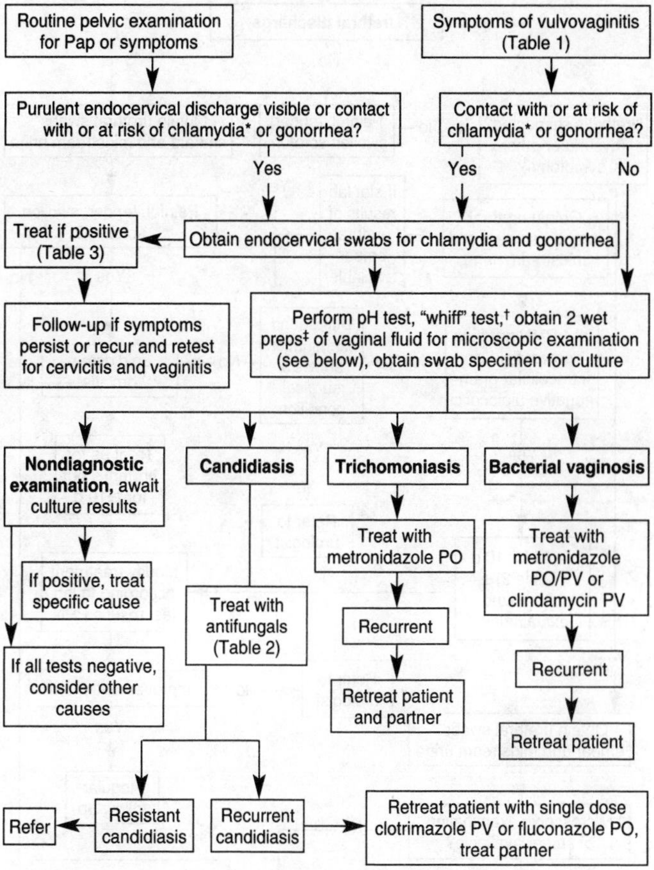
Routine pelvic examination for Pap or symptoms
Symptoms of vulvovaginitis (Table 1)
Purulent endocervical discharge visible or contact with or at risk of chlamydia* or gonorrhea?
Contact with or at risk of chlamydia* or gonorrhea?
Yes
Yes
No
Treat if positive (Table 3)
Obtain endocervical swabs for chlamydia and gonorrhea
Follow-up if symptoms persist or recur and retest for cervicitis and vaginitis
Perform pH test, "whiff" test,† obtain 2 wet preps‡ of vaginal fluid for microscopic examination (see below), obtain swab specimen for culture
Nondiagnostic examination, await culture results
Candidiasis
Trichomoniasis
Bacterial vaginosis
If positive, treat specific cause
If all tests negative, consider other causes
Treat with antifungals (Table 2)
Treat with metronidazole PO
Recurrent
Retreat patient and partner
Treat with metronidazole PO/PV or clindamycin PV
Recurrent
Retreat patient
Refer
Resistant candidiasis
Recurrent candidiasis
Retreat patient with single dose clotrimazole PV or fluconazole PO, treat partner

* *Chlamydial nucleic acid amplification testing (PCR, LCR) of a first voided urine specimen is an option if vaginal examination not possible.*
† *Malodor often intensified after addition of 10% potassium hydroxide (KOH).*
‡ *One sample mixed in a few drops of normal saline; second sample mixed with 10% KOH.*
*Abbreviations: PV = vaginally.*

detect subclinical exophytic and flat lesions, but the clinical utility of this is not proven, and it therefore is not recommended. There is a frustratingly high recurrence rate (approximately 33%) of genital warts 1 year after apparent cure.

## *Hepatitis B (Chapter 44)*

Figure 2: **Management of Urethritis and Epididymo-orchitis**

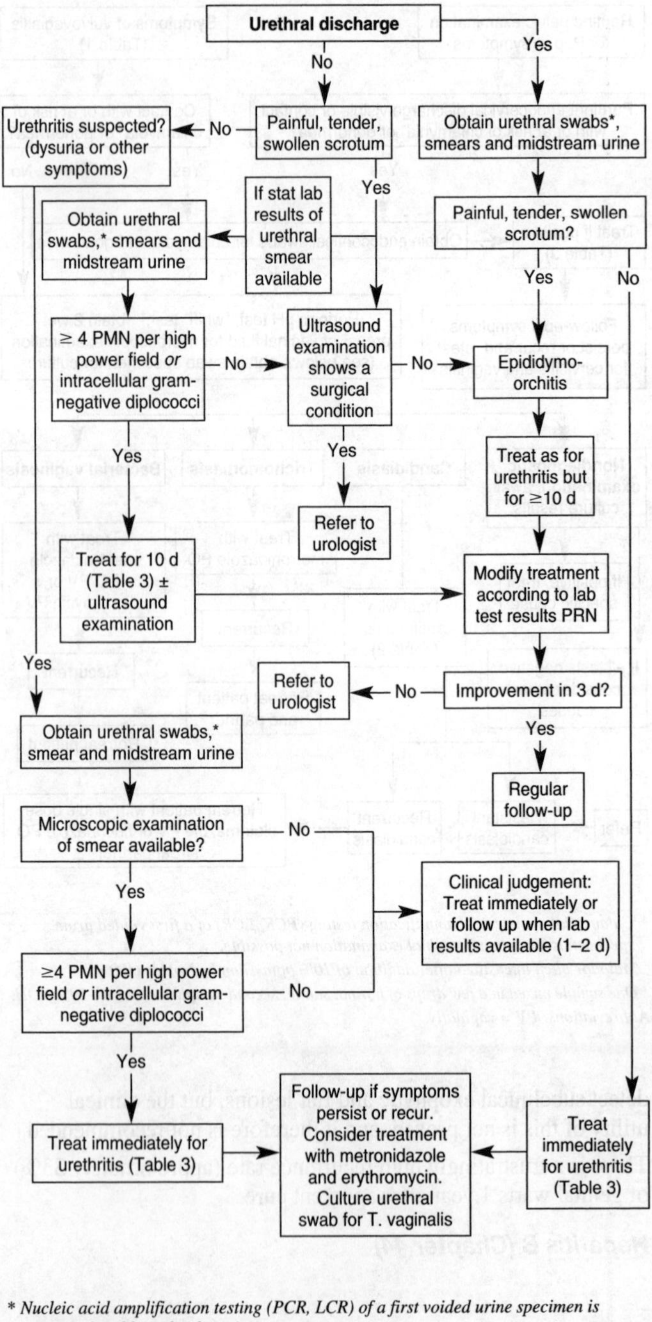
Urethral discharge
No
Yes
Urethritis suspected? (dysuria or other symptoms)
Painful, tender, swollen scrotum
Obtain urethral swabs*, smears and midstream urine
If stat lab results of urethral smear available
Obtain urethral swabs,* smears and midstream urine
Painful, tender, swollen scrotum?
≥ 4 PMN per high power field or intracellular gram-negative diplococci
Ultrasound examination shows a surgical condition
Epididymo-orchitis
Treat as for urethritis but for ≥10 d
Refer to urologist
Treat for 10 d (Table 3) ± ultrasound examination
Modify treatment according to lab test results PRN
Refer to urologist
Improvement in 3 d?
Obtain urethral swabs,* smear and midstream urine
Regular follow-up
Microscopic examination of smear available?
Clinical judgement: Treat immediately or follow up when lab results available (1–2 d)
≥4 PMN per high power field or intracellular gram-negative diplococci
Treat immediately for urethritis (Table 3)
Follow-up if symptoms persist or recur. Consider treatment with metronidazole and erythromycin. Culture urethral swab for T. vaginalis
Treat immediately for urethritis (Table 3)

** Nucleic acid amplification testing (PCR, LCR) of a first voided urine specimen is accurate for chlamydia detection.*

*Abbreviations: PMN = polymorphonuclear leukocytes.*

Table 2: **Drugs Used for Vaginitis and Vaginosis**

| Drug | Dosage | Adverse Effects | Drug Interactions | Use in Pregnancy (P)/Lactation(L) | Cost* |
|---|---|---|---|---|---|
| ***Vulvovaginal Candidiasis*** | | | | | |
| **Imidazoles** | | | | | |
| *clotrimazole*<br>Canesten, generics | 200 mg ovule PV QHS × 3 or 500 mg tab PV (1 dose) | Local hypersensitivity. | | P: with caution.<br>L: not established. | $ |
| *econazole*<br>Ecostatin | 150 mg ovule PV QHS × 3 | | | | $$ |
| *miconazole*<br>Monistat, Micatin, generics | 400 mg PV QHS × 3 | | | | $ |
| *tioconazole*<br>Gynecure | 300 mg ovule or 6.5% oint (1 applicatorful) PV QHS × 1 | | | | $$ |
| **Triazoles** | | | Fluconazole: may ↑ INR with warfarin.<br>May ↓ blood glucose after sulfonylurea administration.<br>May markedly ↑ phenytoin levels.<br>Fluconazole dose should be ↑ 25% when used with rifampin.<br>May ↓ plasma clearance of theophylline (toxicity). | P: terconazole – not in 1st trimester; fluconazole – no.<br>L: not established. | |
| *terconazole*<br>Terazol | 80 mg ovule or 0.8% cream (1 applicatorful) PV × 3 | Local hypersensitivity. | | | $$ |
| *fluconazole*[†]<br>Diflucan, Diflucan-150, generics | 150 mg PO (1 dose) | Dizziness, headache, pruritus, rash, nausea, vomiting, abdominal pain, diarrhea, thrombocytopenia, ↑ transaminase levels, hypokalemia. | | | $$ |

*(cont'd)*

Table 2: **Drugs Used for Vaginitis and Vaginosis** *(cont'd)*

| Drug | Dosage | Adverse Effects | Drug Interactions | Use in Pregnancy (P)/Lactation(L) | Cost* |
|---|---|---|---|---|---|
| **Polyene Macrolides** | | | | | |
| *nystatin* Mycostatin, generics | 100 000 units PV daily × 14 d | None reported. | | P: yes, until 6 wks before term. L: not established. | $ |
| ***Bacterial Vaginosis*** | | | | | |
| *clindamycin* Dalacin Vaginal Cream | Topical: 5 g/d PV × 7 d | Nausea/vomiting, diarrhea, abdominal pain, constipation, heartburn, dizziness, headache, vertigo (< 1% with topical). | | **Topical:** P: yes. | $$$ |
| Dalacin-C | Oral: 300 mg PO BID × 7 d | Oral: pseudomembranous colitis. Topical: candidal vaginitis (10%). | | **Oral:** P: yes. L: with caution. | $$$ |
| *metronidazole* Flagyl, NidaGel | Topical: 5 g (1 applicatorful) PV BID × 5 d<br>Oral: see below | Candidal vaginitis. | | See below. | $$ |
| ***Trichomoniasis or Bacterial Vaginosis*** | | | | | |
| *metronidazole* Flagyl, generics | Oral: 2 g single dose or 500 mg PO BID × 7 d<br>Recurrences: same as above<br>If not effective, 2 g PO daily × 3–5 d | Vertigo, headache, ataxia, abdominal cramps, diarrhea, nausea, vomiting, pseudomembranous colitis, transient leukopenia, candidal vaginitis, taste alterations, gynecomastia. | Disulfiram-like reaction with alcohol.<br>↑ INR with oral anticoagulants.<br>Psychosis/confusion with disulfiram.<br>Barbiturates, phenytoin may ↑ metronidazole metabolism. | P: Safe use in 1st trimester uncertain; may use with caution during 2nd and 3rd trimesters.[‡]<br>L: no. | $<br>$$<br><br>$$ |

[†] *Use with caution in liver dysfunction.*

[‡] *For symptomatic relief of trichomonal vaginitis during the 1st trimester; clotrimazole PV may suppress symptoms until definitive oral treatment can be given simultaneously to woman and partner(s) after 1st trimester.*

* *Cost of indicated course of therapy – includes drug cost only.*
*Legend: $ < $10 $$ $10–20 $$$ $20–30*

Table 3: **Drugs Used in Gonococcal or Chlamydial Cervicitis and Urethritis***

| Drug | Dosage | Comments | Use in Pregnancy (P)/Lactation (L) | Cost† |
|---|---|---|---|---|
| ***Gonococcal Cervicitis and Urethritis‡*** | | | | |
| **Cephalosporins** | | | | |
| *ceftriaxone* Rocephin | 125 mg IM (1 dose) | | P and L: caution. | $ |
| *cefixime* Suprax | 400 mg PO (1 dose) | | P and L: unknown. | $ |
| **Quinolones** | | | | |
| *ciprofloxacin* Cipro | 500 mg PO (1 dose) | | P and L: no. | $ |
| *ofloxacin* Floxin | 400 mg PO (1 dose) | | | $ |
| **Spectinomycin** | | | | |
| Trobicin | 2 g IM (1 dose) | Second-line therapy. Not effective in pharyngeal gonococcal infection. Alternative in pregnant patients allergic to cephalosporins. | P and L: caution. | $$$^{\pi}$ |
| ***Chlamydial Cervicitis and Urethritis‡*** | | | | |
| **Tetracyclines** | | | | |
| *doxycycline* Vibra-Tabs, Vibramycin, generics | 100 mg BID × 7 d | | P: no.<br>L: no. | $ |
| *tetracycline* ◗ generics | 500 mg QID × 7 d | | | $ |

*(cont'd)*

Table 3: **Drugs Used in Gonococcal or Chlamydial Cervicitis and Urethritis*** *(cont'd)*

| Drug | Dosage | Comments | Use in Pregnancy (P)/Lactation (L) | Cost[†] |
|---|---|---|---|---|
| ***Chlamydial Cervicitis and Urethritis*** *(cont'd)* | | | | |
| **Macrolides** | | | | |
| *azithromycin* Zithromax | 1 g PO × 1 dose | May be substituted for doxycycline if tetracycline allergy or intolerance. | P: caution | $$ |
| *erythromycin base* Eryc, Erybid, PCE, Erythromid, generics | 500 mg QID × 7 d; if not tolerated, 250 mg QID × 14 d may be used | Test of cure recommended 3 wks after treatment in pregnancy. | P: yes. L: with caution. | $ |
| **Ofloxacin** ➔ Floxin, generics | 300 mg BID × 7 d | | P: no. L: no. | $$ |
| **Amoxicillin** ➔ Amoxil, generics | 500 mg TID × 10 d | Alternative to erythromycin for pregnant women in 3rd trimester. Test of cure recommended as for erythromycin. | P and L: yes. | $ |

➔ *Dosage adjustment may be required in renal impairment – see Appendix I.*

* *Epididymo-orchitis is treated similarly but for at least 10 d. For PID, see Table 5.*

[‡] *Usually, the results of tests (culture or nucleic acid amplification) for chlamydia and gonorrhea will determine the need for specific treatment. Empirical dual therapy for chlamydia and gonorrhea prior to the results is not recommended unless the likelihood of either infection is high or the patient is unlikely to return for treatment.*

[π] *Available through the Special Access Program, Health Canada.*

[†] *Cost of one course of therapy – includes drug cost only.*

*Legend: $ < $10 $$ $10–25 $$$ $25–50*

## Figure 3: **Management of Pelvic Inflammatory Disease**

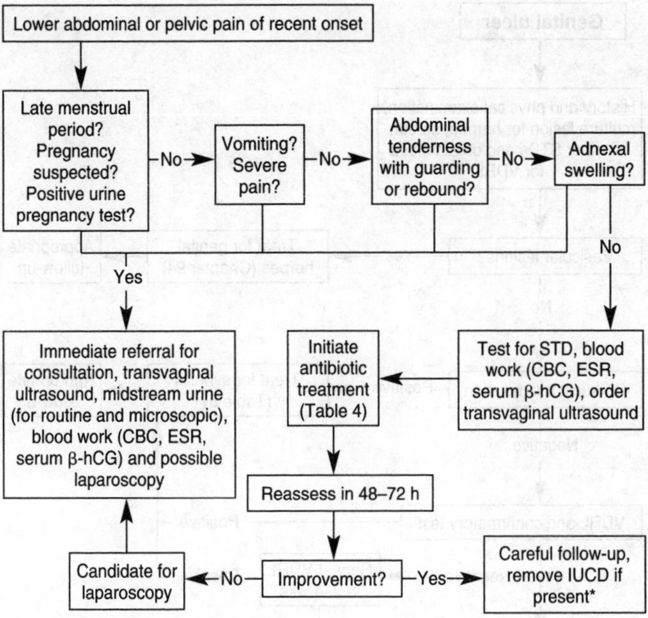

Lower abdominal or pelvic pain of recent onset
Late menstrual period? Pregnancy suspected? Positive urine pregnancy test?
No
Vomiting? Severe pain?
No
Abdominal tenderness with guarding or rebound?
No
Adnexal swelling?
No
Yes
Immediate referral for consultation, transvaginal ultrasound, midstream urine (for routine and microscopic), blood work (CBC, ESR, serum β-hCG) and possible laparoscopy
Initiate antibiotic treatment (Table 4)
Test for STD, blood work (CBC, ESR, serum β-hCG), order transvaginal ultrasound
Reassess in 48–72 h
Candidate for laparoscopy
No
Improvement?
Yes
Careful follow-up, remove IUCD if present*


* ***Note:*** *If the patient has an IUCD in place, it should not be removed until after at least 2 d of antimicrobial therapy has been given.*

## Table 4: **Drugs Used for Outpatient Treatment of PID**

| Drug Regimen | | Cost* |
|---|---|---|
| Ceftriaxone 250 mg IM (single dose) | **plus** doxycycline† 100 mg PO BID | $$$ |
| Cefoxitin‡ 2 g IM + probenecid$^{\pi}$ 1 g PO (single dose) | **plus** doxycycline† 100 mg PO BID | $$ |
| Cefixime 400 mg PO BID | **plus** doxycycline† 100 mg PO BID | $$$$$ |
| Ofloxacin 400 mg PO BID | **plus** metronidazole 500 mg PO BID | $$$ |

***Note:*** *Duration of therapy for all oral agents is 14 d unless otherwise noted.*

† *Erythromycin 500 mg PO QID × 14 d may be used instead of doxycycline if tetracycline allergy, intolerance or pregnancy.*

‡ *Safety in pregnancy is unknown.*

$\pi$ *Not needed if renal impairment is present. Use with caution in pregnancy and lactation.*

*Dosage adjustment may be required in renal impairment – see Appendix I.*

* *Cost of one course of therapy – includes drug cost only.*

*Legend: $ < $10 $$ $10–25 $$$ $25–50 $$$$ $50–75 $$$$$ > $75*

Figure 4: **Management of Genital Ulcers (Herpes, Syphilis)**

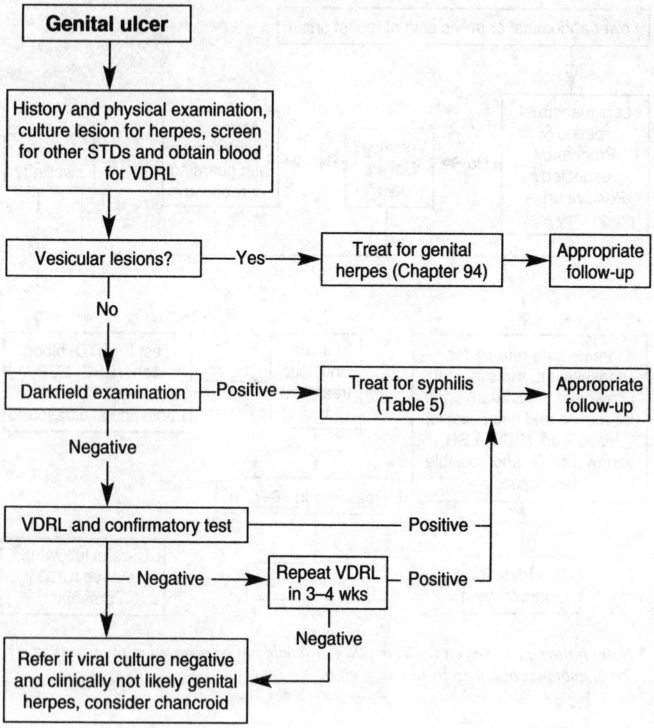
Genital ulcer
History and physical examination, culture lesion for herpes, screen for other STDs and obtain blood for VDRL
Vesicular lesions?
Yes
Treat for genital herpes (Chapter 94)
Appropriate follow-up
No
Darkfield examination
Positive
Treat for syphilis (Table 5)
Appropriate follow-up
Negative
VDRL and confirmatory test
Positive
Negative
Repeat VDRL in 3–4 wks
Positive
Negative
Refer if viral culture negative and clinically not likely genital herpes, consider chancroid

## Therapeutic Tips

- Treatment of sexual partner(s):

| Infection | Treatment Required for Partner(s)? |
|---|---|
| Vulvovaginal candidiasis | Not unless symptomatic, or vaginitis is recurrent |
| Bacterial vaginosis | No |
| Trichomoniasis | Partner(s) always treated |
| Chlamydial or gonorrheal cervicitis, urethritis, epididymo-orchitis, PID | Refer all recent (< 2 months) partners for testing and empirical treatment |
| Primary, secondary and early latent syphilis | Refer all partners in previous 3 mos for testing and empirical treatment. Refer all other partners in previous year for testing. |
| Late latent syphilis | Refer all long-term partners and any of their children who were possibly exposed during pregnancy for testing |
| Genital herpes | No (condoms advised) |
| HPV | No (condoms advised until warts have resolved) |

- Testing and counseling for HIV and STD should be offered, when appropriate, to all patients.
  - patients testing positive for gonorrhea or chlamydia should be screened for syphilis
  - patients with genital herpes should be counseled on how to reduce the risk of transmission
  - the need for regular Pap smears should be emphasized to women with HPV infection

Table 5: **Drugs Used to Treat Syphilis**

| Drug | Dosage | Comments | Cost* |
|---|---|---|---|
| *benzathine penicillin G* Bicillin 1200-LA | **Primary, secondary, early latent (< 1 yr):** 2.4 million units IM once (half in each buttock) | Safe in pregnancy and lactation. May cause Jarisch-Herxheimer reaction in secondary syphilis (chills, fever, headache, myalgia, tachycardia, malaise, sweating, sore throat, hypotension). | $$ |
| | **Late latent (> 1 yr):** 2.4 million units IM weekly × 3 | | $$$ |
| *tetracycline* ➔ generics | **Primary, secondary, early latent (< 1 yr):** Tetracycline: 500 mg PO QID × 14 d | Tetracyclines are alternatives in penicillin-allergic patients. Do not use in pregnancy and lactation. | $ |
| *doxycycline* Vibramycin, Vibra-Tabs, generics | Doxycycline: 100 mg PO BID × 14 d | | $$ |
| | **Late latent (> 1 yr):** Same dosages × 28 d | | $$$ |
| *erythromycin* Eryc, Erybid, Erythromid, PCE, generics | **Primary, secondary, early latent (< 1 yr):** 500 mg PO QID × 14 d | Use only if penicillin desensitization is unsuccessful in pregnant, penicillin-allergic patients. | $ |
| | **Late latent (> 1 yr):** Same dosage × 28 d | | $$ |

➔ *Dosage adjustment may be required in renal impairment – see Appendix I.*

* *Cost of indicated duration – includes drug cost only.*

*Legend: $ < $10 $$ $10–25 $$$ $25–50*

Figure 5: **Management of Anogenital Warts**

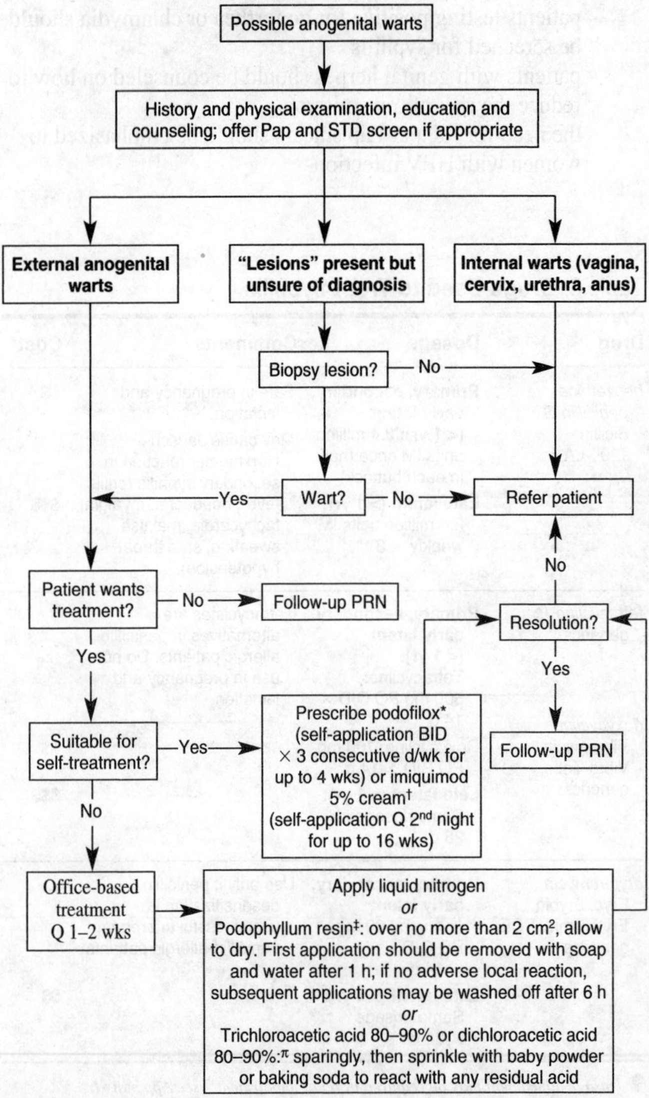
Possible anogenital warts
History and physical examination, education and counseling; offer Pap and STD screen if appropriate
External anogenital warts
"Lesions" present but unsure of diagnosis
Internal warts (vagina, cervix, urethra, anus)
Biopsy lesion?
No
Wart?
Yes
No
Refer patient
No
Patient wants treatment?
No
Follow-up PRN
Yes
Resolution?
Yes
Suitable for self-treatment?
Yes
Prescribe podofilox* (self-application BID × 3 consecutive d/wk for up to 4 wks) or imiquimod 5% cream† (self-application Q 2nd night for up to 16 wks)
Follow-up PRN
No
Office-based treatment Q 1–2 wks
Apply liquid nitrogen
or
Podophyllum resin‡: over no more than 2 cm², allow to dry. First application should be removed with soap and water after 1 h; if no adverse local reaction, subsequent applications may be washed off after 6 h
or
Trichloroacetic acid 80–90% or dichloroacetic acid 80–90%:π sparingly, then sprinkle with baby powder or baking soda to react with any residual acid

*Adverse effects of:*

* ***Podofilox** (Condyline, Wartec): inflammation, burning, erosion, pain, bleeding, pruritus, dizziness, insomnia. Do not use in pregnancy; safety in lactation unknown.*

† ***Imiquimod** (Aldara): mild to moderate erythema, itching and burning. Do not use in pregnancy.*

‡ ***Podophyllum resin** (Podofilm): Systemic: urticaria, fever, paresthesia, polyneuritis, paralytic ileus, blood dyscrasias, coma, death. Local: severe necrosis, scarring, paraphimosis, pseudoepitheliomatous hyperplasia. Do not use in pregnancy; safety in lactation unknown.*

π ***Dichloroacetic acid and trichloroacetic acid:** Inflammation, erosion, pain, burning, ulceration. Safe for use in pregnancy and lactation.*

### *Suggested Reading List*

Anon. Drugs for sexually transmitted infections. *The Med Lett* 1999;41:85–90.

Chernesky MA, Jang D, Lee H, et al. Diagnosis of Chlamydia trachomatis infections in men and women by testing first-void urine by ligase chain reaction. *J Clin Microbiol* 1994;32:2682–2685.

Holmes KK, Sparling PF, Mardh P-A, et al, eds. *Sexually transmitted diseases*. 3rd ed. New York: McGraw-Hill, 1999.

LCDC Expert Working Group on Canadian Guidelines for Sexually Transmitted Diseases. *Canadian STD Guidelines*. 1998 Edition, 1998. (available on the Internet at: http://www.hc–sc.gc.ca/hpb/lcdc/bah)

Sellors JW, Pickard L, Gafni A, et al. Effectiveness and efficiency of selective vs universal screening for chlamydial infection in sexually active young women. *Arch Intern Med* 1992;152:1837–1844.

CHAPTER 91

# Urinary Tract Infection

*Lindsay E. Nicolle, MD*

## Goals of Therapy

- To ameliorate symptoms in acute infection
- To prevent recurrent infection
- To prevent pyelonephritis in pregnancy

## Investigations (Table 1)

*Note:* **Relapse** is recurrence of UTI with the same organism, due to persistence of the organism within the urinary tract, usually in the prostate or kidneys. **Reinfection** is recurrent UTI with a new organism; it generally follows ascension of microorganisms from the periurethral area into the bladder.

## Therapeutic Choices (Figure 1)

### Pharmacologic Choices (Tables 2 and 3)

#### *Co-trimoxazole and Trimethoprim*

These are the drugs of choice for most UTIs. Due to increased antimicrobial resistance, they are less useful for empiric therapy in individuals with complicated UTI. Co-trimoxazole may be used as 3-day therapy for acute uncomplicated UTI. Use of co-trimoxazole is limited by sulfa allergy (trimethoprim alone may be used in sulfa-allergic patients).

#### *Nitrofurantoin*

Nitrofurantoin, a urinary antiseptic, has been widely used to treat UTIs. It may not be as effective as co-trimoxazole for 3-day therapy in the treatment of acute uncomplicated UTI. It is not recommended for treatment of pyelonephritis and is contraindicated in renal failure. Pulmonary and hepatic toxicity may occur, usually with long-term use at full therapeutic doses. Nitrofurantoin macrocrystals may be better tolerated than the standard formulation.

#### *Penicillins*

Resistance of *E. coli* to **amoxicillin** limits its current use. It should be reserved for UTIs with streptococci or enterococci or in selected instances where other agents are not tolerated and the organism is known to be susceptible.

Empiric therapy of uncomplicated UTI with **amoxicillin** will be about 20% less effective than with co-trimoxazole and is not recommended. **Amoxicillin with clavulanic acid** is an effective

Figure 1: **Management of Recurrent Acute, Uncomplicated UTI**

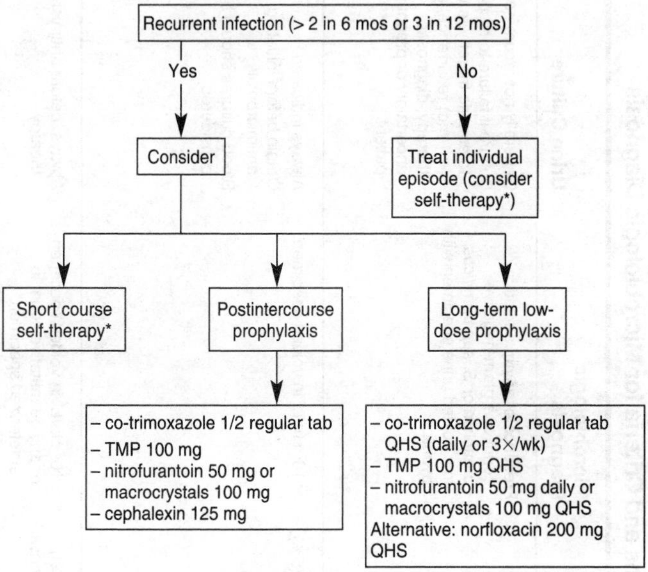
Recurrent infection (> 2 in 6 mos or 3 in 12 mos)
Yes
No
Consider
Treat individual episode (consider self-therapy*)
Short course self-therapy*
Postintercourse prophylaxis
Long-term low-dose prophylaxis
– co-trimoxazole 1/2 regular tab
– TMP 100 mg
– nitrofurantoin 50 mg or macrocrystals 100 mg
– cephalexin 125 mg
– co-trimoxazole 1/2 regular tab QHS (daily or 3×/wk)
– TMP 100 mg QHS
– nitrofurantoin 50 mg daily or macrocrystals 100 mg QHS
Alternative: norfloxacin 200 mg QHS

** 3-day course of treatment, self-administered on appearance of symptoms.*
*Abbreviations: TMP = trimethoprim.*

alternative for resistant organisms, but it is more expensive and is associated with substantial gastrointestinal side effects (10 to 25% incidence). **Pivmecillinam** does not share resistance with other penicillins, and community-acquired isolates show little resistance. The adverse effect spectrum is similar to other penicillins. It is effective as short-course or 7-day therapy for acute cystitis, and is safe for use in pregnancy. It is not indicated for treatment of pyelonephritis.

### *Quinolones*

Use of **nalidixic acid** is limited by development of resistance. The fluoroquinolones (**norfloxacin, ciprofloxacin**, **ofloxacin** and **levofloxacin**) are as effective as co-trimoxazole for treatment of acute uncomplicated UTI due to susceptible organisms but are generally second-line therapy due to cost. Fluoroquinolones are important for treating complicated UTI and for patients infected with resistant organisms. They are **contraindicated** in children and pregnant women because of potential adverse effects on developing cartilage.

### *Cephalosporins*

All the cephalosporins including **cephalexin, cefaclor, cefuroxime axetil** and **cefixime** are effective for the treatment

Table 1: **Clinical Syndromes of UTI, Most Frequent Infecting Organisms and Criteria for Microbiologic Diagnosis**

| Syndrome | Most Common Infecting Organisms* | Microbiologic Diagnosis | Urine Culture |
|---|---|---|---|
| **Acute Uncomplicated UTI (Cystitis)**<br>Occurs in females with normal genitourinary tracts.<br>These women have a genetic predisposition for recurrent UTI.<br>Behavioral factors promoting infection include sexual intercourse and use of spermicides or diaphragm.<br>Usual presenting symptoms include internal dysuria, frequency, suprapubic discomfort and urgency.<br>Recurrences are common but of variable frequency. | *E. coli* (80–90%), *S. saprophyticus* (5–10%), *K. pneumoniae*, *P. mirabilis*, group B *streptococcus*. | Presence of any quantitative count of a gram-negative organism or *S. saprophyticus* in a voided urine specimen with pyuria. | Generally not recommended.<br>Culture if failure to respond to empiric therapy, early (< 1 mo) recurrence following therapy, diagnostic uncertainty or pregnant patient. |
| **Acute Nonobstructive Pyelonephritis**<br>Occurs in women with recurrent uncomplicated UTI but at lower frequency than cystitis.<br>Classic presentation includes fever and flank pain with or without associated irritative urinary symptoms.<br>Patients who present with UTIs with only lower tract symptoms or asymptomatic bacteriuria occasionally have associated "occult" renal infection.<br>Bacteremic infection occurs most frequently in diabetic women or women > 65 yrs. | *E. coli* (80–90%), *P. mirabilis* (5%), *K. pneumoniae* (5%), *S. saprophyticus*. | $\geq 10^7$ cfu/L† in voided specimen. | Always indicated.<br>Obtain before initiating antimicrobials.<br>Blood cultures should be considered. |
| **Complicated UTI**<br>Occurs in individuals with an abnormal genitourinary tract due to structural or functional abnormalities or those with an indwelling catheter. | *E. coli* (50%), *P. mirabilis* (20%), *E. faecalis* (10%), *P. aeruginosa*, *P. stuartii*, *Citrobacter* spp., | $\geq 10^8$ cfu/L† in voided specimen or any quantitative count in catheterized specimen. | Always, before antimicrobial therapy. |

| | | | |
|---|---|---|---|
| Patients may present with cystitis (lower tract) symptoms or fever/pyelonephritis.<br>Management includes search for correctable anomalies; with persistent abnormalities, recurrent infection is common (50% by 6 wks post therapy). | *Enterobacter* spp., *Serratia* spp., group B streptococci, coagulase-negative staphylococci. | | |
| **Bacterial Prostatitis**‡<br>**Acute:** infection usually due to *E. coli* or *S. aureus*. Symptoms include sudden chills, fever, perineal and low back pain, irritative and obstructive voiding. The prostate is tender, swollen, indurated and warm. Prostatic massage is not recommended because it may cause bacteremia.<br>**Chronic:** common, ↑ with age. Symptoms are variable, not diagnostic and may include mild to moderate urgency, frequency, nocturia, dysuria and discomfort in the perineal, suprapubic or genital area. Prostate examination is usually normal. It frequently presents as relapsing UTI in older men. | Enterobacteriaceae, *P. aeruginosa, S. aureus*, others. | Relapsing UTI > $10^8$ cfu/L.†<br>Triple glass test with potential pathogens isolated and pyuria in prostatic massage specimen or postprostatic massage urine specimen. | Voided urine specimen before empiric therapy.<br>Triple glass test. |
| **Asymptomatic Bacteriuria**<br>Microbiologic evidence for UTI in the absence of associated symptoms.<br>Asymptomatic bacteriuria is more common in women, ↑ with age.<br>In pregnancy, screening should be performed for asymptomatic bacteriuria at 12–16 wks. | *E. coli* (60-70%), *P. mirabilis* (coagulase-negative) (10%), group B *streptococcus*, coagulase-negative staphylococci, others. | ≥$10^8$ cfu/L† in 2 consecutive specimens. | Screening of asymptomatic populations recommended only in pregnancy or before invasive genitourinary procedures. |

* *E. coli is the single most frequent organism causing UTI. Individuals with complicated UTI or recent exposure to antimicrobials are more likely to have organisms other than E. coli or organisms of increased antimicrobial resistance.*

† *$10^7$ cfu/L = $10^4$ cfu/mL; $10^8$ cfu/L = $10^5$ cfu/mL.*

‡ *Nonbacterial prostatitis is an inflammatory condition of unknown cause, diagnosed on the basis of prostatic fluid leukocytosis with negative culture. If there is no evidence for inflammation or infection of the prostate (triple glass test) the diagnosis is prostatodynia, which should not be treated with antibiotics.*

of UTI. They are not as well studied as co-trimoxazole or quinolones and may be somewhat less effective, especially with short courses of therapy. Their use is limited by cost. Cephalosporins may be associated with a greater likelihood of vulvovaginal candidiasis.

### Aminoglycosides

Aminoglycosides **(gentamicin, tobramycin, netilmicin and amikacin)** remain the therapy of choice for the treatment of acute pyelonephritis requiring parenteral therapy. Most gram-negative organisms, especially in patients with community-acquired infections, will remain susceptible to these agents. Initial parenteral therapy is switched to oral therapy as soon as symptoms and signs have settled (72 to 96 hours); with such short duration of

Table 2: **Antimicrobials for the Treatment of UTI**

| Antimicrobial | Dose (Adult)❥ | Cost* |
|---|---|---|
| **Oral Agents** | | |
| Amoxicillin/clavulanic acid | 500 mg TID | $$$ |
| Amoxicillin | 500 mg TID | $ |
| Cefaclor | 250 mg TID | $$ |
| Cefixime | 400 mg/d | $$$ |
| Cefuroxime axetil | 250 mg BID | $$ |
| Cephalexin | 500 mg QID | $$ |
| Ciprofloxacin | 250–500 mg BID | $$$ |
| Co-trimoxazole† | 160/800 mg BID | $ |
| Levofloxacin | 250 mg/d | $$$ |
| Nitrofurantoin | 50 mg QID | $$ |
| Nitrofurantoin macrocrystals† | 100 mg QID | $$$ |
| Norfloxacin | 400 mg BID | $$ |
| Ofloxacin | 400 mg BID | $$$ |
| Pivmecillinam | 400 mg BID × 3 d or 200 mg BID × 7 d | $$–$$$ |
| Trimethoprim† | 100 mg BID | $ |
| **Parenteral Agents** | | |
| Gentamicin‡ | 3–5 mg/kg/d | $$ |
| Tobramycin | 3–5 mg/kg/d | $$ |
| Netilmicin | 3–5 mg/kg/d | $ |
| Amikacin | 15 mg/kg/d | $$$$ |
| Ampicillin | 1 g Q6H | $$ |
| Piperacillin | 3 g Q6H | $$$$ |
| Cefazolin | 1 g Q8H | $ |
| Cefuroxime | 750 mg Q8H | $$$ |
| Cefotaxime | 1 g Q8H | $$$ |
| Ceftazidime | 1 g Q8H | $$$$ |
| Ceftriaxone | 1 g Q24H | $$$ |
| Ticarcillin/clavulanate | 1 g Q8H | $$$$$ |

† *First-line agents for acute uncomplicated UTI.*
‡ *First-line parenteral therapy for acute pyelonephritis.*
❥ *Dosage adjustment may be required in renal failure – see Appendix I.*
* *Cost per day – includes drug cost only.*
*Legend:* ***Oral Agents:*** *$ < $1   $$ $1–3   $$$ $3–5   $$$$ > $5*
***Parenteral Agents:*** *$ < $10   $$ $10–25   $$$ $25–50   $$$$ $50–75   $$$$$ > $75*

Table 3: **Duration of Therapy**

| Condition | Duration | Comments |
|---|---|---|
| Acute uncomplicated UTI | 3 d | Generally sufficient unless amoxicillin or nitrofurantoin is used. |
| Use of nitrofurantoin or amoxicillin | 7 d | |
| Therapy in postmenopausal women | 7 d | Longer duration preferred in these populations. |
| Recurrent infection < 1 month | 7 d | |
| Pyelonephritis | 14 d | |
| Complicated UTI | 10–14 d | |
| Prostatitis | 6 wks | Initial therapy; longer courses may be necessary following recurrence.* |

* *Treatment is frequently unsuccessful; long-term suppressive therapy may be needed to prevent recurrences.*

therapy, ototoxicity and nephrotoxicity are unlikely. The aminoglycosides are usually interchangeable for the treatment of UTI; antimicrobial susceptibility and cost determine selection of an individual agent.

## Therapeutic Tips

- Where possible, selection of antimicrobial therapy should be based on urine culture results.
- Antimicrobial susceptibility in populations is dynamic.
- Selection of empiric therapy in symptomatic patients should be based upon anticipated local antimicrobial susceptibilities and an individual patient's recent antimicrobial exposure and tolerance.
- Parenteral therapy should be used for patients who are septic, unable to tolerate oral medications, pregnant with pyelonephritis, or with resistant organisms requiring parenteral therapy.
- Prophylaxis should be considered for women with frequent recurrent uncomplicated UTI.

### *Suggested Reading List*


Nickel JC. Prostatitis. In: Mulholland SG, ed. Antibiotic therapy in urology. Philadelphia: Lippincott-Raven, 1996.

Nicolle LE, Ronald AR. Recurrent urinary tract infection in adult women: diagnosis and treatment. *Infect Dis Clin North Am* 1987;1:793–806.

Nicolle LE. A practical guide to the management of complicated urinary tract infection. *Drugs* 1997;53:583–592.

Stamm WE, Hooton TM. Management of urinary tract infections in adults. *N Engl J Med* 1993;329:1329–1334.

CHAPTER 92

# Malaria Prophylaxis

*W.L. Wobeser, MD, FRCPC and*
*J.S. Keystone, MD, FRCPC*

## Goals of Therapy

- To assess risk of acquisition of malaria
- To provide safe and effective chemoprophylaxis

## Considerations

- Malaria results in 5 million deaths worldwide each year.
- Determinants of acquisition risk include malaria endemicity, season, altitude, degree of rural travel and preventive measures for mosquito bites.
- Additional considerations in choosing prophylaxis include age, pregnancy, allergies and concurrent medications and illnesses.
- The risk of malaria for travelers is *greatest* in sub-Saharan Africa, Papua New Guinea and the Solomon Islands; *intermediate* on the Indian subcontinent and Haiti; and *low* in Southeast Asia and Latin America. There is regional variation of risk within these areas.
- All travelers to an endemic area require prophylaxis.
- When counseling a patient about malaria chemoprophylaxis, check an up-to-date source about the location and extent of drug-resistant *Plasmodium* species. Detailed recommendations for malaria prevention can be obtained from the Centers for Disease Control (CDC) at www.cdc.gov/travel. Health Canada provides travel health information at www.hc-sc.gc.ca/hpb/lcdc/osh/prof_e.html.

## Therapeutic Choices (Figure 1)

### Nonpharmacologic Choices

Malaria transmission by the anopheline mosquito mainly occurs between dusk and dawn; the following measures optimize protection during this time:

- **Insect repellents** containing N,N-diethyl-m-toluamide (DEET) should be used before outdoor activity during the main hours of malarial transmission (evening and nighttime). DEET has been associated (rarely) with neurologic side effects in children exposed to high concentrations (> 35%)

Figure 1: **Malaria Prophylaxis**

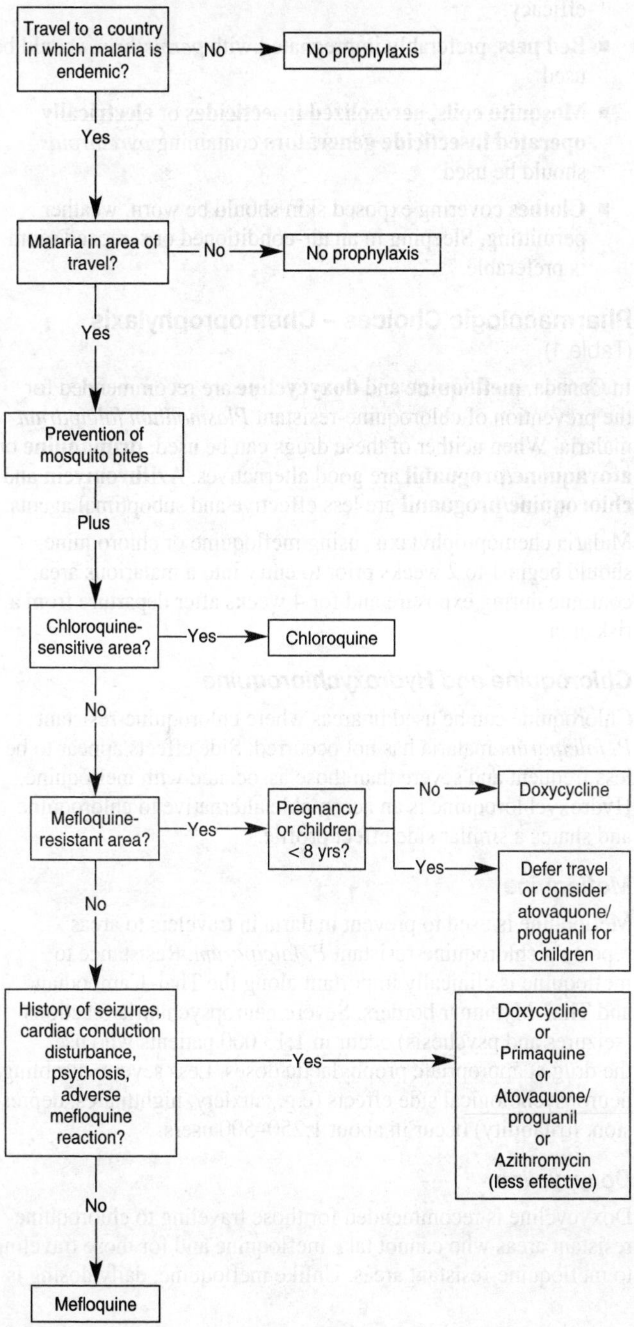
Travel to a country in which malaria is endemic?
No
No prophylaxis
Yes
Malaria in area of travel?
No
No prophylaxis
Yes
Prevention of mosquito bites
Plus
Chloroquine-sensitive area?
Yes
Chloroquine
No
Mefloquine-resistant area?
Yes
Pregnancy or children < 8 yrs?
No
Doxycycline
Yes
Defer travel or consider atovaquone/ proguanil for children
No
History of seizures, cardiac conduction disturbance, psychosis, adverse mefloquine reaction?
Yes
Doxycycline or Primaquine or Atovaquone/ proguanil or Azithromycin (less effective)
No
Mefloquine

and prolonged use. Ultrathon[1] (31.5% DEET) is formulated to reduce percutaneous absorption, thereby prolonging efficacy.

- **Bed nets**, preferably impregnated with *permethrin*, should be used.
- **Mosquito coils, aerosolized insecticides** or **electrically operated insecticide generators** containing *pyrethroids* should be used.
- **Clothes** covering exposed skin should be worn, weather permitting. Sleeping in an air-conditioned or screened room is preferable.

## Pharmacologic Choices – Chemoprophylaxis
(Table 1)

In Canada, **mefloquine** and **doxycycline** are recommended for the prevention of chloroquine-resistant *Plasmodium falciparum* malaria. When neither of these drugs can be used, **primaquine** or **atovaquone/proguanil** are good alternatives. **Azithromycin** and **chloroquine/proguanil** are less effective and suboptimal agents.

Malaria chemoprophylaxis, using mefloquine or chloroquine, should begin 1 to 2 weeks prior to entry into a malarious area, continue during exposure and for 4 weeks after departure from a risk area.

### *Chloroquine and Hydroxychloroquine*

Chloroquine can be used in areas where chloroquine-resistant *P. falciparum* malaria has not occurred. Side effects appear to be less frequent and severe than those associated with mefloquine. Hydroxychloroquine is an acceptable alternative to chloroquine and shares a similar side effect profile.

### *Mefloquine*

Mefloquine is used to prevent malaria in travelers to areas reporting chloroquine-resistant *P. falciparum*. Resistance to mefloquine is clinically important along the Thai–Cambodian and Thai–Myanmar borders. Severe neuropsychiatric reactions (seizures and psychosis) occur in 1:13 000 patients who use the drug at appropriate prophylactic doses. Less severe, disabling, neuropsychological side effects (e.g., anxiety, nightmares, depression, irritability) occur in about 1:250–500 users.

### *Doxycycline*

Doxycycline is recommended for those traveling to chloroquine-resistant areas who cannot take mefloquine and for those traveling to mefloquine-resistant areas. Unlike mefloquine, daily dosing is

---

[1] *Distributed by 3M (1-800-872-8633) and SCS Limited (1-800-749-8425).*

Table 1: **Drugs Used for Malaria Chemoprophylaxis***

| Drug | Adult Dose | Pediatric Dose | Adverse Effects | Cost† |
|---|---|---|---|---|
| *chloroquine phosphate* Aralen, generics | 500 mg (300 mg base) once/wk | < 1 yr: 37.5 mg base<br>1–3 yr: 75 mg base<br>4–6 yr: 100 mg base<br>7–10 yr: 150 mg base<br>11–16 yr: 225 mg base<br>once/wk | For both:<br>Freq: Pruritus, vomiting, headache<br>Occas: Hair depigmentation, skin eruptions, retinopathy (> 100 g base), myopathy, reversible corneal opacity, partial alopecia, blood dyscrasias<br>Rare: nail and mucous membrane discoloration, nerve deafness, photophobia | $ |
| *hydroxychloroquine* Plaquenil | 400 mg (310 mg base) once/wk | | | $ |
| *mefloquine* Lariam | 250 mg once/wk | 15–19 kg: 62.5 mg/wk;<br>20–30 kg: 125 mg/wk;<br>31–45 kg: 187.5 mg/wk;<br>> 45 kg: adult dose | Freq: dizziness, nausea, vomiting, diarrhea, headaches, sinus bradycardia, nightmares, insomnia, mood alteration, anxiety, irritability.<br>Occas: hair loss, skin rash<br>Rare: seizures, psychosis | $$ |
| *doxycycline* Vibra-Tabs, generics | 100 mg once/d | > 8 yrs: 2 mg/kg/d<br>(max.: 100 mg/d) | Freq: GI upset, staining of teeth in children and fetuses<br>Occas: photosensitivity, azotemia in renal disease, enterocolitis<br>Rare: allergic reactions, blood dyscrasias<br>Contraindicated in pregnancy and children < 8 yrs | $$ |
| *atovaquone 250 mg/ proguanil 100 mg* Malarone | 1 tablet daily | 10–20 kg: 1/4 tab<br>21–30 kg: 1/2 tab<br>31–40 kg: 3/4 tab<br>> 40 kg: 1 tab | Occas: GI upset, headache, cough | $$$$$ |

*(cont'd)*

Table 1: **Drugs Used for Malaria Chemoprophylaxis*** *(cont'd)*

| Drug | Adult Dose | Pediatric Dose | Adverse Effects | Cost† |
|---|---|---|---|---|
| *azithromycin*<br>Zithromax | 250 mg once daily | | Occas: abdominal pain, diarrhea, nausea, vomiting | $$$$$ |
| *proguanil (chloroguanide hydrochloride)*<br>Paludrine | 100 mg once daily<br>200 mg in chloroquine-resistant areas | < 2 yr: 25 mg<br>3–6 yr: 50–75 mg<br>7–10 yr: 100 mg once daily (double dose in chloroquine-resistant areas) | Freq: mouth ulcers<br>Occas: anorexia, vomiting, diarrhea<br>Rare: hematuria | $$$ |
| *primaquine phosphate* | Post-exposure:<br>26.3 mg (15 mg base) once/d × 14 d<br>Prophylaxis:<br>52.6 mg (30 mg base) once/d | Post-exposure:<br>0.3 mg/kg/day × 14 d<br>Prophylaxis:<br>0.5 mg/kg/day | Freq: hemolysis with G6PD deficiency<br>Occas: GI upset (take with food) | $ |
| **Self-treatment Regimens** | | | | $ |
| *pyrimethamine 25 mg/ sulfadoxine 500 mg*<br>Fansidar | 3 tabs as a single dose | 2–11 mos: 1/2 tab<br>1–3 yr: 1/2 tab<br>4–8 yr: 1 tab<br>9–14 yr: 2 tabs<br>> 14 yr: 3 tabs | Occas: headache, nausea, vomiting, folate deficiency<br>Rare: Stevens-Johnson syndrome, erythema multiforme, toxic epidermal necrolysis<br>Contraindicated in persons allergic to sulfonamides | |
| *atovaquone 250 mg/ proguanil 100 mg*<br>Malarone | 4 tabs once daily × 3 d | 10–20 kg: 1 tab<br>21–30 kg: 2 tabs<br>31–40 kg: 3 tabs<br>> 40 kg: adult dose | Occas: GI upset, pruritus, cough | $$ |

* *Begin drugs 1 wk before (except doxycycline, which is started 1 to 2 d before) and continue until 4 wks after leaving malarious area.*

† *Cost of 4-wk supply (except primaquine: 2 wks only and Fansidar and Malarone self-treatment regimens: 3 tabs only) – includes drug cost only.*

required. Users are advised to avoid prolonged sun exposure and to use a sunscreen that absorbs UVA radiation (Chapter 61). Doxycycline chemoprophylaxis should begin 1 to 2 days before entry into the area and continue for 4 weeks after departure.

### *Proguanil (Chloroguanide Hydrochloride)*

Proguanil (administered daily) is used as an adjunct to chloroquine for travelers to chloroquine-resistant areas and for those for whom mefloquine is contraindicated (e.g., seizures, psychosis). However, the chloroquine/proguanil combination is considerably less effective than mefloquine and other antimalarials recommended for chloroquine-resistant malaria.

### *Primaquine*

Primaquine is used for terminal prophylaxis ("radical cure") in long-term travelers returning from areas with *P. vivax* and *P. ovale*, both of which have dormant liver forms (hypnozoites). Hypnozoites are not affected by chloroquine or mefloquine. Primaquine may be used as a prophylactic agent against *P. vivax* and chloroquine-resistant *P. falciparum* malaria. It is a very effective prophylactic agent and should be started 1 to 2 days before entry and continue for only 1 week after departure. It should be taken with food.

Primaquine is a potent oxidizing agent which can induce severe hemolytic anemia in those with G6PD deficiency. In risk groups for this enzyme deficiency (blacks, Mediterraneans, Asians and Southeast Asians), a G6PD level is mandatory before primaquine is used. The drug is also contraindicated in pregnancy.

### *Atovaquone/Proguanil (Malarone)*

Malarone, an effective new drug combination, is approved for the treatment of chloroquine-resistant falciparum malaria. Although not yet approved for prevention, several studies have shown the drug to be safe and effective for prophylaxis against chloroquine-resistant malaria. GI upset, headache and cough are uncommon adverse events. Malarone must be taken daily, starting 1 to 2 days before entry to a malarious area and may be discontinued 1 week after departure. Safety data are not available in infants; the drug is not recommended in pregnancy.

### *Azithromycin*

Azithromycin, a macrolide antibiotic, has been shown in 2 small studies to be effective in the prevention of chloroquine-resistant *P. falciparum* malaria. The drug is less effective than other drugs for the prevention of malaria and should be considered a third line agent. Azithromycin must be taken daily, beginning 1 to 2 days before exposure and 4 weeks after departure. Azithromycin is safe for use in pregnancy and children. Cost may be prohibitive.

### *Pyrimethamine/Sulfadoxine (Fansidar)*

Fansidar is carried for self-treatment of a febrile illness when medical care is not immediately available. A single dose is recommended only for areas (e.g., south Asia, west Africa) where the drug is still effective.

### Pregnancy and Infancy

Doxycycline is contraindicated for both groups. Mefloquine has been shown to be safe in the second half of pregnancy and is recommended for children of all ages. Limited data suggest that mefloquine is also safe in the first trimester. The risks of *P. falciparum* malaria in pregnancy far outweigh the potential risks of mefloquine. In sensitive areas, chloroquine with or without proguanil can be recommended for pregnant women and young children. In chloroquine-resistant areas, the addition of proguanil is a suboptimal combination. If a decision is made to travel to areas with intense chloroquine-resistant malaria transmission (e.g., sub-Saharan Africa), women and young children in particular should be strongly encouraged to utilize personal protection measures against mosquito bites.

## Therapeutic Tips

- Mefloquine is not favored as a prophylactic regimen by some physicians in the United Kingdom and developing countries. Travelers may be advised by physicians and travelers from these areas that they are on a dangerous drug. In general, such advice should be accepted politely and ignored.
- No currently available regimen of malaria chemoprophylaxis is ideal and completely effective. Drug-resistant malaria continues to spread.
- All travelers in whom fever develops within 1 year (particularly within 2 months) of return from a malaria-endemic area must be considered to have malaria, regardless of chemoprophylaxis. Thick and thin blood films should be requested from a health care provider to rule out malaria. If negative, they should be repeated twice over 48 hours.

## *Suggested Reading List*


Baird JK, Hoffman SL. Prevention of malaria in travelers. *Med Clin North Am* 1999;83:923–944.

Fradin MS. Mosquitoes and mosquito repellents: A clinician's guide. *Ann Intern Med* 1998;128:931–940.

Lobel HO, Kozarsky PE. Update on prevention of malaria for travelers. *JAMA* 1997;278:1767–1771.

Phillips-Howard PA, Wood D. The safety of antimalarial drugs in pregnancy. *Drug Saf* 1996;14:131–145.

Suh K, Keystone JS. Malaria prophylaxis in pregnancy and children. *Infect Dis Clin Pract* 1996;5:541–546.

CHAPTER 93

# Traveler's Diarrhea

*J. Dick MacLean, MD, FRCPC and*
*David Diemert, MD, FRCPC*

Abdominal pain and diarrhea develop in 20-50% of travelers to less developed countries; fever and bloody stools (dysentery) occur in 5–10% of cases. Traveler's diarrhea is defined as the passage of 3 to 4 unformed stools in a 24-hour period plus at least one symptom of enteric disease, such as abdominal pain or cramps, nausea, vomiting, fever or tenesmus. Most cases are caused by bacteria (predominantly enterotoxigenic *E. coli* as well as *Campylobacter*, *Salmonella* and *Shigella*).

## Goals of Therapy

- To reduce risk of infection in adult travelers
- To limit duration and severity of symptoms while traveling and during the immediate post-travel period

## Investigations

- Patients should be counseled in self-diagnosis: to distinguish mild symptoms (abdominal cramps, malaise, nausea and frequent bowel movements) from the high fever and dysentery of more severe infection requiring urgent antibiotic therapy
- Patients developing symptoms after returning home or presenting with persistent symptoms should be evaluated by:
  – physical examination (abdominal tenderness/guarding)
  – stool for occult blood
  – stool cultures should be especially considered in cases of dysentery, in food handlers and in health- and child-care workers

## Therapeutic Choices

### *Prevention*

### Nonpharmacologic Choices

- Drink only "safe" (boiled, bottled or carbonated) beverages.
- Boil (3 to 5 minutes) or sterilize water (5 drops of 2% tincture of iodine/litre of clear water or iodine water purification tablets or iodinizing resin filters).
- Avoid ice cubes unless made from safe water.

- Eat only fruit (including tomatoes) that has been washed in safe water and peeled. Do not eat watermelon.
- Avoid salads and raw vegetables.
- Eat only thoroughly and recently cooked meats or fish.
- Avoid leftovers and condiments in open bottles.
- Avoid food from street vendors.

### Pharmacologic Choices (Table 1)

#### *Bismuth Subsalicylate (BSS)*

Prophylactic BSS given QID has been shown to decrease attack rates of traveler's diarrhea from 40% to 14% when compared to placebo; BID dosing is less effective. BSS may have antibacterial activity as well as antisecretory and anti-inflammatory properties. Travelers taking anticoagulants or salicylates or who are allergic to salicylates should not take BSS. Side effects are minimal with short-term use (i.e., less than 3 weeks) at recommended doses. However, black stools produced by BSS create diagnostic problems (i.e., confusion with melena).

#### *Antibiotics*

Antibiotic prophylaxis should be given only for short courses (i.e., less than 3 weeks) and only to those at increased health risk (the chronically ill or immunocompromised patient), or for persons who undertake critical travel (e.g., diplomatic missions). Various antibiotics have been shown to significantly reduce the attack rate of traveler's diarrhea in endemic areas. **Co-trimoxazole** and **doxycycline** have in the past been effective in prophylaxis; however, significant bacterial resistance has emerged with both of these antibiotics and their use is no longer recommended. *Fluoroquinolones* **(norfloxacin or ciprofloxacin)** effectively reduce attack rates of traveler's diarrhea by up to 90% and are relatively safe, although bacterial resistance is now being encountered with these antibiotics as well. There is a risk, although low, of *Clostridium difficile*-associated diarrhea in travelers taking antibiotic prophylaxis.

## *Treatment* (Figure 1)

### Nonpharmacologic Choices

- Maintenance of fluid balance (hydration, electrolytes), especially in infants, pregnant women and the frail elderly is the cornerstone of all therapy.
- Travelers with mild diarrhea will benefit from a clear fluid diet of carbonated, non-caffeinated beverages, canned fruit juices, safe water, clear salty soups and salted crackers.

Figure 1: **Treatment of Traveler's Diarrhea**

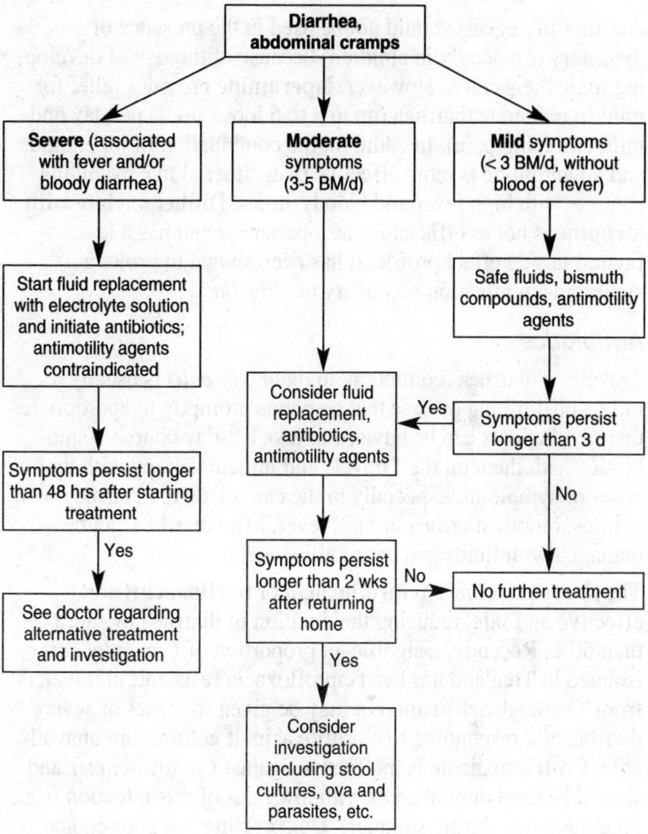
Diarrhea, abdominal cramps
Severe (associated with fever and/or bloody diarrhea)
Moderate symptoms (3-5 BM/d)
Mild symptoms (< 3 BM/d, without blood or fever)
Start fluid replacement with electrolyte solution and initiate antibiotics; antimotility agents contraindicated
Safe fluids, bismuth compounds, antimotility agents
Consider fluid replacement, antibiotics, antimotility agents
Yes
Symptoms persist longer than 3 d
No
Symptoms persist longer than 48 hrs after starting treatment
Yes
See doctor regarding alternative treatment and investigation
Symptoms persist longer than 2 wks after returning home
No
No further treatment
Yes
Consider investigation including stool cultures, ova and parasites, etc.

*Abbreviations: BM = bowel movement*

- Severe diarrhea, especially in infants and pregnant women, requires careful fluid replacement; commercial packets of *oral rehydration salts* (ORS)[1] (care should be taken to use them with safe water) and bottled solutions are available.[2]
- If ORS is unavailable, an emergency but less ideal substitute can be prepared by adding 1 level teaspoon of salt and 8 level teaspoons of sugar to 1 litre of safe water.

[1] *Gastrolyte is available.*

[2] *Enfalac Lytren, Pedialyte, Pediatric Electrolyte are available*

## Pharmacologic Choices (Table 1)

### *Antimotility Agents*

Antimotility agents should not be used in the presence of dysentery (especially in children) because of the risk of developing toxic megacolon. However, **loperamide** provides relief for mild to moderate diarrhea (up to 3 to 5 loose stools per day and mild cramping pain). In addition, the combination of loperamide and an antibiotic is more effective than either alone, excluding patients with high fever and bloody stools. **Diphenoxylate with atropine** is not as efficacious as loperamide and has a less favorable side effect profile. It has been shown to prolong symptoms in infection secondary to *Shigella*.

### *Antibiotics*

Traveler's diarrhea (commonly toxigenic *E. coli*) is usually a mild, self-limiting disease that responds promptly to appropriate therapy. Patients can be advised to take a 3-day course of antibiotics with them on their travels and initiate therapy with the onset of symptoms, especially in the case of severe diarrhea with cramps, bloody diarrhea or high fever. Mild diarrhea can be managed with fluids and antimotility agents.

The *fluoroquinolones* (**ciprofloxacin** or **norfloxacin**) are effective and safe, reducing the duration of diarrhea by more than 50%. Recently, a significant proportion of *Campylobacter* isolated in Thailand has been ciprofloxacin resistant; in travelers from Thailand, **azithromycin** may be given for cases of severe diarrhea not responding to ciprofloxacin, if cultures are unavailable. **Co-trimoxazole** is ineffective against *Campylobacter* and should be used only in areas with low rates of this infection (e.g., inland Mexico during summer). **Doxycycline** is a poor choice because several resistant enteric pathogens have emerged. **Metronidazole** may be useful when diarrhea persists (longer than 14 days) and is associated with weight loss, i.e., to presumptively treat *Giardia lamblia*.

## Therapeutic Tips

- Mild traveler's diarrhea usually resolves within 24 hours with antimotility agents and fluids.
- Discourage the use of over-the-counter agents purchased abroad as they are ineffective for both prophylaxis and treatment. Some foreign products contain chloramphenicol, which may induce aplastic anemia, or iodochlorhydroxyquin, which can cause neurologic damage and optic atrophy with prolonged use.

Table 1: **Drugs Used in Traveler's Diarrhea**

| Drug | Dosage: Treatment | Dosage: Prophylaxis* | Adverse Effects | Comments | Cost† |
|---|---|---|---|---|---|
| **Quinolones** | | | | | |
| *norfloxacin* Noroxin, generics | 400 mg BID × 1–3 d | 400 mg once/d | Infrequently GI disturbance, CNS effects, skin rash. | Not recommended for children. Norfloxacin is less well-absorbed than other quinolones. | $$ |
| *ciprofloxacin* Cipro | 500 mg BID × 1–3 d | 500 mg once/d | | | $$$ |
| *co-trimoxazole* Septra, Bactrim, generics | 160/800 mg BID × 6 doses or 320/1600 mg loading dose, then 160/800 mg × 5 doses | 160/800 mg once/d | GI disturbance, blood dyscrasias, skin reactions (rarely, Stevens-Johnson syndrome). | For regions where co-trimoxazole resistance is uncommon (central Mexico in summer); not first choice in other geographic areas. | $ |
| *metronidazole* Flagyl, generics | 250 mg TID × 7–10 d | | GI disturbance, metallic taste, CNS effects. | For symptoms suggestive of steatorrhea where *Giardia lamblia* infection is common. Avoid alcohol consumption (risk of disulfiram-like reaction). | $ (7d) |
| *azithromycin* Zithromax | 500 mg daily × 7 d | | GI disturbance infrequently. | Not recommended for prophylaxis. | $$$$$ |

*(cont'd)*

Table 1: **Drugs Used in Traveler's Diarrhea** *(cont'd)*

| Drug | Dosage: Treatment | Dosage: Prophylaxis* | Adverse Effects | Comments | Cost† |
|---|---|---|---|---|---|
| *bismuth subsalicylate* Pepto-Bismol, generics | 2 tabs (262 mg/tab) or 30 mL Q 30 min<br>Max.: 8 doses/d | 2 tabs (262 mg/tab) or 30 mL QID (with meals and QHS) | Darkening of tongue and stools, mild tinnitus. | Avoid in patients taking therapeutic doses of salicylates or those in whom salicylates are contraindicated. | $ |
| *loperamide* Imodium, generics | 4 mg STAT, then 2 mg after each loose stool<br>Max.: 16 mg/d | *Prophylactic anti-motility agents have no effect* | Abdominal cramping, rarely dizziness, dry mouth, skin rash. | Do not use if experiencing fever or bloody stools.<br>Do not use longer than 48 h. | $ |

* *Prophylactic treatment should be started on the first day in the area of risk and continued for 1 or 2 d after return home, to a maximum of 3 wks total.*

† *Cost of 3-day treatment unless noted otherwise – includes drug cost only.*
*Legend: $ < $5 $$ $5–10 $$$ $10–20 $$$$ $20–30 $$$$$ > $30*

- Symptoms persisting more than 2 weeks after the return home should be investigated thoroughly. Irritable bowel disease is common, but parasitic infection, antibiotic-associated colitis, disaccharidase deficiency and bowel carcinoma should be considered. Inflammatory bowel disease or celiac disease may be unmasked by an episode of traveler's diarrhea.

## *Suggested Reading List*

Ansdell VE, Ericsson CD. Prevention and empiric treatment of traveler's diarrhea. *Med Clin North Am* 1999;83:945–973.

Committee to Advise on Tropical Medicine and Travel. Statement on travellers' diarrhea. *Can Commun Dis Rep* 1994;20:149–155.

Caeiro JP, DuPont HL. Management of travellers' diarrhoea. *Drugs* 1998;55:73–81.

Ericsson CD. Travelers' diarrhea. *Inf Dis Clin North Am* 1998;12:285–303.

Juckett G. Prevention and treatment of traveler's diarrhea. *Am Fam Physician* 1999;60:119–124.

CHAPTER 94

# Herpesvirus Infections

*Fred Y. Aoki, MD*

The characteristics of some herpesvirus infections such as recurrent genital or orolabial herpes simplex virus (HSV) infection differ when caused by HSV type 1 or 2. However, knowledge of HSV type is not of practical value in guiding selection of drug therapy since both are similarly susceptible to available drugs. Therefore, drug choices can be based on the nature and severity of the disease.

In immunocompromised patients, HSV and varicella-zoster virus (VZV) infections may be more severe and resolve less rapidly than in immunocompetent hosts, but recommended drugs are not different in these two types of patients. The exception is that prolonged treatment of immunocompromised patients (most frequently HIV-infected individuals) with oral acyclovir can lead to drug resistance and therapeutic failure. Resistance is most commonly mediated by a mutation that causes cross-resistance between acyclovir, famciclovir, valacyclovir and ganciclovir. In such patients, foscarnet by injection is the preferred treatment and vidarabine is a less effective but better tolerated alternative.

## Herpes Simplex Virus

### Orolabial and Genital Infection

#### Goals of Therapy

- To ameliorate symptoms
- To prevent outbreaks

*Primary HSV gingivostomatitis* is primarily a disease of children. If the child can swallow, gingivostomatitis of mild to moderate severity can be effectively and safely treated with **acyclovir** oral suspension. Acyclovir 15 mg/kg (0.375 mL/kg) 5 times per day for 7 days[1] or 600 mg/m$^2$ QID for 10 days[2] has been shown to accelerate resolution of orolabial signs and symptoms, fever and reduce the duration of viral shedding. Tolerance was good. If the severity of disease precludes ingestion of medication, IV acyclovir in pediatric doses analogous to those which are efficacious and safe in adults with primary genital herpes (Table 1) can be inferred to be appropriate treatment although no data have been published in support of this recommendation.

---

[1] *BMJ 1997;314:1800–1803.*

[2] *Aoki FY, et al. Acyclovir suspension for the treatment of acute HSV gingivostomatitis in children: a placebo-controlled, double blind trial (Abs). Interscience Conference on Antimicrobial Agents and Chemotherapy. New Orleans: October 1993.*

*Recurrent orolabial herpes* in immunocompetent adults may be treated with oral **acyclovir** 400 mg 5 times per day for 5 days beginning within 1 hour of onset. The duration of pain is reduced by 0.9 days compared to placebo but no other disease parameter is altered. Topical acyclovir ointment is not effective. In immunocompromised hosts, oral and IV acyclovir are effective. **Penciclovir** 1% cream is the first treatment to clearly demonstrate an impact on the course of recurrent orolabial herpes. When it becomes available, patients should be given a prescription and keep the drug close at hand. Treatment should be initiated at the earliest symptom of a recurrence (within 1 hour) and applied every 2 hours while awake for 4 consecutive days.[3]

For individuals in whom *recurrence of labial herpes* is *induced by exposure to sunlight*, oral **acyclovir** 400 mg BID begun 12 hours prior to sun exposure along with frequent **sunscreen** use prevents attacks by 76% compared to placebo. Prophylaxis is continued for the duration of sun exposure. In a strategy analogous to that which is effective in individuals with frequently recurring genital herpes *(vide infra)*, daily oral acyclovir 400 mg BID for up to 4 months *prevents* recurrent cold sores.

*First episodes of genital herpes* in otherwise healthy individuals may range from severe to inapparent. Therapy with IV **acyclovir** (5 mg/kg every 8 hours for 5 to 10 days) is optimal for severe cases. Oral acyclovir 200 mg 5 times daily for 5 to 10 days is approved for this indication as well. Data suggest that, overall, IV treatment is approximately 25% better than PO, depending on the parameter (resolution of local symptoms 50%, systemic symptoms 0%, time to heal 33% and virus shedding 0%). **Famciclovir** 250 mg TID for 7 days and **valacyclovir** 500 to 1000 mg BID for 10 days have comparable efficacy and tolerance to oral acyclovir. The simplicity of the famciclovir and valacyclovir regimens is an advantage.

*Recurrent genital herpes* in immunocompetent and immunocompromised patients can be treated for 5 to 7 days with oral **acyclovir** 200 mg 5 times daily, **famciclovir** 125 mg BID or **valacyclovir** 500 mg BID. Available data do not demonstrate clinically important differences between these drugs. For individuals with frequently recurring disease (6 or more episodes per year), it is important to recommend suppressive therapy because this is much more effective than episodic therapy of individual outbreaks. *Suppression* should be started with **acyclovir** 200 mg TID. If the response is favorable, the dose may be reduced to BID and if unfavorable, increased to 200 mg 5 times daily or 400 mg BID. Suppression should be interrupted periodically to evaluate the need for continued treatment. One

---

[3] *JAMA 1997;227:1374–1379.*

Table 1: **Antivirals for Treatment of Herpesvirus Infections**

| Disease | Dose | Cost* |
|---|---|---|
| ***acyclovir*** – Zovirax, generics | | |
| HSV gingivostomatitis (children) | 15 mg/kg 5 × PO daily × 7 d or<br>600 mg/m² PO QID × 10 d<br>250 mg/m² Q8H IV × 5–10 d | $$<br>$$$<br>$420–840 |
| HSV recurrent orolabial | 400 mg 5 times daily × 5 d | $ |
| Prophylaxis of recurrent orolabial HSV | 400 mg BID 12 h prior to sun exposure × duration of exposure | $ |
| Genital herpes – first episode | 5 mg/kg Q8H IV × 5–10 d<br>200 mg PO 5 times daily × 5–10 d | $750–1500<br>$ |
| recurrent | 200 mg PO 5 times daily × 5–7 d | $ |
| suppression of recurrence | 200 mg BID up to 5 times daily × 3–6 mos | $$$$$ |
| Herpes simplex encephalitis | 10 mg/kg IV Q8H × 10–14 d | $2900–4100 |
| Chickenpox (children)<br>(adults) | 10–20 mg/kg PO QID × 5–7 d<br>800 mg PO 5 times daily × 5 d<br>or 10 mg/kg IV Q8H × 5 d | $<br>$$<br>$1500 |
| Acute herpes zoster | 800 mg PO 5 times daily × 7 d | $$$ |
| ***famciclovir*** – Famvir | | |
| Genital herpes – first episode | 250 mg PO TID × 7 d | $$ |
| recurrent | 125 mg PO BID × 5–7 d | $ |
| suppression of recurrence | 250 mg BID × 3–6 mos. | $$$$$ |
| Acute herpes zoster | 500 mg PO TID × 7 d | $$$ |
| ***valacyclovir*** – Valtrex | | |
| Genital herpes – first episode | 1000 mg PO BID × 10 d | $$$ |
| recurrent | 500 mg PO BID × 5–7 d | $$$ |
| suppression of recurrence | 500 or 1000 mg PO daily (if ≤ 9 or > 9 recurrences/yr) × 3–6 mos. | $$$$$ |
| Acute herpes zoster | 1000 mg PO TID × 7 d | $ |
| ***penciclovir*** *1% cream* – Denavir | | |
| Recurrent orolabial herpes | Apply Q2H while awake × 4 d | † |
| ***trifluridine*** *ophthalmic drops* – Viroptic | | |
| HSV keratoconjunctivitis | 1 drop Q2H while awake (max 9 drops) × 7 d, then 1 drop Q4H while awake (max 5 drops) × 7 d | $ |
| ***idoxuridine*** *ophthalmic drops* – Herplex, Herplex D | | |
| HSV keratoconjunctivitis | 1 drop Q1H while awake and Q2H while sleeping × 5–7 d after healing, or 21 d | $ |

* *Cost per course of treatment – includes drug cost only. Cost of IV acyclovir assumes no wastage.*

*$ <$50  $$ $50–100  $$$ $100–150  $$$$ $150–200  $$$$$ > $200*

† *Expected to be available from SmithKline Beecham Pharma.*

strategy is to stop every 3 to 6 months and to await two recurrences. Only if these two recurrences are close together (maximum of 2 months apart) would another 3- to 6-month course be appropriate. This strategy can be continued almost indefinitely since safety of acyclovir during multiple years of use has been demonstrated. In immunocompromised patients, suppressive therapy will likely lead to resistance and clinical failure. **Famciclovir** 250 mg BID and **valacyclovir** 500 mg daily (for ≤ 9 recurrences per year) or 1000 mg daily (for > 9 recurrences year) are also approved for suppressive therapy of recurrent genital herpes in healthy adults. It is expected that they will be as safe and well tolerated as acyclovir after prolonged use but this has not yet been demonstrated.

## *Encephalitis*

### Goals of Therapy

- To prevent death
- To prevent long-term neurologic sequelae

*Herpes simplex encephalitis* (HSE) is characterized by fever and confusion plus focal neurologic symptoms and signs (behavioral changes, speech disturbances and, less frequently, seizures). A brain abscess is the principal differential diagnostic possibility and antibiotic therapy should be included in the initial treatments prescribed, preferably with the help of an infectious diseases consultant. IV **acyclovir** should be initiated as soon as the diagnosis of HSE is considered. The dose is 10 mg/kg infused IV over not less than 60 minutes to prevent obstructive nephropathy caused by formation of acyclovir crystals in the renal tubular lumen. The dose should be repeated at 8-hour intervals in persons with normal renal function. Because acyclovir is eliminated exclusively through renal excretion by filtration and tubular secretion, dose intervals should be increased in those with renal dysfunction (Appendix I). Duration of treatment is usually 10 days. Rarely, relapse with virologically confirmed recrudescence occurs, necessitating prolonged therapy for 10 to 14 more days.

During therapy, diagnostic testing to demonstrate focal unilateral frontotemporal cerebritis (MRI, EEG, brain scan, CT) and HSV etiology (by detection of HSV in brain biopsy or, more commonly now, of HSV DNA in CSF) should be rapidly effected. Culture of CSF for HSV is uniformly negative. Acute phase serum will contain no HSV antibody in 2 out of 3 patients. A rise in titre will be demonstrated in a convalescent phase serum sample in these patients, indicating primary HSV infection.

Valacyclovir, penciclovir and famciclovir have not been evaluated as treatment for HSE.

### *Keratoconjunctivitis*

### Goals of Therapy

- To ameliorate symptoms
- To prevent corneal injury with vision impairment

HSV can cause keratitis and/or conjunctivitis. Because distinguishing HSV conjunctivitis from bacterial infection can be difficult, and because of the risk of visual impairment, consultation with an ophthalmologist is strongly advised if HSV infection is suspected. Topical **trifluridine** (Viroptic) applied every 2 hours during waking hours for 1 week and every 4 hours during waking hours for the second week is the treatment of choice. Topical **idoxuridine** (Herplex, Herplex-D) is the treatment of second choice. The role of oral acyclovir is controversial. Steroids may be recommended if concurrent uveitis is diagnosed.

## *Varicella-zoster Virus*

### *Chickenpox*

### Goals of Therapy

- To accelerate healing of skin lesions
- To prevent complications

In healthy children and adults, the benefit of **acyclovir** therapy exceeds placebo effects only if initiated within 24 hours of rash onset. For children, the dose should be adjusted for age: 5 to 7 years of age, 20 mg/kg; 8 to 12 years, 15 mg/kg; 13 to 16 years, 10 mg/kg. This dose should be repeated QID for 5 to 7 days. Therapy may lessen the impact on parents by enabling children to return to day care or school earlier. Adults experience complications such as varicella pneumonia more commonly than children, albeit rarely. Oral acyclovir 800 mg 5 times daily for 5 days or IV acyclovir 10 mg/kg every 8 hours for 5 days accelerates healing and is well tolerated. No study of sufficient sample size to rigorously test the hypothesis that acyclovir prevents complications has been described. No data have been published on the utility of the oral prodrug famciclovir or its active moiety, penciclovir, or valacyclovir, for chickenpox therapy.

In immunocompromised hosts, it is intuitively sound to treat chickenpox even if more than 24 hours have elapsed since the rash began. However, available data do not document efficacy in this situation.

### *Acute Herpes Zoster (Shingles)* (Figure 1)

### Goals of Therapy

- To accelerate healing of skin lesions

Figure 1: **Management of Acute Herpes Zoster**

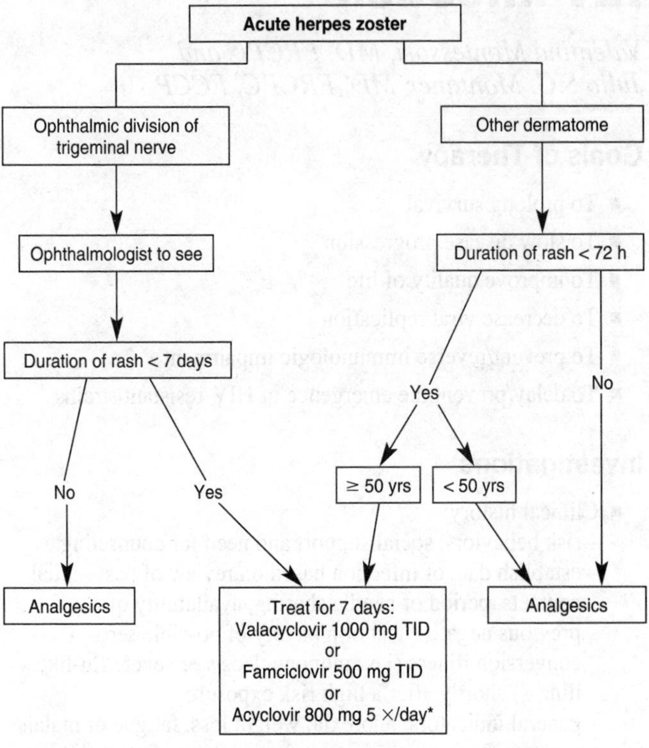
Acute herpes zoster
Ophthalmic division of trigeminal nerve
Other dermatome
Ophthalmologist to see
Duration of rash < 72 h
Duration of rash < 7 days
Yes
No
No
Yes
≥ 50 yrs
< 50 yrs
Analgesics
Treat for 7 days:
Valacyclovir 1000 mg TID
or
Famciclovir 500 mg TID
or
Acyclovir 800 mg 5 ×/day*
Analgesics

* *Only acyclovir is approved for treatment of immunocompromised patients.*

- To prevent post-herpetic neuralgia (Chapter 14)

Glucocorticoids do not reduce the incidence of post-herpetic neuralgia compared to antiherpes drugs prescribed alone.

## *Suggested Reading List*


Corey L. Herpes simplex virus. In: Mandell GL, Bennett JE, Dolin R, eds. *Principles and practice of infectious diseases.* 5th ed. New York: Churchill Livingstone, 2000.

Hyndiuk RA, Tabbara KF, eds. *Infections of the eye.* Boston: Little, Brown, 1986.

Whitley, RJ. Varicella-zoster virus. In: Mandell GL, Bennett JE, Dolin R, eds. *Principles and practice of infectious diseases.* 5th ed. New York: Churchill Livingstone, 2000.

CHAPTER 95

# HIV Infection

*Valentina Montessori, MD, FRCPC and*
*Julio S.G. Montaner, MD, FRCPC, FCCP*

## Goals of Therapy

- To prolong survival
- To slow disease progression
- To improve quality of life
- To decrease viral replication
- To prevent/reverse immunologic impairment
- To delay/prevent the emergence of HIV-resistant strains

## Investigations

- Clinical history:
  - risk behaviors, social support and need for counseling
  - establish date of infection based on review of past sexual contacts, period of needle sharing, availability of a previous negative test or a history of possible seroconversion illness (i.e., mononucleosis or severe flu-like illness) shortly after a high risk exposure
  - general indicators: anorexia, weight loss, fatigue or malaise
  - symptoms of opportunistic infections (e.g., fever, night sweats, cough, dyspnea, diarrhea, headache or skin rashes)
- Past medical history:
  - sexually transmitted diseases (gonorrhea, syphilis, chlamydia, herpes simplex, genital warts)
  - past history or exposure to tuberculosis, hepatitis B or C
  - conditions that may compromise future drug therapy (e.g., kidney stones, peripheral neuropathy, liver disease, pancreatitis, gout)
- Physical examination:
  - focus on signs of immune dysfunction and indications of opportunistic disease
  - specific attention should be directed towards examination of the mental status, skin, visual fields, ocular fundi, oral cavity, lymph nodes, abdomen, rectal and genital exam (including PAP smear in women)
- Laboratory investigations:
  - plasma HIV RNA (also known as plasma viral load or pVL) is the best prognostic marker for progression to AIDS and survival. Plasma viral load ranges vary

according to the test employed. There is no "safe" level. The most sensitive plasma viral load assay currently available has a quantitation limit of 20 HIV-1 RNA copies/mL
- CD4 lymphocyte count and percentage is useful in determining where a patient lies in the continuum of HIV disease and the need for specific intervention (Table 1). Knowledge of the CD4 count can also help to narrow the differential diagnosis in a symptomatic HIV-infected patient. In adults, a CD4 count of 430 to 1360 cells/$mm^3$ (0.43–1.36 Giga/Litre or G/L) is considered normal in most laboratories
- CBC, differential and platelet count
- liver (AST, ALT, alkaline phosphatase, bilirubin) and renal (BUN, creatinine) profiles
- hepatitis B, hepatitis C, syphilis, CMV and toxoplasmosis serologies
- cultures and smears for sexually transmitted diseases as indicated
- sputum cultures and smears for mycobacteria as indicated
- chest x-ray

## Therapeutic Choices

### Nonpharmacologic Choices (Table 1)

### Pharmacologic Choices (Figure 1, Table 2)

#### *Antiretroviral Therapy*

Long-term nonprogression can be expected if plasma viral load is maintained below the level of detection of currently available assays on a long-term basis. When selecting the antiretroviral regimen, use agents with at least additive antiviral effect while minimizing additive toxicities. Also consider issues of cross-resistance, compliance, convenience and cost. Nonadherence to therapy promotes the emergence of drug-resistant strains, representing the single most important challenge remaining. Counseling and support are critical to ensure ongoing compliance.

#### *Postexposure Prophylaxis*

The US Centers for Disease Control and Prevention have summarized recommendations for HIV postexposure prophylaxis (Table 3). When there is increased risk or if the exposure involves HIV-infected blood, prophylaxis is recommended. Other situations require individual decisions.

## Therapeutic Tips

- Develop a long-term treatment strategy ahead of time to deal with drug intolerance and treatment failure due to resistance.

Table 1: **Management of Patients with HIV Infection**

| **CD4 count** (cells/mm³) | |
|---|---|
| **At all times** | • Consider antiretroviral therapy (Figure 1)<br>• General counseling (safer sex, nutrition, etc.)<br>• History and physical examination every 3–6 months<br>• Plasma viral load and CD4 count at least every 3–4 months<br>• Herpes suppression if frequent recurrences (more than 4–6 episodes per year) (Chapter 94)<br>• Syphilis serology<br>• Pneumococcal vaccine<br>• TB skin test and isoniazid prophylaxis if indicated (consider repeating skin test yearly)<br>• Update diphtheria, tetanus and inactivated polio vaccines<br>• Hepatitis B vaccine if appropriate<br>• Consider annual influenza vaccinations |
| **< 500** | • Plasma viral load and CD4 count every 3–4 months<br>• Clinical evaluations and laboratory investigations at least bimonthly if symptomatic, diagnosed with AIDS, or on antiretroviral therapy |
| **< 200** | • Start PCP prophylaxis (Chapter 96) |
| **< 100** | • Start toxoplasmosis prophylaxis if seropositive and not on co-trimoxazole for PCP prophylaxis (Chapter 96) |
| **< 75** | • Consider MAC prophylaxis (Chapter 96) |
| **< 50** | • Screen by an ophthalmologist for early CMV retinitis; to be repeated at 3- to 6-month intervals or consider CMV prophylaxis (Chapter 96) |

- Compliance is the single most critical determinant of therapeutic failure: the simpler the regimen the better.
- Encourage initiation of therapy before immunodeficiency develops. Recognize, however, that antiretroviral therapy works at all stages of the disease and will be required on a long-term basis. Therefore, the best time to start therapy is when the patient is ready to commit to it.
- The current goal of therapy is to suppress plasma viral load below the level of quantitation of the assays (< 50 copies/mL).
- An alternative approach is to use partially suppressive therapy. This is often the only option available to patients who have failed previous courses of therapy. Even short-term decreases in plasma viral load in the order of 0.5 to 1.5 $\log_{10}$ have been associated with substantial (2- to 3-fold) reductions in disease progression and delayed mortality in clinical trials.

## Figure 1: **Approach to Antiretroviral Therapy**

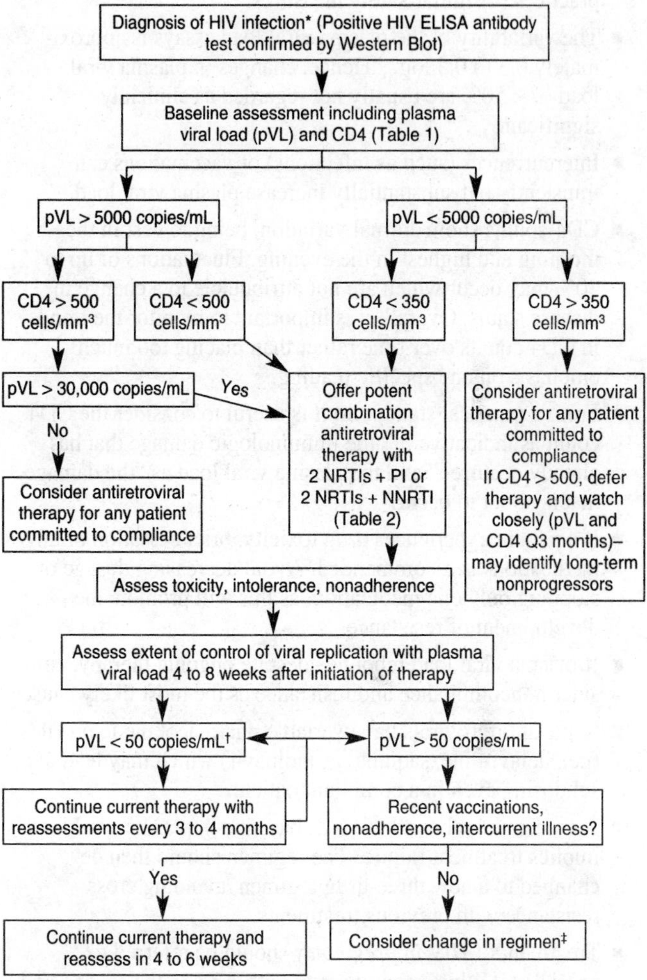
Diagnosis of HIV infection* (Positive HIV ELISA antibody test confirmed by Western Blot)
Baseline assessment including plasma viral load (pVL) and CD4 (Table 1)
pVL > 5000 copies/mL
pVL < 5000 copies/mL
CD4 > 500 cells/mm³
CD4 < 500 cells/mm³
CD4 < 350 cells/mm³
CD4 > 350 cells/mm³
pVL > 30,000 copies/mL
Yes
No
Offer potent combination antiretroviral therapy with 2 NRTIs + PI or 2 NRTIs + NNRTI (Table 2)
Consider antiretroviral therapy for any patient committed to compliance If CD4 > 500, defer therapy and watch closely (pVL and CD4 Q3 months)– may identify long-term nonprogressors
Consider antiretroviral therapy for any patient committed to compliance
Assess toxicity, intolerance, nonadherence
Assess extent of control of viral replication with plasma viral load 4 to 8 weeks after initiation of therapy
pVL < 50 copies/mL†
pVL > 50 copies/mL
Continue current therapy with reassessments every 3 to 4 months
Recent vaccinations, nonadherence, intercurrent illness?
Yes
No
Continue current therapy and reassess in 4 to 6 weeks
Consider change in regimen‡

* *If a patient presents with a history of possible exposure to HIV, with or without a history of a recent mononucleosis-like illness, consider HIV seroconversion. In this setting, the HIV antibody may be negative or "indeterminate", and a p24 antigen may be positive. These patients should be referred to specialists with experience in interpreting these results.*

† *The goal of therapy is to suppress viral replication to prevent the emergence of resistant strains and therefore, prolong the durability of the antiviral response. A goal of pVL < 50 copies/mL is recommended as this is the lower limit of quantitation common to all currently available clinical assays. As the newer, more sensitive assays become available, the goal may be revised.*

‡ *Given the currently available therapeutic alternatives, it is reasonable to delay change in therapy until there is definitive evidence of rebound of viral replication. Full suppression of viral replication represents a very attractive therapeutic strategy. However, if this goal cannot be reached, the interim aim should become partial suppression of viral replication (i.e., pVL below baseline and below 10 000 to 20 000 copies/mL, as long as the CD4 count remains stable and there is no clinical evidence of disease progression).*

*Abbreviations: NRTI = nucleoside reverse transcriptase inhibitors; PI = protease inhibitors; NNRTI = non-nucleoside reverse transcriptase inhibitors.*

- Nonquantifiable levels in plasma do not imply cure, eradication or a reason for complacency with safer sex practices or similar safety measures.
- The variability of the plasma viral load assays is approximately 0.3 to 0.5 $\log_{10}$. Hence, changes in plasma viral load of < 50% are usually not regarded as clinically significant.
- Intercurrences (such as infections) or vaccinations can transiently but substantially increase plasma viral load.
- CD4 counts show diurnal variation, being lowest in the morning and highest in the evening. Fluctuations of up to 30% may occur which are not attributable to a change in disease status. Overall, it is important to monitor the trends in CD4 counts over time rather than placing too much emphasis on one specific reading.
- From a practical standpoint it is useful to consider the CD4 count as indicative of "the immunologic damage that has already occurred" and the plasma viral load as "the damage that is about to occur."
- If a patient experiences drug toxicity, brief cessation of all medications is recommended. Avoid decreasing dosage or stopping only one medication, as this will promote the development of resistance.
- If plasma viral load rebounds despite ongoing therapy, consider noncompliance and resistance as the most likely causes.
- Some antiretrovirals have variable pharmacokinetic profiles (i.e., delavirdine, saquinavir, indinavir) which may lead to subdosing even in a compliant patient.
- A confirmed rebound towards baseline in plasma viral load implies treatment failure. The regimen should then be changed to a new three-drug regimen, avoiding cross resistance with previous treatments.
- Treatment of *HIV in pregnancy* should be referred to specialists. While monotherapy with AZT in the second and third trimesters has resulted in a decrease in vertical transmission of HIV, study into the safety and efficacy of combination antiretroviral therapy in pregnancy is ongoing. Although prevention of HIV in the infant and avoidance of teratogenicity are important considerations in the treatment of HIV-infected pregnant women, at the present time, optimal therapy of the mother should be the primary treatment goal.[1] Furthermore, breast-feeding by HIV-positive women is a recognized risk factor for HIV transmission to the infant and therefore is strongly discouraged.

---

[1] *JAMA 1997;277:1962–1969.*

Table 2: **Antiretroviral Medications**

| Drug | Dosage | Comments | Cost* |
|---|---|---|---|
| **Nucleoside Reverse Transcriptase Inhibitors (NRTI)** | | | |
| *zidovudine* Retrovir (AZT) | 200–300 mg BID | Most common adverse effects: nausea, headache, rash, anemia, leukopenia, elevated liver enzymes and elevated CPK.<br>Should not be combined with stavudine. | $–$$$ |
| *lamivudine* Heptovir, 3TC | 150 mg BID | Most common adverse effect is neutropenia. | $$ |
| *didanosine* (ddI) Videx | ≤ 50 kg: 100 mg BID<br>> 50 kg: 200 mg BID<br>Full daily dose can be given once a day | Most common adverse effects: GI intolerance, pancreatitis, gout, reversible peripheral neuropathy.<br>Should not be combined with zalcitabine. | $ |
| *zalcitabine* (ddC) Hivid | 0.75 mg TID | Most common adverse effects: reversible peripheral neuropathy, mouth ulcers, pancreatitis.<br>Should not be combined with stavudine or didanosine. | $$$ |
| *stavudine* (d4T) Zerit | 40–60 kg: 30 mg BID<br>over 60 kg: 40 mg BID | Reversible peripheral neuropathy.<br>Should not be combined with AZT. | $$ |
| *abacavir* (ABC) Ziagen | 300 mg BID | Most common adverse effect is a hypersensitivity reaction (5%): fever, rash, myalgias, arthralgias, malaise. Reaction may be fatal if medication continued or rechallenged.<br>Pharmacokinetics in renal failure unknown. | $$$ |

*(cont'd)*

Table 2: **Antiretroviral Medications** *(cont'd)*

| Drug | Dosage | Comments | Cost* |
|---|---|---|---|
| **Non-nucleoside Reverse Transcriptase Inhibitors (NNRTI)** | | NNRTIs should be used within a highly suppressive regimen. | |
| *nevirapine* (NVP) Viramune | 200 mg once daily for 2 weeks then increase to 200 mg BID<br>Full daily dose can be given once a day | Most common adverse effects: rash, elevated liver enzymes.<br>Should not be combined with DLV or EFV. | $$ |
| *delavirdine* (DLV) Rescriptor | 400 mg TID | Most common adverse effect is rash.<br>Should not be combined with NVP or EFV. | $$ |
| *efavirenz* (EFV) Sustiva | 600 mg once daily | Most common adverse effects:<br>CNS toxicity (hangover, drowsiness), rash.<br>Should not be combined with nevirapine or delavirdine. | $$$$ |
| **Protease Inhibitors (PI)** | | PIs have multiple drug interactions.<br>PIs are associated with various metabolic effects, i.e., diabetes mellitus, hyperlipidemias, lipodystrophy (limb wasting and accumulation of abnormal fat deposits). | |
| *saquinavir* (FTV) Fortovase | 1200 mg TID | Most common adverse effect is elevated liver enzymes. | $$$$ |

| | | | |
|---|---|---|---|
| *ritonavir* (RTV) Norvir | 300 mg BID × 3d<br>400 mg BID × 4d<br>500 mg BID × 5d, then<br>600 mg BID | Most common adverse effects: GI upset, diarrhea, circumoral paresthesia, elevated liver enzymes, hypertriglyceridemia.<br>Ritonavir acts as a pharmacokinetic enhancer of indinavir, allowing BID dosage; ritonavir 100 mg BID is combined with indinavir 800 mg BID. | $$$$ |
| *indinavir* (IDV) Crixivan | 800 mg TID | Most common adverse effects: elevated liver enzymes, nephrolithiasis.<br>See above for combination with ritonavir. | $$$$ |
| *nelfinavir* (NFV) Viracept | 750 mg TID | Most common adverse effect is GI upset, mostly diarrhea. | $$$$ |

** Cost of 30-day supply – includes drug cost only.*
*Legend: $ $100–200 $$ $200–300 $$$ $300–400 $$$$ $400–500*

Table 3: **Summary of CDC Recommendations for HIV Postexposure Prophylaxis**

| Type of exposure | Action* |
|---|---|
| Massive percutaneous exposure (e.g., deep injury with large-bore needle previously in source patient's vein or artery) or exposure to lesser amount of blood with high HIV titre | Recommend: zidovudine (200 mg tid) and lamivudine (150 mg bid) with or without indinavir† |
| Massive percutaneous exposure (as above) to blood with high HIV titre | Recommend: zidovudine (200 mg tid) and lamivudine (150 mg bid) and indinavir (800 mg tid)‡ |
| Percutaneous exposure to lesser amount of blood with low titre, to fluid containing visible blood or to other potentially infectious fluid (semen; vaginal, cerebrospinal, synovial, pleural, peritoneal, pericardial or amniotic (fluid) or tissue | Offer: zidovudine (200 mg tid) and lamivudine (150 mg bid) |
| Mucous membrane or high-risk skin exposure$^{\pi}$ to blood | Offer: zidovudine (200 mg tid) and lamivudine (150 mg bid) with or without indinavir† |
| Mucous membrane or high-risk skin exposure to fluid containing visible blood or other potentially infectious fluid or tissue | Offer: zidovudine (200 mg tid) with or without lamivudine |
| Percutaneous, mucous membrane or skin exposure to other body fluid (e.g., urine) | Do not offer prophylaxis |

*Note: CDC = US Centers for Disease Control and Prevention.*

* *Start drug therapy as soon as possible after exposure (preferably within 1–2 hours). Continue for 4 weeks.*

† *Possible toxic effects of other drug may outweigh benefit.*

‡ *If indinavir is unavailable, nelfinavir (750 mg tid) may be substituted.*

$^{\pi}$ *High-risk skin exposure = high HIV titre in source patient; prolonged contact; extensive area involved; skin integrity compromised.*

*Adapted with permission from Patrick DM. Can Med Assoc J 1997;156:233.*

## Suggested Reading List

Carpenter CCJ, Fischl MA, Gatell JM, Gazzard BG, Cooper DA, et al. Antiretroviral therapy in adults. Updated recommendations of the international AIDS Society-USA Panel. *JAMA* 2000;283:381–390.

Hogg RS, Yip B, Kully C, et al. Improved survival among HIV-infected patients after initiation of triple-drug antiretroviral regimens. *Can Med Assoc J* 1999;160:659–665.

Mellors JW, Munoz A, Giorgi JV, et al. Plasma viral load and CD4 lymphocytes as prognostic markers of HIV-1 infection. *Ann Intern Med* 1997;126:946–954.

Montaner JSG, Hogg RS, O'Shaughnessy MV. Emerging international consensus for use of antiretroviral therapy. *Lancet* 1997;349:1086.

Pantaleo G, Graziosi C, Demarest JM, et al. HIV infection is active and progressive in lymphoid tissue during the clinically latent stage of disease. *Nature* 1993;362:355–358.

Perelson AS, Neumann AU, Markowitz M, Leonard JM, Ho DD. HIV-1 dynamics in vivo: virion clearance rate, infected cell life-span, and viral generation time. *Science* 1996;271: 1582–1586.

Wei X, Ghosh SK, Taylor ME, et al. Viral dynamics in human immunodeficiency virus type 1 infection. *Nature* 1995;373:117.

CHAPTER 96

# Opportunistic Infections in HIV-positive Patients

*Daniel B. Gregson, MD, FRCPC*

In patients infected with the human immunodeficiency virus (HIV), the frequency of opportunistic infections increases as the CD4 count decreases. Most infections, other than *Mycobacterium tuberculosis* and *Pneumocystis carinii*, occur in patients with CD4 counts < 100 cells/mm$^3$ ($0.1 \times 10^9$/L). Management of common opportunistic infections is outlined; specialist support or other references should be sought for complicated problems.

## Goals of Therapy

- To treat active infections
- To prevent opportunistic infections using prophylactic medications
- To prevent infections with appropriate immunizations
- To restore immune function via inhibition of viral replication (Chapter 95)

## Investigations

The initial evaluation of an HIV-positive patient determines the level of immune dysfunction both from a clinical and a laboratory standpoint and identifies specific risks for opportunistic infections. Baseline tests include:

- HIV seropositivity (if documentation not available)
- CBC, electrolytes, creatinine, liver enzymes
- T-lymphocyte subsets (CD4)
- VDRL
- PPD skin test reactivity
- *Toxoplasma gondii* antibody
- Cytomegalovirus (CMV) antibody
- Hepatitis screening: HBsAb, HBsAg, HAV IgG, HCV IgG
- Chest x-ray
- HIV viral load determination
- Varicella antibody test in patients without a documented history of Varicella

## Therapeutic Choices

### Nonpharmacologic Choices

Patients with HIV infection and immunosuppression should be counselled that their risk of infections can be reduced by following good hygienic practices.

- Good handwashing after contact with contaminated substances (diapers, soil, uncooked meat and produce).
- Avoiding handling sick animals or cat litter.
- Avoiding raw or uncooked meat and eggs (e.g., Caesar salad).
- Drinking from treated water sources only.
- Avoiding cat scratches or cats licking open areas of skin.

### Pharmacologic Choices

Preventive interventions are outlined in Table 1.

## Clinical Syndromes

### Pneumonia

Although many opportunistic pathogens can cause pneumonia in HIV-infected patients, the majority of infections are caused by the agents commonly associated with community-acquired pneumonia or *P. carinii*. Figure 1 outlines an approach to the ambulatory patient.

### Dysphagia

Esophageal candidiasis is the most common cause of dysphagia or odynophagia. This may occur without visible oral candidiasis. Herpes simplex, cytomegalovirus and malignancies are other causes of dysphagia. An empiric trial of oral imidazoles is given initially. If the patient fails to respond after a week, esophagoscopy should be performed.

### CNS Infections

Infectious CNS complications of chronic immunosuppression occur primarily in patients with late-stage HIV infection (CD4 $\leq$ 100 cells/mm$^3$). *Cryptococcus neoformans* and *Toxoplasma gondii* cause the majority of such infections (Figure 2).

### Fever With No Focus of Infection

Patients often present with persistent fever without accompanying organ-specific symptoms. The HIV virus itself can produce fever, night sweats, malaise and weight loss. In patients in whom physical examination shows no focal source, *P. carinii* pneumonia should be considered (Figure 1). If the infection is not identified following routine work-up and blood cultures,

Table 1: **Preventive Interventions for HIV-positive Patients**

| Indications | Condition | Prophylactic Therapy |
|---|---|---|
| Independent of CD4 count | Routine immunizations | Update all vaccines |
| | Bacterial pneumonia | Pneumovax, repeat in 5 years<br>Annual influenza immunization. |
| | Hepatitis | Hepatitis A vaccine for patients with chronic hepatitis C<br>Hepatitis B vaccine for nonimmune individuals |
| | Varicella | Varicella vaccine for asymptomatic children with normal CD4 counts. Post-exposure prophylaxis with IVIG for nonimmune adults |
| | Cervical cancer | Cervical Pap smears Q6 mos × 2, then annually if normal. |
| | Frequent herpes simplex | Acyclovir 200 mg TID or 400 mg BID or Famciclovir 500 mg PO BID |
| | Sexually transmitted disease (STDs) | Patients on antiretroviral therapy can become infected with STDs including resistant HIV strains. Condom use for personal protection is still recommended. |
| Positive PPD (≥ 5mm), independent of CD4 count | *Mycobacterium tuberculosis* | Isoniazid 300 mg/d × 9–12 mos with pyridoxine 50 mg/d<br>or<br>rifampin* 600 mg once daily plus pyrazinamide 20 mg/kg/d × 2 mos |
| CD4 ≤ 200 cells/mm³ or thrush or CD4/CD8 ≤ 0.14 | *Pneumocystis carinii* pneumonia | Co-trimoxazole 160/800 mg/d or QM/W/F, or 80/400 mg/d, or dapsone 100 mg/d with folinic acid 25 mg/wk or atovaquone 1500 mg/d<br>Inhaled pentamidine 300 mg/mo via Respigard inhaler |
| CD4 < 100 cells/mm³ and positive *T. gondii* serology | *Toxoplasma gondii* encephalitis | Co-trimoxazole (PCP dose) or dapsone (PCP dose) + pyrimethamine 50 mg/wk + folinic acid 25 mg/wk<br>or atovaquone 1500 mg/d plus pyrimethamine 50 mg/wk |
| CD4 < 50 cells/mm³ | *Mycobacterium avium* complex | Azithromycin 1250 mg PO once/wk or<br>Clarithromycin 500 mg PO BID or<br>Rifabutin 300 mg PO daily (in order of cost-effectiveness) |
| | Cytomegalovirus | Treatment is not cost effective. Focus should be on restoration of immune system. |
| | Fungal infections | Fluconazole 100–200 mg/d or 400 mg/wk for persons with recurrent thrush or prior esophageal candidiasis |

* *Rifampin should not be administered concurrently with protease inhibitors or non-nucleoside reverse transcriptase inhibitors.*

*Abbreviations: PPD = purified protein derivative (of tuberculin); IVIG = intravenous immune globulin.*

Figure 1: **Management of Pulmonary Symptoms**

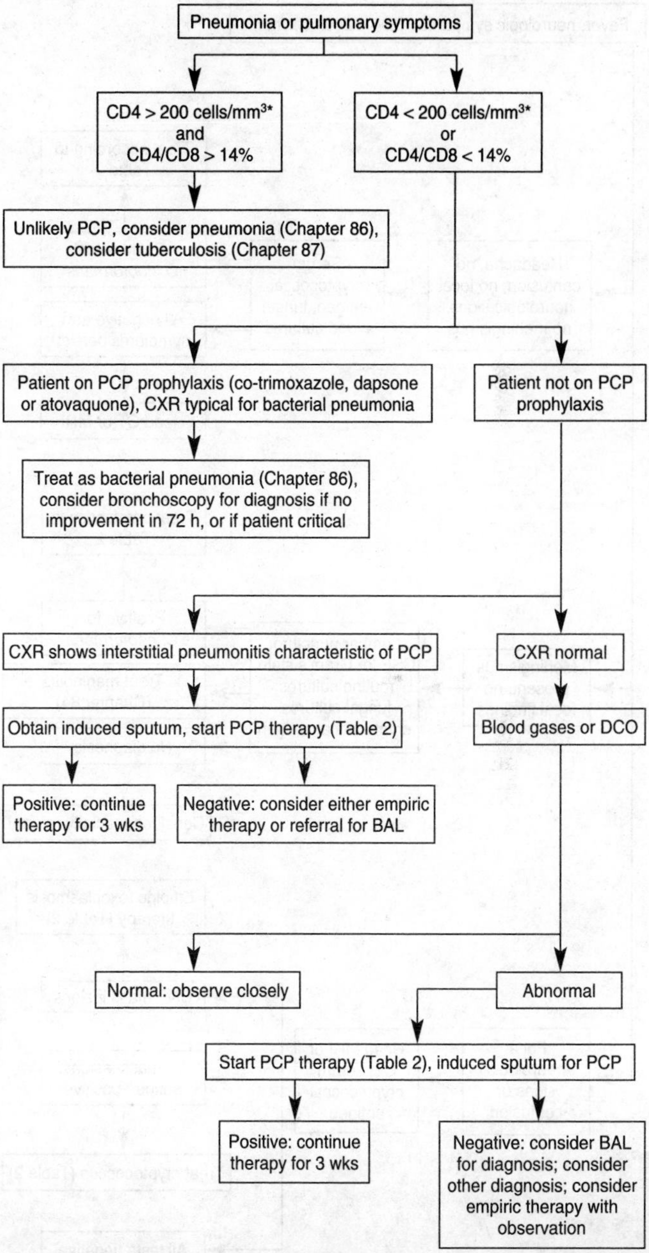
Pneumonia or pulmonary symptoms
CD4 > 200 cells/mm³* and CD4/CD8 > 14%
CD4 < 200 cells/mm³* or CD4/CD8 < 14%
Unlikely PCP, consider pneumonia (Chapter 86), consider tuberculosis (Chapter 87)
Patient on PCP prophylaxis (co-trimoxazole, dapsone or atovaquone), CXR typical for bacterial pneumonia
Patient not on PCP prophylaxis
Treat as bacterial pneumonia (Chapter 86), consider bronchoscopy for diagnosis if no improvement in 72 h, or if patient critical
CXR shows interstitial pneumonitis characteristic of PCP
CXR normal
Obtain induced sputum, start PCP therapy (Table 2)
Blood gases or DCO
Positive: continue therapy for 3 wks
Negative: consider either empiric therapy or referral for BAL
Normal: observe closely
Abnormal
Start PCP therapy (Table 2), induced sputum for PCP
Positive: continue therapy for 3 wks
Negative: consider BAL for diagnosis; consider other diagnosis; consider empiric therapy with observation

** These values apply to adults only. CD4 counts must be adjusted upwards in children.*

*Abbreviations: PCP = Pneumocystis carinii pneumonia; BAL = bronchoalveolar lavage; DCO = diffusing capacity of carbon monoxide; CXR = chest x-ray.*

## Figure 2: **Management of Fever and Neurologic Complaints**

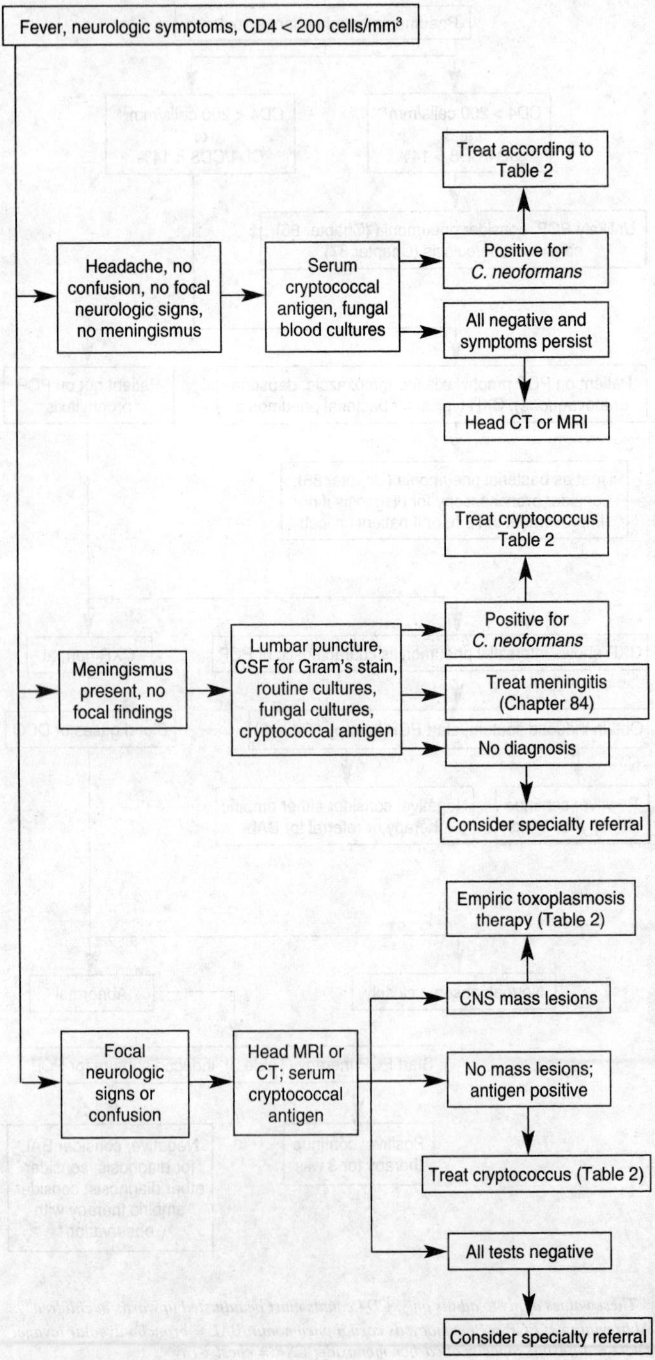
Fever, neurologic symptoms, CD4 < 200 cells/mm³
Headache, no confusion, no focal neurologic signs, no meningismus
Serum cryptococcal antigen, fungal blood cultures
Positive for C. neoformans
Treat according to Table 2
All negative and symptoms persist
Head CT or MRI
Meningismus present, no focal findings
Lumbar puncture, CSF for Gram's stain, routine cultures, fungal cultures, cryptococcal antigen
Positive for C. neoformans
Treat cryptococcus Table 2
Treat meningitis (Chapter 84)
No diagnosis
Consider specialty referral
Focal neurologic signs or confusion
Head MRI or CT; serum cryptococcal antigen
CNS mass lesions
Empiric toxoplasmosis therapy (Table 2)
No mass lesions; antigen positive
Treat cryptococcus (Table 2)
All tests negative
Consider specialty referral

**Table 2: Management of Selected HIV-associated Infections**

| **Infection** | **Treatment** (see also Table 3) |
|---|---|
| ***Candida Species***<br>Mucosal candidal infections: ↑ as CD4 count ↓; initially involve oral and vaginal mucosa; topical therapies used initially; systemic therapy may be required to maintain suppression.<br>Esophageal candidiasis: usually a later manifestation; can occur without oral or vaginal disease.<br>Severe discomfort or esophageal disease requires systemic therapy. | **Thrush, topical therapy:** nystatin suspension 500 000 U QID PO (swish and swallow) or vaginal tablet 100 000 U sucked QID, or clotrimazole vaginal tablet 100 mg sucked 5 ×/d or clotrimazole troche* 10 mg 5×/d.<br>**Vaginal:** miconazole or clotrimazole vaginal cream or suppository.<br>**Systemic oral therapy:** Fluconazole 100–200 mg/d × 2–3 wks is the first choice. Ketoconazole 200–400 mg/d or itraconazole 200 mg/d are alternatives.<br>**Esophageal disease:** start with higher doses then taper when symptoms improved; if failure to respond to fluconazole, amphotericin B 0.3–0.5 mg/kg/d IV × 2–3 wks then weekly when symptoms resolved. Alternatives for patients with less advanced HIV disease are itraconazole 200 mg daily or amphotericin B suspension* 300–500 mg QID. |
| ***Cryptococcus neoformans***<br>Major cause of meningitis in later stages of HIV infection (in 10% of AIDS patients).<br>Diagnosis includes positive serum or CSF cultures or detection of cryptococcal antigen in blood or CSF.<br>Ongoing prophylactic therapy required after treatment of acute infection. | **Induction therapy:** amphotericin B 0.7 mg/kg/d IV × 2–6 wks ± flucytosine 100–150 mg/kg/d Q6H PO × 2 wks, then completion of 12-wk course with fluconazole 400 mg/d PO or IV (fluconazole may be used initially for patients who are well and followed closely).<br>**Maintenance therapy:** fluconazole 200 mg/d PO or amphotericin B 1 mg/kg IV weekly. |
| ***Cytomegalovirus (CMV)***<br>Usually occurs with CD4 counts < 50 cells/mm$^3$.<br>Retinitis with visual disturbances most common manifestation.<br>Enteritis, colitis, pneumonitis, encephalitis, myelitis and neuritis can also occur.<br>Prognosis is poor without therapy.<br>Life-long maintenance therapy required after initial therapy for CMV retinitis. | **Induction therapy:** ganciclovir 5 mg/kg IV Q12H × 14–21 d or foscarnet* 60 mg/kg IV Q8H × 14–21 d (prehydration with saline recommended) or intravitreal ganciclovir implant* (lasts 30–40 wks with 15% risk of early retinal detachment, 50% develop disease in other eye and 25% other visceral disease within 6 mos) or cidofovir* 5 mg/kg IV Q weekly × 2 wks (prehydration and oral probenecid required).<br>**Maintenance therapy:** ganciclovir 5 mg/kg/d IV daily or 6 mg/kg IV 5–7 × per wk or 1 g PO Q8H or 400 µg intravitreal implant (as above) or foscarnet 90–120 mg/kg/d (infused over 2 hours) or cidofovir 5 mg/kg IV Q2 wks. |

*(cont'd)*

Table 2: **Management of Selected HIV-associated Infections** *(cont'd)*

| Infection | Treatment (see also Table 3) |
|---|---|
| ***Mycobacterium avium Complex (MAC)***<br>Occurs with CD4 counts < 100 cells/mm³.<br>Symptoms: fever, weight loss, fatigue, night sweats alone or with diarrhea, anemia, lymphadenopathy, hepatitis.<br>Diagnosis primarily by mycobacterial blood culture or biopsy and culture of involved tissue. | Multidrug regimens: usually include clarithromycin 500 mg BID PO or azithromycin 500 mg/d PO + ethambutol 15 mg/kg/d, ± 1–3 additional drugs (such as rifampin or rifabutin, ciprofloxacin, clofazimine and amikacin).<br>Initial therapy × 2–4 mos, followed by maintenance therapy. |
| ***Pneumocystis carinii***<br>Primary cause of pneumonia (PCP) in HIV-positive patients with CD4 < 200 cells/mm³.<br>All patients at risk of PCP should be receiving prophylaxis (Table 1).<br>Commonly presents as persistent fever with progressive shortness of breath and cough, often with normal chest x-ray.<br>Definitive diagnosis requires induced sputum, bronchoalveolar lavage or lung biopsy. | **Standard therapy:** co-trimoxazole 15–20 mg/kg/d (trimethoprim) IV or PO (divided Q6–8H) × 21 d, or pentamidine 4 mg/kg/d IV × 21 d, or dapsone 100 mg/d PO + trimethoprim 15–20 mg/kg/d PO × 21 d (better tolerated than co-trimoxazole; no IV form), or<br>Other: atovaquone; clindamycin + primaquine; trimetrexate + folinic acid<br>Prednisone (adjunctive) 40 mg BID PO × 5 d, 20 mg BID × 5 d, 20 mg/d to completion of treatment. Addition of prednisone in severe PCP ↓ morbidity and side effects of co-trimoxazole. |
| ***Toxoplasma gondii***<br>Up to 50% of HIV-positive patients with antibodies to this parasite will develop toxoplasma encephalitis as CD4 ↓ below 200 cells/mm³.<br>Most commonly presents as fever with focal neurologic signs; usually a CT scan with contrast or MRI reveals multiple intracranial-enhancing lesions.<br>Patients should be treated empirically; marked clinical response usually within 7 d; if no response, referral to a specialty centre should be considered.<br>Patients with perilesional edema also require dexamethasone.<br>Life-long prophylactic therapy required after acute therapy. | **Standard therapy:** pyrimethamine 100 mg Q12H × 2 doses, then 75 mg/d PO + folinic acid 10–20 mg/d PO + sulfadiazine 100–150 mg/kg Q6H (max. 6 g/d) × 4–8 wks or<br>**Alternatives:** pyrimethamine + folinic acid (doses as above) + clindamycin 600 mg PO or 600–1200 mg IV Q6H or azithromycin 1–1.5 g PO daily or clarithromycin 1 g PO Q12H or dapsone 100 mg daily or atovaquone 750 mg PO Q6H × 4–8 wks.<br>**Maintenance therapy:** pyrimethamine 50 mg/d PO + sulfadiazine 1 g Q12H PO + folinic acid 10 mg/d; or pyrimethamine 50 mg/d PO + clindamycin 300 mg Q6H PO + folinic acid 10 mg/d. |

do fungal and mycobacterial blood cultures and a serum cryptococcal antigen assay. If tests are still negative, consider specialty referral.

### *Diarrhea*

Many pathogens have been associated with diarrhea in HIV-infected patients. Patients with acute symptoms (< 28 days) should have routine stool cultures and blood cultures (× 2 if febrile). Consider *Clostridium difficile* if the patient has taken antibiotics recently. Anti-infectives should be administered as per etiology, including salmonellosis.

Patients with chronic diarrhea (> 28 days) or undiagnosed acute diarrhea should have routine stool cultures, ova and parasite examinations (× 3), modified acid-fast (MAF) stain examination of stool and stool examination for microsporidia. Treat as per etiology. If tests are negative and diarrhea is associated with fever, abdominal pain or blood, do mycobacterial blood cultures and refer the patient for endoscopy with biopsy. Patients with watery nonbloody chronic diarrhea may be treated with loperamide. An empiric trial of **metronidazole** may be warranted.

## Specific Infections

Management of selected infections is outlined in Table 2.

## Discontinuation of Prophylaxis

Prophylaxis can be discontinued for some infections when the immume system recovers following antiviral therapy (Table 4).

Table 4: **Criteria for Discontinuing Prophylaxis of Opportunistic Infections in HIV-positive Patients**

| Opportunistic Pathogen | Criteria for Discontinuing |
|---|---|
| *Pneumocystis carinii* | no prior PCP<br>viral load < 50 copies/mL for 3–6 months<br>CD4 > 200 cells/mm³ for 6 months |
| *Mycobacterium avium* | no prior MAC infection<br>viral load < 50 copies/mL for 3–6 months<br>CD4 > 100 cells/mm³ for 6 months |
| CMV retinitis | non-sight threatening lesion<br>adequate vision in contralateral eye<br>good ophthalmology follow-up<br>viral load < 50 copies/mL for 3–6 months<br>CD4 > 150 cells/mm³ for 6 months |

Table 3: **Drugs Used in HIV-associated Infections**

| Drug | Major or Dose-limiting Toxicities | Comments | Cost* |
|---|---|---|---|
| *amphotericin B* Fungizone | Nephrotoxicity, fever, chills, nausea during infusion, ↑ liver enzymes, bone marrow suppression. | ↑ hemotoxicity of AZT, ↑ nephrotoxicity with nephrotoxic drugs. Should be used in all patients with *Cryptococcus neoformans* infections requiring hospitalization. | $$$ |
| *atovaquone* Mepron | Generally well tolerated. | Should be taken with food (absorption ↑ with food, especially high fat). Less effective than co-trimoxazole for treatment of mild–moderate PCP. | $$ |
| *azithromycin* Zithromax | GI disturbances. | Should be taken on empty stomach. Interchangeable with clarithromycin for MAC therapy. | $ |
| *cidofovir* † Vistide | Nephrotoxicity, ocular hypotony, neutropenia, metabolic acidosis. | Prehydration and probenecid ↓ risk of nephrotoxicity. Avoid other nephrotoxic drugs, e.g., NSAIDs. | † |
| *clarithromycin* Biaxin | Generally well tolerated; diarrhea, vomiting, abdominal pain. | Terfenadine and astemizole should be avoided (↑ risk of arrhythmias). May ↑ carbamazepine and theophylline levels. | $ |
| *clofazimine* ‡ Lamprene | Skin discoloration, peripheral neuropathy. | | ‡ |
| *co-trimoxazole* Bactrim, Septra, generics | Rash, nausea, vomiting and fever (common), leukopenia, thrombocytopenia, hypersensitivity reactions, ↑ liver function tests. | Adverse reactions common, often requiring alternate therapy. ↑ hemotoxicity with AZT, pyrimethamine. ↑ warfarin effect. | PO: $ IV: $$$$–$$$$$ |
| *dapsone* Avlosulfon | Rash, nausea, hemolytic anemia, methemoglobinemia (more common in G6PD deficiency). | Better tolerated than co-trimoxazole in PCP; ↑ hemotoxicity with AZT, pyrimethamine, primaquine, trimethoprim; absorption ↓ by ddI. | $ |

| | | | |
|---|---|---|---|
| *fluconazole* <br>Diflucan, generics | Generally well tolerated; nausea, vomiting, skin rash; ↑ liver function tests. | ↓ levels with carbamazepine, phenytoin, rifampin; ↑ phenytoin levels; ↑ warfarin effect. | PO: $$ <br>IV: $$$$$ |
| *flucytosine* ‡ <br>Ancotil | Bone marrow toxicity, especially with high levels; GI disturbances. | ↑ hemotoxicity with AZT, ganciclovir. | ‡ |
| *foscarnet* ‡ <br>Foscavir | Plasma electrolyte and mineral disturbances (may cause tetany, seizures), nephrotoxicity, anemia, nausea, vomiting, diarrhea, headache. | Prehydrate with normal saline to ↓ nephrotoxicity. Compared to ganciclovir, more difficult to administer. ↑ side effects, but may prolong survival. | ‡ |
| *ganciclovir* <br>Cytovene | Neutropenia, thrombocytopenia, nausea, vomiting, headache, confusion. | ↑ hemotoxicity with AZT; G-CSF can be used to treat neutropenia; ganciclovir-resistant strains of CMV have emerged. | $$$ |
| *itraconazole* <br>Sporanox | Generally well tolerated; nausea, epigastric pain, rash, headache, edema, hypokalemia. | Terfenadine and astemizole should be avoided (risk of arrhythmias). ↓ levels with carbamazepine, $H_2$-blockers, isoniazid, phenytoin, rifampin. ↑ warfarin effect. | $ |
| *ketoconazole* <br>Nizoral | Anorexia, nausea, vomiting, hepatotoxicity. | Absorbed best in acidic environment; ↓ absorption with ddI, antacids, $H_2$-blockers. Terfenadine and astemizole should be avoided (↑ risk of arrhythmias). ↓ levels with carbamazepine, phenytoin, rifampin; ↑ warfarin effect; ↑ hepatoxicity with AZT, co-trimoxazole. | $ |
| *pentamidine* <br>Pentacarinat | Severe hypotension, hypo- and hyperglycemia, nephrotoxicity, cardiac arrhythmias, leukopenia, pancreatitis. | Aerosolized pentamidine well tolerated, but less effective for PCP treatment than IV. Should be injected over 1 h; monitor BP closely. ↑ nephrotoxicity with nephrotoxic drugs. | $$$$ |

*(cont'd)*

Table 3: **Drugs Used in HIV-associated Infections** *(cont'd)*

| Drug | Major or Dose-limiting Toxicities | Comments | Cost* |
|---|---|---|---|
| *pyrimethamine* Daraprim | Bone marrow suppression, blood dyscrasias, hematuria, anorexia, vomiting. | An antifolate agent, thus folinic acid (leucovorin) should be given concurrently to ↓ bone marrow toxicity; ↑ hemotoxicity with sulfonamides, AZT. | $ |
| *rifabutin* Mycobutin | Hepatotoxicity, rash, pruritus, leukopenia, thrombocytopenia. Uveitis at doses > 300 mg/d. | May cause discoloration of urine/feces. | $ |
| *sulfadiazine* ❥ | Hypersensitivity reactions (e.g., rash, pruritus, fever, Stevens-Johnson syndrome); blood dyscrasias. | Used in combination with pyrimethamine. | $ |

* *Cost* ***per day*** *based on dosages in Table 2 for 50 kg person – includes drug cost only.*
*Legend: $ < $10 $$ $10–25 $$$ $25–50 $$$$ $50–100 $$$$$ > $100*
❥ *Dosage adjustment may be required in renal impairment – see Appendix I.*
† *Investigational drug distributed by Upjohn in Canada.*
‡ *Available from Special Access Program, Therapeutic Products Programme, Health Canada.*
*Abbreviations: AZT = zidovudine; ddI = didanosine; G-CSF = granulocyte colony-stimulating factor; G6PD = glucose-6-phosphate dehydrogenase.*

### *Suggested Reading List*

College of Family Physicians of Canada and Health Canada. *Comprehensive guide for the care of persons with HIV disease, Module 1: Adults – men, women, adolescents*. Ottawa: Health Canada, 1993.

Gallant JE, Moore RD, Chaisson RE. Prophylaxis for opportunistic infections in patients with HIV infection. *Ann Intern Med* 1994;120:932–944.

Kovacs JA, Masur H. Prophylaxis against opportunistic infections in patients with human immunodeficiency virus infection. *N Engl J Med* 2000;342:1416–1429.

NIH Conference. Recent advances in the management of AIDS-related opportunistic infections. *Ann Intern Med* 1994;120:945–955.

USPHS/IDSA Prevention of Opportunistic Infections Working Group. 1999 USPHS/IDSA guidelines for the prevention of opportunistic infections in persons infected with human immunodeficiency virus. *MMWR* 1999;48(RR–10):1–66.

CHAPTER 97

# Infections in the Cancer Patient

*Coleman Rotstein, MD, FRCPC, FACP, FIDSA*

Infections are a significant cause of morbidity and mortality in cancer patients despite the progress that has been made in their recognition, therapy and prevention. The expanding armamentarium of antineoplastic chemotherapeutic agents, radiation therapy and immunotherapy has improved the survival of cancer patients, but has simultaneously rendered them more susceptible to infections.

## Goals of Therapy

- To decrease morbidity associated with infection
- To minimize risk of death from infection
- To enhance the supportive care and quality of life of cancer patients by using prophylactic measures to prevent infection and employing outpatient antibiotic management when appropriate

## Investigations

- Thorough history with attention to:
  - the nature of the malignancy and any associated defects in host defenses (e.g., neutropenia, B cell and/or T cell dysfunction)
  - the effects of cytotoxic, myelosuppressive or immunosuppressive therapy employed to treat the patient's cancer; note day of onset of fever relative to the first day of the last cycle of chemotherapy
  - neutropenia (severity and expected duration)
  - the iatrogenic procedures performed on the patient (e.g., splenectomy, placement of venous access devices or other surgical procedures)
  - whether the nature of the malignancy suggests obstruction of natural body passages (e.g., bronchus, bowel, ureter, biliary tree)
  - central nervous system dysfunction
  - occupational and travel history, and exposure to animals
- Complete physical examination with attention to venous access sites
- Laboratory tests:
  - CBC and differential to assess the total neutrophil count

– biochemical profile with attention to renal and liver function
– at least 2 sets of blood cultures and a culture of any other suspected site of infection (e.g., urine, skin)
– radiographic studies appropriate for suspected sites of infection (e.g., chest x-ray for pneumonia, CT scan of the head for encephalitis or cerebral abscess)
– stool for *Clostridium difficile* and other potential pathogens (e.g., *Salmonella, Shigella, Campylobacter* and protozoa) if diarrhea is present
– serological tests, i.e., cytomegalovirus and hepatitis serology if indicated
– when appropriate, biopsy for pathology and culture of skin lesions suspected to be infectious

## Therapeutic Choices

### *Infection Control Measures*

- Infection control measures such as hand washing and use of high efficiency particulate filtration rooms for profoundly neutropenic patients at high risk for filamentous fungal infections.
- Specialized infection control procedures for patients colonized with multiply-resistant organisms (e.g., methicillin-resistant *Staphylococcus aureus* or vancomycin-resistant enterococci).
- For neutropenic patients, avoidance of raw fruits and vegetables, as well as fresh flowers and plants in the patient's room.

## Pharmacologic Choices (Table 1)

### Antibacterial Therapy

- Although neoplasms can cause fevers in cancer patients, an infectious etiology should be sought in all cases of elevated temperature. Fever is defined as a single oral temperature $\geq 38.3^{\circ}$ C or the presence of at least 2 oral temperatures $\geq 38^{\circ}$ C in a 12-hour period in the absence of other causes.
- Most infections are caused by microorganisms that have colonized the patient at or near the site of infection (e.g., the skin, oropharynx or gastrointestinal tract).
- Bacteria are the principal pathogens causing infections in cancer patients, making up > 60% of initially documented episodes of sepsis.
- The choice of antibacterial agents in febrile cancer patients is predicated on the neutrophil count, the patient's clinical status and the site of infection (Figure 1). Neutropenia is

defined as $\leq 1.0 \times 10^9$/L neutrophils. A greater degree of neutropenia (i.e., $< 0.5 \times 10^9$/L) confers a greater risk of developing more severe infection. In addition, the risk of severe infection is directly related to the duration of neutropenia. Because of the high risk of life-threatening bacterial infection, particularly in neutropenic patients, prompt antibiotic therapy must be initiated by the intravenous route. Moreover, in selecting the initial antibiotic regimen and the site of care (i.e., the inpatient or outpatient setting), consider the presence of concurrent comorbid medical illnesses, the control of the cancer and serious medical complications. Outpatient antibiotic therapy may be employed not only for non-neutropenic patients, but also for low-risk neutropenic patients who do not have the aforementioned medical conditions or uncontrolled cancer (Figure 2).

- **Vancomycin** may be incorporated into the initial therapeutic regimen with clinically obvious venous access catheter-related infection, severe mucositis and known colonization with methicillin-resistant *Staphylococcus aureus*. Alternatively, vancomycin may be added once susceptibility testing has been completed.
- Anti-anaerobic coverage (**metronidazole** or **clindamycin**) may be used for presumed anaerobic infection.

### *Antifungal Therapy*

- Non-neutropenic patients who develop *fungal mucositis* (oral and/or esophageal candidiasis) may be treated with a topical agent such as **nystatin** or systemic oral agents such as **ketoconazole**, **fluconazole** or **itraconazole**. Nevertheless, extensive cases may require parenteral therapy with **fluconazole** or **amphotericin B**.
- Parenteral antifungal therapy should be initiated for *documented invasive or disseminated fungal infection* in non-neutropenic and neutropenic cancer patients.
- Treatment of a *documented or suspected fungal infection* in neutropenic patients requires the use of parenteral antifungal therapy with **amphotericin B** most commonly, or **fluconazole** if renal dysfunction exists.
- The **lipid preparations of amphotericin B** have equal efficacy but less nephrotoxicity compared with amphotericin B, and may be used as salvage therapy for fungal infections that fail to respond to amphotericin B or for those patients with amphotericin B toxicity.
- **Itraconazole** (currently only available in an oral formulation) has enhanced activity against *Aspergillus* species.

Figure 1: **Approach to Fever in Cancer Patients**

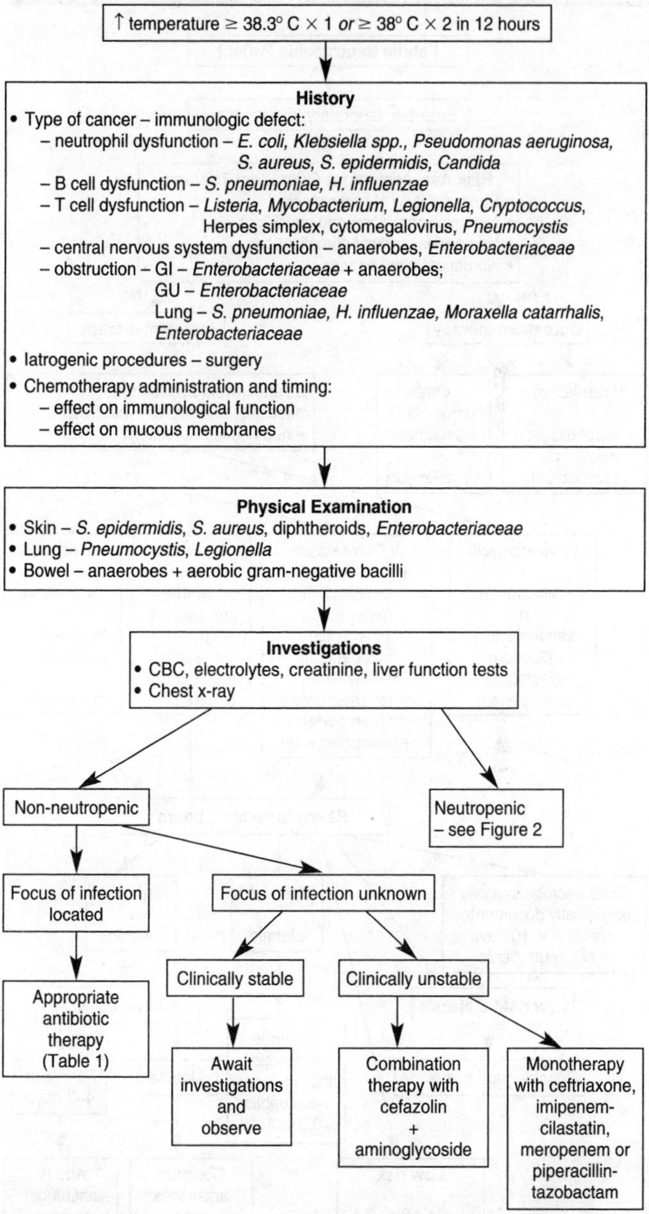
↑ temperature ≥ 38.3° C × 1 *or* ≥ 38° C × 2 in 12 hours
**History**
• Type of cancer – immunologic defect:
– neutrophil dysfunction – *E. coli, Klebsiella spp., Pseudomonas aeruginosa, S. aureus, S. epidermidis, Candida*
– B cell dysfunction – *S. pneumoniae, H. influenzae*
– T cell dysfunction – *Listeria, Mycobacterium, Legionella, Cryptococcus*, Herpes simplex, cytomegalovirus, *Pneumocystis*
– central nervous system dysfunction – anaerobes, *Enterobacteriaceae*
– obstruction – GI – *Enterobacteriaceae* + anaerobes;
GU – *Enterobacteriaceae*
Lung – *S. pneumoniae, H. influenzae, Moraxella catarrhalis, Enterobacteriaceae*
• Iatrogenic procedures – surgery
• Chemotherapy administration and timing:
– effect on immunological function
– effect on mucous membranes
**Physical Examination**
• Skin – *S. epidermidis, S. aureus*, diphtheroids, *Enterobacteriaceae*
• Lung – *Pneumocystis, Legionella*
• Bowel – anaerobes + aerobic gram-negative bacilli
**Investigations**
• CBC, electrolytes, creatinine, liver function tests
• Chest x-ray
Non-neutropenic
Neutropenic – see Figure 2
Focus of infection located
Focus of infection unknown
Clinically stable
Clinically unstable
Appropriate antibiotic therapy (Table 1)
Await investigations and observe
Combination therapy with cefazolin + aminoglycoside
Monotherapy with ceftriaxone, imipenem-cilastatin, meropenem or piperacillin-tazobactam

Figure 2: **Management of Infection in Febrile Neutropenic Cancer Patients**

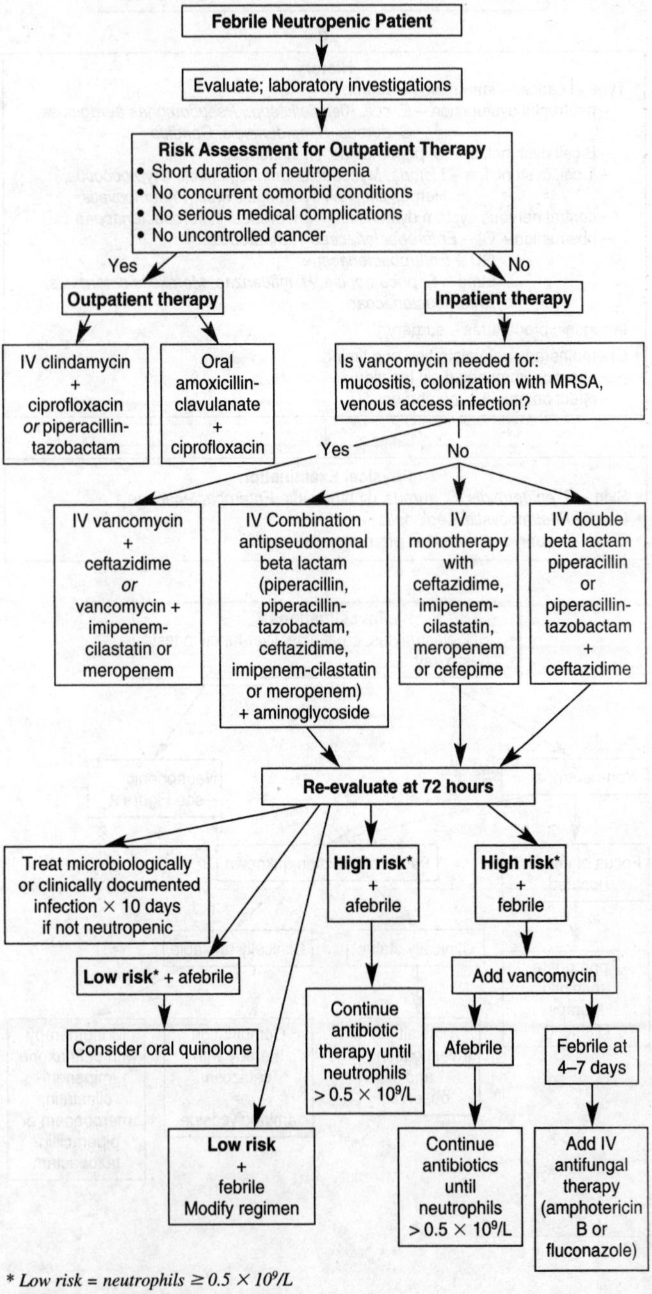
Febrile Neutropenic Patient
Evaluate; laboratory investigations
Risk Assessment for Outpatient Therapy
• Short duration of neutropenia
• No concurrent comorbid conditions
• No serious medical complications
• No uncontrolled cancer
Yes
No
Outpatient therapy
Inpatient therapy
IV clindamycin + ciprofloxacin or piperacillin-tazobactam
Oral amoxicillin-clavulanate + ciprofloxacin
Is vancomycin needed for: mucositis, colonization with MRSA, venous access infection?
Yes
No
IV vancomycin + ceftazidime or vancomycin + imipenem-cilastatin or meropenem
IV Combination antipseudomonal beta lactam (piperacillin, piperacillin-tazobactam, ceftazidime, imipenem-cilastatin or meropenem) + aminoglycoside
IV monotherapy with ceftazidime, imipenem-cilastatin, meropenem or cefepime
IV double beta lactam piperacillin or piperacillin-tazobactam + ceftazidime
Re-evaluate at 72 hours
Treat microbiologically or clinically documented infection × 10 days if not neutropenic
High risk* + afebrile
High risk* + febrile
Low risk* + afebrile
Consider oral quinolone
Continue antibiotic therapy until neutrophils > 0.5 × 10⁹/L
Add vancomycin
Afebrile
Febrile at 4–7 days
Low risk + febrile Modify regimen
Continue antibiotics until neutrophils > 0.5 × 10⁹/L
Add IV antifungal therapy (amphotericin B or fluconazole)

** Low risk = neutrophils $\geq 0.5 \times 10^9$/L*
*High risk = neutrophils $< 0.5 \times 10^9$/L*
*Abbreviations: MRSA = methicillin-resistant S. aureus*

Table 1: **Drugs Used to Treat Infections in Cancer Patients**

| Drug | Dosage | Adverse Effects | Drug Interactions | Cost* |
|---|---|---|---|---|
| **β-lactams** | | Rash, hypersensitivity reactions: interstitial nephritis, neutropenia, hemolytic anemia; thrombocytopenia. | Some penicillins may inactivate aminoglycosides if mixed. | |
| *amoxicillin-clavulanate* Clavulin | One 500/125 tablet PO TID | | | $ |
| *piperacillin* Pipracil | 4 g IV Q6H | | | $$$$ |
| *piperacillin-tazobactam* Tazocin | 12–16 g/1.5–2 g/d IV divided Q6–8H | | | $$$$–$$$$$ |
| *ceftazidime* Ceptaz, Tazidime | 2 g IV Q8H | | | $$$$$ |
| *cefepime* Maxipime | 2 g IV Q8H | Rash, hypersensitivity reactions, hematologic effects. | | $$$$ |
| *ceftriaxone* Rocephin | 1–2 g IV once daily | Pseudocholelithiasis. | | $$–$$$ |
| *imipenem-cilastatin* Primaxin | 500 mg IV Q6H | Imipenem has been associated with seizures at doses of 1 g Q6H. | | $$$$$ |
| *meropenem* Merrem | 1 g IV Q8H | Diarrhea, nausea, rash. | | $$$$$ |
| **Aminoglycosides** | | Ototoxicity (auditory and/or vestibular), nephrotoxicity, neuromuscular paralysis (rare). | Synergistic or additive toxicity if used with vancomycin and/or platinum-derived antineoplastics, amphotericin B and/or other nephrotoxic/ototoxic drugs. | |
| *gentamicin* Garamycin, generics | 5–7 mg/kg once daily† | | | $ |
| *tobramycin* Nebcin | 5–7 mg/kg once daily† | | | $ |
| *amikacin* Amikin | 15–20 mg/kg once daily† | | | $$ |

*(cont'd)*

Table 1: **Drugs Used to Treat Infections in Cancer Patients** *(cont'd)*

| Drug | Dosage | Adverse Effects | Drug Interactions | Cost* |
|---|---|---|---|---|
| *vancomycin* ◗ Vancocin | 15 mg/kg IV Q12H | Shock after rapid IV infusion (over < 1 h), fever, chills, phlebitis, "red-neck" syndrome, tingling and flushing of head, neck, chest, rash (4–5%), transient leukopenia or eosinophilia, ototoxicity. | Nephrotoxicity may be enhanced if given with aminoglycosides or other nephrotoxins. | $$$$ |
| **Macrolides** | | | | |
| *erythromycin* Erythrocin, generics | 1 g IV Q6H | Abdominal pain, nausea, vomiting, diarrhea; thrombophlebitis, transient hearing loss with high doses. | May interfere with metabolism of theophylline, warfarin, carbamazepine, cyclosporine, methylprednisolone, terfenadine, astemizole, cisapride. May ↑ bioavailability of digoxin. | $$$ |
| *azithromycin* Zithromax | 500 mg IV once daily | GI upset | | $ |
| **Miscellaneous** | | | | |
| *ciprofloxacin* Cipro | 500 mg PO BID<br>400 mg IV Q12H | GI upset, rash, CNS toxicity. | Warfarin: ↑ INR.<br>Binds with antacids, iron, sucralfate. | $<br>$$$ |
| *clindamycin* Dalacin C | 600 mg IV Q8H | Diarrhea, minor reversible ↑ liver transaminases, reversible neutropenia, thrombocytopenia, pseudomembranous colitis. | May enhance action of neuromuscular blocking agents. | $$ |
| *metronidazole* Flagyl, generics | 500 mg IV Q12H | GI upset, reversible neutropenia, seizures, peripheral neuropathy (rare), rash, metallic taste. | Disulfiram reaction with alcohol.<br>Potentiation of warfarin effects and other oral coumarin-type anticoagulants. | $ |

| | | | | |
|---|---|---|---|---|
| **Antifungals** | | | | |
| *nystatin* Mycostatin, generics | 3.6 million U PO Q4H | Nausea, vomiting, diarrhea. | | $ |
| *amphotericin B* Fungizone | 0.3–1.5 mg/kg IV Q24H | Rigors, renal dysfunction (azotemia), headache, hypokalemia, phlebitis, thrombocytopenia, anemia, leukopenia (rare), hypotension. | ↑ azotemia when used with other nephrotoxic drugs. | \$\$–\$\$\$ |
| *lipid amphotericin B* AmBisome, Abelcet | 3–5 mg/kg IV Q24H | Less nephrotoxicity than amphotericin B. | | \$\$\$\$\$ |
| *fluconazole* Diflucan | 100–400 mg PO/IV Q24H | Nausea, headache, skin rash, abdominal pain, vomiting, diarrhea. | May cause hepatotoxicity if used with other potentially hepatotoxic drugs.<br>Sulfonylureas, phenytoin, cyclosporine, coumarin-like drugs may require dosage adjustment (monitor).<br>Avoid astemizole, terfenadine and cisapride (↑ risk of cardiac arrhythmias). | PO: \$–\$\$<br>IV: \$\$\$–\$\$\$\$\$ |
| *itraconazole* Sporanox | 100–200 mg PO daily–BID | Nausea, rash, headache, reversible ↑ hepatic enzymes. | Sulfonylureas, phenytoin, coumarin-like drugs, digoxin may require dosage adjustment (monitor).<br>Didanosine, $H_2$-antagonists, rifampin, phenytoin, may ↓ itraconazole levels.<br>Avoid astemizole and terfenadine (↑ risk of cardiac arrhythmias).<br>Itraconazole ↑ levels of lovastatin. | $ |

*(cont'd)*

Table 1: **Drugs Used to Treat Infections in Cancer Patients** *(cont'd)*

| Drug | Dosage | Adverse Effects | Drug Interactions | Cost* |
|---|---|---|---|---|
| **Antiparasitics** | | | | |
| *co-trimoxazole* ❥ Septra, Bactrim, generics | PO/IV: trimethoprim 20 mg/kg/d and sulfamethoxazole 100 mg/kg/d divided QID | Nausea, vomiting, diarrhea; hypersensitivity reactions, leukopenia, thrombocytopenia, hepatitis (rare). | INR may ↑ with warfarin. | PO: $ IV: $$$ |
| **Antivirals** ❥ | | | | |
| *acyclovir* Zovirax, generics | 5–12.4 mg/kg IV Q8H | Phlebitis, rash, hypotension, headache, nausea, tremors, confusion, seizures (1%), renal dysfunction. | Probenecid ↓ renal clearance. | $$$$$ |
| *famciclovir* Famvir | 500 mg TID PO | Headache, nausea, pruritus. | | $ |
| *ganciclovir* Cytovene | Induction: 5 mg/kg IV Q12H<br>Maintenance: 6 mg/kg IV Q24H | Leukopenia, nausea, headache, behavioral changes. | Avoid use with zidovudine (↑ hematological toxicity). | $$ (for maintenance) |
| *valacyclovir* Valtrex | 1 g TID PO | Headache, nausea. | | $ |

† *If appropriate for renal function.*
❥ *Dosage adjustment may be required in renal impairment – see Appendix I.*
* *Cost per day – includes drug cost only. Where doses are expressed in mg/kg, costs were calculated for a 50 kg person.*
*Legend: $ < $25 $$ $25–50 $$$ $50–75 $$$$ $75–100 $$$$$ > $100*

### *Antiviral Therapy*

- There is no indication for the empirical use of antiviral drugs in the treatment of cancer patients without evidence of viral disease.
- Skin or mucous membrane lesions due to Herpes simplex virus or varicella-zoster virus may be treated with **acyclovir** orally or intravenously. Oral **famciclovir** or **valacyclovir** are better absorbed than acyclovir and are alternatives.
- **Foscarnet** intravenously is used for acyclovir-resistant cases of Herpes virus.
- Cytomegalovirus in bone marrow transplant recipients may be treated with **ganciclovir**.

### *Supportive Care Measures*

- The administration of **granulocyte (G-CSF)** and **granulocyte-macrophage (GM-CSF) colony-stimulating factors** may decrease the incidence and duration of neutropenia after chemotherapy. Their use is advocated for patients who remain profoundly neutropenic and have failed to respond to appropriate antimicrobial therapy for documented infection. Once neutrophil counts reach $\geq 1.0 \times 10^9$/L, colony-stimulating factor support should be discontinued.
- As mentioned previously, appropriate infection control measures should be continuously followed in neutropenic and non-neutropenic cancer patients.

### *Prevention of Infection in Cancer Patients*

- For cancer patients with pronounced T cell dysfunction, prophylaxis with **cotrimoxazole** is suggested to prevent *Pneumocystis carinii* pneumonia. Alternative prophylactic agents are inhaled **pentamidine** and **dapsone**.
- Strategies designed to prevent bacterial infection in profoundly neutropenic cancer patients, such as those with acute leukemia, focus on eliminating indigenous microflora and preventing new potential pathogens from being acquired. Potential antimicrobial regimens are fluoroquinolones, cotrimoxazole and oral non-absorbable antibiotics (gentamicin 200 mg, vancomycin 250 mg and nystatin 3.6 million units, all Q4H orally).

  **Ciprofloxacin** significantly decreases febrile morbidity and gram-negative infections, but has shown no effect on mortality. Moreover, there may be a predilection for gram-positive infection when using ciprofloxacin prophylactically. This may be overcome by adding another antibiotic with enhanced gram-positive activity (e.g., a penicillin or macrolide).

- Antifungal prophylaxis with oral **fluconazole** has been demonstrated to prevent invasive fungal infection in allogeneic bone marrow transplant recipients and patients with acute leukemia undergoing remission induction chemotherapy.
- If fluconazole has been employed prophylactically, it should not be used empirically or for therapeutic antifungal therapy for documented fungal infection in neutropenic cancer patients. For these situations, parenteral **amphotericin B** is the drug of choice.

## Therapeutic Tips

- **Aminoglycosides** should be avoided in patients with impaired renal function, particularly those receiving treatment with other nephrotoxic drugs such as cis-platinum, cyclosporine or amphotericin B.
- In deciding on cost-effective empirical therapy, drug acquisition cost by itself is of limited value. Consider the relative effectiveness, side effect profile and overall resource consumption of the available treatments as well.
- Identification of low-risk patients appropriate for outpatient antibiotic management may enhance the patient's quality of life and reduce costs.

## *Suggested Reading List*

Hughes WT, Armstrong D, Bodey GP, et al. 1997 Guidelines for the use of antimicrobial agents in neutropenic patients with unexplained fever. *Clin Infect Dis* 1997;25:551–573.

Rotstein C, Bow EJ, Laverdiere M, Ioannou S, Carr D, Moghaddam N, and The Canadian Fluconazole Prophylaxis Study Group. Randomized placebo-controlled trial of fluconazole prophylaxis for neutropenic cancer patients: Benefit based on purpose and intensity of cytotoxic therapy. *Clin Infect Dis* 1999;28:331–340.

Rotstein C, Mandell LA, Goldberg N. Fluoroquinolone prophylaxis for profoundly neutropenic cancer patients: A meta-analysis. Current Oncology 1997;4(Suppl 2):S2–S7.

Talcott JA, Siegel RD, Finberg R, Goldman L. Risk assessment in cancer patients with fever and neutropenia: A prospective, two-center validation of a prediction rule. *J Clin Oncol* 1992;10:316–322.

Talcott JA, Whalen A, Clark J, et al. Home antibiotic therapy for low-risk cancer patients with fever and neutropenia: A pilot study of 30 patients based on a validated prediction rule. *J Clin Oncol* 1994;12:107–114.

CHAPTER 98

# Nutritional Supplements for Adults

*L. John Hoffer, MD, CM, PhD, FRCPC*

## Goals of Therapy

- To prevent or treat nutritional deficiency disease
- To prevent or treat nondeficiency diseases whose pathophysiology may be mitigated by increased intake of certain nutrients

## Therapeutic Choices

### *Preventive Supplements* (Table 1)

Preventive supplements are vitamin or vitamin/mineral supplements formulated to compensate for inadequacies in the diet of normal persons. They are also useful for patients with excellent diets but increased requirements, mild malabsorption, or increased nutrient losses. Traditionally, these products contained 50 to 150% of the recommended dietary allowance (RDA) for some or many vitamins, but products currently on the market are

Table 1: **Indications For Preventive Supplements**

| |
|---|
| **Clinical evidence of deficient intake*** |
| Voluntary or involuntary weight loss (<1500 kcal/day) |
| History of deficient intake of certain nutrient groups: |
| dairy products and fluid milk (calcium, vitamin D) |
| dark green and deeply colored vegetables and fruits (folic acid, carotenoids, vitamin C) |
| whole grains (folic acid, vitamin $B_6$, vitamin E) |
| **Patient populations at risk of deficient intake or malabsorption*** |
| Prolonged hospital admission |
| Institutionalization |
| Poverty, social isolation |
| GI tract symptoms (nausea, pain, diarrhea, anorexia) |
| GI disease known to be associated with malabsorption |
| Reduced functional and activity status |
| Multiple comorbidities, especially organ failure |
| Swallowing, chewing or dental problems |
| Psychiatric or neurologic disease |
| Chronic substance abuse, especially alcoholism |
| **Increased vitamin/mineral needs** |
| Hemo- or peritoneal dialysis |
| Pregnancy |
| Drug–nutrient interactions |

* *formal dietetic assessment advised*

highly variable, especially with regard to folic acid, vitamin $B_{12}$, vitamin C, vitamin A, iron and zinc.

### *Specific Preventive Supplements*

- **Vitamin A and β-carotene:** The recommended vitamin A intake is 1000 Retinol Equivalents (RE). This can be met by 1 mg of retinol (= 1000 RE = 3333 IU) or 6 mg of its plant-derived precursor, β-carotene (1000 RE = 10 000 IU).
- **Folic acid:** All women of child-bearing potential require a supplement of 0.4 mg/day of folic acid prior to conception, and women with a history of neural tube defect pregnancy require 5 mg/day.
- **Vitamin $B_{12}$:** All persons over age 50 are advised to consume about 2 µg of *synthetic* vitamin $B_{12}$ daily in enriched foods or as a supplement. Synthetic vitamin $B_{12}$ is added to some cold breakfast cereals and soy products.
- **Vitamin D:** Canadians consuming less than ½ liter of fluid milk/day (equivalent to 200 IU vitamin D) are dependent on skin photosynthesis for their vitamin D, but this is absent in winter, prevented by sun block, and decreases greatly with age. Theoretically, 15 minutes of summer sunlight to the hands, arms and face 2 to 3 times/week will meet the requirement of healthy elderly persons; but failing this, healthy persons aged 50 to 70 require 400 IU vitamin D, and those over 70 require 600 IU/day.
- **Calcium:** Children ages 9 to 12 require 1300 mg/day, adults 19 to 50 require 1000 mg/day, and persons over 50 require 1200 mg/day. Most people need supplements to accomplish this. Calcium carbonate (1200 mg provides 500 mg elemental calcium) should be taken with food, in individual divided doses not exceeding 500 mg of calcium, to maximize absorption.
- **Iron:** Because of its potential toxicity, iron supplements at or above the recommended intake (10 mg) should be used only on a case-by-case basis for at risk persons (e.g., adolescents and women with heavy menstrual losses) or people clearly not meeting the recommended intake, until the dietary inadequacy is corrected. Dietary iron deficiency occurs in the elderly but there is a comparable risk of iron storage disease from excessive intake.
- **Pregnancy:** All pregnant women should have taken folic acid prior to conception, and continue it during pregnancy with a standard supplement containing folic acid and a moderate increase in iron during the second and third trimesters. Do not exceed 3300 IU of supplemental retinol (vitamin A).
- **Vegetarian diet:** Both vegans and lacto-ovo-vegetarians should use a vitamin $B_{12}$ supplement providing 2 µg/day. Unless a dietetic evaluation demonstrates otherwise, all

vegans require calcium supplements. Vegetarians are not especially iron deficient and do not routinely require iron supplements.

## Drug-Nutrient Interactions

- The adverse bone effects of **systemic glucocorticoids** are magnified when calcium or vitamin D intake are inadequate.
- **Anticonvulsant drugs** can induce folic acid and vitamin D deficiency. Preventive folic acid and vitamin D supplements should be considered for every patient.
- Depression may not respond to **antidepressant therapy** when folic acid status is marginal or deficient. The nutritional status of depressed patients should be assessed. Unless this is clearly shown to be unnecessary, a multiple vitamin providing the RDA for thiamine, folic acid and synthetic vitamin $B_{12}$ is appropriate.
- **Isoniazid** increases pyridoxine needs and can induce peripheral neuropathy. Patients who require this drug should probably use a preventive supplement. Patients with clinical malnutrition should receive 10 to 50 mg pyridoxine every day.
- Patients receiving **low-dose methotrexate** therapy (as used to treat rheumatoid arthritis) should receive folic acid to reduce the risk of gastrointestinal and liver toxicity (1 to 5 mg/day).
- **Trimethoprim** therapy can unmask marginal folic acid deficiency, but folic acid is not routinely required.
- **Orlistat** induces fat malabsorption; a preventive multivitamin containing the fat soluble vitamins and β-carotene should be used.

### ***Therapeutic Supplements*** (Table 2)

Therapeutic supplements contain 5- to 50-fold excesses of specific vitamins for therapeutic or pharmacologic purposes.

- **Thiamine:** Wernicke's encephalopathy continues to be under-diagnosed in malnourished persons, frequently presenting nonspecifically as confusion or decreased consciousness. All patients at risk (chronic alcoholism, hyperemesis gravidarum, and AIDS) should receive oral thiamine, and those with altered mental status should be treated presumptively with 50 to 100 mg parenterally for 3 days.
- **Antioxidant and vitamin E therapy:** Biologic, epidemiologic and metabolic clinical data indicate that a combination of antioxidant vitamins (plus good diet) may prevent atherosclerotic events. Hard endpoint clinical trials using

Table 2: **Indications For Therapeutic Supplements**

| |
|---|
| Overt deficiency disease |
| Compensation for maldigestion or malabsorption* |
| extensively resected stomach (calcium, folic acid, vitamin $B_{12}$ and iron) |
| absent or diseased terminal ileum (vitamin $B_{12}$) |
| decreased absorptive surface area (most micronutrients) |
| fat maldigestion (fat soluble nutrients: vitamins A,D,E, calcium, magnesium and essential fatty acids) |
| Certain inborn errors of metabolism |
| To treat nutrient-responsive nondeficiency diseases |

* *formal dietetic assessment advised.*

vitamin E alone have had mixed results to date. At present, it is rational to prescribe ascorbic acid 500 mg and vitamin E 400 IU (international units) once or twice daily for patients at cardiovascular risk (including persons with diabetes mellitus[1,2]), or enroll them into a randomized clinical trial. In yet higher doses (1200 IU/day), vitamin E may ameliorate (and hence prevent) tardive dyskinesias. According to new findings, synthetic vitamin E (a racemic mixture of α-tocopherols, usually termed *dl*-α-tocopherol, but more recently termed *all rac*-α-tocopherol) has only one-half the activity/mg of natural vitamin E (*d*-α-tocopherol, now termed *RRR*-α-tocopherol). Moreover, IU of the two forms are no longer considered to have equivalent vitamin E activity. Thus, the recent recommended nutritional adult daily vitamin E intake is 15 mg of *RRR*-α-tocopherol (22 IU), regarded as bioequivalent to 30 mg (67 IU) of *all rac*-α-tocopherol.

- **Plasma homocysteine and vascular risk:** Although not yet assessed in hard endpoint clinical trials, folic acid lowers even "normal" plasma levels of the vascular toxin, homocysteine, potentially preventing coronary artery disease, stroke and deep vein thrombosis (DVT)[3]. A daily 0.4 mg folic acid supplement is rational for most people but should especially be considered for persons at risk of coronary disease, stroke or unexplained DVT whose plasma homocysteine is > 12 to 15 μmol/L. Plasma concentrations > 30 μmol/L without $B_{12}$ deficiency or renal failure mandate referral for detailed investigation.

## Micronutrient Toxicity

- **Iron:** Therapy with iron should be monitored (e.g., to normalize serum ferritin) and/or time limited to avoid iron

[1] *Diabetes Care 1999;22:1245–1251.*
[2] *BMJ 1997;314:1845–1846.*
[3] *JAMA 1998;279:392–393.*

storage disease. There is also theoretical concern that increased tissue iron may catalyze free radical production even in persons without classical iron storage disease. In the absence of an obvious explanation, the diagnosis of iron deficiency should prompt investigation (e.g., GI blood loss, occult celiac disease).

- **Vitamin A:** Except for malabsorption/maldigestion and treating retinitis pigmentosa, there is no current indication for prescribing vitamin A in excess of the recommended daily intake of 3300 IU. Patients with renal failure accumulate retinol and hence are not normally supplemented (special renal failure formulations without vitamin A are used in dialysis centers). Heavy cigarette smokers who used a specially formulated, high-dose β-carotene product (30 mg) had an increased death rate from lung cancer and cardiac causes, although this did not occur in nonsmokers taking high doses of ordinary β-carotene. Despite having low liver retinol stores, patients with chronic liver disease and alcohol abusers are prone to hepatoxicity from retinol and high-dose (30 mg) β-carotene. Retinol consumption ≥ 10 000 IU from fish has been associated with lower bone density and a higher hip fracture rate. Pregnant women require adequate vitamin A, but should not exceed a daily supplement of 3300 IU.
- **Vitamin C:** There is little evidence of toxicity. High-dose vitamin C is an osmotic laxative with predictable effects. Urolithiasis risk is not increased by vitamin C consumption, at least in persons lacking a prior history of oxalate stone formation. Vitamin C can increase iron absorption and interact with it to promote oxidative damage, so large doses should be avoided in persons with iron storage disease. It should also be avoided by persons with end-stage renal disease, who cannot excrete oxalate. "Chewable" vitamin C is still somewhat acidic and if used as a lozenge could promote tooth enamel loss.
- **Vitamin D:** The upper safe daily intake is 2000 IU/day, so adult toxicity with vitamin D is rarely a problem. At risk, however, are some patients with granulomatous diseases (lymphoma, sarcoidosis, tuberculosis) which may be associated with excessive activation of cholecalciferol to the active vitamin, 1,25-dihydroxycholecalciferol. Early toxicity manifests as hypercalciuria, progressing to hypercalcemia.
- **Vitamin E:** There is little evidence of toxicity, but in high doses vitamin E has a mild antiplatelet effect, potentially increasing the risk of hemorrhage. As with aspirin, high doses should be avoided in persons with a bleeding diathesis or uncontrolled hypertension. The combination of aspirin and vitamin E to prevent cerebrovascular events is plausible, but

the corresponding risk of hemorrhage is not known. Some authorities regard concurrent warfarin therapy as a contra-indication to high-dose vitamin E on theoretical grounds and because increased prothrombin times have been reported in some warfarin-treated patients. The one systematic study that examined for this effect failed to show an interaction. The generally regarded as safe upper limit for daily vitamin E intake for adults was recently set as 1000 mg for both the synthetic and natural forms.

- **Folic Acid:** In doses greater than 1 mg/day, folic acid has been reported to mask the hematologic picture of concurrent vitamin $B_{12}$ deficiency, delaying the diagnosis and allowing the neurologic lesion to progress.

## Supplements Sold in Canada

The 6th edition of the *Compendium of Nonprescription Products* (Ottawa: Canadian Pharmacists Association, 1999) lists 608 single entity vitamin or mineral products and over 300 adult oral multiple vitamin compounds. It is recommended to carefully select a well-formulated preventive multiple vitamin/mineral containing the daily iron recommendation for persons who require supplementation or whose diet lacks iron, and an "over 50" product containing 4 mg iron for more general use. The chosen product should provide no more than 1000 RE vitamin A (provided at least partly as β-carotene); about 0.4 mg folic acid; at least 2 μg vitamin $B_{12}$; other B vitamins; 400 IU vitamin D; 10 to 15 mg zinc; 10–100 IU vitamin E.

### *Suggested Reading List*

Anon. Vitamin supplements. *Med Lett Drugs Ther* 1998;40:75–77.

Shils ME, Olson JA, Shike M, Ross AC, eds. *Modern nutrition in health and disease*. 9th ed. Baltimore: Williams & Wilkins, 1999.

Standing Committee on the Scientific Evaluation of Dietary Reference Intakes. *Dietary reference intakes: thiamin, riboflavin, niacin, vitamin $B_6$, folate, vitamin $B_{12}$, pantothenic acid, biotin, and choline*. Washington, DC: National Academy Press, 1998.

Standing Committee on the Scientific Evaluation of Dietary Reference Intakes. *Dietary reference intakes: vitamin C, vitamin E, selenium, and beta-carotene and other carotenoids*. Washington, DC: National Academy Press, 2000.

CHAPTER 99

# Obesity

*David C.W. Lau, MD, PhD, FRCPC*

## Goals of Therapy

- To induce permanent weight loss at a rate not exceeding 1 to 2 kg (2 to 4 pounds) a month
- To prevent weight regain
- To reduce cardiovascular disease morbidity and mortality
- To prevent metabolic comorbidities: diabetes, hypertension and dyslipidemia
- To prevent other medical complications: sleep apnea syndrome, gall bladder disease, gout, degenerative joint disease, and some forms of cancer (colon and endometrial)
- To improve psychosocial well-being and quality of life

## Definition and Classification of Obesity

Obesity is reaching epidemic proportions globally and affects 35% of adult men and 27% of adult women in Canada. The prevalence of metabolic comorbidities such as type 2 diabetes mellitus, dyslipidemia, hypertension and coronary heart disease, is highly correlated with increasing body mass index (BMI). The total direct cost of obesity in Canada in 1997 was conservatively estimated at about $2 billion.

Obesity is characterized by excessive body fat accumulation in adipose tissue to an extent that health may be adversely affected. The body mass index (BMI)[1] is a simple index of weight for height that provides the best anthropometric measure of body fatness in a population.

## Investigations

- Thorough history including life-style (eating and activity) habits, diet readiness to change
- Family history of obesity and comorbidities
- Physical examination
  - weight and height
  - waist circumference and visual inspection of fat distribution
  - blood pressure and heart rate

---

[1] *BMI = weight/height² (kg/m²)*

Table 1: **WHO Weight Classification of Adults Based on Body Mass Index**

| Classification | Body Mass Index (BMI)* ($kg/m^2$) | Risk of Comorbidities† |
|---|---|---|
| **Underweight** | < 18.5 | Low |
| **Normal** | 18.5–24.9 | Average |
| **Overweight** | 25.0–29.9 | Mildly increased |
| **Obese** | ≥ 30.0 | |
| **Class I** | 30.0–34.9 | Moderate |
| **Class II** | 35.0–39.9 | Severe |
| **Class III** | ≥ 40.0 | Very severe |

* *Values are age and gender independent.*

† *Both BMI and a measure of fat distribution (e.g., waist circumference) are important in estimating the risk of comorbidities (type 2 diabetes, hypertension, dyslipidemia). Waist circumference value exceeding 102 cm (40 inches) in men and women below 40 years of age, and 90 cm (35 inches) in men and women 40 to 60 years of age, is associated with increased abdominal fat accumulation and increased cardiovascular disease risks.*

- identify genetic and associated conditions
- target organ damage secondary to complications

■ Determine BMI using nomograms

■ Laboratory tests to screen for diabetes (Chapter 74), dyslipidemia (Chapter 24) and gout (Chapter 54)
- fasting plasma glucose
- fasting lipid profile (total cholesterol, triglycerides, HDL cholesterol and calculated LDL cholesterol)
- serum uric acid
- liver function studies to exclude fatty liver
- routine TSH screening should be discouraged
- pulmonary functions and sleep studies when indicated
- exclude rare known genetic conditions

### Strategies for Healthy Weight

A modest weight loss of 5 to 10% of body weight can lead to health gains. Intervention should be considered for patients with a:
- BMI ≥ 30 $kg/m^2$ in the absence of comorbidities
- BMI ≥ 27 $kg/m^2$ with obesity-related comorbidities or risk factors
- BMI > 25 $kg/m^2$ (overweight individuals) in the presence of two or more obesity-related comorbidities or risk factors

## Goals of Weight Loss

- Recommended optimal rate of weight loss is between 1 to 2 kg (2 to 4 pounds) per month. A kilogram of fat is equivalent to 7780 kcal (3500 kcal/lb)
- Aim for a negative energy balance of 500 kcal/day from the current food intake to achieve a weight loss of a pound per week
- A 500 kcal deficit diet would amount to approximately 20% decrease in food energy intake in men and 30% in women with average daily food energy intake of 2350 kcal/day for men and 1650 kcal/day for women
- Each kg of weight loss is associated with a 0.05 mmol/L and 0.02 mmol/L decrease in total and LDL cholesterol, and a 0.008 mmol/L increase in HDL-cholesterol levels

# Therapeutic Choices

## Nonpharmacologic Choices

### *Nutrition Planning and Diet Composition*

- All weight loss diets must be well-balanced in macronutrient composition and nutritionally adequate to ensure optimal health.
- Ensure an adequate carbohydrate intake of at least 100 g/day (400 kcal/day) to spare protein breakdown, muscle wasting and to avoid large shifts in fluid balance. Complex carbohydrates high in fibre (e.g., kidney beans) are associated with greater satiety and require more time to eat and digest.
- Protein content should be at least 0.8 g/day of high quality mixed proteins to maintain lean body mass and other essential body functions. When energy intakes fall below the level needed for energy balance, protein requirements increase by 1.75 g for every 100 kcal deficit.
- Fat intake should not exceed 30% of total calories, with 10% or less from saturated fat.

### *Physical Activity*

Before engaging in any exercise program, the individual should be assessed to determine the level of fitness. A treadmill stress test should be considered for individuals with cardiovascular risks. Regular physical activity reduces cardiovascular disease risk, enhances a sense of well-being, promotes weight loss, and improves insulin resistance.

- Exercise, when coupled with a judicious caloric-deficit meal plan, accelerates fat loss while maintaining lean body mass, and helps to sustain weight loss over the long term.

- All individuals are encouraged to spend 30 minutes or more of continuous or intermittent (minimum of 10-minute bouts accumulated throughout the day) activities of daily living at least 5 days a week. Initially, physical activity could begin with 5 to 10 minute bouts, with increasing frequency, duration and intensity over a period of time.
- The intensity of physical activity can be defined in a variety of ways, one of the simplest is to estimate the percent of maximum heart rate ($HR_{max}$=220–age). Low intensity values refer to activity that increases heart rate 35 to 54% of $HR_{max}$ and moderate intensity activity increases heart rate 55 to 69% of $HR_{max}$ (Table 2).
- Initial goal is to increase energy expenditure by 700 to 1000 calories a week, or about 100 to 130 calories daily.
- Promote a daily energy expenditure of about 300 kcal and recommend doing a variety of activities, particularly those that are enjoyable and can be continued for life (Table 3).

### Pharmacologic Choices (Table 4)

- Medical therapy is an acceptable adjunct in the short- and long-term management of obesity when life-style measures fail to achieve the desired weight loss.
- Anti-obesity drug therapy, with a target weight loss of 5 to 10%, may be considered as an adjunct to diet, physical activity and behavioral modification.
- The duration of treatment can continue as long as there is continued benefit.
- **Modes of action of anti-obesity drugs:**
  – suppress appetite by reducing food intake
  – increase fat mobilization
  – increase energy expenditure and metabolic rate
  – reduce fat or nutrient absorption
  – alter nutrient partitioning to favor lean body mass.

#### *Appetite Suppressants*

- The majority of anti-obesity drugs available on the market are sympathomimetic noradrenergic appetite suppressants.
- These drugs are readily absorbed and, except for sibutramine, have short half-lives.
- Adverse effects for these drugs are similar and are related to the sympathomimetic properties, including asthenia, dry mouth, constipation and insomnia.
- The stimulant property and modest efficacy of some of these drugs (e.g., phenylpropanolamine and phentermine) limit their use.

Table 2: **Classification of Physical Activity Intensity Based on Activity Lasting up to 60 Minutes***

| Relative Intensity | Heart Rate Reserve (%) | $HR_{max}$ (%) | Absolute Intensity (METs) in Healthy Adults: Young (20–39 yrs) | Middle-aged (40–64 yrs) | Old (65–79 yrs) |
|---|---|---|---|---|---|
| Very low | < 20 | < 35 | < 2.4 | < 2.0 | < 1.6 |
| Low | 20–39 | 35–54 | 2.4–4.7 | 2.0–3.9 | 1.6–3.1 |
| Moderate | 40–59 | 55–69 | 4.8–7.1 | 4.0–5.9 | 3.2–4.7 |
| High | 60–84 | 70–89 | 7.2–10.1 | 6.0–8.4 | 4.8–6.7 |
| Very High | ≥ 85 | ≥ 90 | ≥ 10.2 | ≥ 8.5 | ≥ 6.8 |
| Maximal | 100 | 100 | 12.0 | 10.0 | 8.0 |

*Heart rate reserve and $HR_{max}$ are calculated from the difference between resting and maximum oxygen update ($VO_{2max}$), and resting and maximum heart rate.*

*The intensity of physical activity can be estimated by the percent of maximum heart rate ($HR_{max}$ = 220 – age).*

*Absolute intensities (METs) are approximate mean values. Values for women are about 1–2 METs lower than those for men.*

* *Med Sci Sports Exerc 1998; 30:975.*

- Serotonin-releasing appetite suppressants (fenfluramine and dexfenfluramine) are effective drugs but were withdrawn from the market world wide because of reported association with primary pulmonary hypertension and cardiac valve abnormalities.

### *Lipase Inhibitors*

- The most recent drug approved in Canada for long-term obesity therapy is **orlistat**, a pancreatic lipase inhibitor that exerts its therapeutic activity in the stomach and the gastrointestinal tract by reducing dietary fat absorption by about 30%. It is nonsystemic with less than 2% absorbed, and has a good safety profile.
- In a randomized, placebo-controlled trial, 2-year use of orlistat resulted in an average weight loss of 10.2%, compared with 6.1% body weight loss in the placebo group at the end of the first year.
- Orlistat has been effective in obese subjects with type 2 diabetes, resulting in improvement in glycemic and metabolic control, with favorable changes in lipid and blood pressure profiles.
- Orlistat is administered orally with meals and the recommended dose is 120 mg TID.

Table 3: **Average Energy Consumption Per Hour of Low Intensity Forms of Physical Activity**

| Activity | Average Energy Cost* Kilocalories | Kilojoules |
|---|---|---|
| **Shopping** | 150 | 630 |
| **Light housework (cleaning, vacuuming)** | 220 | 920 |
| **Dancing** | 250 | 1050 |
| **Walking** | | |
| 4 km/h or 2.5 mph | 200 | 840 |
| 6 km/h or 4 mph | 300 | 1260 |

** 1 kilocalorie is approximately 4.2 kilojoules*
*The calories consumed per hour depends on the intensity of the activity, and can range from 150 calories for shopping to just over 300 calories for brisk walking at 6 km/h. Examples of low intensity endurance exercise activity include walking at a brisk pace (6 km/h) for 60 minutes daily (about 50% of* $VO_{2max}$*).*

- Adverse effects are limited mainly to gastrointestinal symptoms (oily spotting, flatus with discharge, fecal urgency, and fatty stools), which relate to orlistat's mode of action. They tend to decrease with use and adherence to a diet with 30% of total energy intake as fat.
- Patients are advised to take a multivitamin that includes fat-soluble vitamins and β-carotene. It should be taken at least two hours before or after orlistat, or at bedtime.

### Sibutramine

- Another anti-obesity agent that will soon be available in Canada is sibutramine (approved and available in the US). It inhibits norepinephrine and serotonin reuptake.
- Sibutramine enhances satiety and decreases hunger. It may also increase thermogenesis and prevent the decline in energy expenditure following weight loss.
- Sibutramine produces a dose-dependent weight loss with an average of 4% for 5 mg/day and 9% of body weight loss for 20 mg/day over a 24-week period, as well as modest improvement in lipid and glucose profiles.
- The recommended starting dose is 10 mg with gradual titration up to a maximum of 20 mg daily.
- Adverse effects include dry mouth, constipation, insomnia, and increased heart rate and blood pressure in some individuals. Unlike dexfenfluramine and fenfluramine, which have been withdrawn from the market, sibutramine is not associated with primary pulmonary hypertension or heart valve abnormalities reported to date.

Table 4: **Drugs Used in the Management of Obesity**

| Drug | Dose | Adverse Effects | Drug Interactions | Comments | Cost* |
|---|---|---|---|---|---|
| **Appetite Suppressants** | | | | | |
| ***Noradrenergic Agents*** | | Dry mouth, constipation, insomnia. | Avoid use with MAOIs (hypertensive crisis). | Phenylpropanolamine and ephedrine/caffeine combinations, commonly used as nonprescription decongestants, are used as appetite suppressants. In Canada they are not approved for use in obesity. | |
| *diethylpropion* Tenuate | 25 mg TID 1 hr AC or 75 mg SR daily, mid-morning | | | | $ |
| *phentermine* Ionamin, Fastin | 15–30 mg daily before breakfast | | | | $ |
| *mazindol* Sanorex | 1 mg TID 1 hr AC or 1–2 mg daily 1 hr before the 1st main meal | | | | $–$$$ |
| ***Serotonergic Agents***[†] | | Nausea, somnolence, sweating, tremor, dry mouth, insomnia. | Avoid use with MAOIs (serotonin syndrome). | Not approved for use in obesity. | |
| *fluoxetine* Prozac, generics | 20–60 mg daily | | | | $–$$$ |
| *sertraline* Zoloft, generics | 25–50 mg daily | | | | $ |
| ***Noradrenergic and Serotonergic*** | | | | | |
| *sibutramine* Meridia | 5–20 mg daily | Dry mouth, constipation, insomnia, may ↑ heart rate and BP. | Avoid using with other serotonergic drugs and MAOIs. | Approval pending in Canada. | |
| **Lipase Inhibitor** | | | | | |
| *orlistat* Xenical | 120 mg daily to TID with each meal containing fat | Oily spotting, flatus with discharge, fecal urgency. | ↓ absorption of fat soluble vitamins. | < 2% of the drug is absorbed systemically. | $$$$$ |

** Cost of 30-day supply – includes drug cost only.*
*Legend: $ < $50   $$ $50–75   $$$ $75–100   $$$$ 100–125   $$$$$ $125–150*

*[†] Fenfluramine (Ponderal) and dexfenfluramine (Redux) were withdrawn from the market because of associated reports of primary pulmonary hypertension and cardiac valve abnormalities.*

### *Investigational Anti-obesity Agents*

- A number of anti-obesity agents with novel mechanisms of action are at different phases of clinical trials. These include appetite suppressants that target the neurotransmitters neuropeptide Y and the agouti-related protein; selective $\beta_3$-adrenergic receptor agonists to increase energy expenditure and fat mobilization via lipolysis; inhibitors of fat digestion and absorption; and nutrient partitioning to favor lean body mass.
- Recent clinical trials using **leptin**, a fat-derived hormone that acts on the hypothalamus to suppress food intake, have yielded only modest weight loss in obese subjects. However, leptin has been shown to be highly effective in a handful of cases of human obesity characterized by leptin deficiency due to genetic mutation.

### *Surgical Choices – Bariatric Surgery*

Other obesity treatment options include bariatric surgery which is usually reserved for people with class 3 obesity (BMI $\geq$ 40 kg/m$^2$). The large scale, prospective, randomized Swedish Obesity Study[1], still under way, has provided encouraging interim data to suggest that weight reduction following bariatric surgery reduced the 2-year incidence of diabetes, hypertension and other health risks by 3- to 32-fold.

## Therapeutic tips

- Assess the patient's readiness for change and focus on successes rather than on failures.
- Aim is to reduce weight for health and not for cosmetic reasons. The recommended rate of weight loss is 1 to 2 kg per month.
- Develop a nutrition program that people can follow over the long term to maintain body weight at a desirable level.
- In addition to being medically safe, any program involving physical activity should be enjoyable, convenient, realistic and structured.
- Physical activity is beneficial for all ages, but as a sole treatment for obesity has only modest effect, with an average weight loss of 0.1 kg/week based on the results of meta-analyses.
- It takes only a few minutes to eat a medium-sized apple or to drink an 8-oz. soft drink, but requires 20 minutes of brisk walking (6 km/h) to consume the 100 kcal ingested.

[1] *Obesity Res 1999;7:477–484.*

- Gradual increments in physical activity are easier to achieve and sustain.
- Even low intensity forms of physical activity are effective in reducing abdominal fat and ameliorating the associated insulin resistance and dyslipidemia.
- Encourage patient to enlist support from peers, spouse and relatives.
- Note: At present there is no evidence that weight loss achieved pharmacologically results in reduced fatal or nonfatal cardiovascular events.

## Suggested Reading List


Clinical guidelines on the identification, evaluation, and treatment of overweight and obesity in adults – the evidence report. *Obes Res* 1998;6(suppl 2):51S–209S.

Guidelines for the approval and use of drugs to treat obesity. A position paper of the North American Association for the Study of Obesity. *Obes Res* 1995;3:473–478.

Lau DCW. Call for action: preventing and managing the expansive and expensive obesity epidemic. *Can Med Assoc J* 1999;160:503–506.

Macdonald SM, Reeder BA, Chen Y, et al. Obesity in Canada: a descriptive analysis. *Can Med Assoc J* 1997;157(1 suppl): S3-S9.

*Obesity. Preventing and managing the global epidemic. Report of a WHO consultation on obesity*. Geneva: World Health Organization, 1998:1–276.

Rabkin S, Chen Y, Leiter LA, et al. Risk factor correlates of body mass index. *Can Med Assoc J* 1997;157(1 suppl):S26–S31.

Willett WC, Dietz WH, Colditz GA. Primary care: guidelines for healthy weight. *N Engl J Med* 1999;341:427–434.

CHAPTER 100

# Eating Disorders

*C. Laird Birmingham, MD, MHSc, FRCPC and*
*Elliot M. Goldner, MD, MHSc, FRCPC*

A disturbance of perception of body image and weight is an essential feature of both anorexia nervosa and bulimia nervosa.

**Anorexia nervosa** is characterized by a refusal to maintain minimally normal body weight. The two subtypes, *restricting* and *binge-eating/purging*, indicate the presence or absence of regular binge eating or purging during the current episode.

**Bulimia nervosa** is characterized by repeated episodes of binge eating followed by inappropriate compensatory behaviors such as self-induced vomiting, misuse of laxatives, diuretics or other medications, fasting or excessive exercise. The two subtypes are *purging* and *nonpurging* (uses inappropriate compensatory behaviors, e.g., fasting or excessive exercise but has not regularly engaged in self-induced vomiting, misuse of laxatives, etc., during the current episode).

## Goals of Therapy

- To assess and treat coexistent deficiencies
- To improve cognitive and emotional function
- To uncover and treat psychiatric comorbidity (e.g., anxiety, depression, family dysfunction, suicidal ideation)
- To develop healthy eating habits
- To treat binge and purge behavior (coexistent in 50% of patients with anorexia nervosa)
- For anorexia nervosa (in addition to above), to achieve a healthy weight (total body fat)

## Investigations

- A thorough history with special attention to:
  - weight, eating habits, binge and purge behavior, menstruation, body image, use of vomiting, laxatives, suppositories, diuretics, ipecac, fasting, and overexercising
  - developmental and psychological history
  - depression, anxiety, suicidal ideation, family dysfunction and sexual abuse
  - symptoms of malnutrition including chest pain, palpitations, seizures, abdominal pain, muscle weakness and cramping
  - dietary history

Figure 1: **Management of Anorexia Nervosa**

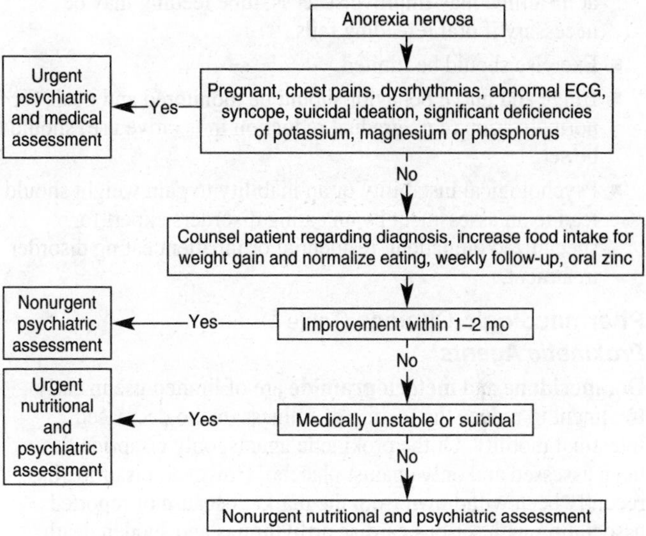
Anorexia nervosa
Pregnant, chest pains, dysrhythmias, abnormal ECG, syncope, suicidal ideation, significant deficiencies of potassium, magnesium or phosphorus
Yes
Urgent psychiatric and medical assessment
No
Counsel patient regarding diagnosis, increase food intake for weight gain and normalize eating, weekly follow-up, oral zinc
Improvement within 1–2 mo
Yes
Nonurgent psychiatric assessment
No
Medically unstable or suicidal
Yes
Urgent nutritional and psychiatric assessment
No
Nonurgent nutritional and psychiatric assessment

- Physical examination for parotid hypertrophy, edema, abnormal dentition; for anorexia nervosa (in addition to above), postural hypotension, heart rate, lanugo hair, hypercarotenemia, height, weight, measurements of body fat, neuromuscular hyperirritability (Chvostek's and Trousseau's signs)
- Laboratory tests:
  – sodium, potassium, chloride, bicarbonate, creatinine, magnesium, calcium, phosphorus, zinc, $B_{12}$, ferritin
  – for anorexia nervosa (in addition to above), ECG, hemoglobin, WBC count, urinalysis, RBC, folate
- For anorexia nervosa, a psychiatric and nutritional assessment if symptoms continue and weight does not normalize after weekly follow-up and counseling

## *Anorexia Nervosa*

### Therapeutic Choices (Figure 1)

#### Nonpharmacologic Choices

- A rapport and therapeutic alliance should be developed and maintained.
- The need for and role of family intervention and treatment should be considered.
- Nutrition should be normalized by setting and maintaining eating goals.

- Nutritional supplements should be used to achieve weight gain if not possible through food. Supportive nursing care at mealtime may improve success; tube feeding may be necessary if oral refeeding fails.
- Exercise should be limited.
- Binge and purge behavior should be monitored and goals for normalization (e.g., gradual reduction in laxative use) should be set.
- Psychological instability or an inability to gain weight should lead to an assessment by an eating disorders expert for specialized outpatient, residential or inpatient eating disorder treatment.

## Pharmacologic Choices (Table 1)

### *Prokinetic Agents*

**Domperidone** and **metoclopramide** are of limited use in early treatment to reduce the feeling of fullness due to decreased intestinal motility. Of the prokinetic agents, only cisapride has been assessed and only against placebo. However, cisapride has recently been withdrawn from the market because of reported association with serious cardiac arrhythmias and sudden death. At present domperidone should be used when effective.

### *Others*

**Anxiolytics** (e.g., clonazepam) should be used for severe anxiety; their use should be minimized due to the potential for dependence. Initiate clonazepam at 0.5 to 1 mg BID and cautiously titrate upward to a maximum dose of 20 mg per day, no more than every 3 days.

**Antidepressants** should be used for coexistent depression (Chapter 5) or purge behavior only, and **only** when cardiac status is stable (no cardiac chest pain, dysrhythmia or abnormal ECG).

**Cyproheptadine** can be tried, particularly in chronic anorexia, to facilitate weight gain.

Oral **zinc supplementation**[1] improves the chance of weight gain irrespective of serum zinc level. Zinc gluconate 100 mg daily for 2 months should be tried.

## Therapeutic Tips

- Normalization of body fat is necessary for psychological treatment to be effective and for cure.
- Treatment refusal is common. A careful reassessment of the treatment plan is necessary.
- Family therapy is an important adjunct to the treatment of children and adolescents.

[1] *Int J Eat Disord 1994;3:251–255.*

Table 1: **Drugs Used in Anorexia Nervosa**

| Drug | Dosage | Adverse Effects | Drug Interactions | Cost* |
|---|---|---|---|---|
| **Prokinetic Agents**† | | Diarrhea, abdominal discomfort, hyperprolactinemia. Drowsiness, restlessness (with metoclopramide). | Metoclopramide: avoid alcohol and other CNS depressants (additive sedative effects). | |
| *domperidone* Motilium, generics | 10–30 mg 1/2H AC | | | $–$$ |
| *metoclopramide* ◗ Maxeran, Reglan, generics | 5–20 mg 1/2H AC | | | $ |
| *cyproheptadine* Periactin | 4–16 mg QHS | Drowsiness (usual), dry mouth (common). | MAOIs; additive effect with other sedatives. | $–$$ |

◗ *Dosage adjustment may be required in renal impairment – see Appendix I.*
*Abbreviations: MAOIs = monoamine oxidase inhibitors; AC = before meals.*
** Cost of 30-day supply – includes drug cost only.*
*Legend: $ < $25 $$ $25–50*

† *Cisapride (Prepulsid) was withdrawn from the market in August 2000 because of reported association with cardiac arrhythmias and sudden cardiac death.*

Figure 2: **Management of Bulimia Nervosa**

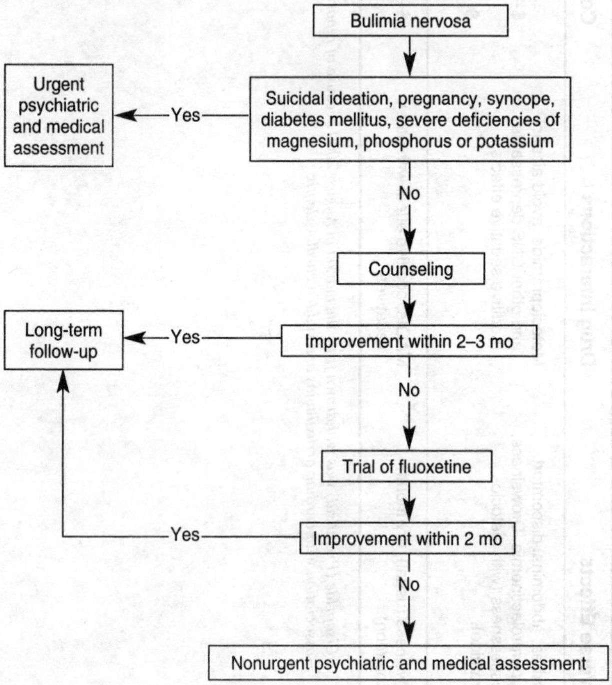
Bulimia nervosa
Suicidal ideation, pregnancy, syncope, diabetes mellitus, severe deficiencies of magnesium, phosphorus or potassium
Yes
Urgent psychiatric and medical assessment
No
Counseling
Improvement within 2–3 mo
Yes
Long-term follow-up
No
Trial of fluoxetine
Improvement within 2 mo
Yes
No
Nonurgent psychiatric and medical assessment

## *Bulimia Nervosa*

### Therapeutic Choices (Figure 2)

### Nonpharmacologic Choices

- Counseling on normal eating behavior and cognitive and emotional issues should be provided and progress followed.
- Patients should be assessed for suicidal ideation and depression; these should be treated if present.
- Psychoeducational groups addressing nutritional and psychological issues can enhance individual therapy.

### Pharmacologic Choices (Table 2)

#### *Antidepressants*

A number of antidepressants have shown some effectiveness in decreasing binge and purge behavior; the only agent currently approved as an antibulimic in Canada is **fluoxetine**.

**Fluoxetine, imipramine, desipramine, phenelzine** and **trazodone** all decrease binge and purge symptoms and may treat concurrent depression. Other SSRIs may be tried after failing

Table 2: **Drugs Used in Bulimia Nervosa**

| Drug | Dosage | Adverse Effects | Drug Interactions | Cost* |
|---|---|---|---|---|
| *fluoxetine* Prozac, generics | 20–60 mg daily<br>(H): ↓ dose | Anxiety, GI discomfort (common).<br>Fluoxetine – less anticholinergic effect than TCAs.<br>Limited experience with fluoxetine overdose indicates that overdose symptoms are mild and usually well tolerated. | Avoid use with MAOIs, L-tryptophan (serotonin syndrome); TCA plasma levels may ↑ therefore decrease TCA dose.<br>Phenytoin serum levels may ↑, monitor. | $$–$$$$ |
| *desipramine* ◗ Norpramin, generics | 50–250 mg daily<br>(H): Use with caution | Anticholinergic effects (e.g., postural hypotension, dizziness, dry mouth, constipation, urinary retention).<br>May prolong cardiac conduction and worsen cardiac dysrhythmias. | Avoid use with clonidine and sympathomimetics.<br>Use extreme caution in combination with MAOIs. | $–$$$ |
| *imipramine* ◗ Tofranil, generics | 50–250 mg daily<br>(H): Use with caution | | | $ |
| *trazodone* Desyrel, generics | 100–500 mg daily in single or divided doses<br>(H): Use with caution | Sedation (common), anticholinergic adverse effects less common than with TCAs. | Avoid use with MAOIs. | $–$$$ |
| *phenelzine* Nardil | 15–75 mg daily in divided doses<br>(H): ↓ dose | Orthostatic hypotension, common and sometimes severe, usually subsides by the fourth week of treatment.<br>Hypertension is uncommon with usual doses and in the absence of drug–food interactions.<br>Drowsiness, dizziness (common). | Avoid use with amphetamines, clomipramine, imipramine, levodopa, meperidine, sumatriptan, sympathomimetics, L-tryptophan. | $–$$ |

◗ *Dosage adjustment may be required in renal impairment – see Appendix I.*
*(H) Dosage adjustment in hepatic impairment.*
*Abbreviations: TCAs = tricyclic antidepressants; MAOIs = monoamine oxidase inhibitors; AC = before meals.*

** Cost of 30-day supply – includes drug cost only.*
*Legend: $ < $25  $$ $25–50  $$$ $50–75  $$$$ $75–100*

one of these agents. Therapy should be maintained for at least 6 months; the usual recommendation is 1 year.

If symptoms persist after a trial of counseling and fluoxetine, treatment by a multidisciplinary team may be necessary.

## Therapeutic Tips

- Antidepressants should be continued for 6 to 12 months if effective. If treatment with one antidepressant fails, another can be tried.
- Cotreatment with more than one antidepressant has no proven advantage and has the potential to increase adverse effects and cost.
- Often during psychological treatment or with significant life stress, a temporary worsening of binge and purge behavior occurs. This does not indicate a worsening in the patient's overall condition.
- Treatment of psychiatric comorbidity is necessary for long-term cure.

## *Suggested Reading List*

Becker AE, Grinspoon SK, Klibanski A, Herzog DB. Eating disorders. *N Engl J Med* 1999;340:1092–1098.

Goldner EM, Birmingham CL. Anorexia nervosa: methods of treatment. In: Mott LA, Lumsden DB, eds. *Understanding eating disorders*. Washington: Taylor and Francis International Publishers, 1994:135–158.

Goldner EM, Birmingham CL, Smye V. Addressing treatment refusal in anorexia nervosa: Clinical, ethical and legal considerations. In: Garner D, Garfinkel PE, eds. *Handbook of treatment for eating disorders*. New York: Guilford Publications, 1997:450–461.

Kim-Sing A, Birmingham CL. Clinical use of magnesium supplementation. *Can J Hosp Pharm* 1990;43(4):161–195.

Leung M, Birmingham CL. The management of anorexia nervosa and bulimia nervosa. *Pharmacy Practice* 1997;13:62–72.

CHAPTER 101

# Chemotherapy-induced Nausea and Vomiting

*Lynne Nakashima, PharmD*

## Goals of Therapy

- To prevent *acute* (starting within 24 hours of chemotherapy), *delayed* (starting > 24 hours after chemotherapy) and *anticipatory* (starting before chemotherapy as a conditioned response) nausea and vomiting to ensure patient compliance with active treatment and to maintain quality of life
- To decrease incidence of nausea and vomiting (once it has occurred) and maintain patient comfort
- To prevent complications (esophageal tears, dehydration, anorexia, malnutrition, weight loss, pathological bone fractures, metabolic alkalosis, chloride and potassium depletion)

## Investigations

- A thorough history including:
  - onset and duration of symptoms
  - timing of nausea and/or retching and/or vomiting
  - description of the vomiting episodes
  - medications the patient is taking
- Physical examination with particular attention to:
  - orthostatic hypotension
  - abdominal pain, distention, constipation, hemorrhage
  - neurologic assessment including cranial nerves, vestibular and pupillary function, extrapyramidal signs
- Laboratory tests:
  - electrolytes: BUN, creatinine, sodium, potassium, chloride (to assess hydration status); calcium, albumin (to assess for hypercalcemia)
  - drug screening, such as for digoxin if suspected as a cause of nausea and vomiting

Although medication is the most likely cause of nausea and vomiting in a patient receiving chemotherapy, other potential causes (e.g., fluid/electrolyte abnormalities, bowel obstruction, central nervous system or hepatic metastases, infections and radiation therapy) should be ruled out. Other drugs (e.g., narcotics, digoxin, antibiotics) may cause or exacerbate nausea and vomiting so a thorough medication history is essential. Some chemotherapeutic agents are more likely to cause nausea and

Table 1: **Emetogenic Potential of Chemotherapy Agents**

| | | |
|---|---|---|
| **High (> 60%)** | | |
| carboplatin | cytarabine (> 500 mg/m$^2$) | lomustine |
| carmustine | dacarbazine | mechlorethamine |
| cisplatin (> 50 mg/m$^2$) | dactinomycin (> 1.5 mg/m$^2$) | streptozocin |
| cyclophosphamide (> 550 mg/m$^2$) | | |
| **Moderate (30–60%)** | | |
| aldesleukin | epirubicin | methotrexate |
| cisplatin (< 50 mg/m$^2$) | idarubicin | mitomycin |
| daunorubicin | ifosfamide | mitoxantrone |
| doxorubicin | irinotecan | procarbazine |
| **Low (< 30%)** | | |
| altretamine | estramustine | progestins |
| aminoglutethimide | estrogens | ralitrexed |
| amsacrine | etoposide | 6-thioguanine |
| anastrozole | fludarabine | tamoxifen |
| androgens | 5-fluorouracil | teniposide |
| L-asparaginase | gemcitabine | thiotepa |
| bleomycin | hydroxyurea | topotecan |
| busulfan | letrozole | vinblastine |
| chlorambucil | melphalan (oral) | vincristine |
| cladribine | mercaptopurine | vindesine |
| docetaxel | paclitaxel | vinorelbine |

vomiting than others (Table 1). Therefore it is important to consider both the emetogenic potential and the expected pattern of emesis of the chemotherapy regimen when choosing antiemetics.

Patient-specific factors such as age less than 50 years, female gender, previous motion sickness or pregnancy-related nausea and vomiting, limited alcohol use and nausea and vomiting with previous chemotherapy regimens may predispose the patient to nausea and vomiting; therefore, antiemetic regimens must also be tailored to the individual patient.

## Therapeutic Choices (Figure 1)

### Nonpharmacologic Choices

- Dietary adjustments
  - try small, light meals several times daily.
  - avoid foods high in fat or those with a heavy aroma.
  - try dry, starchy foods such as crackers.
  - if unable to tolerate solid foods, try ice chips and small sips of clear liquids.
  - avoid food preparation because the smell of food cooking often worsens nausea.

- Behavioral methods
  - relaxation techniques may help decrease physiologic arousal and anxiety.
  - individualized exercise programs may help decrease anxiety and depression.
  - systemic desensitization may be helpful for anticipatory nausea and vomiting.
- Other
  - keep movement to a minimum; rest in bed or a chair to avoid vestibular stimulation.
  - acupuncture and acupressure have been shown to have some effect on chemotherapy-induced emesis.
  - sleep has been shown to protect against chemotherapy-induced nausea and vomiting.

## Pharmacologic Choices (Figure 1 and Table 2)

### *Phenothiazines*

The most commonly used are **prochlorperazine** and **perphenazine**. Considered moderately effective, they are usually used in low emetogenic regimens or as rescue medication. The availability of a wide variety of dosage forms (tablet, suppository, injectable) facilitates prochlorperazine use, especially for outpatients.

### *Metoclopramide*

Metoclopramide blocks the dopaminergic receptors in the chemoreceptor trigger zone and has serotonin antagonistic activity at higher doses. Low doses (10 to 20 mg) are generally as effective as prochlorperazine; however, in high doses (1 to 3 mg/kg), metoclopramide provides significantly greater antiemetic activity. When compared to serotonin antagonists for acute antiemetic efficacy against highly emetogenic chemotherapy, serotonin antagonists are superior and have fewer side effects. For delayed nausea and vomiting, metoclopramide plus a corticosteroid are as effective as a serotonin antagonist plus a corticosteroid and more cost-effective. One limitation is the development of extrapyramidal side effects; diphenhydramine, 25 to 50 mg, should be administered prophylactically to all patients receiving metoclopramide doses ≥ 20 mg PO Q6H.

### *Corticosteroids*

**Dexamethasone** is the most commonly used, although several others including **methylprednisolone** have been studied. The actual mechanism of action is unknown, but the efficacy of corticosteroids is documented. They appear to be effective as single agents, in combination with other antiemetics and for delayed nausea and vomiting. Dexamethasone in combination *with a serotonin antagonist* is the most effective antiemetic

Figure 1: **Management of Nausea and Vomiting Due to Chemotherapy**

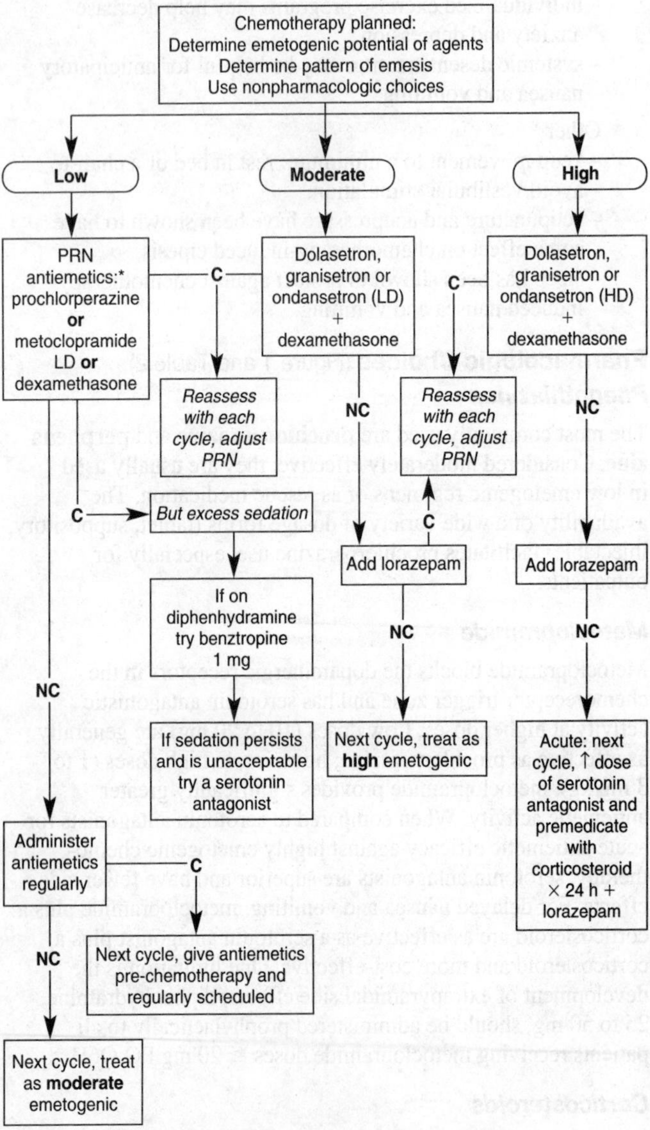
Chemotherapy planned:
Determine emetogenic potential of agents
Determine pattern of emesis
Use nonpharmacologic choices
Low
Moderate
High
PRN antiemetics:* prochlorperazine or metoclopramide LD or dexamethasone
C
Dolasetron, granisetron or ondansetron (LD) + dexamethasone
C
Dolasetron, granisetron or ondansetron (HD) + dexamethasone
Reassess with each cycle, adjust PRN
NC
Reassess with each cycle, adjust PRN
NC
C
But excess sedation
C
Add lorazepam
Add lorazepam
If on diphenhydramine try benztropine 1 mg
NC
NC
NC
If sedation persists and is unacceptable try a serotonin antagonist
Next cycle, treat as high emetogenic
Acute: next cycle, ↑ dose of serotonin antagonist and premedicate with corticosteroid × 24 h + lorazepam
Administer antiemetics regularly
C
NC
Next cycle, give antiemetics pre-chemotherapy and regularly scheduled
Next cycle, treat as moderate emetogenic

*** Add diphenhydramine** *25–50 mg PO with metoclopramide dose.*

*Abbreviations: C = controlled; NC = not controlled; CT = chemotherapy.*

***Doses:***

***Dexamethasone** 10 mg PO/IV pre and 4–8 mg Q12H.*

***Lorazepam** 1 mg S/L pre and Q4H PRN.*

***Ondansetron**: LD (low dose) 8 mg PO/IV pre CT;*
*HD (high dose) 16–32 mg PO/IV pre CT.*

***Metoclopramide:** LD (low dose) 10–20 mg Q6H.*

regimen for *acute nausea and vomiting*. Dexamethasone *alone or in combination with* ***metoclopramide*** appears to be the most effective regimen for *delayed nausea and vomiting*. The optimal dose has not been identified; the usual range is from 4 to 60 mg daily.

### *Serotonin Antagonists*

The serotonin antagonists, **dolasetron**, **granisetron** and **ondansetron** are equivalent in efficacy and toxicity. Single agent efficacy is reported, but in combination with corticosteroids, efficacy is improved and the 2-drug regimen is recommended unless the patient has a contraindication to corticosteroids.[1,2] Serotonin antagonists plus corticosteroids are reported to be no more effective for delayed nausea and vomiting than metoclopramide plus corticosteroids or corticosteroids alone.[3,4] These drugs are well tolerated. The major drawback to their use is cost. However, because of their superior efficacy, serotonin antagonists should be used for the prophylaxis of acute nausea and vomiting for moderate and highly emetogenic regimens. The choice of serotonin antagonist should be based on cost.

### *Benzodiazepines*

Benzodiazepines provide useful antianxiety, amnesic and sedating effects. **Lorazepam** is the most commonly used, usually in combination with other antiemetics.

### *Butyrophenones*

**Haloperidol** and **droperidol** have reported efficacy and are generally used as alternatives to high-dose metoclopramide or ondansetron in refractory nausea and vomiting.

### *Cannabinoids*

**Nabilone** and **dronabinol** are of limited use because they are available only as oral formulations and are associated with several side effects including mood alterations, hallucinations, delusions and increases in heart rate and blood pressure. They are generally used in refractory nausea and vomiting or in combination with other antiemetics.

### *Dimenhydrinate*

An antihistamine useful for treating vomiting due to motion sickness, it is considered no more effective than placebo against chemotherapy-induced nausea and vomiting.

---

[1] *J Clin Oncol 1991;9:675–678.*
[2] *Eur J Cancer 1993;29A (Suppl).*
[3] *Cancer 1995;76:1821–1828.*
[4] *J Clin Oncol 1995;13:2417–2426.*

Table 2: **Drugs Used for Chemotherapy-induced Nausea and Vomiting**

| Drug | Dosage | Adverse Effects | Drug Interactions | Cost* |
|---|---|---|---|---|
| **Benzodiazepines** | | Sedation (up to 80%). | Sedating medications.† | |
| *lorazepam* Ativan, generics | 1 mg PO/SL pre CT, then 1–4 mg Q4H PRN | | | $ |
| **Butyrophenones** | | Sedation, extrapyramidal effects. | Sedating medications.† | |
| *haloperidol* Haldol, generics | Haloperidol:1–2 mg PO/IM pre CT and Q8H | | | $ |
| *droperidol* generics | Droperidol: 0.5–1 mg IV pre CT and Q4H | | | $ |
| **Cannabinoids** | | Sedation (4–89%), dizziness, ataxia (12–65%), psychotropic effects ("high") (27%), tachycardia (7%), orthostatic hypotension (10%), dry mouth (6–62%). | Sedating medications.† | |
| *nabilone* Cesamet | 1 mg PO BID | | | $ |
| *dronabinol* Marinol | 5 mg/m² PO Q2–4H Max: 6 doses/d. May ↑ by 2.5 mg/m² to max 10 mg /m²/dose | | | $$$–$$$$$ |
| **Corticosteroids** | | Mood changes, increased appetite, GI irritation, ulceration, fluid retention, weight gain, may mask signs of infection. | | |
| *dexamethasone* Decadron, Dexasone | 4–10 mg PO pre CT and Q6–12H<br>8–20 mg IV pre CT and Q6–12H | | | PO: $<br>IV: $–$$$ |
| *methylprednisolone* Medrol Solu-Medrol, generics | 0.5–1 mg/kg PO or IV pre CT and Q4 and 8H post CT (max: 4 mg/kg total dose).<br>May also give as single 4 mg/kg dose 30 min pre CT | | | PO: $<br>IV: $–$$ |

| | | | | |
|---|---|---|---|---|
| *metoclopramide*<br>Maxeran, Reglan, generics | Low: 10–20 mg PO Q6H<br>High: 1–3 mg/kg PO/IV Q3H | Sedation (up to 80%), dose-related diarrhea (up to 45%), extrapyramidal effects (3%). | | $–$$$$$ |
| **Phenothiazines** | | Sedation, anticholinergic effects (dry mouth, blurred vision, constipation, nasal congestion, urinary retention), extrapyramidal effects, hypotension, hypersensitivity (1.4%), rare pancytopenia. | Sedating medications.† | |
| *prochlorperazine*<br>Stemetil, generics | Prochlorperazine: 10 mg Q6H | | | $ |
| *perphenazine*<br>Trilafon, generics | Perphenazine: 2–4 mg Q8H | | | $ |
| **Serotonin Antagonists** | | Headache (6–43%) constipation (4–19%), diarrhea (1–16%), sedation (4–10%), transient ↑ in LFTs (< 1–19%), bradycardia (4%), dizziness (3%). | | |
| *dolasetron*<br>Anzemet | 1.8 mg/kg IV pre CT or 100 mg PO pre CT | | | PO: $$<br>IV: $ |
| *granisetron*<br>Kytril | 10 μg/kg IV or 2 mg PO pre CT or 1 mg pre CT and 12 h post | | | PO: $$$<br>IV: $$$$$ |
| *ondansetron*<br>Zofran | low: 8 mg PO/IV pre CT<br>high: 16–32 mg PO/IV pre CT | | | IV and PO: $$–$$$$$ |

† *Additive sedation occurs with, for example, narcotic analgesics, hypnotics, alcohol; avoid or minimize use if possible.*

*Abbreviations: LFTs = liver function tests; CT = chemotherapy.*

*Dosage adjustment may be required in renal impairment – see Appendix I.*

* *Cost per day – includes drug cost only.*

*Legend: $ < $15 $$ $15–30 $$$ $30–45 $$$$ $45–60 $$$$$ > $60*

### *Scopolamine*

Available as a transdermal system placed behind the ear, scopolamine can prevent vomiting related to motion sickness but is generally ineffective in managing nausea and vomiting associated with chemotherapy.

### *Propofol*

Propofol is an anesthetic agent with antiemetic properties. Studies suggest that a continuous infusion at low doses (1 mg/kg/hour) is effective in patients with cisplatin-induced nausea and vomiting that is refractory to serotonin antagonists combined with corticosteroids.[5–7] Its use is still considered investigational; however, propofol use may be considered in severe, refractory vomiting.

## Therapeutic Tips

- Use antiemetic therapy to *prevent* anticipatory nausea and vomiting, which usually worsens with each cycle; up to 30% of patients refuse further chemotherapy because of intolerable nausea and vomiting.
- *Regularly scheduled and administered* antiemetics (i.e., not PRN) are more effective at preventing nausea and vomiting.
- If the patient can tolerate oral antiemetics, this is the recommended route of administration. However, *rectally* administered antiemetics such as prochlorperazine are especially useful in patients who are vomiting or unable to take oral medications and who are at home. For hospitalized patients, the *IV route* of administration is recommended in patients who are vomiting.

## Pharmacoeconomic Considerations

*Jeffrey A Johnson, PhD*

Despite the higher acquisition costs, pharmacoeconomic evaluations suggest that the serotonin antagonists are more cost-effective than metoclopramide in the prevention of acute nausea and vomiting associated with highly emetogenic chemotherapy. Overall cost-savings may be achieved through a reduction in hospital bed days and other costs associated with the management of nausea and vomiting (e.g., nursing time and material costs). Furthermore, the combination of ondansetron and dexamethasone has been shown to be more cost-effective than ondansetron monotherapy in controlling

[5] *Can J Anaesth 1992;39:170–172.*
[6] *Oncology 1993;50:456–459.*
[7] *Anaesth Analg 1992;74:539–541.*

emesis. Pharmacoeconomic evaluations that compare ondansetron with granisetron have generally indicated that granisetron is a more cost-effective choice, depending on the ondansetron dosage regimen that is compared. When compared to a single 8 mg IV dose of ondansetron, IV granisetron is less cost-effective. Pharmacoeconomic evaluations of the less expensive oral granisetron and dolasetron have not been conducted.

For delayed nausea and vomiting, there is no evidence that the serotonin antagonists are more effective than the less expensive combination of metoclopramide plus dexamethasone, therefore implying that the cheaper therapy is more cost-effective.

***Suggested Reading***

*Stewart DJ, Dahrouge S, Coyle D, Evans WK. Costs of treating and preventing nausea and vomiting in patients receiving chemotherapy. J Clin Oncol 1999;17:344–351.*

*Plosker GL, Milne RJ. Ondansetron: a pharmacoeconomic and quality-of-life evaluation of its antiemetic activity in patients receiving cancer chemotherapy. PharmacoEconomics 1992;2:285–304.*

*Plosker GL, Benfield P. Granisetron. A pharmacoeconomic evaluation of its use in the prophylaxis of chemotherapy-induced nausea and vomiting. PharmacoEconomics 1996;9;357–374.*

*Johnson N, Bosanquet N. Cost-effectiveness of 5-hydroxytryptamine receptor antagonists: a retrospective comparison of ondansetron and granisetron. Anticancer Drugs 1995;6:243–249.*

## Suggested Reading List

American Society of Health-System Pharmacists. ASHP therapeutic guidelines on the pharmacologic management of nausea and vomiting in adult and pediatric patients receiving chemotherapy or radiation therapy or undergoing surgery. *Am J Health-System Pharm* 1999;56:729–764.

Gandara DR, Roila F, Warr D, et al. Consensus proposal for 5HT3 antagonists in the prevention of acute emesis related to highly emetogenic chemotherapy. *Support Care Cancer* 1998;6:237–243.

Gregory RE, Ettinger DS. 5HT3 receptor antagonists for the prevention of chemotherapy-induced nausea and vomiting. *Drugs* 1998;53(2):173–189.

Hesketh PJ, Kris MG, Grunberg SM, et al. Proposal for classifying the acute emetogenicity of cancer chemotherapy. *J Clin Oncol* 1997;15:103–109.

National Comprehensive Cancer Network. NCCN antiemesis practice guidelines. *Oncology* 1997;11:57–89.

CHAPTER 102

# Prevention and Treatment of Side Effects of Antineoplastics

*Louis A. Fernandez, MD, FACP, FRCPC*

## Goals of Therapy

- To recognize and provide optimal management of chemotherapy-induced side effects in order to deliver 100% of the recommended dose with curative intent

## Side Effects of Chemotherapy

***Acute*** (Table 1)

- Extravasation
- Thrombophlebitis
- Hypersensitivity reactions
- Rapid tumor lysis syndrome
- Nausea and vomiting (Chapter 101)

***Chronic, Organ-Specific*** (Table 2)

- Skin
- Bone marrow
- Heart
- Lungs
- Nervous system
- Gastrointestinal
- Liver
- Kidneys
- Gonads
- Eyes

## Conclusions

The number of side effects that may occur in a patient is formidable, yet many can be prevented, others are spontaneously reversible and some are treatable. For example, amifostine is a cytoprotective agent which reduces hematologic (anemia, leukopenia, thrombocytopenia) and nonhematologic (mucositis, xerostomia, loss of taste) toxicity in patients treated with antineoplastic agents. In spite of the potential side effects, many patients are able to take most types of chemotherapy in the hope of "cure" or long-term disease-free survival. The ideal chemotherapeutic regimen would be effective if given orally and have no side effects; obviously, we are a long way from the ideal. Researchers have therefore moved their attention to developing biological response modifiers in the hope of controlling malignancies.

Table 1: **Acute Side Effects of Antineoplastic Drugs**

| Acute Side Effect | Investigation(s) | Management | Prevention |
|---|---|---|---|
| **Extravasation**<br>Vesicant drugs:<br>Dactinomycin<br>Daunorubicin<br>Doxorubicin<br>Epirubicin<br>Idarubicin<br>Mechlorethamine<br>Mitomycin<br>Plicamycin<br>Streptozocin<br>Vinblastine<br>Vincristine<br>Vindesine<br>Vinorelbine | Diagnose clinically; burning at the site of infusion. | Stop infusion immediately.<br>Measures such as application of ice, heat, local steroids, IV steroids may provide patient comfort. | Do not insert an IV needle or catheter in the dorsum of the hand or cubital fossa; extravasation in these areas may cause serious damage to tendons.<br>Always try to insert IV lines distally; if unsuccessful move to a proximal site to ensure there is no puncture site proximal to where the IV is finally placed.<br>Do not use force when giving vesicant drugs by IV push.<br>When accessing a Port-A-Cath, be sure that the Huber needle is in the Port-A-Cath receptacle. |
| **Thrombophlebitis** | None specific; diagnosed clinically. | Infuse offending drug slowly. | Peripheral veins may be protected by placing central lines. |
| **Hypersensitivity Reactions**<br>Seen frequently with rituximab (28%) paclitaxel (10%), l-asparaginase (20%) | None helpful.<br>Mechanism of hypersensitivity reactions is unpredictable.<br>Circulating lymphoma cells associated with rituximab reaction. | Stop infusion.<br>Intravascular volume expansion with saline.<br>Administer *steroids.* | When the offending agent is used in future, premedication with *steroids* and *antihistamines* may prevent anaphylaxis.<br>*Erwinia-derived source of l-asparaginase* (not commercially available) may be substituted for *E. coli*-derived source (some cross reactivity) or use *pegaspargase*, a modified form of l-asparaginase which does not cross react. |

*(cont'd)*

Table 1: **Acute Side Effects of Antineoplastic Drugs** *(cont'd)*

| Acute Side Effect | Investigation(s) | Management | Prevention |
|---|---|---|---|
| **Rapid Tumor Lysis Syndrome**<br>Occurs when large numbers of tumor cells are lysed rapidly by chemotherapy.<br>Symptoms are malaise, tetany, oliguria, fluid overload, arrhythmia. | Biochemical profile shows ↓ calcium and ↑ serum phosphate, potassium and uric acid.<br>ECG may show QT interval prolongation. | IV hydration to maintain urine output > 3 L/24 h.<br>Alkalinize urine to pH 7.<br>*Allopurinol* 600 mg/d beginning 24–48 h before chemotherapy for 2–3 d, then 300 mg/d until uric acid levels normal.<br>If metabolic derangements occur, hemodialysis may be needed. | |

Table 2: **Organ-specific Side Effects**

| Organ/System | Goal(s) | Management | Prevention |
|---|---|---|---|
| **Skin/Appendages**<br>Alopecia<br>Nail changes<br>Dry skin<br>Pigmentation changes | Recognize changes in skin and its appendages secondary to chemotherapy. | Wig for alopecia.<br>Most changes in skin and its appendages return to normal after chemotherapy ceases. | Scalp tourniquet is not recommended, particularly for hematological neoplasms due to concerns re: safety and efficacy. |
| **Bone Marrow Suppression** | To titrate dose to avoid prolonged neutropenia and life-threatening thrombocytopenia.<br>To avoid anemia and/or development of myelodysplastic syndrome. | Absolute neutrophil count and platelet count (usually 10 d after chemotherapy) and CBC before next dose of chemotherapy.<br>Macrocytosis is commonly seen due to interference with DNA synthesis. Observe carefully for changes in red cell morphology (poikilocytosis, anisocytosis) that may foretell development of myelodysplastic syndrome.<br>For febrile neutropenia, use broad-spectrum antibiotics (Chapter 97).<br>Platelet transfusions for a platelet count $< 10 \times 10^9$/L if patient not bleeding.[2] If bleeding, transfuse if platelets are 30–40 $\times 10^9$/L.<br>Packed red blood cell transfusions or *erythropoietin* for anemia. | Dose intensity of chemotherapeutic agents causing myelosuppression can be ↑ approximately five-fold if supplemented by use of *granulocyte colony stimulating factor* (G-CSF) and approximately ten-fold if rescued by autologous bone marrow transplantation.[1] Neither survival nor mortality changes with use of G-CSF.<br>Although therapy is costly, prolonged and dangerous neutropenia can be avoided by prophylactic use of G-CSF (usual dose 5 µg/kg SC daily starting 48 to 72 h after chemotherapy and continuing for 10 d). |

[1]*Demetri G. Presented at ASH Satellite Symposium, St. Louis, Mo. Dec 3–7, 1993.*
[2]*Wandt H, et al. Blood 1998;91:3601–3606.*

*(cont'd)*

Table 2: **Organ-specific Side Effects** *(cont'd)*

| Organ/System | Goal(s) | Management | Prevention |
|---|---|---|---|
| **Cardiotoxicity** | Recognize that risk of congestive heart failure (CHF) is dose-related; 0.1% to 1.2% when the cumulative dose of **anthracyclines** is 550 mg/$m^2$, increasing to 50% at 1000 mg/$m^2$.<br>Other cardiac risk factors (if present), combination with other chemotherapeutic agents, monoclonal antibodies such as **trastuzumab** or mediastinal radiation may ↑ the risk of developing CHF. | Look for cardiac risk factors (i.e., hypertension and ischemic heart disease).<br>ECG, serial ejection fractions.<br>If arrhythmias occur during anthracycline infusion, there is no need to discontinue or ↓ the dose of anthracyclines. | *Dexrazoxane* (500 mg/$m^2$–30 min prior to administration of **doxorubicin**) protects against cardiomyopathy.<br>If serial ejection fraction ↓ by 25% from baseline, consider stopping anthracyclines. |
| **Pulmonary Toxicity** | Recognize toxicity and distinguish it from infection; pulmonary toxicity is commonly seen with **bleomycin**, **carmustine**, **cyclophosphamide** and **mitomycin**. | Sputum for Gram's stain, culture and sensitivity, chest x-ray, bronchial washings; possibly gallium scan and lung biopsy.<br>Rule out infections. | *Steroids* may be helpful if damage is due to hypersensitivity and should be given prophylactically when these drugs are used. |
| **Neurotoxicity** | Recognize that neurotoxicity will occur with **vinca alkaloids** and may present as peripheral neuropathy, ileitis, urinary retention, impotence and/or cranial neuropathy.<br>Chemical meningitis, myelopathy with paraplegia and/or leukoencephalopathy are more common with intrathecal administration. | Rule out other causes (e.g., metastatic involvement of the nervous, GI or urinary system).<br>With mild, stable level of toxicity, there is no need to discontinue the drug; however, increasing or severe toxicities mandate discontinuation. | |

| | | | |
|---|---|---|---|
| **Gastrointestinal Toxicity**<br>Mucositis<br>Nausea and vomiting (Chapter 101) | Recognize that mucositis occurs with drugs such as **doxorubicin, methotrexate**, **5-fluorouracil** and **bleomycin** and distinguish it from an infective process. | Rule out infection: swab for Gram's stain; bacterial, fungal, viral cultures.<br>For small ulcers apply *benzocaine in Orabase*.<br>For generalized mucositis, topical rinses such as *lidocaine viscous* (maximum 120 mL/24 h) or *Kaopectate mixed with diphenhydramine* may help; in severe cases pain is relieved by IV morphine.<br>Spicy, salty, acidic, hot, cold or rough foods should be avoided.<br>Caloric intake should be supplemented with milk shakes. If unable to swallow, the patient may be fed by gastric tube or *total parenteral nutrition*. | |
| **Hepatotoxicity** | Recognize that hepatotoxicity may occur with the nitrosoureas (e.g., **carmustine, lomustine**), **cytarabine**, **methotrexate**, **6-mercaptopurine**, **l-asparaginase**, **etoposide**, **plicamycin**, **streptozocin** and **azathioprine**. | Rule out other causes of hepatic damage.<br>No specific treatment; may have to discontinue drug depending upon the severity of liver damage.<br>Liver function tests including bilirubin. Liver biopsy may be needed. | |
| **Nephrotoxicity**<br>Uric acid nephropathy | Prevention, particularly if large number of tumor cells will be lysed. | Serum uric acid, creatinine and BUN. | ↑ hydration such that urine output is > 3 L/24 h.<br>Alkalinize urine to pH > 7.<br>*Allopurinol* 300–600 mg/d PO, 24–48 h before starting chemotherapy. |

(cont'd)

Table 2: **Organ-specific Side Effects** *(cont'd)*

| Organ/System | Goal(s) | Management | Prevention |
|---|---|---|---|
| Other nephrotoxicity | Recognize that drugs such as **cisplatin** and the **nitrosoureas** are nephrotoxic.<br>**Methotrexate** may precipitate in the kidney.<br>**Ifosfamide** and **cyclophosphamide** may cause hemorrhagic cystitis.<br>**Mitomycin** may cause a hemolytic–uremic syndrome. | Urinalysis.<br>Serum creatinine and BUN.<br>Red cell morphology for presence of schistocytes and disseminated intravascular coagulation screen if mitomycin is the offending agent. | The key to prevention of cisplatin-induced nephrotoxicity is hydration: give 2–3 L of *normal saline* IV over 8–12 h.<br>Prophylactic *magnesium supplements.*<br>Methotrexate precipitation may be avoided by ↑ diuresis and alkalinizing urine to pH > 7.<br>*Mesna* is used to prevent ifosfamide-induced hemorrhagic cystitis and may prevent cyclophosphamide-induced hemorrhagic cystitis; mesna should be given at 20% of the ifosfamide dose before and Q4H for 3–5 doses. Rigorous diuresis is also helpful. |
| **Ocular Toxicity** | Recognize effects:<br>**Effect** – **Drug**<br>Cataracts – Busulfan, corticosteroids<br>Optic neuritis – Cisplatin<br>Visual blurring – Cyclophosphamide<br>↑ lacrimation – Doxorubicin<br>Oculomotor palsies, cortical blindness – Vincristine<br>Conjunctivitis – Cytarabine, 5-fluorouracil, methotrexate, 2′-deoxycoformycin | Follow-up by ophthalmologist and may include CT scan of the brain to rule out cortical blindness.<br>Cataract surgery. | Prophylactic *steroid eye drops* may prevent conjunctivitis. |

| | | | |
|---|---|---|---|
| **Gonadal Toxicity** | Prevent sexual dysfunction and infertility. | Baseline sperm count, motility and reproductive hormone levels in males and females (to rule out primary infertility).<br>Assisted reproductive technology. | Sperm banking before chemotherapy and suppression of ovulation during chemotherapy.<br>Counseling against conception while on chemotherapy. |
| **Miscellaneous**<br>Myelodysplastic syndrome (MDS)<br>Secondary malignancy<br>Vascular complications vasospasm, Raynaud's, thromboembolism, cerebral ischemia | | Specific for each (e.g., bone marrow cytology and chromosomal abnormality for MDS).<br>Routine screening methods for diagnosing other malignancies, vascular problems.<br>Successful treatment of secondary MDS and malignancies by standard protocols is disappointing.<br>Standard guidelines for treatment of vascular complications. | |

## *Suggested Reading List*

Hoekman K, van der Vijgh WJF, Vermorken JB. Clinical and preclinical modulation of chemotherapy-induced toxicity in patients with cancer. *Drugs* 1999;57:133–135.

Perry MC, ed. *The chemotherapy source book.* 2nd ed. Baltimore: Williams & Wilkins, 1996.

Perry MC, Yarbro JW, eds. *Toxicity of chemotherapy*. Orlando: Gruenne & Stratton, 1984.

Principles of chemotherapy. In: DeVita VT, Hellman S, Rosenberg SA, eds. *Cancer: Principles and practice of oncology*. 5th ed. Philadelphia: J.B. Lippincott–Raven, 1997.

CHAPTER 103

# Nausea

*C. MacLean, MD, CCFP, FCFP*

Nausea is a common symptom that refers to the unpleasant sensation experienced prior to vomiting. It may be a "simple", transient symptom, secondary to a self-limited condition such as viral gastroenteritis, requiring only symptomatic relief. Nausea may also be a part of a more complex medical problem. Nausea is a symptom and not a diagnosis and the underlying cause should be determined (Table 1). Approaches to nausea and its treatment are dependent on the associated diagnosis (e.g., postoperative nausea and vomiting [PONV], chemotherapy-induced nausea [CIN], metabolic, gastrointestinal, vestibular or neurological causes). This chapter does not address nausea in children or its management in pregnancy (Appendix II). Chemotherapy-induced nausea is reviewed in Chapter 101.

## Goals of Therapy

- To diagnose and treat the underlying cause of the nausea
- To control nausea and provide patient comfort. (Nausea can be more distressing to some patients than actual vomiting.)
- To prevent the development of anticipatory nausea
- To balance the symptomatic treatment with possible adverse effects and cost of medications used
- To avoid complications associated with vomiting, which include dehydration with associated fluid and electrolyte disturbance, acid-base abnormalities and compromised nutritional status
- To control nausea so patients can resume treatment of other conditions

## Investigations

- History:
  - determine if the nausea is acute or chronic
  - explore possible underlying causes – simple versus complex
  - establish onset, progression and temporal sequence of associated events (e.g., surgery) and identify other symptoms (e.g., pain, vertigo)
  - complete an appropriate gastrointestinal functional inquiry
  - inquire about diet history including any new foods, food allergies or intolerances

Table 1: **Common Causes of Nausea**

| | |
|---|---|
| **N** | neurological causes, including central causes, increased intracranial pressure, trauma, CVA, migraine and vestibular causes such as labyrinthitis and motion sickness |
| **A** | alcohol and other drugs, including drug-related adverse effects (e.g., chemotherapy, opioids and antibiotics); drug toxicity (e.g., anticonvulsants, digitalis); drug withdrawal (e.g., benzodiazepines, SSRIs, narcotics) |
| **U** | usually accompanies anesthesia, malignancy including metastasis, migraine, and radiation therapy, pregnancy, noxious odors, pain, fear and medical conditions such as myocardial infarction, congestive heart failure, uremia, Addison's disease and diabetic ketoacidosis |
| **S** | stress and psychiatric causes, including grief, psychogenic nausea, anxiety and depression, and surgical causes such as pseudo obstruction |
| **E** | enteral, which includes gastrointestinal causes such as gastroenteritis, ingestion of irritants and food poisoning, gastroparesis and motility abnormalities, diseases of the liver, gall bladder and pancreas, IBS and constipation |
| **A** | anticipatory nausea, often seen in patients on chemotherapy or in any situation where a patient has been conditioned by a previous experience of nausea and vomiting |

- establish any exposure to or other symptoms of infection such as gastroenteritis
- in all women of reproductive age, rule out pregnancy – inquire about last menstrual period
- obtain a thorough medication history including prescription and nonprescription, herbal, alcohol and other drug use and any history of recent drug changes or withdrawal
- inquire about the patient's feelings, concerns, ideas and functional impairment and expectations of treatment
- explore possible psychosocial stressors, conflicts, sources of emotional pain or loss

■ Physical examination
- vital signs including blood pressure, pulse, respiratory rate and temperature
- determine severity of symptoms and assess hydration including JVP, mucous membranes, skin turgor and postural changes in blood pressure and heart rate
- assess systems related to the probable underlying cause when apparent, e.g., neurological exam for a migraine patient, examine for bowel obstruction if the patient has a malignancy or is postsurgical, check for nystagmus in vertigo-associated nausea
- if no specific cause is identified in the history, the physical exam should be used to rule out other potential causes (e.g., abdominal mass)

■ Other investigations
- laboratory investigations are determined by the history and physical exam

- electrolytes may be indicated if metabolic disturbances are suspected (e.g., test for hypercalcemia in a patient with a malignancy, ketoacidosis in a diabetic, hypokalemia in a patient on diuretics)
- CBC if an infective cause is suspected
- urea/Cr to determine if there is a renal cause and assess degree of dehydration
- x-rays may also be indicated; an abdominal series if a bowel obstruction is suspected or an upper GI with motility studies if gastroesophageal reflux or gastroparesis is suspected. Ultrasound of the liver, gallbladder or pancreas may be useful in some patients.

## Therapeutic Choices

### Nonpharmacologic Choices

- Some forms of complementary therapies have been used (e.g., acupuncture and hypnosis), but require further study.
- Dietary interventions may be important for nausea associated with certain food intolerances.
- Relaxation therapy and cognitive behavior therapies may be useful in the treatment of nausea associated with irritable bowel syndrome and anticipatory nausea respectively.
- Not every patient will want their nausea treated; one therapeutic option is not to give medication but to use watchful waiting.

### Pharmacologic Choices (Table 2)

Although antiemetics are widely prescribed, there is a paucity of randomized controlled trials, except for serotonin (5-HT3) antagonists in the treatment of chemotherapy-induced nausea (Chapter 101) and PONV. In determining treatment, consider if the nausea is acute or chronic, what other medications the patient is taking and the underlying cause of the nausea. Many patients will not be able to tolerate oral medications, and alternative routes of administration (intramuscular, subcutaneous, per rectum or transdermal) will be an important consideration. The management of nausea also can require a preventative approach, and prophylactic administration of antiemetics may be appropriate such as in the nausea associated with motion sickness.

## Therapeutic Tips

- When a more complex cause is suspected, antiemetics may provide some symptomatic relief. However, when possible, determine and treat the underlying cause.

Table 2: **Drugs Used to Treat Nausea***

| Drug (Indications) | Adult Dose | Adverse Effects | Drug Interactions | Cost† |
|---|---|---|---|---|
| **Antacids** (GI-related)<br>Various | 15–30 mL PO Q2–4H PRN | Diarrhea. | May ↓ bioavailability of some drugs (e.g., digoxin); separate dosing by 2h. | \$–\$\$ |
| **Antihistamines** (motion sickness, gastroenteritis, PONV) | | All agents: sedation, anticholinergic effects, confusion. | All agents: additive sedation with alcohol or other sedating medications. | |
| *dimenhydrinate*<br>Gravol, generics | 50–100 mg PO/PR/IM/IV Q4–6H PRN | | | $ PO<br>$$ IV |
| *diphenhydramine*<br>Benadryl, generics | 25–50 mg PO TID–QID PRN<br>10–50 mg IM/IV TID–QID PRN | | | $ PO<br>$$ IV |
| *hydroxyzine*<br>Atarax, generics | 25–100 mg PO/IM TID–QID PRN | | | $ PO<br>$$ IV |
| *promethazine*<br>Phenergan, Histanil, generics | 12.5–25 mg PO/IM/IV Q4–6H PRN | | | $ PO<br>$$$ IV |
| **Anticholinergics** (motion sickness)<br>*scopolamine*<br>Transderm V | 1.5 mg transdermal Q72H PRN | Constipation, dry mouth. Confusion (elderly). | Additive sedation with alcohol or other sedating medications. | $$ |

| | | | | |
|---|---|---|---|---|
| **Antihistamine/Anticholinergic** | | | | |
| (labyrinthitis)<br>*meclizine*<br>Bonamine | 25–50 mg PO Q24H PRN | Sedation, anticholinergic effects. | Additive sedation with alcohol or other sedating medications. | $ |
| **Butyrophenones*** (DIN, PONV) | | All agents: sedation, extrapyramidal effects. | All agents: additive sedation with alcohol or other CNS depressants. | |
| *haloperidol*<br>Haldol, generics | 0.5–5 mg PO/IM/IV Q12H PRN | | | $ PO<br>$$ IV |
| **Dopamine Antagonists** | | All agents: sedation, anticholinergic effects, extrapyramidal effects.<br>Hypotension especially with parenteral chlorpromazine, perphenazine and prochlorperazine.<br>Diarrhea with metoclopramide. | All agents: additive sedation with alcohol or other CNS depressants. | |
| *chlorpromazine*<br>(labyrinthitis)<br>Largactil, generics | 10–25 mg PO Q4–6H PRN<br>50–100 mg PR Q6–8H PRN<br>25–50 mg IM/IV Q3–4H PRN | | | $ PO<br>$$ IV |
| *metoclopramide**<br>(DIN, migraine-related nausea)<br>Maxeran, generics | 10–20 mg PO/SC/IV TID–QID PRN | | | $ PO<br>$$–$$$$ IV |
| *perphenazine**<br>(PONV)<br>Trilafon, generics | 2–4 mg PO/IM/IV Q8H PRN | | | $ |
| *prochlorperazine**<br>(DIN, migraine-related nausea)<br>Stemetil, generics | 5–10 mg PO/PR TID–QID PRN<br>5–10 mg IM/IV BID–TID PRN | | | $ PO<br>$$ IV |

* *See Chapter 101 for treatment of chemotherapy-induced nausea. Includes benzodiazepines, cannabinoids, corticosteroids and serotonin antagonists.*

*Abbreviations: DIN = drug-induced nausea, PONV = postoperative nausea and vomiting.*

*Dosage adjustment may be required in renal impairment – see Appendix I.*

† *Cost per day – includes drug cost only.*

*Legend: $ < $2   $$ $2–4   $$$ $4–6   $$$$ $6–8*

- When prescribing for the elderly – start low and go slow.
- Combination therapy may be required and has been found to be most useful in CIN.
- If current management of a nauseated patient fails to provide some symptomatic relief, reassess the patient and look for other causes.
- Know a few medications well. If one medication fails, try a different class of antinauseant or try an alternate route of administration. Start with less expensive choices.

## Suggested Reading List


Farmer PS. Nausea and vomiting. In: Carruthers-Czyzewski P, ed. *Nonprescription drug reference for health professionals.* Ottawa: Canadian Pharmaceutical Association, 1996:306–309.

Kovac AL. Prevention and treatment of postoperative nausea and vomiting. *Drugs* 2000; 59:213–243.

Pray WS. *Nonprescription product therapeutics*. Philadelphia: Lippincott Williams and Wilkins, 1999.

Taylor AT. Nausea and vomiting. In: DiPiro JT, Talbert RL, Yee GC, et al, eds. *Pharmacotherapy: a pathophysiological approach.* 4th ed. Stamford, CT: Appleton and Lange, 1999:586–597.

Wadibia EC. Antiemetics. *South Med J* 1999; 92:162–165.

CHAPTER 104

# Constipation

*Hugh Chaun, MA, BM, FRCP, FRCP(Ed), FRCPC, FACG*

## Goals of Therapy

- To establish regular bowel function
- To abolish the need to strain and prevent the adverse effects of straining (e.g., hernia, coronary and cerebrovascular dysfunction in the elderly, gastroesophageal reflux)
- To prevent complications (e.g., hemorrhoids, anal fissure, rectal prolapse, stercoral ulcer, fecal impaction, fecal incontinence)
- To treat complications (e.g., fecal impaction, intestinal obstruction)
- To use laxatives wisely and prevent adverse effects of laxative dependence (e.g., cathartic colon)

## Investigations

- Thorough history with special attention to:
  - duration of constipation
  - previous laxative use
  - dietary fibre and fluid
  - physical inactivity or immobilization
  - drugs with constipating effects (e.g., anticholinergics; antidepressants; antiparkinson agents; opioids; antacids containing aluminum and calcium; bismuth; sucralfate; iron supplements; calcium channel blockers; diuretics causing hypokalemia)
  - neuropsychiatric disorders (including depression in the elderly)
  - symptoms of obstructive disease (colonic neoplasm or stricture, anal stricture), painful hemorrhoid or fissure, pregnancy, neurological disease, endocrine disorder (hypothyroidism, diabetes mellitus), collagen vascular disease (progressive systemic sclerosis)
- Physical examination:
  - abdominal mass
- Laboratory tests:
  - CBC
  - stools for occult blood
- Sigmoidoscopy

Figure 1: **Management of Constipation**

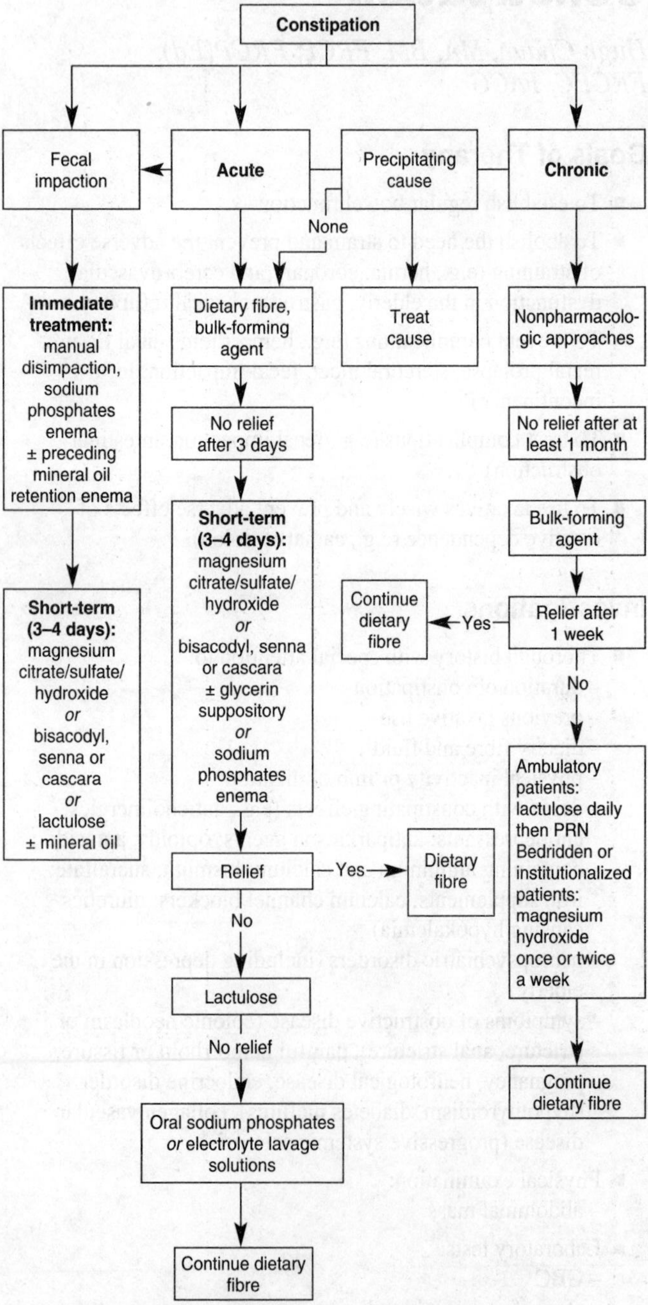
Constipation
Fecal impaction
Acute
Precipitating cause
Chronic
None
Immediate treatment: manual disimpaction, sodium phosphates enema ± preceding mineral oil retention enema
Dietary fibre, bulk-forming agent
Treat cause
Nonpharmacologic approaches
No relief after 3 days
No relief after at least 1 month
Short-term (3–4 days): magnesium citrate/sulfate/hydroxide or bisacodyl, senna or cascara ± glycerin suppository or sodium phosphates enema
Bulk-forming agent
Continue dietary fibre
Yes
Relief after 1 week
Short-term (3–4 days): magnesium citrate/sulfate/hydroxide or bisacodyl, senna or cascara or lactulose ± mineral oil
No
Ambulatory patients: lactulose daily then PRN Bedridden or institutionalized patients: magnesium hydroxide once or twice a week
Relief
Yes
Dietary fibre
No
Lactulose
No relief
Continue dietary fibre
Oral sodium phosphates or electrolyte lavage solutions
Continue dietary fibre

Table 1: **Drugs Used in Constipation**

| Drug | Adult Daily Dosage (oral unless specified) | Approximate Time of Action | Adverse Effects | Comments | Cost* |
|---|---|---|---|---|---|
| **Bulk-forming** | | All agents: | All agents: | All agents: | |
| *psyllium hydrophilic mucilloid* Metamucil, Prodiem plain, generics | 4.5–20 g (psyllium) | 12–72 h | Bloating, abdominal pain, rare allergic reactions. | Increase stool weight; decrease GI transit time; enhance frequency of defecation. | $ |
| *sterculia gum* Normacol | 7–28 g | | | Should be taken with increased fluids. Can be used long term. | $ |
| **Hyperosmotic** | | | | | |
| *glycerin* generics | Suppos: 2.6 g | 15 min–1 h | Rectal discomfort or burning. | Stimulates peristalsis. | $ |
| *lactulose* Duphalac, Lactulax, generics | 15–60 mL (10–40 g) | 24–48 h | Bloating, flatulence, cramps, diarrhea. | Induces bowel water retention. | $ |
| **Lubricant** | | | | Oral dosage form: | |
| *mineral oil* generics | PO: 15–45 mL | 6–8 h | Decreased absorption of fat-soluble vitamins (some drugs). Lipoid pneumonia if aspirated. | Avoid in bedridden patients because of risk of aspiration. Should not be used with stool softeners because ↑ absorption of mineral oil. | $ |
| | Enema: 120 mL | 2–15 min | Seepage from rectum causing pruritus and irritation. | Should be used for short period. | $$$$ |

*(cont'd)*

Table 1: **Drugs Used in Constipation** *(cont'd)*

| Drug | Adult Daily Dosage (oral unless specified) | Approximate Time of Action | Adverse Effects | Comments | Cost* |
|---|---|---|---|---|---|
| **Osmotic/Saline** | | | | All agents: | |
| *magnesium citrate*<br>Citro-Mag (15 g/300 mL) | 4–15 g | 30 min–6 h | Hypermagnesemia in renal dysfunction ($Mg^{++}$ salts). | Stimulate peristalsis. Useful for rapid response | $–$$$ |
| *magnesium hydroxide*<br>Milk of Magnesia, generics | 2.4–4.8 g | 30 min–6 h | | (e.g., preoperatively). | $ |
| *magnesium sulfate*<br>Epsom Salts, generics | 10–30 g | 30 min–6 h | | | $ |
| *sodium phosphates*<br>Fleet Enema, generics<br>Fleet Phospho-Soda, PMS Phosphates | Enema: 120 mL (22 g)<br>Oral: 20 mL (laxative)–45 mL (purgative) | 2–15 min<br>30 min–6 h | Hyperphosphatemia. | Good preparation for colonoscopy. | $$<br>$$ |
| **Stimulant** | | | Abdominal pain, cramps, cathartic colon (all agents). | All agents:<br>Stimulate colonic peristalsis. | |
| *bisacodyl*<br>Dulcolax, generics | PO: 5–15 mg<br>Suppos: 10 mg<br>Micro-enema: 10 mg | 6–12 h<br>15 min–1 h<br>15 min–1 h | Rectal microscopic mucosal changes (bisacodyl suppository, enema). | Most potent purgatives. Usually used short term but may be long term in opioid users. | $<br>$ suppos<br>$$ micro-enema |
| *castor oil*<br>Neoloid, generics | 15–60 mL | 1–3 h | | | $–$$ |
| *senna*<br>Senokot, Glysennid, others | 15–30 mg (sennosides) | 6–12 h | Melanosis coli (anthraquinone derivatives). High sugar content in some senna preparations. | | $ |

| | | | | | |
|---|---|---|---|---|---|
| **Stool Softeners** | | | | | |
| *docusate salts* | | 12–72 h | | Act as surfactants. Used as stool softeners following rectal surgery and in long-term opioid users, but no documented beneficial effects. | |
| Colace, generics | 100–200 mg | | | | $ |
| Surfak, generics | 240 mg | | | | $ |
| **Lavage Solutions** | | | | | |
| *electrolyte solutions* Golytely, Colyte, Klean-Prep, generics | 1000–4000 mL | 30 min–1 h | Retching, nausea, abdominal fullness and bloating. | Contain mainly sodium sulfate and polyethylene glycol. Excellent cleansing for colonoscopy. Klean-Prep is available as 4 × 1 L sachets. | $$$$ |

** Cost per day – includes drug cost only.*
*Legend: $ < $1 $$ $1–2 $$$ $2–3 $$$$ > $3*

- Double contrast barium enema or colonoscopy if recent onset in older patients, severe symptoms, does not resolve with simple measures, cause of rectal bleeding not demonstrated on sigmoidoscopy, weight loss, anemia
- Psychological assessment when appropriate
- Transit study with radiopaque markers, defecography, anorectal manometry in selected patients, e.g., autonomic bowel paresis (diabetes)

## Therapeutic Choices (Figure 1)

### Nonpharmacologic Choices

- When possible, drugs with constipating effects (see Investigations) should be discontinued.
- Dietary fibre (20 to 30 g per day), flax seed, unprocessed bran, whole grains, fruits and vegetables should be encouraged. The daily amount should be increased slowly to minimize side effects.
- Fluid intake should be increased.
- Prune juice, stewed prunes, figs should be tried.
- Regular scheduled time for toilet use should be encouraged, e.g., after breakfast, to develop a conditioned gastrocolic reflex.
- Prolonged straining should be avoided.
- Physical exercise should be encouraged.
- Relaxation exercises for pelvic floor and external anal sphincter muscles in conjunction with biofeedback can be tried.

### Pharmacologic Choices (Table 1)

## Therapeutic Tips

- Constipation is a symptom, not a disease. Establishing the cause, if any, and correcting it should be the primary objective of treatment.
- In general, drug therapy is used only when nonpharmacologic approaches have failed.
- Bulk-forming agents can be safely used for long-term therapy but should be taken with adequate fluids.
- Saline and stimulant laxatives should be used intermittently as needed and as sparingly as possible for short-term therapy, once or twice weekly at most.
- Patient's understanding and cooperation regarding general principles of therapy should be sought, and laxative tolerance should be monitored.

- Lactose-containing dairy products (milk, young cheese) may be the most cost-effective natural cathartic in patients with lactase deficiency.
- To discontinue chronic laxative use, gradually reduce frequency of laxative use over 3 to 4 weeks, while optimizing nonpharmacologic approaches; use an osmotic laxative (e.g., lactulose) intermittently PRN until bowel regularity is achieved.

## Suggested Reading List

Smith MB, Chang EB. Antidiarrheals and cathartics. In: Wolfe MM, ed. *Gastrointestinal pharmacotherapy*. Philadelphia: W.B. Saunders, 1993:139–156.

Tedesco FJ. Laxative use in constipation. *Am J Gastroenterol* 1985;80:303–309.

Velio P, Bassotti G. Chronic idiopathic constipation: pathophysiology and treatment. *J Clin Gastroenterol* 1996;22:190–196.

Wilson JAP. Constipation in the elderly. *Clin Geriatr Med* 1999;15:499–510.

CHAPTER 105

# Diarrhea

*Richard N. Fedorak, MD, FRCPC*

## Definition

Diarrhea is defined as the excretion of fecal matter at a rate greater than 200 g/24 h, with increased loss of fecal water and electrolytes. The increased fecal water content leads to a change in stooling frequency and consistency, which the patient reports as diarrhea. Acute diarrhea occurs for less than 14 days, while diarrhea that persists for more than 14 days is considered chronic.

## Goals of Therapy

- To reduce symptoms and re-establish normal fecal weight (volume)
- To prevent and treat complications, e.g., dehydration, electrolyte depletion, nutrient malabsorption, hemorrhoids, rectal prolapse
- To identify and treat specific etiologies

## Investigations

Prior to the initiation of therapy, 2 key questions must be addressed:

- Is this true diarrhea? Many people who complain of diarrhea actually have a motility disturbance (e.g., irritable bowel syndrome [IBS], Chapter 48). They experience an increased frequency of very small bowel movements, but the 24-hour stool weight does not exceed normal amounts. Measuring fecal fat, osmolarity and bile acid levels can also help determine specific etiologies
- Is the diarrhea acute or chronic? In the absence of fever, dehydration or bloody stools, the management of acute diarrhea should alleviate symptoms rather than provide a specific diagnosis or therapy. **Acute diarrhea** (Figure 1) is usually caused by viral agents, drugs or food toxins and irritants, for which there is no specific therapy, and usually remits spontaneously within 1 week. **Chronic diarrhea** is evaluated as in Figure 2

Figure 1: **Evaluation of Acute Diarrhea**

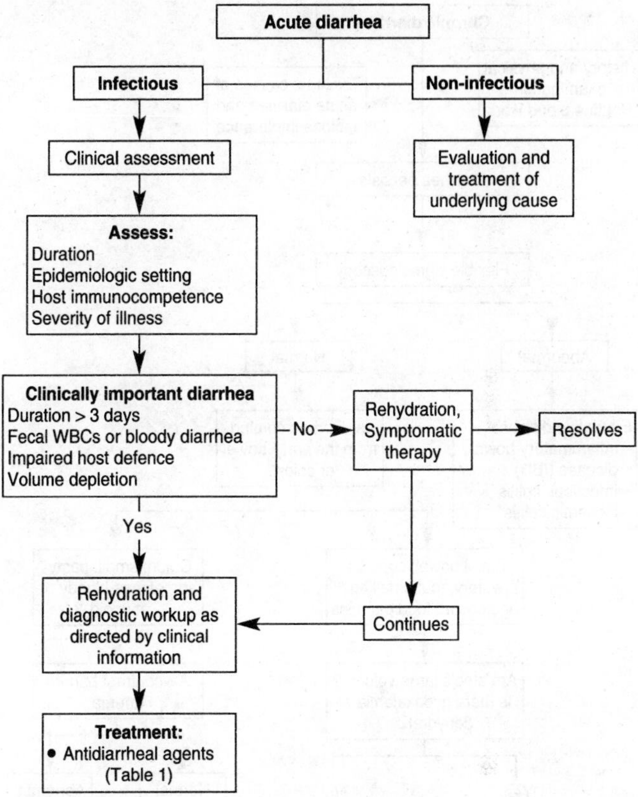
Acute diarrhea
Infectious
Non-infectious
Clinical assessment
Evaluation and treatment of underlying cause
Assess:
Duration
Epidemiologic setting
Host immunocompetence
Severity of illness
Clinically important diarrhea
Duration > 3 days
Fecal WBCs or bloody diarrhea
Impaired host defence
Volume depletion
No
Rehydration, Symptomatic therapy
Resolves
Yes
Rehydration and diagnostic workup as directed by clinical information
Continues
Treatment:
• Antidiarrheal agents (Table 1)

# Therapeutic Choices

## Nonpharmacologic Choices

- Discontinue medications that cause diarrhea (e.g., laxatives, antacids containing magnesium, antibiotics, diuretics, theophylline, cholinergic drugs, promotility agents, prostaglandins)
- Stop ingestion of carbohydrates that are poorly absorbed by the small intestine (e.g., dietetic candies and jams containing sorbitol, mannitol or xylitol; beverages and foods containing fructose; or lactose-containing dairy products). These carbohydrates are poorly absorbed and are fermented in the colon to produce short-chain fatty acids which cause both an osmotic and secretory diarrhea. A 2-week therapeutic trial of a lactose-restricted diet can avoid costly diagnostic work-ups of continued diarrhea caused by lactose malabsorption.

Figure 2: **Evaluation of Chronic Diarrhea**

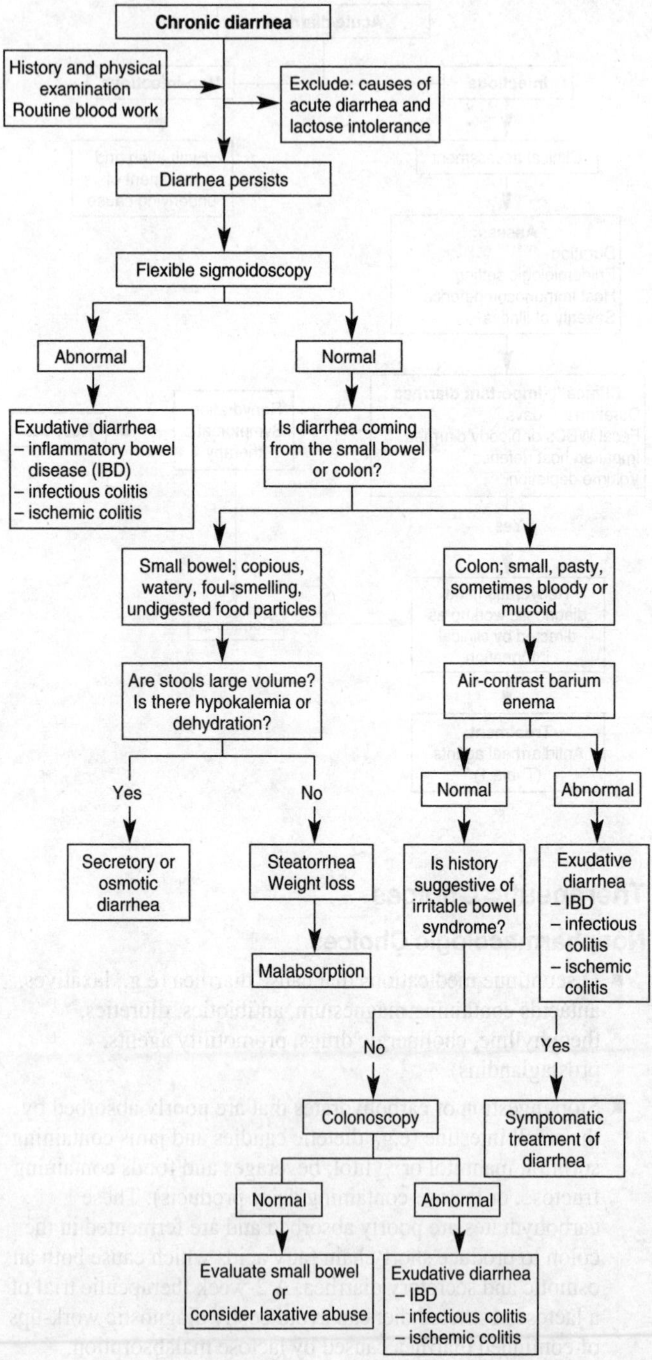
Chronic diarrhea
History and physical examination
Routine blood work
Exclude: causes of acute diarrhea and lactose intolerance
Diarrhea persists
Flexible sigmoidoscopy
Abnormal
Normal
Exudative diarrhea
– inflammatory bowel disease (IBD)
– infectious colitis
– ischemic colitis
Is diarrhea coming from the small bowel or colon?
Small bowel; copious, watery, foul-smelling, undigested food particles
Colon; small, pasty, sometimes bloody or mucoid
Are stools large volume? Is there hypokalemia or dehydration?
Air-contrast barium enema
Yes
No
Normal
Abnormal
Secretory or osmotic diarrhea
Steatorrhea Weight loss
Is history suggestive of irritable bowel syndrome?
Exudative diarrhea
– IBD
– infectious colitis
– ischemic colitis
Malabsorption
No
Yes
Colonoscopy
Symptomatic treatment of diarrhea
Normal
Abnormal
Evaluate small bowel or consider laxative abuse
Exudative diarrhea
– IBD
– infectious colitis
– ischemic colitis

Table 1: **Drugs Used to Treat Diarrhea**

| Drug | Dosage | Adverse Effects | Comments | Cost* |
|---|---|---|---|---|
| **Bismuth** | | | | |
| *bismuth subsalicylate* Pepto-Bismol liquid | 30 mL Q30 min to a max. of 8 doses/d | Salicylate toxicity, black tongue, black stool, bismuth-induced encephalopathy. | Solution: bismuth subsalicylate 17.6 mg/mL. | $† |
| *bismuth subsalicylate with calcium carbonate* Pepto-Bismol tablet | 2 tablets Q30 min to a max. of 8 doses/d | Same as above. Hypercalcemia, hypercalciuria. | Tablet: bismuth subsalicylate 262 mg, calcium carbonate 350 mg. | $† |
| **Hydrophilic Bulking Agents** | | | | |
| *psyllium* Fibrepur, Metamucil, generics | 1 teaspoon (5–6 g) Q12H | Inhaled psyllium powder may cause allergic reactions. | Avoid products containing psyllium mixed with laxatives. | $† |
| *cholestyramine resin* Questran, generics | 4 g Q12H | Nausea, fat soluble vitamin deficiency with long-term use, constipation. | 1 packet contains 4 g and must be mixed with fluids. May bind other drugs in GI tract; do not take within 1 h before or 4 h after other medications. | $ |
| **Opiate Agonists** | | | | |
| *loperamide* Imodium, generics | 2 mg after each loose bowel movement to a max. of 16 mg/d | Sedation, nausea, abdominal cramps. Some addiction potential. | Capsule: 2 mg. Solution: 2 mg/10 mL. After oral administration, absorption is poor (approx. 40% excreted unabsorbed in feces). | $† |
| *diphenoxylate (with atropine sulfate)* Lomotil, generics | 5 mg initially then 2.5 mg after each loose bowel movement to a max. of 20 mg/d | Sedation, nausea, abdominal cramps, dry skin and mucous membranes (from atropine), some addiction potential. | Capsule: diphenoxylate 2.5 mg, atropine 0.025 mg. | $ |

*(cont'd)*

Table 1: **Drugs Used to Treat Diarrhea** *(cont'd)*

| Drug | Dosage | Adverse Effects | Comments | Cost* |
|---|---|---|---|---|
| *codeine*<br>generics | 30–60 mg Q4H PRN | Sedation, nausea, tolerance, potentially addictive. | Tablet: 15 or 30 mg.<br>Solution: 30 or 60 mg/mL. | $ |
| *opium compound*<br>Diban | 1 capsule Q4H PRN | Sedation, nausea, potentially addictive. | Capsule: opium 12 mg, hyoscyamine 52 µg, atropine 10 µg, scopolamine 3 µg, attapulgite 300 mg, pectin 71 mg. | $$ |
| Donnagel PG | 1 capsule Q4H PRN or 15 mL Q4H PRN | Sedation, nausea, potentially addictive. | Capsule: opium 12 mg, pectin 71.4 mg, attapulgite 300 mg.<br>Suspension, per 15 mL: opium 12 mg, pectin 121 mg, kaolin 3 g. | $ |
| *opium camphor (paregoric)* | According to concentration of preparation | Sedation, nausea, potentially addictive. | | $ |
| **Alpha$_2$-adrenergic Agonists** | | | | |
| *clonidine*<br>Catapres, generics | 0.1–0.6 mg Q12H | Centrally mediated sedation and hypotension. | Tablet: 0.1 and 0.2 mg. | $ |
| **Somatostatin** | | | | |
| *octreotide*<br>Sandostatin | 50–500 µg Q12H SC | Pain at injection site. | Ampul: 50, 100, 500 µg.<br>Multidose vial: 200 µg/mL. | $$–$$$$ |
| Sandostatin LAR | 10–30 mg IM monthly | Pain at injection site, nausea, mild diarrhea. | Vial: 10, 20, 30 mg | $$$$–$$$$$ |

** Cost per day – includes drug cost only.*
*Legend: $ < $5 $$ $5–10 $$$ $10–25 $$$$ $25–50 $$$$$ $50–75*

*† Available without prescription; retail mark-up may vary.*

- Reducing oral food intake for 12 to 24 hours will improve symptoms of acute diarrhea. Maintenance of adequate fluid and electrolyte intake is important and a bland diet (low fat, low carbohydrate) can be reintroduced once bowel motions have subsided.

## Pharmacologic Choices (Table 1)

### Oral Rehydration Therapy (ORT)

ORT (Chapters 77, 78) is used to prevent dehydration and electrolyte loss in both acute and chronic diarrhea. It works by enhancing sodium (and thus water) absorption through cotransport of sodium with glucose. ORT should have a balanced sodium to glucose ratio. Solutions that have excess glucose (e.g., Jell-O, soda pop) may aggravate existing diarrhea as a consequence of their osmotic effect. Early use of ORT is essential for young children and the elderly.

### Bismuth

*Antidiarrheal mechanisms:* Bismuth subsalicylate's antisecretory effect is related to the salicylate component; the antimicrobial effect is primarily attributed to the bismuth component. Anti-inflammatory effects are known to occur via a mechanism not related to cyclo-oxygenase inhibition. Bismuth subsalicylate is suspended in clay that may bind enterotoxins.

*Clinical applications:* Bismuth subsalicylate is as effective as loperamide in the management of acute traveler's diarrhea and can be used prophylactically. It has also been used to treat chronic idiopathic diarrhea and diarrhea caused by microscopic colitis. The salicylate component can cause gastric and duodenal mucosal damage, particularly in patients who are also using ASA or NSAIDs. At high doses, the calcium carbonate in the tablet formation can cause hypercalcemia, hypercalciuria and associated metabolic symptoms. Bismuth-related encephalopathy can result from doses 10 times those recommended, or after years of use. Black stools, as a consequence of the bismuth, may be confused with melena.

### Hydrophilic Bulking Agents

*Antidiarrheal mechanisms:* Dietary fibre supplementation may be useful in the management of diarrhea. The ultimate effectiveness of a fibre depends not only on its water-holding capacity but also on its ability to hydrolyze fatty and bile acids which, if not hydrolyzed, directly stimulate intestinal secretion. Bulking agents also increase chyme viscosity and thereby delay gastric emptying and reduce colonic transit times. Psyllium may bind bacterial enterotoxins and prevent direct secretory effects on the gastrointestinal epithelium.

*Clinical application:* **Psyllium** is a hydrophilic agent that increases fecal water-holding capacity and may reduce diarrheal symptoms. Many psyllium-containing products are mixed with laxatives; these products must be avoided in patients with diarrhea.

**Cholestyramine resin**, in addition to its hydrophilic action, has the ability to bind bile acids. Thus, it has a specific usefulness in treating bile acid-induced diarrhea due to malabsorption of bile acids in diseased ileum (e.g., Crohn's disease) or in some cases of IBS where rapid transit results in loss of bile acids into the colon. Cholestyramine's ability to bind luminal bacterial toxins has led to its adjunctive use in toxin-induced diarrhea, e.g., *C. difficile*.

### Opioids

*Antidiarrheal mechanisms:* Opiates act to reduce diarrhea by decreasing intestinal secretion and/or promoting intestinal absorption, reducing intestinal motility and increasing anal sphincter tone.

*Clinical application:* Available opioids include naturally occurring preparations (**paregoric** and **opium alkaloids**) and synthetic preparations (**codeine**, **diphenoxylate** and **loperamide**). These agents are very effective for symptomatic use in both acute and chronic diarrhea; however, side effects limit their acute use and tolerance usually occurs with chronic use. Antimotility effects are not desired if the diarrhea is caused by microorganisms because stasis may enhance their invasion. Diphenoxylate and loperamide have fewer CNS side effects than the other opioids. Diphenoxylate has been combined with atropine to limit its potential for abuse. Loperamide, which has the least number of side effects or abuse potential, is available without prescription. Loperamide has been shown to be effective in patients with radiotherapy- and chemotherapy-induced diarrhea and in patients with ileo-rectal pouch incontinence. Combination of loperamide with simethicone provides faster and more complete relief of acute diarrhea associated with gas-related abdominal discomfort. Codeine may be considered if sedation or analgesia is also required.

### Alpha$_2$-adrenergic Agonists

*Antidiarrheal mechanisms:* Alpha$_2$-adrenergic agonists are potent enhancers of net intestinal absorption, stimulating sodium and chloride absorption and inhibiting bicarbonate and chloride secretion, likely through stimulation of adrenergic receptors at the enterocyte level. In addition, they slow intestinal transit time and may reduce heightened rectal tone in IBS.

*Clinical application:* **Clonidine** is effective against opioid-withdrawal diarrhea and diabetic diarrhea associated with autonomic neuropathy. Unfortunately, the dose required to achieve an antidiarrheal effect is often associated with sedation, dry mouth and symptomatic orthostatic hypotension.

### Somatostatin

*Antidiarrheal mechanisms:* **Somatostatin** and **octreotide** directly reduce intestinal motility, enteric hormone release and gastric and pancreatic secretion; it promotes large and small intestinal water and electrolyte absorption. Indirectly, somatostatin can inhibit the release of peptides that cause diarrhea from neuroendocrine tumors.

*Clinical applications:* **Somatostatin** has a short biological half-life and requires continuous IV infusion, thus limiting its role. **Octreotide**, a long-acting somatostatin analog, can be administered SC daily or a long-acting formulation can be given IM monthly. It has been used to control diarrhea caused by neuroendocrine tumors (VIPoma, carcinoid, medullary carcinoma of the thyroid). Octreotide has also been shown to limit idiopathic and infant secretory diarrhea, as well as diarrhea associated with ileostomy, diabetic neuropathy, chemotherapy, bone marrow transplant, cryptosporidia, graft versus host disease and HIV disease.

## Suggested Reading List

Aranda-Michel J, Giannella RA. Acute diarrhea: a practical review. *Am J Med* 1999;106:670–676.

Fedorak RN. Anti-diarrheal therapy. In: Friedman E, Jacobson ED, McCallum RW, eds. *Gastrointestinal pharmacology and therapeutics*. Philadelphia: Lippincott-Raven, 1997:175–193.

Lennard-Jones JE. Review article: practical management of the short bowel. *Aliment Pharmacol Ther* 1994;8:563–577.

Schiller LR. Review article: anti-diarrhoeal pharmacology and therapeutics. *Aliment Pharmacol Ther* 1995;9:87–106.

Sun WM, Read NW, Verlinden M. Effects of loperamide oxide on gastrointestinal transit time and anorectal function in patients with chronic diarrhoea and faecal incontinence. *Scand J Gastroenterol* 1997;32:34–38.

CHAPTER 106

# Fever in Children

*Joanne M. Langley, MD, MSc, FRCPC*

Fever is a regulated physiologic response in which a new set point for body temperature is established. Temperatures consistently over 38 to 38.1°C can be considered elevated. The febrile response only rarely exceeds 41 to 42°C. The body establishes a new balance of heat loss and production to maintain this homeostasis. Temperature measurement in the rectum, mouth, or tympanic membrane reflects *core* temperature. Axillary temperatures are lower than core, difficult to measure, and not recommended.

Fever itself is not harmful and enhances some host defence mechanisms (lymphocyte transformation, stimulation of T and B lymphocytes). Fever is a different state than disorders of thermoregulation (e.g., heat stroke, malignant hyperthermia) in which heat production exceeds heat loss (Chapter 107).

## Goals of Therapy

- To provide patient comfort
- To relieve parental anxiety
- To avoid potentially harmful secondary effects due to metabolic demands in those with cardiac or pulmonary disorders
- To prevent recurrence of febrile seizure convulsions (although prophylaxis in high risk children was not effective in one study[1])

Nevertheless, there is little evidence for the use of antipyretic therapy.

## Investigations

Fever is a symptom not a diagnosis, and most commonly is an adaptive response to an infective agent. Fever may also occur in malignancy, rheumatologic or immunologic diseases.

- History to ascertain associated symptoms, and physical examination to determine the source of fever
  - clinical judgement determines if the underlying process is benign (e.g., viral respiratory tract infection) or life-threatening (e.g., bacterial meningitis)
  - bacteremia is more likely if the temperature is greater than 41.1°C[2,3]

[1] *Eur J Pediatr 1993;152:747–749.*
[2] *Pediatrics 1994;94:397–399.*
[3] *J Clin Epidemiol 1993;46:349–357.*

- Aggressiveness of the laboratory evaluation depends on clinical assessment of the severity of illness, the age of the child and immune status
  –may include culture of sources of infection (urine, blood, cerebrospinal fluid) or imaging studies
  –because of the low prevalence of bacteremia, nonspecific tests such as the white blood cell count, absolute band count or C-reactive protein are not sufficiently sensitive or specific to be diagnostic in the management of the febrile child[4,5]

## Therapeutic Choices

### Nonpharmacologic Choices

Physical methods for heat reduction use convection, evaporation or conduction. The body aggressively opposes physical cooling by attempting to re-establish a higher temperature by shivering and vasoconstriction, both of which cause patient discomfort. Pharmacologic methods are preferred because they lower the hypothalamic set point.

In the rare instance where core temperatures exceed 41 to 42°C, or where the metabolic demands of fever are a consideration, physical methods may be used in addition to pharmacologic methods. They include :

- **Sponging** with water uses evaporation to dissipate body heat. Alcohol is not recommended as it may be absorbed through the skin, inhaled or accidentally ingested by the child. The colder the water used, the more uncomfortable the patient.
- **Ice packs or cooling (hypothermia) blankets** may be applied to the skin to lower body temperature by conduction. In adult intensive care unit patients, this method is associated with greater temperature fluctuations and more rebound hyperthermia. (Chapter 107)
- **Circulating fans**, sometimes directed over ice before reaching the patient, use convection to transfer heat away from the skin surface.

### Pharmacologic Choices (Table 1)

**Acetaminophen** and **ibuprofen** are the only therapeutic choices available for managing fever in children. They have been well studied and are safe in therapeutic doses. Acetaminophen, because of its safety and long-term use in pediatrics, is recommended over ibuprofen, which is reserved for second-line therapy. Acetylsalicylic acid (ASA) is not recommended in children under 15 years of age because of the risk of Reye's syndrome.

---

[4] *Lancet 1991;337:591–594.*
[5] *Pediatr Child Health 1998;3:273–274.*

Table 1: **Antipyretic Medications in Children**

| Drug* ◗ | Dosage | Adverse Effects | Comments |
|---|---|---|---|
| *acetaminophen* Abenol, Atasol, Tempra, Tylenol, generics | 10–15 mg/kg Q4–6H | Uncommon. Hypersensitivity, agranulocytosis and anemia (rare), chronic use and overdose associated with hepatotoxicity, nephropathy. | Dosage should not exceed 125–150 mg/kg/day. Dehydration enhances risk of renal toxicity. |
| *ibuprofen* Advil, Motrin (Children's), Motrin IB, generics | 5-10 mg/kg Q6–8H | Uncommon. Gastrointestinal intolerance, allergic reactions, tinnitus, visual disturbances, nephropathy. | Not labelled for OTC use in children under 2 years of age. Use with caution in patients with varicella. Inhibits platelet aggregation at normal doses. Dehydration enhances risk of renal toxicity. |

* *Available without prescription. Cost of 1 day supply < $2 – includes drug cost only.*
◗ *Dosage adjustment may be required in renal impairment – see Appendix I.*

## Therapeutic Tips

- Package labelling for acetaminophen and ibuprofen provides dosage based on age; this generally leads to under dosing and should be replaced by a doctor's recommended dosage according to the child's weight.
- Antipyretics should be stored in locked cabinets to prevent unintended access by children.

### *Suggested Reading List*

Baraff L, Bass J, Fleisher G, Klein J, McCracken GH Jr, Powell K, et al. Practice guideline for the management of infants and children 0 to 36 months of age with fever without source. *Pediatrics* 1993;92:1–12.

Drug Therapy and Hazardous Substances Committee. Acetaminophen and ibuprofen in the management of fever and mild to moderate pain in children. *Pediatr Child Health* 1998;3: 273–274.

Kramer M, Naimark L, Leduc D. Parental fever phobia and its correlates. *Pediatrics* 1984;75:1110–1113.

Mackowiak PA, Boulant JA. Fever's glass ceiling. *Clin Infect Dis* 1996;22:525–536.

Plaisance KI, Mackowiak PA. Antipyretic therapy. *Arch Intern Med* 2000;160:449–456.

CHAPTER 107

# Thermoregulatory Disorders in Adults

*Mathieu Simon, MD, FRCPC*

The goal of treating thermoregulatory disorders should most often be directed to the cause of the temperature variance rather than the surrogate thermometer reading.

**Hyperthermia** refers to a symptomatic increase in body temperature above 38.2°C. Unlike fever, hyperthermia is not mediated by the hypothalamus but rather results from inadequate heat dissipation. The distinction between fever and hyperthermia relies on identification of the proper clinical setting. Fever is most often the sign of an underlying infectious or inflammatory process. Hyperthermia occurs predominantly in healthy individuals. Clinical manifestations represent the adverse effects of the increased temperature on various organ systems.

**Hyperpyrexia**, a core temperature above 41°C, results from impairment of both heat loss mechanisms and hypothalamic thermostat setpoint. Hyperpyrexia is most often the sign of an overwhelming infection.

**Hypothermia**, a very common but often unrecognized problem, is defined as a body temperature below 35°C.

## Goals of Therapy

- To recognize and treat the most common thermoregulation disorders (see also Fever, Chapter 106)
- To prevent, diagnose and treat uncommon but lethal complications of these disorders
- To avoid unnecessary, ineffective or dangerous interventions

## Investigations

- Thermoregulation disorders must be considered in the differential of confusion and coma. Clinical awareness and environmental exposure history are essential to the diagnosis
- *Urban hypothermia* is often associated with alcohol/drug intoxication. Hypothermia in this setting may also result from prolonged immobilization of a solitary elderly patient, even at normal room temperature, in association with loss of consciousness, a fall, stroke or fracture
- With hyperthermia, exclude infection and assess hydration status. Inquire about the use of medications (neuroleptic

agents, volatile anesthetics), recreational drugs (cocaine, amphetamines, PCP) and consider intoxication (ASA, tricyclic antidepressant overdose, organophosphates). Endocrinopathies (thyrotoxicosis, pheochromocytoma) may also present with hyperthermia

- Accurate measurement of core temperature is an obvious prerequisite. Electronic devices must be used since standard glass/mercury thermometers will not record temperature below 32°C. Frequent calibration of these instruments is mandatory
- Tests should be ordered according to the clinical setting; blood glucose, electrolytes, renal profile, CBC, creatine kinase (CK), coagulation panel, blood gases, and ECG should be part of the initial evaluation of any unstable patient

## Therapeutic Choices

### *Hyperthermia*

#### Nonpharmacologic Choices

Rest, cooling and rehydration are the mainstay of treatment. Four classical syndromes are described:

- **Heat cramps** occur in muscles following vigorous exercise in the heat. They are caused by salt depletion from excess sweating combined with hypotonic fluid replacement. Core temperature is normal, skin is moist and cool. Treatment includes rest and oral rehydration with a salt-containing solution (1 tsp [5 mL] of salt in 500 mL of water). IV therapy (2 to 3 L of 0.9% sodium chloride [NS] over 4 to 6 hours) is rarely indicated.
- **Heat exhaustion** occurs as a result of both salt and water losses. Patients present with muscle cramps, diaphoresis, headache, nausea and vomiting. Core temperature is minimally increased. Treatment consists of rest in a cool environment, external cooling with a fan and rehydration. The patient should avoid strenuous exercise for 2 to 3 days.
- **Exertional heat stroke** generally occurs acutely with endurance athletes or soldiers submitted to conditions of high heat and humidity without appropriate access to salt and water.
- **Classical heat stroke**, on the contrary, develops slowly during heat waves and affects primarily the elderly or those suffering from chronic illness. Both present with elevated core temperature (classically > 40.5°C) and dry, hot skin. These patients are severely dehydrated and at risk of disseminated intravascular coagulation, rhabdomyolysis, renal failure and seizures. Treatment requires immediate

cooling. The ideal approach is prolonged tepid water misting enhanced by fan evaporation. Tepid water sponging and ice-packs are alternative approaches. Ice-water immersion is impractical and not usually recommended because it induces a peripheral vasoconstriction, which is counterproductive.

### Pharmacologic Choices

Antipyretics are ineffective and dangerous since the hypothalamic thermostat setpoint is normal. Likewise, cooling is of little help in the treatment of fever unless it results in hyperpyrexia. Two distinct syndromes requiring expeditious pharmacologic therapy demand special attention:

- **Malignant hyperthermia** (MH) is a genetic susceptibility to generalized and sustained muscle contraction after exposure to a triggering agent (succinylcholine or volatile anesthetic agents). The sustained muscle contraction results in hyperthermia, metabolic acidosis and increased serum CK. Duchenne's disease and myotonic muscular dystrophy have been associated with an increased incidence of MH. Prompt recognition of the syndrome, interruption of the surgery, cessation of the offending drug, external cooling and administration of a muscle relaxant (e.g., dantrolene 2 mg/kg IV every 5 minutes up to 10 mg/kg) are necessary to reverse this potentially lethal condition. Some experts suggest prevention of recurrence by administering oral dantrolene 2 to 4 mg/kg/day for 2 to 3 days after an episode of MH.
- **Neuroleptic malignant syndrome** (NMS) is a drug-induced idiosyncratic reaction characterized by hyperthermia, altered mentation and muscle rigidity. Drugs implicated are most often phenothiazines (e.g., chlorpromazine) and butyrophenones (e.g., haloperidol) or withdrawal of a dopaminergic agent (e.g., levodopa). Treatment involves cessation of the offending agent, administration of dopaminergic agonists (e.g., bromocriptine 2.5 to 20 mg PO TID), and possibly use of a muscle relaxant (nondepolarizing neuromuscular blockers or dantrolene). Experience in the treatment of this uncommon condition is limited.

## *Hypothermia* (Figure 1)

### Nonpharmacologic Choices

Initial management involves airway, breathing and circulation (ABC) support. Vital signs must be assessed carefully since severe hypothermia may result in barely perceptible pulse and respiration. When these faint signs of life are present and an organized electrical activity is detected, CPR should be withheld because initiating CPR in a nonarrested hypothermic patient may precipitate a fatal arrhythmia. Core temperature below 32°C

Figure 1: **Hypothermia Treatment**

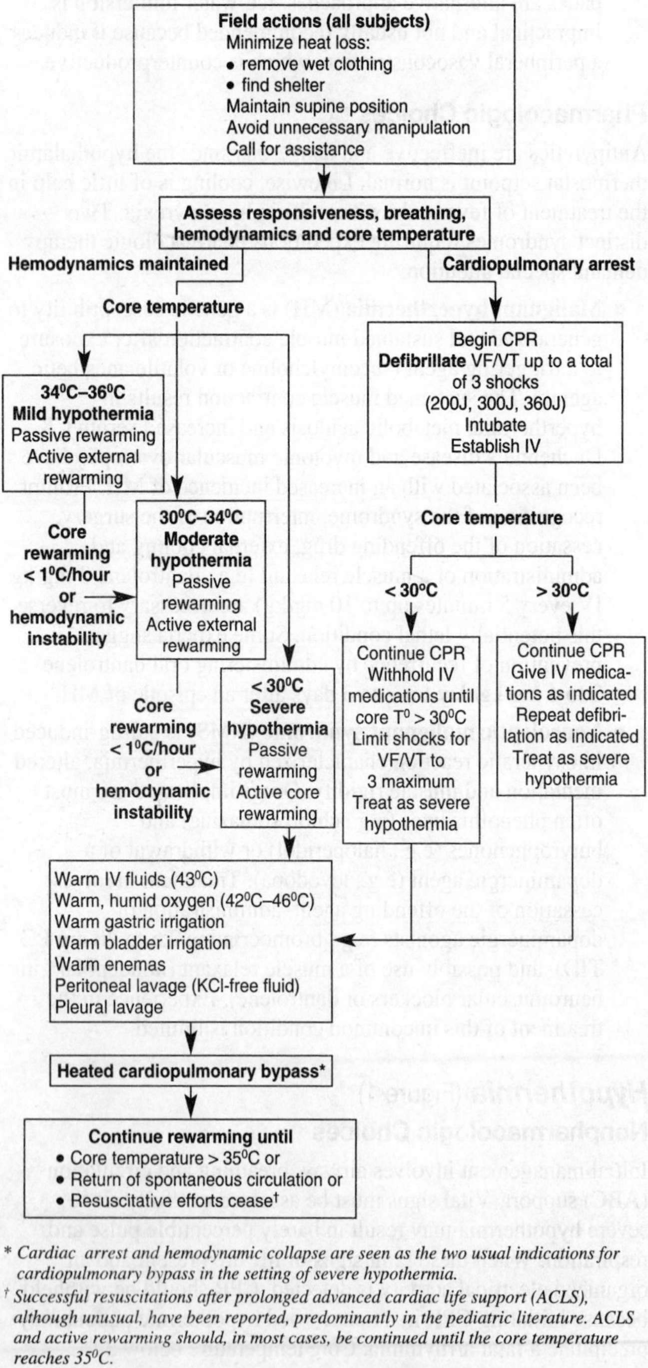
Field actions (all subjects)
Minimize heat loss:
• remove wet clothing
• find shelter
Maintain supine position
Avoid unnecessary manipulation
Call for assistance
Assess responsiveness, breathing, hemodynamics and core temperature
Hemodynamics maintained
Cardiopulmonary arrest
Core temperature
34°C–36°C
Mild hypothermia
Passive rewarming
Active external rewarming
Begin CPR
Defibrillate VF/VT up to a total of 3 shocks (200J, 300J, 360J)
Intubate
Establish IV
30°C–34°C
Moderate hypothermia
Passive rewarming
Active external rewarming
Core rewarming < 1°C/hour or hemodynamic instability
Core temperature
< 30°C
> 30°C
< 30°C
Severe hypothermia
Passive rewarming
Active core rewarming
Core rewarming < 1°C/hour or hemodynamic instability
Continue CPR
Withhold IV medications until core T° > 30°C
Limit shocks for VF/VT to 3 maximum
Treat as severe hypothermia
Continue CPR
Give IV medications as indicated
Repeat defibrillation as indicated
Treat as severe hypothermia
Warm IV fluids (43°C)
Warm, humid oxygen (42°C–46°C)
Warm gastric irrigation
Warm bladder irrigation
Warm enemas
Peritoneal lavage (KCl-free fluid)
Pleural lavage
Heated cardiopulmonary bypass*
Continue rewarming until
• Core temperature > 35°C or
• Return of spontaneous circulation or
• Resuscitative efforts cease†

* *Cardiac arrest and hemodynamic collapse are seen as the two usual indications for cardiopulmonary bypass in the setting of severe hypothermia.*

† *Successful resuscitations after prolonged advanced cardiac life support (ACLS), although unusual, have been reported, predominantly in the pediatric literature. ACLS and active rewarming should, in most cases, be continued until the core temperature reaches 35°C.*

predisposes to ventricular fibrillation (VF) which could be preceded by ECG changes such as QT-interval prolongation, T-wave inversion and Osborne waves. Trivial manoeuvres such as endotracheal intubation or simply moving the patient could be sufficient triggers. Electrical defibrillation for VF is less effective at core temperatures below 30$^0$C but should be attempted. If 3 shocks at 200, 300 and 360J respectively are unsuccessful in restoring an organized rhythm, shift efforts to aggressive rewarming while continuing advanced cardiac life support protocol (Figure 1). Recovery following prolonged resuscitation is well described and it is suggested that hypothermia victims should not be pronounced dead until warm and dead.

Controversies still exist on the utility of *temperature correcting* arterial pH and blood gases relative to the hypothermia. *Uncorrected* pH, $pO_2$ and $pCO_2$ values are more physiologic and more valuable to the clinician.

Following ABC support, rewarming takes precedence. There are 3 progressive modalities:

- **Passive rewarming** consists of minimizing heat loss by removing wet or frozen clothing, keeping the patient dry and covered with warm blankets. Passive rewarming relies on the patient's ability to shiver, which is lost below 32$^0$C. It is an essential first-line intervention but additional steps should be taken in more severe hypothermia.
- **Active external rewarming** refers to the use of warming blankets or warm water immersion. This approach should only be used in stable patients with minimal metabolic abnormalities since paradoxical acidosis and worsening of core hypothermia may result. This is due to the peripheral vasodilatation induced by external rewarming while the central organs remain cold. If used, active external rewarming should be limited to the body trunk.
- **Active core rewarming** is the favored approach in severe hypothermia. Heated IV crystalloids (40$^0$C to 42$^0$C) should be administered through a peripheral IV line. If a blood warmer is not available, IV solutions could be heated in a microwave oven but only if they do not contain dextrose and the temperature is monitored before administration. Blood cannot be heated in a microwave.
  Mechanical ventilation using heated oxygen (40$^0$C to 45$^0$C) is another simple and effective technique. Heated peritoneal lavage, administered through a temporary catheter using 2000 mL of dialysate at 44°C, exchanged every 20 minutes, can increase core temperature by up to 2°C per hour. Disseminated intravascular coagulation, intra-abdominal bleeding and electrolyte imbalance are the most common complications. Heated enemas, nasogastric lavage, bladder

irrigation, open and closed thoracic lavage have all been tried with mixed results.

Heated cardiopulmonary bypass provides the fastest and most physiologic method of active core rewarming. This technique is usually limited to the management of patients suffering cardiac arrest or those with unstable hemodynamics and arrhythmias. The transfer of these patients to a hospital where the technique is available should be considered.

## Pharmacologic Choices

- Since hypothermia is often associated with alcohol intoxication, **thiamine** supplementation is part of the supportive therapy. **Glucose** and **naloxone** (if opioid overdose is suspected) should probably also be administered. Other sources of intoxication and appropriate therapy should be considered.
- **Prophylactic antibiotic** therapy is controversial. Some authors advocate wide-spectrum antibiotic coverage for the first 3 days but there are no clinical trial data to support this recommendation.
- Hypothermic patients will usually require **fluid resuscitation** with warm isotonic solutions. Vasopressors should be avoided since they are usually ineffective and could precipitate arrhythmia.
- Pharmacologic management of cardiac arrest in hypothermic patients is difficult. Most antiarrhythmic agents, with the notable exception of **bretylium**, are considered ineffective until rewarming. Bretylium (5 mg/kg IV) is the drug of choice for VF. Procainamide should be avoided.

## Therapeutic Tips

- Hyper and hypothermia are more commonly signs of an underlying illness than primary problems. Establishing the appropriate diagnosis and instituting definitive therapy are more important in these circumstances than treating the thermometer reading.
- Nonpharmacologic management is the basis for therapy of true thermoregulation disorders.
- Hypothermic patients are prone to cardiac arrhythmia; ECG monitoring is mandatory. Aggressive resuscitation and rewarming are warranted.

## *Suggested Reading List*

Cummins RO, ed. *Advanced cardiac life support*. 2nd ed. Dallas: American Heart Association, 1997.

Hanania NA, Zimmerman JL. Accidental hypothermia. *Crit Care Clin* 1999;15:235–249.

Kirkpatrick AW, Chun R, Brown R, Simons RK. Hypothermia and the trauma patient. *Can J Surg* 1999;42:333–343.

Leikin JB, Aks SE, Andrews S, Auerbach PS, et al. Environmental injuries. *Dis Mon* 1997;43:809–916.

## CHAPTER 108

# Cough

*Tony R. Bai, MD, FRACP, FRCPC*

## Goals of Therapy

- To choose appropriate therapy based on cough etiology
- To decrease or abolish a nonproductive or distressing cough
- To resist nonspecific cough suppression therapy which may delay diagnosis of a curable cause

## Investigations

- Clinical history including:
  – potential causes (Tables 1 and 2)
  – duration of cough – acute vs chronic (cough > 3 weeks)
  – presence and nature of sputum (blood-tinged, purulence)
  – timing and nature of cough (day or night)
  – associated diseases (sinusitis, gastroesophageal reflux, asthma)
  – smoking habits
  – ACE inhibitor (ACEI) use; all ACEIs may cause cough (two-fold greater prevalence in women)
- Investigations of **acute cough** are guided by the presence and nature of sputum. In **chronic cough**, sequential investigation, including empiric therapy, is the most cost-effective approach (Figure 1)

## Therapeutic Choices

### Nonpharmacologic Choices

- Avoid stimuli causing cough: cigarette smoking, cold air, exercise, pungent chemicals.
- Stop or reduce dose of drugs causing cough (e.g., ACEIs) if possible.
- In acute exacerbations of suppurative lung disease, postural drainage (physiotherapy referral) may help.

Table 1: **Causes of Acute Cough**

| |
|---|
| Infections: upper and lower respiratory tract |
| Asthma |
| Exacerbations of chronic bronchitis |
| Bronchogenic carcinoma |
| Foreign body inhalation |
| Gastroesophageal reflux with aspiration |
| Left heart failure |

Figure 1: **Management of Chronic Cough***

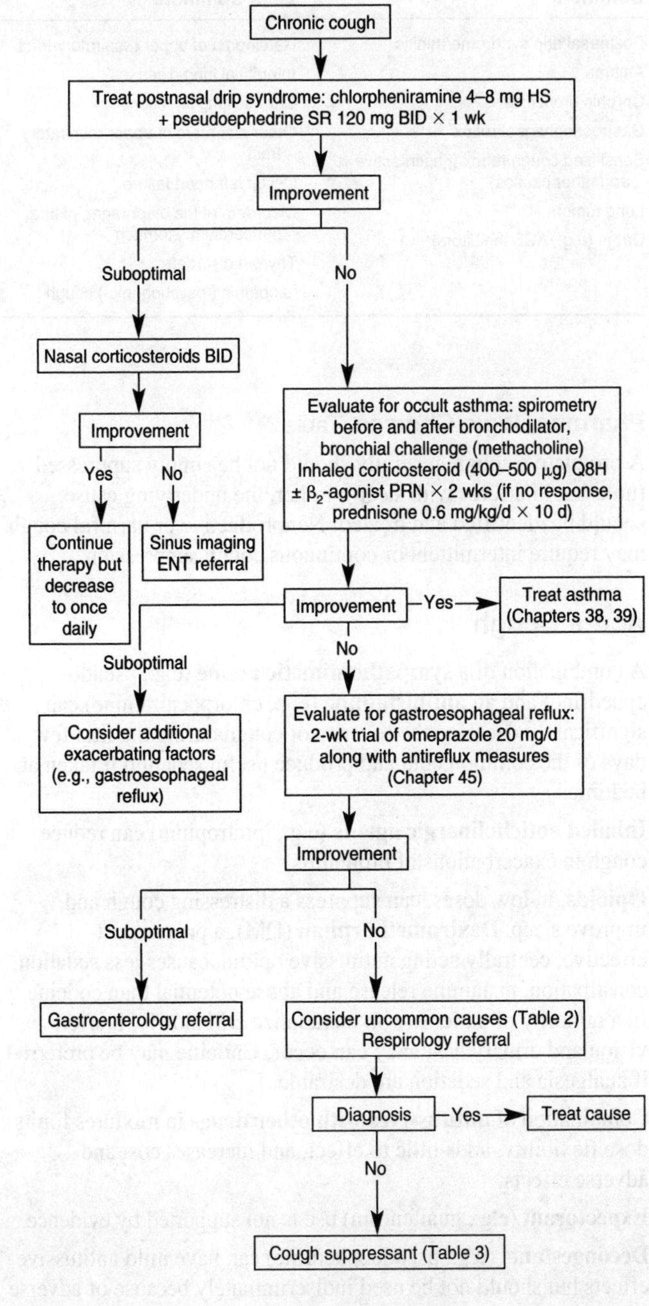
Chronic cough
Treat postnasal drip syndrome: chlorpheniramine 4–8 mg HS + pseudoephedrine SR 120 mg BID × 1 wk
Improvement
Suboptimal
No
Nasal corticosteroids BID
Improvement
Yes
No
Continue therapy but decrease to once daily
Sinus imaging ENT referral
Evaluate for occult asthma: spirometry before and after bronchodilator, bronchial challenge (methacholine) Inhaled corticosteroid (400–500 µg) Q8H ± β2-agonist PRN × 2 wks (if no response, prednisone 0.6 mg/kg/d × 10 d)
Improvement
Yes
Treat asthma (Chapters 38, 39)
No
Suboptimal
Consider additional exacerbating factors (e.g., gastroesophageal reflux)
Evaluate for gastroesophageal reflux: 2-wk trial of omeprazole 20 mg/d along with antireflux measures (Chapter 45)
Improvement
Suboptimal
No
Gastroenterology referral
Consider uncommon causes (Table 2) Respirology referral
Diagnosis
Yes
Treat cause
No
Cough suppressant (Table 3)

* *Algorithm assumes the chest x-ray is normal, and smoking has been discontinued for 4 weeks.*

Table 2: **Causes of Chronic Cough**

| Common | Less Common |
|---|---|
| Postnasal drip syndrome/rhinitis | Carcinoma of upper respiratory tract |
| Asthma | Interstitial lung diseases |
| Chronic bronchitis | Chronic lung infections |
| Gastroesophageal reflux | Other disorders of upper respiratory tract |
| Sensitized cough reflex (postinfective and other causes) | Occult left heart failure |
| Lung tumors | Disorders of the diaphragm, pleura, pericardium, stomach |
| Drugs (e.g., ACE inhibitors) | Thyroid disorders |
| | Idiopathic ("psychogenic") cough |

### Pharmacologic Choices (Table 3)

A productive cough generally should not be simply suppressed (unless it interferes with sleep); rather, the underlying cause should be identified and treated. Nonproductive or harmful cough may require intermittent or continuous cough suppression.

## Acute Cough

A combination of a **sympathomimetic amine** (e.g., pseudoephedrine) and an **antihistamine** (e.g., chlorpheniramine) can significantly decrease the severity of cough during the first few days of the common cold and produce useful sedation if taken at bedtime.

**Inhaled anticholinergic agents** (e.g., ipratropium) can reduce cough in exacerbations of bronchitis.

**Opioids**, in low doses, can suppress a distressing cough and improve sleep. **Dextromethorphan** (DM), a proven cost-effective, centrally acting antitussive opioid, causes less sedation, constipation, histamine release and abuse potential than codeine. In a minority of patients who metabolize DM slowly, blurred vision and urinary hesitancy can occur. **Codeine** may be preferred if analgesia and sedation are desirable.

Combination of **antitussives with other drugs** in mixtures limits dose flexibility, adds little to effect, and increases cost and adverse effects.

**Expectorant** (e.g., guaifenesin) use is not supported by evidence.

**Decongestants** (e.g., pseudoephedrine) can have mild antitussive effects but should not be used indiscriminately because of adverse effects (e.g, sleep disturbance, increased blood pressure). They reduce nasal congestion when applied topically.

Table 3: **Drugs Used in Cough Suppression**

| Drug | Dosage | Adverse Effects | Cost* |
|---|---|---|---|
| **Antitussives** | | | |
| *dextromethorphan*<br>Benylin DM, Formula 44, Delsym (sustained release), others | Adult:<br>15–30 mg Q6–8H<br>60 mg Q12H (sustained release)<br>Pediatric:<br>< 2 yrs: 1 mg/kg/d divided Q6–8H<br>2–5 yrs: 2.5–5 mg Q4H to 7.5 mg Q6–8H up to 30 mg/d<br>6–11 yrs: 5–10 mg Q4H to 15 mg Q6–8H up to 60 mg/d<br>12+ yrs: 10–20 mg Q4H to 30 mg Q6–8H up to 120 mg/d | Drowsiness, GI upset, blurred vision and urinary hesitancy in patients who metabolize DM slowly. | $† |
| *codeine* (if analgesia and sedation desired)<br>generics | Adult:<br>5–20 mg Q4–8H<br>Pediatric:<br>< 2 yrs: 0.8–1.2 mg/kg/d divided Q4–6H<br>2–5 yrs: 0.25 mg/kg Q4–6H PRN up to 20 mg/d<br>6–11 yrs: 0.25 mg/kg Q4–6H PRN up to 60 mg/d<br>≥12 yrs: 0.25 mg/kg Q4–6H PRN up to 120 mg/d | Constipation, drowsiness, nausea. | $ |
| **Anticholinergics** | | | |
| *ipratropium*<br>Atrovent | 2–4 puffs QID | Dry mouth, metallic taste. | $$/inhaler |
| **Antihistamines** | | | |
| various agents, e.g., *chlorpheniramine*<br>Chlortripolon, generics | Adult: 4–8 mg HS<br>Pediatric: 1–2 mg HS | Mild sedation, decreases with tolerance. | $† |

* *Cost of 100 mL or 15 tablets – includes drug cost only.*
† *Available without prescription – retail mark-up may vary.*

*Legend:* $ < $10 $$ $10–20

**Antihistamines** act indirectly as antitussives by reducing swelling, nasal discharge and itchiness.

**Demulcent preparations** (e.g., 5 to 10 mL simple syrup containing 125 mg citric acid monohydrate per 5 mL) or cough lozenges are soothing, largely because of their sugar content, which probably coats sensory endings in the hypopharynx. Their effect lasts only a few minutes.

## Therapeutic Tips

- In most patients with chronic cough, treatment of the identifiable cause will resolve the symptom.
- Patients with a recurrence of cough within 3 months after treatment require chronic or episodic therapy.
- More than one cause of chronic cough may occur in the same individual.
- The cough reflex can become "sensitized", with a reduced threshold for sensory nerve activation following a variety of insults. This leads to a prolonged cough requiring prolonged antitussive therapy (e.g., DM) or nebulized lidocaine. Psychogenic cough is a diagnosis of exclusion; patients recognize emotional stress as a frequent trigger and nocturnal cough is absent. Psychiatrist/psychologist referral may be appropriate.
- If for medical reasons an ACEI that is inducing cough cannot be discontinued or must be readministered because alternative therapies (e.g., angiotensin II antagonists) have failed, inhaled sodium cromoglycate can be helpful.[1]
- Oral codeine and morphine remain the gold standard antitussives in cough associated with malignant or terminal respiratory disease. Oral DM is the nonaddictive gold standard for most other chronic coughs in which analgesia/sedation is not required.
- The increased cough and mucus production in acute exacerbations of asthma, COPD, cystic fibrosis and bronchiectasis should respond to appropriate treatment of the underlying cause; cough suppressants in such patients could lead to retention of mucus and deterioration in the underlying disease.
- Older antihistamines (e.g., chlorpheniramine) have been found to be more efficacious than the newer, relatively nonsedating group in treating postnasal drip syndrome. This may be attributed to their mild anticholinergic effect.

---

[1] *Lancet 1995;345:13–16.*

- The use of multi-ingredient cough mixtures is not advised.
- The antitussive effect of inhalations of warm water vapor with menthol and eucalyptus has not been adequately evaluated. Hypo-osmolar solutions can provoke cough.

## Suggested Reading List

ACCP consensus conference: managing cough as a defense mechanism and as a symptom. *Chest* 1998;114:133S–181S.

Carney IK, Gibson PG, Murree-Allen K, et al. A systematic evaluation of mechanisms in chronic cough. *Am J Respir Crit Care* 1997;156:211–216.

Fuller RW, Jackson DM. Physiology and treatment of cough. *Thorax* 1990;45:425–430.

Ing AJ, Ngu MC. Cough and gastro-oesophageal reflux. *Lancet* 1999;353:944–946.

Pratter MR, Bartter T, Akers S, et al. An algorithmic approach to chronic cough. *Ann Intern Med* 1993;119:977–983.

CHAPTER 109

# Persistent Hiccoughs

*James M. Wright, MD, PhD, FRCPC*

Persistent or intractable hiccoughs are unusual but distressing. They may cause insomnia, weight loss or depression and are associated with metabolic causes and abnormalities of the CNS, ear, throat, thorax and abdomen.

## Goals of Therapy

- To decrease or stop hiccoughs
- To prevent recurrence

## Investigations

- Complete history (including medication and alcohol use) and physical examination to provide clues for further investigations
- If no abnormalities, it is reasonable to do a CBC, electrolytes, creatinine and chest x-ray
- Further investigations depend on findings of the history, physical and baseline investigations: upper GI tract endoscopy, CT brain scan, abdominal ultrasound, etc.

If all investigations are negative or etiological treatment is impossible, a therapeutic trial to stop the hiccoughs is warranted.

## Therapeutic Choices

### Nonpharmacologic Choices

- Drug-induced persistent hiccoughs are uncommon. Alcohol, corticosteroids and benzodiazepines are the drug classes most frequently implicated.[1]
- Vagal stimulation (e.g., posterior pharyngeal wall stimulation, Valsalva manoeuvre, digital rectal massage, etc.) may be helpful.
- Gastric aspiration is effective in gastric distention.
- Phrenic nerve disruption is reserved for cases where all else has failed.

[1] *Prescrire Internat 1999;8:23.*

### Pharmacologic Choices

The condition is rare; hence, only two randomized, controlled trials were identified. The first was in 51 patients who developed hiccoughs during anesthesia;[2] patients were randomized to receive methylphenidate or saline injection in a double-blind protocol. Equal numbers of cures were found in the two groups. The second was a cross-over trial comparing baclofen with placebo (see below). Most of the treatment recommendations are based on case reports/open trials in small numbers of patients.

#### *Dopamine Antagonists*

**Chlorpromazine** historically has been the drug of choice.[3] It has been used IV (25 to 50 mg over 0.5 to 1 hour) in the emergency room. A trial of 50 to 100 mg PO daily for 2 to 3 days is also reasonable. **Haloperidol**, 2 to 5 mg IM or 5 to 15 mg PO, has also been effective in some cases.

**Metoclopramide**, 10 mg IV or IM followed by 10 to 20 mg QID PO, has been successful. It may act as a dopamine antagonist or by enhancing gastric emptying.

#### *Baclofen*

Baclofen has been reported effective in cases of intractable hiccoughs, with maintenance therapy required in at least one half. A randomized, double blind, cross-over trial in 4 patients with intractable hiccoughs demonstrated that baclofen was unable to eliminate the hiccoughs, but did provide dose-related symptomatic relief.[4] Starting with 5 mg BID, the dose is increased gradually every 2 to 3 days to a maximum daily dose of 75 mg. If effective, baclofen should not be discontinued suddenly. The minimum maintenance dose can be determined by gradually reducing the dose over time. Mild side effects (drowsiness, weakness, nausea and fatigue) are relatively frequent.

#### *Calcium Channel Blockers*

**Nifedipine** (30 to 60 mg daily) was shown to be effective in 4 of 7 patients with persistent hiccoughs[5]. In a recent report (2 patients), IV **nimodipine** was also successful.[6]

Many other drugs have been reported effective in a small number of case reports. However, the data are insufficient to recommend any of them. There are no pharmacoeconomic studies for this rare disorder.

---

[2] *Anesthesiology 1969;31:89–90.*
[3] *JAMA 1955;157:309–310.*
[4] *Am J Gastroenterol 1992;87:1789–1791.*
[5] *Neurology 1990;40:531–532.*
[6] *Am J Med 1999;106:600.*

## Therapeutic Tips

- When a drug is effective, hiccoughs generally stop abruptly within a few hours; in some cases, the frequency and amplitude may slowly decrease.
- Attempts should be made to withdraw treatments gradually; maintenance therapy may be required in some cases.
- Benzodiazepines should be avoided as worsening of hiccoughs has been reported.
- When a drug is ineffective, there is no need to continue treatment for more than 3 days.

## *Suggested Reading List*

Friedman NL. Hiccoughs: A treatment review. *Pharmacotherapy* 1996;16:986–995.

Launois S, Bizec JL, Whitelaw WA, et al. Hiccough in adults: an overview. *Eur Respir J* 1993;6:563–575.

Walker P, Watanabe S, Bruera E. Baclofen, a treatment for chronic hiccough. *J Pain Symptom Manage* 1998;16: 125–132.

## APPENDIX I

# Dosage Adjustment in Renal Impairment

*James McCormack, BSc(Pharm), PharmD, Bruce Carleton, BPharm, PharmD and Janet Cooper, BSc(Pharm)*

Careful dosage adjustment may reduce the risk of drug toxicity in patients with impaired renal function. The following is an approach to empiric dosage adjustments (dose and/or interval) in adult patients based on an estimate of renal function (Figure 1, Table 1). This approach does not apply to patients on dialysis (consult specialized references).

## Patient/Drug Considerations

The following questions should be answered prior to making empiric dosage adjustments. Table 2 provides drug-specific information.

**Is the patient's renal function impaired?**

Use the following formula[1] to estimate the **weight-corrected creatinine clearance** (ClCr) and to guide empiric dosage adjustments:

$$\text{Males: ClCr (mL/s/70 kg)} = \frac{(140 - \text{age}) \times 1.5}{\text{serum creatinine } (\mu\text{mol/L})}$$

$$\text{Females: ClCr (mL/s/70 kg)} = 0.85 \times \text{above equation}$$

Many clinicians may be more familiar with a ClCr formula which includes weight. When using formulas to estimate ClCr, first identify the reason for the ClCr determination. If an estimate of the patient's true ClCr (in mL/second) is needed, then use a ClCr formula which includes weight. However, if the estimate of the degree of renal impairment is to guide dosage adjustments, use a weight-corrected estimate of ClCr rather than the patient's actual ClCr. This weight-corrected estimate is then compared to a "normal" ClCr for a 72 kg male (1.8 to 2 mL/s) to approximate the degree of renal dysfunction. Charts which suggest empiric dosage adjustments are usually based on the assumption that the baseline or normal ClCr is 1.8 to 2 mL/s. In addition, a weight-corrected ClCr is easier to calculate.

---

[1] *McCormack JP, Cooper J, Carleton B. Simple approach to dosage adjustment in patients with renal impairment. Am J Health-Sys Pharm 1997;54:2505–2509.*

Elderly (older than 65) or malnourished patients may have relatively low muscle mass and therefore produce less creatinine. If the actual serum creatinine for such patients is used, the formula can often overestimate renal function. A rule of thumb in such patients is not to use a serum creatinine < 100 μmol/L in the above formula.

In general, if ClCr estimates are > 1 mL/s/70 kg, empiric dosage adjustments are not required because changes in ClCr from 2 to 1 mL/s/70 kg are associated with relatively small changes in the half-life of a drug or its active metabolite. However, as ClCr falls below 1 mL/s/70 kg, empiric dosage adjustments should be based on the following questions.

**Is the drug effective/safe in patients with renal impairment?** (Table 2, column 1)
Some drugs are ineffective or potentially toxic in patients with significant renal dysfunction (ClCr < 0.5 mL/s/70 kg) and should be avoided.

**Is the drug nephrotoxic?** (Table 2, column 2)
A number of drugs have the potential to worsen renal function and an alternative non-nephrotoxic agent should be used if possible.

**Is an immediate clinical effect required?**
When failure to elicit an immediate response (e.g., life-threatening conditions or severe pain) poses a significant risk of mortality or morbidity, drug dosing should be aimed at obtaining a therapeutic response within minutes or hours irrespective of renal function. In an attempt to achieve a rapid response, usual initial doses should be used, followed by empiric dosage adjustments once the patient has responded.

**If an immediate effect is not required can the dose be titrated?** (Table 2, column 3)
Many conditions do not require an immediate or maximal effect and dose titration can often be used to determine the lowest effective dose. To identify the correct dose for any patient, but particularly in patients with renal impairment, start with a low dose (e.g., 1/4 or 1/2 of the typically recommended dose), and titrate up to a clinical effect.

**Is the drug > 50% renally eliminated or does it have active or toxic metabolites?** (Table 2, columns 4–7)
Drugs that are primarily eliminated by the kidney (> 50%) require empiric dosage adjustments based on an estimate of renal function. In addition, some drugs are metabolized to active or toxic metabolites which may be excreted by the kidney and may need dosage adjustments. Some drugs should be avoided in patients with compromised renal function if toxic metabolites can accumulate (e.g., meperidine).

## Approach to Empiric Dosage Adjustments

When dose titration is not possible or desired, empiric dosage adjustments should be made on the basis of estimates of renal function.

### Interval vs Dose Adjustment

For drugs given intermittently, the dose or the dosing interval can be adjusted based on the desired goal. Often a combination of extending the interval and reducing the dose is effective and convenient. If the aim is to achieve steady-state maximum/peak and minimum/trough concentrations (e.g., aminoglycosides) similar to those seen in patients with normal renal function, the interval between doses should be extended. If a relatively constant steady-state concentration is desired (e.g., anti-hypertensives), the dose should be reduced.

### Drugs Eliminated ≥ 75% by the Kidney (Table 2, column 6)

Guidelines for the dosage of these drugs, based on the usual dosing interval, are provided in Table 1. For frequently administered drugs (e.g., Q4H–Q12H), extending the interval may decrease the cost of administration or adherence problems.

### Drugs Eliminated 50–74% by the Kidney (Table 2, column 5)

These drugs have a significant proportion of non-renal clearance and therefore empiric dosage adjustments are generally not required until renal function estimates are < 0.75 mL/s/70 kg (Table 1).

### Drugs Eliminated < 50% by the Kidney (Table 2, column 4)

For drugs eliminated < 50% by the kidneys, empiric dosage adjustments are generally not required, assuming the drug has no active or toxic metabolites. However, these drugs may require dosage adjustment in patients with significant liver dysfunction.

### Drugs with Active or Toxic Metabolites (Table 2, column 7)

Empiric dosage adjustments for drugs with active or toxic metabolites which are dependent on renal elimination should be made as if the drug was 75–100% renally eliminated.

## Further Dosage Adjustments Based on Clinical Response

All of the above recommendations are for empiric dosage adjustments, and further dosage changes must always be made based on a patient-specific assessment of efficacy and toxicity. Serum drug concentration monitoring may guide dosage adjustments for certain drugs (Table 2, column 8).

## Figure 1: Empiric Dosage Adjustment Based on Renal Function (Adults)

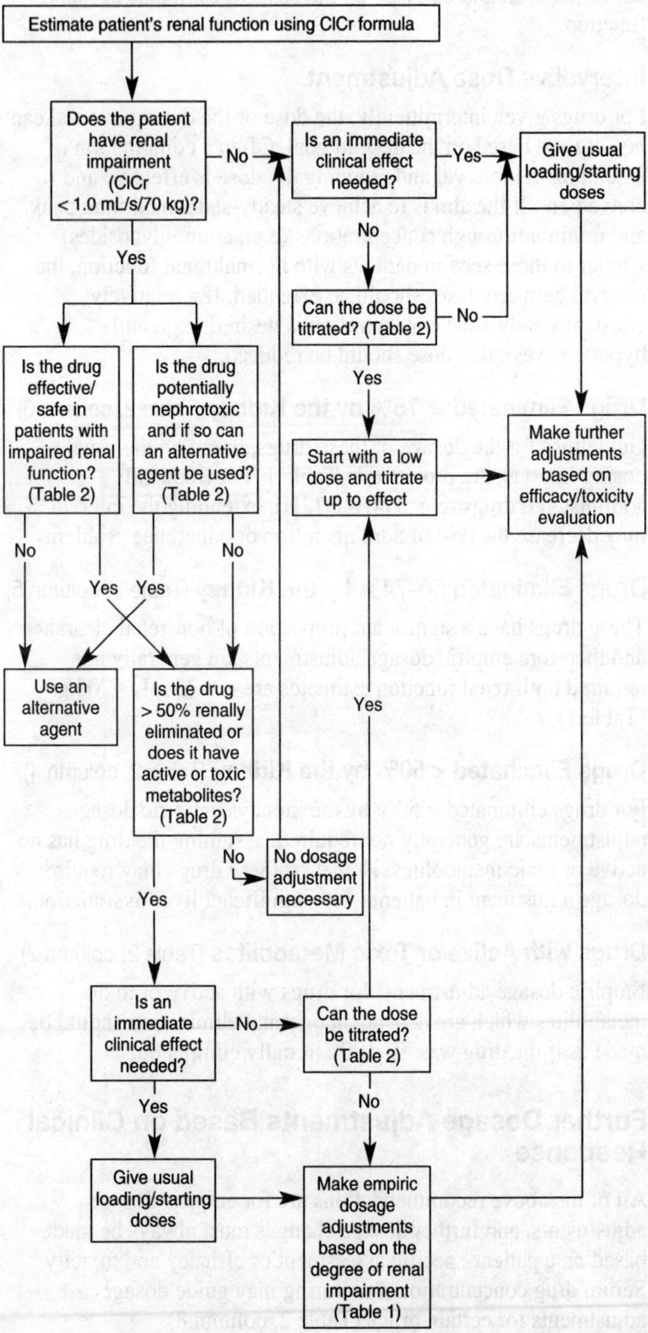
Estimate patient's renal function using ClCr formula
Does the patient have renal impairment (ClCr < 1.0 mL/s/70 kg)?
No
Is an immediate clinical effect needed?
Yes
Give usual loading/starting doses
No
Can the dose be titrated? (Table 2)
No
Yes
Start with a low dose and titrate up to effect
Make further adjustments based on efficacy/toxicity evaluation
Yes
Is the drug effective/ safe in patients with impaired renal function? (Table 2)
Is the drug potentially nephrotoxic and if so can an alternative agent be used? (Table 2)
No
No
Yes
Yes
Use an alternative agent
Is the drug > 50% renally eliminated or does it have active or toxic metabolites? (Table 2)
Yes
No
No dosage adjustment necessary
Yes
Is an immediate clinical effect needed?
No
Can the dose be titrated? (Table 2)
Yes
No
Give usual loading/starting doses
Make empiric dosage adjustments based on the degree of renal impairment (Table 1)

Table 1: **Suggested Empiric Dosage Adjustments in Adults for Drugs Primarily Renally Eliminated**
(based on percentage renal elimination and estimated creatinine clearance [normal ClCr = 2.0 mL/s/70 kg])

**How to Use Table 1:**

**1:** Estimate renal function (ClCr), *e.g., a patient with an estimated ClCr of 0.42 mL/s/70 kg is receiving IV ampicillin.*

**2:** Determine percentage renal elimination of drug (Table 2), *e.g., ampicillin is 75–100% renally eliminated, according to Table 2.*

**3:** Determine normal dosing interval, *e.g., usual dosing interval for ampicillin is Q6H.*

**4:** Using above information, determine empiric dosage adjustment, *e.g., the patient's ClCr is between 0.25–0.5 mL/s/70 kg. Therefore, the empiric dosing adjustment is to administer the ampicillin Q12H.*

| | | | Normal Dosing Interval | | | | |
|---|---|---|---|---|---|---|---|
| **% Renal Elimination of Drug:** | **75–100%** | **50–74%** | **Q4H** | **Q6H** | **Q8H** | **Q12H** | **Q24H** |
| | > 1.0 | > 0.75 | none | none | none | none | none |
| **Estimated ClCr (mL/s/70 kg)** | 0.5–1.0 | 0.33–0.75 | Q6H | Q8H | Q12H | Q24H | ↓D 25%* |
| | 0.25–0.5 | 0.16–0.33 | Q8H | Q12H | Q24H | Q24H and ↓D 25% * | ↓D 50%* |
| | < 0.25 | < 0.16 | Q12H | Q24H | Q24H and ↓D 25% * | Q24H and ↓D 50% * | ↓D 75%* |

**none** = *no dosage adjustment necessary;* **↓D** = *decrease usual dose by indicated percentage.*

* *For certain drugs, decreasing the dose is not appropriate, or one may need to extend interval > Q24H if available dosage forms do not permit specific dose reductions.*

Table 2: **Dosage Adjustment in Renal Impairment—Adults***

| Drug | Avoid | Nephrotoxic | Titrate | % Renal Elimination < 50% | % Renal Elimination 50–74% | % Renal Elimination ≥ 75% | AM | SDCM |
|---|---|---|---|---|---|---|---|---|
| abacavir | | | | • | | | | |
| acarbose | | | • | • | | | — | |
| acebutolol | | | • | | • | | ■ | |
| acetaminophen | | | • | • | | | | |
| acetazolamide | • | | | | | • | | |
| acitretin | | | | • | | | | |
| acyclovir | | | | | | • | | |
| alendronate | • | | | • | | | | |
| allopurinol | | | • | • | | | ■ | |
| alprazolam | | | • | • | | | | |
| amantadine[1] | | | • | | | • | | |
| amikacin | | • | | | | • | | • |
| amiloride | • | | • | | • | | | |
| 5-aminosalicylic acid | | | | • | | | | |
| amiodarone | | | • | • | | | — | |
| amitriptyline | | | • | • | | | — | |
| amlodipine | | | • | • | | | | |
| amoxapine | | | | • | | | — | |
| amoxicillin | | | | | • | | | |
| amoxicillin/ clavulanate | | | | | • | | | |
| amphotericin | | • | | • | | | | |
| ampicillin | | | | | | • | | |
| anileridine | | | • | • | | | | |
| anistreplase | | | | • | | | — | |
| antacids: magnesium/ aluminum[2] | • | | • | • | | | | |
| ASA | | • | • | • | | | | |
| astemizole | | | • | • | | | | |
| atenolol | | | • | | | • | | |
| atorvastatin | | | • | • | | | — | |
| atovaquone | | | | • | | | | |
| auranofin | • | • | | • | | | | |
| azathioprine | | | • | • | | | ■ | |
| azithromycin | | | | • | | | | |
| aztreonam | | | | | | • | | |
| bacampicillin | | | | | | • | | |
| baclofen | | | • | | | • | | |
| beclomethasone | | | | • | | | | |
| benazepril | | | • | • | | | ■ | |
| benztropine[3] | | | • | | | | | |
| bezafibrate | | | • | | • | | | |
| bismuth subsalicylate | | | | • | | | | |
| bisoprolol | | | • | | • | | | |
| bretylium | | | • | | | • | ■ | |

[1] *Administer amantadine Q48–72H for ClCr 0.25–1.0 mL/s/70 kg, once weekly for ClCr < 0.25 mL/s/70 kg.*
[2] *Aluminum and/or magnesium may accumulate in renal impairment.*
[3] *Route of elimination for benztropine unknown.*

Table 2: **Dosage Adjustment in Renal Impairment—Adults*** *(cont'd)*

| Drug | Avoid | Nephro-toxic | Titrate | % Renal Elimination < 50% | 50–74% | ≥ 75% | AM | SDCM |
|---|---|---|---|---|---|---|---|---|
| bromocriptine | | | | • | | | | |
| bumetanide | | | • | • | | | | |
| buprenorphine | | | • | • | | | | |
| bupropion | | | • | • | | | ■ | |
| buspirone | | | • | • | | | ■ | |
| candesartan | | | • | • | | | | |
| capreomycin | | • | | | • | | | |
| captopril | | | • | | • | | | |
| carbamazepine | | | • | • | | | — | • |
| carbidopa | | | • | • | | | | |
| carvedilol | | | • | • | | | — | |
| cefaclor | | | | | • | | | |
| cefadroxil | | | | | | • | | |
| cefamandole | | | | | | • | | |
| cefazolin | | | | | | • | | |
| cefepime | | | | | | • | | |
| cefixime | | | | | • | | | |
| cefoperazone | | | | • | | | | |
| cefotaxime | | | | | • | | ■ | |
| cefotetan | | | | | | • | | |
| cefoxitin | | | | | | • | | |
| cefprozil | | | | | • | | | |
| ceftazidime | | | | | | • | | |
| ceftizoxime | | | | | | • | | |
| ceftriaxone | | | | • | | | | |
| cefuroxime | | | | | | • | | |
| celecoxib | | • | • | • | | | | |
| cephalexin | | | | | | • | | |
| cerivastatin | | | | • | | | | |
| cetirizine | | | • | | • | | | |
| chloral hydrate | • | | • | • | | | ■ | |
| chloramphenicol | | | | • | | | — | |
| chlordiazepoxide | | | • | • | | | ■ | |
| chloroquine | | | | | • | | | |
| chlorpheniramine | | | • | • | | | | |
| chlorpromazine | | | • | • | | | — | |
| chlorpropamide | • | | • | • | | | ■ | |
| chlorthalidone | • | | • | | • | | | |

**Avoid** = *Avoid drug if ClCr < 0.5 mL/s/70 kg as drug may be ineffective or toxic.*

**Nephrotoxic** = *Potentially nephrotoxic drug: avoid if possible as may worsen renal function.*

**Titrate** = *Start with a low dose and titrate to desired effect, regardless of renal function.*

**AM** = *Drug metabolized to active or toxic metabolites:*

■ = *dosage reduction required (calculated as if drug was 75–100% renally eliminated);*

— = *no dosage reduction required.*

**SDCM** = *Serum drug concentration monitoring may help guide dosage adjustments.*

**Omission of a drug from this table does not imply that dosage adjustment is NOT required in renal impairment. Refer to specific references for dosing in dialysis.*

Table 2: **Dosage Adjustment in Renal Impairment—Adults*** *(cont'd)*

| Drug | Avoid | Nephro-toxic | Titrate | % Renal Elimination < 50% | % Renal Elimination 50–74% | % Renal Elimination ≥ 75% | AM | SDCM |
|---|---|---|---|---|---|---|---|---|
| cholestyramine | | | • | • | | | | |
| choline magnesium trisalicylate | | • | • | • | | | | |
| cidofovir | • | • | | | | • | ■ | |
| cilazapril | | | • | • | | | ■ | |
| cimetidine | | | • | | • | | | |
| ciprofloxacin | | | | | • | | | |
| cisapride | | | • | • | | | | |
| citalopram | | | • | • | | | | |
| clarithromycin | | | | • | | | ■ | |
| clindamycin | | | | • | | | | |
| clodronate | • | • | | | | • | | |
| clofibrate | • | | • | • | | | | |
| clomiphene | | | | • | | | | |
| clonazepam | | | • | • | | | | |
| clonidine | | | • | • | | | | |
| cloxacillin | | | | • | | | | |
| clozapine | | | • | • | | | — | |
| codeine | | | • | • | | | | |
| colchicine | • | | • | • | | | | |
| co-trimoxazole | | | | | • | | | |
| cyclosporine | | • | • | • | | | — | • |
| cyproheptadine | | | • | • | | | | |
| cyproterone acetate | | | | • | | | | |
| danazol | | | | • | | | | |
| delavirdine | | | | • | | | | |
| desipramine | | | • | • | | | | |
| dexamethasone | | | | • | | | | |
| diazepam | | | • | • | | | | |
| diclofenac | | • | • | • | | | | |
| dicloxacillin | | | | • | | | | |
| dicyclomine | | | • | | | • | | |
| didanosine | | | | • | | | ■ | |
| diethylpropion | | | | • | | | | |
| diflunisal | | • | • | • | | | | |
| digoxin | | | • | | | • | | • |
| diltiazem | | | • | • | | | | |
| dimenhydrinate | | | • | • | | | | |
| diphenhydramine | | | • | • | | | | |
| disopyramide | | | | | • | | | |
| dolasetron[4] | • | | | • | | | — | |
| domperidone | | | • | • | | | | |
| donepezil | | | • | • | | | — | |
| doxazosin | | | • | • | | | | |
| doxepin | | | • | • | | | — | |
| doxycycline | | | | • | | | | |

[4] *Dolasetron is not recommended in severe renal impairment because of possibility of prolonged $QT_c$ intervals and other cardiac conduction abnormalities due to ↑ hydrodolasetron levels.*

## Table 2: **Dosage Adjustment in Renal Impairment—Adults*** *(cont'd)*

| Drug | Avoid | Nephro-toxic | Titrate | % Renal Elimination | | | AM | SDCM |
|---|---|---|---|---|---|---|---|---|
| | | | | < 50% | 50–74% | ≥ 75% | | |
| efavirenz | | | | • | | | | |
| enalapril | | | • | • | | | ■ | |
| eptifibatide | | | | • | | | | |
| erythromycin | | | | • | | | | |
| esmolol | | | | • | | | | |
| estrogens | | | • | • | | | | |
| ethacrynic acid | • | | • | • | | | | |
| ethambutol | | | | | • | | | |
| ethopropazine[5] | | | • | | | | | |
| ethosuximide | | | | • | | | | |
| etidronate | | • | | | • | | | |
| etodolac | | • | • | • | | | | |
| famciclovir | | | | • | | | ■ | |
| famotidine | | | • | | | • | | |
| felodipine | | | • | • | | | | |
| fenofibrate | | | • | • | | | ■ | |
| fenoprofen | | • | • | • | | | | |
| fentanyl | | | | • | | | | |
| fexofenadine[6] | | | • | • | | | | |
| fluconazole | | | | | • | | | |
| fludrocortisone | | | • | • | | | | |
| flucytosine | | | | | | • | | |
| flunarizine | | | • | • | | | | |
| flupenthixol | | | • | • | | | | |
| fluphenazine | | | • | • | | | | |
| fluoxetine | | | • | • | | | — | |
| flurazepam | | | • | • | | | — | |
| flurbiprofen | | • | • | • | | | | |
| fluvastatin | | | • | • | | | | |
| foscarnet | • | • | | | | • | | |
| fosinopril | | | • | • | | | — | |
| furosemide[7] | | | • | | • | | | |
| gabapentin | | | • | | | • | | |
| ganciclovir | | | | | | • | | |
| gemfibrozil | | | • | • | | | ■ | |

[5] *Route of elimination for ethopropazine unknown.*

[6] *Clearance of fexofenadine is ↓ in renal impairment; reduce dose to once daily.*

[7] *In severe renal impairment, larger doses of furosemide than those used in patients with normal renal function may be required.*

**Avoid** = *Avoid drug if ClCr < 0.5 mL/s/70 kg as drug may be ineffective or toxic.*

**Nephrotoxic** = *Potentially nephrotoxic drug: avoid if possible as may worsen renal function.*

**Titrate** = *Start with a low dose and titrate to desired effect, regardless of renal function.*

**AM** = *Drug metabolized to active or toxic metabolites:*

■ = *dosage reduction required (calculated as if drug was 75–100% renally eliminated);*

— = *no dosage reduction required.*

**SDCM** = *Serum drug concentration monitoring may help guide dosage adjustments.*

**Omission of a drug from this table does not imply that dosage adjustment is NOT required in renal impairment. Refer to specific references for dosing in dialysis.*

Table 2: **Dosage Adjustment in Renal Impairment—Adults*** *(cont'd)*

| Drug | Avoid | Nephro-toxic | Titrate | % Renal Elimination < 50% | 50–74% | ≥ 75% | AM | SDCM |
|---|---|---|---|---|---|---|---|---|
| gentamicin | | • | | | | • | | • |
| gliclazide | | | • | • | | | | |
| glyburide | • | | • | • | | | | |
| gold sodium thiomalate | • | • | | | • | | | |
| goserelin | | | | • | | | | |
| granisetron | | | | • | | | | |
| haloperidol | | | • | • | | | | |
| heparin | | | | • | | | | |
| hydralazine | | | • | • | | | | |
| hydrochlorothiazide | • | | • | | | • | | |
| hydrocortisone | | | • | • | | | | |
| hydromorphone | | | • | • | | | | |
| hydroxyurea | | • | | | • | | | |
| hydroxyzine | | | | • | | | — | |
| hyoscyamine | | | • | | | • | | |
| ibuprofen | | • | • | • | | | | |
| imipenem/cilastatin | | | | | • | | | |
| imipramine | | | • | • | | | — | |
| indapamide | • | | • | • | | | | |
| indinavir | | | | • | | | | |
| indomethacin | | • | • | • | | | | |
| infliximab[8] | | | | | | | | |
| insulin | | | • | • | | | | |
| interferon alfa-2b | | | | • | | | | |
| irbesartan | | | • | • | | | | |
| isoniazid | | | | • | | | | |
| isosorbide | | | • | • | | | — | |
| itraconazole | | | | • | | | | |
| kanamycin | | • | | | | • | | • |
| ketoconazole | | | | • | | | | |
| ketoprofen | | • | • | • | | | | |
| ketotifen | | | | • | | | | |
| labetalol | | | • | • | | | | |
| lamivudine | | | | | • | | ■ | |
| lamotrigine | | | • | • | | | | |
| lansoprazole | | | • | • | | | | |
| leflunomide | • | | • | • | | | — | |
| leuprolide | | | • | • | | | | |
| levodopa | | | • | • | | | — | |
| levofloxacin | | | | | | • | | |
| levonorgestrel | | | | • | | | | |
| levothyroxine | | | • | • | | | | |
| lidocaine | | | • | • | | | — | |
| lisinopril | | | • | | | • | | |
| lithium | | • | | | | • | | • |
| loratadine | | | • | • | | | — | |

[8] *How infliximab is metabolized and excreted is unknown.*

Table 2: **Dosage Adjustment in Renal Impairment—Adults*** *(cont'd)*

| Drug | Avoid | Nephro-toxic | Titrate | % Renal Elimination | | | AM | SDCM |
|---|---|---|---|---|---|---|---|---|
| | | | | <50% | 50–74% | ≥75% | | |
| lorazepam | | | • | • | | | | |
| losartan | | | • | • | | | — | |
| lovastatin | | | | • | | | | |
| loxapine | | | • | • | | | | |
| maprotiline | | | • | • | | | — | |
| medroxyprogesterone | | | | • | | | | |
| mefenamic acid | | • | • | • | | | | |
| mefloquine | | | | • | | | | |
| megestrol | | | | • | | | | |
| meperidine | • | | • | • | | | ■ | |
| mercaptopurine | | | | • | | | ■ | |
| meropenem | | | | | • | | | |
| mesoridazine | | | • | • | | | | |
| metformin | • | | • | | | • | | |
| methadone | | | | • | | | | |
| methazolamide | • | | | • | | | | |
| methotrexate | • | • | | | | • | | |
| methotrimeprazine | | | • | • | | | — | |
| methyldopa | | | • | • | | | ■ | |
| methylphenidate | | | • | • | | | | |
| methylprednisolone | | | | • | | | | |
| metoclopramide | | | • | | • | | | |
| metolazone[9] | | | • | | • | | | |
| metoprolol | | | • | • | | | | |
| metronidazole | | | | • | | | — | |
| mexiletine | | | • | • | | | — | |
| miconazole | | | | • | | | | |
| midazolam | | | • | • | | | | |
| midodrine | | | • | • | | | ■ | |
| minocycline | | | | • | | | | |
| minoxidil | | | • | • | | | | |
| misoprostol | | | • | • | | | | |
| moclobemide | | | • | • | | | | |
| montelukast | | | • | • | | | | |
| morphine | | | • | • | | | ■ | |
| nabumetone | | • | • | • | | | ■ | |
| nadolol | | | • | | | • | | |

[9] *Dosage reduction of metolazone not necessary in renal impairment.*

**Avoid** = *Avoid drug if ClCr < 0.5 mL/s/70 kg as drug may be ineffective or toxic.*

**Nephrotoxic** = *Potentially nephrotoxic drug: avoid if possible as may worsen renal function.*

**Titrate** = *Start with a low dose and titrate to desired effect, regardless of renal function.*

**AM** = *Drug metabolized to active or toxic metabolites:*

■ = *dosage reduction required (calculated as if drug was 75–100% renally eliminated);*

— = *no dosage reduction required.*

**SDCM** = *Serum drug concentration monitoring may help guide dosage adjustments.*

**Omission of a drug from this table does not imply that dosage adjustment is NOT required in renal impairment. Refer to specific references for dosing in dialysis.*

Table 2: **Dosage Adjustment in Renal Impairment—Adults*** *(cont'd)*

| Drug | Avoid | Nephro-toxic | Titrate | % Renal Elimination | | | AM | SDCM |
|---|---|---|---|---|---|---|---|---|
| | | | | < 50% | 50–74% | ≥ 75% | | |
| nadroparin | | | | | | • | | |
| nafcillin | | | | • | | | | |
| nalidixic acid | • | | | • | | | ■ | |
| naltrexone | | | | • | | | — | |
| naproxen | | • | • | • | | | | |
| naratriptan | | | | | • | | | |
| nelfinavir | | | | • | | | | |
| netilmicin | | • | | | | • | | • |
| nevirapine | | | | • | | | | |
| niacin | | | • | • | | | | |
| nicardipine | | | • | • | | | | |
| nifedipine | | | • | • | | | | |
| nimodipine | | | • | • | | | | |
| nitrofurantoin | • | | | • | | | ■ | |
| nitroglycerin | | | • | • | | | | |
| nizatidine | | | • | | • | | | |
| norethindrone | | | | • | | | | |
| norfloxacin | | | | | | • | | |
| nortriptyline | | | | • | | | — | |
| ofloxacin | | | | | | • | | |
| olanzapine | | | • | • | | | | |
| olsalazine | | | • | • | | | | |
| omeprazole | | | • | • | | | | |
| ondansetron | | | • | • | | | | |
| orlistat | | | | • | | | | |
| oxaprozin | | • | • | • | | | | |
| oxazepam | | | • | • | | | | |
| oxprenolol | | | • | • | | | | |
| oxycodone | | | | • | | | | |
| pamidronate | | • | | | • | | | |
| pantoprazole | | | • | • | | | | |
| paroxetine | | | • | • | | | | |
| pemoline | | | • | | • | | | |
| penicillamine | • | • | | • | | | | |
| penicillin G/V | | | | | • | | | |
| pentamidine | | • | | • | | | | |
| pentazocine | | | • | • | | | | |
| pentoxifylline | | | | • | | | | |
| pergolide | | | • | • | | | | |
| perindopril | | | • | • | | | ■ | |
| perphenazine | | | • | • | | | | |
| phenelzine | | | • | • | | | | |
| phenobarbital | | | • | • | | | — | |
| phentermine | | | • | | | • | | |
| phenylbutazone | | • | • | • | | | | |
| phenytoin | | | • | • | | | | • |
| pimozide | | | • | • | | | | |
| pinaverium bromide | | | • | • | | | | |
| pindolol | | | • | • | | | | |

Table 2: **Dosage Adjustment in Renal Impairment—Adults*** *(cont'd)*

| Drug | Avoid | Nephro-toxic | Titrate | % Renal Elimination < 50% | 50–74% | ≥ 75% | AM | SDCM |
|---|---|---|---|---|---|---|---|---|
| pioglitazone | | | • | • | | | | |
| piperacillin | | | | | | • | | |
| piroxicam | | • | • | • | | | | |
| pivmecillinam | | | | | • | | | |
| plicamycin | | • | | | | • | | |
| pramipexole | | | • | | | • | | |
| pravastatin | | | • | • | | | | |
| prazosin | | | • | • | | | | |
| prednisone | | | • | • | | | | |
| primaquine | | | | • | | | | |
| primidone | | | • | • | | | — | |
| probenecid | • | | | • | | | | |
| procainamide | | | | | • | | ■ | • |
| progesterone | | | • | • | | | | |
| proguanil | | | | • | | | — | |
| promethazine | | | • | • | | | | |
| propafenone | | | | • | | | | |
| propantheline | | | | • | | | | |
| propoxyphene | • | | • | • | | | ■ | |
| propranolol | | | • | • | | | | |
| propylthiouracil | | | | • | | | | |
| protriptyline | | | | • | | | — | |
| pyrazinamide | • | | | • | | | | |
| pyrimethamine | | | | • | | | | |
| quinapril | | | • | • | | | ■ | |
| quinidine | | | | • | | | — | |
| quinine | | | | • | | | | |
| rabeprazole | | | | • | | | | |
| raloxifene | | | | • | | | | |
| ramipril | | | • | • | | | ■ | |
| ranitidine | | | • | | • | | | |
| ranitidine bismuth citrate | | | | | • | | | |
| repaglinide | | | • | • | | | | |
| reserpine | | | • | • | | | | |
| ribavirin | | | | • | | | ■ | |
| rifampin | | | | • | | | — | |
| risedronate | • | | | | | • | | |

**Avoid** = *Avoid drug if ClCr < 0.5 mL/s/70 kg as drug may be ineffective or toxic.*
**Nephrotoxic** = *Potentially nephrotoxic drug: avoid if possible as may worsen renal function.*
**Titrate** = *Start with a low dose and titrate to desired effect, regardless of renal function.*
**AM** = *Drug metabolized to active or toxic metabolites:*
■ = *dosage reduction required (calculated as if drug was 75–100% renally eliminated);*
— = *no dosage reduction required.*
**SDCM** = *Serum drug concentration monitoring may help guide dosage adjustments.*
**Omission of a drug from this table does not imply that dosage adjustment is NOT required in renal impairment. Refer to specific references for dosing in dialysis.*

Table 2: **Dosage Adjustment in Renal Impairment—Adults*** *(cont'd)*

| Drug | Avoid | Nephro-toxic | Titrate | % Renal Elimination | | | AM | SDCM |
|---|---|---|---|---|---|---|---|---|
| | | | | < 50% | 50–74% | ≥ 75% | | |
| risperidone | | | • | • | | | ■ | |
| ritonavir | | | | • | | | — | |
| rivastigmine | | | • | • | | | | |
| rizatriptan | | | | • | | | — | |
| rofecoxib | | • | • | • | | | | |
| ropinirole | | | • | • | | | | |
| rosiglitazone | | | • | • | | | | |
| salbutamol | | | • | • | | | | |
| salsalate | | • | • | • | | | ■ | |
| saquinavir | | | | • | | | | |
| secobarbital | | | | • | | | | |
| selegiline | | | | • | | | — | |
| sertraline | | | • | • | | | | |
| sibutramine | | | | • | | | — | |
| sildenafil | | | • | • | | | | |
| simvastatin | | | • | • | | | | |
| sodium fluoride | | | | | | • | | |
| sotalol | | | • | | • | | | |
| spironolactone | • | | • | • | | | ■ | |
| stavudine | | | | • | | | ■ | |
| streptomycin | | • | | | | • | | • |
| sucralfate[10] | | | | • | | | | |
| sulfadiazine | | • | | | • | | | |
| sulfadoxine/ pyrimethamine[11] | | | | | | • | | |
| sulfasalazine | | | | • | | | — | |
| sulfinpyrazone | • | • | • | • | | | | |
| sulfisoxazole | | | | | • | | | |
| sulindac | | • | • | • | | | — | |
| sumatriptan | | | | • | | | | |
| tamsulosin | | | | • | | | | |
| teicoplanin | | • | | | • | | | |
| telmisartan | | | • | • | | | | |
| temazepam | | | • | • | | | | |
| tenoxicam | | • | • | • | | | | |
| terazosin | | | • | • | | | | |
| terfenadine | | | | • | | | | |
| testosterone undecanoate | | | • | • | | | — | |
| tetracycline | | • | | | • | | | |
| theophylline | | | | • | | | | • |
| thioridazine | | | • | • | | | — | |
| thiothixene | | | • | • | | | | |
| tiaprofenic acid | | • | • | | | • | | |
| tibolone | | | | • | | | — | |

[10] *Aluminum may accumulate in renal impairment.*

[11] ***Antimalarial prophylaxis with sulfadoxine/pyrimethamine is contraindicated in severe renal insufficiency.***

Table 2: **Dosage Adjustment in Renal Impairment—Adults*** *(cont'd)*

| Drug | Avoid | Nephro-toxic | Titrate | % Renal Elimination | | | AM | SDCM |
|---|---|---|---|---|---|---|---|---|
| | | | | < 50% | 50–74% | ≥ 75% | | |
| ticarcillin | | | | | | • | | |
| ticarcillin/clavulanate | | | | | • | | | |
| ticlopidine | | | | • | | | | |
| timolol | | | • | • | | | | |
| tirofiban | | | | | • | | | |
| tizanidine | | | • | • | | | | |
| tobramycin | | • | | | | • | | • |
| tolbutamide | | | | • | | | | |
| tolcapone | | | | • | | | | |
| tolmetin | | • | • | • | | | | |
| tolterodine | | | • | • | | | — | |
| topiramate | | | • | | | • | | |
| torsemide | | | • | • | | | | |
| trandolapril | | | • | • | | | ■ | |
| trazodone | | | • | • | | | | |
| triamterene | • | • | • | • | | | ■ | |
| triazolam | | | • | • | | | | |
| trifluoperazine | | | • | • | | | | |
| trimebutine | | | | • | | | | |
| troglitazone | | | • | • | | | | |
| L-tryptophan | | | • | • | | | | |
| valacyclovir | | | | • | | | ■ | |
| valproic acid | | | • | • | | | | |
| valsartan | | | • | • | | | | |
| vancomycin | | • | | | | • | | • |
| venlafaxine | | | • | • | | | ■ | |
| verapamil | | | • | • | | | — | |
| vigabatrin | | | • | | | • | | |
| vitamin E | | | | • | | | | |
| warfarin | | | • | • | | | | |
| yohimbine[12] | • | | • | • | | | | |
| zafirlukast | | | • | • | | | | |
| zalcitabine | | | | • | | | ■ | |
| zaleplon | | | • | • | | | | |
| zidovudine | | | | • | | | | |
| zolmitriptan | | | | • | | | — | |

[12] *Route of elimination for yohimbine unknown.*

**Avoid** = *Avoid drug if ClCr < 0.5 mL/s/70 kg as drug may be ineffective or toxic.*

**Nephrotoxic** = *Potentially nephrotoxic drug: avoid if possible as may worsen renal function.*

**Titrate** = *Start with a low dose and titrate to desired effect, regardless of renal function.*

**AM** = *Drug metabolized to active or toxic metabolites:*

■ = *dosage reduction required (calculated as if drug was 75–100% renally eliminated);*

— = *no dosage reduction required.*

**SDCM** = *Serum drug concentration monitoring may help guide dosage adjustments.*

**Omission of a drug from this table does not imply that dosage adjustment is NOT required in renal impairment. Refer to specific references for dosing in dialysis.*

## APPENDIX II

# Drug Exposure During Pregnancy and Lactation

*Orna Diav-Citrin, MD and*
*Gideon Koren, MD, FRCPC*

Many pregnant women are exposed to a variety of medications that may exert therapeutic, toxic or teratogenic effects on the fetus. Since the thalidomide disaster, many physicians and pregnant women tend to withhold any medication during pregnancy, although the risk of teratogenic effect from most drugs in therapeutic doses is nonexistent. Major congenital defects occur in 1 to 3% of the general population at birth. Of the major defects, about 25% are of genetic origin (genetically inherited diseases, new mutations and chromosomal abnormalities) and 65% are of unknown etiology (multifactorial, polygenic, spontaneous errors of development and synergistic interactions of teratogens). Only 2 to 3% of malformations is thought to be associated with drug treatment. The remaining defects are related to other environmental exposures including infectious agents, maternal disease states, mechanical problems and irradiation.

Proper prescribing in pregnancy is a challenge and should provide maximal safety to the fetus as well as therapeutic benefit to the mother. To date, very few drugs are proven teratogens in humans. However, drug-induced malformations are important because they are potentially preventable.

Maternal physiologic changes during pregnancy may alter the pharmacokinetics of drugs. Clearance rates of many drugs increase during late pregnancy due to increases in both renal and hepatic elimination (e.g., digoxin, phenytoin), while in others the clearance rate decreases (e.g., theophylline). Generally, little is known about the relationship between maternal serum drug concentration and risk of teratogenicity.

The importance of **timing of drug exposure** is better understood; the effect produced by a teratogenic agent depends upon the developmental stage in which the conceptus is exposed. Several important phases in human development are recognized:

- The "**all or none**" **period**, the time from conception until somite formation. Insults to the embryo in this phase are likely to result in death and miscarriage or intact survival. The embryo is undifferentiated and repair and recovery are possible through multiplication of the still totipotential cells. Exposure to teratogens during the presomitic stage usually does not cause congenital malformations unless the agent persists in the body beyond this period.

- The **embryonic period**, from 18 to 60 days after conception when the basic steps in organogenesis occur. This is the period of maximum sensitivity to teratogenicity since tissues are differentiating rapidly and damage becomes irreparable. Exposure to teratogenic agents during this period has the greatest likelihood of causing a structural anomaly. The pattern of anomalies produced depends on which systems are differentiating at the time of teratogenic exposure.
- The **fetal phase**, from the end of the embryonic stage to term, when growth and functional maturation of formed organs and systems occurs. Teratogen exposure in this period will affect fetal growth (e.g., intrauterine growth restriction) and the size or function of an organ, rather than cause gross structural anomalies. The term fetal toxicity is commonly used to describe such an effect. The potential effect of psychoactive agents (e.g., antidepressants, antiepileptics, alcohol and other drugs of abuse) on the developing central nervous system has lead to a new field of behavioral teratology.

Many organ systems continue structural and functional maturation long after birth. Most of the adenocarcinomas associated with first trimester exposure to diethylstilbestrol occurred many years later.

Teratogens must reach the developing conceptus in sufficient amounts to cause their effects. Large molecules with a molecular weight greater than 1000 (e.g., heparin) do not easily cross the placenta into the embryonic-fetal bloodstream. Other factors influencing the rate and extent of placental transfer of xenobiotics include polarity, lipid solubility and the existence of a specific protein carrier.

In an attempt to provide the practitioner, who is considering treatment of the pregnant woman, with a better assessment of fetal risk, the FDA developed a classification of fetal risk in 1979. These categories initially appeared logical but were *not* found to be very *helpful* in counseling individual patients. Drug manufacturers may have legal rather than scientific reasons for assigning particular designations. The classification frequently resulted in ambiguity and even false alarm. For example, oral contraceptives are denoted as X (i.e., contraindicated in pregnancy), despite failure of two meta-analyses to show increased teratogenic risk. In 1994 the Teratology Society stated that the FDA ratings are inappropriate and should be replaced by narrative statements that summarize and interpret available data regarding hazards of developmental toxicity and provide estimates of teratogenic risk.

Table 1: **Possible Teratogenic Drugs in Humans**

| Drug | Adverse Effects |
|---|---|
| D-penicillamine | High dose treatment: connective tissue disorders (cutis laxa) [case reports]. |
| Methimazole | Scalp defects (aplasia cutis congenita) [case reports and an epidemiological study in which methimazole had been added to animal feeds as a weight enhancer and in those areas a higher incidence of aplasia cutis congenita was found]. |

## Teratogenic Counseling*

- Ascertain the clinical facts regarding the nature of the exposure: the length, dosage, and timing during pregnancy, as well as other exposures of concern (e.g., alcohol, cigarette smoking, herbal remedies).
- Collect all available current data regarding the agent and draw conclusions regarding the risk of exposure.
- Counseling should include background human baseline risk for major malformations, whether the fetus is at increased risk, which anomaly has been associated with the agent in question, a risk assessment, methods of prenatal detection when available, limitations in our knowledge, and limitations of prenatal diagnostic capabilities.
- Additional aspects include the potential risk of the medical condition for which a drug is prescribed, known interactions (in both directions) between the disease state and the pregnancy, and preventive measures when applicable (e.g., folic acid supplementation in carbamazepine exposure).
- Because more than 50% of pregnancies are unplanned, teratogenic risk assessment should be started prior to pregnancy.

Table 1 lists possible teratogenic drugs with yet insufficient evidence for teratogenicity in humans. Table 2 lists drugs with sufficient evidence to prove their teratogenic effect in humans. They should be avoided, when possible, in pregnancy. Table 3 presents drugs of choice during gestation for common maternal conditions.

## Drug Use During Lactation*

The extent of drug exposure in the infant depends on several factors: the pharmacokinetic properties of the drug in the infant

* *Antenatal drug/chemical risk counseling or information on safety of drug use during lactation is available from the Motherisk Program, Hospital for Sick Children, Toronto. Tel: (416) 813-6780; e-mail: momrisk@sickkids.on.ca; website: www.motherisk.org*

Table 2: **Proven Teratogenic Drugs in Humans**

| Drug | Adverse Effects |
|---|---|
| **Alcohol** | Fetal alcohol syndrome: growth impairment, developmental delay, and dysmorphic facies. Cleft palate and cardiac anomalies may occur. Full expression of the syndrome occurs with chronic daily ingestion of 2 g alcohol per kg (8 drinks per day) in about 1/3 and partial effects in ¾ of offspring. |
| **Angiotensin converting enzyme inhibitors (ACEI) and angiotensin II antagonists** | Adverse effects related to hemodynamic effects of ACEI and angiotensin II antagonists on the fetus, teratogenic risk with first trimester exposure appears to be low. In late pregnancy, ACEI fetopathy: intrauterine renal insufficiency, neonatal hypotension, oliguria with renal failure, hyperkalemia, complications of oligohydramnios (i.e., fetal limb contractures, lung hypoplasia, and craniofacial anomalies), prematurity, intrauterine growth restriction and fetal death. |
| **Carbamazepine** | First trimester exposure: 1% risk of neural tube defects (10 times baseline risk). A pattern of malformations similar to the fetal hydantoin syndrome has also been associated. |
| **Chemotherapeutic agents** | A significant increase in the incidence of various fetal malformations and early miscarriages following first trimester exposure. |
| **Cocaine** | Abruptio placenta, prematurity, fetal loss, decreased birth weight, microcephaly, limb defects, urinary tract malformations, and poorer neurodevelopmental performance. Methodological problems make the findings difficult to interpret. Cocaine abuse is often associated with poly-drug abuse, alcohol consumption, smoking, malnutrition and poor prenatal care. Human epidemiology indicates the risk of major malformation from cocaine is probably low, but the anomalies may be severe. |
| **Coumarin anticoagulants** | First trimester exposure (6–9 wks gestation): fetal warfarin syndrome (nasal hypoplasia and calcific stippling of the epiphyses). Intrauterine growth retardation and developmental delay, eye defects and hearing loss. Warfarin embryopathy is found in 1/3 of the cases where a coumarin derivative was given throughout pregnancy. Associated with high rate of miscarriage. After the first trimester: risk of CNS damage due to hemorrhage. |
| **Diethylstilbestrol** | Vaginal clear cell adenocarcinoma in offspring exposed in utero before 18th wk (> 90% of the cancers occurred after 14 years of age). High incidence of benign vaginal adenosis. Increased miscarriage rate and preterm delivery. In males exposed in utero: no signs of malignancy but genital lesions in 27% and pathologic changes in spermatozoa in 29%. |
| **Folic acid antagonists: aminopterin and methotrexate** | Fetal aminopterin syndrome: CNS defects, craniofacial anomalies, abnormal cranial ossification, abnormalities in first branchial arch derivatives, intrauterine growth restriction and mental retardation after first trimester exposure. |
| **Hydantoins (phenytoin)** | Fetal hydantoin syndrome: craniofacial dysmorphology, anomalies and hypoplasia of distal phalanges and nails, growth restriction, mental deficiency and cardiac defects. |
| **Lithium** | Small increase in risk for major anomalies and a specific risk for cardiac teratogenesis in early gestation. The risk of Ebstein's anomaly exceeds spontaneous rate of occurrence. Fetal echocardiography if exposed in first trimester. |

*(cont'd)*

Table 2: **Proven Teratogenic Drugs in Humans** *(cont'd)*

| Drug | Adverse Effects |
|---|---|
| **Misoprostol** | First trimester exposure: limb defects and Moebius sequence. Absolute teratogenic risk: probably low. |
| **Retinoids (acitretin, isotretinoin) and megadoses of vitamin A** | Systemic exposure: potent human general and behavioral teratogen. Retinoic acid embryopathy: craniofacial anomalies, cardiac defects, abnormalities in thymic development and alterations in CNS development. Risk for associated miscarriage: 40%. |
| **Tetracyclines** | Discoloration of the teeth after 17 wks gestation when deciduous teeth begin to calcify. Close to term: crowns of permanent teeth may be stained. Oxytetracycline and doxycycline associated with a lower incidence of enamel staining. |
| **Thalidomide** | Malformations limited to tissues of mesodermal origin, primarily limbs (reduction defects), ears, cardiovascular system, and gut musculature. Critical period: 34th–50th day after the beginning of the last menstrual period. A single dose of < 1 mg per kg has produced the syndrome. Embryopathy found in about 20% of pregnancies exposed in the critical period. |
| **Valproic acid** | First trimester exposure: neural tube defects with 1–2% risk of meningomyelocele, primarily lumbar or lumbosacral. Fetal valproate syndrome: craniofacial dysmorphology, cardiovascular defects, long fingers and toes, hyperconvex fingernails and cleft lip, has been delineated by some investigations. |

and mother; milk composition; the amount of milk consumed; the physiology of the breast and the infant's suckling pattern. The susceptibility of an infant to adverse effects from drugs depends on the extent of exposure and the infant's sensitivity. Adverse drug reactions can be dose-related, and reflect the pharmacologic effect of the drug, or idiosyncratic (rarely).

Most drugs taken by the breast-feeding mother are excreted into the milk. The amount of drug consumed by the infant is usually less than 5% of the maternal dose (weight adjusted). When maternal drug therapy is indicated, the agent with minimal risk to the infant should be chosen. The infant should be monitored for potential adverse effects. When toxicity is likely, drug concentration in the milk and infant's plasma may sometimes be measured.

### *Drugs Usually Contraindicated During Breast-feeding*

- **Antineoplastic drugs** — potential risk for toxicity.
- **Ergot alkaloids** (ergotamine, bromocriptine) — potential risk of suppression of lactation and adverse effects in infant.
- **Lithium** — drug reaches one-third to one-half therapeutic blood concentration in infant; long-term effects of infant exposure unknown.

Table 3: **Drugs of Choice for Selected Conditions During Pregnancy**

| Condition | Drugs of Choice | Alternative | Comments |
|---|---|---|---|
| **Allergy** | antihistamines: chlorpheniramine, diphenhydramine, dimenhydrinate | | |
| **Anticoagulation** | heparin and low molecular weight heparins | warfarin (in cases where benefit justifies risk) | |
| **Asthma** | inhaled bronchodilators (salbutamol, terbutaline or ipratropium bromide) and inhaled corticosteroids (beclomethasone, budesonide) | systemic corticosteroids and theophylline | |
| **Anxiety** | benzodiazepines | | Watch neonate for possible withdrawal when high doses used close to term. |
| **Bacterial infections** | penicillins, cephalosporins, erythromycin, co-trimoxazole | aminoglycosides, quinolones | |
| **Bipolar affective disorder** | lithium | carbamazepine, valproic acid | With lithium, fetal echocardiography. With carbamazepine and valproic acid, periconceptional folate supplementation and level II ultrasound for NTD prevention. |
| **Constipation** | bulk-forming agents (i.e., methylcellulose, psyllium hydrophilic mucilloid) | lubricants (i.e., paraffin oil, glycerin) or osmotic agents (i.e., magnesium salts, lactulose) | |

*(cont'd)*

Table 3: **Drugs of Choice for Selected Conditions During Pregnancy** *(cont'd)*

| Condition | Drugs of Choice | Alternative | Comments |
|---|---|---|---|
| **Cough** | antihistamines, codeine (when indicated) | | Avoid high doses of codeine close to term (risk of neonatal opioid withdrawal). |
| **Depression** | tricyclic antidepressants, fluoxetine | other selective serotonin reuptake inhibitors | |
| **Diabetes mellitus** | human insulin | | Important to achieve strict glycemic control before conception and during the 1st trimester. |
| **Diarrhea** | bulk forming agents (i.e., methylcellulose, psyllium hydrophilic mucilloid), kaolin, pectin | loperamide | |
| **Dyspepsia** | alginic acid compound – Gaviscon, antacids – numerous aluminum hydroxide combinations | $H_2$-antagonists, omeprazole | |
| **Epilepsy** | carbamazepine | benzodiazepines, valproic acid, phenytoin | With carbamazepine and valproic acid, periconceptional folate supplementation and level II ultrasound for NTD prevention. |
| **Fever and pain** | acetaminophen | ASA, NSAIDs | Avoid full anti-inflammatory dose of NSAIDs in 3rd trimester. |
| **Herpetic infections** | acyclovir | | |

| | | | |
|---|---|---|---|
| **Hypertension** | methyldopa, hydralazine | calcium channel blockers, beta-blockers | With beta-blockers, reduced birth weight and persistent beta-blockade possible in newborn. |
| **Hyperthyroidism** | propylthiouracil | methimazole | Fetal ultrasound near term for goitre detection. |
| **Migraine** | acetaminophen | ASA, NSAIDs, sumatriptan | Avoid full anti-inflammatory dose of NSAIDs in 3rd trimester. |
| **Nausea/vomiting** | doxylamine/pyridoxine – Diclectin | dimenhydrinate, metoclopramide | |
| **Schizophrenia** | phenothiazines | haloperidol | Watch neonate for possible adverse effects if taken close to term. |
| **Vaginal candidiasis** | vaginal: nystatin, miconazole, clotrimazole | fluconazole: single systemic dose of 150 mg | |

- **Drugs of abuse** — potential hazard to nursing infant and concern that a mother using these substances may not be capable of proper infant care.
- **Gold** — potential adverse effects and long half-life in infant.
- **Oral contraceptives** — not recommended in early lactation, may change milk composition and decrease yield.
- **Radioactive compounds** — potential exposure of the nursing infant to excessive radioactivity.
- **Iodine-containing compounds** — iodine is transported into breast milk and may induce goitre and hypothyroidism.

## Suggested Reading List

Bennett PN. *Drugs and human lactation: A comprehensive guide to the content and consequences of drugs, micronutrients, radiopharmaceuticals, and environmental and occupational chemicals in human milk.* 2nd ed. Amsterdam: Elsevier, 1996.

Briggs GG, Freeman RK, Yaffe SJ. *Drugs in pregnancy and lactation: A reference guide to fetal and neonatal risk.* 5th ed. Baltimore: Williams and Wilkins, 1998.

Committee on drugs. The transfer of drugs and other chemicals into human milk. *Pediatrics* 1994;93:137–150.

Hale TW. *Medications and mother's milk.* 8th ed. Amarillo: Pharmasoft Medical Publishing, 1999.

Koren G, ed. *Maternal fetal toxicology: A clinician's guide.* 2nd ed. New York: Marcel Dekker, 1994.

## APPENDIX III

# Pharmacoeconomic Considerations

*Jeffrey A. Johnson, PhD*

The economic impact of the choices made in a therapeutic area is an increasingly important consideration for health care systems and for individual clinicians. **Pharmacoeconomics is the application of economic evaluation techniques in the study of drug therapy.** Increasingly, studies are published incorporating economic evaluations of therapeutic choices for a variety of conditions. Where such evidence is available, some of the chapters in this edition provide information regarding the pharmacoeconomic considerations for that therapeutic area. This Appendix will provide some general guidance when considering the pharmacoeconomic impact of your therapeutic choices.

**Pharmacoeconomic evaluations are concerned with comparing the dollars spent on treatment alternatives for the outcomes achieved.** It is important to remember that in choosing among many alternatives in a therapeutic area, both sides of the equation must be considered. Drug acquisition costs, while an important component, only provide one side of the cost-outcome story and only a part of that story. At the end of most chapters in this edition, a summary table indicates the relative cost of each therapeutic choice. It is also important to consider the relative effectiveness of each choice.

Consider the following hypothetical example. There are three drug choices in a given therapeutic area, Drugs X, Y and Z. Drugs X and Y are older and are less expensive; Drug Z is newer and provides improved clinical outcomes, but is also more expensive.

| Drug | Cost | Outcomes |
|---|---|---|
| X | $$ | + |
| Y | $$ | + |
| Z | $$$ | +++ |

Although Drug Z costs $$$, it provides +++ level of outcomes, whereas Drug X costs $$ but provides only + level of outcomes. This would imply that, in general, Drug Z is more cost effective than Drug X.

However, defining what is a meaningful outcome is often difficult as *outcomes* have taken on many different forms. For this edition of *Therapeutic Choices*, it was not possible to reconcile all different outcome measures and provide a relative ranking for all therapeutic areas. Instead, we have attempted to draw attention to the issue and remind the reader to consider all possible and relevant treatment costs, not just drug acquisition costs, and also to consider the relative effectiveness of the choices where such information is available.

## Cost Issues

### *Direct Costs*

When considering the cost of drug therapy, it is important to recognize the impact of drug therapy choices on *downstream* costs. Such costs are often outside the drug budget, and may include additional laboratory tests required to monitor for adverse side effects, but may also include reduced costs for physician visits or hospitalizations for conditions that were not adequately controlled on previous therapeutic choices. Cost of resources used in the treatment of diseases or conditions is referred to as *direct medical costs*.

The following health care resources are all associated with direct medical costs. Any number of these resources may be important to consider when any therapeutic choice is made. That is, when one drug is chosen over another, it is important to consider what impact that treatment may have on any or all of the following:

- Hospitalizations
- Laboratory/radiological tests
- Emergency room/medical center visits
- Drug therapy
- Home care services
- Long-term care

### *Indirect Costs*

Important cost considerations may also include *downstream* costs to society as a result of disease or medical interventions that are outside of the health care system and health care budgets. Such costs include lost or reduced productivity in the workplace due to death or illness. For example, if a drug therapy for migraine headaches is able to reduce the frequency of headaches and consequently reduce the number of days of work missed, this has a positive impact on the overall productivity of the employer and therefore society in general. These costs are referred to as *indirect costs*. The impact of health care on indirect costs is often difficult to quantify and may not always be included in economic evaluations, but is also an important consideration in making therapeutic choices.

### *Perspective on Costs*

The perspective used in determining the important and relevant costs is also important. Who would be burdened with what costs? Pharmacoeconomic evaluations may assume the viewpoint of a single provider, an insurer, the provincial health care system, or society as a whole. Depending on the perspective, the total *costs* of a therapeutic choice may differ.

Consider a patient who moves through various levels of care from a hospital, to an extended care facility, to home. In the hospital's view, its relevant costs are those incurred during the hospital stay. For instance, the hospital would welcome any therapeutic choice that reduces the length of stay and/or other services during the stay. An earlier discharge, however, may mean that more intensive and more costly nursing home care is required. This is relevant from the perspective of the nursing home and the provincial or regional health care system; it is irrelevant to the hospital. Finally, when the patient is transferred home, a family member may assume the role of caregiver. From society's perspective, the caregiver's time is a cost; however, this cost is outside the realm of the health care system and outside the coverage of provincial health plans.

## Outcomes

The bottom line in pharmacoeconomic considerations is the ratio of net dollars spent per outcome achieved. Outcomes or consequences of drug therapy can be valued in a number of different ways. The choice of which outcome is best depends on the information available and the condition being evaluated. The following are some commonly used approaches in pharmacoeconomic evaluations:

### *Dollars spent per clinical outcome*

- Outcomes are some recognized unit of clinical effect (e.g., cost per year of life saved; cost per case of nephrotoxicity avoided).
- Referred to as a **cost-effectiveness analysis**.
- This approach is probably the most commonly used in pharmacoeconomic evaluations.

### *Dollars spent for dollars saved*

- Outcomes given a dollar value.
- Referred to as a **cost-benefit analysis**.
- This approach often requires the economic valuation of a human life, which presents many difficulties, methodological and philosophical.

### *Dollars spent for quality of life outcomes*

- Outcomes are measured as Quality Adjusted Life Years (QALYs) gained.
- Referred to as a **cost-utility analysis**.
- This approach is used when the impact on health-related quality of life is an important outcome of the condition or its treatment.
- Theoretically, the use of a common outcome measure such as QALYs gained, would allow for comparison of cost-outcome relationships across different therapeutic areas (see Laupacis et al., 1992). However, because of differences in study methodologies, this is not always possible.

## Patient Risk and Pharmacoeconomic Considerations

In assessing the economic impact of therapeutic choices, it is also important to consider the selection of patients in terms of level of risk. The economic benefits of drug therapies follow on the clinical benefits. A drug has to be clinically effective to be cost-effective and the more effective a drug is, the more cost-effective it is likely to be. As with clinical considerations, the economic impact of a treatment is likely to improve for patients who are at greater risk. The same therapeutic choice is not necessarily cost-effective in all patients. This information is not always available when economic evaluations are based on clinical trials.

### *Suggested Reading List*

Destky AS, Naglie IG. A clinician's guide to cost-effectiveness analysis. *Ann Intern Med* 1990;113:147–154.

Laupacis A, Feeny D, Detsky AS, Tugwell PX. How attractive does a new technology have to be to warrant adoption and utilization? Tentative guidelines for using clinical and economic evaluations. *Can Med Assoc J* 1992;146:473–481.

APPENDIX IV

# Glossary of Abbreviations

| | |
|---|---|
| ABG | arterial blood gases |
| AC | before meals |
| ACE | angiotensin-converting enzyme |
| ADHD | attention deficit hyperactivity disorder |
| ADL | activities of daily living |
| AFB | acid fast bacilli |
| ALP | alkaline phosphatase |
| ALT | alanine transaminase |
| ANA | antinuclear antibody |
| Anti HBe | antibody to HBeAg |
| Anti HCV | antibody to HCV |
| AOM | acute otitis media |
| APSAC | anisoylated plasminogen streptokinase activator complex |
| aPTT | activated partial thromboplastin time |
| ARDS | acute respiratory distress syndrome |
| ASA | acetylsalicylic acid |
| ASOT | antistreptolysin-o titer |
| AST | aspartate transaminase |
| BAL | bronchoalveolar lavage |
| BCG | bacillus Calmette-Guérin |
| BDZ | benzodiazepine |
| BID | two times per day |
| BMI | body mass index |
| BP | blood pressure |
| BPH | benign prostatic hyperplasia |
| BSS | bismuth subsalicylate |
| C&S | culture and sensitivity |
| CABG | coronary artery bypass graft |
| CAD | coronary artery disease |
| cAMP | cyclic adenosine monophosphate |
| CBC | complete blood count |
| CBT | cognitive behavioral therapy |
| CCB | calcium channel blocker |
| cfu/L | colony-forming units/litre |
| cGMP | cyclic guanosine monophosphate |
| CHF | congestive heart failure |
| CK | creatine kinase |
| ClCr | creatinine clearance |
| CMV | cytomegalovirus |
| CNS | central nervous system |
| COPD | chronic obstructive pulmonary disease |

| | |
|---|---|
| CPAP | continuous positive airways pressure |
| CPK | creatine phosphokinase |
| CRP | C-reactive protein |
| CSF | cerebrospinal fluid |
| CT | computed tomography |
| CTD | connective tissue diseases |
| CVA | cerebrovascular accident |
| CVD | cardiovascular disease |
| CVP | central venous pressure |
| CXR | chest x-ray |
| d | day |
| DHE | dihydroergotamine |
| DIC | disseminated intravascular coagulation |
| DM | dextromethorphan |
| DRE | digital rectal examination |
| DTs | delirium tremens |
| DU | duodenal ulcer |
| DVT | deep vein thrombosis |
| DXA | dual energy x-ray densitometry |
| ECF | extracellular fluid |
| ECG | electrocardiogram |
| ECL | enterochromaffin-like |
| ECT | electroconvulsive therapy |
| EGD | esophagogastroduodenoscopy |
| EHT | endoscopic hemostatic therapy |
| ENT | ear, nose & throat |
| ERCP | endoscopic retrograde cholangiopancreatography |
| ESR | erythrocyte sedimentation rate |
| ESRD | end stage renal disease |
| FCH | familial combined hyperlipidemia |
| FEV | forced expiratory volume |
| FHTG | familial hypertriglyceridemia |
| FSH | follicle-stimulating hormone |
| GAD | generalized anxiety disorder |
| GERD | gastroesophageal reflux disease |
| GGT | gamma glutamyl transpeptidase |
| GI | gastrointestinal |
| GTN | nitroglycerin |
| GTT | glucose tolerance test |
| GU | genitourinary |
| HAV | hepatitis A virus |
| HBeAg | hepatitis Be antigen |
| HBIG | hepatitis B immune globulin |
| HBsAg | hepatitis B surface antigen |
| HBV | hepatitis B virus |
| HCV | hepatitis C virus |

| | |
|---|---|
| HDL-C | high-density lipoprotein cholesterol |
| HDV | hepatitis D (delta) virus |
| hFH | heterozygous familial hypercholesterolemia |
| Hgb | hemoglobin |
| HPN | high-potency neuroleptic |
| HPV | human papilloma virus |
| $H_2RA$ | $H_2$-receptor antagonist |
| HRQOL | health-related quality of life |
| HS | bedtime |
| HSG | hysterosalpingogram |
| 5HT | 5-hydroxytryptamine |
| IBD | inflammatory bowel disease |
| IBS | irritable bowel syndrome |
| IBW | ideal body weight |
| ICF | intracellular fluid |
| ICU | intensive care unit |
| IFNa | interferon alfa |
| IL-1 | interleukin-1 |
| IM | intramuscular |
| INR | International Normalized Ratio |
| IOP | intraocular pressure |
| ISA | intrinsic sympathomimetic activity |
| ISDN | isosorbide dinitrate |
| IU | international unit |
| IUCD | intra-uterine contraceptive device |
| IV | intravenous |
| IVIG | intravenous immune globulins |
| IVP | intravenous pyelogram |
| j | joule |
| JVP | jugular venous pressure |
| LBBB | left bundle branch block |
| LDH | lactic dehydrogenase |
| LDL-C | low-density lipoprotein cholesterol |
| LFT | liver function test |
| LH | luteinizing hormone |
| LMWH | low-molecular-weight heparins |
| LP | lumbar puncture |
| LPN | low-potency neuroleptic |
| LRTI | lower respiratory tract infection |
| MAC | mycobacterium avium complex |
| MAO | monoamine oxidase |
| MAOI | monoamine oxidase inhibitor |
| MCV | mean corpuscular volume |
| MDI | metered-dose inhaler |
| MDS | myelodysplastic syndrome |
| MI | myocardial infarction |

| | |
|---|---|
| MMI | methimazole |
| MMSE | mini-mental state examination |
| MODY | maturity onset diabetes of the young |
| MOFS | multiple organ failure syndrome |
| MRA | magnetic resonance angiography |
| MRI | magnetic resonance imaging |
| MSK | musculoskeletal |
| NE | norepinephrine |
| NG | nasogastric |
| NS | normal saline |
| NSAIDs | nonsteroidal anti-inflammatory drugs |
| NTD | neural tube defects |
| NYHA | New York Heart Association |
| OA | osteoarthritis |
| OC | oral contraceptive |
| OCD | obsessive–compulsive disorder |
| OCP | oral contraceptive pill |
| ORT | oral rehydration therapy |
| OTC | over-the-counter |
| PC | after meals |
| PCP | *Pneumocystis carinii* pneumonia |
| PCR | polymerase chain reaction |
| PD | panic disorder |
| PDA | panic disorder with agoraphobia |
| PE | pulmonary embolism |
| PEEP | positive end-expiratory pressure |
| PEFR | peak expiratory flow rates |
| PFT | pulmonary function test |
| PG | prostaglandin |
| PG inhibitors | prostaglandin synthetase inhibitors |
| $PGE_1$ | prostaglandin $E_1$ |
| PID | pelvic inflammatory disease |
| PMN | polymorphonucleocyte |
| PO | by mouth |
| PPD | purified protein derivative (of tuberculin) |
| PPI | proton pump inhibitors |
| PR | rectally |
| PRN | when necessary |
| PRP | primary Raynaud's phenomenon |
| PSA | prostate specific antigen |
| PT | prothrombin time |
| PTCA | percutaneous transluminal coronary angioplasty |
| PTH | parathyroid hormone |
| PTSD | post-traumatic stress disorder |
| PTT | partial thromboplastin time |
| PTU | propylthiouracil |

| | |
|---|---|
| PUD | peptic ulcer disease |
| PUVA | psoralen-ultraviolet light (treatment) |
| QHS | each bedtime |
| QID | four times per day |
| RBC | red blood cell |
| RE | retinol equivalents |
| RIMA | reversible inhibitors of monoamine oxidase A |
| RNA | ribonucleic acid |
| RNI | recommended nutrient intake |
| RP | Raynaud's phenomenon |
| rtPA | recombinant tissue plasminogen activator (alteplase) |
| SAD | seasonal affective disorder |
| SAH | subarachnoid hemorrhage |
| SBT | serum bactericidal titer |
| SC | subcutaneous |
| SIADH | syndrome of inappropriate antidiuretic hormone |
| SK | streptokinase |
| SL | sublingual |
| SLE | systemic lupus erythematosus |
| SLR | straight leg raise |
| SMBG | self-monitored blood glucose |
| SRP | secondary Raynaud's phenomenon |
| SSRI | selective serotonin reuptake inhibitor |
| SSSS | staphylococcal scalded skin syndrome |
| STD | sexually transmitted disease |
| SVT | supraventricular tachycardia |
| TCA | tricyclic antidepressant |
| TD | tardive dyskinesia |
| TENS | transcutaneous electrical nerve stimulation |
| TIA | transient ischemic attack |
| TIBC | total iron binding capacity |
| TID | three times per day |
| TIPS | transjugular intrahepatic portosystemic shunt |
| TNF | tumor necrosis factor |
| TPN | total parenteral nutrition |
| TSH | thyroid-stimulating hormone |
| TTKG | transtubular K concentration gradient |
| TUIP | transurethral incision of the prostate |
| TURP | transurethral resection of the prostate |
| UBT | urea breath test |
| UGIB | upper gastrointestinal bleeding |
| UK | urokinase |
| UTI | urinary tract infection |
| UVA | ultraviolet-A |
| UVB | ultraviolet-B |

| | |
|---|---|
| VAS | vasoactive substances |
| VDRL | Venereal Disease Research Laboratories |
| VF | ventricular fibrillation |
| VLDL | very low-density lipoprotein |
| VMO | vastus medialis obliquus |
| VMS | vasomotor symptoms |
| VSST | visual sexual stimulation tests |
| VT | ventricular tachycardia |
| VTE | venous thromboembolism |
| WBC | white blood cell |

APPENDIX V

# Microorganism Abbreviations Used in *Therapeutic Choices*

| Abbreviation | Full Name |
|---|---|
| **Bacteria** | |
| *B. fragilis* | *Bacteroides fragilis* |
| *C. pneumoniae* | *Chlamydia pneumoniae* |
| *C. trachomatis* | *Chlamydia trachomatis* |
| *C. difficile* | *Clostridium difficile* |
| *C. diphtheriae* | *Corynebacterium diphtheriae* |
| *E. aerogenes* | *Enterobacter aerogenes* |
| *E. cloacae* | *Enterobacter cloacae* |
| *E. faecalis* | *Enterococcus faecalis* |
| *E. coli* | *Escherichia coli* |
| *F. necrophorum* | *Fusobacterium necrophorum* |
| *H. influenzae* | *Haemophilus influenzae* |
| *H. pylori* | *Helicobacter pylori* |
| *K. pneumoniae* | *Klebsiella pneumoniae* |
| *L. pneumophila* | *Legionella pneumophila* |
| *L. monocytogenes* | *Listeria monocytogenes* |
| *M. catarrhalis* | *Moraxella catarrhalis* |
| *M. tuberculosis* | *Mycobacterium tuberculosis* |
| *M. pneumoniae* | *Mycoplasma pneumoniae* |
| *N. gonorrhoeae* | *Neisseria gonorrhoeae* |
| *N. meningitidis* | *Neisseria meningitidis* |
| *N. asteroides* | *Nocardia asteroides* |
| *P. acnes* | *Propionibacterium acnes* |
| *P. mirabilis* | *Proteus mirabilis* |
| *P. stuartii* | *Providencia stuartii* |
| *P. aeruginosa* | *Pseudomonas aeruginosa* |
| *S. typhi* | *Salmonella typhi* |
| *S. marcescens* | *Serratia marcescens* |
| *S. aureus* | *Staphylococcus aureus* |
| *S. epidermidis* | *Staphylococcus epidermidis* |
| *S. saprophyticus* | *Staphylococcus saprophyticus* |
| *S. pneumoniae* | *Streptococcus pneumoniae* |
| *S. pyogenes* | *Streptococcus pyogenes* |
| *S. viridans* | *Streptococcus viridans* |

| Abbreviation | Full Name |
|---|---|
| **Blood Parasites** | |
| *P. falciparum* | *Plasmodium falciparum* |
| *P. malariae* | *Plasmodium malariae* |
| *P. ovale* | *Plasmodium ovale* |
| *P. vivax* | *Plasmodium vivax* |
| **Fungi** | |
| *C. albicans* | *Candida albicans* |
| *C. neoformans* | *Cryptococcus neoformans* |
| **Protozoa/Parasites** | |
| *E. histolytica* | *Entamoeba histolytica* |
| *G. lamblia* | *Giardia lamblia* |
| *P. carinii* | *Pneumocystis carinii* |
| *T. gondii* | *Toxoplasma gondii* |
| *T. vaginalis* | *Trichomonas vaginalis* |
| **Viruses** | |
| CMV | Cytomegalovirus |
| HAV | Hepatitis A virus |
| HBV | Hepatitis B virus |
| HCV | Hepatitis C virus |
| HIV | Human immunodeficiency virus |
| HPV | Human papillomavirus |
| HSV | Herpes simplex virus |

# Index

Italic entries indicate a generic drug name. Bold entries indicate that the item receives detailed treatment in the text. An italic *t* beside the page number refers to a table.


3TC *see* lamivudine

## A

*abacavir*, HIV infection 793*t*
ABC *see* abacavir
Abenol *see* acetaminophen
absolute alcohol 393
*acamprosate*, alcohol withdrawal 69
*acarbose*, diabetes 619, 621*t*, 622
Accolate *see* zafirlukast
Accupril *see* quinapril
Accutane *see* isotretinoin
*acebutolol*
  angina 218*t*
  hypertension 183*t*
  myocardial infarction 210*t*
ACE inhibitors
  causing hyperkalemia 664, 674*t*
  CHF 233, 234*t*, 239
  claudication 283
  diabetes 628
  hypertension 182, 183*t*, 185-86*t*, 187
  induced cough 189, 896
  myocardial infarction 204*t*, 205, 207, 211*t*, 214
*acetaminophen*
  acute pain 102-3, 104*t*
  acute stroke 268*t*
  Bell's palsy 134
  causing headache 89
  chronic fatigue syndrome 437*t*
  fever 883, 884*t*
  fibromyalgia 432*t*, 433
  headache in adults 82, 84*t*
  headache in children 93-94, 96*t*
  hypercalcemia 672
  osteoarthritis 469, 470*t*, 471, 472*t*
  otitis media 685
  postoperative cataract 160
  rheumatoid arthritis 465
  rhinitis 308
  streptococcal sore throat 695
  sunburn 512
*acetaminophen* with *codeine*
  back pain 114, 115*t*
  Bell's palsy 134
*acetazolamide*, glaucoma 165*t*, 166
Acetoxyl *see* benzoyl peroxide
acetylsalicylic acid *see* ASA
*acitretin*, psoriasis 532, 534*t*
**acne 493-500**, 577
Acnex *see* salicylic acid
ACTH *see* adrenocorticotropic hormone
Acthar *see* adrenocorticotropic hormone
Actifed 310*t*
Activase rtPA *see* alteplase
Actonel *see* risedronate
Actos *see* pioglitazone
Acular *see* ketorolac
*acyclovir*
  Bell's palsy 134-35, 136*t*
  herpesvirus infections 120, 782-83, 784*t*, 785-87
  HIV-associated infections 800*t*
  infections in cancer patients 818*t*, 819
  red eye 171*t*
  varicella 545*t*
Adalat preparations *see* nifedipine
*adapalene*, acne 495*t*, 495
Adderall, ADHD 20
adenoma, toxic 629
*adenosine*, SVT 250*t*, 250
ADHD *see* **attention deficit hyperactivity disorder**
Adrenalin *see* epinephrine
*adrenocorticotropic hormone*, gout 446, 450*t*
Advil *see* ibuprofen
African plum tree, prostatic hyperplasia 416
Aggrastat *see* tirofiban
Aggrenox *see* dipyridamole
**agitation** *see also* **anxiety disorders 1-6**
A-Hydrocort *see* hydrocortisone
Airomir *see* salbutamol
akathisia 60, 61*t*
Albalon *see* naphazoline
Albalon A 171*t*
*albumin*, hypercalcemia 668*t*
**alcoholic liver disease 354, 356**
alcohol withdrawal syndrome 63-65, 66-68*t*
Alcomicin *see* gentamicin
Aldactone *see* spironolactone
*aldesleukin*, adverse effects 844*t*
Aldomet *see* methyldopa
*alendronate*
  bone loss prevention 442
  osteoporosis 479, 481*t*, 483, 485
Alesse 575*t*
alginates, GERD 376, 377*t*, 379*t*
Algosteril, pressure ulcers 526*t*
Allegra *see* fexofenadine
*allethrins*, pediculosis 555*t*
Allevyn, pressure ulcers 526*t*
*allopurinol*
  antineoplastic side effects 854*t*, 857*t*

gout 451*t*, 452-53
Alomide *see* lodoxamide
alopecia 855*t*
*alosetron*, IBS 411, 412*t*
*alpha₁ antitrypsin protein*, COPD 336
alpha-blockers
hypertension 183*t*, 184, 185*t*
prostatic hyperplasia 416, 418*t*, 420
Raynaud's phenomenon 287, 288*t*
*9-alpha-fludrocortisone*, hypoaldosteronism 679
Alphagan *see* brimonidine
5 alpha-reductase inhibitors, prostatic hyperplasia 416-17, 418*t*
alpha tocopherol *see* vitamin E
Alphosyl *see* coal tar and derivatives
*alprazolam*
akathisia 61*t*
anxiety disorders 10, 12*t*
benzodiazepine withdrawal 72*t*
*alprostadil*, erectile dysfunction 606, 607*t*
Altace *see* ramipril
*alteplase*
acute stroke 264, 267*t*-68*t*, 270
myocardial infarction 212*t*, 213-14
thromboembolism 296
thrombosis 278
*altretamine*, causing nausea and vomiting 844*t*
*aluminum chloride hexahydrate*, skin infections 559
Alupent *see* orciprenaline
Alzheimer's disease 25-27, 31
*amantadine*
akathisia 60
cocaine withdrawal 69, 71*t*
Parkinson's disease 61*t*, 140*t*, 142, 145
Amatine *see* midodrine
AmBisone *see* amphotericin B
*amcinonide*, dermatitis 540*t*
Amerge *see* nazatriptan
*amifostine*, antineoplastic side effects 852
*amikacin*
bacterial meningitis 700*t*
HIV-associated infections 804*t*
infections in cancer patients 815*t*
septic shock 742-43*t*
tuberculosis 726-27*t*
UTI 766*t*, 766
Amikin *see* amikacin
*amiloride*
CHF 237*t*
edema 663*t*, 664
hypokalemia 682*t*, 682
*aminoglutethimide*, adverse effects 844*t*
*aminophylline*, asthma in adults 314, 315*t*
*5-aminosalicylic acid*
Crohn's disease 403
IBD 397, 400*t*
ulcerative colitis 404-5
ulcerative proctitis 406
*amiodarone*
atrial fibrillation/flutter 247*t*
CHF 232, 238
SVT 249, 251*t*
ventricular tachycardia 256, 261*t*
*amitriptyline*
anxiety disorders 11
back pain 116*t*
chronic fatigue syndrome 437*t*
depression 36*t*, 38, 40
fibromyalgia 432*t*, 433
headache in adults 87*t*, 88-90
headache in children 93, 98*t*, 100
herpes zoster 120
IBS 411, 412*t*
neuralgia 121, 122*t*
pain control in palliative care 131*t*
*amlodipine*
angina 217, 219*t*, 224*t*
CHF 239
hypertension 183*t*, 185*t*
Raynaud's phenomenon 288*t*
*amoxapine*, depression 39
*amoxicillin*
acute osteomyelitis 732, 733-34*t*
bacterial endocarditis prophylaxis 708-9*t*
chlamydial infection 756*t*
COPD 336
infections in cancer patients 815*t*
otitis media 686-87, 688*t*-89*t*
pneumonia 715-16*t*
PUD 388, 389*t*
skin infections 560, 564*t*
UTI 762-63, 766*t*
*amoxicillin-clavulanate*
acute osteomyelitis 732, 733-34*t*
infections in cancer patients 815*t*
otitis media 689*t*
pneumonia 715*t*-16*t*
UTI 762-63, 766*t*
Amoxil *see* amoxicillin
amphetamines
causing agitation 6
withdrawal from 63
*amphotericin B*
causing hypokalemia 674*t*
HIV-associated infections 803*t*, 806*t*
infections in cancer patients 812, 817*t*, 820

*ampicillin*
bacterial endocarditis prophylaxis 708-9*t*
bacterial meningitis 700*t*, 702-3*t*
cholestatic disease 354
otitis media 687
UTI 762, 766*t*
Ampicin *see* ampicillin
*amsacrine*, causing nausea and vomiting 844*t*
anabolic steroids, osteoporosis 484
Anafranil *see* clomipramine
analgesics
acute pain 101-3, 104*t*-5*t*, 107-9
Bell's palsy 134
burns 519
causing headache 88
chronic fatigue syndrome 437*t*
fibromyalgia 432*t*, 433
headache in adults 82-83, 84*t*, 87*t*, 88-89
headache in children 92-94, 96*t*, 100
pain control in palliative care 127-28, 129*t*-31*t*
sports injuries 487
Anaprox *see* naproxen
*anastrozole*, causing nausea and vomiting 844*t*
Ancef *see* cefazolin
Ancotil *see* flucytosine
androgens
causing nausea and vomiting 844*t*
low sexual desire 610, 611*t*
osteoporosis 484
**anemias 639-47**
**anemias which respond to erythropoietin 639, 646-47**
**angina pectoris**
pharmacoeconomic considerations 227-28
postmyocardial infarction 204-5
**stable 215-20**
**unstable 220-28**
angioneurotic edema 339
angiotensin converting enzyme inhibitors *see* ACE inhibitors
angiotensin II receptor blockers
CHF 233
hypertension 182, 183*t*, 185*t*
*anileridine*, pain control in palliative care 128, 130*t*
*anistreplase*, myocardial infarction 204*t*, 211*t*
ankle sprain 488*t*-89*t*
anogenital warts *see* genital warts
**anorexia nervosa 836-39**
Ansaid *see* flurbiprofen
antacids
GERD 375-76, 377*t*, 379*t*
nausea 864*t*
ulcers 385, 386*t*, 740
*antazoline*, red eye 171*t*
anterior knee pain syndrome 488*t*
anthracyclines, adverse effects 856*t*
Anthraforte *see* anthralin
*anthralin*, psoriasis 533*t*, 535
anthranilates, as sunscreen 511*t*
Anthranol *see* anthralin
antiarrhythmics
atrial fibrillation/flutter 243, 246*t*-47*t*, 248-50
CHF 232, 238
antibacterials
infections in cancer patients 811-12, 819
red eye 170*t*, 173
skin infections 561, 563, 564*t*-67*t*
anticholinergics
asthma in adults 314, 315*t*
asthma in children 323, 324*t*
causing agitation 2
COPD 331-32, 333*t*
cough 894, 895*t*
enuresis 426, 428*t*
incontinence 424, 427*t*
nausea 864*t*-65*t*
Parkinson's disease 140*t*, 142
rhinitis 308, 310*t*, 311
anticoagulants
acute stroke 269
angina 223*t*, 226
atrial fibrillation/flutter 248, 249*t*, 249
CHF 232, 238
in pregnancy 278, 921*t*
ischemic stroke prevention 176, 177*t*, 178
myocardial infarction 211*t*
thromboembolism 296
thrombosis 276-78, 280
anticonvulsants
adverse effects 823, 862*t*
headache in children 95, 99
neuralgia 122*t*
seizures 155, 740
antidepressants *see* also monoamine oxidase inhibitors; selective serotonin reuptake inhibitors; tricyclic antidepressants
ADHD 21*t*, 23
adverse effects 161, 823
agitation 5-6
alcohol withdrawal 69
anorexia nervosa 838
anxiety disorders 10-11, 15
bulimia nervosa 841*t*, 842
dementia 29-31
depression 33, 38-40
insomnia 41
neuralgia 122*t*

psychoses 60
smoking cessation 348
antidiabetic agents 619, 620*t*-22*t*, 622
antidiarrheals 401, 403
antidiuretics, enuresis 428*t*
antiemetics
headache in children 94-95, 96*t*, 100
nausea and vomiting 845-47, 848*t*-49*t*, 850, 863, 864*t*-65*t*
pharmacoeconomic considerations 850-51
antiepileptics
headache in adults 86*t*-87*t*
in pregnancy 155
lactation 155
seizures 147, 149, 151*t*-54*t*, 151, 157
antifungals, infections in cancer patients 812, 817*t*, 820
antihistamines
causing glaucoma 161, 166
cough 894, 895*t*, 896
dermatitis 539
dermatographism 545*t*
headache in children 95, 99*t*
in pregnancy 549, 921*t*
nausea 864*t*-65*t*
pruritus 353, 546, 547*t*-48*t*, 549-51, 554
red eye 171*t*
rhinitis 300-301, 302-3*t*, 304, 308, 311
urticaria 545*t*
urticaria pigmentosa 545*t*
antihypertensives, hypertension 183*t*, 184
antihyperuricemic agents, gout 447-48, 452-53
anti-inflammatory drugs *see also* nonsteroidal anti-inflammatory drugs
asthma in adults 313-14, 317-18
asthma in children 323, 326
bacterial meningitis 702, 705
postoperative, cataract 160
red eye 172*t*
antimalarials, rheumatoid arthritis 462*t*
antimetabolites, in pregnancy 403
antimotility agents, traveler's diarrhea 778
antinauseants, headache in adults 83
**antineoplastics**
**adverse effects 509*t*, 852-60,** 862*t*
hypercalcemia 669
anti-obesity agents 830-34
antioxidants, therapeutic 823-24
antiparasitics, infections in cancer patients 818*t*
antiparkinson agents 60, 61*t*
antiplatelet agents
angina 223*t*, 226
ischemic stroke prevention 175-76, 177*t*
myocardial infarction 211*t*-12*t*
antiprogestins, endometriosis 593
antipsychotics *see also* neuroleptics 55, 56*t*-57*t*, 58-62
agitation 2-4
antiresorptive agents
hypercalcemia 670*t*-71*t*
osteoporosis 479
antiretroviral agents
HIV-associated infections 800*t*
HIV infection 789-92, 793*t*-95*t*
antirheumatic drugs, disease-modifying 454-55, 459-61, 462*t*-64*t*, 465
antiseptics, skin infections 559-60
antispasmodics
causing glaucoma 161
enuresis 426, 428*t*
incontinence 427*t*
antitussives, cough 894, 895*t*, 896
antivirals
Bell's palsy 134-35
infections in cancer patients 818*t*, 819
Anturan *see* sulfinpyrazone
**anxiety disorders** *see also* **agitation 7-15**
generalized anxiety disorder 8*t*, 12-14*t*, 15
obsessive-compulsive disorder 8*t*, 11, 12-13*t*
panic disorder 8*t*, 10, 12-13*t*
panic disorder with agoraphobia 10, 12-13*t*
post-traumatic stress disorder 8*t*, 11, 12-13*t*
social phobia 8*t*, 10-11, 12-14*t*
specific phobia 8*t*, 11
anxiolytics
alcohol withdrawal 69
anorexia nervosa 838
Anzemet *see* dolasetron
appetite suppressants 830-31, 833*t*, 834
*apraclonidine*, glaucoma 165*t*, 166
Apresoline *see* hydralazine
Aquacel, pressure ulcers 526*t*
Aquacort *see* hydrocortisone
Aquasite 171*t*
Aralen *see* chloroquine
Arava *see* leflunomide
Aredia *see* pamidronate
Aricept *see* donepezil
Aristocort preparations *see* triamcinolone
Aristospan *see* triamcinolone
**arthritis**
**gouty 444-47**
**osteoarthritis 467-75**
**rheumatoid 454-66**

ASA
acute pain 103, 104*t*
acute stroke 269, 271
aggravating pruritus 545
angina 217, 223*t*
arrhythmias 238
atrial fibrillation/flutter 249*t*
causing headache 89
claudication 283
dementia 30
fibromyalgia 432*t*, 433
headache in adults 82, 84*t*, 88-89
headache in children 93-94, 96*t*
ischemic stroke prevention 175-76, 177*t*, 178
myocardial infarction 206-7, 211*t*, 213-14
rheumatoid arthritis 457*t*, 459
sports injuries 487
thrombosis 269
Asacol *see* 5-aminosalicylic acid
**ascites 350-51, 357*t***
*ascomycin*, dermatitis 541
ascorbic acid *see* Vitamin C
*l-asparaginase*, adverse effects 844*t*, 853*t*, 857*t*
aspiration pneumonia 268
Aspirin *see* ASA
**asthma**
**adults 312-19**
pharmacoeconomic considerations 319
**children 320-28**
in pregnancy 921*t*
with hypertension 186*t*
Atacant *see* candesartan
Atarax *see* hydroxyzine
Atasol *see* acetaminophen
*atenolol*
angina 218*t*, 224*t*, 244*t*
headache in adults 86*t*, 90
hypertension 183*t*
myocardial infarction 210*t*
SVT 251*t*
Ativan *see* lorazepam
*atorvastatin*, dyslipidemias 196*t*, 198*t*
*atovaquone*
HIV-associated infections 800*t*, 804*t*, 806*t*
malaria prophylaxis 770, 771*t*-72*t*, 773
pregnancy 773
Atromid-S *see* clofibrate
*atropine*
diarrhea 877*t*
rhinitis 307
traveler's diarrhea 778
Atrovent *see* ipratropium
**attention deficit hyperactivity disorder 16-24**
*auranofin*, rheumatoid arthritis 461
Aureomycin *see* chlortetracycline
*aurothioglucose*, rheumatoid arthritis 461, 463*t*
*aurothiomalate*, rheumatoid arthritis 460-61, 463*t*
Avandia *see* rosiglitazone
Avapro *see* irbesartan
Avaxim *see* hepatitis A vaccine
Aventyl *see* nortriptyline
Avlosulfon *see* dapsone
*avobenzone*, as sunscreen 511*t*
Axid *see* nizatidine
*azatadine*, pruritus 548*t*
*azathioprine*
causing hepatotoxic reactions 857*t*
hepatitis, autoimmune chronic active 354, 359*t*
IBD 398, 400*t*
polymyalgia rheumatica 442
rheumatoid arthritis 461, 463*t*
*azelaic acid*, acne 499
*azithromycin*
bacterial endocarditis prophylaxis 708*t*
chlamydial infection 756*t*
HIV-associated infections 800*t*, 804*t*, 806*t*
infections in cancer patients 816*t*
malaria prophylaxis 770, 772*t*, 773
otitis media 687, 690*t*
pneumonia 717*t*
pregnancy 756*t*
skin infections 561, 565*t*
streptococcal sore throat 696*t*
traveler's diarrhea 778, 779*t*
Azmacort *see* triamcinolone
Azopt *see* brinzolamide
AZT *see* zidovudine

# B

Baciguent *see* bacitracin
Bacitin *see* bacitracin
*bacitracin*
burns 518*t*
red eye 170*t*
skin infections 563, 567*t*
**back pain 111-17**
*baclofen*
neuralgia 122*t*
persistent hiccoughs 899
spasticity 74-75, 76*t*, 78
trigeminal neuralgia 120
bacteriuria 765*t*
Bactrim *see* co-trimoxazole
Bactroban *see* mupirocin

Balnetar *see* coal tar and derivatives
band ligation, esophageal varices 393
barbiturates
  in lactation 155
  insomnia 47
  seizures 155
Baygam *see* immune globulins
Bayhep B *see* hepatitis B immune globulin
Beben *see* betamethasone
*beclomethasone*
  asthma in adults 314, 316*t*
  asthma in children 323, 325*t*, 326
  COPD 332, 334*t*
  dermatitis 540*t*
  rhinitis 301, 303*t*
Beconase preparations *see* beclomethasone
**Bell's palsy 133-36**
Benadryl *see* diphenhydramine
*benazepril*, hypertension 183*t*
Benemid *see* probenecid
**benign prostatic hyperplasia 414-20**
  pharmacoeconomic considerations 420
*benserazide*, Parkinson's disease 138, 139*t*
Bentylol *see* dicyclomine
Benylin DM *see* dextromethorphan
Benzamycin *see* benzoyl peroxide 495*t*
*benzathine penicillin G*
  streptococcal sore throat 696*t*
  syphilis 759*t*
*benzocaine*
  acute pain 108
  mucositis 857*t*
benzodiazepines
  adverse effects 862*t*
  agitation 4-6
  akathisia 59-60, 61*t*
  anxiety disorders 10-11, 12*t*, 15
  behavioral problems 30
  causing agitation 2
  insomnia 45-47, 50
  nausea and vomiting 847, 848*t*
  spasticity 77*t*, 78
  withdrawal from 66*t*, 70, 72
benzophenones, as sunscreen 511*t*
*benzoyl peroxide*, acne 495*t*, 495, 499
*benztropine*
  agitation 5*t*
  parkinsonism 61*t*
  Parkinson's disease 140*t*
Berotec preparations see fenoterol
beta-agonists
  asthma in adults 314, 315*t*, 318
  asthma in children 320, 322-23, 324*t*, 326, 328
  COPD 331, 333*t*-34*t*
  hyperkalemia 678
  septic shock 739
beta-blockers
  adverse effects 194*t*, 312, 674*t*
  angina 217, 218*t*, 220, 224*t*, 226
  atrial fibrillation/flutter 243, 244*t*
  behavioral problems 30
  causing syncope 289*t*
  CHF 235, 238*t*
  esophageal varices 394
  glaucoma 162-63, 164*t*, 166
  headache in adults 86*t*, 88
  headache in children 95, 98*t*
  hypertension 182, 183*t*, 185-86*t*, 187, 189
  hyperthyroidism 631
  myocardial infarction 204*t*, 204-5, 207, 210*t*, 213-14
  postoperative, cataract 160
  postural orthostatic tachycardia syndrome 293
  rhinitis 309*t*
  SVT 250, 251*t*, 251
  thyroid storm 632
  vasovagal syncope 293
  ventricular tachycardia 260*t*
*beta-carotene*
  deficiency 823
  recommended daily intake 822, 826
  toxicity 825
Betadine *see* povidone-iodine
Betagan *see* levobunolol
Betaloc *see* metoprolol
*betamethasone*
  dermatitis 540*t*
  IBD 399*t*
  pruritus 554
  psoriasis 530, 533*t*
*betaxolol*, glaucoma 162, 164*t*
Betnesol *see* betamethasone
Betnovate *see* betamethasone
Betoptic preparations *see* betaxolol
*bezafibrate*, dyslipidemias 197*t*, 199
Bezalip preparations *see* bezafibrate
Biaxin *see* clarithromycin
Bicillin *see* benzathine penicillin G
*bioallethrin*, pediculosis 555*t*
Biobrane, burns 517
Biocclusive, pressure ulcers 526*t*
Biquin Durules *see* quinidine
*bisacodyl*, constipation 131, 870*t*
*bismuth subsalicylate*
  diarrhea 877*t*, 879
  PUD 389*t*
  traveler's diarrhea 776, 780*t*
*bisoprolol*, hypertension 183*t*
bisphosphonates
  bone loss prevention 442, 594
  bone pain 131*t*

hypercalcemia 669, 672
osteoporosis 479, 481*t*, 484-85
*bleomycin*, adverse effects 844*t*, 856-57*t*
Blocadren *see* timolol
blood, hypovolemia 657
Bonamine *see* meclizine
Bonefos *see* clodronate
breast-feeding *see* lactation
*bretylium*
hypothermia 890
ventricular tachycardia 256
Brevicon 575*t*
Bricanyl *see* terbutaline
*brimonidine*, glaucoma 165*t*, 166
*brinzolamide*, glaucoma 163, 164*t*
*bromazepam*, benzodiazepine withdrawal 72*t*
*bromocriptine*
cocaine withdrawal 69, 71*t*
hyperthermia 887
Parkinson's disease 139*t*, 141
psychoses 60
*brompheniramine*
pruritus 547*t*
rhinitis 304, 310*t*
Bronalide *see* flunisolide
bronchodilators
asthma in adults 313-14
asthma in children 324*t*
COPD 331
*budesonide*
asthma in adults 314, 316*t*
asthma in children 323, 325*t*
COPD 332, 334*t*
croup 341*t*
IBD 398, 399*t*
rhinitis 301, 303*t*
**bulimia nervosa** 39, **836, 840-42**
bulking agents
constipation 869*t*
diarrhea 877*t*, 879-80
bullous impetigo 558, 563
bullous pemphigoid 545*t*
*bumetanide*
CHF 236*t*
edema 662*t*
hypertension 182
*bupivacaine*, acute pain 108
*buprenorphine*
cocaine withdrawal 69
opioid withdrawal 70, 71*t*
*bupropion*
ADHD 23
depression 37*t*, 39
Parkinson's disease 144
smoking cessation 347*t*, 348
Burinex *see* bumetanide
**burns 513-19**
Buspar *see* buspirone
*buspirone*
anxiety disorders 14*t*, 15
behavioral problems 30
benzodiazepine withdrawal 72
depression 40
psychoses 59
*busulfan*, adverse effects 844*t*, 858*t*
*butalbital*
headache in adults 82, 84*t*
headache in children 94, 96*t*
*butorphanol*, headache in adults 83
butylmethoxy-dibenzoylmethane, as sunscreen 511*t*
butyrophenones, nausea and vomiting 847, 848*t*, 865*t*

# C

Cafergot preparations, headache in adults 84*t*
*caffeine*, headache in children 94, 96*t*
calamine, pruritus 546
Calcimar *see* calcitonin
*calcipotriol*, psoriasis 532, 534*t*, 535
*calcitonin*
hypercalcemia 670*t*, 672
osteoporosis 482*t*, 483-86
*calcitriol*, osteoporosis 484
*calcium*
deficiency 823
hypercalcemia 668*t*
hyperkalemia 676, 677*t*
menopause 596
osteoarthritis 468
osteoporosis 478-79, 480*t*, 484-86
recommended daily intake 822
therapeutic supplement 824*t*
*calcium carbimide*, alcohol withdrawal 65
calcium channel blockers
angina 217, 219*t*, 220, 224*t*, 226
arrhythmias 238-39
atrial fibrillation/flutter 243, 245*t*
claudication 283
headache in adults 86*t*, 88
headache in children 95, 98*t*
hypertension 183*t*, 184, 185-86*t*
myocardial infarction 204*t*, 204-5, 207
Raynaud's phenomenon 287, 288*t*
SVT 250, 251*t*, 251
Caltine *see* calcitonin
*camphor*, pruritus 546
cancer
associated infections 810-20
causing hypercalcemia 669, 672
in HIV-positive patients 800*t*
*candesartan*, hypertension 183*t*

candidiasis *see also* thrush
HIV patients 803*t*
vulvovaginal 749, 751, 753*t*, 803*t*
Canesten *see* clotrimazole
cannabinoids, nausea and vomiting 847, 848*t*
Capastat Sulfate *see* capreomycin
Capoten *see* captopril
*capreomycin*, tuberculosis 726*t*
*capsaicin*
neuralgia 123
osteoarthritis 470*t*, 471, 472*t*
*captopril*
CHF 234*t*
hypertension 182, 183*t*
myocardial infarction 211*t*
*carbachol*, glaucoma 165*t*, 166
*carbamazepine*
agitation 4-5
behavioral problems 30
depression 34*t*
headache in adults 89
headache in children 95
neuralgia 122*t*
pain control in palliative care 131*t*
seizures 151-52*t*, 157
trigeminal neuralgia 120
*carbidopa*, Parkinson's disease 138, 139*t*
Carbolith *see* lithium
carbonic anhydrase inhibitors, glaucoma 163, 164*t*-65*t*, 166
*carboplatin*, causing nausea and vomiting 844*t*
*carboxymethylcellulose*, red eye 171*t*
carbuncles 559, 563
Cardene *see* nicardipine
cardiac conduction disturbances 60
cardioversion
atrial fibrillation/flutter 232
SVT 248
ventricular tachycardia 255-56
Cardizem preparations *see* diltiazem
Cardura *see* doxazosin
*carmustine*, adverse effects 844*t*, 856-57*t*
*carvedilol*
CHF 235, 238*t*
hypertension 185*t*
*cascara*, constipation 131
*castor oil*, constipation 870*t*
Catapres *see* clonidine
**cataract surgery, postoperative care 158-60**
catechol-O-methyl-transferase inhibitors *see* COMT inhibitors
cation-exchange resins, hyperkalemia 678-79
Caverject *see* alprostadil
Ceclor *see* cefaclor
Cedocard SR *see* isosorbide dinitrate
*cefaclor*
otitis media 689*t*
pneumonia 716*t*
UTI 763, 766*t*
*cefadroxil*
bacterial endocarditis prophylaxis 708*t*
skin infections 561, 564*t*
*cefazolin*
acute osteomyelitis 734*t*
bacterial endocarditis prophylaxis 708*t*
skin infections 565*t*
UTI 766*t*
*cefepime*, infections in cancer patients 815*t*
*cefixime*
acute osteomyelitis 733-34*t*
gonococcal infection 755*t*
otitis media 689*t*
PID 757*t*
pneumonia 716*t*
UTI 763, 766*t*
Cefizox *see* ceftizoxime
*cefotaxime*
acute osteomyelitis 730*t*, 733-34*t*
bacterial meningitis 700*t*, 701, 702-3*t*
croup 341*t*
otitis media 687
peritonitis 357*t*
pneumonia 715-16*t*
septic shock 742-43*t*
spontaneous bacterial peritonitis 352
UTI 766*t*
*cefoxitin*, PID 757*t*
*cefprozil*
otitis media 690*t*
pneumonia 716*t*
*ceftazidime*
acute osteomyelitis 733-34*t*
bacterial meningitis 700*t*, 703*t*
infections in cancer patients 815*t*
pneumonia 716*t*
septic shock 742-43*t*
UTI 766*t*
Ceftin *see* cefuroxime
*ceftizoxime*, septic shock 742-43*t*
*ceftriaxone*
bacterial meningitis 700*t*, 701, 702-3*t*, 705
gonococcal infection 755*t*
infections in cancer patients 815*t*
in pregnancy 755*t*
peritonitis 352, 357*t*
PID 757*t*
pneumonia 715-16*t*
septic shock 742-43*t*
UTI 766*t*

*cefuroxime*
acute osteomyelitis 733-34*t*
croup 341*t*
otitis media 690*t*
pneumonia 716*t*
skin infections 565*t*
UTI 763, 766*t*
Cefzil *see* cefprozil
Celebrex *see* celecoxib
*celecoxib*
osteoarthritis 471, 472*t*
rheumatoid arthritis 458*t*, 459
Celestoderm V *see* betamethasone
Celexa *see* citalopram
Cellufresh *see* carboxymethylcellulose
cellulitis 558, 562, 568
Celluvisc *see* carboxymethylcellulose
*cephalexin*
acute osteomyelitis 733, 734*t*
bacterial endocarditis prophylaxis 708*t*
skin infections 561, 563, 564*t*
streptococcal sore throat 697*t*
UTI 763, 766*t*
cephalosporins
gonococcal infection 755*t*
otitis media 687
pneumonia 715*t*-16*t*
septic shock 741*t*
skin infections 561, 563, 564*t*-65*t*
streptococcal sore throat 695, 697*t*
UTI 763, 766
Ceptaz *see* ceftazidime
cerebral ischemia *see* **stroke**
*cerivastatin*, dyslipidemias 196*t*, 198*t*
cervical cancer, HIV-positive patients 800t
cervical cap 571*t*
cervical radiculopathy 120-21
cervicitis 749-51, 755*t*-56*t*
C.E.S. *see* estrogen
Cesamet *see* nabilone
Cetamide *see* sulfacetamide
Cetaphil *see* methoxsalen
*cetirizine*, pruritus 548*t*, 549
chemotherapy *see* antineoplastics
CHF *see* **congestive heart failure**
chickenpox 784*t*, 786
chlamydial infection 749-50, 755*t*-56*t*
*chloral hydrate*, insomnia 47
*chlorambucil*
causing nausea and vomiting 844*t*
rheumatoid arthritis 461
*chloramphenicol*
bacterial meningitis 701
red eye 170*t*
skin infections 565*t*
*chlordiazepoxide*
alcohol withdrawal 67*t*
benzodiazepine withdrawal 72*t*
pruritus 550
*chlorhexidine*
scabies 554
skin infections 559
chloroguanide *see* proguanil
Chloromycetin *see* chloramphenicol
*chloroquine*
malaria prophylaxis 744, 770, 771*t*
rheumatoid arthritis 460, 462*t*
*chlorpheniramine*
cough 894, 895*t*, 896
pruritus 547*t*
rhinitis 308
*chlorpromazine*
adverse effects 887
headache in adults 83
headache in children 94, 96*t*
nausea 865*t*
persistent hiccoughs 899
psychoses 55, 56*t*, 62
*chlorpropamide*, diabetes 620*t*
*chlortetracycline*, red eye 170*t*
*chlorthalidone*
CHF 236*t*
edema 662*t*
hypertension 182, 183*t*
Chlor-Tripolon *see* chlorpheniramine
Chlor-Tripolon Decongestant 310*t*
cholangitis, primary sclerosing 353
Choledyl *see* oxtriphylline
**cholestatic disease 353-54, 358*t***
*cholestyramine*
diarrhea 403, 877*t*, 880
dyslipidemias 195, 196*t*
IBS 412*t*
pruritus 354, 358*t*, 550
*choline magnesium trisalicylate*
acute pain 103
osteoarthritis 472*t*
rheumatoid arthritis 457*t*, 459
cholinergic agonists, glaucoma 163, 165*t*, 166
cholinesterase inhibitors, dementia 27
*chondroitin sulfate*, osteoarthritis 471
**chronic fatigue syndrome 435-38**
**chronic obstructive pulmonary disease 329-37**
**chronic tophaceous gout 453**
Chronovera *see* verapamil
*cidofovir*, HIV-associated infections 803*t*, 806*t*
Cidomycin *see* gentamicin
*cilazapril*
CHF 234*t*
hypertension 183*t*
myocardial infarction 211*t*
Ciloxan *see* ciprofloxacin

*cimetidine*
GERD 376, 377*t*
PUD 386*t*
cinnamates, as sunscreen 511*t*
Cinoxate *see* ethoxyethyl p-methoxycinnamate
Cipro *see* ciprofloxacin
*ciprofloxacin*
acute osteomyelitis 730*t*, 732, 733-34*t*
bacterial meningitis 705
cholangitis 353
gonococcal infection 755*t*
HIV-associated infections 804*t*
infections in cancer patients 816*t*, 819
pneumonia 717*t*
pregnancy 755*t*
red eye 170*t*
septic shock 741-42*t*, 744*t*
skin infections 565*t*
traveler's diarrhea 778, 779*t*
traveler's diarrhea prophylaxis 776
tuberculosis 727*t*
UTI 763, 766*t*
cirrhosis, primary biliary 353, 359*t*
*cisapride*
eating disorders 838
GERD 376
*cisplatin*, adverse effects 844*t*, 858*t*
*citalopram*
anxiety disorders 10, 13*t*
depression 35*t*, 38
Citro-Mag *see* magnesium citrate
*cladribine*, causing nausea and vomiting 844*t*
Claforan *see* cefotaxime
*clarithromycin*
bacterial endocarditis prophylaxis 708*t*
HIV-associated infections 800*t*, 804*t*, 806*t*
otitis media 691*t*
pneumonia 717*t*
PUD 388, 389*t*
skin infections 561, 563, 565*t*
streptococcal sore throat 696*t*
Claritin *see* loratadine
**claudication, intermittent 281-84**
Clavulin *see* amoxicillin-clavulanate 564*t*
Clearsite, pressure ulcers 526*t*
*clemastine fumarate*, pruritus 547*t*
Climara *see* estradiol
*clindamycin*
acne 495*t*, 495
acute osteomyelitis 730*t*, 732, 733-34*t*
bacterial endocarditis prophylaxis 708*t*
HIV-associated infections 804*t*
infections in cancer patients 812, 816*t*
in pregnancy 754*t*
septic shock 744*t*
skin infections 561, 563, 565*t*
streptococcal sore throat 698
vaginosis 754*t*
*clobazam*, seizures 151-52*t*
*clobetasol*, dermatitis 540*t*
*clobetasone*, dermatitis 540*t*
*clodronate*, hypercalcemia 670*t*, 672
*clofazimine*, HIV-associated infections 804*t*, 806*t*
*clofibrate*, dyslipidemias 197*t*, 199
Clomid *see* clomiphene
*clomiphene*, endometriosis 586, 588*t*
*clomipramine*
anxiety disorders 10-11, 12*t*
depression 36*t*, 38
*clonazepam*
agitation 5
akathisia 61*t*
anorexia nervosa 838
anxiety disorders 10, 12*t*
spasticity 77*t*, 78
trigeminal neuralgia 120
*clonidine*
ADHD 20, 22*t*, 23
diarrhea 878*t*, 880-81
hypertension 183*t*, 184, 186*t*
opioid withdrawal 70, 71*t*
psychoses 59
*clopidogrel*
acute stroke 271
claudication 283
ischemic stroke prevention 176, 177*t*
myocardial infarction 207, 212*t*
Clopixol-Acuphase *see* zuclopenthixol
*clorazepate*, benzodiazepine withdrawal 72*t*
*clotrimazole*
HIV-associated infections 803*t*
in pregnancy 753*t*
vulvovaginal candidiasis 753*t*
*cloxacillin*
acute osteomyelitis 730*t*, 733*t*, 733, 735*t*
bacterial meningitis 700*t*, 703*t*
croup 341*t*
pneumonia 715-16*t*
skin infections 560-61, 563, 564*t*
*clozapine*
Parkinson's disease 144
psychoses 55, 57*t*, 58-61
Clozaril *see* clozapine
*coal tar* and derivatives, psoriasis 530, 532, 533*t*, 535
*cocaine*
acute pain, topical 108
causing agitation 6
withdrawal from 63, 66*t*, 69, 71*t*

*codeine*
acute pain 105*t*, 107
back pain 115*t*
burns 519
cough 894, 895*t*, 896
diarrhea 878*t*, 880
headache in adults 82, 84*t*
headache in children 94
IBD 401
osteoarthritis 469
pain control in palliative care 127, 129*t*
Cogentin *see* benztropine
coital timing, contraception 571*t*
Colace *see* docusate salts
*colchicine*
alcoholic liver disease 354
gout 446-47, 449*t*
Colestid *see* colestipol
*colestipol*
dyslipidemias 195, 196*t*
pruritus 550
**colitis,** HIV-positive patients 803*t*
**colitis, ulcerative 403-6**
Collagenase, pressure ulcers 526*t*
*colloidal oatmeal*, pruritus 545
colloids, hypovolemia 657-58
Colyte *see* electrolyte solutions
Combivent 334*t*
Comfeel, pressure ulcers 526*t*
complex regional pain syndrome (CRPS) 121
COMT inhibitors, Parkinson's disease 143
condoms
contraception 571*t*
STD protection 569, 575-76, 800*t*
Congest *see* estrone
**congestive heart failure** 185*t*, 205, **229-40**
conjunctivitis 858*t*
**constipation 867-73**
in pregnancy 921*t*
Contac Cold 310*t*
continuous positive airways pressure, CHF 195
**contraception 569-77**
emergency postcoital 574*t*, 576
contraceptives, injectable 570, 573*t*
contraceptives, oral
causing hyperlipidemia 194*t*
contraception 569-70, 573*t*, 575*t*, 576-77
dysmenorrhea 580, 582*t*, 583
endometriosis 589*t*, 591, 593-94
COPD *see* **chronic obstructive pulmonary disease**
Cordarone *see* amiodarone
Coreg *see* carvedilol
Corgard *see* nadolol
coronary angioplasty, myocardial infarction 204*t*
Cortate *see* hydrocortisone
Cortenema *see* hydrocortisone
corticosteroids *see also* steroids
adverse effects 161, 194*t*, 442, 674*t*, 858*t*
antineoplastic side effects 853*t*, 856*t*, 858*t*
asthma in adults 314, 316*t*, 317
asthma in children 320, 322-23, 325*t*, 326, 328
Bell's palsy 134-35
bullous pemphigoid 545*t*
COPD 332, 334*t*-35*t*, 336
Crohn's disease 401, 403
dermatitis 539, 540-42*t*, 541, 545*t*
gout 446, 450*t*
headache in adults 83
hepatitis, alcoholic 356
hypercalcemia 669
IBD 397-98, 399*t*
lateral epicondylitis 490*t*
lichen diseases 545*t*
myocardial infarction 206
nausea and vomiting 845, 847, 848*t*
osteoarthritis 470*t*, 474
plantar fasciitis 491*t*
polymyalgia rheumatica 441-43
postoperative, cataract 160
prurigo nodularis 545*t*
pruritus 550, 554
psoriasis 530, 532, 533*t*
rheumatoid arthritis 461, 465
rhinitis 301, 303*t*, 304
septic shock 746
sunburn 512
ulcerative proctitis 406
Corticreme *see* hydrocortisone
Cortifoam *see* hydrocortisone
Cosopt 164*t*
*co-trimoxazole*
causing hyperkalemia 674*t*
COPD 336
HIV-associated infections 800*t*
infections in cancer patients 818*t*, 819
otitis media 687, 688*t*
peritonitis 357*t*
pneumonia 717*t*, 804*t*, 806*t*
skin infections 566*t*
spontaneous bacterial peritonitis 352
traveler's diarrhea 776, 778, 779*t*
UTI 762, 766*t*
**cough 892-97**
in pregnancy 922*t*
Coumadin *see* warfarin
Coversyl *see* perindopril

COX-2 inhibitors
acute pain 103
dysmenorrhea 582*t*
osteoarthritis 471, 472*t*
rheumatoid arthritis 458*t*, 459
Crixivan *see* indinavir
**Crohn's disease 401-3**
cromoglycate *see* sodium cromoglycate
Cromolyn *see* sodium cromoglycate
*crotamiton*
pruritus 546
scabies 556*t*
**croup 338-42**
CRPS *see* complex regional pain syndrome
Cryptococcus neoformans 803*t*
Crystapen *see* penicillin
Cuprimine *see* penicillamine
cyanocobalamin *see* vitamin $B_{12}$
Cyclen 575*t*
*cyclobenzaprine*
back pain 115*t*
fibromyalgia 432*t*, 433
Cyclocort *see* amcinonide
Cyclomen *see* danazol
cyclo-oxygenase inhibitors *see* COX-2 inhibitors
*cyclopentolate*, postoperative, cataract 160
*cyclophosphamide*
adverse effects 844*t*, 856*t*, 858*t*
rheumatoid arthritis 461
*cycloserine*, tuberculosis 725*t*
*cyclosporine*
causing hyperkalemia 674*t*
dermatitis 541
IBD 400*t*
rheumatoid arthritis 461, 464*t*
ulcerative colitis 406
Cylert *see* pemoline
*cyproheptadine*
anorexia nervosa 838, 839*t*
headache in children 95, 99*t*, 100
pruritus 548*t*
*cyproterone*, acne 496
cystitis 764*t*
*cytarabine*, adverse effects 844*t*, 857-58*t*
cytomegalovirus 800*t*, 803*t*
cytoprotective agents, ulcers 740
Cytotec *see* misoprostol
Cytovene *see* ganciclovir

# D

d4T *see* stavudine
*dacarbazine*, causing nausea and vomiting 844*t*
*dactinomycin*, adverse effects 844*t*, 853*t*
Dalacin preparations *see* clindamycin
*dalteparin*
angina 223*t*
myocardial infarction 211*t*
thrombosis 276, 277*t*
*danazol*, endometriosis 589*t*, 591-92, 594
Dantrium *see* dantrolene
*dantrolene*
hyperthermia 887
psychoses 60
spasticity 76*t*, 78
*dapsone*
dermatitis herpetiformis 545*t*
HIV-associated infections 800*t*, 804*t*, 806*t*
infections in cancer patients 819
Daraprim *see* pyrimethamine
*daunorubicin*, adverse effects 844*t*, 853*t*
Daypro *see* oxaprozin
DDAVP *see* desmopressin
ddC *see* zalcitabine
ddI *see* didanosine
Debrisan, pressure ulcers 526*t*
Decadron *see* dexamethasone
decarboxylase inhibitors, Parkinson's disease 138
Decongest *see* xylometazoline
decongestants
causing glaucoma 161
cough 894
red eye 170*t*, 173
rhinitis 300-301, 302*t*, 306, 308, 309*t*-10*t*, 311
decubitus ulcers *see* **pressure ulcers**
DEET *see* N,N-diethyl-m-toluamide
*deferoxamine*, hemochromatosis 356, 359*t*
defibrillators
atrial fibrillation/flutter 248
CHF 238
ventricular tachycardia 262
**dehydration, children 648-54** *see also* **hypovolemia**
*delavirdine*, HIV infection 794*t*
delirium 2-3
Delsym *see* dextromethorphan
Deltasone *see* prednisone
**dementia** 3-4, **25-32**
pharmacoeconomic considerations 31-32
Demerol *see* meperidine
Demulen 575*t*
Denavir *see* penciclovir
Depakene *see* valproic acid
Depen *see* penicillamine
Depo-Medrol *see* methylprednisolone
Depo-Provera *see* medroxyprogesterone
deprenyl *see* selegiline

**depression 33-42**
agitated 5-6
in pregnancy 922*t*
pharmacoeconomic considerations 41
Dermasone *see* clobetasol
**dermatitis**
**atopic 538-42**, 545*t*
contact 545*t*
herpetiformis 545*t*
dermatographism 545*t*, 551
Dermazin *see* silver sulfadiazine
Dermovate *see* clobetasol
Desferal *see* deferoxamine
*desipramine*
ADHD 22*t*, 23
anxiety disorders 10, 12*t*
back pain 116*t*
bulimia nervosa 840, 841*t*
chronic fatigue syndrome 437*t*
cocaine withdrawal 69, 71*t*
dementia 29
depression 36*t*, 38, 40
neuralgia 121, 122*t*
*desmopressin*, enuresis 428*t*, 429
Desocort *see* desonide
*desogestrel*, contraception 569, 575*t*
*desonide*, dermatitis 540*t*
*desoximetasone*, dermatitis 540*t*
Desquam-X *see* benzoyl peroxide
Desyrel *see* trazodone
Detrol *see* tolterodine
*dexamethasone*
bacterial meningitis 702, 705*t*, 705
croup 341*t*
hyperthyroidism 635*t*
nausea and vomiting 845, 847, 848*t*, 850-51
pain control in palliative care 131*t*
postoperative, cataract 160
red eye 172*t*
Dexasone *see* dexamethasone
*dexbrompheniramine*, rhinitis 310*t*
*dexchlorpheniramine*, pruritus 547*t*
Dexedrine *see* dextroamphetamine
Dexiron *see* iron
*dexrazoxane*, cardiomyopathy 856*t*
*dextran*, red eye 171*t*
*dextroamphetamine*, ADHD 18, 20, 21*t*
*dextromethorphan*, cough 894, 895*t*, 896
*dextrose*
dehydration in children 653*t*
hypovolemia 656, 657*t*, 658
seizures 156*t*
Diaßeta *see* glyburide
**diabetes mellitus** 186*t*, **612-28**
in pregnancy 922*t*
pharmacoeconomic considerations 627-28
diabetic foot 732*t*, 733
diabetic neuropathy 121, 123
Diabinese *see* chlorpropamide
Diamicron *see* gliclazide
Diamox preparations *see* acetazolamide
Diane-35, acne 496, 498*t*
diaphragm, contraceptive 571*t*
**diarrhea** 805, **874-81**
**traveler's 775-81**
*diazepam*
alcohol withdrawal 67*t*-68*t*
anxiety disorders 10
benzodiazepine withdrawal 72*t*, 72
myoclonus 131
pruritus 550
spasticity 77*t*, 78
Diban 878*t*
dibenzoylmethanes, as sunscreen 511*t*
Dicetel *see* pinaverium
*diclofenac*
acute pain 103
dysmenorrhea 582*t*
postoperative, cataract 160
red eye 172*t*
rheumatoid arthritis 457*t*
*dicyclomine* 427*t*-28*t*
IBS 411, 412*t*
*didanosine*, HIV infection 793*t*
Didrocal *see* etidronate
Didronel *see* etidronate
*dienestrol*, menopause 598*t*
*N,N-diethyl-m-toluamide*, malaria prophylaxis 768, 770
*diethylpropion*, obesity 833*t*
Differin *see* adapalene
*diflorasone*, dermatitis 540*t*
Diflucan *see* fluconazole
*diflucortolone*, dermatitis 540*t*
*diflunisal*
acute pain 103
rheumatoid arthritis 457*t*
*digoxin*
adverse effects 674*t*, 676
atrial fibrillation/flutter 242*t*, 243, 244*t*
CHF 235
myocardial infarction 205
SVT 250*t*, 250, 251*t*, 251
*dihydroergotamine*
headache in adults 82, 85*t*, 89
headache in children 94, 97*t*
Dilantin *see* phenytoin
Dilaudid preparations *see* hydromorphone
*diltiazem*
angina 217, 219*t*, 220, 224*t*, 227
atrial fibrillation/flutter 242*t*, 243, 245*t*
CHF 239
hypertension 183*t*, 184, 185*t*
myocardial infarction 205, 207

Raynaud's phenomenon 288*t*
SVT 250*t*-51*t*
*dimenhydrinate*
headache in adults 83
nausea and vomiting 131, 847, 864*t*
Dimetane *see* brompheniramine
Dimetapp Liqui-Gels 310*t*
Diomycin *see* erythromycin
Diovan *see* valsartan
dioxybenzone, as sunscreen 511*t*
Dipentum *see* olsalazine
*diphenhydramine*
dermatitis 539
mucositis 857*t*
nausea 864*t*
parkinsonism 61*t*
pruritus 547*t*, 554
*diphenoxylate*
diarrhea 877*t*, 880
IBD 398, 401
traveler's diarrhea 778
*dipivefrin*, glaucoma 165*t*, 166
Diprolene Glycol *see* betamethasone
Diprosone *see* betamethasone
*dipyridamole*
acute stroke 271
ischemic stroke prevention 176, 177*t*, 178
Disalcid *see* salsalate
Disipal *see* orphenadrine
*disopyramide*
atrial fibrillation/flutter 246*t*
myocardial infarction 205
ventricular tachycardia 259*t*
disseminated intravascular coagulation 740
*disulfiram*, alcohol withdrawal 65
Ditropan *see* oxybutynin
diuretics
adverse effects 509*t*, 674*t*
ascites 350
CHF 235, 236*t*
edema 661, 662*t*-63*t*, 664-65
hypertension 182, 183*t*, 185*t*, 187, 190
in pregnancy 661
myocardial infarction 205
*divalproex*
dementia 30
headache in adults 86*t*, 88
seizures 154*t*
DLV *see* delavirdine
DMARD *see* antirheumatic drugs, disease-modifying
*dobutamine*
CHF 239
septic shock 742
docetaxel, causing nausea and vomiting 844*t*
*docusate* salts, constipation 131, 871*t*
*dolasetron*, nausea and vomiting 847, 849*t*
Dolobid *see* diflunisal
*domperidone*
anorexia nervosa 838, 839*t*
GERD 376, 378*t*-79*t*
headache in adults 83
nausea 143
*donepezil*, dementia 27, 28*t*, 31
Donnagel PG 878*t*
*dopamine*
CHF 239
septic shock 742
dopamine agonists
cocaine withdrawal 69, 71*t*
hyperthermia 887
Parkinson's disease 138, 139*t*, 141-42, 144-45
dopamine antagonists
nausea 865*t*
persistent hiccoughs 899
*dorzolamide*, glaucoma 163, 164*t*
Dovonex *see* calcipotriol
*doxazosin*
hypertension 183*t*, 184
prostatic hyperplasia 416, 418*t*, 419
*doxepin*
anxiety disorders 11
depression 36*t*, 38
dermatitis 539
headache in adults 87*t*, 88
pruritus 546, 550
*doxorubicin*, adverse effects 844*t*, 853*t*, 856-58*t*
*doxycycline*
acne 497*t*
chlamydial infection 755*t*
in pregnancy 755*t*
malaria prophylaxis 770, 771*t*, 773
PID 757*t*
pneumonia 715*t*, 717*t*
pregnancy 774
rosacea 503, 504*t*
syphilis 759*t*
traveler's diarrhea 776, 778
DPE *see* dipivefrin
dressings
burns 517
pressure ulcers 525, 526*t*
Drisdol *see* vitamin D
Dristan *see* oxymetazoline
Drixoral 310*t*
*dronabinol*, nausea and vomiting 847, 848*t*
*droperidol*, nausea and vomiting 847, 848*t*
drug eruptions, pruritus 545*t*, 551

**drug withdrawal syndromes**
alcohol 63-65, 66-68*t*
benzodiazepines 66*t*, 70, 72-73
cocaine 66*t*, 69, 71*t*
opioids 66*t*, 70, 71*t*
Dulcolax *see* bisacodyl
DuoDerm
burns 517
pressure ulcers 526*t*
Duolube 171*t*
Duovent UDV 334*t*
Duphalac *see* lactulose
Duragesic *see* fentanyl
Duricef *see* cefadroxil
Dyrenium *see* triamterene
**dyslipidemias** 185*t*, **191-201**
pharmacoeconomic considerations 199-200
**dysmenorrhea 578-83**
dysphagia, HIV-positive patients 799
dysrhythmias 205
dysthymia 34*t*
dystonias 60

# E

**eating disorders 836-42**
anorexia nervosa 836-39
bulimia nervosa 39, 836, 840-42
*echinacea*, rhinitis 308
*echothiophate*, glaucoma 165*t*, 166
*econazole*, vulvovaginal candidiasis 753*t*
Ecostatin *see* econazole
Edecrin *see* ethacrynic acid
**edema 659-65**, 740
EES *see* erythromycin
*efavirenz*, HIV infection 794*t*
Effexor *see* venlafaxine
EFV *see* efavirenz
Elavil *see* amitriptyline
Eldepryl *see* selegiline
electrolyte replacement 651*t*, 653*t*, 656-58, 776-77, 879
electrolyte lavage solutions, constipation 871*t*
Elocom *see* mometasone
Eltor *see* pseudoephedrine
Eltroxin *see* levothyroxine
Emadine *see* emedastine
embolism, pulmonary *see* **thromboembolism, venous**
*emedastine*, red eye 171*t*
Eminase *see* anistreplase
EMLA, acute pain 108
*enalapril*
CHF 234*t*
hypertension 182, 183*t*
myocardial infarction 211*t*
encephalitis 784*t*, 785, 800*t*, 803-4*t*
**encephalopathy, hepatic 352, 358*t***
**endocarditis, bacterial 707-10**
**endometriosis 584-94**
Enfalac *see* oral rehydration therapy
Engerix-B *see* hepatitis B vaccine
*enoxaparin*
angina 223*t*
myocardial infarction 211*t*
thrombosis 276, 277*t*
*entacapone*, Parkinson's disease 143
enteritis, HIV-positive patients 803*t*
Entex LA *see* phenylpropanolamine
Entocort *see* budesonide
Entrophen *see* ASA
**enuresis 425-29**
enzymes, ulcer débridement 524
Epaxal Berna *see* hepatitis A vaccine
epicondylitis, lateral 490*t*
epididymo-orchitis 750, 752
epiglottitis 338-39, 341*t*
Epilock, pressure ulcers 526*t*
*epinephrine*
acute pain 108
asthma in adults 314
croup 341*t*
GI bleeding 393
*epirubicin*, adverse effects 844*t*, 853*t*
Epival *see* divalproex
epsom salts *see* magnesium sulfate
*eptifibatide*
angina 223*t*, 226
myocardial infarction 207, 212*t*
**erectile dysfunction 602-8**
ergoloid mesylates, dementia 27
Ergomar *see* ergot derivatives
*ergotamine*, headache in adults 82, 84*t*
ergot derivatives
causing headache 89
headache in adults 82, 84*t*-85*t*
headache in children 94, 97*t*
Erybid *see* erythromycin
Eryc *see* erythromycin
erysipelas 558, 562, 568
Erysol *see* erythromycin
erythrasma 558
Erythrocin *see* erythromycin
Erythromid *see* erythromycin
*erythromycin*
acne 495*t*, 495-96, 497*t*
chlamydial infection 756*t*
COPD 336
infections in cancer patients 816*t*
in pregnancy 756*t*
otitis media 691*t*
pneumonia 717*t*
red eye 170*t*
rosacea 503, 505*t*
septic shock 745*t*
skin infections 561, 563, 565*t*

streptococcal sore throat 695, 696*t*
syphilis 759*t*
*erythropoietin*, anemia 646, 647*t*, 855*t*
*esdepallethrin*, scabies 556*t*
esophageal varices 393-94
Estalis 481*t*, 599*t*
Estrace *see* estradiol
Estracomb 481*t*, 599*t*
Estraderm *see* estradiol
*estradiol*
acne 496, 498*t*
menopause 598*t*-99*t*
osteoporosis 480*t*-81*t*
*estramustine*, causing nausea and vomiting 844*t*
Estring *see* estradiol
Estrogel *see* estradiol
estrogens
acne 496
adverse effects 194*t*, 844*t*
after hysterectomy 587
contraception 569-70, 573*t*, 575*t*
hypercalcemia 669
incontinence 424, 427*t*
menopause 596, 598*t*-600*t*, 600-601
osteoarthritis 468
osteoporosis 479, 480*t*-81*t*, 483, 485-86
*estrone*
menopause 598*t*
osteoporosis 480*t*
*estropipate*
menopause 598*t*
osteoporosis 480*t*
*etanercept*, rheumatoid arthritis 465
*ethacrynic acid*
CHF 236*t*
edema 662*t*
*ethambutol*
HIV-associated infections 804*t*
tuberculosis 725*t*, 727*t*, 727-28
*ethanolamine*, esophageal varices 393
*ethinyl estradiol*
contraception 570, 574-75*t*, 576
menopause 598*t*
*ethionamide*, tuberculosis 726*t*
*ethopropazine*, Parkinson's disease 140*t*
*ethosuximide*, seizures 149, 151-52*t*
*2-ethoxyethyl p-methoxycinnamate*, as sunscreen 511*t*
*ethynodiol diacetate*, contraception 575*t*
Etibi *see* ethambutol
*etidronate*
bone loss prevention 442
hypercalcemia 670*t*, 672
osteoporosis 479, 481*t*, 483, 485
*etodolac*, rheumatoid arthritis 457*t*
*etoposide*, adverse effects 844*t*, 857*t*
Euglucon *see* glyburide
Eumovate *see* clobetasone
Eurax *see* crotamiton
eutectic mixture of local anesthetics *see* EMLA
Evista *see* raloxifene
Exelon *see* rivastigmine
extravasation, antineoplastic drugs 852, 853*t*
Eyestil *see* sodium hyaluronate

## F

factitious hyperthyroidism 629
*famciclovir*
herpesvirus infections 120, 782-83, 784*t*, 785, 787
HIV-associated infections 800*t*
infections in cancer patients 818*t*, 819
*famotidine*
GERD 376, 377*t*
PUD 386*t*
Famvir *see* famciclovir
Fansidar, malaria prophylaxis 772*t*
Fastin *see* phentermine
Feldene *see* piroxicam
*felodipine*
angina 217
hypertension 183*t*, 185*t*
Raynaud's phenomenon 288*t*
*fenofibrate*, dyslipidemias 197*t*, 199
*fenoprofen*, rheumatoid arthritis 457*t*
*fenoterol*
asthma in adults 314, 315*t*
asthma in children 322, 324*t*
COPD 331, 333*t*-34*t*
*fentanyl*
acute pain 106*t*, 108
burns 519
neuralgia 122*t*
pain control in palliative care 128, 130*t*
ferrous compounds *see* iron
**fever** *see also* **thermoregulatory disorders**
HIV-positive patients 799, 802, 805
**in children 882-84**
in pregnancy 922*t*
*feverfew*, headache in adults 88
*fexofenadine*
pruritus 548*t*, 549
rhinitis 300
fibrates, dyslipidemias 197*t*, 199
Fibrepur *see* psyllium
**fibrillation**
**atrial 242-49**
**ventricular 253-56, 258-62**
**fibromyalgia 430-34**
*finasteride*, prostatic hyperplasia 416-17, 418*t*, 419-20

Fiorinal preparations
headache in adults 84*t*
headache in children 96*t*
Flagyl *see* metronidazole
Flamazine *see* silver sulfadiazine
Flarex *see* fluorometholone
*flavoxate*, incontinence and enuresis 427*t*-28*t*
*flecainide*
atrial fibrillation/flutter 247*t*, 249
CHF 238
myocardial infarction 205
SVT 251*t*
ventricular tachycardia 260*t*
Fleet preparations *see* sodium phosphates
Flexeril *see* cyclobenzaprine
Flomax *see* tamsulosin
Flonase *see* fluticasone
Florinef *see* fludrocortisone
Florone *see* diflorasone
Flovent *see* fluticasone
Floxin *see* ofloxacin
Fluanxol *see* flupenthixol
*fluconazole*
HIV-associated infections 800*t*, 803*t*, 807*t*
infections in cancer patients 812, 817*t*, 820
in pregnancy 753*t*
vulvovaginal candidiasis 753*t*
*flucytosine*, HIV-associated infections 803*t*, 807*t*
*fludarabine*, causing nausea and vomiting 844*t*
*fludrocortisone*
hypotension 143
orthostatic hypotension 293
postural orthostatic tachycardia syndrome 293
vasovagal syncope 291, 292*t*
*flunarizine*
headache in adults 86*t*, 88
headache in children 95, 98*t*, 100
*flunisolide*
asthma in adults 314
asthma in children 323
COPD 334*t*
rhinitis 303*t*
*fluocinolone*, dermatitis 540*t*
*fluocinonide*, dermatitis 540*t*
Fluoderm *see* fluocinolone
*fluoride*, osteoporosis 484
*fluorometholone*
postoperative, cataract 160
red eye 172*t*
*fluoroquinolone*
pneumonia 715*t*
postoperative, cataract 160
*5-fluorouracil*, adverse effects 844*t*, 857-58*t*
Fluotic *see* fluoride
*fluoxetine*
anxiety disorders 10, 13*t*
bulimia nervosa 840, 841*t*
chronic fatigue syndrome 437*t*
depression 35*t*, 40
obesity 833*t*
psychoses 60
smoking cessation 348
*flupenthixol*, psychoses 56*t*, 59*t*
*fluphenazine*, psychoses 56*t*, 59*t*
*flurazepam*
benzodiazepine withdrawal 72*t*
insomnia 47
*flurbiprofen*
dysmenorrhea 581*t*
endometriosis 588*t*
postoperative, cataract 160
red eye 172*t*
rheumatoid arthritis 457*t*
*fluticasone*
asthma in adults 314, 316*t*
asthma in children 323, 325*t*
COPD 332, 334*t*
rhinitis 303*t*
*fluvastatin*, dyslipidemias 196*t*, 198*t*
*fluvoxamine*
anxiety disorders 10, 13*t*
depression 35*t*
FML preparations *see* fluorometholone
folate *see* folic acid
*folic acid*
anemia 643, 645*t*
deficiency 642-43, 823
recommended daily intake 822, 826
therapeutic supplement 824*t*, 824
to treat methotrexate side effects 460
toxicity 826
*folinic acid*
HIV-associated infections 804*t*
to treat methotrexate side effects 460
folliculitis 545*t*, 558, 560-61, 563
Foradil *see* formoterol
foreign body obstruction, airway 339
*formoterol*
asthma in adults 314, 315*t*
asthma in children 322, 324*t*
COPD 331, 333*t*
Formula 44 *see* dextromethorphan
Fortaz *see* ceftazidime
Fortovase *see* saquinavir
Fosamax *see* alendronate
*foscarnet*
herpesvirus infections 782
HIV-associated infections 803*t*, 807*t*
infections in cancer patients 819
Foscavir *see* foscarnet

*fosinopril*
CHF 234*t*
hypertension 183*t*
myocardial infarction 211*t*
fracture, stress, tibia/fibula 489*t*-90*t*
Fragmin *see* dalteparin
*framycetin*
burns 518*t*
red eye 170*t*
skin infections 563, 567*t*
Fraxiparine *see* nadroparin
Frisium *see* clobazam
Froben *see* flurbiprofen
FTV *see* saquinavir
Fucidin *see* fusidic acid
Fungizone *see* amphotericin B
*furosemide*
ascites 350, 357*t*
CHF 237*t*, 240
edema 661, 662*t*, 664
hypercalcemia 669
hyperkalemia 677*t*
hypertension 182
furuncles 558, 563, 568
*fusidic acid*
burns 518*t*
skin infections 563, 567*t*

# G

*gabapentin*
seizures 151-52*t*
trigeminal neuralgia 120-21, 122*t*
gamma benzene hexachloride *see* lindane
*ganciclovir*
herpesvirus infections 782
HIV-associated infections 803*t*, 807*t*
infections in cancer patients 818*t*, 819
Garamycin *see* gentamicin
**gastroesophageal reflux disease 373-81**
pharmacoeconomic considerations 380
**gastrointestinal bleeding, upper 390-95**
Gastrolyte *see* oral rehydration therapy
*gemcitabine*, causing nausea and vomiting 844*t*
*gemfibrozil*, dyslipidemias 197*t*, 199
genital herpes *see* herpes, genital
genital ulcers 758
genital warts 750-51, 760
*gentamicin*
acute osteomyelitis 730*t*, 733*t*, 735*t*
bacterial endocarditis prophylaxis 709*t*
bacterial meningitis 700*t*, 702*t*, 704*t*
cholestatic disease 353
infections in cancer patients 815*t*, 819
pneumonia 717*t*
postoperative, cataract 160
red eye 170*t*
septic shock 742-43*t*
skin infections 563, 567*t*
UTI 766*t*, 766
Genteal *see* hydroxypropyl methylcellulose
GERD *see* **gastroesophageal reflux disease**
*gestodene*, contraception 569
GI bleeding *see* **gastrointestinal bleeding, upper**
gingivostomatitis 782, 784*t*
**glaucoma 161-67**
*gliclazide*, diabetes 620*t*
glucocorticoids
adverse effects 823
hepatitis, autoimmune chronic active 354
hypercalcemia 672
hyperthyroidism 631
thyroid storm 632
ulcerative colitis 405
GlucoNorm *see* repaglinide
Glucophage *see* metformin
*glucosamine sulfate*, osteoarthritis 471
*glucose*
hyperkalemia 677*t*, 678
hypothermia 890
*glyburide*, diabetes 620*t*
*glycerin*, constipation 869*t*
glycopeptides, septic shock 742*t*, 744*t*
glycoprotein IIb/IIIa inhibitors
acute stroke 269
angina 223*t*-24*t*, 227
myocardial infarction 212*t*
Glysennid *see* senna
**goitre 636-37**
toxic multinodular 629
*gold*
asthma in adults 317
rheumatoid arthritis 459-61, 463*t*
Golytely *see* electrolyte lavage solutions
gonadotropin-releasing hormone analogues 590*t*, 592-94
gonococcal infection 749-50, 755*t*
*goserelin*, endometriosis 590*t*, 592
**gout** 186*t*, **444-53**
*gramicidin*
red eye 170*t*
skin infections 563
*granisetron*, nausea and vomiting 847, 849*t*, 851
*granulocyte colony-stimulating factor*
infections in cancer patients 819
neutropenia 855*t*
*granulocyte-macrophage colony-stimulating factor*, infections in cancer patients 819

granulomatous diseases, hypercalcemia 669
Graves' disease 629
Gravol *see* dimenhydrinate
GTN *see* nitroglycerin
Gynecure *see* tioconazole
Gyne-T *see* intrauterine device

# H

$H_1$ blockers, pruritus 546
$H_2$ antagonists
GERD 376, 377*t*, 379*t*, 379
GI bleeding 393
pruritus 550
PUD 384-85, 386*t*
ulcers 388, 740
Habitrol *see* nicotine
*halcinonide*, dermatitis 540*t*
Halcion *see* triazolam
Haldol *see* haloperidol
hallucinogens, causing agitation 2, 6
*halobetasol*, dermatitis 540*t*
Halog *see* halcinonide
*haloperidol*
adverse effects 887
agitation 2-4, 5*t*, 6, 131
alcohol withdrawal 67*t*
behavioral problems 29-30
confusion 131
nausea and vomiting 131, 847, 848*t*, 865*t*
persistent hiccoughs 899
psychoses 55, 56*t*, 59*t*, 59, 62
Havrix *see* hepatitis A vaccine
**headache**
**adults 80-91**
**children 92-100**
drug-induced 89
pharmacoeconomic considerations 90-91
rebound 89
heat cramps 886
heat exhaustion 886
heat stroke 886-87
**hemochromatosis 356, 359*t***
hemodialysis, hyperkalemia 679
Hepalean *see* heparin
*heparin*
angina 221, 223*t*
anticoagulation in pregnancy 278, 921*t*
atrial fibrillation/flutter 248
causing hyperkalemia 674*t*
ischemic stroke prevention 176, 177*t*, 178
myocardial infarction 204*t*, 211*t*
thrombocytopenia 740
thromboembolism 296
thrombosis 269, 274*t*, 277*t*, 277
heparins, low molecular weight
angina 223*t*
in pregnancy 277
ischemic stroke prevention 178
thrombosis 274*t*, 276, 277*t*, 279-80
hepatic dysfunction 740
**hepatitis**
**alcoholic 356**
**autoimmune chronic active 354, 359*t***
HIV-positive patients 800*t*
**viral 362-72**
hepatitis A 364, 368*t*-69*t*
*hepatitis A vaccine* 364, 368*t*
HIV-associated infections 800*t*
**hepatitis B** 362-64, **364-67**, 368*t*-69*t*
*hepatitis B immune globulin* 364-65, 369*t*
*hepatitis B vaccine* 364-65, 368*t*
HIV-associated infections 800*t*
**hepatitis C** 362-64, **367**, 369*t*, **371**
hepatitis D 365-66
Heptovir *see* lamivudine
*heroin*, pain control in palliative care 128
herpes simplex
encephalitis 784*t*, 785
genital 758-59, 782-85, 784*t*
HIV-positive patients 800*t*
keratoconjunctivitis 784*t*, 786
orolabial 782-85, 784*t*
**herpesvirus infections 782-87**
herpes simplex virus 782-86, 800*t*
varicella-zoster virus 786-87
herpes zoster, acute 119-20, 784*t*, 786-87
Herplex *see* idoxuridine
*hexachlorophene*, skin infections 559
**hiccoughs, persistent 898-900**
Histanil *see* promethazine
Hivid *see* zalcitabine
**HIV infection** 759, **788-97**
**HIV-positive patients**
candidiasis 803*t*
central nervous system infections 799
cervical cancer 800*t*
colitis 803*t*
diarrhea 805
dysphagia 799
encephalitis 800*t*, 803-4*t*
enteritis 803*t*
fever 799, 802, 805
fungal infections 800*t*
hepatitis 800*t*
herpes simplex virus 800*t*
meningitis 803*t*
myelitis 803*t*
neuritis 803*t*

odynophagia 799
**opportunistic infections 798-809**
pneumonia 799, 800*t*, 801, 804*t*
pneumonitis 803*t*
retinitis 803*t*
STDs 800*t*
tuberculosis 800*t*
varicella 800*t*
HIV postexposure prophylaxis 789, 796*t*
HMG CoA reductase inhibitors, dyslipidemias 195, 196*t*, 198*t*, 198
homomenthyl salicylate *see* homosalate
*homosalate*, as sunscreen 511*t*
hormone replacement therapy *see* estrogens
Humalog *see* insulin
Humulin preparations *see* insulin
hyaluronans, osteoarthritis 470*t*, 473*t*, 474
Hycort *see* hydrocortisone
Hyderm *see* hydrocortisone
*hydralazine*
CHF 235
hypertension 183*t*, 184, 185-86*t*
*hydrochlorothiazide*
CHF 236*t*
edema 661, 662*t*, 664
hypertension 182, 183*t*
*hydrocodone*, acute pain 107
*hydrocortisone*
dermatitis 540*t*
hypercalcemia 669
hyperthyroidism 635*t*
IBD 398, 399*t*
psoriasis 531, 533*t*, 535
septic shock 746
thyroid storm 632
HydroDiuril *see* hydrochlorothiazide
Hydromorph Contin *see* hydromorphone
*hydromorphone*
neuralgia 122*t*
pain control in palliative care 127-28, 129*t*-30*t*
Hydrosorb, pressure ulcers 526*t*
hydroxocobalamin *see* vitamin $B_{12}$
*hydroxychloroquine*
malaria prophylaxis 770, 771*t*
rheumatoid arthritis 459-61, 462*t*
*hydroxymorphone*, acute pain 107
*hydroxypropyl methylcellulose*, red eye 171*t*
*hydroxyurea*, causing nausea and vomiting 844*t*
*hydroxyzine*
dermatitis 539
nausea 864*t*
pruritus 354, 548*t*
Hygroton *see* chlorthalidone
*hyoscyamine*, IBS 411, 412*t*
**hypercalcemia 666-73**
hypercholesterolemia, heterozygous familial 194
hyperchylomicronemia, familial 194
hyperkalemia 674*t*, **675-79**
hyperlipidemia, familial combined 194
hypernatremic dehydration 651, 652*t*
hyperparathyroidism 669
**hypertension 180-90**, 205
in pregnancy 923*t*
pharmacoeconomic considerations 190
**hyperthermia 885-87, 890**
**hyperthyroidism** 194*t*, **629-31,** 923*t*
hypertriglyceridemia, familial 194
**hyperuricemia 444, 447-48, 452-53**
hypnotics, insomnia 45-47, 50
hypoglycemia 617
**hypokalemia** 674*t*, **679-83**
hyponatremic dehydration 652*t*, 652
Hypotears see polyvinyl alcohol
hypotension, orthostatic 293
**hypothermia 885, 887-90**
**hypothyroidism 632-33, 636**
**hypovolemia 655-58** see *also* **dehydration**
Hytrin *see* terazosin

# I

$^{131}$I *see* iodine (radioactive)
iatrogenic hyperthyroidism 629
IBD *see* **inflammatory bowel disease**
IBS *see* **irritable bowel syndrome**
*ibuprofen*
acute pain 103, 104*t*
back pain 115*t*
Bell's palsy 134
chronic fatigue syndrome 437*t*
dysmenorrhea 581*t*
endometriosis 588*t*
fever 883, 884*t*
fibromyalgia 432*t*, 433
headache in adults 84*t*
headache in children 94, 96*t*
osteoarthritis 469, 471, 472*t*
rheumatoid arthritis 457*t*
rhinitis 308
septic shock 746
sunburn 512
*ibutilide*, atrial fibrillation/flutter 242*t*
*idarubicin*, adverse effects 844*t*, 853*t*
idiopathic edema 664
*idoxuridine*
herpesvirus infections 784*t*, 786
red eye 171*t*
IDV *see* indinavir
*ifosfamide*, adverse effects 844*t*, 858*t*
Iletin preparations *see* insulin

*iloprost*, Raynaud's phenomenon 287
Ilosone *see* erythromycin
Imdur *see* isosorbide-5-mononitrate
imidazoles, vulvovaginal candidiasis 753*t*
*imipenem-cilastatin*
acute osteomyelitis 730*t*, 733*t*, 735*t*
infections in cancer patients 815*t*
pneumonia 716*t*
septic shock 742-43*t*
*imipramine*
ADHD 22*t*, 23
anxiety disorders 10, 12*t*
bulimia nervosa 840, 841*t*
cocaine withdrawal 69
depression 36*t*, 38, 40
enuresis 428*t*
headache in adults 90
incontinence 427*t*, 429
pain control in palliative care 131*t*
psychoses 60
Imitrex preparations *see* sumatriptan
immune globulins
hepatitis A 364, 369*t*
septic shock 746
immunosuppressives
bullous pemphigoid 545*t*
IBD 398, 400*t*
polymyalgia rheumatica 442
ulcerative colitis 405
immunotherapy, septic shock 746
Imodium *see* loperamide
Imovane *see* zopiclone
impetigo 558-59, 561, 563
impotence *see* **erectile dysfunction**
Imuran *see* azathioprine
Inapsine *see* droperidol
**incontinence, urinary 422-24, 427*t***
*indapamide*
edema 662*t*
hypertension 183*t*
Inderal preparations *see* propranolol
*indinavir*
HIV infection 795*t*
HIV prophylaxis 796*t*
Indocid *see* indomethacin
*indomethacin*
acute pain 103
dysmenorrhea 581*t*
gout 446-47, 449*t*
headache in adults 83
orthostatic hypotension 293
rheumatoid arthritis 457*t*
septic shock 746
sunburn 512
**infections in cancer patients 810-20**
Infergen *see* interferon alfa
Inflamase *see* prednisolone
**inflammatory bowel disease 396-407**
*infliximab*
Crohn's disease 403
IBD 398, 400*t*
rheumatoid arthritis 465
*influenza vaccine*, HIV-associated infections 800*t*
Infufer *see* iron
Inhibace *see* cilazapril
**injuries, sports 487-92**
Innohep *see* tinzaparin
inotropes, CHF 239
insect bites, pruritus 545*t*
insect repellants, malaria prophylaxis 768, 770
**insomnia 43-51**
*insulin*
adverse effects 618-19
diabetes mellitus 612, 614-19, 622-23, 627-28
hyperkalemia 676, 677*t*, 678
insulin resistance 619
Intal *see* cromoglycate
Integrilin *see* eptifibatide
*interferon alfa*
hepatitis B 365-66, 366*t*, 369*t*
hepatitis C 369*t*-70*t*, 371-72
**intermittent claudication 281-84**
IntraSite Gel, pressure ulcers 526*t*
intrauterine device 572*t*, 576
Intron A *see* interferon alfa
*iodine*, hyperthyroidism 631, 634*t*
*iodine (radioactive)*
hyperthyroidism 630, 634*t*
thyroid cancer 638
Ionamine *see* phentermine
Iopidine *see* apraclonidine
*ipratropium*
asthma in adults 314, 315*t*, 318
asthma in children 323, 324*t*, 326
COPD 331-32, 333*t*-34*t*
cough 894-95*t*
rhinitis 304, 308
*irbesartan*, hypertension 183*t*
*irinotecan*, adverse effects 844*t*
*iron*
anemia 641-42, 644*t*-45*t*
recommended daily intake 822
therapeutic supplement 824*t*
toxicity 824-25
**iron deficiency anemia 639, 641-42, 644*t*-45*t***
**irritable bowel syndrome 408-13**
ischemic heart disease 185*t*
ISDN *see* isosorbide dinitrate
Ismo *see* isosorbide-5-mononitrate
isonatremic dehydration 651, 652*t*
*isoniazid*
adverse effects 823
HIV-associated infections 800*t*

tuberculosis 722, 724*t*, 727*t*, 727-28
*isoproterenol*
asthma in adults 314
septic shock 742
Isoptin preparations *see* verapamil
Isopto Carbachol *see* carbachol
Isopto Carpine *see* pilocarpine
Isopto Tears *see* hydroxypropyl methylcellulose
Isordil *see* isosorbide dinitrate
*isosorbide-5-mononitrate*, angina 217, 218*t*
*isosorbide dinitrate*
angina 217, 218*t*, 224*t*, 227
CHF 233
myocardial infarction 210*t*
*isosorbide mononitrate*, myocardial infarction 210*t*
Isotamine *see* isoniazid
*isotretinoin*
acne 495*t*, 495-96, 497*t*, 500
in pregnancy 499
rosacea 505*t*
Isotrex *see* isotretinoin
*itraconazole*
HIV-associated infections 803*t*, 807*t*
infections in cancer patients 812, 817*t*
IUD 572*t*, 576
*ivermectin*, scabies 554

## J

Jectofer *see* iron

## K

K-10 *see* potassium chloride
Kadian *see* morphine
Kaltostat, pressure ulcers 526*t*
*kanamycin*, tuberculosis 726*t*
Kantrex *see* kanamycin
Kaochlor *see* potassium chloride
*kaolin*, as sunscreen 510
Kaon *see* potassium gluconate
Kayexalate *see* sodium polystyrene sulfonate resin
K-Dur *see* potassium chloride
Keflex *see* cephalexin
Kefurox *see* cefuroxime
Kefzol *see* cefazolin
Kemadrin *see* procyclidine
Kenalog *see* triamcinolone
keratoconjunctivitis herpesvirus 784*t*, 786
*ketanserin*, Raynaud's phenomenon 287
ketoacidosis 618-19
*ketoconazole*
HIV-associated infections 803*t*, 807*t*
infections in cancer patients 812
psoriasis 535
*ketoprofen*
dysmenorrhea 581*t*
endometriosis 588*t*
rheumatoid arthritis 457*t*
*ketorolac*
acute pain 103, 105*t*, 107
headache in adults 83, 84*t*
postoperative, cataract 160
red eye 172*t*
*ketotifen*
asthma in children 325*t*, 326
pruritus 550
Klean-Prep *see* electrolyte lavage solutions
K-Lyte *see* potassium citrate
K-Lyte/Cl *see* potassium chloride
Kwellada-P *see* permethrin
Kytril *see* granisetron

## L

*labetalol*, hypertension 183*t*
Lacrilube 171*t*
Lacri-Lube S.O.P. 171*t*
lacrimation 858*t*
lactation
antiepileptics 155
barbiturates 155
contraception 576-77
**drug exposure 918, 920, 924**
HIV infection 792
tuberculosis 728
Lactulax *see* lactulose
*lactulose*
constipation 131, 869*t*
hepatic encephalopathy 352, 358*t*
IBS 412*t*
Lamictal *see* lamotrigine
*lamivudine*
hepatitis B 366*t*, 366-67, 369*t*
HIV infection 793*t*
HIV prophylaxis 796*t*
*lamotrigine*, seizures 151*t*, 153*t*
Lamprene *see* clofazimine
Lanoxin *see* digoxin
*lansoprazole*
GERD 378*t*
PUD 386*t*
Largactil *see* chlorpromazine
Lariam *see* mefloquine
laryngotracheobronchitis 338, 341*t*
Lasix *see* furosemide
*latanoprost*, glaucoma 163, 164*t*, 166
laxatives
causing hypokalemia 674*t*
constipation 869*t*-71*t*, 872-73
*leflunomide*, rheumatoid arthritis 464*t*, 465

*leptin*, obesity 834
Leritine *see* anileridine
Lescol *see* fluvastatin
*letrozole*, adverse effects 844*t*
leukotriene antagonists
  asthma in adults 316*t*, 317-18
  asthma in children 325*t*, 326
  rhinitis 301
*leuprolide*, endometriosis 590*t*, 592
Levaquin *see* levofloxacin
*levobunolol*, glaucoma 162, 164*t*
*levocabastine*
  red eye 171*t*
  rhinitis 301, 303*t*, 304
*levodopa*
  Parkinson's disease 138, 139*t*, 141-45
  withdrawal 887
*levofloxacin*
  pneumonia 715*t*, 717*t*
  septic shock 742*t*, 744*t*
  UTI 763, 766*t*
*levonorgestrel*, contraception 574-75*t*, 576
*levothyroxine*
  goitre 637
  hypothyroidism 633, 635*t*, 636
  myxedema coma 636
  thyroid cancer 638
Levsin *see* hyoscyamine
Lewy body disease 25, 30
Licetrol *see* pyrethrins
lichen planus 545*t*
lichen simplex chronicus 545*t*
Lidex *see* fluocinonide
*lidocaine*
  acute pain 108
  mucositis 857*t*
  myocardial infarction 204*t*
  neuralgia 123
  ventricular tachycardia 256
*lindane*
  pediculosis 555*t*
  scabies 556*t*
Lioresal *see* baclofen
lipase inhibitors, obesity 831-32, 833*t*
Lipidil preparations *see* fenofibrate
Lipitor *see* atorvastatin
Liquifilm preparations *see* polyvinyl alcohol
Liquor Carbonis Detergens *see* coal tar and derivatives
*lisinopril*
  CHF 234*t*
  hypertension 183*t*
  myocardial infarction 211*t*
Lithane *see* lithium
*lithium*
  agitation 5
  behavioral problems 30
  depression 34*t*, 39
  headache in adults 87*t*, 89
  hyperthyroidism 631
liver capsular stretch 125
**liver diseases, chronic**
  **alcoholic liver disease 354, 356**
  **ascites 350-51, 357*t***
  **cholestatic disease 353-55, 358*t***
  **hemochromatosis 356, 359*t***
  **hepatic encephalopathy 352, 358*t***
  **hepatitis, autoimmune chronic active 354, 359*t***
  **spontaneous bacterial peritonitis 352, 357*t***
  **Wilson's disease 356, 360*t***
Livial *see* tibolone
Livostin *see* levocabastine
LMWH *see* heparins, low molecular weight
*lodoxamide*
  red eye 171*t*
  rhinitis 304
Loestrin 575*t*
Lomotil
  diarrhea 877*t*
  IBD 401
*lomustine*, adverse effects 844*t*, 857*t*
Loniten *see* minoxidil
loop diuretics
  CHF 236*t*-37*t*
  edema 661, 662*t*, 665
  hypercalcemia 669, 672
  hyperkalemia 679
*loperamide*
  diarrhea 877*t*, 880
  IBD 401
  IBS 411, 412*t*
  traveler's diarrhea 778, 780*t*
Lopid *see* gemfibrozil
Lopresor *see* metoprolol
*loratadine*
  pruritus 548*t*, 549
  rhinitis 304
*lorazepam*
  agitation 4-6
  alcohol withdrawal 67*t*
  anxiety disorders 10-11
  behavioral problems 30
  benzodiazepine withdrawal 72*t*
  insomnia 46-47, 48*t*
  myoclonus 131
  nausea and vomiting 847, 848*t*
  pruritus 550
  seizures 156*t*
*losartan*, hypertension 182, 183*t*
Losec *see* omeprazole
Lotensin *see* benazepril
Lotronex *see* alosetron
*lovastatin*, dyslipidemias 196*t*, 198*t*

Lovenox *see* enoxaparin
Loxapac *see* loxapine
*loxapine*
  agitation 4-5, 5*t*
  behavioral problems 29
  psychoses 55, 56*t*, 58
Lozide *see* indapamide
Ludiomil *see* maprotiline
Lugol's solution *see* iodine
lumbar radiculopathy 120-21
Lupron Depot *see* leuprolide
Luvox *see* fluvoxamine
Lyderm *see* fluocinonide
Lyofoam, pressure ulcers 526*t*
Lytren *see* oral rehydration therapy

# M

*magnesium*
  constipation 131
  headache in adults 88
  therapeutic supplement 824*t*
  ventricular tachycardia 256
*magnesium citrate*, constipation 870*t*
*magnesium hydroxide*, constipation 870*t*
*magnesium silicate*, as sunscreen 510
*magnesium sulfate*
  constipation 870*t*
  myocardial infarction 204*t*
**malaria prophylaxis 768-74**
Malarone, malaria prophylaxis 771*t*-72*t*, 773
malignant hyperthermia 887
malnutrition, with stroke 268
Manerix *see* moclobemide
mania 5
MAOIs *see* monoamine oxidase inhibitors
*maprotiline*
  depression 36*t*, 38
  neuralgia 121, 122*t*
Marinol *see* dronabinol
Marvelon 575*t*
mast cell stabilizers, red eye 171*t*
Mavik *see* trandolapril
Maxalt *see* rizatriptan
Maxeran *see* metoclopramide
Maxidex *see* dexamethasone
Maxipime *see* cefepime
*mazindol*, obesity 833*t*
*mechlorethamine*, adverse effects 844*t*, 853*t*
*meclizine*, nausea 865*t*
Medrol preparations *see* methylprednisolone
*medroxyprogesterone*
  contraception 570, 573*t*
  endometriosis 589*t*, 591, 593-94
  menopause 599*t*
  osteoporosis 481*t*
*mefenamic acid*, dysmenorrhea 581*t*
*mefloquine*, malaria prophylaxis 770, 771*t*, 774
**megaloblastic anemia 639, 642-43, 645*t***
*megestrol*, endometriosis 589*t*
Megral, headache in adults 84*t*
*melanin*, as sunscreen 510
*melatonin*, insomnia 50
Mellaril *see* thioridazine
*melphalan*, causing nausea and vomiting 844*t*
**meningitis**
  **bacterial 699-706**
  HIV-positive patients 803*t*
  viral 705*t*
**menopause 595-601**
*menthol*, pruritus 546
*menthyl anthranilate*, as sunscreen 511*t*
*meperidine*
  acute pain 106*t*, 107
  Bell's palsy 134
  headache in adults 83
  pain control in palliative care 128, 130*t*
Mepron *see* atovaquone
*mercaptopurine*
  adverse effects 844*t*, 857*t*
  IBD 398, 400*t*
Meridia *see* sibutramine
*meropenem*
  infections in cancer patients 815*t*
  pneumonia 716*t*
  septic shock 742*t*-43*t*
Merrem *see* meropenem
Mesasal *see* 5-aminosalicylic acid
M-Eslon preparations *see* morphine
*mesna*, antineoplastic side effects 858*t*
*mestranol*, contraception 575*t*
metalloproteinase inhibitors 471
Metamucil *see* psyllium
*metformin*, diabetes 619, 621*t*
*methadone*, opioid withdrawal 70, 71*t*
*methazolamide*, glaucoma 165*t*, 166
*methicillin*, pneumonia 715*t*
*methimazole*
  hyperthyroidism 631, 634*t*
  thyroid storm 632
*methocarbamol*, fibromyalgia 432*t*, 433
*methotrexate*
  adverse effects 823, 844*t*, 857*t*-58*t*
  asthma in adults 317
  cholestatic disease 353
  IBD 398, 400*t*
  in pregnancy 403
  polymyalgia rheumatica 442
  psoriasis 534*t*
  rheumatoid arthritis 459-61, 462*t*
*methotrimeprazine*, psychoses 56*t*

*methoxsalen*, psoriasis 532, 534*t*, 535
*methylbenzylidene camphor*, as sunscreen 511*t*
*methylcellulose*, red eye 171*t*
*methyldopa*, hypertension 183*t*, 184, 186*t*
*methylphenidate*
ADHD 18, 20, 21*t*
depression 40
*methylprednisolone*
acne 495*t*
dermatitis 540*t*
gout 446, 450*t*
IBD 399*t*
nausea and vomiting 845, 848*t*
osteoarthritis 473*t*
polymyalgia rheumatica 442
methylxanthines, asthma in children 323
*methysergide*
contraindicated in children 95
headache in adults 83, 87*t*, 88
*metoclopramide*
anorexia nervosa 838, 839*t*
GERD 376, 378*t*-79*t*
headache in adults 83
headache in children 94, 96*t*
nausea and vomiting 131, 845, 847, 849*t*, 850-51, 865*t*
persistent hiccoughs 899
*metolazone*
ascites 350, 357*t*
CHF 236*t*
edema 662*t*
hypertension 182, 183*t*
*metoprolol*
angina 218*t*, 224*t*
atrial fibrillation/flutter 242*t*, 244*t*
CHF 235, 238*t*
headache in adults 86*t*, 88
hypertension 183*t*, 185*t*
myocardial infarction 204*t*, 210*t*
SVT 250-51*t*
syncope 292*t*
Metrocream *see* metronidazole
Metrogel *see* metronidazole
*metronidazole*
cholestatic disease 353
hepatic encephalopathy 352, 358*t*
HIV-associated diarrhea 805
IBD 401
infections in cancer patients 812, 816*t*
in pregnancy 401, 754*t*
PID 757*t*
PUD 388-89, 389*t*
rosacea 503, 504*t*
septic shock 741*t*, 744*t*
skin infections 566*t*
traveler's diarrhea 778, 779*t*
trichomoniasis 754*t*
vaginosis 754*t*
Mevacor *see* lovastatin
*mexiletine*, ventricular tachycardia 260*t*
Mexitil *see* mexiletine
Mexoryl SX *see* terephthalylidene dicamphor sulfonic acid
Miacalcin *see* calcitonin
Micardis *see* telmisartan
Micatin *see* miconazole
Miconal *see* anthralin
*miconazole*
HIV-associated candidiasis 803*t*
vulvovaginal candidiasis 753*t*
Micro-K *see* potassium chloride
Micronor *see* norethindrone
Midamor *see* amiloride
*midazolam*, myoclonus 131
*midodrine*
hypotension, Parkinson's disease 143
orthostatic hypotension 293
postural orthostatic tachycardia syndrome 293
vasovagal syncope 291, 292*t*, 293
*mifepristone*, endometriosis 593
migraine *see* **headache**
Migranal preparations *see* dihydroergotamine
miliaria 545*t*
Milk of Magnesia *see* magnesium hydroxide
*milrinone*, CHF 239
mineralocorticoids, hypoaldosteronism 679
*mineral oil*
constipation 131, 869*t*
red eye 171*t*
minerals *see also specific mineral* 821-26
Minestrin 575*t*
Minipress *see* prazosin
Minitran *see* nitroglycerin
Minocin *see* minocycline
*minocycline*
acne 496, 497*t*
rheumatoid arthritis 465
rosacea 503, 504*t*
Min-Ovral 575*t*
*minoxidil*, hypertension 183*t*, 184, 187
Mirapex *see* pramipexole
Mireze *see* nedocromil
*mirtazapine*, depression 39
*misoprostol*
bone pain 131*t*
GI bleeding 459
NSAID-associated ulcers 390
osteoarthritis 471
PUD 387*t*
Mithracin *see* plicamycin
mithramycin *see* plicamycin

*mitomycin*, adverse effects 844*t*, 853*t*, 856*t*, 858*t*
*mitoxantrone*, causing nausea and vomiting 844*t*
MMI *see* methimazole
Mobiflex *see* tenoxicam
*moclobemide*
  anxiety disorders 11, 14*t*
  depression 37*t*, 38-39
  Parkinson's disease 144
Modecate *see* fluphenazine
Moditen *see* fluphenazine
Modulon *see* trimebutine
*mometasone*
  dermatitis 540*t*
  rhinitis 303*t*
Monistat *see* miconazole
Monitan *see* acebutolol
monoamine oxidase inhibitors
  anxiety disorders 10-11, 13*t*
  depression 35*t*, 38, 40
Monopril *see* fosinopril
*montelukast*
  asthma in adults 316*t*, 317
  asthma in children 325*t*, 326
mood stabilizers
  agitation 5
  depression 34*t*
*morphine*
  acute pain 106*t*, 107
  back pain 114, 115*t*
  Bell's palsy 134
  burns 519
  cough 896
  neuralgia 122*t*
  pain control in palliative care 127-28, 129*t*
Morphine HP *see* morphine
Morphitec *see* morphine
M.O.S. preparations *see* morphine
Motilium *see* domperidone
Motrin *see* ibuprofen
MS Contin *see* morphine
MS•IR *see* morphine
mucositis 857*t*
*mupirocin*
  burns 518*t*
  skin infections 563, 567*t*
Murocel *see* methylcellulose
**muscle cramps 78-79**
muscle relaxants
  back pain 114, 115*t*
  fibromyalgia 432*t*, 433
  hyperthermia 887
  incontinence 424
  septic shock 739
Myambutol *see* ethambutol
Mycifradin *see* neomycin
Myclo *see* clotrimazole
Mycobacterium avium complex 800*t*, 804t
Mycobutin *see* rifabutin
Mycostatin *see* nystatin
Mydfrin *see* phenylephrine
myelitis, HIV-positive patients 803*t*
myelodysplastic syndrome 859*t*
**myocardial infarction**
  **acute 202-5, 210*t*-12*t***
  pharmacoeconomic considerations 213-14
  prevention 174
Myochrysine *see* aurothiomalate
Mysoline *see* primidone
myxedema coma 636

## N

*nabilone*, nausea and vomiting 847, 848*t*
*nabumetone*, rheumatoid arthritis 457*t*
*nadolol*
  angina 218*t*, 244*t*
  headache in adults 86*t*, 88
  hypertension 183*t*
  myocardial infarction 210*t*
  orthostatic hypotension 293
*nadroparin*
  ischemic stroke prevention 178
  thrombosis 276, 277*t*
*nafarelin*, endometriosis 590*t*, 592
*nafcillin*, skin infections 560
nail changes 855*t*
Nalfon *see* fenoprofen
*nalidixic acid*, UTI 763
*naloxone*
  acute pain 108-9
  hypothermia 890
  septic shock 746
*naltrexone*
  alcohol withdrawal 65, 68*t*
  opioid withdrawal 70, 71*t*
*nandrolone*, osteoporosis 484
*naphazoline*, red eye 170-71*t*
Naphcon *see* naphazoline
Naphcon-A 171*t*
Naprosyn *see* naproxen
*naproxen*
  acute pain 103, 105*t*
  back pain 115*t*
  dysmenorrhea 581*t*
  endometriosis 588*t*
  gout 446-47, 449*t*
  headache in adults 84*t*
  headache in children 95, 96*t*, 99*t*, 100
  osteoarthritis 469
  pain control in palliative care 131*t*
  rheumatoid arthritis 458*t*
narcotics, adverse effects 862*t*
Nardil *see* phenelzine

Nasacort preparations *see* triamcinolone
Nasonex *see* mometasone
**nausea 861-66**
in pregnancy 923*t*
**nausea and vomiting, chemotherapy-induced 843-51**
*nazatriptan*
headache in adults 82-83, 85*t*, 91
headache in children 97*t*
Nebcin *see* tobramycin
necrotizing fasciitis 558, 560, 562
*nedocromil*
asthma in adults 316*t*, 317
asthma in children 325*t*, 326
red eye 171*t*
*nefazodone*
chronic fatigue syndrome 437*t*
depression 37*t*, 39
*nelfinavir*, HIV infection 795*t*
Neoloid see castor oil
Neo-Medrol Acne Lotion 495*t*
*neomycin*
acne 495*t*
hepatic encephalopathy 352, 358*t*
red eye 170*t*
skin infections 563, 567*t*
Neoral *see* cyclosporine
Neosporin 170*t*
Neovisc *see* hyaluronans
Neptazane *see* methazolamide
Nerisone *see* diflucortolone
*netilmicin*, UTI 766*t*, 766
Netromycin *see* netilmicin
**neuralgia 118-24**, 125
acute (herpes zoster) 119-20
chronic peripheral neuropathic pain 120-21, 123
postherpetic 121, 123
recurrent (trigeminal) 120
neuritis, HIV-positive patients 803*t*
neuroleptic malignant syndrome 59-60, 887
neuroleptics *see also* antipsychotics
ADHD 22*t*, 23
agitation 5*t*, 6
behavioral problems 29, 31
depression 34*t*
psychoses 55, 59*t*, 59
Neurontin *see* gabapentin
neuropathic pain *see* **neuralgia**
neuropathy, diabetic 121, 123
*nevirapine*, HIV infection 794*t*
NFV *see* nelfinavir
*niacin*, dyslipidemias 197*t*
*nicardipine*
angina 217
hypertension 183*t*
Nicoderm *see* nicotine
Nicorette preparations *see* nicotine
*nicotine*
smoking cessation 346, 347*t*, 348
withdrawal from 63
nicotinic acid *see* niacin
Nicotrol *see* nicotine
*nicoumalone*, ischemic stroke prevention 177*t*, 178
NidaGel *see* metronidazole
*nifedipine*
angina 217, 219*t*
atrial fibrillation/flutter 243
hypertension 183*t*, 184
persistent hiccoughs 899
Raynaud's phenomenon 287, 288*t*
Niferex *see* iron
*nimodipine*, persistent hiccoughs 899
nitrates
angina 217, 218*t*, 220, 223*t*, 226-27
causing syncope 289*t*
CHF 233, 235
myocardial infarction 204, 210*t*
*nitrazepam*
benzodiazepine withdrawal 72*t*
insomnia 47
Nitro-Dur *see* nitroglycerin
*nitrofurantoin*, UTI 762, 766*t*
*nitroglycerin*
angina 217, 218*t*, 223*t*
CHF 239
myocardial infarction 204*t*, 210*t*
Nitrol *see* nitroglycerin
Nitrolingual Spray *see* nitroglycerin
Nitrong SR *see* nitroglycerin
nitrosoureas, adverse effects 857*t*-58*t*
Nitrostat *see* nitroglycerin
*nitrous oxide*, acute pain 108
Nix preparations *see* permethrin
*nizatidine*
GERD 376, 377*t*
PUD 386*t*
Nizoral *see* ketoconazole
non-nucleoside reverse transcriptase inhibitors, HIV infection 794*t*
nonsteroidal anti-inflammatory drugs *see also* anti-inflammatory drugs
acute pain 103, 107
adverse effects 389-90, 509*t*, 664, 674*t*
back pain 114, 115*t*
burns 517
dysmenorrhea 580, 581*t*, 583
endometriosis 588*t*, 591
gout 446-47, 449*t*, 453
headache in children 93, 95, 99*t*
hypertension 189
myocardial infarction 206
neuralgia 120
orthostatic hypotension 293
osteoarthritis 470*t*, 471, 472*t*

pain control in palliative care 131*t*
postoperative, cataract 160
red eye 172*t*
rheumatoid arthritis 455-56, 457*t*-58*t*, 459
sports injuries 487
thrombosis 275
*norepinephrine*, septic shock 746
*norethindrone*
contraception 575*t*
menopause 599*t*
osteoporosis 481*t*
*norfloxacin*
peritonitis 357*t*
red eye 170*t*
spontaneous bacterial peritonitis 352
traveler's diarrhea 776, 778, 779*t*
UTI 763, 766*t*
Norgesic, headache in children 96*t*
*norgestimate*
acne 496, 498*t*
contraception 575*t*
*d-norgestrol*, contraception 575*t*
Norinyl 575*t*
Noritate *see* metronidazole
Normacol *see* sterculia gum
Noroxin *see* norfloxacin
Norpace preparations *see* disopyramide
Norplant *see* levonorgestrel
Norpramin *see* desipramine
*nortriptyline*
dementia 29
depression 36*t*, 38, 40
headache in adults 87*t*, 88
neuralgia 121, 122*t*
Norvasc *see* amlodipine
Norvir *see* ritonavir
Nova-T *see* intrauterine device
Novolin preparations *see* insulin
Nozinan *see* methotrimeprazine
NSAIDs *see* nonsteroidal anti-inflammatory drugs
N-Terface, pressure ulcers 526*t*
nucleoside reverse transcriptase inhibitors, HIV infection 793*t*
Nu-Gel, pressure ulcers 526*t*
**nutritional supplements, adults 821-26**
NVP *see* nevirapine
*nystatin*
HIV-associated candidiasis 803*t*
infections in cancer patients 812, 817*t*, 819
pregnancy 754*t*
vulvovaginal candidiasis 754*t*

# O

**obesity 827-35**
obsessive-compulsive disorder 8*t*, 11, 12-13*t*
*octocrylene*, as sunscreen 511*t*
*octreotide*
diarrhea 878*t*, 881
GI bleeding 394
orthostatic hypotension 294
*octyl salicylate*, as sunscreen 511*t*
Ocuclear *see* oxymetazoline
Ocufen *see* flurbiprofen
Ocuflox *see* ofloxacin
ocular lubricants, red eye 171*t*
oculomotor palsies 858*t*
odynophagia, HIV-positive patients 799
Oesclim *see* estradiol
Oestrilin *see* estrone
*ofloxacin*
chlamydial infection 756*t*
gonococcal infection 755*t*
PID 757*t*
pregnancy 756*t*
red eye 170*t*
tuberculosis 727*t*
UTI 763, 766*t*
Ogen *see* estropipate
oil retention enemas, constipation 131
*olanzapine*
agitation 4
Parkinson's disease 144
psychoses 55, 57*t*, 58-59, 61-62
*olopatadine*, red eye 171*t*
*olsalazine*, IBD 397, 399*t*
*omeprazole*
GERD 378*t*, 379-80
GI bleeding 393
osteoarthritis 471
PUD 386*t*
*ondansetron*, nausea and vomiting 847, 849*t*, 850-51
Opcon-A 171*t*
Ophtrivin-A 171*t*
opioids
acute pain 102-3, 105*t*-6*t*, 107-9
adverse effects 862*t*
aggravating pruritus 545
back pain 114, 115*t*
causing headache 89
cough 894
diarrhea 877*t*-78*t*, 880
headache in adults 84*t*
herpes zoster 120
IBD 397, 401
neuralgia 118, 121, 122*t*, 123-24
pain control in palliative care 127-28, 131*t*
withdrawal from 66*t*, 70, 71*t*
*opium*, diarrhea 878*t*
OpSite, pressure ulcers 526*t*
Opticrom *see* sodium cromoglycate
Optimine *see* azatadine
oral rehydration therapy 653, 656, 879

Oramorph SR *see* morphine
Orap *see* pimozide
Orbenin *see* cloxacillin
*orciprenaline*, asthma in adults 314, 315*t*
Orinase *see* tolbutamide
*orlistat*
 adverse effects 823
 obesity 831, 833*t*
Ornade 310*t*
*orphenadrine*
 back pain 115*t*
 headache in children 96*t*
ORT *see* oral rehydration therapy
Ortho Diaphragm Coil 571*t*
Ortho preparations
 contraception 575*t*
 menopause 598*t*
orthostatic hypotension 293
Orudis *see* ketoprofen
Ostac *see* clodronate
**osteoarthritis 467-75**
**osteomyelitis, acute 729-36**
osteopenia 478
**osteoporosis 476-86**
 pharmacoeconomic considerations 485-86
Ostoforte *see* vitamin D
**otitis media, acute, in children 684-93**
Otrivin *see* xylometazoline
Ovral 575*t*
*oxaprozin*, rheumatoid arthritis 458*t*
*oxazepam*
 behavioral problems 30
 benzodiazepine withdrawal 72*t*
 insomnia 47, 48*t*
Oxeze *see* formoterol
*oxprenolol*, hypertension 183*t*
Oxsoralen *see* methoxsalen
*oxtriphylline*, asthma in adults 314, 315*t*
*oxybenzone*, as sunscreen 511*t*
*oxybutynin*, incontinence and enuresis 427*t*-28*t*
*oxycodone*
 acute pain 107
 neuralgia 122*t*
OxyContin *see* oxycodone
oxygen, COPD 336
*oxymetazoline*
 red eye 170*t*
 rhinitis 309*t*

# P

PABA esters *see* para-aminobenzoic acid esters
pacemakers
 atrial fibrillation/flutter 248-49
 CHF 238
*paclitaxel*, adverse effects 844*t*, 853*t*
*padimate O*, as sunscreen 511*t*
**pain** *see* also **headache**
 **acute 101-9**
 **back 110-17**
 bone 125
 **in palliative care 125-32**
 menstrual *see* **dysmenorrhea**
 muscular *see* **fibromyalgia**
 **neuropathic 118-24**, 125
 sports injuries 488*t*-90*t*
Palafer *see* iron
Paludrine *see* proguanil
*pamidronate*, hypercalcemia 670*t*, 672
Panectyl *see* trimeprazine tartrate
panic disorder 8*t*, 10, 12-13*t*
 with agoraphobia 10, 12-13*t*
PanOxyl *see* benzoyl peroxide
Pantoloc *see* pantoprazole
*pantoprazole*
 GERD 378*t*
 GI bleeding 393
 PUD 387*t*
para-aminobenzoic acid esters, as sunscreen 511*t*
Para preparations *see* pyrethrins
parkinsonism 60, 61*t*
**Parkinson's disease 137-46**
Parlodel *see* bromocriptine
Parnate *see* tranylcypromine
*paroxetine*
 anxiety disorders 10, 13*t*
 depression 35*t*
 syncope 292*t*
Parsitan *see* ethopropazine
Parsol 1789, as sunscreen 511*t*
Patanol *see* olopatadine
patellofemoral syndrome 488*t*
Paxil *see* paroxetine
PCE *see* erythromycin
PCP *see* phencyclidine
Pedialyte *see* oral rehydration therapy
Pediatric Electrolyte *see* oral rehydration therapy
Pediazole, otitis media 691*t*
**pediculosis 552-57**
pelvic inflammatory disease 750, 757*t*, 757
*pemoline*, ADHD 18, 20, 21*t*
*penciclovir*, herpesvirus infections 783, 784*t*
*penicillamine*
 rheumatoid arthritis 461
 Wilson's disease 356, 360*t*
*penicillin*
 acute osteomyelitis 733*t*, 735*t*
 bacterial meningitis 702-3*t*
 causing hypokalemia 674*t*
 otitis media 687
 pneumonia 715*t*-16*t*

septic shock 741*t*
skin infections 560-61, 563, 564*t*, 568
streptococcal sore throat 695, 696*t*, 698
syphilis 759*t*
UTI 762-63
Pentacarinat *see* pentamidine
*pentamidine*
causing hyperkalemia 674*t*
HIV-associated infections 800*t*, 804*t*, 807*t*
infections in cancer patients 819
Pentamycetin *see* chloramphenicol
Pentasa *see* 5-aminosalicylic acid
*pentastarch*, hypovolemia 657
*pentazocine*, acute pain 107
*pentoxifylline*
claudication 283-84
dementia 30
septic shock 746
Pen-Vee *see* penicillin
Pepcid *see* famotidine
**peptic ulcer disease 382-90**
Pepto-Bismol *see* bismuth subsalicylate
Percocet *see* oxycodone
Percodan *see* oxycodone
*pergolide*
cocaine withdrawal 71*t*
Parkinson's disease 139*t*, 141
Periactin *see* cyproheptadine
pericarditis 206
*perindopril*, hypertension 183*t*
**peritonitis, spontaneous bacterial 352, 357*t***
peritonsillar abscess 339
Permax *see* pergolide
*permethrin*
pediculosis 554, 555*t*
scabies 545*t*, 554, 556*t*
*perphenazine*
agitation 4
nausea and vomiting 845, 849*t*, 865*t*
psychoses 56*t*
*petrolatum*
as sunscreen 510
red eye 171*t*
$PGI_2$ analogues, Raynaud's phenomenon 287
phantom limb pain 121, 123
**pharmacoeconomic considerations 925-28**
acute stroke 271
allergic rhinitis 301, 304
angina pectoris 227-28
asthma in adults 319
benign prostatic hyperplasia 420
chemotherapy-induced nausea and vomiting 850-51
dementia 31-32
depression 41
diabetes mellitus 627-28
dyslipidemias 199-200
GERD 380
headache 90-91
hypertension 190
myocardial infarction 213-14
osteoporosis 485-86
postmyocardial infarction 213-14
psychoses 61-62
thrombosis 279-80
*phencyclidine*, causing agitation 6
*phenelzine*
anxiety disorders 10-11, 13*t*
bulimia nervosa 840, 841*t*
depression 35*t*, 38
Phenergan *see* promethazine
*pheniramine*, red eye 171*t*
phenobarbital, seizures 149, 151*t*, 153*t*, 156*t*, 157
phenothiazines
adverse effects 887
headache in adults 83
nausea and vomiting 845, 849*t*
pruritus 547*t*
psychoses 60
*phentermine*, obesity 830, 833*t*
*phenylephrine*
postoperative, cataract 160
red eye 170*t*
*phenylpropanolamine*
incontinence 424, 427*t*
obesity 830
rhinitis 304, 310*t*
*phenytoin*
alcohol withdrawal 68*t*
headache in adults 89
neuralgia 122*t*
seizures 149, 151*t*, 153*t*, 156*t*, 157
trigeminal neuralgia 120
phobia 8*t*, 10-11, 12-14*t*
phosphate enemas, constipation 131
phosphates, hypercalcemia 669
Phospholine Iodide *see* echothiophate
phototherapy
dermatitis 541
pruritus 550
psoriasis 532, 535-36
phototoxic reactions 509*t*
Phyllocontin *see* aminophylline
PID *see* pelvic inflammatory disease
*pilocarpine*, glaucoma 164*t*, 166
Pilopine HS *see* pilocarpine
*pimozide*, psychoses 56*t*, 59
*pinaverium*, IBS 411, 412*t*
*pindolol*
behavioral problems 30
depression 40
hypertension 183*t*

*pioglitazone*, diabetes 621*t*, 622
*piperacillin*
infections in cancer patients 815*t*
pneumonia 716*t*
septic shock 742-43*t*
UTI 766*t*
*piperacillin-tazobactam*
infections in cancer patients 815*t*
pneumonia 716*t*
septic shock 742-43*t*
*piperonyl butoxide*
pediculosis 555*t*
scabies 556*t*
Piportil *see* pipotiazine
*pipotiazine*, psychoses 59*t*
Pipracil *see* piperacillin
*piroxicam*
dysmenorrhea 582*t*
rheumatoid arthritis 458*t*
*pivampicillin*, otitis media 688*t*
*pivmecillinam* 763, UTI 766*t*
pizotifen *see* pizotyline
*pizotyline*
headache in adults 87*t*, 88
headache in children 95, 98*t*, 100
Plan B *see* levonorgestrel
plantar fasciitis 491*t*
Plaquenil *see* hydroxychloroquine
Plavix *see* clopidogrel
Plendil *see* felodipine
*plicamycin*
adverse effects 853*t*, 857*t*
hypercalcemia 671*t*, 672
PMS Phosphates *see* sodium phosphates
Pneumocystis carinii 800*t*, 804*t*
**pneumonia**
aspiration 268
**community-acquired 711-18**
HIV-positive patients 799, 800*t*, 801, 804*t*
pneumonitis 803*t*
Pneumovax, HIV-associated infections 800*t*
Polaramine *see* dexchlorpheniramine
*polidocanol*, gastrointestinal bleeding 393
Polycidin 170*t*
Polycitra-K *see* potassium citrate
*polyethylene glycol*, red eye 171*t*
**polymyalgia rheumatica 439-43**
*polymyxin B*
red eye 170*t*
skin infections 563, 567*t*
*polysorbate*, red eye 171*t*
Polysporin
postoperative, cataract 160
red eye 170*t*
Polytrim *see* polymyxin B
*polyvinyl alcohol*, red eye 171*t*
Pondocillin *see* pivampicillin
Ponstan *see* mefenamic acid
portal hypertension *see* **ascites**
**postmyocardial infarction 205-14**
pharmacoeconomic considerations 213-14
post-traumatic stress disorder 8*t*, 11, 12-13*t*
postural orthostatic tachycardia syndrome 293
*potassium*
causing hyperkalemia 674*t*
dehydration in children 653*t*
edema 661
hypovolemia 658
*potassium bicarbonate*, hypokalemia 680, 681*t*
*potassium chloride*, hypokalemia 680, 681*t*
*potassium citrate*, hypokalemia 680, 681*t*
**potassium disturbances 674-83**
hyperkalemia 674*t*, 675-79
hypokalemia 674*t*, 679-83, 681*t*, 682-83
*potassium gluconate*, hypokalemia 681*t*
*potassium phosphate*, hypokalemia 682
potassium-sparing diuretics
CHF 237*t*
edema 661, 663*t*, 664-65
hypokalemia 682-83
*povidone-iodine*
burns 518*t*
skin infections 559
PPI *see* proton pump inhibitors
*pramipexole*, Parkinson's disease 139*t*, 141-42
Pramox *see* pramoxine
*pramoxine*, pruritus 546
Prandase *see* acarbose
Pravachol *see* pravastatin
*pravastatin*, dyslipidemias 196*t*, 198*t*
*prazosin*
hypertension 183*t*, 184
Raynaud's phenomenon 287, 288*t*
Pred *see* prednisolone
*prednisolone*
postoperative, cataract 160
red eye 172*t*
*prednisone*
Bell's palsy 134-35, 136*t*
COPD 332, 335*t*, 336
Crohn's disease 401, 403
gout 446, 450*t*
hepatitis, autoimmune chronic active 354, 359*t*
hypercalcemia 669, 672
IBD 397-98, 399*t*
pneumonia 804*t*
polymyalgia rheumatica 441-42

rheumatoid arthritis 461
ulcerative colitis 406
ulcerative proctitis 406
Prefrin *see* phenylephrine
pregnancy
allergy 921*t*
anemia 641*t*, 643
anticoagulants 278, 921*t*
antiepileptics 155, 922*t*
antihistamines 549, 921*t*
anxiety 921*t*
asthma 317-18
atovaquone 773
azithromycin 756*t*
bacterial infections 921*t*
bipolar affective disorder 921*t*
ceftriaxone 755*t*
ciprofloxacin 755*t*
clindamycin 754*t*
clotrimazole 753*t*, 923*t*
constipation 921*t*
cough 922*t*
depression 922*t*
diabetes 614, 623-27, 922*t*
diuretics 661
doxycycline 755*t*, 774
**drug exposure 916-24**
dyslipidemias 194*t*, 195
dyspepsia 922*t*
edema 659
erythromycin 756*t*
fever 922*t*
fluconazole 753*t*
gestational diabetes 612, 614
heparins, low molecular weight 278, 922*t*
herpetic infections 922*t*
HIV infection 792
hypertension 186*t*
hyperthyroidism 923*t*
isotretinoin 499
malaria prophylaxis 774
mefloquine 773
methotrexate 403
metronidazole 401, 754*t*
migraine 923*t*
nausea and vomiting 923*t*
nystatin 754*t*
ofloxacin 756*t*
pain 922*t*
pruritic urticarial papules 545*t*
psychoses 58
purine antimetabolites 403
pyrazinamide 727-28
quinolones 763
schizophrenia 923*t*
sexually transmitted diseases 753*t*-56*t*, 759*t*
spectinomycin 755*t*
terconazole 753*t*
tetracycline 496
thrombosis 278
tuberculosis 727-28
vaginal candidiasis 923*t*
vitamin and mineral requirements 821*t*, 822, 825
Premarin *see* estrogens
Prepulsid *see* cisapride
pressor amines *see* alpha agonists
**pressure ulcers 520-29**
Prevacid *see* lansoprazole
Preven 574*t*
priapism 605-6, 608
*prilocaine*, acute pain 108
*primaquine*
malaria prophylaxis 770, 772*t*, 773
pneumocystis carinii 804*t*
primary hyperparathyroidism 669
Primaxin *see* imipenem-cilastatin
*primidone*, seizures 151*t*, 153*t*, 157
Prinivil *see* lisinopril
*probenecid*
gout 451*t*, 452
HIV-associated infections 803*t*
PID 757*t*
*procainamide*
arrhythmias 238
atrial fibrillation/flutter 242*t*, 246*t*, 249, 250*t*
myocardial infarction 205
ventricular tachycardia 256, 259*t*
*procaine*, acute pain 108
Procan SR *see* procainamide
*procarbazine*, causing nausea and vomiting 844*t*
*prochlorperazine*
headache in adults 83
headache in children 94, 96*t*
nausea and vomiting 845, 849*t*, 865*t*
**proctitis, ulcerative 406-7**
*procyclidine*, Parkinson's disease 61*t*, 140*t*
Prodiem preparations *see* psyllium
*progesterone*, osteoporosis 479, 481*t*, 485
progestins
causing nausea and vomiting 844*t*
contraception 569, 575*t*, 576-77
endometriosis 589*t*, 591
menopause 596, 599*t*
osteoporosis 481*t*
*proguanil*, malaria prophylaxis 770, 771*t*-72*t*, 773
prokinetic agents
anorexia nervosa 838, 839*t*
GERD 376, 378*t*
Prolopa, Parkinson's disease 138, 139*t*
*promethazine*

nausea 864*t*
pruritus 547*t*
Prometrium *see* progesterone
Pronestyl preparations *see* procainamide
Pronto Lice Killing Shampoo Kit *see* pyrethrins
Propaderm *see* beclomethasone
*propafenone*
arrhythmias 238
atrial fibrillation/flutter 247*t*
myocardial infarction 205
SVT 251*t*
ventricular tachycardia 260*t*
Propine *see* dipivefrin
*propofol*
nausea and vomiting 850
seizures 156*t*
*propoxyphene*, acute pain 107
*propranolol*
akathisia 59-60, 61*t*
angina 218*t*
anxiety disorders 11, 14*t*
atrial fibrillation/flutter 242*t*, 244*t*
headache in adults 86*t*, 88-90
headache in children 93, 98*t*, 100
hypertension 183*t*
hyperthyroidism 631, 635*t*
myocardial infarction 210*t*
orthostatic hypotension 293
SVT 251*t*
thyroid storm 632
*propylthiouracil*
alcoholic liver disease 354
hyperthyroidism 631, 634*t*
thyroid storm 632
Propyl-Thyracil *see* propylthiouracil
Proscar *see* finasteride
prostaglandin analogs, glaucoma 163, 165*t*, 166
prostaglandin $E_1$ *see* alprostadil
**prostatic hyperplasia, benign 414-20**
pharmacoeconomic considerations 420
prostatitis 765*t*, 767*t*
protease inhibitors, HIV infection 794*t*-95*t*
Protectaid Sponge 571*t*
proton pump inhibitors
GERD 376, 378-79*t*, 379
GI bleeding 393-94, 459
NSAID-associated ulcers 390
PUD 384-85, 386*t*-87*t*, 388-89, 389*t*
septic shock 740
*protriptyline*, depression 36*t*, 38
Provera *see* medroxyprogesterone
Proviodine *see* povidone-iodine
Prozac *see* fluoxetine
prurigo nodularis, pruritus 545*t*
**pruritus 543-51**
cholestatic 354, 358
*pseudoephedrine*
cough 894
rhinitis 300, 302*t*, 309*t*-10*t*
psoralens
phototoxic reactions 509*t*
psoriasis 532
**psoriasis 530-37**
**psychoses 52-62**
pharmacoeconomic considerations 61-62
psychostimulants, causing agitation 2
*psyllium*
constipation 869*t*
diarrhea 877*t*, 879-80
IBS 411, 412*t*
PTU *see* propylthiouracil
PUD *see* **peptic ulcer disease**
Pulmicort *see* budesonide
purine antimetabolites
in pregnancy 403
ulcerative colitis 406
Purinethol *see* 6-mercaptopurine
PVF K *see* penicillin
pyelonephritis 764*t*, 767*t*, 767
*pyrazinamide*
HIV-associated infections 800*t*
in pregnancy 727-28
tuberculosis 725*t*, 727*t*, 727
pyrethrins, pediculosis 555*t*
*pyridoxine*
deficiency 823
HIV-associated infections 800*t*
tuberculosis 728
Wilson's disease 356
*pyrimethamine*
HIV-associated infections 800*t*, 804*t*, 808*t*
malaria prophylaxis 772*t*, 773


# Q


Questran preparations *see* cholestyramine
*quetiapine*, Parkinson's disease 144
Quibron-T/SR *see* theophylline
*quinapril*
CHF 234*t*
hypertension 183*t*
myocardial infarction 211*t*
*quinidine*
arrhythmias 238
atrial fibrillation/flutter 246*t*
myocardial infarction 205
ventricular tachycardia 259*t*
*quinine sulfate*, muscle cramps 79
quinolones
COPD 336
skin infections 561
Quintasa *see* 5-aminosalicylic acid
Qvar *see* beclomethasone

## R


R & C *see* pyrethrins
radioactive iodine *see* iodine (radioactive)
radioactive yttrium-90, osteoarthritis 474
Rafton *see* alginates
*ralitrexed*, causing nausea and vomiting 844*t*
*raloxifene*, osteoporosis 482*t*, 483-86
*ramipril*
  CHF 234*t*
  hypertension 183*t*
  myocardial infarction 211*t*
*ranitidine*
  GERD 376, 377*t*, 380
  PUD 386*t*, 388-89, 389*t*
rapid tumor lysis syndrome 852, 854*t*
**Raynaud's phenomenon 285-88**, 859*t*
Reactine *see* cetirizine
Reality (female condom) 571*t*
Rebetron 370*t*
*reboxetine*, depression 39
recombinant tissue plasminogen activator *see* alteplase
Recombivax HB *see* hepatitis B vaccine
**red eye 168-73**
*red veterinary petrolatum*, as sunscreen 510
Refresh *see* polyvinyl alcohol
Reglan *see* metoclopramide
rehydration therapy
  intravenous 656-58
  oral 653, 656, 879
Relafen *see* nabumetone
Remicade *see* infliximab
**renal impairment**
  acute 740
  **dosage adjustment 901-15**
Renedil *see* felodipine
*repaglinide*, diabetes 620*t*, 622
Requip *see* ropinirole
Rescriptor *see* delavirdine
*reserpine*, hypertension 183*t*, 184
resins, dyslipidemias 195, 196*t*
*resorcinol*, acne 495
respiratory distress syndrome, acute 739
Restore, pressure ulcers 526*t*
Restoril *see* temazepam
*reteplase*, myocardial infarction 212*t*
Retavase *see* reteplase
Retin-A *see* tretinoin
retinitis 803*t*
retinoids
  acne 495*t*, 495, 497*t*, 499
  adverse effects 509*t*
  psoriasis 532
retinol *see* vitamin A
Retisol-A *see* tretinoin
retropharyngeal abscess 339
Retrovir *see* zidovudine
reversible inhibitors of monoamine oxidase-A
  anxiety disorders 14*t*
  depression 38-40
**rheumatoid arthritis 454-66**
Rheumatrex *see* methotrexate
Rhinalar *see* flunisolide
**rhinitis**
  **allergic 298-305**
  pharmacoeconomic considerations 301, 304
  **viral 306-11**
rhinitis medicamentosa 302*t*
Rhinocort preparations *see* budesonide
Rhodis *see* ketoprofen
*ribavirin*, hepatitis C 370*t*, 371-72
*riboflavin*, headache in adults 88
*rifabutin*, HIV-associated infections 800*t*, 804*t*, 808*t*
Rifadin *see* rifampin
*rifampin*
  bacterial meningitis 701, 705
  HIV-associated infections 800*t*, 804*t*
  pneumonia 717*t*
  pruritus 354
  streptococcal sore throat 698
  tuberculosis 724*t*, 727*t*, 727-28
*rimexolone*
  postoperative, cataract 160
  red eye 172*t*
*risedronate*, osteoporosis 481*t*, 483, 485
Risperdal *see* risperidone
*risperidone*
  agitation 4
  dementia 28*t*, 29
  psychoses 55, 57*t*, 58-59, 61-62
Ritalin preparations *see* methylphenidate
*ritonavir*, HIV infection 795*t*
*rituximab*, adverse effects 843*t*
*rivastigmine*, dementia 27, 28*t*
Rivotril *see* clonazepam
*rizatriptan*
  headache in adults 82-83, 85*t*, 91
  headache in children 97*t*
Robaxacet 432*t*
Robaxisal 432*t*
Rocaltrol *see* calcitriol
Rocephin *see* ceftriaxone
Rofact *see* rifampin
*rofecoxib*
  dysmenorrhea 582*t*
  osteoarthritis 471, 472*t*
Roferon-A *see* interferon alfa
*ropinirole*, Parkinson's disease 139*t*, 141-42
**rosacea 501-6**
*rosiglitazone*, diabetes 621*t*, 622
Roychlor *see* potassium chloride

rt-PA *see* alteplase
RTV *see* ritonavir
Rubramin *see* vitamin $B_{12}$
Rythmodan preparations *see* disopyramide
Rythmol *see* propafenone

# S

Sabril *see* vigabatrin
SalAc *see* salicylic acid
Salazopyrin *see* sulfasalazine
*salbutamol*
- asthma in adults 314, 315*t*
- asthma in children 322, 324*t*
- COPD 331, 333*t*-34*t*
- hyperkalemia 677*t*, 678

salicylates, as sunscreen 511*t*
salicylates, nonacetylated, osteoarthritis 470*t*, 471, 472*t*
*salicylic acid*
- acne 495*t*, 495
- psoriasis 530

*saline*
- burns 516
- hyperkalemia 677*t*
- hypovolemia 656-57
- osteoarthritis 474
- pressure ulcers 524
- seizures 156*t*

*salmeterol*
- asthma in adults 314, 315*t*
- asthma in children 322, 324*t*
- COPD 333*t*

*salmon calcitonin*
- hypercalcemia 670*t*
- osteoporosis 482*t*, 484, 486

Salofalk *see* 5-aminosalicylic acid
*salsalate*
- osteoarthritis 471, 472*t*
- rheumatoid arthritis 458*t*, 459

Sandimmune *see* cyclosporine
Sandomigran *see* pizotyline
Sandostatin *see* octreotide
Sans-Acne *see* erythromycin
Sansert *see* methysergide
*saquinavir*, HIV infection 794*t*
Sarna-P *see* pramoxine
*saw palmetto*, prostatic hyperplasia 416
Scabene *see* esdepallethrin
**scabies** 545*t*, 551, **552-57**
schizophrenia 4-5, 52, 55, 58, 60
sclerosing agents
- esophageal varices 393
- GI bleeding 393

*scopolamine*, nausea and vomiting 131, 850, 864*t*
Sectral *see* acebutolol
**seizures** 60, **147-57**
Select 575*t*
selective estrogen receptor modulators 482*t*, 483
selective serotonin reuptake inhibitors
- ADHD 23
- adverse effects 862*t*
- anxiety disorders 10-11, 13*t*
- chronic fatigue syndrome 437*t*
- dementia 29
- depression 34*t*, 34, 35*t*, 38-41
- headache in adults 87*t*, 88
- headache in children 95, 98*t*
- nausea and vomiting 847, 849*t*, 850-51
- neuralgia 123
- Parkinson's disease 144
- Raynaud's phenomenon 287
- vasovagal syncope 293

*selegiline*
- dementia 29
- Parkinson's disease 140*t*, 142-43

*senna*, constipation 870*t*
*sennosides*, constipation 131
Senokot *see* senna
sepsis syndrome 737*t*, 741-42*t*
**septic shock 737-47**
Septra *see* co-trimoxazole
Serax *see* oxazepam
Serevent *see* salmeterol
Seromycin *see* cycloserine
Serophene *see* clomiphene
Seroquel *see* quetiapine
serotonin-norepinephrine reuptake inhibitors
- anxiety 13*t*
- depression 39-40

serotonin antagonists *see* selective serotonin reuptake inhibitors
*sertraline*
- anxiety disorders 10, 13*t*
- chronic fatigue syndrome 437*t*
- depression 35*t*
- obesity 833*t*

Serzone *see* nefazodone
**sexual dysfunction**
- men **602-8**
- women **608-11**

**sexually transmitted diseases 748-61**
- *see also* **hepatitis B; HIV infection**
- cervicitis 749-51, 755*t*-56*t*
- epididymo-orchitis 750, 752
- genital herpes 758-59
- genital ulcers 758
- genital warts 750-51, 760
- HIV-positive patients 800*t*
- pelvic inflammatory disease 750, 757*t*, 757
- syphilis 750, 758-59, 759*t*
- trichomoniasis 751, 754*t*

urethritis 749-50, 752, 755*t*-56*t*
vaginitis 749*t*, 749, 751, 753*t*-54*t*
vaginosis 749*t*, 753*t*-54*t*
vulvovaginal candidiasis 749, 751, 753*t*
shingles *see* herpes zoster, acute
shin splints 489*t*
Sibelium *see* flunarizine
*sibutramine*, obesity 832, 833*t*
*sildenafil*, erectile dysfunction 143, 606, 607*t*
*silver sulfadiazine*
burns 518*t*
skin infections 563, 567*t*
*simvastatin*, dyslipidemias 196t, 198*t*, 199-200
Sinemet preparations, Parkinson's disease 138, 139*t*, 141
Sinequan *see* doxepin
**single thyroid nodule 637-38**
Singulair *see* montelukast
Sintrom *see* nicoumalone
**skin infections, bacterial 558-68**
Slo-Bid *see* theophylline
Slow-K *see* potassium chloride
**smoking cessation 343-49**
social phobia 8*t*, 10-11
*sodium*
dehydration in children 653*t*
hypercalcemia 668
hypovolemia 657*t*, 657
psychoses 60
*sodium bicarbonate*
hyperkalemia 677*t*, 678
pruritus 545
*sodium chloride*
postural orthostatic tachycardia syndrome 293
syncope 292*t*
*sodium cromoglycate*
asthma in adults 316*t*, 317
asthma in children 323, 325*t*, 326
cough 896
red eye 171*t*
rhinitis 301, 302*t*, 304
*sodium hyaluronate*, red eye 171*t*
*sodium ipodate*, hyperthyroidism 631
*sodium phosphates*, constipation 870*t*
*sodium polystyrene sulfonate resin*, hyperkalemia 677*t*, 678-79
Sodium Sulamyd *see* sulfacetamide
*sodium tetradecyl sulfate*, esophageal varices 393
sodium valproate *see* valproic acid
Soframycin *see* framycetin
Sofra-tulle *see* framycetin
Solganol *see* aurothioglucose
Solu-Cortef *see* hydrocortisone
Solu-Medrol *see* methylprednisolone
*somatostatin*, diarrhea 878*t*, 881
*sorbitol*, red eye 171*t*
Sorbsan, pressure ulcers 526*t*
Soriatane *see* acitretin
Sotacor *see* sotalol
*sotalol*
atrial fibrillation/flutter 247*t*
CHF 232, 238
SVT 251*t*
ventricular tachycardia 260*t*
**spasticity 74-78**
*spectinomycin*
gonococcal infection 755*t*
in pregnancy 755*t*
spermicides 572*t*, 576
*spironolactone*
acne 499
ascites 350, 357*t*
CHF 235, 237*t*
edema 663*t*, 664
hypokalemia 682*t*, 682
sponge, contraceptive 571*t*
**spontaneous bacterial peritonitis 352, 357*t***
Sporanox *see* itraconazole
**sports injuries 487-92**
sprains 487, 488*t*-89*t*
SSD *see* silver sulfadiazine
SSRIs *see* selective serotonin reuptake inhibitors
staphylococcal scalded skin syndrome 558
Starnoc *see* zaleplon
Statex *see* morphine
Staticin *see* erythromycin
status epilepticus 155-56
*stavudine*, HIV infection 793*t*
Stelazine *see* trifluoperazine
Stemetil *see* prochlorperazine
*sterculia gum*, constipation 869*t*
steroids *see also* corticosteroids
acne 499-500
osteoporosis 484
red eye 172*t*, 173
rhinitis 301, 304
StieVa-A *see* tretinoin
Stievamycin 495*t*
stimulant laxatives, constipation 131
stimulants, ADHD 18, 20, 21*t*
stool softeners, constipation 131, 871*t*
strains 487
Streptase *see* streptokinase
**streptococcal sore throat 694-98**
*streptokinase*
myocardial infarction 204*t*, 212*t*, 213-14
thrombosis 278
*streptomycin*, tuberculosis 725*t*, 727*t*, 727

*streptozocin*, adverse effects 844*t*, 853*t*, 857*t*
stress fracture, tibia/fibula 489*t*-90*t*
**stress incontinence 422-24, 427*t***
**stroke, acute 263-72**
pharmacoeconomic considerations 271
**stroke, ischemic**
**prevention 174-79**, 859*t*
*sucralfate*
PUD 387*t*
septic shock 740
Sudafed *see* pseudoephedrine
Sulcrate *see* sucralfate
*sulfacetamide*, red eye 170*t*, 172*t*
*sulfadiazine*, HIV-associated infection 804*t*, 808*t*
*sulfadoxine*, malaria prophylaxis 772*t*, 773
*sulfasalazine*
Crohn's disease 403
IBD 397, 399*t*
rheumatoid arthritis 461, 463*t*
ulcerative colitis 405
*sulfinpyrazone*, gout 451*t*, 452
*sulfisoxazole*, otitis media 691*t*
sulfonamides, glaucoma 166
sulfonylureas
adverse effects 509*t*
diabetes 619, 620*t*
*sulfur*
acne 495
scabies 556*t*
*sulindac*
acute pain 103
rheumatoid arthritis 458*t*
*sumatriptan*
headache in adults 82-83, 85*t*
headache in children 97*t*
**sunburn 507-12**
sunscreens 508-10, 511*t*, 512
Suplasyn *see* hyaluronans
supraglottitis 338-39, 341*t*
Suprax *see* cefixime
Surfak *see* docusate salts
Surgam *see* tiaprofenic acid
Surmontil *see* trimipramine
Sustiva *see* efavirenz
SVT *see* **tachycardia, supraventricular**
Symmetrel *see* amantadine
sympatholytics, hypertension 184
sympathomimetics
causing agitation 2
cough 894
Synalar *see* fluocinolone
Synarel *see* nafarelin
**syncope 289-94**
Synphasic 575*t*
Synthroid *see* levothyroxine
Synvisc *see* hyaluronans
syphilis 750, 758-59, 759*t*
Syprine *see* trientine

# T

$T_4$ *see* levothyroxine
**tachyarrhythmias**
**ventricular fibrillation 253-56, 258-62**
**ventricular tachycardia 253-62**
**tachycardia**
**supraventricular 241-52**
**ventricular 253-62**
*tacrolimus*, dermatitis 541
Tagamet *see* cimetidine
talc
as sunscreen 510
heat rash 545*t*
Tambocor *see* flecainide
*tamoxifen*, causing nausea and vomiting 844*t*
*tamsulosin*, prostatic hyperplasia 416, 418*t*, 419
Tapazole *see* methimazole
tar *see* coal tar and derivatives
tardive dyskinesia 59
Tasmar *see* tolcapone
Tavist *see* clemastine fumarate
*tazarotene*
acne 495*t*
psoriasis 532, 533*t*, 535
Tazidime *see* ceftazidime
Tazocin *see* piperacillin-tazobactam
Tazorac *see* tazarotene
Tear-Gel 171*t*
Tears Encore *see* polysorbate
Tebrazid *see* pyrazinamide
Tegaderm
burns 517
pressure ulcers 526*t*
*tegaserod*, IBS 411
Tegopen *see* cloxacillin
Tegretol preparations *see* carbamazepine
*teicoplanin*, septic shock 742*t*, 744*t*
Telfa, pressure ulcers 526*t*
*telmisartan*, hypertension 183*t*
*temazepam*
benzodiazepine withdrawal 72*t*
dementia 30
insomnia 46, 48*t*
Tempra *see* acetaminophen
*teniposide*, causing nausea and vomiting 844*t*
tennis elbow 490*t*
Tenormin *see* atenolol
*tenoxicam*, rheumatoid arthritis 458*t*
Tenuate *see* diethylpropion
Terazol *see* terconazole

*terazosin*
hypertension 183*t*, 184
prostatic hyperplasia 416, 418*t*, 419
*terbutaline*
asthma in adults 314, 315*t*
asthma in children 322, 324*t*
COPD 331, 333*t*
*terconazole*
in pregnancy 753*t*
vulvovaginal candidiasis 753*t*
*terephthalylidene dicamphor sulfonic acid*, as sunscreen 511*t*
*testosterone*, low sexual desire 610, 611*t*
*tetracaine*, acute pain 108
*tetracycline*
acne 496, 497*t*
chlamydial infection 755*t*
COPD 336
in pregnancy 496
pneumonia 717*t*
PUD 389*t*, 389
rosacea 503, 504*t*
syphilis 759*t*
Tetracyn *see* tetracycline
*tetrahydrozoline*, red eye 170*t*
Theo-Dur *see* theophylline
*theophylline*
asthma in adults 314, 315*t*
asthma in children 323
COPD 332, 335*t*, 336
**thermoregulatory disorders in adults 885-91**
hyperthermia 885-87, 890
hypothermia 885, 887-90
*thiamine*
alcohol withdrawal 67*t*
deficiency 823
hypothermia 890
seizures 156*t*
therapeutic supplement 823
thiazide diuretics
causing hyperlipidemia 194*t*
CHF 236*t*
edema 661, 662*t*, 664-65
hypertension 182, 183*t*, 185-86*t*, 190
*6-thioguanine*, causing nausea and vomiting 844*t*
*thiopental*, seizures 156*t*
*thioridazine*
ADHD 22*t*
behavioral problems 29
psychoses 56*t*, 58
*thiotepa*, causing nausea and vomiting 844*t*
thrombocytopenia, septic shock 740
**thromboembolism, systemic 295-97**
**thromboembolism, venous 273-80,** 859*t*
pharmacoeconomic considerations 279-80
with stroke 269
thrombolytics
myocardial infarction 212*t*
thrombosis 278
thrombophlebitis 843*t*, 852
thrombosis, deep vein *see* **thromboembolism, venous**
thrush 803*t*
**thyroid disorders 629-38**
goitre 636-37
hyperthyroidism 629-31
hypothyroidism 632-33, 636
single thyroid nodule 637-38
thyroid storm 632
thyroiditis 629
**thyroid storm 632**
Tiamol *see* fluocinonide
*tiaprofenic acid*, rheumatoid arthritis 458*t*
Tiazac *see* diltiazem
*tibolone*, low sexual desire 611*t*
Ticar *see* ticarcillin
*ticarcillin*
acute osteomyelitis 730*t*, 733*t*, 735*t*
septic shock 743*t*
UTI 766*t*
Ticlid *see* ticlopidine
*ticlopidine*
ischemic stroke prevention 176, 177*t*
myocardial infarction 207, 212*t*
Tilade *see* nedocromil
Timentin, septic shock 743*t*
*timolol*
glaucoma 162, 164*t*
hypertension 183*t*
myocardial infarction 210*t*
orthostatic hypotension 293
Timoptic preparations *see* timolol
Timpilo 164*t*
*tinzaparin*, thrombosis 276, 277*t*
*tioconazole*, vulvovaginal candidiasis 753*t*
*tirofiban*
angina 224*t*, 226
myocardial infarction 207, 212*t*
*titanium dioxide*, as sunscreen 510
*tizanidine*, spasticity 74-75, 76*t*, 78
*tobramycin*
bacterial meningitis 700*t*
infections in cancer patients 815*t*
pneumonia 717*t*
postoperative, cataract 160
red eye 170*t*
septic shock 742-43*t*
UTI 766*t*, 766
Tobrex *see* tobramycin
Tofranil *see* imipramine
*tolbutamide*, diabetes 620*t*

*tolcapone*, Parkinson's disease 140*t*, 143
Tolectin *see* tolmetin
*tolmetin*
acute pain 103, 105*t*
rheumatoid arthritis 458*t*
*tolterodine* 427*t*-28*t*
Topamax *see* topiramate
Topicort *see* desoximetasone
Topilene *see* betamethasone
*topiramate*, seizures 151*t*, 153*t*
Topisone *see* betamethasone
*topotecan*, causing nausea and vomiting 844*t*
Toradol *see* ketorolac
Toxoplasma gondii 800*t*, 804*t*
tracheitis, bacterial 338, 341*t*
Trandate *see* labetalol
*trandolapril*
CHF 234*t*
hypertension 183*t*
myocardial infarction 211*t*
transcutaneous nerve stimulation
fibromyalgia 433
osteoarthritis 468
pain control in palliative care 126
Transderm-Nitro *see* nitroglycerin
Transderm V *see* scopolamine
*tranylcypromine*
anxiety disorders 10-11, 13*t*
depression 35*t*, 38
Trasicor *see* oxprenolol
*trastuzumab*, adverse effects 856*t*
**traveler's diarrhea 775-81**
*trazodone*
agitation 4
bulimia nervosa 840, 841*t*
chronic fatigue syndrome 437*t*
dementia 28*t*, 29
depression 39
Trecator *see* ethionamide
*tretinoin*, acne 495*t*, 495
*triamcinolone*
acne 500
asthma in adults 314, 316*t*
asthma in children 323, 325*t*
COPD 334*t*
dermatitis 540*t*
gout 450*t*
lateral epicondylitis 490*t*
plantar fasciitis 491*t*
psoriasis 533*t*
rhinitis 303*t*
Triaminic *see* pseudoephedrine
*triamterene*
CHF 237*t*
edema 663*t*, 664
hypokalemia 682*t*, 682
*triazolam*
benzodiazepine withdrawal 72*t*
insomnia 46-47, 48*t*
trichomoniasis 751, 754*t*
*triclosan*, skin infections 559
Tri-Cyclen 575*t*
acne 496, 498*t*
tricyclic antidepressants *see also* antidepressants
anxiety disorders 10-11, 12*t*
back pain 116*t*, 117
chronic fatigue syndrome 437*t*, 790
depression 34*t*, 36*t*, 38, 40-41
enuresis 428*t*, 429
fibromyalgia 432*t*, 433
headache in children 98*t*
IBS 412*t*
incontinence 427*t*
neuralgia 121
pain control in palliative care 131*t*
Parkinson's disease 144
Tridesilon *see* desonide
*trientine*, Wilson's disease 356, 360*t*
*triethanolamine salicylate*, as sunscreen 511*t*
*trifluoperazine*, psychoses 56*t*
*trifluridine*
herpesvirus infections 784*t*, 786
red eye 171*t*
trigeminal neuralgia 120
*trihexyphenidyl*, Parkinson's disease 61*t*, 140*t*
*triiodothyronine*, depression 40
Trilafon *see* perphenazine
Trilisate *see* choline magnesium trisalicylate
*trimebutine*, IBS 411, 412*t*
*trimeprazine tartrate*, pruritus 547*t*
*trimethoprim*
adverse effects 823
causing hyperkalemia 674*t*
HIV-associated infections 804*t*
UTI 762, 766*t*
*trimetrexate*, HIV-associated infections 804*t*
*trimipramine*, depression 36*t*, 38
Trinipatch *see* nicotine
Triphasil 575*t*
*triprolidine*, rhinitis 310*t*
triptans, headache in adults 82-83, 85*t*, 89
Triptil *see* protriptyline
Triquilar 575*t*
Trobicin *see* spectinomycin
*tropicamide*, postoperative, cataract 160
Trusopt *see* dorzolamide
Tryptan *see* L-tryptophan
*L-tryptophan*
depression 40
insomnia 47, 49*t*, 50
T-Stat *see* erythromycin

tubal ligation 572*t*
**tuberculosis 719-28**, 800*t*
Twinrex, viral hepatitis 368*t*
Tylenol *see* acetaminophen 84*t*
Tylenol with Codeine, headache in adults 84*t*

# U

**ulcerative colitis 403-6**
**ulcerative proctitis 406-7**
ulcers *see also* **peptic ulcer disease; pressure ulcers**
  NSAID-associated 389-90
  stress 740
Ultradol *see* etodolac
UltraMOP *see* methoxsalen
Ultravate *see* halobetasol
Uniphyl *see* theophylline
**upper gastrointestinal bleeding** *see* **gastrointestinal bleeding, upper**
urethritis 749-50, 752, 755*t*-56*t*
**urge incontinence 422, 424, 427*t***
uric acid nephropathy 857*t*
uricosurics, gout 451*t*, 452
**urinary tract infection 762-67**
Urispas *see* flavoxate
*urokinase*
  thromboembolism 296
  thrombosis 278
Urso *see* ursodeoxycholic acid
*ursodeoxycholic acid*, cholestatic disease 353, 359*t*
urticaria 545*t*, 550-51
urticaria pigmentosa 545*t*
UTI *see* **urinary tract infection**
UVA absorbers, as sunscreen 511*t*
UVB absorbers, as sunscreen 511*t*

# V

vacuum device, erectile dysfunction 605
vaginitis 749*t*, 749, 751, 753*t*-54*t*
vaginosis 749*t*, 751, 753*t*-54*t*
*valacyclovir*
  herpesvirus infections 120, 782-83, 784*t*, 785, 787
  red eye 171*t*
Valium *see* diazepam
valproate *see* valproic acid
*valproic acid*
  agitation 4-5
  depression 34*t*
  headache in adults 86*t*, 88
  headache in children 95, 99*t*
  seizures 151*t*, 154*t*, 157
  trigeminal neuralgia 120
*valsartan*, hypertension 182, 183*t*
Valtrex *see* valacyclovir
Vancenase *see* beclomethasone
Vanceril *see* beclomethasone
Vancocin *see* vancomycin
*vancomycin*
  bacterial endocarditis prophylaxis 709*t*
  bacterial meningitis 700*t*, 701, 702*t*, 704*t*
  infections in cancer patients 812, 816*t*, 819
  pneumonia 715*t*
  septic shock 741*t*-42*t*, 744*t*
  skin infections 561
*vancyclovir*, infections in cancer patients 818*t*, 819
Vaponefrin *see* epinephrine
Vaqta *see* hepatitis A vaccine
varicella 545*t*
  HIV-positive patients 800*t*
*varicella vaccine*, HIV-associated infections 800*t*
**varicella-zoster virus 786-87**
vascular dementia 25, 30
vasectomy 572*t*
Vasocidin 172*t*
Vasocon *see* naphazoline
Vasocon-A 171*t*
vasoconstrictors, red eye 170*t*, 173
vasodilators, causing syncope 289*t*
vasopressin, esophageal varices 394
vasopressors, septic shock 742
vasospasm 859*t*
Vasotec *see* enalapril
V-Cillin *see* penicillin
vegetarians, nutritional supplements 822-23
*venlafaxine*
  anxiety disorders 13*t*, 15
  chronic fatigue syndrome 437*t*
  depression 37*t*, 39
  Parkinson's disease 144
Ventodisk *see* salbutamol
Ventolin *see* salbutamol
*verapamil*
  angina 217, 219*t*, 220, 225*t*
  arrhythmias 239
  atrial fibrillation/flutter 242*t*, 243, 245*t*
  headache in adults 86*t*, 88
  hypertension 183*t*, 184, 185*t*
  myocardial infarction 205, 207
  SVT 250-51*t*, 251
Verelan *see* verapamil
Vexol *see* rimexolone
Viagra *see* sildenafil
Vibramycin *see* doxycycline
Vibra-Tabs *see* doxycycline
Videx *see* didanosine

*vigabatrin*, seizures 151*t*, 154*t*
Vigilon, pressure ulcers 526*t*
*vinblastine*, adverse effects 844*t*, 853*t*
vinca alkaloids, causing neurotoxic reactions 856*t*
*vincristine*, adverse effects 844*t*, 853*t*, 858*t*
*vindesine*, adverse effects 844*t*, 853*t*
*vinorelbine*, adverse effects 844*t*, 853*t*
Vioxx *see* rofecoxib
Viracept *see* nelfinavir
viral exanthem, pruritus 545*t*
**viral hepatitis 362-72**
Viramune *see* nevirapine
Viroptic *see* trifluridine
Visine *see* tetrahydrozoline
Visken *see* pindolol
Vistide *see* cidofovir
*vitamin A*
 cholestatic disease 354, 358*t*
 recommended daily intake 822, 826
 therapeutic supplement 824*t*
 toxicity 825
vitamin A acid *see* tretinoin
*vitamin* $B_{12}$
 anemia 643, 645*t*, 646
 deficiency 642-43, 823
 recommended daily intake 822, 826
 therapeutic supplement 824*t*
vitamin $B_1$ *see* thiamine
vitamin $B_6$ *see* pyridoxine
*vitamin C*
 rhinitis 307
 toxicity 825
*vitamin D*
 cholestatic disease 354, 358*t*
 deficiency 823
 menopause 596
 osteoarthritis 468
 osteoporosis 479, 480*t*, 485
 recommended daily intake 822, 826
 therapeutic supplement 824*t*
 toxicity 825
vitamin deficiencies
 cholestatic disease 354, 358*t*
 drug-induced 823
*vitamin E*
 as sunscreen 510
 dementia 27, 28*t*, 29
 recommended daily intake 826
 sunburn 511-12
 therapeutic supplement 823-24, 824*t*
 toxicity 825-26
*vitamin K*
 cholestatic disease 354, 358*t*
 seizures 155
vitamins *see also specific vitamin* 821-26
Vivelle *see* estradiol
Voltaren preparations *see* diclofenac
vomiting *see* **nausea and vomiting**
VT *see* **tachycardia, ventricular**
VTE *see* **thromboembolism, venous**

## W

*warfarin*
 acute stroke 269
 anticoagulation in pregnancy 278, 921*t*
 atrial fibrillation/flutter 248, 249*t*
 CHF 238
 drug interactions 279*t*
 ischemic stroke prevention 177*t*, 178
 myocardial infarction 207, 211*t*
 thromboembolism 296
 thrombosis 274*t*, 276-77, 280
Warfilone *see* warfarin
Wellbutrin *see* bupropion
Wellferon *see* interferon alfa
Wernicke's encephalopathy 823
Westcort *see* hydrocortisone
**Wilson's disease 356, 360*t***
Winpred *see* prednisone
withdrawal *see* **drug withdrawal syndromes**

## X

Xalatan *see* latanoprost
Xanaflex *see* tizanidine
Xanax *see* alprazolam
xanthine oxidase inhibitors, gout 451*t*, 452
Xenical *see* orlistat
xerosis, pruritus 545*t*
*xylocaine*, plantar fasciitis 491*t*
*xylometazoline*
 red eye 171*t*
 rhinitis 309*t*

## Y

*yohimbine*
 orthostatic hypotension 293
 syncope 292*t*

## Z

Zaditen *see* ketotifen
*zafirlukast*
 asthma in adults 316*t*, 317
 asthma in children 325*t*, 326
*zalcitabine*, HIV infection 793*t*
*zaleplon*, insomnia 45, 47, 48*t*
Zantac preparations *see* ranitidine
Zarontin *see* ethosuximide
Zaroxolyn *see* metolazone

Zelmac *see* tegaserod
Zerit *see* stavudine
Zestril *see* lisinopril
Ziagen *see* abacavir
*zidovudine*
  HIV infection 792, 793*t*
  HIV prophylaxis 796*t*
Zinacef *see* cefuroxime
*zinc* (oral)
  anorexia nervosa 838
  viral rhinitis 308
  supplementation 826
  Wilson's disease 356, 360*t*
*zinc oxide*, as sunscreen 510
Zithromax *see* azithromycin
Zocor *see* simvastatin
Zofran *see* ondansetron
Zoladex *see* goserelin
*zolmitriptan*
  headache in adults 82-83, 85*t*, 91
  headache in children 97*t*
Zoloft *see* sertraline
Zomig *see* zolmitriptan
Zonalon *see* doxepin
*zopiclone*
  fibromyalgia 432*t*, 433
  insomnia 46-47, 49*t*
Zostrix *see* capsaicin
Zovirax *see* acyclovir
*zuclopenthixol*, psychoses 59*t*
Zyban *see* bupropion
Zyloprim *see* allopurinol
Zyprexa *see* olanzapine